# Instructional
# Course Lectures

Volume 57 2008

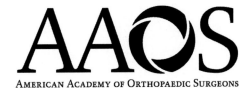

AMERICAN ACADEMY OF ORTHOPAEDIC SURGEONS

# Instructional
# Course Lectures

Volume 57 2008

*Edited by*
Paul J. Duwelius, MD
Adjunct Associate Professor of Orthopaedics, OHSU
Clinical Attending, St. Vincent Hospital and Medical Center
Orthopaedic and Fracture Clinic
Portland, Oregon

Frederick M. Azar, MD
Professor
Residency Program Director
Sports Medicine Fellowship Director
University of Tennessee - Campbell Clinic
Department of Orthopaedic Surgery
Memphis, Tennessee

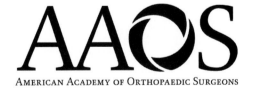

AMERICAN ACADEMY OF ORTHOPAEDIC SURGEONS

*Published 2008 by the*

American Academy
of Orthopaedic Surgeons
6300 North River Road
Rosemont, IL 60018

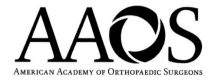

**AMERICAN ACADEMY OF ORTHOPAEDIC SURGEONS**

**Instructional Course Lectures Volume 57**
American Academy of Orthopaedic Surgeons

The material presented in *Instructional Course Lectures 57* has been made available by the American Academy of Orthopaedic Surgeons for educational purposes only. This material is not intended to present the only, or necessarily best, methods or procedures for the medical situations discussed, but rather is intended to represent an approach, view, statement, or opinion of the author(s) or producer(s), which may be helpful to others who face similar situations.

Some drugs or medical devices demonstrated in Academy courses or described in Academy print or electronic publications have not been cleared by the Food and Drug Administration (FDA) or have been cleared for specific uses only. The FDA has stated that it is the responsibility of the physician to determine the FDA clearance status of each drug or device he or she wishes to use in clinical practice.

Furthermore, any statements about commercial products are solely the opinion(s) of the author(s) and do not represent an Academy endorsement or evaluation of these products. These statements may not be used in advertising or for any commercial purpose.

Some of the authors or the departments with which they are affiliated have received something of value from a commercial or other party related directly or indirectly to the subject of their chapter.

ISBN 10: 0-89203-414-9
ISBN 13: 978-0-89203-414-7

Printed in the USA

Library of Congress Cataloging-in-Publication Data

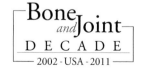

# Contributors

**Roy K. Aaron, MD,** Professor, Orthopaedics, Director, Center for Restorative and Regenerative Medicine, Department of Orthopaedics, Brown Medical School, Providence, Rhode Island

**Christopher S. Ahmad, MD,** Assistant Professor, Orthopaedic Surgery, Department of Orthopaedic Surgery, Columbia University, New York, New York

**Todd J. Albert, MD,** Chairman and Professor, Orthopaedic Surgery – Rothman Institute, Thomas Jefferson University, Philadelphia, Pennsylvania

**A. Herbert Alexander, MD,** Professor, Department of Surgery, Uniformed Services University of the Health Sciences, Bethesda, Maryland

**Ian J. Alexander, MD, FRCS(C),** Orthopaedic Surgery, Summa Health System, Akron, Ohio

**Geoffrey T. Anders, JD, CPA, CHBC,** President, The Health Care Group, Inc., Plymouth Meeting, Pennsylvania

**LTC Romney C. Anderson, MD, MC, USA,** Director, Orthopaedic Traumatology, National Naval Medical Center, Bethesda, Maryland

**Jeffrey O. Anglen, MD, FACS,** Professor and Chairman, Department of Orthopaedics, Indiana University, Indianapolis, Indiana

**Robert A. Arciero, MD,** Professor, Orthopaedics, Department of Orthopaedics, University of Connecticut, Farmington, Connecticut

**Elizabeth A. Arendt, MD,** Professor and Vice Chair, Orthopaedic Surgery, University of Minnesota, Minneapolis, Minnesota

**David D. Aronsson, MD,** Professor, Department of Orthopaedics and Rehabilitation, University of Vermont College of Medicine, Burlington, Vermont

**B. Sonny Bal, MD,** Assistant Professor, Department of Orthopaedic Surgery, University of Missouri – Columbia, Columbia, Missouri

**F. Alan Barber, MD, FACS,** Plano Orthopaedic and Sports Medicine Center, Plano, Texas

**Michael R. Baumgaertner, MD,** Professor, Chief, Orthopaedic Trauma Service, Orthopaedic Department, Yale University School of Medicine, New Haven, Connecticut

**Ryan T. Bicknell, MD, MSc, FRCSC,** Department of Orthopaedics and Sports Medicine, University of Washington, Seattle, Washington

**Yaw Boachie-Adjei, MD,** Resident Physician, Department of Orthopaedic Surgery, University of Virginia, Charlottesville, Virginia

**Pascal Boileau, MD,** Professor, Orthopaedic Surgery and Sports Traumatology, L'Archet 2 Hospital, Nice, France

**Christopher M. Bono, MD,** Chief, Orthopaedic Spine Service, Brigham and Women's Hospital, Assistant Professor, Harvard Medical School, Boston, Massachusetts

**James V. Bono, MD,** Clinical Professor of Orthopaedic Surgery, Department of Orthopaedic Surgery, Tufts University, Boston, Massachusetts

**Christopher T. Born, MD, FAAOS, FACS,** Professor of Orthopaedic Surgery, The Warren Alpert Medical School of Brown University, Chief, Orthopaedic Trauma, Rhode Island Hospital, Department of Orthopaedics, Brown University / Rhode Island Hospital, Providence, Rhode Island

**Michael J. Botte, MD,** Clinical Professor, Department of Orthopaedic Surgery, UCSD School of Medicine, Division of Orthopaedic Surgery, Scripps Clinic, La Jolla, California

**Kevin J. Bozic, MD, MBA,** Assistant Professor in Residence, Department of Orthopaedic Surgery, University of California, San Francisco, San Francisco, California

**Gert J. Breur, DVM, PhD, DACVS,** Professor of Small Animal Orthopaedics and Neurosurgery, Department of Veterinary Clinical Services, Purdue University, West Lafayette, Indiana

**Robert H. Brophy, MD,** Fellow, Sports Medicine / Shoulder, Hospital for Special Surgery, New York, New York

**Thomas E. Brown, MD,** Associate Professor, Department of Orthopaedic Surgery, University of Virginia, Charlottesville, Virginia

**Jason H. Calhoun, MD, FACS,** Chairman and J. Vernon Luck Distinguished Professor, Department of Orthopaedic Surgery, University of Missouri – Columbia, Columbia, Missouri

**Barbara J. Campbell, MD,** Director, Somerset Hospital Bone Health Clinic, AAOS Women's Health Issues Advisory Board, WHIAB Liason to AAOS Council of Education, Somerset Central Medical Associates, Ltd., Somerset, Pennsylvania

**Cordelia W. Carter, MD,** Resident, Department of Orthopaedic Surgery, Columbia University Medical Center, New York, New York

**Michael J. Christie, MD,** Director, Southern Joint Replacement Institute, Nashville, Tennessee

**Gustavo X. Cordero, MD,** Orthopaedic Resident, Department of Orthopaedic Surgery and Rehabilitation, University of Nebraska Medical Center, Omaha, Nebraska

**CAPT Dana C. Covey, MD, MC, USN,** Chairman, Department of Orthopaedic Surgery, Naval Medical Center, San Diego, California

**Quanjun Cui, MD, MS,** Assistant Professor, Department of Orthopaedic Surgery, University of Virginia, Charlottesville, Virginia

**Bradford L. Currier, MD,** Professor, Orthopaedic Surgery, Vice Chairman for Practice Department of Orthopaedics, Department of Orthopaedic Surgery, Mayo Clinic, Rochester, Minnesota

**Timothy A. Damron, MD, FACS,** David G. Murray Endowed Professor of Orthopaedic Surgery, Department of Orthopaedics, SUNY Upstate Medical University, Syracuse, New York

**James K. DeOrio, MD,** Associate Professor, Duke Orthopaedics, Department of Orthopaedics, Duke University Medical Center, Durham, North Carolina

**Mohammad Diab, MD,** Associate Professor, Department of Orthopaedic Surgery, UCSF, San Francisco, California

**Lawrence D. Dorr, MD,** Director, Arthritis Institute, Inglewood, California

**Clive P. Duncan, MD,** Professor, Department of Orthopaedics, University of British Columbia, Vancouver, British Columbia, Canada

**Andrew Dutton, MD, FRCS,** Clinical Fellow, Department of Orthopaedic Surgery, Massachusetts General Hospital, Boston, Massachusetts

**Paul J. Duwelius, MD,** Adjunct Associate Professor of Orthopaedics, OHSU, Clinical Attending, St. Vincent Hospital and Medical Center, Orthopaedic and Fracture Clinic, Portland, Oregon

**Mark E. Easley, MD,** Assistant Professor, Department of Orthopaedics, Duke University Medical Center, Durham, North Carolina

**Jason C. Eck, DO, MS,** Resident, Department of Orthopaedic Surgery, Memorial Hospital, York, Pennsylvania

**Thomas A. Einhorn, MD,** Professor and Chairman, Department of Orthopaedic Surgery, Boston University Medical Center, Boston, Massachusetts

**Bassem Elhassan, MD,** Department of Orthopedics, Mayo Clinic, Rochester, Minnesota

**Nathan K. Endres, MD,** Fellow, Harvard Shoulder Service, Department of Orthopaedics, Harvard University, Boston, Massachusetts

**Thomas K. Fehring, MD,** Ortho Carolina Hip and Knee Center, Ortho Carolina, Charlotte, North Carolina

**COL James R. Ficke, MD, MC, USA,** Orthopaedic Consultant, US Army Surgeon General, Department of Orthopaedics and Rehabilitation, Brooke Army Medical Center, Fort Sam Houston, Texas

**Larry D. Field, MD,** Co-Director, Upper Extremity Service, Mississippi Sports Medicine and Orthopaedic Center, Jackson, Mississippi

**Frank J. Frassica, MD,** Professor and Chair, Department of Orthopaedic Surgery, Johns Hopkins University, Baltimore, Maryland

**LTC H. Michael Frisch, MD, MC, USA,** Director of Orthopaedic Traumatology, Department of Orthopaedics and Rehabilitation, Walter Reed Army Medical Center, Washington, DC

**John P. Fulkerson, MD,** Clinical Professor, University of Connecticut and Orthopaedic Associates of Hartford P.C., Farmington, Connecticut

**Seth C. Gamradt, MD,** Shoulder and Sports Medicine Fellow, Hospital for Special Surgery, New York, New York

**Reinhold Ganz, MD,** Professor Emeritus, Consultant, Orthopaedics Department, Balgrist University Hospital, Zurich, Switzerland

**Kevin L. Garvin, MD,** L. Thomas Hood Professor and Chair, Department of Orthopaedic Surgery and Rehabilitation, University of Nebraska Medical Center, Omaha, Nebraska

**Harris Gellman, MD,** Adjunct Clinical Professor, University of Miami, Department of Orthopaedic Surgery, Miami, Florida, Adjunct Clinical Professor, University of Arkansas, Department of Orthopaedic Surgery, Little Rock, Arkansas

**Christian Gerber, MD, FRCSEd (Hon),** Professor and Chairman, Department of Orthopaedics, Balgrist University Hospital, Zurich, Switzerland

**Alexander J. Ghanayem, MD,** Professor, Department of Orthopaedic Surgery and Rehabilitation, Chief, Division of Spine Surgery, Department of Orthopaedic Surgery and Rehabilitation, Loyola University Medical Center, Maywood, Illinois

Gregory J. Golladay, MD, Clinical Assistant Professor, MSU, Orthopaedic Associates of Grand Rapids, PC, Spectrum Health, Grand Rapids, Michigan

Frank Gottschalk, MB.BCh, FRCSEd, Professor, Orthopaedic Surgery, Department of Orthopaedic Surgery, U.T. Southwestern Medical Center, Dallas, Texas

Letha Yurko Griffin, MD, PhD, Georgia State University, Adjunct and Clinical Faculty, Peachtree Orthopaedic Clinic, Atlanta, Georgia

Kenneth Gustke, MD, Florida Orthopaedic Institute, Tampa, Florida

Sharon L. Hame, MD, Associate Clinical Professor, Department of Orthopaedic Surgery, UCLA School of Medicine, Los Angeles, California

Jo A. Hannafin, MD, PhD, Professor of Orthopaedic Surgery, Weill Medical College of Cornell University, Director of Orthopaedic Research, Hospital for Special Surgery, New York, New York

COL Roman A. Hayda, MD, MC, USA, Chief, Orthopaedic Trauma, Department of Orthopaedics and Rehabilitation, Brooke Army Medical Center, Fort Sam Houston, Texas

David A. Heck, Clinical Scholar, Baylor Institute for Health Care Research and Improvement, Dallas, Texas

Laurence D. Higgins, MD, Chief, Sports Medicine, BWH Chief, Harvard Shoulder Service, Brigham and Women's Hospital, Boston, Massachusetts

Alan E. Hillard, MD, Radiologist, Boone Imaging Center, Columbia, Missouri

Serena S. Hu, MD, Professor, Department of Orthopaedic Surgery, University of California, San Francisco, San Francisco, California

Jean-Yves Jenny, MD, Senior Consultant, Knee Surgery Unit, University Hospital, Strasbourg, France

Richard E. Jones, MD, Chief, Total Joint Restoration, Orthopaedic Specialists, Dallas, Texas

W. Ben Kibler, MD, Medical Director, Department of Orthopaedic Surgery / Sports Medicine, Lexington Clinic Sports Medicine Center, Lexington, Kentucky

Ira H. Kirschenbaum, MD, Assistant Clinical Professor, Department of Orthopaedic Surgery, New York University / Hospital for Joint Diseases, New York, New York

Kenneth A. Krackow, MD, Professor and Vice Chairman, Department of Orthopaedic Surgery, State University of New York at Buffalo, Department Head, Department of Orthopaedic Surgery, Kaleida Health, Department of Orthopaedic Surgery – Lower Extremity Reconstruction, Buffalo, New York

Paul F. Lachiewicz, MD, Professor, Department of Orthopaedics, University of North Carolina School of Medicine, Chapel Hill, North Carolina

Carlos J. Lavernia, MD, Medical Director, Orthopaedic Institute, Mercy Hospital, Miami, Florida

Michael Leunig, MD, Senior Orthopaedic Surgeon, Department of Orthopaedics, Schulthess Clinic, Zurich, Switzerland

Lawrence Scott Levin, MD, FACS, Chief, Division of Plastic and Reconstructive Surgery, Professor of Plastic and Orthopaedic Surgery, Duke University Medical Center, Durham, North Carolina

William N. Levine, MD, Vice Chairman and Associate Professor, Department of Orthopaedic Surgery, Columbia University Medical Center, New York, New York

Randall T. Loder, MD, Garceau Professor of Orthopaedic Surgery, Director of Pediatric Orthopaedics, James Whitcomb Riley Children's Hospital, Indianapolis, Indiana

William T. Long, MD, Arthritis Institute, Inglewood, California

Jason A. Lowe, MD, Resident Physician, Department of Orthopaedics, University of Missouri, Columbia, Missouri

Jay D. Mabrey, MD, Chief, Department of Orthopaedics, Baylor University Medical Center, Dallas, Texas

Steven J. MacDonald, MD, FRCSC, Associate Professor of Orthopaedic Surgery, Chief of Surgery, Chief of Orthopaedics, University of Western Ontario, University Hospital, London, Ontario, Canada

Abhijit Manaswi, MD, MS, FRCS, Fellow, Adult Reconstruction, Department of Orthopaedic Surgery, University of Virginia, Charlottesville, Virginia

Carole J. Mankin, MSLS, Research Librarian, Treadwell Library and Smith-Peterson Library, Massachusetts General Hospital, Boston, Massachusetts

Henry J. Mankin, MD, Edith M. Ashley Professor of Orthopaedics Emeritus, Harvard Medical School, Department of Orthopaedic Surgery, Massachusetts General Hospital, Boston, Massachusetts

Satyajit V. Marawar, MD, Fellow, Department of Orthopaedic Surgery, Medical College of Wisconsin, Milwaukee, Wisconsin

Randall E. Marcus, MD, Charles N. Herndon Professor and Chairman, Department of Orthopaedics, Case Western Reserve University and University Hospitals, Case Medical Center, Cleveland, Ohio

J. Bohannon Mason, MD, Ortho Carolina Hip and Knee Center, Ortho Carolina, Charlotte, North Carolina

**Frederick A. Matsen III, MD,** Chair, Professor, Department of Orthopaedics and Sports Medicine, University of Washington, Seattle, Washington

**CDR Michael T. Mazurek, MD, MC, USN,** Director, Orthopaedic Trauma, Tumor and Reconstructive Service, Department of Orthopaedic Surgery, Naval Medical Center, San Diego, California

**James P. McAuley, MD, FRCSC,** Associate Professor, Department of Orthopaedic Surgery, London Health Sciences Center, University of Western Ontario, London, Ontario, Canada

**William M. Mihalko, MD, PhD,** Associate Professor, Department of Orthopaedic Surgery, Department of Mechanical and Aerospace Engineering, University of Virginia, Charlottesville, Virginia

**Allan Mishra, MD,** Adjunct Clinical Assistant Professor, Department of Orthopaedic Surgery, Menlo Medical Clinic, Stanford University, Menlo Park, California

**Chris Moros, BS,** Research Assistant, Department of Orthopaedics, Shoulder, Elbow, and Sports Medicine, Columbia University, New York, New York

**Rhys Morris, PhD,** Senior Medical Physicist / Honorary Research Fellow, Department of Medical Physics and Clinical Engineering, University Hospital of Wales, Cardiff, Wales, United Kingdom

**Sandeep Munjal, MCh (Orth), MD,** Attending Orthopaedic Surgeon, Department of Orthopaedics, Physician's Clinic of Iowa, Cedar Rapids, Iowa

**MAJ Clinton K. Murray, MD, MC, USA,** Infectious Disease Fellowship Program Director, Department of Medicine, Brooke Army Medical Center, Fort Sam Houston, Texas

**Mark W. Pagnano, MD,** Associate Professor of Orthopaedics, Mayo College of Medicine, Mayo Clinic, Rochester, Minnesota

**Guy D. Paiement, MD,** Senior Faculty Surgeon, Division of Orthopaedic Surgery, Cedars-Sinai Health System, Los Angeles, California

**Sebastien Parratte, MD,** Research Fellow, Mayo Clinic, Rochester, Minnesota

**Javad Parvizi, MD,** Associate Professor, Director, Clinical Research, Department of Orthopaedic Surgery, Rothman Institute at Thomas Jefferson University, Philadelphia, Pennsylvania

**Jay Patel, MD, MS,** Resident, Department of Orthopaedic Surgery, University of California, Irvine, Orange, California

**Michael J. Patzakis, MD,** Professor and Chairman, Department of Orthopaedic Surgery, Keck School of Medicine of USC, LA County and USC Medical Center, Los Angeles, California

**Vincent D. Pellegrini, Jr, MD,** James L. Kernan Professor and Chair, Department of Orthopaedics, University of Maryland School of Medicine, Baltimore, Maryland

**Matthew J. Phillips, MD,** Assistant Professor of Orthopaedics, State University of New York at Buffalo, University Orthopaedics Services, Kaleida Health – Buffalo General Hospital, Buffalo, New York

**Marco Antonio Guedes de Souza Pinto, MD,** Orthopaedic Workshop of the Lar Escola Sao Francisco, Universidade Federal de Sao Paulo, Sao Paulo, Brazil

**Michael S. Pinzur,** MD, Professor of Orthopaedic Surgery and Rehabilitation, Department of Orthopaedic Surgery and Rehabilitation, Loyola University Medical Center, Maywood, Illinois

**Kornelis A. Poelstra, MD, PhD,** Assistant Professor of Orthopaedics, Department of Orthopaedics, University of Maryland – Shock Trauma, Baltimore, Maryland

**Col Elisha T. Powell IV, MD, MC, USAF,** Commander and Orthopaedic Surgeon, Department of Orthopaedic Surgery, 3rd Medical Group, Elmendorf Air Force Base, Alaska

**Charles T. Price, MD,** Associate Program Director, Orthopaedic Residency Program, Director of Orthopaedic Research, Medical Education Faculty Practice – Pediatric Orthopaedic Surgery, Orlando Regional Medical Center / Arnold Palmer Hospital for Children, Orlando, Florida

**Matthew T. Provencher, MD,** Assistant Director, Shoulder and Sports Service, Department of Orthopaedic Surgery, Naval Medical Center, San Diego, California

**Wael A. Rahman, MD, MSc,** Orthopaedic Reconstruction Fellow, Department of Orthopaedics, University of British Columbia, Vancouver, British Columbia, Canada

**Raj Rao, MD,** Associate Professor, Director of Spine Surgery, Department of Orthopaedic Surgery, Medical College of Wisconsin, Milwaukee, Wisconsin

**Michael A. Rauh, MD,** Orthopaedic Surgical Fellow, Department of Orthopaedic Surgery, Sports Health, Cleveland Clinic, Cleveland, Ohio

**Charles E. Rhoades, MD,** Clinical Professor of Orthopaedic Surgery, Dickson Diveley Orthopaedic Clinic, Kansas City Orthopaedic Institute, Leawood, Kansas

**Corey J. Richards, MD, MASc, FRCSC,** Orthopaedic Reconstruction Fellow, Department of Orthopaedics, University of British Columbia, Vancouver, British Columbia, Canada

**Col Mark W. Richardson, MD, MC, USAF,** Chairman, Department of Orthopaedic Surgery, Chief, Orthopaedic Traumatology, Wilford Hall Medical, San Antonio, Texas

**Michael D. Ries, MD,** Professor of Orthopaedic Surgery, Chief of Arthroplasty, University of California, San Francisco, San Francisco, California

**Anthony A. Romeo, MD,** Director, Shoulder and Elbow Service, Department of Orthopaedic Surgery, Rush University, Chicago, Illinois

**Harry E. Rubash, MD,** Chief of Orthopaedic Surgery, Massachusetts General Hospital, Edith M. Ashley Professor, Harvard Medical School, Boston, Massachusetts

**Richard K.N. Ryu, MD,** Private Practice, Santa Barbara, California

**Khaled J. Saleh, MD,** Associate Professor and Division Head, Adult Reconstruction, Department of Orthopaedic Surgery, University of Virginia, Charlottesville, Virginia

**V. James Sammarco, MD,** Cincinnati Sports Medicine and Orthopaedic Center, Cincinnati, Ohio

**Aaron Sciascia, MS, ATC,** Program Coordinator, Department of Orthopaedics / Sports Medicine, Lexington Clinic Sports Medicine Center, Lexington, Kentucky

**Thomas P. Schmalzried, MD,** Associate Medical Director, Joint Replacement Institute, Los Angeles, California

**Andrew H. Schmidt, MD,** Associate Professor, University of Minnesota, Hennepin County Medical Center, Minneapolis, MN

**Edward M. Schwarz, PhD,** Professor, Department of Orthopaedics, University of Rochester, Rochester, New York

**Nigel E. Sharrock, MD, ChB,** Senior Scientist and Clinical Professor, Attending Anesthesiologist, Department of Anesthesiology, Hospital for Special Surgery, New York, New York

**Naomi N. Shields, MD,** Clinical Associate Professor, Department of Orthopaedic Surgery, University of Kansas School of Medicine, Wichita, Kansas

**Franklin H. Sim, MD,** Professor of Orthopaedic Surgery, Department of Orthopaedic Surgery, Mayo Clinic, Rochester, Minnesota

**Theddy Slongo, MD,** Consultant, Children's University Hospital, Department of Pediatric Surgery, Bern, Switzerland

**James D. Slover, MD, MS,** Department of Orthopaedic Surgery, Massachusetts General Hospital, Boston, Massachusetts

**Douglas G. Smith, MD,** Professor, Department of Orthopaedics and Sports Medicine, Harborview Medical Center / University of Washington, Seattle, Washington

**Wade R. Smith, MD,** Director of Orthopaedic Surgery, Denver Health Medical Center, University of Colorado, Denver, Colorado

**Jeffrey T. Spang, MD,** University of Connecticut, Sports Medicine Fellow, University of Connecticut Orthopaedics, University of Connecticut Hospital, Farmington, Connecticut

**Bryan D. Springer, MD,** Ortho Carolina Hip and Knee Center, Charlotte, North Carolina

**Philip F. Stahel, MD,** Denver Health Medical Center, Denver, Colorado

**David R. Steinberg, MD,** Associate Professor, Director of Hand Fellowship, Department of Orthopaedic Surgery, University of Pennsylvania, Philadelphia, Pennsylvania

**James B. Stiehl, MD,** Associate Clinical Professor, Department of Orthopaedic Surgery, Medical College of Wisconsin, Milwaukee, Wisconsin

**Nirmal C. Tejwani, MD,** Associate Professor, Department of Orthopaedics, New York University Hospital for Joint Diseases, New York, New York

**Kimberly J. Templeton, MD,** Associate Professor of Orthopaedic Surgery, University of Kansas Medical Center, Kansas City, Kansas

**Debra J. Thomas, MD,** Arthritis Institute, Inglewood, California

**Paul Tornetta III, MD,** Professor and Vice Chairman, Program Director, Department of Orthopaedic Surgery, Boston University and Boston Medical Center, Boston, Massachusetts

**Laura L. Tosi, MD,** Director, Bone Health Program, Division of Orthopaedics, Children's National Medical Center, Washington, DC

**Clifford B. Tribus, MD,** Associate Professor, Department of Orthopaedics and Rehabilitative Medicine, University of Wisconsin – Madison, Madison, Wisconsin

**Peter Tsai, MD,** Department of Orthopaedic Surgery, University of Pennsylvania, Philadelphia, Pennsylvania

**Andrew G. Urquhart, MD,** Assistant Professor, Department of Orthopaedic Surgery, Chief, LER Division, University of Michigan Medical Center, Ann Arbor, Michigan

**Gilles Walch, MD,** Orthopaedic Surgeon, Department of Shoulder Surgery, Centre Orthopédique Santy, Lyon, France

**Samuel R. Ward, PT, PhD,** Assistant Professor, Department of Radiology, University of California San Diego, San Diego, California

**Jon J.P. Warner, MD,** Chief, The Harvard Shoulder Service, Professor of Orthopaedic Surgery, Massachusetts General Hospital, Harvard Medical School, Boston, Massachusetts

**David J. Warwick, MD, FRCS, FRCS Orth, EDipHS,** Consultant, Orthopaedic Surgeon, Department of Orthopaedic Surgery, University of Southampton, Southampton, United Kingdom

**Peter M. Waters, MD,** Professor of Orthopaedic Surgery, Associate Chief of Orthopaedic Surgery, Department of Orthopaedic Surgery, Children's Hospital Boston, Harvard Medical School, Boston, Massachusetts

**Kristy Weber, MD,** Associate Professor, Departments of Orthopaedics and Oncology, Johns Hopkins University, Baltimore, Maryland

**Stuart L. Weinstein, MD,** Ignacio V. Ponseti Chair and Professor, Department of Orthopaedic Surgery, University of Iowa, Iowa City, Iowa

**Joseph C. Wenke, PhD,** Research Physiologist, US Army Institute of Surgical Research, San Antonio, Texas

**Clifford R. Wheeless III, MD,** Orthopaedic Surgeon, Oxford, North Carolina

**David R. Whiddon, MD,** Otto E. Aufranc Adult Reconstruction Fellow, New England Baptist Hospital, Boston, Massachusetts

**Riley J. Williams III, MD,** Associate Professor and Attending Surgeon, Department of Sports Medicine and Shoulder Service, Hospital for Special Surgery – Weill Cornell Medical College, New York, New York

**Richard L. Wixson, MD,** Department of Orthopaedics, Northwestern University Feinberg School of Medicine, Chicago, Illlinois

**Philip Wolinsky, MD,** Professor, Orthopaedic Surgery, University of California at Davis, Sacramento, California

**George W. Wood II, MD,** Professor of Orthopaedic Surgery, Staff, Campbell Clinic, University of Tennessee, Memphis, Tennessee

**Charalampos G. Zalavras, MD,** Associate Professor, Department of Orthopaedic Surgery, LAC and USC Medical Center, University of Southern California, Los Angeles, California

**Bruce H. Ziran, MD,** Director of Orthopaedic Trauma, Associate Professor of Orthopaedics, Neoucom, St. Elizabeth Health Center, Youngstown, Ohio

# Preface

Instructional courses are the cornerstone of education at the Annual Meeting of the American Academy of Orthopaedic Surgeons. These instructional courses have outstanding faculty who update the members on timely topics in their various areas of expertise. Each course is carefully selected by the subspecialty societies and has passed peer review from the Instructional Courses Committee. Lectures included in this volume have been deemed excellent by course attendees and were selected for inclusion in this volume by the Committee.

It has been my privilege to serve as the Chairman of the AAOS Instructional Courses Committee for the 2007 annual meeting at the request of the Academy's president, Richard Kyle, MD, and to serve as editor for this publication.

I would like to thank my assistant editor, Frederick Azar, MD, who reviewed all the sports medicine chapters for this volume. Members of the Instructional Courses Committee include Frederick Azar, MD; Dempsey Springfield, MD; James Heckman, MD; Mary O'Connor, MD; J. Lawrence Marsh, MD; Terry Light, MD; and Kenneth Egol, MD, all whom have done an outstanding job in reviewing and selecting courses, which ultimately are published in this volume. I also want to thank Dempsey Springfield and James Heckman who helped select instructional course lectures for presentation in the *Journal of Bone and Joint Surgery*.

Volume 57 includes 57 chapters written by more than 150 authors and noted scholars in their field who have devoted time and extraordinary commitment in teaching the AAOS membership—I deeply appreciate their commitment. This volume concentrates on new topics that are extremely timely and revisits topics that continue to educate the membership on more general aspects of orthopaedic knowledge and basic science.

The publication of Instructional Course Lectures, volume 57, would be impossible without the efforts of the AAOS editors and supporting staff, including Marilyn L. Fox, PhD, director of the AAOS publications department, Lisa Claxton Moore, managing editor for the Instructional Course Lectures series, and Kathleen Anderson, associate senior editor. Reid L. Stanton, manager of electronic media at AAOS, organized and edited the DVD material, which is an outstanding addition to recent editions. I also particularly want to thank Kathy Niesen for her support and guidance in directing my efforts as a member of the Academy's Instructional Courses Committee. I could not have done my job without the great support she provided.

On behalf of all the contributors to this volume and to those who provided the background support, I hope that you, the AAOS members and readers, find volume 57 to be a worthy continuation of this long-lasting series of publications. This edition provides further expansion of the fascinating field of orthopaedic surgery, and it is the Committee's wish that you enjoy the publication and find it to be educational.

As we pass through our careers in this wonderful field of orthopaedic surgery we have many mentors. John Connolly, MD, who was Chairman at the University of Nebraska and Creighton's Orthopedic Residency program during my training, was one of my great mentors and educators. Dr. Connolly passed away this year. I dedicate this volume to the contributions that he made in the field of orthopaedic surgery and research.

Paul J. Duwelius, MD
Portland, Oregon

# Table of Contents

## Section 4 Adult Reconstruction: Hip

## Section 5 Adult Reconstruction: Knee

## Section 6 Foot and Ankle

## Section 7 Spine

## Section 10 Orthopaedic Medicine

## Section 11 Practice Management

# Trauma

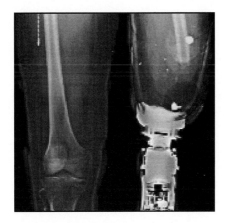

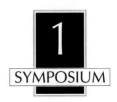

# The Changing Face of Orthopaedic Trauma: Locked Plating and Minimally Invasive Techniques

Nirmal C. Tejwani, MD
*Philip Wolinsky, MD

## Abstract
*Rapid advances in the field of orthopaedic trauma have improved treatment options while keeping pace with the changing characteristics of the trauma population. The availability of locking implants has changed the approach to treating fractures in older patients with osteoporotic bones as well as in those with comminuted and complex injuries. Minimally invasive approaches have allowed the preservation and protection of soft tissues while allowing adequate reduction and fixation of fractures. This biologically friendly approach coupled with newer implants and instruments will improve early and long-term outcomes in trauma care.*

**Instr Course Lect 2008;57:3-9.**

During the past decade, significant changes have occurred in the field of orthopaedic trauma, including advances in implant technology and the advent of minimally invasive techniques and the use of biologic therapies in fracture care.

In elderly, osteoporotic patients, advances in implant technology, such as the development of locked plating systems, have enhanced the surgeon's ability to manage fragility fractures with a stable fixation construct. Improved technology has facilitated the introduction of minimally invasive reduction and fixation techniques to minimize soft-tissue dissection and disruption of the environment at the fracture site. A better understanding of the biology of fracture healing has led to the development of new biologic therapies. An examination of these evolving ideas and techniques will provide a framework for a better understanding of the changing face of orthopaedic trauma care.

## Locked Plating

Locked plates involve a simple design change from nonlocking plates. Because the undersides of the screw heads and the screw holes are threaded, the screws can thread into (or lock into) the plate. This change completely alters the biomechanical behavior of the fixation system; the use of locked plating alters strain at the fracture site, which has a direct effect on bone healing.

### Strain: Concept Review

Strain is defined as the change in the length of the fracture gap divided by the length of the fracture gap ($\Delta L/L$). It can be thought of as the deformation that occurs at a fracture site when a force is applied to it. Very small amounts of strain induce callus formation. Strain of less than 2% is tolerated by lamellar bone, 2% to 10% is tolerated by woven bone, and bone resorption prevails at levels of 10% to 30%. Strain determines the type of tissue that forms at the fracture site. Primary bone healing can occur with strain levels of less than 2% and secondary bone healing with callus strain levels of 2% to 10%; however, with strain levels of more than 10%, no bone healing can occur. By controlling the strain at the fracture site, the type of bone healing and whether bone healing occurs can both be controlled.[1]

By manipulating the stability of

*Philip Wolinsky, MD or the department with which he is affiliated has received research or institutional support from Synthes and Zimmer.*

the fracture fixation and the reduction of the fracture, the amount of strain at the fracture site can be controlled. Small fracture gaps will result in high local strain with no bone formation, whereas larger gaps cause lower strain levels and the formation of repair tissue. Because primary bone healing requires a strain of less than 2%, compression at the fracture site must be obtained. Splints, casts, intramedullary nails, bridging plates, and external fixation lead to strain levels of 2% to 10% and to secondary (callus, enchondral ossification) bone healing.

Strain within the fracture gap can be reduced by increasing the length of the gap (by fracture comminution, an imperfect reduction, or bony resorption at the fracture site) or by decreasing motion within the gap, which is dependent on the stiffness of the fixation construct.[2]

## Plating Methods and Mechanics
### Conventional Plating

Conventional plates rely on direct bony contact and friction between the plate and bone for stability. The torque used to insert the screws generates an axial preload and results in friction between the plate and bone. The plate must be perfectly contoured to sit directly on the bone. Because the screws can toggle in the plate, bicortical screw fixation is required to generate the high forces required to prevent this motion.[1,3] Good bone quality is required to achieve solid fixation.

The surgical approach used to apply the plate may damage the blood supply to the fracture site, and the plate may also damage the blood supply to the part of the bone that is compressed beneath it. The total biologic injury to the fracture is a combination of the original trauma and the surgical injury.

### Bridge Plating

Bridge plating or "internal external fixation" provides flexible fracture fixation and is typically used for the fixation of multifragmented shaft fractures. The plate is tunneled extraperiosteally and anchored remotely from the fracture site. This technique is believed to reduce vascular damage to the bone. The flexible fixation leads to healing with callus formation, which may be more rapid than that achieved with standard open fixation because there is less damage to the vascular supply at the fracture site.[4,5]

### Locked Screw Plating

Locking plates provide angular and axial stability by fixing the screws to the plate via a threaded interface. Each screw-plate interface contributes angular stability because the screws act like threaded bolts and maintain the position between the plate and the bone. Because the screws do not press the plate against the bone, there is no need for axial preloading of the screws. The bone plate contact area is minimized, which is less deleterious to the blood supply. Because the plate does not need to touch the bone, the plate does not have to be perfectly contoured to exactly fit the surface of the bone. Guides can be used to make percutaneous screw insertion easier because intraoperative plate contouring is not needed.

Locking screws have a larger core diameter than conventional screws because they transfer more bending load. When loaded perpendicularly to the long axis of the bone, the thinner threads will cut less into the surrounding bone.[4,5]

### How to Apply Plates

Building the plate-fracture construct essentially impacts the management of strain at the fracture site.

The stresses on the plate and screws should be designed to allow fracture healing before the hardware fails. One of the key factors to consider is the fracture type. It is important to determine if there is a large gap, where the fracture ends are too far apart to touch when loaded (often defined as > 6 mm), or a small gap (< 2 mm).

### Screw Position: Effect on Fracture Site Stiffness

The working length of a plate is defined as the distance from the first screw to the fracture site. When screws are placed close to the fracture site, the working length is short. If there are empty screw holes close to the fracture site, the working length is long. The working length affects axial stiffness and the torsional rigidity of the fixation construct. By omitting the screw closest to the fracture site, flexibility increases by 60% in compression and by 30% in torsion. Locking compression plate fatigue tests showed that when a small fracture gap (1 mm) was present, no construct failed; however, when a large gap (6 mm) was present, only the construct with the shortest working length lasted for 1 million test cycles.[6]

### Stress on the Plate and the Two Screws Closest to the Fracture Site

Leaving the screw hole closest to the fracture site empty (longer working length) increases the stress on the plate by 133%. When a large gap (6 mm) is present, the innermost two screws should be placed as close to the fracture site as possible.[6,7]

When a small fracture gap (1 mm) is present, plate stresses decrease when the working length increases because as the screws are spaced out, the plate becomes more flexible. This allows the fracture ends to contact and protects the plate. If the hole closest to the fracture gap is left empty, a 10% reduction in plate stress and a 63% reduction in stress on the screws occurs. If two holes are left empty, the plate stress decreases by 45% and the screw stress by 78%. When small gaps are present, the screws should be spread out, and two to three screws closest to the fracture site should be left out to make the plate more flexible.[6-8]

### Number of Screws

Inserting more than three screws does not increase axial stability, and more than four screws will not increase torsional stability. Screw position does not affect torsional stability but does affect axial stiffness. The closer an additional screw is placed to the fracture site, the stiffer the screw-plate construct becomes in axial compression. When using bridging plates for a lower extremity fracture, two to three screws on either side of the fracture are recommended. In theory, two unicortical screws per fragment are the bare minimum; however, this construct will fail if one screw breaks or if the screw-bone interface undergoes bone resorption. Unicortical screws should be used only in patients with excellent bone quality and when there is confidence that both screws are correctly placed. A minimum of three screws is recommended to ensure that at least two screws are "good" screws. For upper extremity fractures, three to four screws are recommended to resist the higher torsional forces present in the upper extremities.[6,8]

### Plate-to-Bone Distance

Increasing the distance the plate sits off the bone decreases stability because a longer portion of a screw is exposed and unsupported between the plate and bone; greater screw deformation can occur.[6]

### Plate Length

Screw pull-out force is inversely proportional to the distance between the fulcrum at the fracture site and the screw position. For the same bending moment, longer plates will produce less pull-out force. A construct with a shorter plate will have a reduction in axial stiffness; however, a change in plate length does not affect torsional stiffness. In practice, plate length is based on the plate span width and the plate screw density. Plate span width is defined as the length of the plate divided by the length of the fracture. A value of 2 to 3 is used for comminuted fractures, and a value of 8 to 10 is used for simple fractures. Screw density is defined as the number of screws divided by the number of screw holes in the plate. A value of 0.5 to 0.4 is recommended—meaning that less than one half of the screw holes are filled.[1,8]

### Unicortical Screws

Unicortical locking screws can be used because the screw heads lock to the plate. Because the metaphysis and the diaphyseal cortex of osteoporotic bone have a thin cortex, the working length of a unicortical screw in these situations will be very small. Therefore, a bicortical screw should be used to improve the working length of the screw. Unicortical locked screws are typically used in the diaphyseal segment (thick cortex) of a patient with good bone quality.[4,8]

### Hybrid Techniques

Hybrid fixation refers to using locked and nonlocked screws in the same plate. Most plating systems allow the insertion of both types of screw either in adjacent holes or through the same holes. A plate can be used as a compression plate, a locked internal fixator, or as a combination of both. If the plate has been well contoured, a regular screw can be inserted to pull the bone to the plate and complete the reduction of the fracture. If needed, locking screws then can be added to contribute points of angular stability. Another concern with pure locking plates is that they can only generate compression with an external compression device. Screws can be only inserted perpendicular to the plate, which means that no lag screws can be placed through the plate. Because locked screws cannot be angled in the plate, the screws may "miss" a fragment.[8]

A study evaluating the use of hybrid fixation in an osteoporotic distal humerus model showed that hybrid fixation did not decrease torsional stiffness; therefore, if a nonlocking screw is placed for a reduction, it does not need to be replaced with a locking screw.[3]

### Plate Placement in Osteoporotic Bone

Axial loads result in shear stresses at the plate-bone interface that are resisted by the frictional force between the plate and the bone. The magnitude of this frictional force depends on (1) the frictional coefficient between the plate and bone and (2) the normal force (applied at 90°) to the plate. This normal force is equal to the axial force generated by the torque used when inserting screws and is approximately 3 to 5 Nm for 3.5-mm screws placed in a nonosteopenic femur. The screw placed with the most torque will bear the largest load. When axial loads are applied to osteopenic bone, the bone

## Table 1
### Errors That Can Lead to Failure of Locking Plate Fixation

| Error | Details |
|-------|---------|
| Failure to lock the screw to the plate when the screw is inserted because of screw-plate malalignment | Locked screws will tolerate up to 5° of screw-insertion angle deviation. Deviation of more than 5° results in decreased stability because of the mismatch between the threads in the plate and the threads in the screw heads. Using an aiming device when inserting the locking screw can help to prevent this error. |
| Placing lag screws (absolute stability) in a fracture segment that is being bridged (relative stability) | This technique mixes two opposing fracture fixation techniques; the lag screws can interfere with the motion that is needed for secondary healing. |
| Not placing the locking screw in bone | Locking screws offer "good bite" only when placed in bone. |
| Improper placement of a locking screw in a fragment | Once a locking screw is placed in a fragment, a nonlocked screw cannot be used to fine-tune the reduction. |
| A locking screw cold welds to the plate. | To prevent this error, a torque-limiting screwdriver should be used for insertion. This error occurs less often when stainless steel plates are used compared with titanium plates. |
| An implant causes a problem with the path of the fixed screw. | This error occurs when there is screw "traffic" after articular fixation, or if a total joint arthroplasty is present. New polyaxial plates allow some variation in the path of locked screws. |
| The locking plate is placed too far off the bone. | Symptoms can result if locking plates are placed too far off the bone: plate prominence. |

may not be able to resist the shear forces generated by the advancing screw threads. This results in the feeling of "no bite" or "bad bite." Approximately 3 Nm can be generated in osteopenic bone, and this may allow motion with as little as 500 N of load. When an axial load that overcomes the frictional force is applied, the cortex closest to the plate provides axial screw control. When the shear stresses exceed the strength of the cortical bone, the bone is either compressed or resorbed; both conditions lead to screw loosening. Loosening of the fixation construct will lead to high fracture gap strain and a lack of healing.

When bending loads are applied to nonlocking screws, the bone captured by the screw threads resists shear stresses. The screw-bone interface is the weak link. The force needed to move a screw is equal to the stress resistance of the bone multiplied by its contact area with the screw. As the force increases, the screw heads rotate in the plate until they become parallel to the applied force.

The stability of a construct applied to osteopenic bone can be improved by several methods. Stress reduction at the screw-bone interface can be accomplished by increasing the contact area between the screw and the bone (such as by injection of polymethylmethacrylate or using a cancellous screw with wider threads). Stability of the construct can also be improved by using locking screws that change shear stress to compressive stress because bone is much better able to resist compressive stresses. In a locked system, the fixation strength is related to all of the screw-bone interfaces rather than the single best standard screw. Stability also is improved by increasing the frictional coefficient

between the plate and bone.[2]

### Current Indications for Using Locking Plates

Locking plates are indicated for patients with osteopenic bone. Because locking screws do not depend on a "good bite" for fixation, it may be possible to insert the screws at multiple angles through periarticular plates to better resist pull-out from the bone. Other advantages of locking plate systems include the better resistance of locking screws to bending and torsion forces; the decreased risk of stripping screws during insertion because the plate does not have to be compressed against the bone for stability; the larger core diameter of locking screws better resists cantilever and bending forces at the screw-cortex junction; and locking screws cannot toggle in the plate. Locking plates also are indicated for use in short fracture segments because the plates allow placement of multiple fixed-angle screws. Locking plates can also be used to stabilize two-column fractures when fixation on only one column is used (distal radius, distal femur and tibia, proximal tibia—there is no need to reconstruct the opposite column in comminuted fractures). Long bridge plates are useful for indirect fracture reduction because the plates do not have be perfectly contoured. Locking plates also are used to treat malunions and nonunions, in which disuse osteopenia or the presence of prior screw holes prevents the placement of standard nonlocking screws, and in periprosthetic fractures with short fracture segments that are osteoporotic.[2,9]

Errors that can lead to failures of locking plate fixation[9,10] are shown in Table 1. From an economic standpoint, locking plates and screws are more expensive than nonlocking hardware.

## Minimally Invasive Techniques

Percutaneous or minimally invasive techniques have transformed surgical indications and patient care, especially in injuries resulting from high-energy, soft-tissue trauma. Over the past few years, there has been increased use of biologic methods to minimize iatrogenic surgical trauma, decrease blood loss, and avoid the disruption of fracture biology associated with traditional open approaches. Newer implants have facilitated these improvements with precontoured plates and instruments designed for fracture reduction and percutaneous implant placement. Biologic internal fixation does not compromise the restoration of early and complete function of the limb and allows painless function and reliable healing.

Three-dimensional CT and MRI have led to a better understanding of fracture anatomy without exposing the entire fracture area. Percutaneous or minimally invasive techniques may be used for almost all periarticular fractures and proximal femur and humerus fractures. These techniques also have been adopted for nailing long bone fractures, allowing significantly smaller incisions than those of traditional methods.

### Biology

The goal of periarticular fracture surgery is anatomic articular reduction with acceptable metadiaphyseal alignment. The original AO principles of respecting soft tissues, stable fracture fixation, and early postoperative rehabilitation still apply to treatment of these injuries.

The blood supply to a long bone is composed of the nutrient arteries supplying the inner two thirds of the cortex and the periosteal arteries supplying the outer third of the cortex. In high-energy trauma, the blood supply to the fractured area may be almost completely disrupted, and some bony fragments may have a tenuous blood supply. Enhanced periosteal circulation derived from surrounding muscles becomes the primary source of blood supply at the fracture site. Treatment with traditional open reduction and internal fixation involving soft-tissue dissection and subperiosteal plating disperses the fracture hematoma, further strips the bone of its blood supply, and may result in bone necrosis and infection.

The use of principles of indirect reduction, minimal or no periosteal stripping with submuscular plating, smaller incisions, and less soft-tissue dissection with decreased vascular disruption leads to faster fracture healing, minimizes the infection rate, and decreases the need for bone grafting. In areas with high vascularity, such as acetabulum fractures, the use of minimally invasive approaches reduces the morbidity and blood loss associated with extensive approaches.

### Implants

A variety of implants are available that allow minimally invasive fracture fixation. These plates or nails usually are available with insertion guides that allow more precise implant placement, including screw placement distally or proximally to the fracture. Commercially available precontoured plates match the anatomy of the bone and can facilitate fracture reduction. These plates are designed for open plating; however, they can be used percutaneously with fluoroscopy or insertion guides. There is increasing use of precontoured locking plates, with screw heads that thread onto the plate, allowing a rigid construct. Because the locking screw plate construct is biomechanically stronger, it obviates the need for double plates and incisions, thereby reducing iatrogenic soft-tissue trauma and periosteal injury. It is important to remember that the fracture cannot be reduced to the locking plate and must be reduced anatomically before hardware placement.

Standard plates also may be contoured to fit the fractured bone by using radiographs and bone models. These plates can then be inserted percutaneously or with a small incision. A selection of instruments allowing percutaneous insertion of intramedullary nails is available, including those with longer nail insertion guides and longer sleeves for locking bolts.

### Techniques and Considerations

The technique for minimally invasive or percutaneous approaches is exacting and has a definite learning curve. Preoperative planning is essential to determine fracture patterns, implant selection and positioning, and incision placement.

Patient factors and fracture patterns must be carefully considered. Certain patient populations with poor blood circulation, significant bone and soft-tissue loss, and those who have had previous surgeries may not be amenable to indirect reduction and percutaneous techniques. Certain fracture patterns with significant joint compression or articular comminution will require an open approach for the articular reduction, followed by minimal incisions proximally or distally for implant placement.

A temporizing joint-spanning external fixator is useful for articular fracture alignment, regaining leg length, and for soft-tissue and pain management. External fixator pin placements must be such that they are proximal or distal to the expected plate length. Open fractures can be débrided and compartments released as needed with the fixator in place. Associated vascular injuries, if present, also can be treated. After the soft-tissue envelope is ready (usually 1 to 3 weeks after the initial injury), the definitive surgical procedure can be undertaken.

It is important to understand the characteristics of implant options; some allow fracture manipulation and reduction using the plate, whereas others require fracture reduction before plate application.

The use of percutaneous plates has been well described in the literature, with the use of locking plates for proximal tibial and distal femoral fractures. The use of this technique has been described for almost all fractures in the human body, including spine, calcaneus, and hip fractures.[11-15]

Fractures with significant joint compression and articular comminution may require arthrotomy to allow visualization of the fracture of the articular surface. Judicious use of large, pointed, bone reduction clamps and Kirschner wires is recommended for articular reduction. The articular depression can be elevated using bone tamps and supported with bone graft or substitutes, using the same mini incision. The periarticular screws for compression should be inserted as a "raft" to hold up the articular elevation. Direct visualization of the joint does not preclude a percutaneous approach to the rest of the bone, which can be fixed using these techniques; thus, the incision is re-stricted to the articular part of the bone as in a traditional approach.

Fluoroscopy is essential to confirm adequate reduction and extra-articular hardware placement and can help in guiding the location of the plate and the screws. Views must be orthogonal to the screws to confirm that they are correctly placed. Assessment of limb alignment and rotation can be difficult without direct visualization. At the knee, comparative radiographs from the contralateral side allow comparison of tibial plateau slope. The knee hyperextension test and fluoroscopy to check cortical diameter match is suggested to confirm accurate reduction.[16]

Proximal humerus fractures are amenable to percutaneous techniques, with the use of pins or plates. Percutaneous plating also has been described for humeral shaft fractures.[17] Certain acetabulum fractures and pelvic fractures also may be treated by judicious use of percutaneous techniques, including the use of sacroiliac screws.[18]

The emerging use of computer-guided navigation systems will allow more accurate placement of percutaneous screws and hardware and will decrease radiation exposure from fluoroscopy.[19,20]

## Outcomes

Stannard and associates[21] presented a study of 39 tibial plateau fractures treated with Less Invasive Stabilization System plates (LISS, Synthes, Paoli, PA). Most fractures healed without complications; 90% of patients had anatomic fracture reduction with the use of percutaneous techniques.[21] Cole and associates[22] evaluated 77 proximal tibia fractures treated with locked plates and a minimally invasive approach and reported a 97% union rate and malunion rate of less that 10%. The infection rate in both studies was low (Stannard, 6%; Cole, 4%) despite a 25% rate of open fractures. In a study of 23 patients with high-energy tibial plateau fractures treated with limited incisions and external fixation, Weigel and associates[23] found excellent results in 24 knees at an average follow-up of 8 years. The average knee range of motion was 120° of flexion; no patient required a reconstructive procedure. The authors noted that the articular cartilage was tolerant of the injury and mild residual articular displacement.

Brandt and associates[15] reported decreased surgical time and blood loss with a percutaneous hip fracture fixation using a specific implant. Kregor and associates[24] reported excellent results with 93% healing rates using LISS plate fixation in 103 distal femur fractures. No loss of fixation occurred, and a low infection rate (3%) was achieved using this minimally invasive technique.

## Summary

Improvements in implant technology, such as locked plating systems, and the use of minimally invasive techniques is changing the face of orthopaedic trauma care. Minimally invasive techniques allow better soft-tissue preservation and thereby lessen wound complications in high-energy fractures. The fracture biology remains undisturbed, leading to faster fracture healing and a decrease in the need for bone grafting. New implants allow improved fixation by changing plate-screw biomechanics and allowing better fracture fixation in patients with poor quality bone. A good understanding of bone and fracture anatomy will increase the use of improved implants and minimally invasive surgical techniques. The expanded use of computer navigation systems may be the next step to improve minimally invasive techniques and orthopaedic trauma care.

## References

1. Perren SM: Evolution of the internal fixation of long bone fractures. *J Bone Joint Surg Br* 2002;84:1093-1110.

2. Egol K, Kubiak EN, Fulkerson E, et al: Biomechanics of locked plates and screws. *J Orthop Trauma* 2004;18:488-493.

3. Gardner MJ, Griffith MH, Demetrakopoulos D, et al: Hybrid locked plating of osteoporotic fractures of the humerus. *J Bone Joint Surg Am* 2006;88:1962-1966.

4. Perren SM: Evolution and rationale of locked internal fixator technology introductory remarks. *Injury* 2001;32(suppl 2):B3-9.

5. Wagner M: General principles for the clinical use of the LCP. *Injury* 2003;34(suppl 2):B31-42.

6. Stoffel K, Dieter U, Stachowiak G, et al: Biomechanical testing of the LCP: How can stability in locked internal fixators be controlled? *Injury* 2003;34 (suppl 2):B11-B19.

7. Ellis T, Bourgeault CA, Kyle RF: Screw position affects dynamic compression plate strain in an in vitro fracture model. *J Orthop Trauma* 2001;15:333-337.

8. Gautier E, Sommer C: Guidelines for the clinical application of the LCP. *Injury* 2003;34:(suppl 2):B63-B76.

9. Haidukewych GJ: Innovations in locked plating technology. *J Am Acad Orthop Surg* 2004;12:205-212.

10. Kaab MJ, Frenk A, Schmeling A, et al: Locked internal fixator sensitivity of screw plate stability to the correct insertion angle of the screw. *J Orthop Trauma* 2004;18:483-487.

11. Truumees E, Hilibrand A, Vaccaro AR: Percutaneous vertebral augmentation. *Spine J* 2004;4:218-229.

12. Alvarez L, Alcaraz M, Pérez-Higueras A, et al: Percutaneous vertebroplasty: Functional improvement in patients with osteoporotic compression fractures. *Spine* 2006;31:1113-1118.

13. Talarico LM, Vito GR, Zyryanov SY: Management of displaced intraarticular calcaneal fractures by using external ring fixation, minimally invasive open reduction, and early weight-bearing. *J Foot Ankle Surg* 2004;43:43-50.

14. Alobaid A, Harvey EJ, Elder GM, Lander P, Guy P, Reindl R: Minimally invasive dynamic hip screw: Prospective randomized trial of two techniques of insertion of a standard dynamic fixation device. *J Orthop Trauma* 2004;18:207-212.

15. Brandt SE, Lefever S, Janzing HM, Broos PL, Pilot P, Houben BJ: Percutaneous compression plating (PCCP) versus the dynamic hip screw for pertrochanteric hip fractures: Preliminary results. *Injury* 2002;33:413-418.

16. Krettek C, Miclau T, Grün O, Schandelmaier P, Tscherne H: Intraoperative control of axes, rotation and length in femoral and tibial fractures: Technical note. *Injury* 1998;29 (suppl 3):C29-C39.

17. Apivatthakakul T, Arpornchayanon O, Bavornratanavech S: Minimally invasive plate osteosynthesis (MI-

PO)of the humeral shaft fracture: Is it possible?: A cadaveric study and preliminary report. *Injury* 2005;36:530-538.

18. Crowl AC, Kahler DM: Closed reduction and percutaneous fixation of anterior column acetabular fractures. *Comput Aided Surg* 2002;7:169-178.

19. Chong KW, Wong MK, Rikhraj IS, Howe TS: The use of computer navigation in performing minimally invasive surgery for intertrochanteric hip fractures: The experience in Singapore. *Injury* 2006;37:755-762.

20. Tonetti J, Carrat L, Lavalleé S, Pittet L, Merloz P, Chirossel JP: Percutaneous iliosacral screw placement using image guided techniques. *Clin Orthop Relat Res* 1998;354:103-110.

21. Stannard JP, Wilson TC, Volgas DA, Alonso JE: The less invasive stabilization system in the treatment of complex fractures of the tibial plateau: Short-term results. *J Orthop Trauma* 2004;18:552-558.

22. Cole PA, Zlowodzki M, Kregor PJ: Treatment of proximal tibia fractures using the less invasive stabilization system: Surgical experience and early clinical results in 77 fractures. *J Orthop Trauma* 2004;18:528-535.

23. Weigel DP, Marsh JL: High-energy fractures of the tibial plateau: Knee function after longer follow-up. *J Bone Joint Surg Am* 2002;84-A:1541-1551.

24. Kregor PJ, Stannard JA, Zlowodzki M, Cole PA: Treatment of distal femur fractures using the less invasive stabilization system: Surgical experience and early clinical results in 103 fractures. *J Orthop Trauma* 2004;18:509-520.

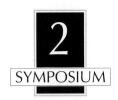

# The Changing Face of Orthopaedic Trauma: Fragility and Periprosthetic Fractures

*Andrew H. Schmidt, MD

## Abstract

*Because fragility fractures and periprosthetic fractures represent an increasingly common source of morbidity for the elderly population, all orthopaedic surgeons should be prepared to care for such injuries in their practice. Fractures in elderly patients appear to heal more slowly because of decreased numbers and responsiveness of osteoprogenitor stem cells, and stable fixation is more difficult to achieve. It is important to review the mechanical and biologic considerations relevant to the treatment of these challenging injuries.*

**Instr Course Lect 2008;57:11-16.**

Fractures related to osteoporosis (referred to as fragility fractures) and periprosthetic fractures are increasingly common. It is estimated that 200 million people worldwide are at risk for a fragility fracture, and 40% of women and 14% of men older than 50 years will experience a fragility fracture.[1,2] Many people who have had a fragility fracture will have another fragility fracture later in life. In fact, a history of previous fracture is associated with a twofold increase of fragility fracture in women.[3] Other risk factors for fragility fracture include diabetes in both genders and mental health disorders in men.[3] The number of patients who fracture their hip, a common form of fragility fracture, is expected to in-

crease 66% from 2000 to 2021 and by 190% from 2000 to 2051.[4] The cost of treating these fractures alone may overwhelm the health care systems of some countries.[4] The orthopaedic surgeon is in a unique position to help patients by referring those with fragility fractures for treatment of osteoporosis.

Fragility fractures and periprosthetic fractures typically occur in elderly patients. These fractures are difficult to stabilize for many reasons, including the presence of pre-existing implants in patients with periprosthetic fractures and decreased bone mineral density in those with fragility fractures. By definition, a fragility fracture occurs in osteopenic bone that has thin trabe-

culae and decreased capacity to support internal fixation devices. Fragility fractures are usually the result of low-energy injuries and often involve the metaphyseal segments of bone. In men, fragility fractures typically involve the spine, ribs, and the wrist, whereas in women fragility fractures most often occur in the spine, ribs, wrist, humerus, and femur. Although surgical treatment is not always needed, successful internal fixation may be challenging when surgery is indicated.

Periprosthetic fractures occur through stress risers related to the associated implant and often involve osteolytic lesions that may not have been recognized. The associated implant limits options for internal fixation of the fracture and impairs the function of the local immune system. Both of these factors contribute to the increased risk of complications during the management of periprosthetic fractures with regard to both fracture healing and infection.

## Biomechanical and Biologic Consequences of Osteoporosis

Osteoporotic bone has distinct morphologic characteristics that in-

*Andrew H. Schmidt, MD or the department with which he is affiliated has received research or institutional support from Smith and Nephew and serves as a consultant or employee for Smith and Nephew.*

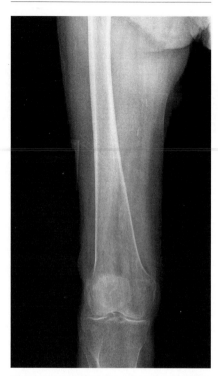

**Figure 1** AP radiograph of the distal femur of a 98-year-old woman. Note the thinning of the cortex and the medullary expansion of the distal femur. These changes result in what is often described as the "stove-pipe femur."

fluence its biomechanical properties and therefore the choices and techniques for internal fixation. The diaphysis undergoes both endosteal cortical resorption and medullary expansion. The result is a thinning of the cortex and an overall increase in the diameter of the bone (Figure 1). Mechanically, these changes are adaptive and serve to maintain the flexural rigidity of the bone by increasing its moment of inertia, thus counterbalancing the increased cortical porosity (decreased density) that would otherwise weaken it. In the metaphysis, the primary finding in patients with osteoporosis is decreased bone mineral density, which affects the compressive strength of cancellous bone and increases the likelihood of articular impaction. These changes make it difficult to insert internal fixation.

The effects of aging on the bone must be considered in terms of both mechanical and biologic changes. From a mechanical perspective, decreased bone density and decreased cortical thickness diminish the holding power of screws; at the same time, changes in bone morphology affect the mechanical strength of the bone as a whole. Decreased bone mineral density means that the applied load at the bone-implant interface can exceed the mechanical tolerance of the bone, leading to fatigue failure of the bone, resorption of damaged bone, and ultimately to loosening of the implant.

From a biologic perspective, it is known that there are decreased numbers of osteoprogenitor stem cells in elderly patients, and remaining cells demonstrate a decreased proliferative response to normal stimuli. Although fracture healing proceeds through normal mechanisms in elderly patients, the process is much slower than in younger patients. In elderly patients, there is a confluence of factors—prolonged fracture healing, less secure fixation, and a patient who is less able to tolerate changes in function or protect the injured limb—that make the treatment of fragility and periprosthetic fractures a challenge.

## Fragility Fractures

Indications for surgery in most fractures are well defined and include consideration of the patient's functional demands and expectations, as well as the fracture characteristics, including the degree of articular impaction and fracture displacement.

In general, load-sharing implants (such as intramedullary nails) are preferred to load-bearing devices (such as plates). When fixing osteoporotic fractures, devices offering relative stability (such as bridge plates, buttress plates, and nails) are preferred to devices that rely on absolute stability (such as lag screws or compression plates). Because of decreased bone mineral density, bone augmentation with materials such as polymethylmethacrylate or one of the calcium phosphate cements should be considered.[5] It is also important to protect the entire bone to avoid secondary fracture.[6] Fixed-angle devices such as blade plates or the newer locking plates should be used if possible. Plates using locked screws will decrease stress on the bone by shifting the primary forces from the screw-bone interface to the screw-plate interface; these devices do not fail unless the entire volume of bone fails.

Arthroplasty may be better than internal fixation for specific fractures, such as those about the shoulder, elbow, and hip.[7-9]

### Proximal Humerus Fractures
Hemiarthroplasty of the shoulder has traditionally been recommended for the treatment of displaced, comminuted proximal humerus fractures in elderly patients.[10] However, recent studies question the role of surgery for many of these patients because functional outcomes are similar with surgical and nonsurgical treatment in three-part fractures, and results of internal fixation and arthroplasty are similar for those with four-part fractures.[11] In its most recent review of this topic, the Cochrane Database of Systematic Reviews was unable to establish a definitive conclusion concerning the management of proximal humerus fractures.[12]

Recent literature supports both internal fixation and hemiarthroplasty of the shoulder for displaced proximal humerus fractures in elderly patients. There has been increased interest in new methods of repairing these fractures, with some investigators reporting successful outcomes with locking plates.[13] In one study (M Torchia, MD, Minneapolis, MN, unpublished data presented at the Minnesota Orthopedic Society annual meeting, 2006) a technique using "balanced-compression" was used to repair displaced proximal humerus fractures in 10 elderly patients (age range, 77 to 90 years). Four patients had two-part fractures, five had three-part fractures, and one patient had a four-part fracture based on the Neer classification system. All patients were treated with balanced compression using a locking plate, bone grafting, and tension band fixation. Active motion was delayed for 3 months; all fractures healed, and all patients regained normal function.

Robinson and associates[10] reported the results of a 13-year observational study of 163 consecutive patients treated with shoulder hemiarthroplasty for a proximal humerus fracture. At 1 year, 138 patients were available for a functional assessment. The median modified Constant score was 64 at the 1-year assessment; patients typically had a good pain score but poorer scores for function, motion, and muscle power. Prosthetic survival was 93.9% at 10 years, with revision as an evaluation end point. In this study, patient age, the presence of a neurologic deficit, the need for revision surgery, radiographic displacement of the prosthetic head from the central axis of the glenoid, and displacement of the tuberosities were significant predictive factors of the 1-year Constant score ($P < 0.05$).

For proximal humerus fractures requiring surgery, both hemiarthroplasty and internal fixation are good treatment options. The preference and skills of the surgeon should determine the treatment choice.

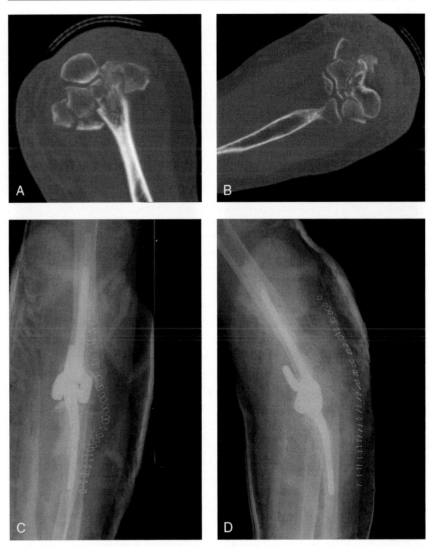

**Figure 2**   Comminuted distal humerus fracture in a 70-year-old woman. AP **(A)** and lateral **(B)** two-dimensional CT reconstructions of the elbow showing severe comminution of the articular surface. Postoperative AP **(C)** and lateral **(D)** radiographs of the elbow after primary total elbow arthroplasty.

### Distal Humerus Fractures

Distal humeral fractures in elderly patients can be associated with severe comminution and difficulty with internal fixation. Although internal fixation seems to produce better results than nonsurgical treatment, more complications occur in elderly patients than in younger patients.[14] If internal fixation is used to treat these fractures, the use of locked plates, the increased use of bone grafts, and more conservative rehabilitation should be considered. Alternatively, total elbow replacement is viewed as a good option for these patients (Figure 2). In a retrospective review, Frankle and associates[8] studied women older than 65 years who sustained a distal humerus fracture. Patients treated with immediate total elbow replacement had improved Mayo Elbow Performance scores and needed no revision surgery, which was necessary in 25% of the patients who were treated with internal fixation.

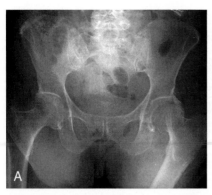
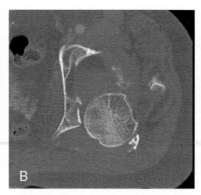
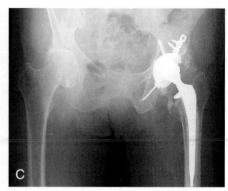

**Figure 3**    A posterior hip fracture-dislocation in a 80-year-old woman was treated with acute open reduction and internal fixation of the acetabulum, with immediate total hip arthroplasty. **A,** AP radiograph of the pelvis showing the dislocated left hip. **B,** Axial CT cut showing fracture of the posterior wall of the acetabulum with severe marginal impaction. **C,** Postoperative radiograph after reconstruction. The patient was doing well at 5-year follow-up.

### Distal Radius Fractures

Volar locked plating has been favored for the internal fixation of distal radius fractures. Interestingly, bone density has been shown to influence the outcome of distal radius fractures more than radiographic parameters.[15] Orbay and Fernandez[16] published a review of patients older than 75 years with a distal radius fracture who were treated using volar locked plating. In this study, patients had no significant loss of reduction or plate failures. Overall arm and hand function was good, and grip strength was 77% of that in the noninjured hand.

Another study examined the use of calcium-phosphate cement in augmenting bone and preventing the collapse of distal radius fractures treated with more conservative measures.[17] In 52 osteoporotic women, treatment with percutaneous pinning, injection of calcium phosphate cement, and 3 weeks of casting was compared with percutaneous pinning and 6 weeks of cast treatment. The group with the augmented regimen of calcium phosphate cement had better functional outcome, range of motion, and grip strength ($P < 0.001$).[17] In contrast, loss of reduction was significantly higher in the control (nonaugmented) group ($P < 0.001$).

### Acetabular Fractures

Poor results have been reported in osteopenic patients with acetabular fractures who were treated with standard open reduction and internal fixation. Immediate total hip arthroplasty (THA) may be a good treatment choice in centers experienced with this surgery (Figure 3). The rationale for acute THA is that it may avoid a likely second surgery in an elderly patient with a compromised medical condition. It must be determined, however, if acute THA can be done safely and without an increased risk of hip dislocation or acetabular component loosening. At the author's institution, a candidate for acute THA would be an elderly patient with an injury following low-energy trauma; with impaction of the femoral head, acetabular roof, and/or anterior or posterior wall; an incongruent reduction; and poor bone quality.

### Proximal Femoral Fractures

Fractures of the upper end of the femur are very common in elderly patients. Most surgeons still treat nondisplaced and/or impacted femoral neck fractures with multiple screws. The treatment of displaced femoral neck fractures is controversial; internal fixation, hemiarthroplasty, and THA all are appropriate in specific situations. Extracapsular fractures are usually managed with internal fixation. Stable fracture patterns, defined as those fractures without loss of the posteromedial buttress and/or lateral wall, may be easily treated with a traditional sliding hip screw. The current consensus is that unstable fractures are better treated with an intramedullary device.[18]

### Distal Femoral Fractures

Supracondylar femur fractures are common in elderly patients. Most patients benefit from stabilization of these injuries so that knee motion and functional abilities can be maintained. Although a variety of plates or retrograde intramedullary nails can be used successfully in these fractures, locked distal femoral periarticular plates are a popular treatment option. Current techniques include initial reconstruction of the femoral condyles with interfragmentary lag screws as needed using an anterolateral approach, followed by stabilization of the distal segment to the femoral shaft with a submuscular plate. Fixation of the plate to the shaft can be percutaneous or done through a second incision in the lateral thigh. No studies have demonstrated a benefit to percutaneous techniques.

Locking distal femoral nails are becoming available, which will cause renewed debate about the ideal method to manage these fractures. Tejwani and associates[19] studied the biomechanical effect of locked distal screws in retrograde nailing of osteoporotic distal femur fractures. In seven matched pairs of embalmed cadaveric femora, a 2.5-cm gap in the supracondylar region of the distal femur was stabilized with a 12-mm diameter retrograde nail with or without locking screws. Constructs with a locked distal screw exhibited less collapse, less anterior and medial translation of the nail at the fracture site, and less varus angulation than the unlocked distal screw nails. Properly designed comparative trials of periarticular locked plating versus retrograde nailing are needed before it can be determined if these new implants improve results compared with traditional techniques and implants.

Severely comminuted distal femoral fractures in elderly patients also can be treated with primary total knee arthroplasty. Most authors have reported on the use of hinged implant designs, with complete resection of the distal femur below the fracture site.[20] These patients typically have low functional demands, and have a shortened life expectancy. Immediate arthroplasty allows for rapid mobilization and may decrease the risk of fixation failure and reoperation that exists when any form of internal fixation is attempted.

## Periprosthetic Fractures

Risk factors for periprosthetic fractures include weakened bone from stress risers related to the existing implant, periprosthetic osteolysis, screw holes, cortical perforations, and trauma. Treatment goals are to achieve fracture union, maintain the function of the associated prosthesis, and avoid the "succession of fractures" that often occurs when a second fracture occurs adjacent to the implant used to stabilize the first. When treating a periprosthetic fracture, several factors must be considered, including the health of the patient, the patient's use of tobacco, the presence of any systemic disease, and whether the patient is immunocompromised. Other factors to consider include whether the patient has been treated with previous irradiation, the degree of osteoporosis and/or osteolysis that is present about the fracture site, the type of implant present (press-fit versus cemented, short-stem versus long-stem), whether there is more than one implant, and whether there have been previous fractures or if other stress risers are in the bone.

Nonsurgical treatment options include traction or bracing, which are appropriate for stable, minimally displaced fractures and are rarely indicated. External fixation is similarly rarely used because of the poor fixation achieved and the risk of infection. Cerclage wire alone can be used for trochanteric fractures or long spiral fractures. Plating is the most common method of fracture stabilization about functioning prostheses. Plating seems to be more reliable when a fixed-angle device is used in the distal half of the femur and when long plates are used with screw fixation at each end.[21] Cortical struts are useful to augment fixation, although their routine use has been questioned.[22] Alternatively, for fem-

oral fractures about total hip stems, long-stem revision is an approach that is applicable to all fractures, but it is usually reserved only for those about a failed (loose, worn, or malpositioned) stem.

For fracture at the tip of the femoral stem, the dilemma is whether to revise or proceed with fracture reduction and fixation. Slightly better results seem to be achieved with long-stem revision THA than with internal fixation of these fractures.[23,24] Stable implants require only fixation, whereas unstable implants require revision and fixation.

## Summary

Fragility fractures, including periprosthetic fractures, are becoming more common as the population ages and as more elderly patients undergo arthroplasty. Management of these fractures is complicated by delayed fracture healing and the impaired biomechanical quality of osteopenic bone. These fractures demand special consideration, including consideration of alternative methods of fracture fixation. Such methods include the use of intramedullary nails instead of plates when possible, the use of locking screws when plating is necessary, consideration of bone augmentation, and possibly, the use of biophysical stimulation. The literature does not provide definitive evidence that these theoretic measures are of clinical benefit.

## References

1. Cummings SR, Kelsey JL, Nevitt MC, O'Dowd KJ: Epidemiology of osteoporosis and osteoporotic fractures. *Epidemiol Rev* 1985;7:178-208.

2. Eastell R, Lambert H: Strategies for skeletal health in the elderly. *Proc Nutr Soc* 2002;61:173-180.

3. Holmberg AH, Johnell O, Nilsson PM, Nilsson J, Berglund G, Akesson K: Risk factors for fragility fracture in middle age: A prospective population-based study of 33,000 men and women. *Osteoporos Int* 2006; 17:1065-1077.

4. Chipchase LS, McCaul K, Hearn TC: Hip fracture rates in South Australia: Into the next century. *Aust N Z J Surg* 2000;70:117-119.

5. Collinge C, Merk B, Lautenschlager EP: Mechanical evaluation of fracture fixation augmented with tricalcium phosphate in a porous osteoporotic cancellous bone model. *J Orthop Trauma* 2007;21:124-128.

6. Patton JT, Cook RE, Adams CI, Robinson CM: Late fracture of the hip after reamed intramedullary nailing of the femur. *J Bone Joint Surg Br* 2000; 82:967-971.

7. Mighell MA, Kolm GP, Collinge CA, Frankle MA: Outcomes of hemiarthroplasty for fractures of the proximal humerus. *J Shoulder Elbow Surg* 2003;12:569-577.

8. Frankle MA, Herscovici D, Di Pasquale TG, Vasey MB, Sanders RW: A comparison of open reduction and internal fixation and primary total elbow arthroplasty in the treatment of intraarticular distal humerus fractures in women older than age 65. *J Orthop Trauma* 2003;17:473-480.

9. Healy WL, Iorio R: Total hip arthroplasty: Optimal treatment for displaced femoral neck fractures in elderly patients. *Clin Orthop Relat Res* 2004;429:43-48.

10. Robinson CM, Page RS, Hill RM, Sanders DL, Court-Brown CM, Wakefield AE: Primary hemiarthroplasty for treatment of proximal humeral fractures. *J Bone Joint Surg Am* 2003;85-A:1215-1223.

11. Misra A, Kapur R, Maffuli N: Complex proximal humeral fractures in adults: A systematic review of management. *Injury* 2001;32:363-372.

12. Handoll HH, Gibson JN, Madhok R: Interventions for treating proximal humeral fractures in adults. *Cochrane Database Syst Rev* 2003;4:CD000434.

13. Fankhauser F, Boldin C, Schippinger G, Haunschmid C, Szyszkowitz R: A new locking plate for unstable fractures of the proximal humerus. *Clin Orthop Relat Res* 2005;430:176-181.

14. Srinivasan K, Agarwal M, Matthews SJ, Giannoudis PV: Fractures of the distal humerus in the elderly: Is internal fixation the treatment of choice? *Clin Orthop Relat Res* 2005;434:222-230.

15. Hollevoet N, Verdonk R: Outcome of distal radius fractures in relation to bone mineral density. *Acta Orthop Belg* 2003;69:510-514.

16. Orbay JL, Fernandez DL: Volar fixed-angle plate fixation for unstable distal radius fractures in the elderly patient. *J Hand Surg Am* 2004;29:96-102.

17. Zimmermann R, Gabl M, Lutz M, Angermann P, Gschwentner M, Pechlaner S: Injectable calcium phosphate bone cement Norian SRS for the treatment of intra-articular compression fractures of the distal radius in osteoporotic women. *Arch Orthop Trauma Surg* 2003;123:22-27.

18. Utrilla AL, Reig JS, Munoz FM, Tufanisco CB: Trochanteric gamma nail and compression hip screw for trochanteric fractures: A randomized, prospective, comparative study in 210 elderly patients with a new design of the gamma nail. *J Orthop Trauma* 2005;19:229-233.

19. Tejwani NC, Park S, Iesaka K, Kummer F: The effect of locked distal screws in retrograde nailing of osteoporotic distal femur fractures: A laboratory study using cadaver femurs. *J Orthop Trauma* 2005;19:380-383.

20. Appleton P, Moran M, Houshian S, Robinson CM: Distal femoral fractures treated by hinged total knee replacement in elderly patients. *J Bone Joint Surg Br* 2006;88:1065-1070.

21. Duwelius PJ, Schmidt AH, Kyle RF, Talbott V, Ellis TJ, Butler JB: A prospective, modernized treatment protocol for periprosthetic femur fractures. *Orthop Clin North Am* 2004;35: 485-492.

22. Ricci WM, Bolhofner BR, Loftus T, Cox C, Mitchell S, Borrelli J: Indirect reduction and plate fixation, without grafting, for periprosthetic femoral shaft fractures about a stable intramedullary implant. *J Bone Joint Surg Am* 2005;87:2240-2245.

23. Mont MA, Maar DC: Fractures of the ipsilateral femur after hip arthroplasty: A statistical analysis of outcome based on 487 patients. *J Arthroplasty* 1994;9:511-519.

24. Jukkala-Partio K, Partio EK, Solovieva S, Paavilainen T, Hirvensalo E, Alho A: Treatment of periprosthetic fractures in association with total hip arthroplasty: A retrospective comparison between revision stem and plate fixation. *Ann Chir Gynaecol* 1998;87: 229-235.

# Technical Tips in Fracture Care: Fractures of the Hip

*Jeffrey O. Anglen, MD
Michael R. Baumgaertner, MD
Wade R. Smith, MD
Paul Tornetta III, MD
*Bruce H. Ziran, MD

## Abstract

*Hip fracture is an increasingly common and clinically significant injury with substantial economic impact. Associated risk factors are age, gender, race, bone density, activity level, and medical disorders. Prevention efforts include treatment of osteoporosis and programs to reduce the risks of a fall.*

*Nondisplaced or impacted fractures of the femoral neck can be treated with screw fixation. Displaced femoral neck fractures in younger, more active patients may be treated with reduction and fixation. In physiologically older patients, joint arthroplasty is indicated for displaced fractures. In patients with systemic arthritis or preexisting hip disease, total hip arthroplasty may be an appropriate treatment choice.*

*Intertrochanteric fractures are treated with reduction and fixation using either a sliding hip screw and side plate or intramedullary nail with cephalic interlock. Key technical points for successful outcomes include proper patient positioning, using a correct starting point for the nail, achieving acceptable reduction before fixation, and the use of various reduction techniques and aids.*

**Instr Course Lect 2008;57:17-24.**

Fractures of the hip joint include fractures of the acetabulum, femoral head, and proximal femur. This chapter will examine fractures of the femoral neck and intertrochanteric area of the proximal femur.

## Etiology, Incidence, and Risk Factors

Hip fracture can occur in patients of any age. In younger patients, such fractures are usually the result of high-energy trauma, such as a motor vehicle crash. In these patients, multiple system injuries or associated orthopaedic injuries often occur. In elderly patients, injury usually results from a lower energy mechanism such as a fall; older patients often have multiple medical comorbidities.

Hip fracture in elderly patients is extremely common. Current statistics show that more than 250,000 such injuries occur annually in the United States, with an expected increase to 350,000 by 2020.[1] Projections for the worldwide incidence of hip fracture are as high as 6.5 million annually by 2050.[2] A 50-year-old Caucasian woman currently has a 17.5% lifetime risk of hip fracture; for men of the same age, the risk is 6%. In the United States, the annual cost for the care of patients with hip fractures is more than $14 billion and may increase to $250 billion by 2040. Risk factors for hip fracture in elderly patients are shown in Table 1.

## Outcome

Hip fracture is a significant event with potentially negative outcomes. Twenty percent of elderly patients with hip fractures die within 1 year of the fracture. The relative risk of death within that period is increased 3.3 times for women and 4.2 times for men with hip fracture, compared with age-matched control subjects who have not had a hip fracture. Ap-

*Jeffrey Anglen, MD or the department with which he is affiliated has received royalties from EBI and serves as a consultant or employee for Eli Lilly. Bruce Ziran, MD or the department with which he is affiliated has received miscellaneous nonincome support, commercially derived honoraria, or other nonresearch-related funding from Stryker and Synthes.

**Table 1**
**Risk Factors for Hip Fracture in Elderly Patients**

Age: the incidence of hip fracture increases for each decade of life from the sixth to the ninth.

Gender: 80% of hip fractures occur in women, although the rate of increase may be higher in men according to some studies.

Race: Caucasian women have 2.4 times the risk of hip fracture compared with African-American women. The highest incidence of hip fracture occurs in Scandinavian women.

Bone mineral density: each standard deviation below the age-adjusted average doubles the risk of hip fracture.

Previous wrist fracture

Previous fall or other fracture

High transfer dependence

Dementia

Visual impairment

Neuromuscular impairment

Lower extremity weakness

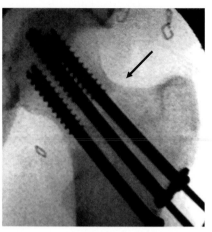

**Figure 1** Placement of cannulated screws in parallel orientation with all threads crossing the fracture site results in compression of the fracture line (*arrow*). The use of washers in metaphyseal areas facilitates compression.

proximately one half of the patients with hip fracture never regain their premorbid level of ambulation, and approximately 17% who were community ambulators prior to the hip fracture will be institutionalized after the fracture.

## Prevention

The prevention of hip fractures involves the use of dietary supplements and medications to treat patients with osteoporosis, reducing the risk of falls through exercise to improve balance and physical strength, behavioral instruction, environmental modifications, and the use of hip protectors in selected patients.[3-5] Information about reducing the risks of falls is available on the American Academy of Orthopaedic Surgeons Website.[6]

## Treatment

In most patients, fractures of the hip require surgical treatment. Nonsurgical treatment is occasionally appropriate for bedridden or non-ambulatory patients, those with extremely limited life expectancy, those with severe neurologic im-

pairment, or patients who are unable to tolerate surgery.

### Femoral Neck Fractures

The timing of surgery for a patient with a femoral neck fracture depends on many factors. In young patients, a femoral neck fracture is considered by most surgeons to be an emergent condition, with the risk of developing osteonecrosis of the femoral head increasing with any delay in treatment. However, a recent meta-analysis by Damany and associates[7] did not show strong evidence for this position. In elderly patients, optimization of the patient's medical condition may require surgery to be delayed; however, delays of more than 48 hours have been shown to increase the length of hospitalization, and delays in surgery of more than 4 to 5 days increase patient mortality.[8,9]

Fractures of the femoral neck have been classified by the Garden system into four types. In a Garden type 1 fracture, the femoral neck is impacted into the femoral head in a valgus position; a Garden type 2 fracture is a nondisplaced, nonim-

pacted fracture; a Garden type 3 is a displaced fracture with an offset of less than 50% of the neck width; and a Garden type 4 fracture has more than 50% displacement.

The appropriate surgical treatment for Garden type 1 and 2 fractures is fixation in situ with percutaneous, partially threaded, cannulated screws. The screws should be placed parallel and peripheral along the cortical bone of the neck to prevent postoperative displacement (Figure 1). Three screws are sufficient.[10] One screw is placed inferiorly along the medial aspect of the neck (calcar) and the other two screws are placed in an inverted triangular arrangement anterior and posterior. Correct positioning of the screws along the cortex of the femoral neck, particularly inferior and posterior, leads to a significant improvement in the rate of union. The more superior screws in the metaphysis should have washers to allow compression. Threads should not cross the fracture site.

For displaced fractures in younger patients, reduction and fixation preserve the hip joint. The most important surgeon-controlled factor in outcome is the quality of reduction. An open reduction is often required to achieve anatomic alignment. The patient is positioned supine on a fracture table to facilitate fluoroscopic visualization of the femoral neck. Good biplanar C-arm images should be confirmed before the patient is prepared for surgery. Either the Smith Petersen (anterior) or the Watson Jones (anterolateral) surgical approach can be used. The anterolateral approach makes it easier to insert fixation screws. An anterior arthrotomy is gently performed to preserve blood supply; it is done in a manner that allows closure of the capsule at the end.

Tips for achieving proper reduction include inducing full muscle relaxation in the patient and the use of joysticks. This procedure is commonly performed with a 4.5-mm Schanz screw in the femoral shaft, and a 2.5-mm terminally threaded Kirschner wire in the femoral head. Provisional reduction is held with multiple smooth Kirschner wires, while the reduction is evaluated with direct vision and fluoroscopy. The contour of the femoral head and neck should make a smooth, lazy S outline along superior, inferior, anterior, and posterior borders (Figure 2). Fixation is performed with three large, cannulated lag screws, as previously described.

In an elderly patient with a displaced femoral neck fracture, the surgeon and patient should discuss the options of treatment with open reduction and internal fixation or with hip joint arthroplasty. If joint replacement is chosen, hemiarthroplasty (bipolar or unipolar) or total hip arthroplasty may be performed. With either method, the stem may be cemented or cementless.

Internal fixation results in less blood loss, shorter surgical time, a lower infection rate, and a lower overall complication rate; however, the rate of resurgery is significantly higher.[11] Differences in the mortality rate have not been clearly established; however, a recent meta-analysis suggests a slightly higher mortality rate for patients treated with arthroplasty.[12] A study using cost analysis methodology suggested that arthroplasty was the most cost-effective treatment when complications, mortality, and the rate of resurgery were considered at 2 years postoperatively. However, the best functional results were obtained in patients with a healed femoral neck with no osteonecrosis after open reduction and internal fixation.[13] A reasonable approach is to perform arthroplasty in any patient older than 75 years, or older than 55 years if there are significant comorbidities, such as neurologic disease, lower extremity weakness, significant osteoporosis, and preexisting arthritis, or if the patient is sedentary with a limited activity level. Reduction and fixation may be a worthwhile treatment choice in healthy, active patients who are younger than 60 years, do not have arthritis, have good bone quality, and have limited comminution. For patients who do not fit into either group, treatment options should be carefully discussed with the patient.

If arthroplasty is selected, total hip arthroplasty is indicated in patients with preexisting arthritis, acetabular damage, or in patients with systemic arthritic disease, even if the hip is relatively spared. Some surgeons believe that better functional results are achieved with total hip arthroplasty for all patients.[14] In a recent prospective, randomized study of 81 elderly patients with displaced

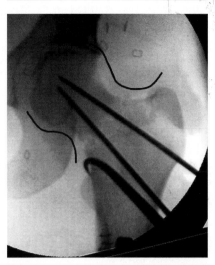

**Figure 2**  Accurate reduction of the femoral neck results in a smooth S outline of the head and neck in both AP and lateral projections.

femoral neck fractures, patients treated with total hip arthroplasty reported walking farther and had better hip scores than patients treated with hemiarthroplasty. There were no significant differences in mortality rates or complications in the two groups.[15] Dislocations occurred in three patients treated with total hip arthroplasty. Some studies have shown higher dislocation rates with total hip arthroplasty (more than 10% in some studies).[16] No consistent clinical differences have been found in several studies comparing bipolar with unipolar hemiarthroplasty; however, bipolar prostheses have a significantly higher cost.[17-20] In studies comparing cemented with cementless stems, results showed better functional results and less pain with the use of cemented stems, although most of these studies included patients with older stem designs.[21-24] The comparison of posterior and lateral surgical approaches have shown no differences in outcome.[25] The use of general and regional anesthesia has also resulted in similar outcomes.[26,27]

### Intertrochanteric Fractures

Intertrochanteric (pertrochanteric) fractures in ambulatory patients are treated with reduction and fixation. This procedure is best performed on a fracture table (Figure 3). Verification of C-arm visualization is recommended before the patient is prepared and draped for surgery.

Reduction is performed with longitudinal traction and rotation, which is usually internal. The use of crutch support of the distal fragment is often helpful (Figure 4); occasionally, a percutaneous ball-tipped spike or Schanz screw is used to assist in the reduction (Figures 5 and 6). These devices are often placed through a small anterior stab incision to correct a flexed proximal fragment.

Fixation options for these frac-tures include a sliding compression screw and side plate, intramedullary hip screws, 95°-blade plates or a screw and side plates, and specialized plates such as the Medoff plate or a locking proximal femur plate. In most instances, a sliding compression screw or an intramedullary screw will be equally effective, and both can be placed through relatively small incisions. A sliding compression screw with a two-hole side plate is adequate fixation for simple two-part fractures. A meta-analysis of the literature suggests that intraoperative complications and postoperative femoral fractures more commonly occur with intramedullary hip screws; however, the more recent literature suggests that intramedullary screws may allow earlier ambulation.[28-30] If there is comminution of the lateral cortex,

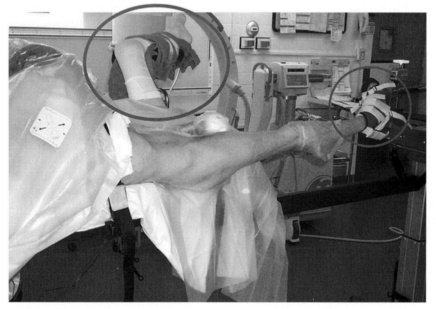

**Figure 3**   The patient is positioned on the fracture table with the foot (on the injured side) slightly internally rotated to facilitate reduction. Note the position of the leg and foot (*circled areas*). The hemilithotomy position, which should only be used for short periods (< 2 hours), is shown.

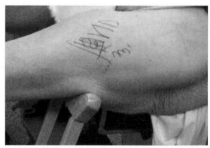
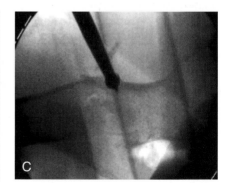

**Figure 4**   A crutch can be used to support the leg and reduce posterior sag.

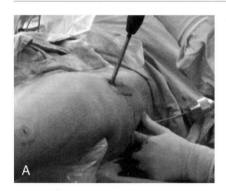
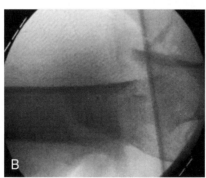
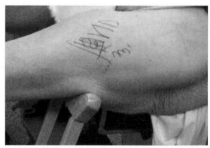

**Figure 5**   **A,** A percutaneous ball-tipped spike is used to improve reduction by resisting flexion of the proximal fragment. **B,** Fluoroscopic view showing apex anterior angulation at the fracture site caused by flexion of the proximal fragment. **C,** Fluoroscopic view showing correction of the malreduction using a percutaneous ball-tipped spike.

or reverse obliquity of the fracture line, an intramedullary screw or 95°-device is necessary to resist displacement.[31,32] Use of a standard compression hip screw in fractures of this type will often result in shortening and medial displacement.

A sliding compression hip screw can be placed through a minimal incision for simple, stable (lateral cortex intact) fractures. The guide pin is placed percutaneously through a poke hole with fluoroscopic control, using a 130° or larger angle guide that is determined based on preoperative planning. The ideal position of the guide pin is central and deep on both views. This placement results in a final screw position with a tip-apex distance of less than 2 cm, which decreases the risk of screw cutout.[33] An incision from skin to bone is made from the guidewire distally 2 or 3 cm. Reaming, measuring, tapping, and screw placement are done in standard fashion through this incision. A two-hole short barrel plate is inserted through the incision and bluntly worked to the bone; after verification of position, it is attached with cortical screws (Figure 7).

Intramedullary hip screw or nail placement begins with proper positioning to allow access to the starting point without introducing varus malalignment. The trunk of the patient should be leaned or angled toward the opposite side. An adequate incision must be made in obese patients to allow the insertion handle to be used without undue lateral pressure from the soft tissues proximal to the hip; this results in fracture distraction (Figure 8). As with any intramedullary device, the starting point is the key factor in good technique. The most common error is using a starting point too far lateral, which results in varus malalign-

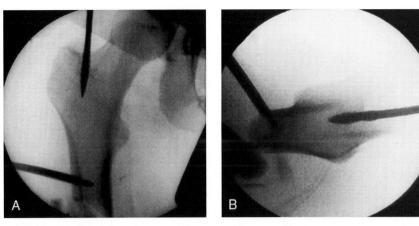

**Figure 6** Percutaneous placement of a Schanz pin may be useful in controlling the proximal fragment in many fractures of the proximal femur. **A,** AP fluoroscopic view showing use of a percutaneous unicortical Schanz pin to resist abduction of the short proximal fragment. **B,** Lateral fluoroscopic view showing correct alignment of the T-handled awl.

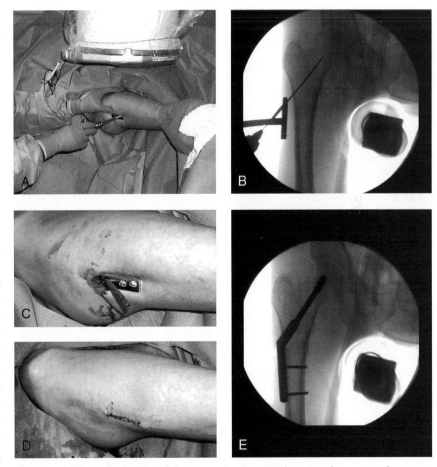

**Figure 7** Photograph **(A)** and fluoroscopic view **(B)** showing placement of a percutaneous guide pin for minimal incision hip screw insertion. **C,** After reaming and placement of the lag screw through a small (4 cm) incision, the two-hole plate can be inserted and attached by mobilizing the skin and soft tissues. **D,** Final incision for a three-hole plate. **E,** Fluoroscopic view showing the final reduction and plate position.

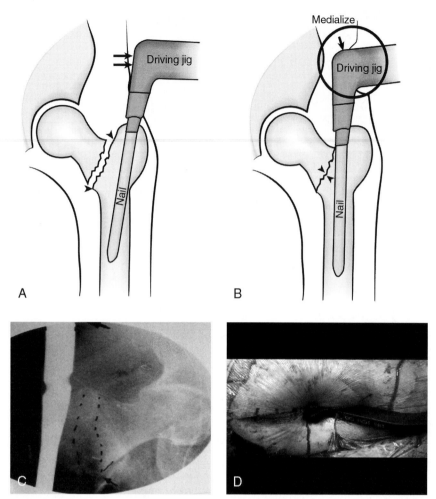

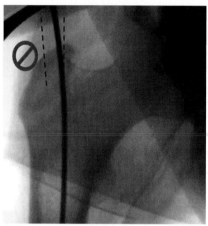

**Figure 9**  An excessively lateral starting point, which will result in varus, should be avoided. This fluoroscopic view shows a guidewire in good position. Dashed lines indicate the correct entry window. The circle with a bar indicates a starting zone that is too far lateral.

**Figure 8**  Illustration showing a potential complication that may occur during intramedullary nail placement in patients with large hips. **A,** A small incision in the hip allows only the nail to go through the skin and subcutaneous tissue. In patients with large hips, this causes the soft tissue to resist the medial positioning of the insertion driving handle. This lateral force is indicated by the two arrows. That resistance forces the nail laterally and can create a distraction force at the intertrochanteric fracture site resulting in a gap (*arrowheads*). **B,** To prevent this complication, a larger skin incision has been made in the hip, and the subcutaneous tissue is divided. This larger incision allows the driving handle to move through and past the skin level, to go more medially, and prevents lateral pressure against the intertrochanteric region. The distraction force at the fracture site is relaxed. Note that the gap has been closed at the intertrochanteric fracture site (*arrowheads*). Lateral distraction is caused by impingement of soft tissues on the driving handle and can be prevented by making an adequate incision. **C,** Fluoroscopic image showing lateral distraction of the fracture site. **D,** Clinical photograph showing the insertion handle in the soft tissues.

ment (Figure 9). Adequate reduction of the fracture before fixation is essential; the device will not correct malreduction. Some techniques to achieve reduction include percutaneous placement of ball-tipped spikes or Schanz pins used as a joystick. Temporary Kirschner wire stabilization of the fragments in reduced position may be helpful. In some very unstable fractures, temporarily pinning the proximal frag-

ment to the acetabulum with transarticular smooth pins may be necessary (Figure 10). Care should be taken to keep all joysticks or temporary fixation out of the path of the definitive fixation hardware.

Hip screws, whether connected to the shaft by means of a plate or an intramedullary nail, have the common complication of screw cutout of the head and subsequent loss of fixation and joint destruction (Figure 11). The risk of this complication is reduced by correct screw placement in the head, which is central and deep in both AP and lateral radiographic views. This position is described by the tip-to-apex distance.[33] The sum of the measured distances from the tip of the screw to the apex of the femoral head on both views should be less than 2 cm.

## Summary

Hip fractures, which can occur in patients of any age, are common and have a significant economic and per-

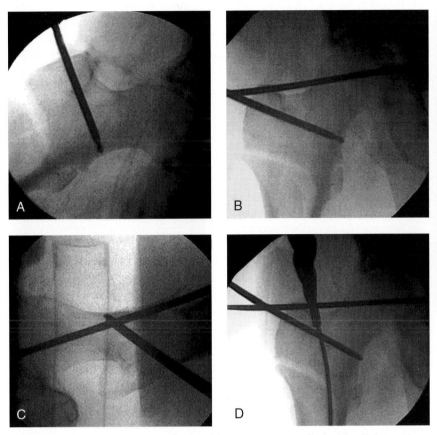

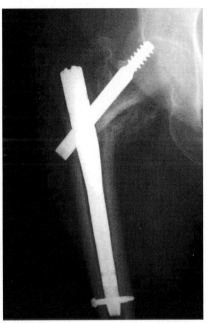

**Figure 11** Lag screw cutout is prevented by placing the screw central and deep, as indicated by a cumulative tip-apex distance of less than 2.5 cm.

**Figure 10** **A,** A very unstable proximal fragment is controlled with a Schanz pin as a joystick. After using the joystick for reduction, the proximal fragment is pinned to the acetabulum with a smooth pin placed out of the way of definitive intramedullary fixation. AP **(B)** and lateral **(C)** fluoroscopic views of the short proximal fragment pinned to the pelvis. **D,** The guidewire and reamer are passed with the temporary stabilization in place.

sonal impact on the patient. Treatment is based on the type of fracture, the location of the fracture, and the patient's age and medical comorbidities. Nondisplaced or impacted fractures of the femoral neck can be treated with screw fixation, and displaced femoral neck fractures can be treated with reduction and fixation or with hip arthroplasty. Intertrochanteric fractures are treated with reduction and fixation. To ensure the best outcomes for patients, various techniques and aids should be used, including proper patient positioning, choosing the correct starting point for nail insertion, and achieving acceptable reduction before fixation.

## References

1. National Center for Injury Prevention and Control Website. Available at: http://www.cdc.gov/ncipc/factsheets/falls.htm. Accessed November 2006.

2. Riggs BL, Melton L: The worldwide problem of osteoporosis: Insights afforded by epidemiology. *Bone* 1995;17:505S-511S.

3. Chapuy MC, Arlot ME, Duboeuf F, et al: Vitamin $D_3$ and calcium to prevent hip fractures in the elderly women. *N Engl J Med* 1992;327:1637-1642.

4. Tinetti ME, Baker DI, McAvay G, et al: A multifactorial intervention to reduce the risk of falling among elderly people living in the community. *N Engl J Med* 1994;331:821-827.

5. Kannus P, Parkkari J, Niemi S, et al: Prevention of hip fracture in elderly people with use of a hip protector. *N Engl J Med* 2000;343:1506-1513.

6. How to reduce your risks of falling. American Academy of Orthopaedic Surgeons Website. Available at: http://orthoinfo.aaos.org/fact/thr_report.cfm?thread_id=78&topcategory=Injury%20Prevention. Accessed June 13, 2007.

7. Damany DS, Parker MJ, Chojnowski A: Complications after intracapsular hip fractures in young adults: A meta-analysis of 18 published studies involving 564 fractures. *Injury* 2005;36:131-141.

8. Siegmeth AW, Guruswamy K, Parker MJ: Delay to surgery prolongs hospital stay in patients with fractures of the proximal femur. *J Bone Joint Surg Br* 2005;87:1123-1126.

9. Moran CG, Wenn RT, Sikand M, Taylor AM: Early mortality after hip fracture: Is delay before surgery im-

portant? *J Bone Joint Surg Am* 2005;87: 483-489.

10. Swiantkowski MF, Harrington RM, Kella TS, Van Patten PK: Torsion and bending analysis of internal fixation techniques for femoral neck fractures: The role of implant design and bone density. *J Orthop Res* 1987;3:433-444.

11. Masson M, Parker MJ, Fleischer S: Internal fixation versus arthroplasty for intracapsular proximal femoral fractures in adults. *Cochrane Database Syst Rev* 2003;2:CD001708.

12. Bhandari M, Devereaux PJ, Swiontkowski MF, et al: Internal fixation compared with arthroplasty for displaced fractures of the femoral neck: A meta-analysis. *J Bone Joint Surg Am* 2003;85-A:1673-1681.

13. Iorio R, Healy WL, Lemos DW, Appleby D, Lucchesi CA, Saleh KJ: Displaced femoral neck fractures in the elderly: Outcomes and cost effectiveness. *Clin Orthop Relat Res* 2001; 383:229-242.

14. Healy WL, Iorio R: Total hip arthroplasty: Optimal treatment for displaced femoral neck fractures in elderly patients. *Clin Orthop Relat Res* 2004;429:43-48.

15. Baker RP, Squires B, Gargan MF, Bannista GC: Total hip arthroplasty and hemiarthroplasty in mobile, independent patients with a displaced intracapsular fracture of the femoral neck: A randomized controlled trial. *J Bone Joint Surg Am* 2006;88:2583-2589.

16. Lee BP, Berry DJ, Harmsen WS, Sim FH: Total hip arthroplasty for the treatment of an acute fracture of the femoral neck: Long-term results. *J Bone Joint Surg Am* 1998;80:70-75.

17. Calder SJ, Anderson GH, Jagger C, Harper WM, Gregg PJ: Unipolar or bipolar prosthesis for displaced intracapsular hip fracture in octogenarians: A randomized prospective study. *J Bone Joint Surg Br* 1996;78: 391-394.

18. Raia FJ, Chapman CB, Herrera MF, Schweppe MW, Michelson CB, Rosenwasser MP: Unipolar or bipolar hemiarthroplasty for femoral neck fractures in the elderly? *Clin Orthop Relat Res* 2003;414:259-265.

19. Wathne RA, Koval KJ, Aharenoff GB, Zuckerman JD, Jones DA: Modular unipolar versus bipolar prosthesis: A prospective evaluation of functional outcomes after femoral neck fracture. *J Orthop Trauma* 1995;9:298-302.

20. Cornell CN, Levine D, O'Doherty J, Lyden J: Unipolar versus bipolar hemiarthroplasty for the treatment of femoral neck fractures in the elderly. *Clin Orthop Relat Res* 1998;348:67-71.

21. Emery RJ, Broughton NS, Desai K, Bulstrode CJ, Thomas TL: Bipolar hemiarthroplasty for subcapital fracture of the femoral neck: A prospective randomized trial of cemented Thompson and uncemented Moore stems. *J Bone Joint Surg Br* 1991;73: 322-324.

22. Lo WH, Chen WM, Huang CK, Chen TH, Chiu FY, Chen CM: Bateman bipolar hemiarthroplasty for displaced intracapsular femoral neck fractures: Cemented versus uncemented. *Clin Orthop Relat Res* 1994; 302:75-82.

23. Khan RJK, MacDowell A, Crossman P, Keene GS: Cemented or uncemented hemiarthroplasty for displaced intracapsular fractures of the hip: A systematic review. *Injury* 2002; 33:13-17.

24. Parker MJ, Gurusamy K: Arthroplasties (with and without bone cement) for proximal femoral fractures in adults. *Cochrane Database Syst Rev* 2004;2:CD001706.

25. Parker MJ, Pervez H: Surgical approaches for inserting hemiarthroplasty of the hip. *Cochrane Database Syst Rev* 2002;3:CD001707.

26. O'Hara DA, Duff A, Berlin JA, et al: The effect of anesthetic technique on postoperative outcomes in hip fracture repair. *Anesthesiology* 2000;92: 947-957.

27. Felsenthal G, Magaziner J: Spinal anesthesia versus general anesthesia for hip fracture repair: A longitudinal observation of 741 elderly patients during 2-year follow-up. *Am J Orthop* 2000;29:25-35.

28. Utrilla AL, Reig JS, Munoz FM, Tufanisco CB: Trochanteric gamma nail and compression hip screw for trochanteric fractures: A randomized, prospective, comparative study in 210 elderly patients with a new design of the gamma nail. *J Orthop Trauma* 2005;19:229-233.

29. Pajarinen J, Lindahl J, Michelsson O, Savolainen V, Hirvensalo E: Pertrochanteric femoral fractures treated with a dynamic hip screw or a proximal femoral nail: A randomized study comparing post-operative rehabilitation. *J Bone Joint Surg Br* 2005;87: 76-81.

30. Parker MJ, Handoll H: Gamma and other cephalocondylic intramedullary nails versus extramedullary implants for extracapsular hip fractures in adults. *Cochrane Database Syst Rev* 2005;4:CD000093.

31. Templeman D, Baumgaertner MR, Leighton RK, Lindsey RW, Moed BR: Reducing complications in the surgical treatment of intertrochanteric fractures. *Instr Course Lect* 2005; 54:409-415.

32. Sadowski C, Lubbeke A, Saudan M, Riand N, Stern R, Hoffmeyer P: Treatment of reverse oblique and transverse intertrochanteric fractures with use of an intramedullary nail or a 95 degrees screw-plate: A prospective, randomized study. *J Bone Joint Surg Am* 2002;84-A:372-381.

33. Baumgaertner MR, Solberg BD: Awareness of tip-apex distance reduces failure of fixation of trochanteric fractures of the hip. *J Bone Joint Surg Br* 1997;79:969-971.

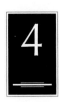

# Locking Plates: Tips and Tricks

Wade R. Smith, MD
*Bruce H. Ziran, MD
*Jeffrey O. Anglen, MD
Philip F. Stahel, MD

## Abstract

*Locking plates are fracture fixation devices that allow the insertion of fixed-angle/angular-stable screws or pegs and do not require friction between the plate and bone. The clinical care impetus for the development of these plates has been a combination of factors, including the increasing survival of patients with high-energy injuries, aging Western European and North American populations with an increasing rate of fragility fractures, and dissatisfaction of patients and surgeons with the outcomes of treatment of specific periarticular fractures. Nonclinical factors likely include a push by industry for new technology and new markets as well as the general interest of the public in "minimally invasive" surgery.*

*Instr Course Lect 2008;57:25-36.*

Locking plates are fracture fixation devices with threaded screw holes, which allow screws to thread to the plate and function as a fixed-angle device.[1-3] These plates may have a mixture of holes that allow placement of both locking and traditional nonlocking screws (so-called combi plates).[4,5] The first locking plates were introduced about two decades ago for use in spinal and maxillofacial surgery.[6-8] In the late 1980s and into the 1990s, experimentation with various types of internal fixation devices led to the development

of locking plates for fracture care.[9-11] The initial emphasis was on developing stable fixation that would not require extensive soft-tissue stripping or disruption.[12]

Although locking plates have been used for years in specialized research trials, they have been available in North America for general orthopaedic applications only in the last 6 or 7 years.[13-15] Currently, numerous companies offer a variety of locking plate systems for treatment of extremity fractures. Many of these systems have been on the mar-

ket for only a couple of years. Given the increased expense of these plates compared with that of traditional nonlocking equipment and the short time that they have been available for general use, it would seem fair to ask: What are the advantages and disadvantages of locking plates? What are the indications and contraindications? How do we use them effectively? How can failures be avoided? The objective of this review will be to address these questions and provide practical information and tips for the practicing orthopaedic surgeon.

## What Is a Locking Plate?

Any plate that allows the insertion of fixed-angle/angular-stable screws or pegs can be used as a locking plate. The main biomechanical difference from conventional plates is the fact that conventional plates require compression of the plate to the bone and rely on friction at the bone-plate interface. With increasing axial loading cycles, the screws can begin to toggle, which decreases the friction force and leads to plate loosening. If this occurs prematurely, fracture instability will occur, leading to

*Bruce H. Ziran, MD or the department with which he is affiliated has received miscellaneous nonincome support, commercially-derived honoraria, or other nonresearch-related funding from Stryker and Synthes and Jeffrey O. Anglen MD or the department with which he is affiliated has received royalties from EBI and is a consultant or employee for Eli Lilly.*

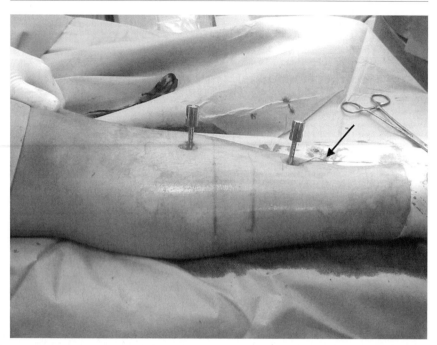

**Figure 1** Minimally invasive, percutaneous locking plate fixation. The locking drill sleeves are attached to the proximal and distal ends of the locking plate through a skin incision and counterincision. These drill sleeves serve as joysticks and provide a frame in which to move the plate into perfect position under fluoroscopic control. The plate is attached to a strong suture (*arrow*) to pull it through the submuscular plane and to help remove it if that is required during surgery.

implant failure. Thus, the more difficult it is to achieve and maintain tight screw fixation (as for example, in metaphyseal and osteoporotic bone), the more difficult it is to maintain stability.

This biomechanical prerequisite of conventional plates is associated with biologic pitfalls due to compression of periosteal blood supply and compromise of the vascularity of the fracture. Thus, conventional plate osteosynthesis with rigid fixation (interfragmentary compression and lag screws) has been associated with a substantial complication rate, including infection, hardware failure, delayed union, and nonunion.[12,16]

In contrast, locking plates follow the biomechanical principle of external fixators and do not require friction between the plate and bone.

They are considered to be internal fixators from a biomechanical standpoint because the angular-stable interface between the screws and the plate allows placement of the plate without any contact to the bone.[1,3,14,15,17] In essence, however, locking plates can be considered to be external fixators placed underneath the skin envelope, although they are more stable as a result of the shorter distance between the plate and the bone. Many conventional plates now have locking counterparts. There is an increasing trend by manufacturers to supply anatomy-specific plates with locking options. Examples include anatomically preshaped plates for the proximal and distal parts of the femur, proximal and distal parts of the tibia, proximal and distal parts of the humerus, and calcaneus.[18-22] In many

instances, the design of the plate allows substantially less contact between the plate and bone, in an attempt to preserve the periosteal blood supply and bone perfusion. Increasingly, locking plate systems have special features such as outriggers, jigs, and blunted ends to enhance the surgeon's ability to pass the plate in a submuscular or subcutaneous manner for a minimally invasive application[23-27] (Figure 1).

## Principles of Locking Plate Fixation

Comminuted intra-articular fractures, such as bicondylar tibial plateau and distal femoral fractures, are highly unstable. After an anatomic joint reduction is achieved, the articular segment must be reconnected to the shaft while appropriate alignment is maintained. Achieving adequate stability for fracture healing is difficult in the presence of metaphyseal or metaphyseal-diaphyseal comminution. An additional medial buttress in the form of a plate or an external fixator may be required when a conventional laterally-based plate is used. Locking plates potentially provide increased stability in these instances to a degree that a second plate is not required. The increased stability is the result of the difference in the mechanics of conventional plate and locking plate fixation.[3,14,17,28-30] As mentioned above, locking plates do not depend on the bone-plate interface. Stability is maintained at the angular-stable, screw-plate interface. As a result of this stable monoblock of the locking internal fixator, the pullout strength of locking head screws is substantially higher than that of conventional screws.[3,14,17,28-30] Because the screws are locked to the plate, it is difficult for one screw to pull out or fail unless all adjacent screws fail.

The increase in stability provided by locking plates is most helpful to surgeons treating a fracture in poor-quality bone, a comminuted bicondylar fracture, or any highly unstable fracture for which a single plate may not provide adequate stability. Also, because only a single plate is needed and the plate does not depend on a tight fit to the bone for stability, substantially less soft tissue dissection may be required, thus preserving the local blood supply and enhancing fracture healing.[12,28,31]

The biomechanical and biologic advantages of locking plate systems, compared with conventional plates, have led to a widespread use of these new implants in recent years.[23,26,32-41] However, the effective and successful use of locking plates and of minimally invasive techniques remains highly challenging and is associated with a substantial learning curve. The uncritical use of locking plates for a broad range of undifferentiated indications is associated with substantial pitfalls and has led to new patterns of failure of fracture fixation in recent years.[42-46] Thus, the surgeon working with locking plates must be well aware of the indications and contraindications, technical tricks, advantages and limitations, and typical pitfalls and adverse events associated with these new implants.[2,13,28,47]

## Disadvantages of Locking Plates

Locking plates are substantially more expensive than conventional plates. They are also unnecessary for many fractures. Locking plates are more difficult to use for achieving an adequate reduction. Particularly with specialty plates, which have only locking holes, fracture reduction must be achieved primarily, be-

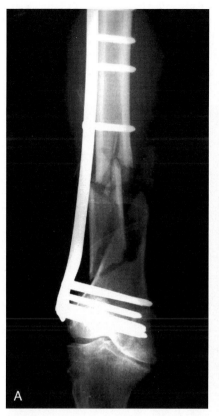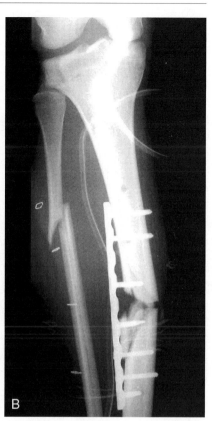

**Figure 2**    Primary malreduction with the use of a locking plate for fixation of a distal femoral fracture (**A**) and a tibial shaft fracture (**B**). A fundamental biomechanical difference between locking plates and conventional plates is that locking head screws do not pull the bone to the plate but lock into the plate in the identical position. These two examples of malreduced fractures emphasize the notion that adequate reduction has to be achieved before a fracture is fixed with a locking plate.

fore plate fixation. Once a locking screw has been placed through the plate into bone, this particular bone segment can no longer be manipulated by insertion of additional screws or by using compression devices. This makes the sequence of screw placement critical to avoid fracture malreduction (Figure 2). Surgeons who use locking plates need a variety of reduction techniques, such as "no-hands" traction, femoral distractors, and percutaneous clamps.[48] The surgeon must keep in mind that, despite the advanced technology of expensive locking plates, they do not improve fracture reduction and cannot help a

poorly reduced fracture to heal. For example, if the final fracture construct is too stiff, particularly when a bridging technique is used, nonunion may occur. The combination of a stiff plate, stiff screws, and fracture distraction is a formula for nonunion (Figure 3).

## Indications

Most fractures undergoing surgical treatment do not require a locking plate. Most heal with conventional plates or intramedullary nails, provided that the principles of safe surgery are followed. There are specific fractures, however, that are associated with a higher risk of loss of reduction and plate or screw failure with subsequent nonunion. These are often termed "unsolved" or "problem" fractures and include comminuted intra-articular frac-tures, short-segment periarticular fractures, and fractures in osteopen-ic bone. These injury patterns repre-sent the typical spectrum of indica-tions for locking plates.

However, decision making re-garding the use of a locking plate must include precise preoperative consideration of the exact principle by which the locking plate will be used. ("What's your plan?") The main indications for the use of a locking plate include four "classic" principles:[47] (1) the compression principle, for osteoporotic diaphy-seal fractures; (2) the neutralization principle, also for osteoporotic dia-physeal fractures; (3) the bridging principle ("locked internal fixator" principle), for comminuted diaphy-seal or metaphyseal extra-articular fractures; and (4) the combination principle ("combi plate" principle), for comminuted metaphyseal intra-articular fractures.

The surgeon using a locking plate for fracture fixation must be well aware of the exact indication, ac-cording to these four principles, for which the angular-stable implant will be used (Table 1). For simple, noncomminuted diaphyseal frac-tures in osteoporotic bone requiring an open reduction and rigid internal fixation, locking plates offer the ad-

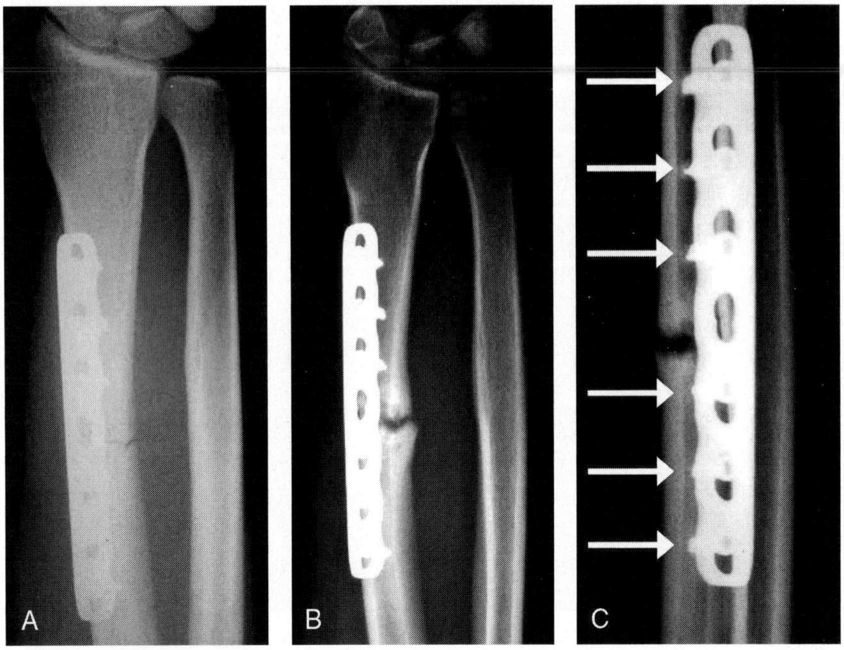

**Figure 3**  **A** through **C,** Locking plate fixation of a simple fracture of the radial shaft, leading to nonunion. The use of locking plates is contraindicated for simple fractures that require interfragmentary compression. In **C,** three locking head screws were used on each side of the fracture (*arrows*), whereas the dynamic compression holes of the combi plate were left empty. This stiff construct led to a nonunion within a few months after surgery.

**Table 1**
**Indications for Locking Plates**

| Indication | Biomechanical Principle | Technique | Bone Quality | Typical Anatomic Location |
|---|---|---|---|---|
| Comminuted shaft fractures | Bridging | Locked internal fixator | Normal or osteopenic | Femur, tibia, humeral shaft |
| Comminuted metaphyseal intra-articular fractures | Combination | Combined (lag screws for articular fixation, locking head screws for metaphyseal bridging) | Normal or osteopenic | Distal part of femur, distal part of tibia |
| Short-segment metaphyseal fractures | Bridging or combination | Locked internal fixator | Normal or osteopenic | Proximal part of humerus, distal part of humerus, distal part of radius, proximal part of tibia |
| Simple fractures in osteoporotic bone | Compression | Dynamic compression with eccentric screw placement or a compression device; locking head screws for shaft; tension device with locking head screws only | Osteopenic | Osteoporotic forearm |
| Simple fractures in osteoporotic bone | Neutralization | Conventional lag screw; locking head screws for neutralization plate | Osteopenic | Osteoporotic ankle |

vantage of increased pullout resistance of the locking head screws compared with that of conventional screws. Thus, for these fractures, locking plates can be applied according to the compression principle through eccentric placement of screws in the dynamic compression unit of the "combi hole" or by the use of a compression device after initial placement of one locking head screw on the other side of the fracture. On the basis of the same rationale, locking plates also can be used according to the neutralization principle to protect a lag screw in osteoporotic bone, with increased pullout resistance of the locking head screws. However, it is crucial to understand that locking head screws can never provide interfragmentary compression. Compression can be achieved only by the use of a compression device or by eccentric placement of conventional screws in the combi hole of a combination locking plate (lag first, then lock).[5,28,30,47]

The classic and ideal indications for fracture fixation with locking plates are represented by the bridging principle and the combination principle (Table 1). Both concepts apply to fixation of fractures with substantial comminution—either high-energy fractures in young patients or low-energy osteoporotic fractures in elderly patients. The bridging principle is typically represented by the concept of minimally invasive percutaneous plate fixation, whereby the angular-stable plate is used as an internal splint that bridges the comminuted fracture. With this method, indirect reduction is performed by ensuring adequate axial alignment, length, and rotation of the extremity while the fracture fragments are not exposed or directly reduced. In contrast to the com-

pression and neutralization principles, which provide absolute rigid stability leading to primary (direct) fracture healing, the bridging concept provides relative, elastic fixation that leads to secondary (indirect) fracture healing by callus formation. For adequate bridge plate fixation, three or four holes of the plate should be left empty at the level of the fracture, as discussed below.

The combination principle refers to a biomechanical mixture of compression and bridging with only one implant. Although the original locking plates available for fracture fixation, such as the point contact fixator (PC-Fix) and the less invasive stabilization system (LISS), provided all of the innovative biomechanical and biologic properties of angular-stable devices, surgeons expressed the desire to use a combination of both concepts, locking and compression plate fixation, with only one implant. This option was made available for the first time in the early 21st century by the locking compression plate (LCP), which was designed by Robert Frigg (Bettlach, Switzerland) on the basis of an idea from Prof. Michael Wagner (Vienna, Austria).[4,5,15,28]

The combination technique is indicated for fixation of fractures with a simple pattern (for example, an intra-articular split) at one level

and comminution (for example, metaphyseal-diaphyseal comminution) at a different level. Under these circumstances, the plate can be used to achieve interfragmentary compression of the simple fracture pattern by means of a dynamic compression technique or placement of a lag screw through the dynamic compression unit of the plate. Thereafter, the plate can be used as a locked internal fixator to align the articular fragment to the shaft in a bridging manner. The combination principle is feasible only with plates that allow placement of both locking head screws and conventional compression screws in one implant.[47]

## Contraindications

Despite the widespread use of locking plates and their wide range of indications, a few contraindications must be acknowledged and respected (Table 2). The uncritical use of locking plates may lead to failure of fixation and to nonunion, particularly if the above-mentioned standard principles for use of locking plates are violated. A typical contraindication to the use of a locking plate as a locked internal fixator is a simple fracture pattern that requires interfragmentary compression. For example, simple diaphyseal fractures of the forearm fixed with a plate with a locked internal fixation tech-

**Table 2**
**Contraindications for Locking Plates**

| Contraindication | Wrong Technique | Example | Expected Adverse Outcome |
|---|---|---|---|
| Simple fractures | Locked internal fixator | Simple forearm or humeral shaft fracture | Nonunion |
| Simple fractures | Minimally invasive percutaneous plate fixation | Simple distal tibial fracture | Nonunion |
| Displaced intra-articular fractures | Locked internal fixator | Tibial pilon fracture | Malunion, arthritis |

nique are prone to nonunion (Figure 3). Similarly contraindicated is the percutaneous locking plate fixation of simple fractures with use of a minimally invasive technique. This concept violates the principle of the fracture gap width in relation to strain and thus leads to nonunion, as described in the literature.[12] Finally, indirect reduction and locking-plate fixation are contraindicated for displaced intra-articular fractures because these injuries require anatomic open reduction and rigid interfragmentary compression.

Because of their cost, locking plates are relatively contraindicated for fractures that can be stabilized satisfactorily with conventional plates. For example, diaphyseal forearm fractures have healing rates in excess of 90% with conventional plates. Although there are some claims that, theoretically, the use of unicortical locking plates should increase healing rates because of the lack of soft-tissue stripping, this has not been validated in any type of controlled trial, to our knowledge. Overuse of these plates in some health care systems may negatively impact overall patient care by consuming resources that could be better used elsewhere.

## Tips, Tricks, and Pitfalls
Successful use of locking plates depends on adherence to established principles of surgical fracture care and learning the tricks of the specific technology. Gautier and Sommer[47] recently presented prudent guidelines that may improve the individual learning curve of surgeons who are less familiar with these new implants.

In general, successful use begins with a formal preoperative drawing. The advent of digitized radiography at many centers requires that digital

templates be available. If plain radiographs are used, the use of tracing paper is still the most effective way to draw a preoperative plan. The sequence of screw placement, the length and position of the plate, and the surgical approach are all critical to success. A precise preoperative plan reduces the guesswork and increases the likelihood of technical success. The preoperative plan also ensures that the surgeon will have all necessary implants available at the time of surgery.

Correct positioning of the patient is vital, particularly if the plan calls for minimally invasive or percutaneous insertion of the implant. The surgeon should ensure that all necessary images are obtainable before preparing and draping the patient. A radiolucent table is very helpful. Tightly rolled bumps of different sizes fashioned before the operation can aid in fracture reduction as well as visualization, particularly in the lateral plane. Fracture reduction can be challenging with locking plates because the locking screws do not pull the plate to the bone in the manner of conventional screws. Therefore, it is essential that the surgeon have a preoperative plan for fracture reduction. Combinations of traction to correct length and alignment in the anteroposterior plane and placement of bumps under the extremity to correct lateral plane deformities can successfully permit reductions with minimal direct manipulation of the fracture fragments. Specialized reduction clamps can be used judiciously with percutaneous long-bone and periarticular reductions. Conventional screws or "whirlybird" push-pull types of devices can be used to pull the bone to the plate initially to secure fracture reduction. Once the fracture is reduced, then locking screws can be

added as needed to provide stability.

Effective use of locking plates requires an understanding of the potential pitfalls of usage. Locking holes offer minimal opportunity for screw angulation. More than 5° of angulation between the screw and the locking hole can cause the screw to eventually fail. Careful technique is necessary to ensure that the screw is perfectly lined up with the axis of the screw threads in the plate. This may be quite difficult in a minimally invasive procedure. Malaligned screw threads can lead to loose screws and loss of reduction (Figure 4). The weakest part of the combi locking plate (for example, the LCP) is the dynamic compression unit. This is the part of the plate that should be used for bending, if required, and it is the part that breaks when there is increased stress concentration and strain on the plate.[17,42] For this reason, when a bridge plate is used to fix a comminuted fracture, at least three or four plate holes should be left empty at the level of the fracture, to achieve a larger area of stress distribution on the plate [42,47,49] (Figure 5). In contrast to conventional plates, which fail at the interface between the screws and the plate—often leading to breakage of conventional screw heads—the interface of the locking head screw with the threaded locking hole is the strongest part of the locking plate system. Locking screw heads are less likely to break because the difference between the core diameters of the screw shaft and head is much smaller than it is with conventional screws. Nevertheless, locking head screws can break in cases of chronic instability and increased strain as a result of rotational forces, as is exemplified by proximal humeral nonunion shown in Figure 4, B.

Locking plates allow the use of

both bicortical and unicortical locking head screws. The choice of screw type (self-drilling/self-tapping or self-tapping only) and screw length (unicortical or bicortical) needs to be based on defined principles to avoid complications. As a general rule, self-drilling/self-tapping screws, as are used in minimally invasive locking plates (such as the LISS), should be used exclusively in a unicortical fashion. The main reason is that self-drilling screws have sharp tips that may cause neurovascular and/or soft-tissue damage across the far cortex. Furthermore, drilling of the far cortex with self-drilling/self-tapping screws may lead to simultaneous disruption of the tapped thread in the near cortex and thus reduce the overall purchase of the locking head screws. Similarly, a pitfall with unicortical placement of self-tapping screws is the selection of an inadequate screw length. If the screw is too short, the threads in the near cortex will not have enough purchase, and the locking monoblock frame is prone to failure by pullout with cyclic loading (Figure 6). In contrast, if the unicortical screw is slightly too long, the nondrilling screw tip will push off from the far cortex, thus destroying the tapped thread in the near cortex.

The pullout resistance of unicortical locking head screws is almost identical to that of similar-diameter bicortical conventional screws and about 70% of that of bicortical locking head screws. Thus, how much pullout strength is needed? There is no way to objectively judge this, nor is it necessarily important, because these constructs rarely fail through pullout per se. Two factors are essential for decision making with regard to the use of unicortical or bicortical locking head screws. These

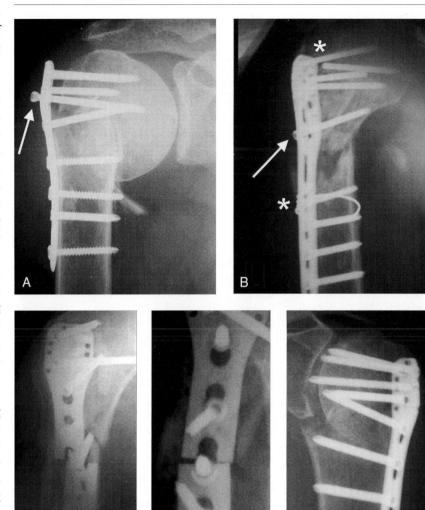

**Figure 4**   Typical patterns of failure of locking plate fixation of proximal humerus fractures. Although the locking plate technique has revolutionized the surgical fixation of this fracture in recent years, typical failure patterns occur with locking plates whenever basic concepts and technical principles are not respected. **A** and **B,** Secondary loss of reduction with varus collapse can occur as a result of use of screws of inadequate length in the humeral head fragment and inappropriate fixation of locking head screws in the plate (*arrows*). The interfaces between the locking head screws and the threaded plate holes should not fail if the screws are inserted at the perfect angle and attached with a torque-limiting screw driver. Increased strain in a construct with too much stiffness and exposure to high rotational forces will lead either to breakage of the plate in the dynamic compression part of the combi hole, which is the weakest part of this construct (**C** and **D**) or, more rarely, to a failure at the screw-plate interface (**B**) with breakage of the screws (*asterisks*). If the locking screws in the head part of the fracture are too long, they may protrude into the glenohumeral joint, because locking head screws cannot recede backward, as conventional screws can. This failure pattern is particularly frequent if the fracture is malreduced in varus (**E**).

are, first, the quality of the cortical bone and, second, the extent of rotational forces applied to the fractured bone. Cortical thickness is of great

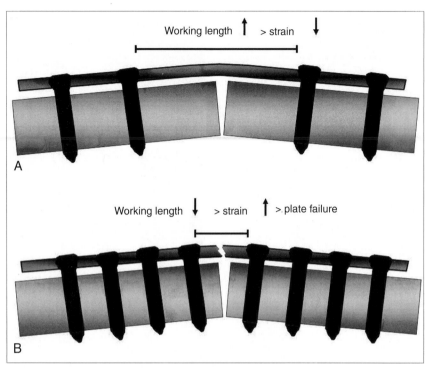

**Figure 5** Relationship of working length and strain at the level of the fracture for the locked internal fixator principle. When a fracture is bridged with a locking plate, three or four plate holes should be left empty at the level of the fracture to increase the working length and decrease the strain and stress concentration on the plate **(A)**. In contrast, if a locking construct is made too stiff with too many screws at the level of the fracture **(B)**, the short working length will lead to increased strain and stress concentration with loading and torsional forces, causing the plate to break.

importance in determining the adequacy of the working length of unicortical screws.[47] The working length of a unicortical screw in good-quality cortical bone usually provides sufficient pullout resistance equaling the pullout strength of a bicortical conventional screw, as mentioned previously. In contrast, in metaphyseal bone and osteoporotic cortical bone, the cortex is usually very thin, thus rendering the working length of unicortical screws insufficient. This reduction in pullout strength is of particular importance when osteoporotic bone is mainly loaded by torsional forces such as occurs in the humerus. Under these conditions, an adequate working length must be achieved by using bicortical locking head screws, as outlined in Table 3.

For these reasons, bicortical fixation is recommended for osteoporotic bone in general and for metaphyseal fractures in bone of normal quality. Also, unicortical screws should not be used in anatomic locations exposed to high rotational forces, such as the humeral shaft. In fact, the only advantage of using unicortical screws may be the lack of penetration of the bone and periosteum on the far side of the bone, and this advantage is highly debatable as far as its true impact on fracture healing. Additionally, unicortical screws are less stiff than bicortical locking screws. Unicortical screws are indicated for periarticular fractures in which the screws are placed in the direction of an articular surface, such as in the proximal part of the humerus.

Locking head screws have some peculiar differences from conventional screws. Although these differences may seem intuitively obvious, they have implications with regard to clinical application. The first difference is that a torque-limiting screwdriver is useful during placement of the locking head screw. The advantage of the use of a torque-limiting device is that, as long as the screw is centered in the hole, the thread cannot be stripped or overtightened. Deformation of the screw heads by overtightening or cross-threading (cold welding) into the plate can make hardware removal very difficult. This happens more often with the minimally invasive technique, which can result in stripping of the screw heads and angulation of the screws because of the difficulty in judging orientation without direct visualization. In contrast to the situation with conventional screws, the purchase of the screw in the bone cannot be felt, because locking head screws always feel tight. Unfortunately, the tight feel is deceptive. Many surgeons, through years of experience and training, have developed a tactile feedback loop based on how the screw "feels" as it tightens down. The fixation can still fail despite "tightness" of the screws, particularly if there is substantial malreduction (Figure 2) or if the screws are cross-threaded or not adequately locked in the plate (Figure 4, A and B).

One strategy that is used to overcome this problem is to carefully place perpendicular 2.0-mm Kirschner wires in the most distal and proximal plate holes before screw insertion. To ensure that the wires are truly perpendicular, they should be placed through the locking drill guides. Alignment can then be checked by looking for the round "bull's-eye" of the drill guide in the locking hole on the lateral radiograph. These wires will maintain length and can also serve as a reference for subsequent placement of screws. Alternatively, a drill bit can be left in place through the drill sleeve to hold the plate in place temporarily, until an adequate reduction is achieved.

Although minimally invasive techniques have been improved in recent years by the introduction of locking plates, achieving and maintaining an adequate reduction remain sources of pitfalls and failures. Sliding any minimally invasive plate in the submuscular plane along the bone can be challenging. There are several strategies for aligning the plate along the bone percutaneously. Kirschner wires can be inserted manually just anterior and posterior to the bone to mark the boundaries for plate passage. The plate is then passed between the wires, and the wires will prevent posterior or anterior deviation of the plate. Another tactic is to make 4- to 6-cm incisions at the proximal and distal sites of the plate. With use of blunt dissection down to bone, the plate can be directly visualized as it passes into the wound. Locking drill sleeves should be attached to the most proximal and distal holes of the plate to form a

frame for easier positioning of the plate on the bone as depicted in Figure 1. In this way, the plate can be centered on the bone at each end and anchoring screws can be placed under direct visualization. If the fracture is well reduced with regard to length, alignment, and rotation, then the plate will be appropriately positioned along the entire length of bone when it is centered at each end. The plate must be held to the bone

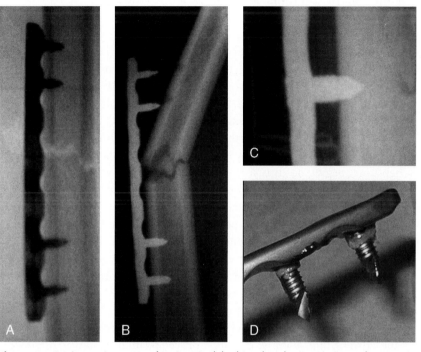

**Figure 6** Inappropriate use of unicortical locking head screws. Several errors in concept and technique led to failure of the fixation of this simple humeral shaft fracture. **A,** The plate was used as a bridging locked internal fixator, holding the fracture in distraction and rendering it prone to nonunion. **B,** This inadequate locking plate fixation failed early after the surgery. The fracture was fixed by only two unicortical locking head screws on each side, which is insufficient for fixation of a humeral shaft fracture exposed to high rotational forces. Some unicortical screws that were placed without sufficient purchase in the near cortex had no pullout resistance at all **(C)**. A conventional compression plate was used for revision fixation. The fracture healed fully within 3 months. It is important to emphasize that locking plates usually fail as a monoblock if the locking head screws are properly attached to the threaded plate holes **(D)**.

**Table 3**
**Decision Making for the Use of Unicortical or Bicortical Locking Head Screws**

| Screw Placement | Bone Quality | Fracture Location | Working Length | Comments |
|---|---|---|---|---|
| Unicortical | Normal | Diaphysis | Adequate | Except for fractures exposed to high rotational forces; eg, in humerus |
| Bicortical | Normal and osteopenic | Diaphysis and metaphysis | Adequate | Use self-tapping but not self-drilling screws for bicortical fixation |
| Unicortical | Normal | Metaphysis | Inadequate | Except for minimally invasive use of self-drilling/self-tapping screws or short-segment metaphyseal fractures (eg, in proximal part of humerus) |
| Unicortical | Osteopenic | Diaphysis and metaphysis | Inadequate | Contraindication for unicortical screws |

by first placing a conventional screw or a "whirlybird" tool because the placement of a self-drilling/self-tapping screw will push the plate away from the bone and may cold weld the screw head to the plate. Because the incisions are distant to the fracture site, the principle of minimally invasive fixation is preserved, as the fracture fragments and soft-tissue attachments are undisturbed.

Locking plates, particularly the specialized so-called all-locking plates, require an approach to fracture reduction that is completely different from what most orthopaedic surgeons have practiced. When one begins to use locking plates, a good approach is to "start easy." One should consider initially using combination plates that permit the use of traditional reduction techniques. Lost in the current enthusiasm for this new technology is the recollection that 10 years ago almost no surgeons in the world were using locking plates routinely. Most of the current high-volume experts in this field started by practicing on sawbones and attending workshops. This is a good approach for anyone starting to use these techniques.

Malreduction can result in failure regardless of whether the plate is conventional or locking. Common complications include varus in the proximal part of the humerus and distal part of the femur and distraction in diaphyseal fractures (Figures 2, 3, and 4). In many instances, locking plates are used as bridge plates in the presence of substantial comminution. Plates that are very stiff or stiff fracture constructs with too many screws can lead to nonunion and eventually plate failure (Figure 5). Bridge plates must be longer, and fewer screws are needed. For the treatment of periarticular fractures, few screws are needed in the diaphysis, but more screws may be required near the articular surface. The precise length of the bridge plate and the number of screws needed for a specific fracture remain controversial. In general, the length of the plate should be more than two times the length of the fracture zone. Screws should be spread evenly, and ideally there should be at least one empty hole between each pair of holes filled with screws. As mentioned previously, when the bridging principle is used, three or four screw holes should be left empty at the level of the fracture to avoid a local stress concentration, which may lead to breakage of the plate.[42] The even distribution of force over a long working plate length with relatively few screws appears to provide a stable stimulus for indirect bone healing and callus formation.

## Summary

Locking plate technology offers improved fixation stability in osteopenic bone and for comminuted and periarticular fractures. The additional stability per screw compared with that of conventional, nonlocking fixation enhances the application of minimally invasive fracture techniques such as use of bridge plates and percutaneous fracture stabilization. The application of locking plates is somewhat more difficult than the placement of conventional plates. Fracture reductions are often done indirectly, the locking screw must be carefully aligned along the axis of the receiving hole to ensure proper tightness, and the length of the plate must be selected carefully. Despite the necessity of mastering these nuances, the use of locking plates will likely increase, particularly with the increasing prevalence of fragility fractures in the aging population and the increase in high-energy fractures in younger patients surviving severe trauma. Although a substantial amount of biomechanical and animal data have been published, few studies have validated the long-term advantages of fixation with locking plates. The initial results in studies that included a variety of fractures are encouraging, although it is increasingly apparent that failures do occur. The causes of failure should be examined carefully in both the literature and one's own practice to learn from mistakes and refine techniques.

## References

1. Greiwe RM, Archdeacon MT: Locking plate technology: Current concepts. *J Knee Surg* 2007;20:50-55.

2. Cantu RV, Koval KJ: The use of locking plates in fracture care. *J Am Acad Orthop Surg* 2006;14:183-190.

3. Egol KA, Kubiak EN, Fulkerson E, Kummer FJ, Koval KJ: Biomechanics of locked plates and screws. *J Orthop Trauma* 2004;18:488-493.

4. Frigg R: Locking Compression Plate (LCP): An osteosynthesis plate based on the Dynamic Compression Plate and the Point Contact Fixator (PC-Fix). *Injury* 2001;32(suppl 2):63-66.

5. Frigg R: Development of the locking compression plate. *Injury* 2003;34(suppl 2):B6-B10.

6. Morscher E, Sutter F, Jenny H, Olerud S: Anterior plating of the cervical spine with the hollow screw-plate system of titanium. *Chirurg* 1986;57:702-707.

7. Arnold W: Initial clinical experiences with the cervical spine titanium locking plate. *Unfallchirurg* 1990;93:559-561.

8. Söderholm AL, Lindqvist C, Skutnabb K, Rahn B: Bridging of mandibular defects with two different reconstruction systems: An experimental study. *J Oral Maxillofac Surg* 1991;49:1098-1105.

9. Miclau T, Remiger A, Tepic S, Lindsey R, McIff T: A mechanical comparison of the dynamic compression plate, limited contact-dynamic compression plate, and point contact fixator. *J Orthop Trauma* 1995;9:17-22.

10. Kolodziej P, Lee FS, Patel A, et al: Biomechanical evaluation of the schuhli nut. *Clin Orthop Relat Res* 1998;347:79-85.

11. Borgeaud M, Cordey J, Leyvraz PE, Perren SM: Mechanical analysis of the bone to plate interface of the LC-DCP and of the PC-FIX on human femora. *Injury* 2000;31(suppl 3): C29-C36.

12. Perren SM: Evolution of the internal fixation of long bone fractures: The scientific basis of biological internal fixation: Choosing a new balance between stability and biology. *J Bone Joint Surg Br* 2002;84:1093-1110.

13. Sommer C, Gautier E, Müller M, Helfet DL, Wagner M: First clinical results of the Locking Compression Plate (LCP). *Injury* 2003;34(suppl 2): B43-B54.

14. Schütz M, Südkamp NP: Revolution in plate osteosynthesis: New internal fixator systems. *J Orthop Sci* 2003;8: 252-258.

15. Wagner M, Frenk A, Frigg R: New concepts for bone fracture treatment and the locking compression plate. *Surg Technol Int* 2004;12:271-277.

16. Broos PL, Sermon A: From unstable internal fixation to biological osteosynthesis: A historical overview of operative fracture treatment. *Acta Chir Belg* 2004;104:396-400.

17. Stoffel K, Dieter U, Stachowiak G, Gächter A, Kuster MS: Biomechanical testing of the LCP: How can stability in locked internal fixators be controlled? *Injury* 2003;34(suppl 2): B11-B19.

18. Stoffel K, Booth G, Rohrl SM, Kuster M: A comparison of conventional versus locking plates in intraarticular calcaneus fractures: A biomechanical study in human cadavers. *Clin Biomech (Bristol, Avon)* 2007;22: 100-105.

19. Haidukewych G, Sems SA, Huebner D, Horwitz D, Levy B: Results of polyaxial locked-plate fixation of periarticular fractures of the knee. *J Bone Joint Surg Am* 2007;89:614-620.

20. Fankhauser F, Boldin C, Schippinger G, Haunschmid C, Szyszkowitz R: A new locking plate for unstable fractures of the proximal humerus. *Clin Orthop Relat Res* 2005;430:176-181.

21. Kettler M, Biberthaler P, Braunstein V, Zeiler C, Kroetz M, Mutschler W: Treatment of proximal humeral fractures with the PHILOS angular stable plate: Presentation of 225 cases of dislocated fractures. *Unfallchirurg* 2006; 109:1032-1040.

22. Hasenboehler EA, Agudelo JF, Morgan SJ, Smith WR, Hak DJ, Stahel PF: Treatment of complex proximal femur fractures by the proximal femur locking compression plate. *Orthopedics* 2007;30:618-623.

23. Hasenboehler E, Rikli D, Babst R: Locking compression plate with minimally invasive plate osteosynthesis in diaphyseal and distal tibial fracture: A retrospective study of 32 patients. *Injury* 2007;38:365-370.

24. Haidukewych GJ: Innovations in locking plate technology. *J Am Acad Orthop Surg* 2004;12:205-212.

25. Gardner MJ, Griffith MH, Dines JS, Lorich DG: A minimally invasive approach for plate fixation of the proximal humerus. *Bull Hosp Jt Dis* 2004; 62:18-23.

26. Lill H, Hepp P, Rose T, König K, Josten C: The angle stable locking-proximal-humerus-plate (LPHP) for proximal humeral fractures using a small anterior-lateral-deltoid-splitting-approach: Technique and first results. *Zentralbl Chir* 2004;129:43-48.

27. Imatani J, Noda T, Morito Y, Sato T, Hashizume H, Inoue H: Minimally invasive plate osteosynthesis for comminuted fractures of the metaphysis of the radius. *J Hand Surg Br* 2005;30: 220-225.

28. Wagner M: General principles for the clinical use of the LCP. *Injury* 2003;34 (suppl 2):B31-B42.

29. Gutwald R, Alpert B, Schmelzeisen R: Principle and stability of locking plates. *Keio J Med* 2003;52:21-24.

30. Niemeyer P, Südkamp NP: Principles and clinical application of the locking compression plate (LCP). *Acta Chir Orthop Traumatol Cech* 2006; 73:221-228.

31. Sommer CH, Gautier E: Relevance and advantages of new angular stable screw-plate systems for diaphyseal fractures (locking compression plate versus intramedullary nail). *Ther Umsch* 2003;60:751-756.

32. Sommer C: Fixation of transverse fractures of the sternum and sacrum with the locking compression plate system: Two case reports. *J Orthop Trauma* 2005;19:487-490.

33. Wong KK, Chan KW, Kwok TK, Mak KH: Volar fixation of dorsally displaced distal radial fracture using locking compression plate. *J Orthop Surg (Hong Kong)* 2005;13:153-157.

34. Rikli DA, Babst R: New principles in the surgical treatment of distal radius fractures: Locking implants. *Ther Umsch* 2003;60:745-750.

35. Stahel PF, Infanger M, Bleif IM, Heyde CE, Ertel W: Palmar angular-stable plate osteosynthesis: A new concept for treatment of unstable distal radius fractures. *Trauma Berufskrankh.* 2005;7(suppl 1):S27-S32.

36. Schaller TM, Roehr B: Salvage of a failed opening wedge tibial osteotomy using a locking plate. *Orthopedics* 2007; 30:161-162.

37. Rose PS, Adams CR, Torchia ME, Jacofsky DJ, Haidukewych GG, Steinmann SP: Locking plate fixation for proximal humeral fractures: Initial results with a new implant. *J Shoulder Elbow Surg* 2007;16:202-207.

38. Larson AN, Rizzo M: Locking plate technology and its applications in upper extremity fracture care. *Hand Clin* 2007;23:269-278.

39. Murakami K, Abe Y, Takahashi K: Surgical treatment of unstable distal radius fractures with volar locking plates. *J Orthop Sci* 2007;12:134-140.

40. Weinraub GM: Midfoot arthrodesis using a locking anterior cervical plate as adjunctive fixation: Early experience with a new implant. *J Foot Ankle Surg* 2006;45:240-243.

41. Gallentine JW, Deorio JK, Deorio MJ: Bunion surgery using locking-plate fixation of proximal metatarsal chevron osteotomies. *Foot Ankle Int* 2007;28:361-368.

42. Sommer C, Babst R, Müller M, Hanson B: Locking compression plate loosening and plate breakage: A report of four cases. *J Orthop Trauma* 2004;18:571-577.

43. Arora R, Lutz M, Hennerbichler A, Krappinger D, Espen D, Gabl M: Complications following internal fixation of unstable distal radius fracture with a palmar locking-plate. *J Orthop Trauma* 2007;21:316-322.

44. Arora R, Lutz M, Zimmermann R, Krappinger D, Gabl M, Pechlaner S: Limits of palmar locking-plate osteosynthesis of unstable distal radius fractures. *Handchir Mikrochir Plast Chir* 2007;39:34-41.

45. Namazi H, Mozaffarian K: Awful considerations with LCP instrumentation: A new pitfall. *Arch Orthop Trauma Surg* 2007;127:573-575.

46. Phisitkul P, McKinley TO, Nepola JV, Marsh JL: Complications of locking plate fixation in complex proximal tibia injuries. *J Orthop Trauma* 2007; 21:83-91.

47. Gautier E, Sommer C: Guidelines for the clinical application of the LCP. *Injury* 2003;34(suppl 2):B63-B76.

48. Pallister I, Iorwerth A: Indirect reduction using a simple quadrilateral frame in the application of distal tibial LCP-technical tips. *Injury* 2005;36: 1138-1142.

49. Lill H, Hepp P, Korner J, et al: Proximal humeral fractures: How stiff should an implant be? A comparative mechanical study with new implants in human specimens. *Arch Orthop Trauma Surg* 2003;123:74-81.

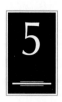

# External Fixation: How to Make It Work

*Bruce H. Ziran, MD
Wade R. Smith, MD
*Jeffrey O. Anglen, MD
Paul Tornetta III, MD

## Abstract

*The external fixator has been in use for more than a century. Wutzer (1789-1863) used pins and an interconnecting rod-and-clamp system. Parkhill (1897) and Lambotte (1900) used devices that were unilateral with four pins and a bar-clamp system. By 1960, Vidal and Hoffmann had popularized the use of an external fixator to treat open fractures and infected pseudarthroses. The complications associated with the use of external fixation in the late 20th century were predominantly caused by a lack of understanding of the principles of application, the principles of fracture healing with external fixation, and old technology. Its use was reserved for the most severe injuries and for cases complicated by infection. Thus, pin problems, nonunions, and malunions were common. Better technology and understanding have since allowed for greater versatility and better outcomes. Simultaneous with developments in the Western world, Ilizarov developed the principles of external fixation with use of ring and wire fixation. It was not until the late 1980s and early 1990s, when more interaction and exchange between the West and East (Russia) became possible, and with the help of Italians who embraced the philosophy of external fixation, that the use of external fixation was proven to be successful. Several variations of external fixation have been developed, and its use is now widespread. However, in the United States, all but a minority of surgeons still have substantial apprehension about the use of external fixation.*

*Instr Course Lect 2008;57:37-49.*

This chapter reviews the principles of external fixation and describes healing under these conditions. Existing technology with specific attention to pin design, modular designs, and aspects of ring fixation for the general practitioner also is reviewed. The paradigm of using the external fixator for bone healing is outlined, and the different types of external fixator applications, including damage-control frames and configurations of hybrid frames for the tibia, are discussed. Pin care issues are reviewed, and pin care techniques that work are presented.

## Principles of External Fixation

External fixation is a minimally invasive technique whose application and management have been refined so that it is now another valuable tool in the management of fractures and other complicated musculoskeletal conditions. From pin care to frame mechanics, the fixator can be applied and adjusted to meet the needs in each clinical context, and many of the problems previously associated with its use can be circumvented. Even so, it is not a panacea and should not be used in situations in which plates or nails are more suitable. Currently the external fixator has two common treatment configurations: the damage-control orthopaedic frame, which was designed to be a temporary device, and the definitive-treatment frame, which was designed to be used for definitive management of fractures and for posttraumatic reconstruction. These two applications are

*Bruce H. Ziran, MD or the department with which he is affiliated has received miscellaneous noncome support, commercially-derived honoraria, or other nonresearch-related funding from Stryker and Synthes. Jeffrey O. Anglen, MD or the department with which he is affiliated has received royalties from EBI and is a consultant or employee for Eli Lilly.*

based on different principles of treatment. When the damage-control frame is used, the impact of the fixator on the systemic state of the patient and on the definitive intervention that may follow (plate or nail fixation) must be considered. Also, it may become necessary to use the external fixator as the definitive treatment, so it is important to know how to convert the damage-control frame to the definitive-treatment frame configuration. When the definitive-treatment frame configuration is used, it is critical to understand how to modulate the mechanical properties of the fixator in response to the bone being treated. Thus, an understanding of how to "read the bone" is important, as is an understanding of the techniques of application that allow long-term use of the fixator. Finally, because some frames will need to be in place for a prolonged period (those used for limb-lengthening and salvage), effective management of routine issues (pin tracts, discomfort, and walking) is necessary.

## Damage-Control Frames

The early damage-control frames were used primarily for severe open fractures because these fractures were not amenable to the fracture fixation techniques available at the time. Because external fixation was used in the most extreme cases, it was associated with the most complications, such as infection and nonunion. Furthermore, effective principles of soft-tissue management and ways to obtain healing in the presence of exposed bone and bone loss were just being learned. Nonetheless, for lack of a better option, external fixation was used. As plate and nail fixation methods improved, fractures in most multiple-trauma patients were stabilized with

definitive fixation immediately (in less than 24 to 48 hours). This has been described as the era of early total care. Subsequently, although early total care was reasonable for the bone, it was not always optimal for every patient because of numerous systemic issues. The evolution of collaborative management of the trauma patient, for whom orthopaedic treatment is performed within the context of the "big picture," heralded the modern era of damage-control orthopaedics. In this era, there is appropriate stabilization of the essential bone injuries (usually with a damage-control orthopaedic frame), until the patient's systemic condition becomes optimized, at which point definitive fracture stabilization is undertaken, usually with nails or plates. Although there remains controversy about the timing of fixation, which is beyond the scope of this chapter, a definitive indication has been established for external fixation as a method with which to stabilize the skeleton during the early stages of multiple trauma.

In this chapter, the application of a damage-control orthopaedic frame for the pelvis and extremities will be described. Simple-to-remember anatomic windows and simple frame constructs that can be applied to most fractures will be presented. With the use of battery-powered drills, a single "damage-control tray" can be assembled to simplify application.

## Definitive-Treatment Frames

When external fixation is used as definitive treatment, it should first be applied in a configuration that provides the maximum stability (a rigid construct) to the fresh fracture environment. This is the best environment for healing of the soft tissues as well as for the early stages of bone

healing. However, this environment should not be maintained indefinitely because it will result in excessive stress-shielding of the fracture site and can lead to an osteopenic nonunion. This type of nonunion is one of the most challenging to treat because there is not only a problem with healing but also challenges with regard to obtaining a stable construct because of the changes in bone quality. Over time, the external fixator should be changed or modulated to allow a progressive load transfer or destiffening of the construct to help stimulate bone healing.

Once there is evidence of biologic activity (early fracture callus), there should be a slow and progressive load transfer to the healing callus. As hypothesized by Pauwels[1] and later explained in different terms by Perren[2] (with his interfragmentary strain theory), pure compression and hydrostatic pressure will stimulate the mesenchymal cells to differentiate toward chondrogenesis and subsequently endochondral ossification. Strain will result in the formation of collagenous tissue and subsequent intramembranous ossification. Combinations of these two temporally spaced events (compression then strain) can manifest themselves as callus healing or, as is the case with use of the Ilizarov principle, regenerate formation.[2] All of this, however, depends on adequate blood flow because, in its absence, there will be no bone healing, regardless of the type of fracture fixation. Thus, as the initial construct with the stiff fixator begins to demonstrate some biologic activity, the fixator undergoes a "controlled destiffening" so that there is a slow but definitive transfer of load bearing from the fixator to the bone. This load sharing will gradually stimulate the developing callus until solid bone healing has occurred.

Several authors have examined both theoretic and practical methods of analyzing healing in association with the use of external fixation.[2-10] Factors that contribute to the nature and speed of osseous healing include the location of the fracture, the nature of the blood supply, and the method of fixation (pin or wire configuration). Although the experience has not been well documented in the English language literature, those who have visited the center in Russia established by Ilizarov have seen remarkable work, all done with fine wire fixation. Metaphyseal healing within 3 to 4 weeks, massive reconstructions, and eradication of infection have all been demonstrated (personal communication). Again, as a result of the historic geopolitical issues, such information has not been well disseminated in the Western literature. What the Russians have demonstrated clearly is that appropriate concern regarding the biology of the soft tissues as well as that of the bone, along with stable frame configurations and physiologic loading, can result in reliable healing with use of external fixation. Usually, frame constructs start out stiff and progressively transfer load to healing bone.

However, two crucial elements are not well known: how to optimize the load transfer (destiffening) and how to know when it is complete and the fracture has healed. Still, the goal of external fixation is to provide what has been called flexible stability. The stability is provided by the frame and the construct while the flexibility is added by manipulating the components. Incidentally, this is the same principle on which modern plate fixation techniques are based. As constructs began to include longer plate spans with fewer screws, the introduction of locked plates essentially resulted in an internalized fixator. Now it is commonplace to use longer plate spans with a few widely spaced locked screws to obtain a flexible (long-span) but stable (locked-screw) construct.

The ring fixator is based on the same principles, in that initial stability is achieved with multidirectional wires or pins and little initial weight bearing is allowed to obtain a stable environment. Then, as weight bearing is initiated, there is a controlled axial micromotion that provides the stimulus for fracture healing. Because the device is inherently flexible and yet stable, it achieves the same end result. In fact, as tensioned wires are loaded, they often loosen and serendipitously transfer more load to the construct. If this occurs too quickly, the subsequent excessive instability will result in pin-related problems and discomfort; hence, the saying among experienced users of ring and wire fixators has been: "A stable frame is a comfortable frame, and a comfortable frame is a stable frame."

Because the use of ring and wire fixators is complex, in this chapter, only the simpler hybrid frame will be discussed. With this frame, the principles that should be followed include beginning with a rigid frame construct. As the construct with the stiff fixator begins to demonstrate some biologic activity (fracture callus equals evidence of vascularity), the fixator undergoes a "controlled destiffening," so that there is a slow but definitive transfer of load from the fixator to the bone during weight-bearing activities. In theory, this load sharing gradually stimulates the developing callus until healing has occurred. If there is no evidence of biologic activity or vascularity (that is, no callus), an intervention such as bone grafting or resection and transport should be considered. An atrophic nonunion will not heal regardless of the device that is used.

## Pin Technology, Design, and Method of Application

There are many different pin designs, and there remains a philosophical rift among surgeons with regard to the best way to place pins. What has been learned is that mechanical chipping and thermal necrosis of the bone are deleterious to pin longevity and that the most important factor may be the management of the soft tissues around the pin. Older pins were designed either to be placed after predrilling or to be self-drilling and threading. There are advantages and disadvantages to both methods. With predrilling, the cutting should be done with sharp, well-designed drills, and the thermal necrosis and mechanical issues are minimized. (It is important for the surgeon to check the drills to ensure a sharp bit.) However, there is definitely a wobble during the subsequent hand placement of the pins. This wobble can result in a small but meaningful conical deformation of the near cortex, which reduces the initial stability of the pin in the near cortex and increases the stress in the far cortex. On the other hand, the older spade-tipped pin (also called a trocar), which was drilled directly into the bone, resulted in chipping of the bone and sufficient heat generation to cause necrosis of the bone. Thus, their poor design defeated their advantage (except in metaphyseal bone).

Subsequently, pin designs have included a modified drill point with flutes along with threads with a cutting lead edge for tapping, followed by threads for fixation. This allows one-step placement of pins that minimizes thermal and mechanical complications. The pins can be placed with a motorized device, and the controlled axial motion of insertion minimizes the wobble of hand placement. Critics of one-step insertion point to the difficulty in feeling the far cortex as well as the theoretical possibility of stripping the near-cortex threads when the cutting tip encounters the endosteal surface of the far cortex. However, the use of appropriate cutting tips as well as an appropriately designed thread pitch allow the advancement speed of the pin (determined by the thread pitch) to be controlled such that the pin engages and cuts through the far cortex without difficulty. Furthermore, as a result of the brief resistance of the pin tip as it encounters the far cortex, there is usually an audible and palpable drain on the drill motor at such an instant. This alerts the surgeon that the far cortex has been reached so that overpenetration can be avoided.

Such theoretic advantages were demonstrated in a study of dogs by Seitz and associates,[11] who found a 22% decrease in the pull-out strength of self-drilling pins placed with motorized power as well as a substantial wobble with pins placed by hand. Because pull-out is rarely a mode of failure and loose pins are a frequent cause of pin and/or soft-tissue problems, the potential downside of wobble makes power insertion an attractive option. The downside of power insertion is mainly related to the use of improper technique.

The issue of heat generation with self-drilling pins was studied with thermocouples used near each cortex and measurement of heat generation during several modes of pin insertion and was determined to depend on numerous factors.[12] In that study, comparison of predrilling with hand insertion, hand insertion of self-cutting pins, and power insertion revealed no apparent differences among the three methods of insertion. In fact, power insertion appeared to generate less heat. The obvious question is why would the placement of self-cutting, self-tapping pins with power generate less heat than the other methods? The most likely conclusion would be that the time in contact with bone causes frictional heat during insertion. Thus, although power insertion appears more aggressive, because it involves less time of frictional contact with the bone it theoretically creates less heat. Modern self-drilling pins placed with power have been in use clinically for many years and have demonstrated good performance. One compromise is to predrill the holes with a sharp drill and use power to place the pins to avoid the wobble that can occur with manual placement.

Since the late 1990s, battery-powered drills have been used to place self-drilling, self-tapping half-pins (thus, there has been no hand insertion or predrilling), but diligent attention has been paid to soft-tissue care. It is important to feel and listen during pin insertion. Usually, there is a brief delay as the drill point cuts through the near cortex, after which it steadily progresses. Then there is a slight sensation of resistance and a change in the drill-motor pitch when the far cortex is reached. The advance should be stopped at that point. If resistance is encountered and excessive drilling is required, something is wrong, and the pin may need to be repositioned.

Another recent advance has been the use of pin coatings both to enhance fixation and to reduce infection. Silver-coated pins have been shown to be associated with less bacterial colonization than uncoated pins, but their clinical performance has not been found to be definitively superior to that of uncoated pins. There is also a potential for systemic silver absorption with their use.[13] Hydroxyapatite-coated pins have had an excellent track record with regard to fixation and longevity and have outperformed standard titanium pins with regard to both infection and longevity.[14] Finally, tapered pins were developed to increase radial preload and insertion torque, both of which have been found to improve pin longevity. However, if the pins are backed up, even a slight amount, their benefit is lost because of the taper, and they need to be well monitored. As a result of these issues as well as the successful performance of other designs, the practical value of tapered pins is questionable at this juncture.

## Fixator Designs: Comparison of Modular, All-in-One, and Hybrid Designs

There are various designs of external fixators. Outdated, single-bar devices had difficulty in maintaining fracture alignment. The improved manufacturing and design of clamps have led to newer modular designs that are very user friendly and adaptable to a wide variety of clinical scenarios. The modern so-called unilateral alternatives, such as those with multidirectional connections and clustered pin clamps on each side, have had an equal amount of success when used properly and have even been expanded to be more modular. To date, no single study demonstrates clinical superiority of any one design. Modular designs are preferable because they are light, are easy to apply, and provide the maximal versatility in most clinical situations. Their application will be outlined below.

The circular fixator has a long history and was popularized by those who followed Ilizarov's philosophy. Because of a long learning curve, maintenance problems, and other difficulties, this device was accepted by only a minority of orthopaedic surgeons. In response, the hybrid frame was developed to provide some of the advantages of the ring design with the ease of application of standard fixators, particularly for periarticular fractures. The hybrid frame was initially popular and then quickly fell out of favor because of high rates of complications and failures. If the literature is critically reviewed, it is apparent that most of the failures of ring fixators, both Ilizarov and hybrid devices, occurred in the treatment of more severe injuries. Use of such methods to treat severely disrupted soft tissues and highly comminuted articular segments was doomed to fail. In short, the application of these frame designs was pushed beyond their abilities. Thus, it was less the fixator and more the indication or application that was at fault. If applied for the proper indication, hybrid frame designs can work well.[15] Furthermore, application of these fixators is not like insertion of a plate or nail (passive management) because it requires active (but simple) management. The recommended application and management of a hybrid frame (Figure 1) will be outlined later.

## External Fixators and MRI

A new issue that has arisen is the safety of external fixator parts during MRI of either the limb or other body parts. MRI-safe means that a

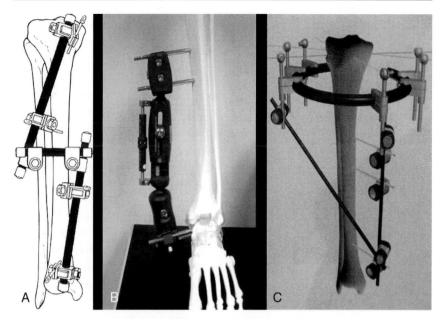

**Figure 1**  Representation of different types of fixator constructs. **A,** Modular half-pin. **B,** Unibody, monolateral. **C,** Hybrid.

fixator does not generate any deleterious effects (no known hazards) in any magnetic resonance environment. MRI-conditional means that the individual parts do not generate any deleterious effects in specifically defined (for example, 1.5-T) magnetic resonance environments. There are three issues related to safety during MRI:

1. The magnetic field causes a direct force on magnetic materials. It is not an issue with nonmagnetic steel, aluminum, carbon, or plastic.

2. Induced electric currents can be produced in a magnetic field. Most modern fixator components are not individually magnetic, but when the components are linked together, as in a standard fixator frame, a closed circuit is created, and an electric current can be induced by the magnetic field. This is true even when carbon fiber or other nonmetallic material is used because virtually all elements have some degree of conductivity and inductivity. A circuit of MRI components with

carbon rods and a loop into the patient can generate clinically relevant currents.[16,17]

3. Heating of materials can occur. The induced current can cause heating of the device and perhaps local tissue damage. There are few to no clinical data regarding this phenomenon, and the US Food and Drug Administration has yet to rule on what is considered "safe." Currently, there is no industry standard for what is considered MRI-safe or what is clinically safe. Only one company to date has attempted to "insulate" the construct against any inductive currents, but there is still a known temperature gradient that forms.

The resultant interaction of the frame with the machine itself can disturb the calibration of the magnetic resonance machine, which can be damaging and costly to repair. Finally, even when it is possible to perform MRI on a patient with an external fixator, clamps located near the field being scanned, even when several centimeters from the skin, can result in enough interference to make the scan meaningless. Judicious use of MRI, with the fixator clamps placed as remote from the area of interest as possible, is recommended.[18] In addition, it should be remembered that MRI safety with regard to the individual components of the fixator does not ensure safety of MRI when the frame is assembled into a closed circuit, and one should beware of misleading marketing claims in this regard.

## Use of the External Fixator as Definitive Fixation

The external fixator is an ideal device with which to obtain healing because it is one of the only devices that provides a stable construct in which the mechanical parameters (rigidity and alignment) can be modulated as needed throughout treatment. The frame is usually applied to create as much stability as possible at the fracture site. Later, with minimal adjustments, the system can be made more flexible to allow micromotion or macromotion to help stimulate healing of the fracture. Furthermore, if problems develop with parts other than the pins or wires, those parts are easily replaced. With modern designs, there have been very few reported failures or broken parts, although exceptions do occur with some of the ball-cam designs. In these designs, a ball is eccentrically turned to lock an interference fit into place, but if there is even minimal loosening the entire mechanism may suddenly release; therefore, locking mechanisms other than the ball-cam design are preferable.

The technique for definitive fixation is based on the concept of the stable base (J Hutson, MD, personal communication). With this method,

each fixation segment has a stable configuration of pins or wires and an external fixation module (ring, clamp, or bar). Then individual stable bases are connected to each other in the desired orientation. Frequently, a common bar or clamp can be used for more than one segment (transport frames), but ensuring that each independent segment has a stable configuration is important. We prefer to place at least three or four fixation wires or half-pins (for a metaphyseal segment) or three half-pins (for a diaphyseal segment) so that one or two can be removed if necessary without destabilizing the construct. In the event that the fracture does not heal or another problem requires removal, the frame should be removed and the fracture should be controlled with external bracing for 1 to 2 weeks before internal fixation. The infection rate associated with intramedullary nailing after external fixation is relatively low (8%) in the absence of a true pin-tract infection, but most traumatologists recommend an interval of frame removal, pin-tract curettage, and perhaps antibiotic coverage before placement of the intramedullary nail. We recommend drilling and curettage of the pin tracts to remove any colonized or necrotic tissue that could increase the risk of infection. The patient is treated with a broad-spectrum antibiotic for 1 or 2 weeks before placing the internal fixation. Although there is little evidence on which to base this recommendation, it is believed that the morbidity and costs of a subsequent infection justify the use of such a protocol.[19]

There have been several studies in which the different healing patterns of fractures have been measured while the extremity was in an external fixator.[3-6] In these studies,

the stiffness and strain of the fracture callus were measured during the healing process and how healing occurs is outlined. The common finding of these studies is that, if the fracture is to heal, a proper load transfer from the external fixator to the developing callus is necessary. As noted previously, the first stage of application of the external fixation should achieve a rigid construct to allow the earliest stages of the fracture-healing process to begin as well as to allow the soft tissues to recover. Once there is early callus formation, the frame needs to be progressively "destiffened" to transfer more and more load to the developing callus. If the construct is made too flexible too early, the resultant strain may exceed the local limits of the developing callus and produce a nonunion. In contrast, if there is insufficient load transfer, there will be inadequate callus formation, bone resorption, and disuse osteopenia. Both of these situations are undesirable. Removing bars, adjusting the locations of bars, or removing pin and/or wire components can destiffen the construct in a systematic way to achieve fracture healing.

With use of ring designs, the load transfer is usually a repetitive stimulus that occurs with increased physiologic loading. As healing progresses, wires and half-pins can be removed or support struts can be loosened. Finally, intervening struts can be removed altogether, and the patient can have a trial of weightbearing. This is done so that, if pain occurs with weight bearing, the struts can be reapplied with the presumption that healing is incomplete and a repeat trip to the operating room to reapply removed "stable bases" is not required.

If a modular or monolateral design is used in the tibia, the key element is the anteromedial stabilizer because the center of gravity is medial during single-limb stance. Having main fixator struts or bars near the center of gravity minimizes the cantilever load on the fixator pins. With a true monolateral system, the frame is placed in the anteromedial quadrant of the leg, and, as healing progresses, the fixator is either manually compressed or progressively dynamized. In modular hybrid constructs, there is an anteromedial strut and a secondary bar that connects to the lateral side of the leg and creates a triangular or delta-shaped construct. In these configurations, the delta bars are the first to be removed. This is followed by moving the anteromedial bar farther from the skin or by reducing the number of pins and/or wires in each segment. Although there are several methods available to decrease stiffness and allow load transfer to the healing callus, these actions are done only when there is ample radiographic and clinical evidence of healing (callus progression and pain-free function). Before complete dynamization occurs, a trial of disconnection with weight bearing

(usually in the physician's office or for 1 week) is performed to ensure that clinical healing is occurring (Figure 2).

## External Fixator Configurations for Damage-Control Frames

These are the simplest of frames, and many configurations are possible. The ones described here allow percutaneous placement (away from vital structures) while providing adequate initial stability and wound access and minimizing the risks associated with delayed internal fixation.

Humerus: Five-mm pins should be placed in the anterolateral quadrant of the proximal part of the humerus and in the posterolateral quadrant of the distal part of the humerus. Fine wires and 4-mm pins can be used in very distal fragments (Figure 3).

Forearm: In most of the forearm, the subcutaneous border of the ulna can be used as a suitable landmark, but only 3-mm (distal) or 4-mm (proximal) pins should be used. The radius is not as suitable for percutaneous fixation, and an open ap-

proach is recommended if such fixation is used.

Pelvis: The anterior superior iliac spine is an excellent landmark, and 5-mm pins should be directed medially and posteriorly. If the fixator is

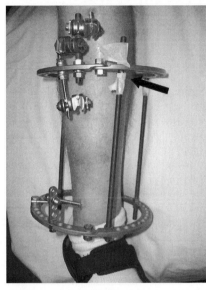

**Figure 2** Clinical photograph of a ring fixator in the completely dynamic mode. The inner nuts are turned back a few millimeters when the fracture is thought to be almost completely healed. This maneuver dynamizes the fixator and stimulates maturation of the healing callus. Note that tape (*arrow*) has been applied to the nuts to prevent drift.

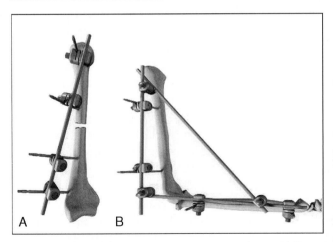
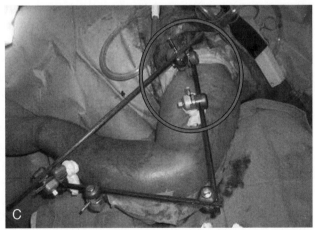

**Figure 3** Schematic illustrations of humeral (**A**) and elbow (**B**) frames. **C,** Clinical photograph of an elbow damage-control frame.

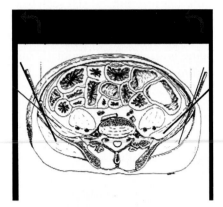

**Figure 4** Diagram of pin placement into the pelvis. The bold lines demonstrate the direction of desired pin placement (in the case of imperfect pin placement) for two fracture types. If the pelvis is being "closed" (right part of picture), then pin placement should not traverse the ilium to the outside (nonbold lines) but instead should traverse to the inside. The forces on the pin-bone interface during reduction are better resisted in this fashion. Likewise, on the left side, the pelvis is being "opened," and the opposite is true. This situation is relatively rare.

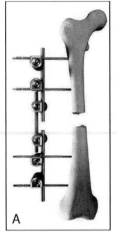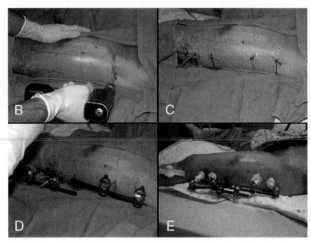

**Figure 5** **A,** Schematic of a femoral frame. **B** through **E,** Montage of external fixator placement in the intensive care unit for damage-control. Local preparation and sterile technique are used to place pins percutaneously (**B** and **C**). Two stable bases are created (**D**) and connected to stabilize the femur (**E**).

to be used to reduce an "open-book" type of pelvic fracture (for example, internal rotation of the hemipelvic segments), the pin should not exit the iliac wing laterally because, with manipulation of the displaced pelvic fracture, the pins can just rotate in the iliac crest, leaving the fracture unreduced. Also, such pins will become loose and contribute to skin problems. In these cases, it is preferable to err with the pin exiting the inner table so that, during the reduction maneuver, pin rotation is resisted by the inner table of the ilium (Figure 4). Conversely, if the fixator will be used to "open" the pelvis, as in the treatment of a lateral compression injury, pin placement should err to the outer cortex for similar mechanical and soft-tissue reasons. If needed, a superior acetabular pin can be placed 5 to 10 cm

proximal to the tip of the greater trochanter in line with the femur to provide fixation. Care should be taken that this pin does not penetrate into the soft tissues of the pelvis. Alternatively, through an open approach, the anterior inferior iliac spine can be used for pin placement with the pin directed posteriorly. We recommend against placing pins in the greater trochanter because of the high risk of infection.

Femur: Along the entire length of the femur, the anterolateral quadrant is best suited for placement of 5-mm pins. The anterolateral aspect of the thigh contains no vital structures, and the pin tracks do not interfere with subsequent surgical approaches (Figure 5).

Tibia: The anteromedial quadrant is best suited for 5-mm pins, as there is little soft tissue and easy access. The pins are placed perpendicular to the anteromedial face of the tibial cortex (Figure 6).

Knee: The knee can be stabilized with placement of pins into the anteromedial aspect of the tibia and the anterolateral aspect of the femur to

create a stable base in each segment. A single large bar should be connected to each pin pair with adequate length to connect to another bar. An intercalary bar completes the zigzag or z construct (Figure 7).

Ankle: The ankle can be stabilized with use of a single 4- or 5-mm transfixion pin across the calcaneus, with or without the addition of 4-mm midfoot or metatarsal pins. Because of problems with loosening of transfixion pins in the calcaneus, the use of two posterior calcaneal pins attached to a U-shaped bar or ring is preferable. These pins seem to create fewer problems. We caution against placing two transverse pins into the calcaneus because of the risk of damage to vital structures on the medial side, such as the flexor tendons and the neurovascular bundle[20,21] (Figure 8).

### Stable Base

When building an external fixation frame, one should first create a stable base in each bone segment. To achieve this, a single bar is placed between the two pins in each fragment. Then another bar (an intercalary bar) is connected to the bars in each base. For example, when two pins are placed into the femoral fragments, there should be a bar that connects the two pins in each fragment, and then an additional bar is used to stabilize the fracture. If the intercalary bar is connected to only one of the two pins in each base, the resultant stability of the construct may be inadequate because the holding power and the stability of a bar-to-bar connection is greater than that of a bar-to-pin connection. Another strong recommendation is to place the compartment, through which a pin is passing, on stretch during insertion. For example, if a wire is passing across the distal part of the femur from posterior-lateral to anterior-medial, the knee is straightened (to place the posterior muscle-tendon units on stretch) during initial insertion; then, as the pin exits anteromedially, the knee is flexed (to place the medial quadriceps muscle-tendon units on stretch). This maneuver not only helps maintain motion around the adjacent joint but also minimizes irritation by the pin during such motion. This can help minimize irritation of the tissues and facilitate pin care.

## Application of a Hybrid Frame to the Tibia

The application of a hybrid frame to either the proximal or the distal part of the tibia is relatively simple (Figure 9). The hybrid frame is best used for extra-articular or very simple fractures (C1 according to the AO/Orthopaedic Trauma Association classification system). Originally, one would use two or three wires and/or one or two half-pins in the articular segment with a longitudinally parallel support member in the

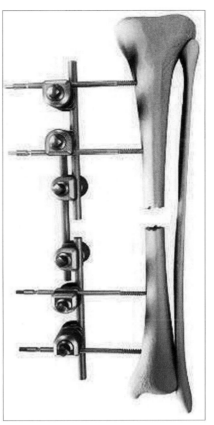

**Figure 6** Schematic of a tibial frame. Note that pins are placed anteromedially when possible.

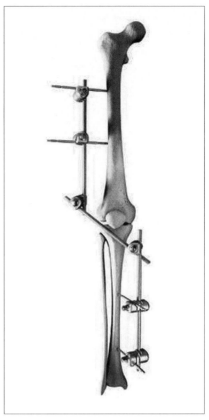

**Figure 7** Schematic of a knee frame. The femoral pins are anterolateral, and the tibial pins are anteromedial.

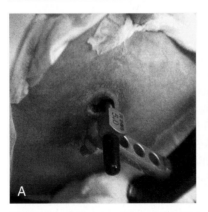

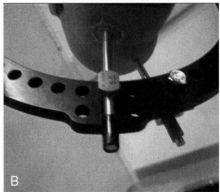

**Figure 8** A loose calcaneal transfixion pin associated with infection (**A**) and a pin inserted posteriorly and attached to a U-shaped bar or ring (**B**).

anteromedial quadrant of the leg and a delta support bar. As soft tissues stabilize and weight bearing is initiated, the surgeon monitors the radiographs for evidence of healing. If callus is present (at approximately

2 to 4 weeks), load transfer is initiated by one of several methods. Having the patient bear weight statically while the delta bar is loosened and then retightened resets the load on the bar and effectively transfers

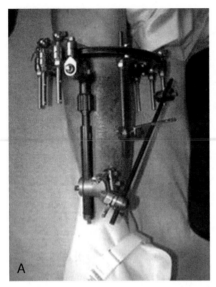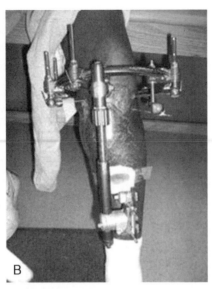

**Figure 9** **A,** Example of initial hybrid application with use of an anteromedial strut and a delta bar. This configuration established initial rigidity for both soft-tissue healing and initiation of the fracture-healing cascade. **B,** After 2 to 4 weeks, when there are some radiographic signs of callus formation, the fracture is progressively loaded in a controlled fashion. The fixator is destiffened with use of one of several methods. These include removal of the delta bar; changes in the bar-bone distance (farther equals less stiff); removal of pins or wires; or, in the present example, use of a dynamic axial bar that allows controlled, spring-loaded axial micromotion.

some load to the bone. Removal of a wire or pin will also destiffen the construct, but we do not recommend this method in case any problems develop with the remaining pins. If a dynamic component has been used, it can be dynamized as described below. In the absence of a dynamic component, another more practical method is to move the bar farther from the skin (bone), which would effectively decrease the stiffness of the frame and result in greater load transfer at the site of callus.

Progressive weight bearing increases load transfer. When a dynamic device is used, as is preferred, load transfer can be started by dialing 1 mm of axial motion into the system. As healing progresses (at approximately 6 weeks), more load is transferred by increasing weight bearing further and by removing the delta bar. With dynamic compo-

nents, more motion can be dialed in. This process is continued so that, by 12 weeks, some half-pins can be removed and/or more motion can be dialed in. At 16 weeks, if the radiographs and clinical status warrant it, the components are disengaged while the metaphyseal and diaphyseal stable bases are maintained. This allows full load transfer while keeping the frame components in the leg but not connected in case healing is incomplete and more time in the fixator is required. The remainder of the device is removed 1 week later if the patient has no symptoms and the fracture remains aligned. With use of this algorithm, if there is satisfactory initial reduction, progressive physiologic loading, and progressive dynamization (load transfer), fracture healing can frequently be expected. In our experience with a series of proximal and

distal tibial fractures, this method was well tolerated and resulted in a healing rate of greater than 95%.[15] It should be noted, however, that this method is indicated for only specific fracture types. To avoid the problems reported in the past with use of a hybrid device, it is important to understand the appropriate indications for its use. As the saying goes, one needs "the right tool for the right job."

## Pin Care

Localized pin tract infection has been the nemesis of external fixation and one of the primary reasons many surgeons avoid its use. The anatomic sites that are most prone to pin-related complications are those with a large soft-tissue sleeve and those subject to motion of the soft tissues. Excessive motion of the muscle and skin around the bone results in local inflammation that leads to a pin-tract infection, which in turn can progress to infect the bone. What appears to be clear to most experienced surgeons is that the most important parameter is the control of soft-tissue motion. Stabilizing the soft tissues around the pin to prevent motion is probably more important than the method or agent of cleaning. There are numerous methods with which to stabilize the skin. One of the best is application of a gentle compressive dressing between the bar and skin. With this method, it is important to avoid excessive pressure and skin necrosis.

Pin-care protocols range from doing nothing to washing the site of entry three times a day with cotton swabs and peroxide. Temple and Santy[22] performed a comprehensive review of studies on pin care in the literature. They found one randomized, controlled study in which saline solution, alcohol, and no cleaning were compared, and no cleaning resulted in fewer infections. Another study demonstrated no difference between daily and weekly pin care.[23] There is now sufficient evidence that elaborate pin care is not necessary and that simple and occasional attention to the pins may be sufficient. Most practitioners recommend daily pin care performed for personal hygiene reasons. There is no evidence that any one modality or chemical works better than another, but a nontissue-toxic cleaner such as soap is recommended. It would seem that pin site irritation leading to inflammation is a probable mechanism that results in infection and, finally, loosening of the pin. Therefore, minimizing mechanical skin motion may be more important than the frequency of cleaning or type of cleaning agents[24] (Figure 10).

We developed a pin-care protocol that has served us well but is not based on scientific data. As described previously, when a pin is being inserted, the soft-tissue compartment should be placed on stretch, and the skin should be released if needed so that there is no skin tension. The pin sites are covered and, to ensure that there is no pistoning of the soft tissue, we use bolsters, spacers, or sponges to stabilize it. The pin sites are left covered and are not inspected for as long as the patient is in the intensive care unit. If the pins are cleaned during the inpatient stay, we use saline solution or alcohol and do not probe the tracts with cotton swabs. Nursing staff and aides do not provide pin care. The pin sites are gently wiped with an alcohol pledget and then covered. The surrounding skin is stabilized by placing a bolster between the bar and the skin that applies gentle pressure to the skin

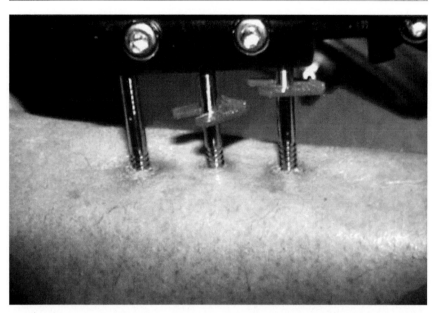

**Figure 10**    Three pins, with no associated infection, with pin clips that were used to hold the dressings in place.

and prevents motion with routine activity.

The patient is instructed to shower daily after he or she is discharged and to clean the fixator with soap and water in the shower as part of a daily routine. The skin and pins are dried with a clean towel, and the pin sites are wiped with an alcohol pledget. The skin is then stabilized as described previously. Bath water, fresh water lakes, and seawater are avoided.

Problems with pin tract infection should be managed as quickly as they are identified. We use the classification of Checketts and associates.[25,26] Although the literature often describes relatively high rates of "pin tract infection," close inspection will demonstrate that most pin-related problems fall into the Checketts grade I and II categories, which are very mild. A problematic pin is one associated with ongoing exudates or purulent discharge with surrounding inflammation and subsequent loosening. When a pin site

looks irritated, we first assess the nature of the pin care being provided. We then check the stability of the pin in bone and of the entire construct. If the pin or construct is loose, any and all pin care will usually be futile. We stratify our pin problems in two ways, according to stability and inflammation. Any pin that is unstable and associated with inflammation is removed. Pins associated with inflammation and transudate that are stable (Checketts grades I and II) are retained.[25] We begin by ensuring proper skin stability, and we frequently apply Bactroban (mupirocin) ointment. Pins that are associated with inflammation and purulence are at greater risk. In addition to all of the interventions provided for grade I and II problems, we add oral antibiotics in adequate doses (Keflex [cephalexin], 500 mg four times a day, or Levaquin [levofloxacin], 500 mg daily) because suboptimal antibiotics are not only ineffective but also can lead to the development of resistant or-

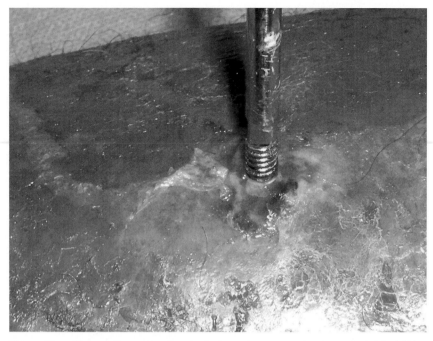

**Figure 11** Suppuration around a pin that requires aggressive treatment. Modalities include more frequent cleaning, the application of mupirocin cream, and a full dose of oral antibiotics. The pin should be tested for tightness. If it is loose, it should be removed or replaced.

ganisms (Figure 11). We also increase the frequency of cleaning if there is accumulation of dried exudates. If after such interventions there is no improvement, we then check the stability of the pin again, and if it is loose we remove it. Also, as noted previously in our description of the method of application, the use of three or four fixation points in each segment provides the latitude of being able to remove one or two pins during treatment without compromising the outcome or necessitating a return to the operating room. With this methodology, we have substantially limited the need to revise pins, and patients have tolerated fixators very well.

## Summary

The external fixator is a useful tool for several applications, from damage control to definitive treatment.

Advanced applications can be used to treat deformity, infection, and fractures that are not healing. The poor reputation of external fixation, especially in the United States, is the result of misunderstandings, misapplication, and mismanagement. The principles of application and management are fairly straightforward and versatile. The technique does require more attention than internal fixation, and careful clinical and radiographic monitoring is needed. External fixation is not the best treatment of the typical fracture, but its use can be of benefit in well-selected situations.

## References

1. Pauwels F: A new theory on the influence of mechanical stimuli on the differentiation of supporting tissue. The tenth contribution to the functional anatomy and causal morphology of the supporting structure. *Z Anat Entwicklungsgesch* 1960;121:478-515.

2. Perren SM: Evolution of the internal fixation of long bone fractures: The scientific basis of biological internal fixation: Choosing a new balance between stability and biology. *J Bone Joint Surg Br* 2002;84:1093-1110.

3. Aro HT, Chao EY: Biomechanics and biology of fracture repair under external fixation. *Hand Clin* 1993;9:531-542.

4. Aro HT, Chao EY: Bone-healing patterns affected by loading, fracture fragment stability, fracture type, and fracture site compression. *Clin Orthop Relat Res* 1993;293:8-17.

5. Egger EL, Gottsauner-Wolf F, Palmer J, Aro HT, Chao EY: Effects of axial dynamization on bone healing. *J Trauma* 1993;34:185-192.

6. Bourgois R, Burny F: Measurement of the stiffness of fracture callus in vivo: A theoretical study. *J Biomech* 1972;5:85-91.

7. Hinsenkamp M, Burny F, Dierickx M, Donkerwolcke M: Modifications of electric potentials of the pins of Hoffman's "fixateur externe" during fracture healing. *Acta Orthop Belg* 1978;44:732-737.

8. Huiskes R, Chao EY: Guidelines for external fixation frame rigidity and stresses. *J Orthop Res* 1986;4:68-75.

9. Burny F, Bourgois R: Biomechanical study of the Hoffman external fixation device. *Acta Orthop Belg* 1972;38:265-279.

10. Seide K, Weinrich N, Wenzl ME, Wolter D, Jurgens C: Three-dimensional load measurements in an external fixator. *J Biomech* 2004;37:1361-1369.

11. Seitz WH Jr, Froimson AI, Brooks DB, Postak P, Polando G, Greenwald AS: External fixator pin insertion techniques: Biomechanical analysis and clinical relevance. *J Hand Surg Am* 1991;16:560-563.

12. Wikenheiser MA, Markel MD, Lewallen DG, Chao EY: Thermal re-

sponse and torque resistance of five cortical half-pins under simulated insertion technique. *J Orthop Res* 1995; 13:615-619.

13. Masse A, Bruno M, Bosetti M, Biasibetti A, Cannas M, Gallinaro P: Prevention of pin track infection in external fixation with silver coated pins: Clinical and microbiological results. *J Biomed Mater Res* 2000;53:600-604.

14. Pommer A, Muhr G, David A: Hydroxyapatite-coated Schanz pins in external fixators used for distraction osteogenesis: A randomized, controlled trial. *J Bone Joint Surg Am* 2002;84:1162-1166.

15. Varsalona R, Ziran B, Avondo S, Mollica Q: The use of hybrid fixators in proximal tibia fractures, in *Proceedings of the Eighteenth Annual Meeting of the Orthopaedic Trauma Association*. Toronto, Ontario, Canada, 2002.

16. Nyenhuis JA, Park SM, Kamondetdacha R, Amjad A, Shellock FG, Rezai AR: MRI and implanted medical devices: Basic interactions with an emphasis on heating. *IEEE Trans Dev Mater Reliab.* 2005;5:467-480.

17. Luechinger R, Boesiger P, Disegi JA:. Safety evaluation of large external fixation clamps and frames in a magnetic resonance environment. *J Biomed Mater Res B Appl Biomater* 2006;2007;82:17-22

18. ASTM F2503-05: Standard practice for marking medical devices and other items for safety in the magnetic resonance environment. *ASTM International* 2005.

19. Bhandari M, Zlowodzki M, Tornetta P III, Schmidt A, Templeman DC: Intramedullary nailing following external fixation in femoral and tibial shaft fractures. *J Orthop Trauma* 2005; 19:140-144.

20. Casey D, McConnell T, Parekh S, Tornetta P III: Percutaneous pin placement in the medial calcaneus: Is anywhere safe? *J Orthop Trauma* 2004; 18(8 suppl):S39-S42.

21. Santi MD, Botte MJ: External fixation of the calcaneus and talus: An anatomical study for safe pin insertion. *J Orthop Trauma* 1996;10: 487-491.

22. Temple J, Santy J: Pin site care for preventing infections associated with external bone fixators and pins. *Cochrane Database Syst Rev* 2004;1: CD004551.

23. W-Dahl A, Toksvig-Larsen S, Lindstrand A: No difference between daily and weekly pin site care: A randomized study of 50 patients with external fixation. *Acta Orthop Scand* 2003;74: 704-708.

24. Mahan J, Seligson D, Henry SL, Hynes P, Dobbins J: Factors in pin tract infections. *Orthopedics* 1991;14: 305-308.

25. Checketts RG, Otterburn M: Pin tract infection: Definition, prevention, incidence, in *Abstracts of the 2nd Riva Congress: Current Perspectives in External and Intramedullary Fixation*. Riva di Garda, Italy, 1992, pp 98-99.

26. Checketts RG, Moran CG, MacEachern AG, Otterburn M: Pin track infection and the principles of pin site care, in De Bastiani G, Apley AG, Goldberg AAJ (eds): *Orthofix External Fixation in Trauma and Orthopaedics*. London, UK, Springer-Verlag, 2000, pp 97-103.

# Management of Open Fractures and Subsequent Complications

*Charalampos G. Zalavras, MD
Randall E. Marcus, MD
Lawrence Scott Levin, MD
Michael J. Patzakis, MD

## Abstract

*Early, systemic, wide-spectrum antibiotic therapy is necessary for the treatment of open fractures. The bead pouch technique delivers antibiotics locally and prevents secondary wound contamination. The open fracture wound should be thoroughly débrided. To avoid the complication of gas gangrene, the wound should not be closed. Extensive soft-tissue damage may necessitate the use of local or free flaps. Techniques of fracture stabilization depend on the anatomic location of the fracture and the characteristics of the injury. Early bone grafting and supplemental procedures may be needed to achieve healing. Management of the infected open fracture is based on radical débridement, skeletal stabilization, microbial-specific antibiotics, soft-tissue coverage, and reconstruction of bone defects.*

**Instr Course Lect 2008;57:51-63.**

Open fractures are associated with an increased risk of infection and healing complications. Management of open fractures is based on the following principles: assessment of the patient, classification of the injury, antibiotic therapy, débridement and wound management, fracture stabilization, early bone grafting, and supplemental procedures to achieve healing.

## Assessment, Classification, and Antibiotic Therapy

Open fractures usually are the result of high-energy trauma and should alert the treating physician to the possibility of associated injuries. Therefore, detailed evaluation and appropriate resuscitation of the patient are necessary. The neurovascular status of the injured extremity should be carefully assessed, and the development of compartment syndrome should not be overlooked.[1] The soft-tissue injury should be evaluated to determine the size and location of the wound, the degree of muscle damage, and the presence of contamination.

The Gustilo and Anderson classification system,[2] which was subsequently modified by Gustilo and associates,[3] is widely used to grade open fractures. In this system, type I indicates a puncture wound of 1 cm or less with minimal contamination or muscle crushing. Type II indicates a laceration of more than 1 cm in length with moderate soft-tissue damage and crushing; bone coverage is adequate and comminution is minimal. A type IIIA open fracture involves extensive soft-tissue damage, often due to a high-energy injury with a severe crushing component. Massively contaminated wounds and severely comminuted or segmental fractures are included in this subtype. Soft-tissue coverage of the bone is adequate. Type IIIB indicates extensive soft-tissue damage with periosteal stripping and bone exposure, usually with severe

*Charalampos G. Zalavras, MD or the department with which he is affiliated has received research or institutional support from Synthes and Smith & Nephew and miscellaneous nonincome support, commercially-derived honoraria, or other nonresearch-related funding from Smith & Nephew.*

contamination and bone comminution. Flap coverage is required to provide soft-tissue coverage. A type IIIC fracture is associated with an arterial injury requiring repair.

The reliability of this classification has been questioned. In a study in which orthopaedic surgeons had been asked to classify open fractures of the tibia on the basis of videotaped case presentations, the average agreement among the observers was 60% overall, which was deemed to be moderate to poor.[4] Therefore, classification of the open fracture should be done only in the operating room, after wound exploration and débridement. The degree of contamination and soft-tissue crushing are important factors in the classification of an open fracture, but they may be mistakenly overlooked in a wound of small size.

As most open fractures are contaminated with microorganisms, antibiotics are used not for prophylaxis but rather to treat wound contamination. To prevent a clinical infection, immediate antibiotic administration, wound débridement, soft-tissue coverage, and fracture stabilization are necessary. Tetanus prophylaxis may be necessary, depending on the patient's immunization status. The risk of a clinical infection depends on the severity of the injury and ranges from 0% to 2% for type I open fractures, 2% to 10% for type II, and 10% to 50% for type III.

The rate of infection of open fractures is associated with the fracture characteristics, antibiotic therapy variables, and host parameters.[5,6] Infection rates progressively increased from 1.4% (7 of 497 fractures) for type I open fractures to 3.6% (25 of 695 fractures) for type II open fractures to 22.7% (45 of 198 fractures) for type III.[5] The location of the fracture is also important,

with the infection rate for open tibial fractures being twice that for open fractures in other locations.[5]

The administration of antibiotics before débridement decreased the infection rate (2 of 84 fractures) compared with that found when no antibiotics had been given (11 of 79 fractures).[7] The antibiotics should cover both gram-positive and gram-negative organisms, and they should be given as soon as possible, preferably within 3 hours after the injury.[5] The duration of antibiotic therapy, the time between the injury and the surgery, and the type of wound closure do not seem to be significant variables.[5,8]

Even though the infection rates associated with primary and secondary closure are the same, gas gangrene may occur after primary closure of wounds contaminated with clostridial organisms. The partial closure technique, in which the traumatic wound is left open and the surgical extension of the wound is closed (Figure 1), is recommended for type I and II open fractures.[9]

The usefulness of cultures of wound specimens is controversial because they often fail to identify the organism that subsequently causes the infection.[10-12] Cultures of wound specimens obtained before wound débridement are no longer recommended because of their poor predictive value. However, the results of cultures of postdébridement specimens and sensitivity testing may help in the selection of the best agents for subsequent procedures or in the treatment of an early infection.

Although some authors have recommended cephalosporin as a single agent for patients with a type I or II open fracture, the antibiotic therapy should target both the gram-positive and the gram-negative pathogens

contaminating the wound.[13] A commonly used regimen consists of a first-generation cephalosporin (for example, cefazolin), which is active against gram-positive organisms, combined with an aminoglycoside (for example, gentamicin or tobramycin), which is active against gram-negative organisms. Substitutes for aminoglycosides include quinolones,[10] aztreonam, third-generation cephalosporins, or other antibiotics with gram-negative coverage. Systemic administration of aminoglycosides may not be necessary if aminoglycoside-impregnated beads are used for local antibiotic delivery.

Clostridial myonecrosis (gas gangrene) is a particular concern when an injury is contaminated with anaerobic organisms (for example, farm injuries) or there is a vascular injury that may create conditions of ischemia and low oxygen tension.[14] Therefore, in such cases, ampicillin or penicillin should be added to the antibiotic regimen to provide coverage against anaerobes.

Antibiotic administration should be started promptly, as a delay of more than 3 hours has been shown to increase the risk of infection.[5] The recommended duration of therapy is 3 days.[5,13,15] An additional 3 days of administration of antibiotics—selected on the basis of the results of initial cultures—is recommended for subsequent surgical procedures, such as wound coverage and bone grafting.

Local therapy with antibiotic-impregnated polymethylmethacrylate cement has been used as an adjunct to systemic antibiotic therapy in the treatment of open fractures (Figure 2) and has been shown to reduce the infection rate. Ostermann and associates[16] reported an infection rate of 3.7% in a group that received combined treatment with

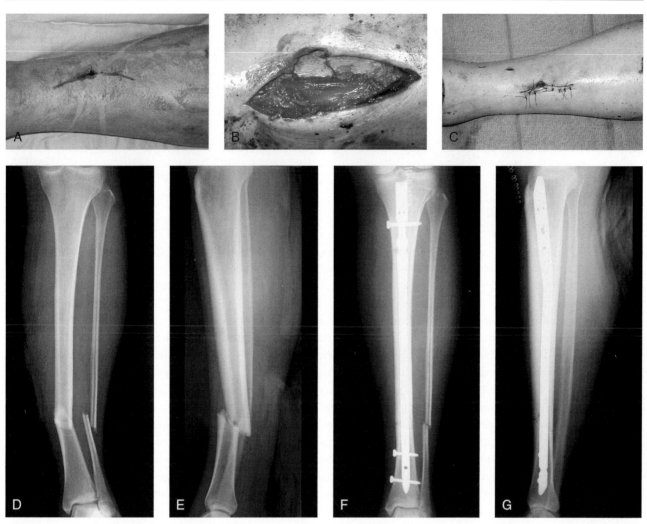

**Figure 1**    **A,** Type I open fracture of the tibia with a small (< 1 cm) traumatic wound. The surgical extension of the wound, necessary for débridement, is marked on the skin. **B,** Following surgical extension of the wound, the open fracture site was débrided, and the fracture was fixed. **C,** The wound was managed with the partial closure technique, in which the surgical extension of the wound is closed and the traumatic wound is left open. This minimizes the risk of gas gangrene without requiring a repeat surgical procedure for wound closure. Preoperative AP **(D)** and lateral **(E)** radiographs of the fractured tibia and fibula. Postoperative AP **(F)** and lateral **(G)** radiographs following intramedullary nailing of the tibia.

both systemic antibiotics and antibiotic beads. This rate was considerably lower than the 12% infection rate associated with open fractures treated with systemic antibiotics alone.

Polymethylmethacrylate powder is mixed with the antibiotic in powder form, polymerized, and then formed into beads, which are incorporated on a 24-gauge wire; usually 3.6 g of tobramycin is mixed with 40 g of polymethylmethacrylate cement.[17] Aminoglycosides are common choices for the antibiotic because of their broad spectrum of activity, heat stability, and low allergenicity. Vancomycin is not recommended as an initial agent because of concerns of overuse leading to development of resistant microorganisms.

The bead pouch technique achieves a high local concentration of antibiotics; minimizes systemic toxicity; and seals the wound from the external environment with a semipermeable barrier, thereby preventing secondary contamination by nosocomial pathogens and at the same time maintaining an aerobic wound environment.

## Soft-Tissue Management
Open fractures are always associated with a soft-tissue injury, and they

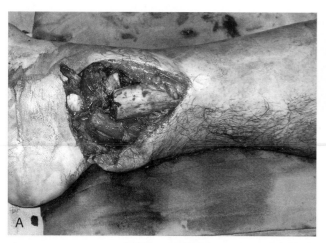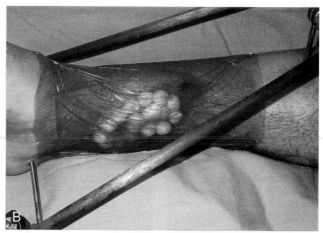

**Figure 2**    **A,** Type IIIB open fracture of the distal part of the tibia. **B,** Antibiotic beads were placed in the wound, which was then sealed with a semipermeable membrane until the time of the soft-tissue coverage procedure.

can be thought of as a soft-tissue injury that includes a fracture. The management of both the bone and the soft tissues is the major determinant of fracture healing and functional restoration of the traumatized extremity. An integrated approach, the so-called orthoplastic approach, takes into account the importance of early and definitive treatment of both aspects of the injury.[18] Important issues related to the management of the fracture include when to provide coverage, how coverage should be provided, who should provide coverage, and where coverage should be provided.

Mechanisms of injury include electrical burns, crushing, avulsion, blasts, and degloving.[19] Management of these injuries requires an understanding of the personalities of soft-tissue injuries, which helps to guide decision making. For example, soft-tissue degloving, which is frequently seen in deceleration injuries, particularly in elderly individuals, often results in avulsion of perforating vessels to the overlying skin.[20] This is commonly seen in the pelvis, where it is called a *Morel-Lavallée lesion.* The same pathologic entity is found in the

extremities and can progress to necrosis of the skin envelope with the exposure of hardware and bone.[21]

It is vital to recognize that, in addition to the variety of mechanisms that can cause an acute soft-tissue injury, a variety of underlying morbidities can be associated with an open fracture. These include diabetes mellitus,[22] peripheral vascular disease, collagen vascular disease and chronic venous insufficiency with underlying venous stasis, immunocompromise, previous fractures or surgical incisions, and nutritional deficiencies.

Appropriate débridement is critical.[23] A tourniquet should be used during the débridement to distinguish blood-stained tissue from normal tissue, as local hemorrhage obscures debris and dirt that must be removed.[24] Loop magnification may be needed. Sharp débridement is essential, and it should be done in a centripetal fashion. Liberal use of fasciotomies facilitates wound inspection and releases compromised muscle compartments. Radical excision of necrotic tissue, as proposed by Godina,[25] should be performed so that all nonviable tissue, including bone, is removed. The

wound should look healthy and, when there is doubt, all questionable tissue should be removed.

New techniques for débridement such as use of the Versajet device (Smith and Nephew, Memphis, TN) have shown the benefit of reducing tissue loss during initial or second-look procedures. Usually, coverage should be obtained with one or two formal débridements; if more débridements are required, then radical débridement has not been performed.

After débridement, one must decide if the soft-tissue deficiency associated with the open fracture can be managed by the orthopaedic traumatologist.[26] If not, it is essential that a microvascular surgeon be consulted as soon as possible. If the local surgical community cannot handle the soft-tissue problem, then the patient should be referred to another institution as soon as possible for definitive wound coverage.

Vascularity is the single most important determinant of complications after an open fracture. Vascularity includes arterial, venous, and lymphatic conduits. Knowledge of the angiosomes helps the surgeons to avoid improper placement of incisions and surgical approaches that can further compromise watershed areas, leading to soft-tissue necrosis following open reduction and external fixation.[27] The concept of perforators must be understood as well.[28] These are side branches from the main arterial vessels that give rise to skin angiosomes. Tissue necrosis is the result of compromised perforators and the watershed areas lying between angiosomes.

Evaluation of the blood supply in skin includes hands-on examination as well as palpation of pulses and appreciation of temperature differences along cutaneous surfaces. Skin that has venous discoloration suggests venous insufficiency, whereas slow refill indicates an arterial-side insufficiency. Doppler examinations, formal arteriography, digital subtraction arteriography, and at times venography are important ways to ascertain the vascular status of an extremity. Without an anterior tibial artery,[29] anterolateral skin territories may be compromised and incisions in this region should be avoided.

A soft-tissue closure plan must be formulated during the initial wound assessment and the initial fixation of fractures. This is not a consecutive process, nor does planning occur after skeletal fixation. There are multiple options for the treatment of the wound before closure; these include the placement of antibiotic beads, and recently the wound vacuum-assisted closure (KCI, San Antonio, TX) has been used as a bridging technique before definitive coverage takes place several days later. Other techniques that can be used before closure include the application of Epigard (Parke-Davis, Detroit, MI)[27] or Adaptic gauze (Johnson and Johnson, Raynham, MA) over the wound, porcine allograft, or antibiotic beads. The goals of wound coverage are to prevent desiccation of tissue, optimize antibiotic delivery, optimize patient comfort, and seal the wound from the external environment. At the same time as débridement or initial fracture management is performed, tetanus toxoid prophylaxis, as indicated, and the appropriate antibiotics should be administered. Incisions that have been used to extend the initial wounds can be closed to decrease the exposure of deeper tissues.[9,30]

Open fractures should never be closed primarily because of the risk of gas gangrene. Although microsurgeons are able to do an immediate free tissue transfer,[31] this method remains controversial. In our opinion, there is no rationale for performing definitive closure immediately; returning to the operating room in 24 to 48 hours is a time-tested method, and the data reported by Godina do not indicate a difference between wounds closed at the first surgical setting and those closed 72 hours later.[25]

Most open wounds can be covered with split-thickness skin grafts. Local or regional flaps may involve more morbidity because transposed skin flaps or muscles may be compromised, particularly in high-energy injuries, and free tissue transfer may be more reliable. Free tissue transfer is often the most definitive form of treatment.

## Fracture Management

Stabilizing the open fracture protects the soft tissues from further injury by fracture fragments, facilitates the host response to microbes despite the presence of implants,[32] improves wound care, and allows early motion of adjacent joints and early mobilization of the patient.

The choice of fracture fixation depends on the bone that is fractured, the location of the fracture (intra-articular, metaphyseal, or diaphyseal), the extent of soft-tissue injury and contamination, and the physiologic status of the patient. Fixation can be definitive or provisional, and techniques include intramedullary nailing, external fixation, and plate fixation. More than one technique may be applicable to a specific injury.

Intramedullary nailing is widely used for stabilization of diaphyseal fractures of the lower extremity.[33-35] External fixation is indicated for fractures associated with extensive contamination and soft-tissue damage and when there is a need for rapid fracture stabilization or minimal interference with the patient's physiologic response to the injury (so-called damage control),[36] as in the case of a type IIIC fracture in a multiply injured patient whose condition is unstable. Plate fixation is indicated for periarticular fractures and for diaphyseal fractures of the upper extremity.

The method of stabilizing an open tibial diaphyseal fracture is controversial. Both unreamed intramedullary nailing and external fixation have been used successfully in the management of open tibial fractures. In two prospective, randomized studies comparing the two techniques, half-pin external fixators were associated with malalignment in 31% of the cases, and with pin tract infection in 50%,[34] but there were no differences in fracture site infection and bone healing rates between the two methods.[34,35] The severity of the soft-tissue injury rather than the choice of implant appeared to be the main factor influencing infection and bone healing.[34] A meta-analysis of the management of open tibial fractures demonstrated that unreamed intramedullary nailing reduced the risks of a revision, malunion, and superficial infection compared with the risks associated with external fixators.[37] Intramedullary nailing does not require the same high level of patient compliance, but an external fixator may be particularly useful for patients with vascular injury or extensive soft-tissue damage and contamination.

The endosteal blood supply is preserved to a greater degree with unreamed nailing than it is with reamed nailing.[34,35,38-40] Thus, unreamed nailing may be preferable to reamed nailing for open tibial fractures, where periosteal vascularity may already be compromised by the traumatic insult. Reamed nailing, on the other hand, allows insertion of larger-diameter implants, improves stability at the fracture site, and helps reduce the implant failure rate. Moreover, the cortical circulation that is disrupted during reaming is gradually reconstituted, although this may occur more slowly than it does with unreamed nailing.[39]

Reamed nailing of open tibial fractures was compared with unreamed nailing in two prospective, randomized studies.[41,42] Neither established a significant difference in infection rates (1 of 40 and 1 of 26 with unreamed nailing compared with 2 of 45 and 1 of 19 with reamed nailing). There were fewer screw failures in the reamed-nailing group in both studies.

Some complications associated with external fixation are due to the transition to another form of fixation, and external fixation can be successfully used as definitive treatment.[43-45] In a prospective study of 101 type II and III fractures treated with external fixation, Marsh and associates[45] reported that 96 fractures healed. There were six fracture-site infections. Early bone grafting of fractures with bone defects treated with external fixation reduces healing complications.[46]

Delayed conversion of external fixation to intramedullary nailing can increase the prevalence of infection to as high as 50%.[12,47] On the other hand, Blachut and associates[48] showed that early conversion of the fixator to a nail (at a mean of 17 days) in the absence of pin tract infection was associated with an infection rate of only 5%. Conversion to an intramedullary nail can be done safely if the fixator had been in place for a short period of time and in the absence of pin tract infection. Otherwise, the fixator should be maintained until the fracture heals.

Reamed intramedullary nailing is the preferred fixation technique for open diaphyseal femoral fractures, but external fixation for provisional fracture stabilization is an option in unstable patients.[49-51] Brumback and associates[33] found no infections after the treatment of 62 type I, II, and IIIA open femoral fractures with reamed intramedullary nailing and only 3 infections (11%) after such treatment of 27 type IIIB open femoral fractures.

Plate fixation is the preferred method of treatment of open forearm and humeral fractures.[52-54] Intramedullary nailing is an option for open diaphyseal fractures of the humerus, but there are concerns regarding shoulder pain and stiffness. External fixation can be useful in the presence of severe soft-tissue injury and contamination.[55,56]

One option for managing open periarticular fractures is provisional spanning external fixation (with the addition of limited internal fixation with screws to restore articular congruency in intra-articular fractures) with plate fixation performed later.[57] Alternatively, these fractures can be treated definitively with use of either a ring fine-wire fixator (with limited internal fixation if needed)[58,59] or plate fixation.[60] The development of locking plates and minimally invasive osteosynthesis techniques have shown promise recently.[61,62]

Open fractures associated with a vascular injury require special considerations. The order of fracture fixation and arterial repair is controversial. Available options include (1) fracture fixation first followed by arterial repair,[63] (2) arterial repair first followed by fracture fixation,[64] and (3) use of an arterial intraluminal shunt.[65] Decision making depends on an individualized assessment of the characteristics of each case in consultation with the vascular surgeon. Important factors to be considered are the ischemia time that has already elapsed (muscle will not tolerate ischemia for more than 6 hours) and the complexity of the fracture pattern (definitive fixation may be time consuming).

## Bone Grafting and Other Techniques to Promote Healing

Bone grafting can help in fracture repair or the reconstruction of skeletal defects. The basic types of bone grafts used in fracture treatment are autogenous cancellous bone, autogenous cortical bone, vascularized corticocancellous bone, and bone graft substitutes. Autogenous cancellous bone is the gold standard for providing osteoconduction, osteoinduction, and osteogenesis. This bone delivers an osteoconductive matrix made of both hydroxyapatite and collagen. Furthermore, it delivers an abundance of growth factors as well as stromal cells to the fracture site. It has the obvious advantage of histocompatibility and it revascularizes quickly, but it lacks structural integrity.[66] In 1952, Urist showed that structural integrity becomes normal at approximately 1 year.[67] The limited quantity of autogenous cancellous bone available and donor site morbidity are disadvantages. To improve osteocyte survival when obtaining autogenous cancellous bone, the surgeon should keep the donor cells moist and chilled in a blood-soaked sponge.

Vascularized corticocancellous grafts provide excellent osteoconduction, osteoinduction, and stromal cells to the fracture site. These grafts have the advantage of providing good structural integrity, and they can be used in defects of more than 6 cm in size. They usually consist of vascularized fibular or iliac crest grafts that maintain the viability of the bone cells while not undergoing extensive resorption; they also provide new blood supply to the fracture site.[68]

Allografts, bone graft substitutes, ceramics, demineralized bone matrix, bone marrow, and composite grafts are often used in closed fractures, but they are less useful in open fractures because of the decreased vascularity and the contamination often seen in these complex fractures.

The timing of bone grafting is important, particularly for open fractures. Bone grafting is usually not performed at the initial open reduction and internal fixation procedure, except when the surgeon is dealing with intra-articular defects. In Gustilo-Anderson type I and II open fractures, bone grafting can usually be performed safely at the time of the delayed primary closure. In type III fractures, bone grafting should be performed only after

successful closure, usually at 6 to 9 weeks after the injury.[12]

Electrical stimulation of the bone can be accomplished with three clinical modalities: direct-current stimulation (implanted electrodes); electromagnetic stimulation by inductive coupling, with time-varying magnetic fields (noninvasive); and capacitive coupling stimulation with external electrodes (noninvasive). A double-blinded, randomized clinical study of the use of pulsed electromagnetic fields on delayed tibial unions demonstrated a 45% union rate compared with a 14% union rate with use of a placebo device.[69] In another study, involving capacitively coupled electromagnetic fields, Scott and King[70] reported a 60% success rate at 21 weeks compared with a 0% success rate with a placebo. Brighton and associates[71] compared 167 fractures treated with direct current with 56 treated with capacitively coupled electrical current and with 48 treated with conventional bone grafting. There were no significant differences among the three groups. As the number of risk factors such as open fracture, cigarette smoking, and peripheral vascular disease increased, the healing rate decreased in all three groups in this unblinded study. Electrical stimulation plays a role in promoting bone healing and probably works as well as conventional bone grafting, but its effects are directly affected by the local and systemic host biology, a situation similar to that seen with bone grafting.

Over the past 50 years, ultrasound has also been studied in relation to the stimulation of bone callus.[72] In a prospective, randomized trial of closed and type I open tibial fractures treated with low-intensity ultrasound (30 mW/cm² for 20 minutes per day), the time to healing was reduced by

24%.[73,74] Other studies have also demonstrated benefits.[75,76]

In 1965, Urist[77] reported his discovery of bone morphogenetic protein (BMP) in bone matrix, which is responsible for osteoinduction. Subsequently, 16 different proteins (BMP-1 through BMP-16) have been identified in bone matrix. All of these, except BMP-1, are in the family of transforming growth factor-β (TGF-β). Furthermore, all play a role during embryogenesis and tissue repair in postnatal life.[78-84] It is believed that osteoinduction is mediated by BMP-2 through BMP-7 and BMP-9, which provide primordial signals for the differentiation of mesenchymal stem cells into osteoblasts.[85] BMP-2, BMP-6, and BMP-9 all have been shown to be more effective when pluripotent cells are present.

Clinical research has revealed that recombinant BMP (rhBMP) can be used successfully as a supplemental agent to achieve bone healing. In the BESTT study, rhBMP-2 was used in an open-fracture setting.[86] One hundred forty-seven fractures were treated with open reduction and internal fixation without the use of rhBMP, while 145 open tibial fractures were treated with open reduction and internal fixation with the addition of either 0.75 mg/mL of rhBMP-2 or 1.50 mg/mL of rhBMP-2. The group treated with 1.50 mg/mL of BMP-2 had a 44% reduction in the need for secondary intervention compared with the control group. A Canadian study of 124 open tibial fractures randomized either to receive rhBMP-7 or to a control group demonstrated that rhBMP-7 therapy reduced the need for secondary intervention from 27% to 12%.[87] In another study, rhBMP-7 bound to type 1 collagen was compared with conventional autogenous bone grafting for the treatment of tibial nonunions.[88] Similar union rates were found, both clinically and radiographically.

In summary, the use of rhBMP therapy as a supplemental procedure to achieve bone healing is safe and effective as a treatment of delayed union or nonunion of fractures and it is probably equivalent to autogenous bone grafting. There is no conclusive evidence that the use of rhBMP in fresh fractures will increase the healing rate.[89] Problems encountered with the use of rhBMP are its short biologic half-life and difficulties in retaining the product at the fracture site. Often, a large bolus dose is required, and the release of growth factors is not uniform. Finally, the high cost of rhBMP is a factor that limits its use.

In the future, gene transfer therapy may be used to deliver growth factors to the fracture site. Osteogenic proteins can be encoded directly to the fracture site, allowing a sustained local concentration and dose of growth factors. Furthermore, endogenous synthesized proteins are more effective than recombinant synthesized proteins, and the in vivo transfer is minimally invasive and less expensive than rhBMP therapy. Investigators have used a direct percutaneous gene delivery technique to enhance the healing of segmental bone defects in a rat model.[90] The genetically modified osteoprogenitor cells were delivered directly to the segmental bone defects with a single intralesional injection of adenovirus carrying BMP-2. At 8 weeks, the osseous union rate was 75% in the treated animals compared with 4% in control animals. The authors showed that a single percutaneous injection of adenovirus carrying BMP-2 can

induce healing of critical-size defects in rats at 8 weeks and that the tissue repair is by trabecular bone with normal mineral content.

Although the use of gene transfer therapy is an exciting possibility for the future enhancement of fracture healing, there remain considerable safety concerns regarding the injection of adenovirus with osteoinduction genes and the fear of transgenic expression.[91]

## Management and Reconstruction of Infected Fractures

The management of chronic osteomyelitis with a limb-salvage protocol consists of débridement, systemic and local antibiotic treatment, skeletal stabilization, soft-tissue coverage, and bone grafting and/or reconstructive procedures for treatment of ununited fractures and existing bone defects. These principles can be incorporated in a staged protocol, often implemented by a multidisciplinary team consisting of an orthopaedic surgeon, an infectious disease specialist, and a microvascular surgeon.

When there is an infection, several factors must be evaluated carefully to develop a detailed management plan. Imaging studies should be reviewed to assess the status of bone healing, the location and extent of cortical and medullary bone involvement, and the status and integrity of existing implants. The quality and integrity of the soft-tissue envelope, and the need for flap coverage, should be evaluated. The neurovascular status of the extremity should be determined. Cultures and sensitivity tests allow the selection of appropriate antibiotics for local delivery with antibiotic beads and for systemic therapy. Subsequent cultures of intraoperative specimens

should be performed, and the results may indicate that a different antibiotic is required. The medical status of the patient should be assessed to ensure that it allows the safe execution of a complex reconstructive plan. Interventions, such as nutritional support and cessation of smoking, will help to optimize the patient's condition before surgery.

Radical débridement of all nonviable tissue, including skin, soft tissue, and bone, is necessary. Débridement proceeds until bleeding, viable tissue is seen at the resection margins, to ensure that all foci of infection are removed.[92,93] Viable bone is characterized by punctuate bleeding, known as the paprika sign. Débridement should not be limited by concerns about the osseous or soft-tissue defects. Specimens of purulent fluid, soft tissue, and bone from the affected area should be sent for aerobic and anaerobic cultures; it is especially important to perform cultures for mycobacteria and fungi when the patient is immunocompromised or has a chronic infection.[92,94] The wound should be irrigated with a copious amount of saline solution, and antibiotics may be added to the terminal liter of the irrigation fluid.

The dead space that results from débridement is filled with physician-made polymethylmethacrylate antibiotic-impregnated beads. The pathogen must be susceptible to the eluted antibiotic. If wound closure is not possible, the wound containing antibiotic beads is sealed with a semipermeable membrane so that the eluted antibiotic(s) remain in the involved area to achieve a high local concentration.[17]

When a nonunion is associated with infection, subsequent procedures for wound management and bone grafting are planned, and the beads can be removed at that time. In the future, biodegradable delivery systems will eliminate the need for this surgical removal.[95]

The type of systemic antibiotic therapy is chosen on the basis of the results of the preoperative cultures, but it can be modified based on the results of the intraoperative culture and sensitivity tests. Administration of antibiotics is a key part of the management, but it will fail without adequate débridemur. Intravenous antibiotics are generally given for 4 to 6 weeks.[96] Although antibiotic-resistant organisms are a problem, vancomycin is useful for oxacillin-resistant *Staphylococcus aureus* infections, and the recently introduced antibiotics linezolid and quinupristin/dalfopristin have been used for oxacillin-resistant *S aureus* and vancomycin-resistant *Enterococcus* infections.[97]

The decision to retain or remove implants from the site of an infected fracture must be individualized and depends on the time since the fracture fixation, bone-healing status, stability provided by the hardware, and fracture location.[92] If the fracture has healed, the internal fixation device should be removed. When the fracture has not healed, the internal fixation device should be left in place as long as it is stabilizing the fracture. Loose hardware that is not providing stability should be removed. If the fracture has not healed and the hardware is removed, the fracture should be stabilized with another device; our preference is to use an external fixator for diaphyseal nonunions of the tibia and an intramedullary rod for diaphyseal nonunions of the femur.

In cases with an adequate soft-tissue envelope, delayed or primary closure can be performed depending on the extent of the infection. If soft tissues are compromised, coverage should be achieved with local or free muscle flaps. Soft-tissue coverage is usually performed at 3 to 7 days after the initial débridement.[98-100] The staged coverage allows the treatment of organisms with specific antibiotics based on the results of cultures of deep-tissue specimens taken during the first débridement and permits a repeat débridement before flap transfer.

Autogenous iliac crest bone grafting can be used to manage bone defects up to 6 cm in size. Bone grafting techniques for the tibia include anterior, posterolateral, and free vascularized grafting of the defect site.[98,101-103] Bone grafting is performed when the soft-tissue envelope has healed, flap viability has been determined, and infection has been controlled, usually 6 to 8 weeks after the muscle transfer or when the soft tissues are healed.[92] For anterior tibial defects and most nonunions, the muscle flap is elevated and the graft is placed at the nonunion or defect site. Posterolateral bone grafting is an alternative if infection control has been established (on the basis of no anterior sequestra and no need for anterior débridement), there is no anterior defect, and there is no need for a soft-tissue transfer.

Bone defects longer than 6 cm require specialized reconstructive procedures, such as vascularized bone grafting or distraction osteogenesis. The free vascularized fibular graft is a versatile flap that, in addition to bone, can include muscle, skin, and fascia.[104] It is particularly useful for combined bone and soft-tissue defects and in patients opposed to having an external fixator. Distraction osteogenesis is a useful method for reconstruction of infected bone defects and for correction of malalign-ment and large limb-length discrepancies.[105]

Limb salvage based on the described principles can be achieved with eradication of infection and osseous union in 67% to 100% of cases.[99,106-109] Siegel and associates[109] reported that, at a mean of 5.1 years postoperatively, limb salvage had been accomplished in all of 46 patients with chronic tibial osteomyelitis and all but 2 had clinical and radiographic evidence of union. Thirty-nine patients were able to walk independently, whereas the others used assistive devices. Thirty-eight of 42 patients who had been working were able to return to work within 6 months after union, and 23 of 37 patients who had been participating in recreational and sports activities were able to resume those activities. Smoking, advanced age, and intra-articular involvement were found to adversely affect the outcome.

## Summary

The goals in the management of open fractures are prevention of infection, fracture union, and restoration of function. Management of chronic posttraumatic osteomyelitis and infected nonunion of the tibia is challenging; however, infection control, osseous union, and a satisfactory functional outcome can be achieved with use of the aforementioned principles.

## References

1. Blick SS, Brumback RJ, Poka A, Burgess AR, Ebraheim NA: Compartment syndrome in open tibial fractures. *J Bone Joint Surg Am* 1986;68: 1348-1353.

2. Gustilo RB, Anderson JT: Prevention of infection in the treatment of one thousand and twenty-five open frac-

tures of long bones: Retrospective and prospective analyses. *J Bone Joint Surg Am* 1976;58:453-458.

3. Gustilo RB, Mendoza RM, Williams DN: Problems in the management of type III (severe) open fractures: A new classification of type III open fractures. *J Trauma* 1984;24:742-746.

4. Brumback RJ, Jones AL: Interobserver agreement in the classification of open fractures of the tibia: The results of a survey of two hundred and forty-five orthopaedic surgeons. *J Bone Joint Surg Am* 1994;76:1162-1166.

5. Patzakis MJ, Wilkins J: Factors influencing infection rate in open fracture wounds. *Clin Orthop Relat Res* 1989;243:36-40.

6. Bowen TR, Widmaier JC: Host classification predicts infection after open fracture. *Clin Orthop Relat Res* 2005;433:205-211.

7. Patzakis MJ, Harvey JP Jr, Ivler D: The role of antibiotics in the management of open fractures. *J Bone Joint Surg Am* 1974;56:532-541.

8. Skaggs DL, Friend L, Alman B, et al: The effect of surgical delay on acute infection following 554 open fractures in children. *J Bone Joint Surg Am* 2005;87:8-12.

9. Patzakis MJ, Wilkins J, Moore TM: Considerations in reducing the infection rate in open tibial fractures. *Clin Orthop Relat Res* 1983;178:36-41.

10. Patzakis MJ, Bains RS, Lee J, et al: Prospective, randomized, double-blind study comparing single-agent antibiotic therapy, ciprofloxacin, to combination antibiotic therapy in open fracture wounds. *J Orthop Trauma* 2000;14:529-533.

11. Lee J: Efficacy of cultures in the management of open fractures. *Clin Orthop Relat Res* 1997;339:71-75.

12. Fischer MD, Gustilo RB, Varecka TF: The timing of flap coverage, bone-grafting, and intramedullary nailing in patients who have a fracture of the tibial shaft with extensive soft-tissue injury. *J Bone Joint Surg Am* 1991;73:1316-1322.

13. Templeman DC, Gulli B, Tsukayama DT, Gustilo RB: Update on the management of open fractures of the tibial shaft. *Clin Orthop Relat Res* 1998;350:18-25.

14. Patzakis MJ: Clostridial myonecrosis. *Instr Course Lect* 1990;39:491-493.

15. Zalavras CG, Patzakis MJ: Open fractures: Evaluation and management. *J Am Acad Orthop Surg* 2003;11:212-219.

16. Ostermann PA, Seligson D, Henry SL: Local antibiotic therapy for severe open fractures: A review of 1085 consecutive cases. *J Bone Joint Surg Br* 1995;77:93-97.

17. Zalavras CG, Patzakis MJ, Holtom P: Local antibiotic therapy in the treatment of open fractures and osteomyelitis. *Clin Orthop Relat Res* 2004;427:86-93.

18. Levin LS: The reconstructive ladder: An orthoplastic approach. *Orthop Clin North Am* 1993;24:393-409.

19. Levin LS, Nunley JA: The management of soft-tissue problems associated with calcaneal fractures. *Clin Orthop Relat Res* 1993;290:151-156.

20. Heitmann C, Khan FN, Levin LS: Vasculature of the peroneal artery: An anatomic study focused on the perforator vessels. *J Reconstr Microsurg* 2003;19:157-162.

21. Baumeister S, Levin LS, Erdmann D: Literature and own strategies concerning soft-tissue reconstruction and exposed osteosynthetic hardware. *Chirurg* 2006;77:616-621.

22. Oishi SN, Levin LS, Pederson WC: Microsurgical management of extremity wounds in diabetics with peripheral vascular disease. *Plast Reconstr Surg* 1993;92:485-492.

23. Levin LS: Soft tissue coverage options for ankle wounds. *Foot Ankle Clin* 2001;6:853-866.

24. Erdmann D, Lee B, Roberts CD, Levin LS: Management of lawnmower injuries to the lower extremity in children and adolescents. *Ann Plast Surg* 2000;45:595-600.

25. Godina M: Early microsurgical reconstruction of complex trauma of the extremities. *Plast Reconstr Surg* 1986;78:285-292.

26. Heitmann C, Levin LS: The orthoplastic approach for management of the severely traumatized foot and ankle. *J Trauma* 2003;54:379-390.

27. Levin LS: New developments in flap techniques. *J Am Acad Orthop Surg* 2006;14(10 suppl):S90-S93.

28. Erdmann D, Sweis R, Wong MS, et al: Vascular endothelial growth factor expression in pig latissimus dorsi myocutaneous flaps after ischemia reperfusion injury. *Plast Reconstr Surg* 2003;111:775-780.

29. Heller L, Levin LS: Lower extremity microsurgical reconstruction. *Plast Reconstr Surg* 2001;108:1029-1041.

30. Heitmann C, Patzakis MJ, Tetsworth KD, Levin LS: Musculoskeletal sepsis: Principles of treatment. *Instr Course Lect* 2003;52:733-743.

31. Gopal S, Majumder S, Batchelor AG, Knight SL, De Boer P, Smith RM: Fix and flap: The radical orthopaedic and plastic treatment of severe open fractures of the tibia. *J Bone Joint Surg Br* 2000;82:959-966.

32. Worlock P, Slack R, Harvey L, Mawhinney R: The prevention of infection in open fractures: An experimental study of the effect of fracture stability. *Injury* 1994;25:31-38.

33. Brumback RJ, Ellison PS Jr, Poka A, Lakatos R, Bathon GH, Burgess AR: Intramedullary nailing of open fractures of the femoral shaft. *J Bone Joint Surg Am* 1989;71:1324-1331.

34. Henley MB, Chapman JR, Agel J, Harvey EJ, Whorton AM, Swiontkowski MF: Treatment of type II, IIIA, and IIIB open fractures of the tibial shaft: A prospective comparison of unreamed interlocking intramedullary nails and half-pin external fixators. *J Orthop Trauma* 1998;12:1-7.

35. Tornetta P III, Bergman M, Watnik N, Berkowitz G, Steuer J: Treatment of grade-IIIb open tibial fractures: A prospective randomised comparison of external fixation and non-reamed locked nailing. *J Bone Joint Surg Br*

1994;76:13-19.

36. Roberts CS, Pape HC, Jones AL, Malkani AL, Rodriguez JL, Giannoudis PV: Damage control orthopaedics: Evolving concepts in the treatment of patients who have sustained orthopaedic trauma. *Instr Course Lect* 2005; 54:447-462.

37. Bhandari M, Guyatt GH, Swiontkowski MF, Schemitsch EH: Treatment of open fractures of the shaft of the tibia. *J Bone Joint Surg Br* 2001;83: 62-68.

38. Shepherd LE, Costigan WM, Gardocki RJ, Ghiassi AD, Patzakis MJ, Stevanovic MV: Local or free muscle flaps and unreamed interlocked nails for open tibial fractures. *Clin Orthop Relat Res* 1998;350:90-96.

39. Schemitsch EH, Kowalski MJ, Swiontkowski MF, Senft D: Cortical bone blood flow in reamed and unreamed locked intramedullary nailing: A fractured tibia model in sheep. *J Orthop Trauma* 1994;8:373-382.

40. Schemitsch EH, Kowalski MJ, Swiontkowski MF, Harrington RM: Comparison of the effect of reamed and unreamed locked intramedullary nailing on blood flow in the callus and strength of union following fracture of the sheep tibia. *J Orthop Res* 1995;13:382-389.

41. Keating JF, Blachut PA, O'Brien PJ, Meek RN, Broekhuyse H: Reamed nailing of open tibial fractures: Does the antibiotic bead pouch reduce the deep infection rate? *J Orthop Trauma* 1996;10:298-303.

42. Finkemeier CG, Schmidt AH, Kyle RF, Templeman DC, Varecka TF: A prospective, randomized study of intramedullary nails inserted with and without reaming for the treatment of open and closed fractures of the tibial shaft. *J Orthop Trauma* 2000;14: 187-193.

43. Edwards CC, Simmons SC, Browner BD, Weigel MC: Severe open tibial fractures: Results treating 202 injuries with external fixation. *Clin Orthop Relat Res* 1988;230:98-115.

44. Behrens F, Searls K: External fixation of the tibia: Basic concepts and prospective evaluation. *J Bone Joint Surg Br* 1986;68:246-254.

45. Marsh JL, Nepola JV, Wuest TK, Osteen D, Cox K, Oppenheim W: Unilateral external fixation until healing with the dynamic axial fixator for severe open tibial fractures. *J Orthop Trauma* 1991;5:341-348.

46. Blick SS, Brumback RJ, Lakatos R, Poka A, Burgess AR: Early prophylactic bone grafting of high-energy tibial fractures. *Clin Orthop Relat Res* 1989; 240:21-41.

47. McGraw JM, Lim EV: Treatment of open tibial-shaft fractures: External fixation and secondary intramedullary nailing. *J Bone Joint Surg Am* 1988;70: 900-911.

48. Blachut PA, Meek RN, O'Brien PJ: External fixation and delayed intramedullary nailing of open fractures of the tibial shaft: A sequential protocol. *J Bone Joint Surg Am* 1990;72:729-735.

49. Harwood PJ, Giannoudis PV, van Griensven M, Krettek C, Pape HC: Alterations in the systemic inflammatory response after early total care and damage control procedures for femoral shaft fracture in severely injured patients. *J Trauma* 2005;58:446-454.

50. Nowotarski PJ, Turen CH, Brumback RJ, Scarboro JM: Conversion of external fixation to intramedullary nailing for fractures of the shaft of the femur in multiply injured patients. *J Bone Joint Surg Am* 2000;82:781-788.

51. Scalea TM, Boswell SA, Scott JD, Mitchell KA, Kramer ME, Pollak AN: External fixation as a bridge to intramedullary nailing for patients with multiple injuries and with femur fractures: Damage control orthopedics. *J Trauma* 2000;48:613-623.

52. Chapman MW, Gordon JE, Zissimos AG: Compression-plate fixation of acute fractures of the diaphyses of the radius and ulna. *J Bone Joint Surg Am* 1989;71:159-169.

53. Moed BR, Kellam JF, Foster RJ, Tile M, Hansen ST Jr: Immediate internal fixation of open fractures of the di-

aphysis of the forearm. *J Bone Joint Surg Am* 1986;68:1008-1017.

54. Vander Griend R, Tomasin J, Ward EF: Open reduction and internal fixation of humeral shaft fractures: Results using AO plating techniques. *J Bone Joint Surg Am* 1986;68:430-433.

55. Mostafavi HR, Tornetta P III: Open fractures of the humerus treated with external fixation. *Clin Orthop Relat Res* 1997;337:187-197.

56. Marsh JL, Mahoney CR, Steinbronn D: External fixation of open humerus fractures. *Iowa Orthop J* 1999;19: 35-42.

57. Sirkin M, Sanders R, DiPasquale T, Herscovici D Jr: A staged protocol for soft tissue management in the treatment of complex pilon fractures. *J Orthop Trauma* 1999;13:78-84.

58. Watson JT: High-energy fractures of the tibial plateau. *Orthop Clin North Am* 1994;25:723-752.

59. Tornetta P III, Weiner L, Bergman M, et al: Pilon fractures: Treatment with combined internal and external fixation. *J Orthop Trauma* 1993;7:489-496.

60. Benirschke SK, Agnew SG, Mayo KA, Santoro VM, Henley MB: Immediate internal fixation of open, complex tibial plateau fractures: Treatment by a standard protocol. *J Orthop Trauma* 1992;6:78-86.

61. Kregor PJ, Stannard JA, Zlowodzki M, Cole PA: Treatment of distal femur fractures using the less invasive stabilization system: Surgical experience and early clinical results in 103 fractures. *J Orthop Trauma* 2004;18: 509-520.

62. Stannard JP, Wilson TC, Volgas DA, Alonso JE: The less invasive stabilization system in the treatment of complex fractures of the tibial plateau: Short-term results. *J Orthop Trauma* 2004;18:552-558.

63. Seligson D, Ostermann PA, Henry SL, Wolley T: The management of open fractures associated with arterial injury requiring vascular repair. *J Trauma* 1994;37:938-940.

64. Ashworth EM, Dalsing MC, Glover

JL, Reilly MK: Lower extremity vascular trauma: A comprehensive, aggressive approach. *J Trauma* 1988;28: 329-336.

65. Reber PU, Patel AG, Sapio NL, Ris HB, Beck M, Kniemeyer HW: Selective use of temporary intravascular shunts in coincident vascular and orthopedic upper and lower limb trauma. *J Trauma* 1999;47:72-76.

66. Stringa G: Studies of the vascularisation of bone grafts. *J Bone Joint Surg Br* 1957;39:395-420.

67. Urist MR, McLean FC: Osteogenetic potency and new-bone formation by induction in transplants to the anterior chamber of the eye. *J Bone Joint Surg Am* 1952;34:443-476.

68. Dell PC, Burchardt H, Glowczewskie FP Jr: A roentgenographic, biomechanical, and histological evaluation of vascularized and non-vascularized segmental fibular canine autografts. *J Bone Joint Surg Am* 1985;67:105-112.

69. Sharrard WJ: A double-blind trial of pulsed electromagnetic fields for delayed union of tibial fractures. *J Bone Joint Surg Br* 1990;72:347-355.

70. Scott G, King JB: A prospective, double-blind trial of electrical capacitive coupling in the treatment of nonunion of long bones. *J Bone Joint Surg Am* 1994;76:820-826.

71. Brighton CT, Shaman P, Heppenstall RB, Esterhai JL Jr, Pollack SR, Friedenberg ZB: Tibial nonunion treated with direct current, capacitive coupling, or bone graft. *Clin Orthop Relat Res* 1995;321:223-234.

72. Corradi C, Cozzolino A: [The action of ultrasound on the evolution of an experimental fracture in rabbits]. *Minerva Ortop* 1952;55:44-45.

73. Cook SD, Ryaby JP, McCabe J, Frey JJ, Heckman JD, Kristiansen TK: Acceleration of tibia and distal radius fracture healing in patients who smoke. *Clin Orthop Relat Res* 1997; 337:198-207.

74. Heckman JD, Ryaby JP, McCabe J, Frey JJ, Kilcoyne RF: Acceleration of tibial fracture-healing by non-invasive, low-intensity pulsed ultra-sound. *J Bone Joint Surg Am* 1994;76: 26-34.

75. Rubin C, Bolander M, Ryaby JP, Hadjiargyrou M: The use of low-intensity ultrasound to accelerate the healing of fractures. *J Bone Joint Surg Am* 2001;83:259-270.

76. Duarte LR, Xavier CA, Choffie M, McCabe JM: Review of nonunions treated by pulsed low-intensity ultrasound. *Proceedings of the 1996 Meeting of the Societe Internationale de Chirurgie Orthopaedique et de Traumatologie (SICOT)*. Amsterdam, SICOT, 1996, p 110.

77. Urist MR: Bone: Formation by autoinduction. *Science* 1965;150:893-899.

78. Wozney JM, Rosen V, Celeste AJ, et al: Novel regulators of bone formation: molecular clones and activities. *Science* 1988;242:1528-1534.

79. Celeste AJ, Iannazzi JA, Taylor RC, et al: Identification of transforming growth factor beta family members present in bone-inductive protein purified from bovine bone. *Proc Natl Acad Sci USA* 1990;87:9843-9847.

80. Ozkaynak E, Schnegelsberg PN, Jin DF, et al: Osteogenic protein-2: A new member of the transforming growth factor-beta superfamily expressed early in embryogenesis. *J Biol Chem* 1992;267:25220-25227.

81. Barnes GL, Kostenuik PJ, Gerstenfeld LC, Einhorn TA: Growth factor regulation of fracture repair. *J Bone Miner Res* 1999;14:1805-1815.

82. Gerstenfeld LC, Cullinane DM, Barnes GL, Graves DT, Einhorn TA: Fracture healing as a post-natal developmental process: Molecular, spatial, and temporal aspects of its regulation. *J Cell Biochem* 2003;88:873-884.

83. Glienke J, Schmitt AO, Pilarsky C, et al: Differential gene expression by endothelial cells in distinct angiogenic states. *Eur J Biochem* 2000;267:2820-2830.

84. Wozney JM, Rosen V: Bone morphogenetic protein and bone morphogenetic protein gene family in bone formation and repair. *Clin Orthop Relat Res* 1998;346:26-37.

85. Cheng H, Jiang W, Phillips FM, et al: Osteogenic activity of the fourteen types of human bone morphogenetic proteins (BMPs). *J Bone Joint Surg Am* 2003;85:1544-1552.

86. Govender S, Csimma C, Genant HK, et al: BMP-2 Evaluation in Surgery for Tibial Trauma (BESTT) Study Group: Recombinant human bone morphogenetic protein-2 for treatment of open tibial fractures: A prospective, controlled, randomized study of four hundred and fifty patients. *J Bone Joint Surg Am* 2002;84: 2123-2134.

87. McKee MD: Recombinant human bone monohogenic protein-7: Applications for clinical trauma. 2005; 19(suppl 10):526-528.

88. Friedlaender GE, Perry CR, Cole JD, et al: Osteogenic protein-1 (bone morphogenetic protein-7) in the treatment of tibial nonunions. *J Bone Joint Surg Am* 2001;83(suppl 1(pt 2)): S151-S158.

89. Termaat MF, Den Boer FC, Bakker FC, Patka P, Haarman HJ: Bone morphogenetic proteins. Development and clinical efficacy in the treatment of fractures and bone defects. *J Bone Joint Surg Am* 2005;87:1367-1378.

90. Betz OB, Betz VM, Nazarian A, et al: Direct percutaneous gene delivery to enhance healing of segmental bone defects. *J Bone Joint Surg Am* 2006;88: 355-365.

91. Baltzer AW, Lattermann C, Whalen JD, et al: Genetic enhancement of fracture repair: Healing of an experimental segmental defect by adenoviral transfer of the BMP-2 gene. *Gene Ther* 2000;7:734-739.

92. Patzakis MJ, Zalavras CG: Chronic posttraumatic osteomyelitis and infected nonunion of the tibia: Current management concepts. *J Am Acad Orthop Surg* 2005;13:417-427.

93. Tetsworth K, Cierny G III: Osteomyelitis debridement techniques. *Clin Orthop Relat Res* 1999;360:87-96.

94. Patzakis MJ, Wilkins J, Kumar J, Holtom P, Greenbaum B, Ressler R:

Comparison of the results of bacterial cultures from multiple sites in chronic osteomyelitis of long bones: A prospective study. *J Bone Joint Surg Am* 1994;76:664-666.

95. McKee MD, Wild LM, Schemitsch EH, Waddell JP: The use of an antibiotic-impregnated, osteoconductive, bioabsorbable bone substitute in the treatment of infected long bone defects: Early results of a prospective trial. *J Orthop Trauma* 2002; 16:622-627.

96. Patzakis MJ: Management of acute and chronic osteomyelitis, in Chapman MW, Szabo RM, Marder RA, et al (eds): *Chapman's Orthopaedic Surgery,* ed 2. Philadelphia, PA, Lippincott Williams and Wilkins, 2000, pp 3533-3559.

97. Rao N, Ziran BH, Hall RA, Santa ER: Successful treatment of chronic bone and joint infections with oral linezolid. *Clin Orthop Relat Res* 2004; 427:67-71.

98. Patzakis MJ, Abdollahi K, Sherman R, Holtom PD, Wilkins J: Treatment of chronic osteomyelitis with muscle flaps. *Orthop Clin North Am* 1993;24: 505-509.

99. Gayle LB, Lineaweaver WC, Oliva A, et al: Treatment of chronic osteomyelitis of the lower extremities with debridement and microvascular muscle transfer. *Clin Plast Surg* 1992;19: 895-903.

100. Swiontkowski MF, Hanel DP, Vedder NB, Schwappach JR: A comparison of short- and long-term intravenous antibiotic therapy in the postoperative management of adult osteomyelitis. *J Bone Joint Surg Br* 1999;81:1046-1050.

101. Reckling FW, Waters CH III : Treatment of non-unions of fractures of the tibial diaphysis by posterolateral cortical cancellous bone-grafting. *J Bone Joint Surg Am* 1980;62: 936-941.

102. Han CS, Wood MB, Bishop AT, Cooney WP III: Vascularized bone transfer. *J Bone Joint Surg Am* 1992;74: 1441-1449.

103. Esterhai JL Jr , Sennett B, Gelb H, et al: Treatment of chronic osteomyelitis complicating nonunion and segmental defects of the tibia with open cancellous bone graft, posterolateral bone graft, and soft-tissue transfer. *J Trauma* 1990;30:49-54.

104. Malizos KN, Zalavras CG, Soucacos PN, Beris AE, Urbaniak JR: Free vascularized fibular grafts for reconstruction of skeletal defects. *J Am Acad Orthop Surg* 2004;12:360-369.

105. Paley D, Maar DC: Ilizarov bone transport treatment for tibial defects. *J Orthop Trauma* 2000;14:76-85.

106. Anthony JP, Mathes SJ, Alpert BS: The muscle flap in the treatment of chronic lower extremity osteomyelitis: Results in patients over 5 years after treatment. *Plast Reconstr Surg* 1991; 88:311-318.

107. Zalavras CG, Patzakis MJ, Thordarson DB, Shah S, Sherman R, Holtom P: Infected fractures of the distal tibial metaphysis and plafond: Achievement of limb salvage with free muscle flaps, bone grafting, and ankle fusion. *Clin Orthop Relat Res* 2004;427:57-62.

108. Weiland AJ, Moore JR, Daniel RK: The efficacy of free tissue transfer in the treatment of osteomyelitis. *J Bone Joint Surg Am* 1984;66:181-193.

109. Siegel HJ, Patzakis MJ, Holtom PD, Sherman R, Shepherd L: Limb salvage for chronic tibial osteomyelitis: An outcomes study. *J Trauma* 2000; 48:484-489.

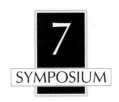

# 7

## SYMPOSIUM

# Orthopaedic War Injuries: From Combat Casualty Care to Definitive Treatment: A Current Review of Clinical Advances, Basic Science, and Research Opportunities

CAPT Dana C. Covey, MD, MC, USN; Roy K. Aaron, MD
Christopher T. Born, MD; Jason H. Calhoun, MD, FACS
*Thomas A. Einhorn, MD; *COL Roman A. Hayda, MD, MC, USA
Lawrence Scott Levin, MD, FACS; CDR Michael T. Mazurek, MD, MC, USN
MAJ Clinton K. Murray, MD, MC, USA; Col Elisha T. Powell IV, MD, MC, USAF
*Edward M. Schwarz, PhD; Joseph C. Wenke, PhD

## Abstract

*Musculoskeletal war wounds often involve massive injury to bone and soft tissue that differ markedly in character and extent compared with most injuries seen in civilian practice. These complex injuries have challenged orthopaedic surgeons to the limits of their treatment abilities on the battlefield, during medical evacuation, and in subsequent definitive or reconstructive treatment. Newer methodologies are being used in the treatment of these wounds to prevent so-called second hit complications, decrease complications associated with prolonged medical evacuation, reduce the incidence of infection, and restore optimal function. Basic science advances hold the promise of providing foundations for future treatment options that may improve both bone and soft-tissue healing. Research on the treatment of these often devastating wounds also will have broad applicability to trauma resulting from acts of terrorism or from natural disasters.*

**Instr Course Lect 2008;57:65-86.**

More than 26,000 US military personnel have been wounded in the ongoing wars in Iraq and Afghanistan,[1] approximately 70% of whom have sustained musculoskeletal trauma.[2] These injuries are often extensive in scope, involve profound bone and soft-tissue loss, and are severely contaminated. Most of those wounded in action have injuries resulting from exploding ordnance such as mortars, rockets, and roadside bombs (also known as improvised explosive devices [IEDs]). Despite the lethality of the weapons involved in the current conflicts, the percentage of military personnel who survive their wounds is increasing because of advances in personal protection, training, battlefield surgical treatment, and rapid evacuation. As a result, military service members are surviving with devastating musculoskeletal injuries that would not have been survivable in previous wars.

This chapter examines clinical and basic science issues germane to injuries to the musculoskeletal system caused by war trauma and identifies clinical complications associated with combat-related orthopaedic injuries,

*Thomas A. Einhorn, MD or the department with which he is affiliated has received research or institutional support from Stryker and Wyeth Research and is a consultant or employee for Stryker. Col Roman A. Hayda, MD, MC, USA or the department with which he is affiliated has received research or institutional support from Zimmer. Edward M. Schwarz, MD or the department with which he is affiliated has received research or institutional support from the US Army Reserve Acquisition Activity.*

**Table 1**
**Distribution of Terrorist Tactics by Incidents, Injuries, and Fatalities, 1998-2005**

| Tactic | Incidents | Injuries | Fatalities |
|---|---|---|---|
| Armed attack | 3,545 | 4,915 | 6,060 |
| Arson | 693 | 169 | 291 |
| Assassination | 1,607 | 772 | 2,289 |
| Barricade/Hostage | 51 | 1,408 | 598 |
| Bombing* | 9,928 | 48,381 | 13,230 |
| Hijacking | 29 | 5 | 26 |
| Kidnapping | 1,058 | 82 | 776 |
| Other | 146 | 418 | 113 |
| Unconventional attack | 47 | 2,435 | 3,004 |
| Unknown | 318 | 240 | 391 |
| Total | 17,422 | 58,825 | 26,778 |

*Bombings represent 57% of total incidents, 82% of injuries, and 49% of fatalities.
Data from Rand-MIPT Terrorism Incident Database project. Available at:
http://www.rand.org/ise/projects/terrorismdatabase and http://ww.tkb.org/IncidentTacticModule.jsp. Accessed March 12, 2007.

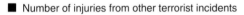
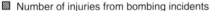
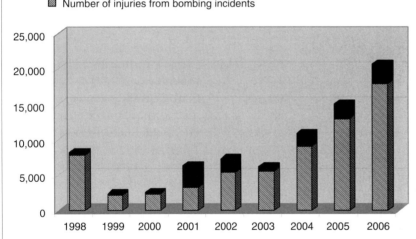

■ Number of injuries from other terrorist incidents

▨ Number of injuries from bombing incidents

**Figure 1**   Bar graph showing worldwide injuries caused by terrorist incidents from 1998 to 2006.

vices are the preferred weapons of terrorists because these inexpensive munitions are readily designed, assembled, transported, and detonated. Recent studies suggest that at the close of 2005, bomb blasts accounted for 82% of all injuries worldwide caused by terrorists, and this statistic is continuing to trend upward (Table 1 and Figures 1 and 2).[4-6] Explosions of overwhelming proportions also can occur outside the military or political environment.[7-9]

Blast injury may be considered a fourth weapon of mass destruction. In a membership survey conducted by the Eastern Association for the Surgery of Trauma, only 73% of trauma surgeon respondents had an understanding of the pathophysiology and classification of blast injuries.[10] Because of necessity, the military medical community has continued to expand its understanding and ability to manage blast-related injuries; however, the civilian medical community remains quite unprepared.

### Blast Physics
Bomb detonation is the rapid chemical transformation of a solid or liquid into a gas. The gas expands radially outward as a high-pressure shock wave that exceeds the speed of sound. Air is highly compressed on the leading edge of the blast wave, creating a shock front. The body of the wave, including the associated mass outward movement of air (sometimes called the blast wind) follows this front. In an open area, the overpressure that results from the blast generally follows a well-defined pressure/time curve (Friedlander wave) with an initial near-instantaneous spike in the ambient air pressure[11] (Figure 3). This overpressure rapidly decays and is followed by a negative pressure wave,

specific treatments currently available, and possible promising future treatments.

### Blast Injury: Pathophysiology and Injury Patterns
Disaster response plans have centered on mitigating the effects of injury from natural disasters and the

potential sequelae of terrorist-promoted catastrophes involving nuclear, chemical, and biologic agents. However, within the current geopolitical environment, explosions and bombings are the primary disasters to which both civilian and military medical/surgical personnel routinely respond.[3] Explosive de-

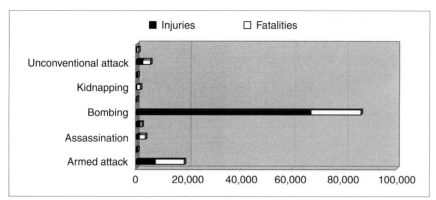

**Figure 2**    Bar graph showing worldwide injuries and fatalities from terrorist incidents from 1998 to 2006.

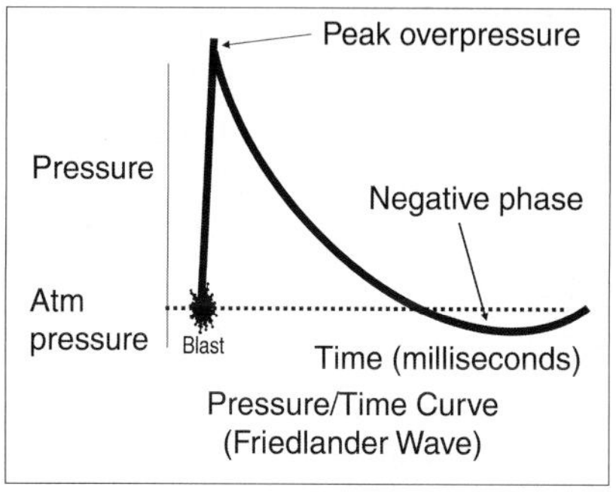

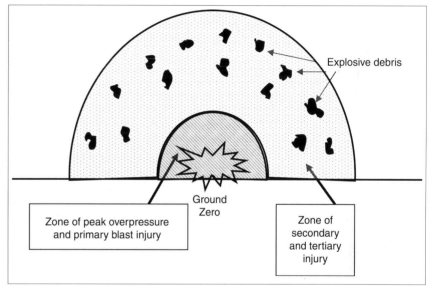

**Figure 3**    Friedlander wave depicting the pressure-time relationship of a bomb blast. Note the rapid peak and decline to the negative pressure wave.

which sucks debris into the area. In an open air blast, the wave rapidly decays as the inverse cube of the radius. The pressure/time curves can vary depending on the local topography, the presence of walls or solid objects, and whether the blast is detonated indoors or outside. The blast wave can reflect off and flow around solid surfaces. Reflected waves can be magnified eight to nine times, causing substantially greater injury.[12,13] Blasts that occur in buildings and other confined spaces can be more devastating and lethal because of the increased energy of the complex and reflected waves.[14,15]

The velocity, duration, and magnitude of the overpressure from the blast wave are dependent on several factors, including the physical size and explosive component of the charge being detonated. High-energy explosives, such as trinitrotoluene (TNT) and nitroglycerin, are much more powerful than ordinary gunpowder. The latter tends to produce conflagrations with a higher thermal output. The medium through which the blast wave moves also is a factor. Water with its increased density allows for faster propagation and a longer duration of positive pressure, accounting for the increased severity of injury in that environment. The

**Figure 4**    Schematic of blast injury zones. After the blast event, the area of blast overpressure rapidly expands but decays in strength. Primary blast injury occurs proximate to ground zero, whereas secondary and tertiary injury can extend far beyond the area of the primary blast.

distance from the explosion's epicenter also is a factor, with pressure-wave decay occurring roughly as the inverse cube of the distance.[12,16]

### Categories of Blast Injury

Injury results from three primary components as they interface either directly or indirectly with the victim. These include the high-pressure shock front and associated blast wave as well as thermal components from the detonation. Classically, the injuries have been divided into three categories (primary, secondary, and tertiary) (Figure 4). Several quaternary elements have recently been recognized.

### Primary Blast Injuries

Primary blast injury occurs as the shock front and blast wave move through the body. Differences in densities of the body's anatomic components (particularly at air/fluid interfaces) are susceptible to spalling, implosion, and inertial mismatches as well as pressure differentials. Spalling describes the forcible, explosive movement of fluid from more dense to less dense tissues, such as in the lungs. Implosion relates to areas of gas that are rapidly compressed at the time of shock-front impact but then rapidly reexpand after it passes, causing a rebound expansion with attendant shearing and injury; this frequently occurs in the ear/tympanic membrane and intestine. Acceleration/deceleration can cause tearing of organ pedicles and mesentery when there is an inertial difference between organ structures. Pressure differentials occur wherever there is a liquid-gas interface and incompressible, water-filled organs (such as vessels) have fluid forced into the less compressible adjacent structure.

The most susceptible organs to primary blast injury are the ears, lungs, and gastrointestinal tract. The ear is the organ most sensitive to blast injury, and tympanic membrane rupture is a marker of overpressure exposure. The lungs are moderately more resistant; however, with enough energy exposure, disruption of the capillary-alveolar interface that leads to parenchymal hemorrhage can occur as well as destruction of the alveolar walls. Emphysematous spaces can be created in addition to pneumothorax. The interstitial changes of blast lung can lead to acute respiratory distress syndrome. Infiltrates can be seen on a chest radiograph within 90 minutes of the blast.[17] In rare instances, air embolism of the vascular tree is believed to lead to sudden death.[18,19] The gastrointestinal tract, as a gas-filled organ, can be injured by implosion and rupture. The mucosal wall can become bruised. Shearing injuries can occur as a result of

acceleration/deceleration relative to more solid, adjacent structures. Other organ systems have varying degrees of response to injury from primary blast, and models have been developed to better study the overall pathophysiologic effects.[12,20-22] The lungs tend to be the predominant nonauditory system injured in most air blasts, whereas the gastrointestinal tract is more susceptible to underwater blasts. Markers are being sought to better diagnose and treat blast overpressure injury.[13,23]

Amputations are not common but are important as a marker for a lethal injury when they occur. Amputations primarily occur through the shaft rather than as disarticulations and are believed to be the result of direct coupling of the blast wave into the tissues. Fracture results from axial stress to the long bone, and flailing of the extremity from the flow of the blast wind gas completes the amputation, although there is some controversy on this theory.[16,24] Improved knowledge in this area has resulted in the development of more effective body armor. Amputation infrequently results from laceration by projectiles formed secondary to the blast.

### Secondary Blast Injuries
Secondary blast injury results from the victim being struck by missiles that are propagated by the explosion (fragments). These can be intentionally embedded into the explosive device to cause wounding. Missiles such as nails, screws, nuts, and bolts are often used by terrorists. Some fragments may be part of the bomb's housing, or fragments may be local material that became airborne because of proximity to the explosion. Glass is common. Most penetrating injuries caused by blast-driven projectiles should be considered as contaminated, and appropri-

ate prophylaxes such as antibiotics and tetanus vaccinations should be used. Small entry holes may be misleading, and decisions regarding which wounds to explore and débride may be difficult. Radiographs should be liberally used to detect the presence of foreign bodies. There have been reports of the wounding of victims by bone fragments from the bodies of suicide terrorists or other blast victims; these injuries require special management.[25,26]

### Tertiary and Quaternary Injuries
Tertiary injury is caused by the victim's body being thrown as a projectile by the blast and can result in fractures, head trauma, and other blunt injury. Quaternary injury can result from structural collapse or burns secondary to the detonation. Crush, traumatic amputation, compartment syndrome injuries, and other blunt and penetrating injuries can be common sequelae of structural collapse. Flash burns to exposed skin can occur as a result of the thermal component of the detonation. Secondary fires can cause additional burns as well as injury from smoke inhalation.

## First Response Considerations
First responders and other providers must exercise due caution when attempting to render aid to blast victims. In addition to dangers imposed by structures affected by the blast, the terrorist may deliberately target the responders with a second explosion. Another potential tool for inducing more casualties is the use of a so-called dirty bomb, in which the bomb is seeded with chemical, biologic, or radioactive material to contaminate the area, causing additional deaths and injuries. First responders must try to ensure that victims and the blast scene are not contami-

nated. If contamination is not recognized, responders and the medical facility to which patients are transported will be compromised.

Any response to blast events requires an organized and educated response in spite of the inherent confusion. Prognostic factors used to determine the severity of blast casualties include the blast magnitude, blasts within enclosed spaces, distance from ground zero, urban environment, elapsed time to initial care, accuracy of triage, and building collapse. Traumatic amputation, blast lung, torso injury, and multisystem injuries that include head injury are associated with poor survival. Understanding the pathophysiology of blasts, accurate triage, and preparation are vital for effective management of an inherently chaotic event.[27]

## Battlefield Damage Control: Prevention of the Second Hit

During World War II, the likelihood of US personnel surviving their battlefield wounds was nearly 70%, and by the end of the Vietnam conflict this statistic had increased to more than 76%.[28] In 2007, the survivability from battlefield injury in the Iraq War is a remarkable 89.3%, a number that has remained relatively constant throughout the conflict despite fluctuations in combat intensity.[1] The first hit is defined as the patient's initial traumatic injury. In the case of civilian trauma, improvements in injury prevention and survival of vehicular trauma have occurred with the advent of automobile crumple zones, airbags, seatbelt laws, child car seats, and maturation of civilian trauma systems.[29] Prevention of injury from the first hit on the battlefield has also improved because of personal body armor, better armored vehi-

cles, intense training of military personnel, and the availability of initial surgical capability positioned within minutes of active combat.

The second hit represents an insult to the traumatized patient that occurs during treatment, and one that the surgeon can modulate. In the current civilian model, the goal is preventing multisystem organ failure and acute respiratory distress syndrome.[30]

## Treatment Strategies for Polytraumatized Patients

The past two decades have witnessed a continued evolution in the treatment of polytraumatized patients. In 1989, Bone and associates[31] published the results of a prospective, randomized trial of early versus delayed intramedullary nailing of femur fractures. In a study by Baker and associates,[32] the authors determined that if the patient's injury severity score was 18 or less, it did not matter in terms of morbidity and mortality whether early or late stabilization was used. However, patients with an injury severity score greater than 18 who were stabilized late (> 48 hours) had longer intensive care unit (ICU) stays, longer hospitalization, and more pulmonary complications. From this finding, the concept of early total care (ETC) was developed and advocated for the most severely injured patients. However, soon thereafter, reports of patients who had thoracic injury and who were treated with early intramedullary fixation began to show higher rates of acute respiratory distress syndrome and mortality when principles of ETC were applied compared with patients who underwent delayed stabilization. This finding brought into question the safety of ETC for certain polytraumatized patient groups.

Damage control is a term coined by the US Navy that refers to "the capacity of a ship to absorb damage and maintain mission integrity."[33] Using this terminology, Rotondo and associates[34] established a strategy called damage control surgery (DCS) for treating civilian patients who sustained multivisceral injuries from penetrating abdominal trauma.[35] This concept was advocated for patients in extremis and was performed in three phases: (1) rapid initial stabilization surgery; (2) a period in the ICU for physiologic optimization; and (3) return to the operating room when the patient is able to withstand prolonged surgery for definitive treatment (Figure 5). The concept of damage control orthopaedics (DCO) originated from the concept of DCS.[36-38] Similarly, the goal is to limit the physiologic insult to patients in extremis and provide rapid provisional stabilization (usually with external fixation), followed by physiologic optimization and late definitive reconstruction after the patient is stabilized (Figure 6). In an attempt to quantify this second hit, Pape and associates[39] examined interleukin (IL) levels in patients treated with early intramedullary nailing versus those provisionally stabilized and treated with late intramedullary nailing. They found a significant increase in IL-6 levels at 7, 24, and 48 hours and increased IL-8 at 7 hours in the group treated with early intramedullary nailing compared with the group that was stabilized and treated with delayed intramedullary fixation. Although the authors did not correlate IL levels with complications, they found a systemic inflammatory response associated with early definitive treatment (such as intramedullary nailing) that could represent a second hit.

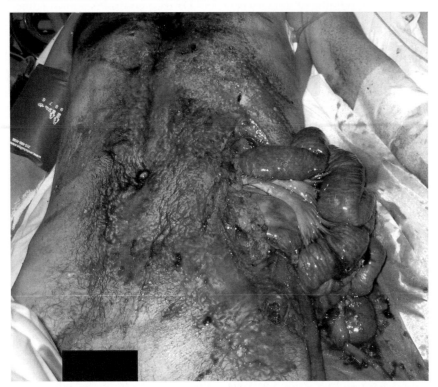

**Figure 5** Photograph of a patient injured by an IED. The patient's abdominal contents were eviscerated. Because the zone of injury will likely continue to demarcate over time, resection of necrotic segments of bowel with reanastomosis would be an unwise initial treatment.

## Battlefield Surgery

The earliest level of surgical capability on the battlefield is provided at locations offering level II care (Figure 7). Care is provided by units called forward resuscitative surgical systems and forward surgical teams in the US Marine Corps and US Army, respectively. These units are designed to be light and mobile and were located in tents during the early stages of the Iraq War. Because of the changing character of the Iraq War, most of these units have become stationary and now work from buildings of opportunity or other structures. Unfortunately, these locations do not have operating rooms with laminar airflow or a substerile entrance, which results in an environment that is barely clean and certainly not sterile. Although well suited for emergency surgical stabilization and resuscitation of wounded personnel, this environment is not well suited for providing definitive care. This and other factors have resulted in the "level II doctrine" that calls for hemorrhage control, stabilization of abdominal and thoracic injury, débridement of contamination, provisional stabilization of fractures, rapid revascularization when indicated, liberal use of fasciotomies, administration of prophylactic antibiotics, and rapid transport to facilities providing higher levels of care with greater capabilities such as an ICU. In essence, DCS and DCO are the practices used at level II care facilities.

To determine if current battlefield damage control techniques are effective, the US Army Institute of Surgical Research analyzed the results of the first 485 autopsies from the conflicts in Iraq and Afghanistan and found that only 17.5% of injuries were believed to be potentially survivable. Of the 85 fatalities that were salvageable, only 6% died of multiple system organ failure, viewed as one of the major final adverse outcomes of the second hit (JB Holcomb, MD, Washington, DC, unpublished data presented at the American Academy of Orthopaedic Surgeons' symposium, Extremity War Injuries II, 2007). This finding suggests that current battlefield damage control techniques are effective.

An important question is whether the battlefield second hit is the same as the second hit that occurs in civilian trauma patients. DCS was developed for patients who sustained thoracic and abdominal trauma as a result of penetrating injury. As this concept has evolved in civilian trauma centers, DCS and DCO have been applied as strategies for patients with blunt polytrauma. Most trauma that occurs on the battlefield is penetrating trauma (recognizing that a substantial proportion of blast injuries have a blunt component) and is likely more applicable to what damage control techniques were initially applied. Therefore, the battlefield second hit is not quite the same as the second hit in the civilian setting because in combat-injured patients, it is most important to prevent the so-called lethal triad. This triad is a cascade of events characterized by a drop in the patient's core body temperature (below 35°C) because of open body cavities and administration of excess fluids; acidosis caused by hypovolemia and lactate overproduction; and coagulopathy.[40] Current strategy focuses on prevention of this lethal triad

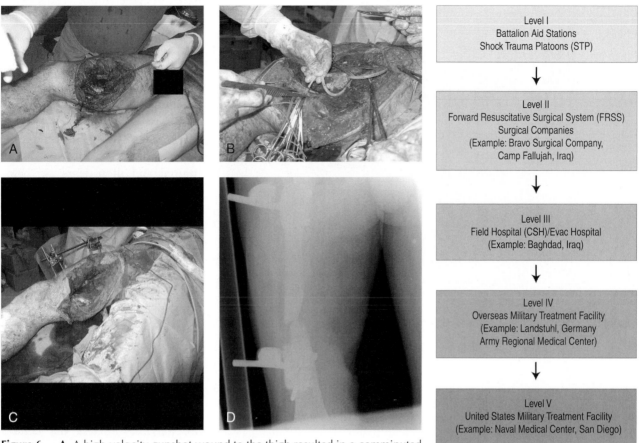

**Figure 6** **A,** A high-velocity gunshot wound to the thigh resulted in a comminuted femur fracture and segmental loss of femoral artery. **B,** The femoral artery was rapidly shunted. **C,** The patient was treated with hemorrhage control, revascularization, débridement, and provisional stabilization. **D,** AP radiograph of the stabilized femur.

**Figure 7** Levels of casualty care from the most basic (level I) to the most advanced (level V).

Level I
Battalion Aid Stations
Shock Trauma Platoons (STP)

Level II
Forward Resuscitative Surgical System (FRSS)
Surgical Companies
(Example: Bravo Surgical Company,
Camp Fallujah, Iraq)

Level III
Field Hospital (CSH)/Evac Hospital
(Example: Baghdad, Iraq)

Level IV
Overseas Military Treatment Facility
(Example: Landstuhl, Germany
Army Regional Medical Center)

Level V
United States Military Treatment Facility
(Example: Naval Medical Center, San Diego)

through hemorrhage control and rapid surgical treatment to stabilize and prevent the patient from becoming cold and acidotic, followed by swift transport to places providing higher levels of care (such as an ICU) for physiologic optimization.

### Far Forward Hemorrhage Control

Hemorrhage control at level II is divided into compressible and noncompressible components. For a compressible hemorrhage, a tourniquet has often been applied in the field and is removed by the surgeon. Once surgical hemostasis is obtained, the extremity is evaluated for perfusion. If the extremity is not perfused because of a lost segment of artery and/or vein, the preferred technique at this level of care is placement of a temporary vascular shunt. This technique, which involves placement of a silicone tube to bypass a missing segment of blood vessel, can be performed by general and orthopaedic surgeons and can rapidly restore blood flow with less blood loss and physiologic insult. Recent data from a US Marine Corps level II surgical unit in Iraq showed 100% patient survival in 20 patients treated with 27 temporary vascular shunts; only 6 shunts failed (clotted during transportation), although perfusion was maintained; 3 patients ulti-

mately required amputations.[41] For noncompressible hemorrhage, two types of hemostatic dressings have been used—HemCon (HemCon Medical Technologies, Portland, OR) and QuikClot (Z-Medica, Wallingford, CT). Both types of hemostatic dressings are effective in animal models in stopping noncompressible hemorrhage such as from liver lacerations and groin wounds.[42-45] See chapter 8 for more information on vascular shunts and hemostatic dressings.

Two techniques that have been helpful on the battlefield to prevent ongoing hemorrhage, metabolic derangements, and dilutional coagulopathy are hypotensive resuscita-

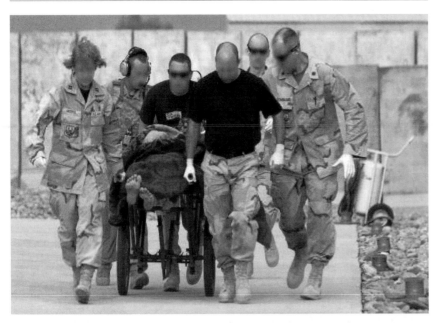

**Figure 8**    Photograph of a patient being moved at Balad Air Base, Iraq.

tion and the use of fresh whole blood. In hypotensive resuscitation, rebleeding occurs after clot formation at certain levels of arterial pressure.[46] In a porcine model, Sondeen and associates[47] demonstrated a rebleed effect at a systolic blood pressure of greater than 80 mm Hg and mean arterial pressure greater than 60 mm Hg after control of an aortic laceration. By resuscitating patients below this threshold, intravascular volume can be preserved, and the adverse effects of dilution and hypothermia mitigated. At facilities providing level II care, the only available blood products are packed red blood cells (which are in limited supply), and fresh whole blood from a "walking blood bank" of prescreened blood donors who supply blood to patients requiring massive transfusions. Kauvar and associates[48] analyzed data from the initial phase of the Iraq War, including all patients requiring massive transfusions both at level II and III facilities, and showed similar mortality

and complication rates in patients receiving individual blood products compared with those receiving fresh whole blood. This finding suggests that fresh whole blood can be an effective lifesaving means to transfuse exsanguinating patients on the battlefield, where blood products are limited or impractical. Once stabilized on the battlefield, patients can then be rapidly moved to places offering higher levels of care with a more robust ICU capability.

Improved survivability on the battlefield is a result of many factors, some of which have been learned from previous conflicts and experience with civilian trauma. The current Middle East conflicts have provided a large volume of data on DCS and DCO, from which knowledge for enhanced trauma care can be extrapolated. The direction of future research in this area should focus on establishing more objective parameters for defining when a patient can safely undergo definitive care that is both

injury specific (blunt versus penetrating trauma) and treatment specific (plate versus nail fixation and early versus late fixation). The ultimate goal of research is to improve patient survivability and maximize functional outcome.

## Aeroevacuation Challenges and Advances

Injured and ill patients are being moved out of the combat zone much faster than they were 10 to 15 years ago (Figure 8). The average time for patients injured in Iraq and Afghanistan to be transported to Landstuhl Regional Medical Center (LRMC) in Germany, and on to the United States has decreased from 10 to 14 days (the average time during the 1991 Persian Gulf War) to 3 days currently. The doctrine has changed from stable patient care to critical patient care—moving sicker patients sooner rather than holding them in hospitals in or near the combat zone. The development of Critical Care Air Transport Teams has facilitated increased critical care patient movement[49] (Figure 9).

Care for the wounded begins on the battlefield with level I care—basic first aid provided by nonmedical service members, buddy aid, or by a trained combat lifesaver. Wounded personnel who are unable to return to duty are then rapidly transported through five levels or echelons of care, each more advanced and sophisticated, until they reach hospitals located in the United States. Level II care provides surgical resuscitation by small, highly mobile surgical teams. Level III care is provided at an Air Force theater hospital or combat support hospital (Figure 10). These modular facilities provide the highest level of medical, surgical, and trauma care available within the combat zone; have a capability similar to a US civilian trauma center; and often receive casualties directly from the battlefield. Level IV care for all casualties who undergo aeromedical evacuation from Iraq or Afghanistan is provided at LRMC. This Department of Defense Medical Center is the first echelon where definitive surgical treatment can be provided outside the combat zone. Most patients stay no longer than 72 hours at LRMC before being evacuated to a level V facility in the United States. Level V care is the final stage of the aeromedical evacuation process and is delivered at one of the major military treatment facilities in the United States.[50] New advances, as well as challenges, have arisen from this revolutionary change in how patients are transported and cared for through the aeromedical evacuation system. See chapter 8 for more information on levels of casualty care.

### Negative Pressure Wound Management in the Air

Negative pressure wound therapy has revolutionized the treatment of soft-tissue wounds resulting from both traumatic and nontraumatic injuries. This treatment augments wound granulation and healing, promotes wound contraction, controls wound secretions, decreases wound edema, reduces skin maceration, and improves pain management.[51-58] Ongoing experience using negative pressure wound therapy in the operating room on the traumatic wounds of Iraqi nationals has reproduced many of the previously mentioned benefits.[59] Because of aeromedical limitations and other concerns, negative pressure wound therapy has not been routinely applied in the management of soft-tissue wounds before an evacuated casualty arrives in the United States.

A commercially produced wound treatment system has completed air

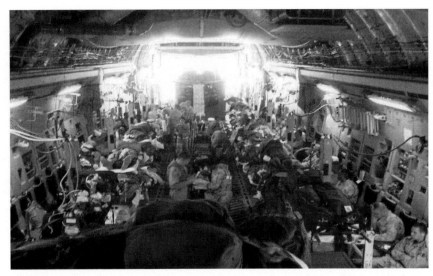

**Figure 9**  Photograph of the interior of a C-17 aircraft during an aeromedical evacuation mission to Germany.

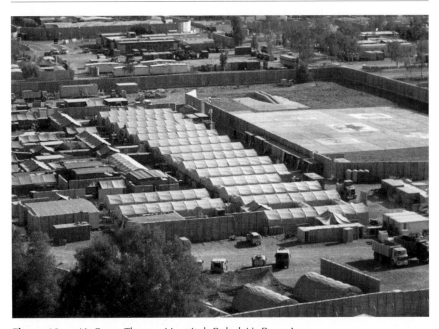

**Figure 10**  Air Force Theater Hospital, Balad Air Base, Iraq.

worthiness testing by the US Air Force and is available for use. A feasibility study of using this system in the aeromedical evacuation system is now underway. If proven to be safe and feasible, early negative pressure wound therapy using appropriate equipment and trained medical support for selected soft-tissue wounds in US casualties may improve outcomes. The use of the transportable negative pressure wound system during aeromedical evacuation has the potential to improve pain management, facilitate wound healing, and simplify in-flight wound care. Specifically, medical attendants may be able to dispense fewer medications to these patients and spend less time reinforcing saturated wound dressings.

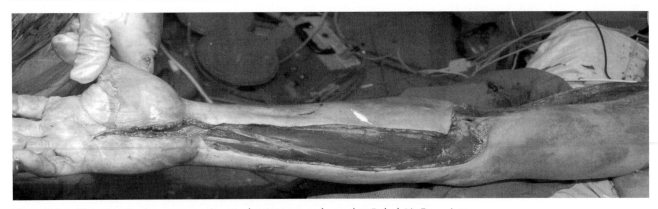

**Figure 11**  Photograph of an upper extremity fasciotomy performed at Balad Air Base, Iraq.

By initiating this wound therapy at level II and III medical treatment facilities close to the battlefield, it may be possible to definitively close wounds more quickly at the level IV facility in Germany (LRMC) and level V facilities in the United States, potentially shortening hospital stays and overall recovery times.[50]

## Compartment Syndrome Management

Extremity compartment syndromes are a concern as severely injured patients are rapidly transported from the combat theater to LRMC and then on to the United States (Figure 11). Patients arrive at LRMC and the United States as early as 24 to 72 hours after injury. This cohort represents a physically fit group of patients before injury who are now extremely ill as a result of very high-energy injuries.

Over 3,000 patients with traumatic injuries to the extremities were retrospectively evaluated at LRMC between January 2005 and August 2006. Three hundred thirty-seven patients underwent 685 fasciotomies during the first 3 days after injury in Iraq and Afghanistan. Some of these fasciotomies were not performed until arrival at LRMC, and a group of these patients had

muscle necrosis and long-term morbidity (COL WC Dorlac, MD, USAF, MC, LRMC, Germany, personal communication, 2007). Forty-six percent (315 of 685) fasciotomies were to the leg, and 22% (150 of 685) were to the forearm. Patients who underwent a fasciotomy revision had higher rates of muscle necrosis (240 or 35% versus 62 or 9%) and mortality (137 or 20% versus 27 or 4%) than those who did not receive a revision ($P < 0.01$). The anterior compartment of the leg was most commonly missed. Patients who underwent fasciotomy after evacuation had significantly higher rates of muscle necrosis (77 or 23% versus 33 or 10%) and mortality (64 or 19% versus 17 or 5%) than patients who were treated with fasciotomies in the combat theater ($P < 0.01$). Hypotension, hypoxia, pressor use, and elevated creatinine and lactate levels were associated with muscle necrosis and mortality ($P < 0.05$) (COL WC Dorlac, MD, USAF, MC, LRMC, Germany, personal communication, 2007).

Some combination of four criteria (IED blast, extremity injury, resuscitation with ≥ 5 L crystalloid solution, and/or transfusion with ≥ 5 units of fresh frozen plasma) in conjunction with aspects of the air

evacuation process (such as intravenous fluid rates; litter immobility; relative decrease in ambient oxygen; relative decrease in humidity, vibration, and cabin pressure at altitude) may lead to the occult development/evolution of extremity compartment syndrome that can cause life-threatening complications. As a result, a new protocol was developed by the Joint Theater Trauma System to address this challenge (COL DH Jenkins, MD, USAF, MC, Balad, Iraq, personal communication, 2007). Ongoing research and data collection may determine if rapid aeromedical evacuation is possibly the fifth factor leading to the development of occult compartment syndrome. However, it is possible that these compartment syndromes may occur as the injury evolves in the first 24 to 72 hours after blast, thermal, or penetrating injury and may not be affected by rapid aeromedical transport.

## Deep Venous Thrombosis

Explosive injuries commonly occur during war and are infrequent occurrences in the civilian environment. The effects of a high-energy blast may cause an increased risk of deep venous thrombosis (DVT) and pulmonary embolism in combat casualties. There is an increasing recognition of DVT in individuals who complete an extended period of travel on an airplane. One randomized study found a 10% prevalence (in 12 of 116 passengers) of asymptomatic DVT in individuals on flights of 8 or more hours.[60] DVT is often a factor before the patient enters the aeromedical evacuation system. Other than data on immobility, no data exist on other aeroevacuation-related stressors (such as accelerative/ decelerative forces, lower ambient oxygen tension, dehydration, vibration, immobility for extended periods during the evacuation process, and elevation in thrombin-antithrombin complex) that may exacerbate rates of DVT and pulmonary embolism.

The Joint Theater Trauma System staff has developed a treatment protocol for patients at highest risk for DVT and pulmonary embolism to include those undergoing emergency trauma surgical procedures with major orthopaedic injuries of the extremities, spine, and pelvis; those with ongoing coagulopathy; or patients with a prohibitive risk of bleeding. Enoxaparin therapy and the use of sequential compression devices and inferior vena cava filters are all options based on the guideline. No pulmonary embolisms have occurred in patients at LRMC since the protocol was instituted (COL WC Dorlac, MD, USAF, MC, LRMC, Germany, personal communication, 2007).

Flight testing is ongoing for a pneumatic sequential compression device for aeromedical use. DVT and pulmonary embolisms can be prevented in 90% or more of surgical and trauma patients without additional risk factors by using a systematic preventive strategy.

Since October 2001, more than 44,000 patients have been safely transported in the US military aeromedical evacuation system. Of these patients, more than 9,373 had battle injuries. In 2006, 1,796 patients were evacuated from Iraq or Afghanistan to facilities in Germany offering higher levels of care.[61] The aeromedical system has been overwhelmingly successful because of the dedication and sacrifice of countless military health care professionals.

## Evolving Technologies for Enhanced Care
### Repair of Segmental Bone Defects

Most orthopaedic surgeons have experience treating musculoskeletal injuries sustained in a civilian setting. These injuries include fractures (such as hip fractures, distal radius fractures), skeletal injuries sustained as a result of blunt trauma, and penetrating injuries such as those from low-velocity gunshot wounds. However, in modern-day warfare, sophisticated weapons now increase the force and resultant devastation produced by explosive ordinances and other military devices. As a consequence, battlefield wounds are produced by high-velocity missiles (speeds greater than 2,000 feet per second), blasts, and land mines. Treatment of these injuries requires a recognition and understanding of the wounding mechanisms. For example, the type of trauma produced by high-velocity missiles includes not only the laceration and crushing of bone and soft tissues but also the damage produced by the shock wave and cavitation resulting from the energy transfer.[62] Blast injuries are discussed in detail in the "Blast Injury: Pathophysiology and Injury Patterns" section of this chapter. With more than 100 million land mines planted in 71 countries worldwide, almost

2,000 people are injured by these devices every month (1 victim every 20 minutes). New experimental models must be developed to simulate the soft- and skeletal-tissue damage produced by battlefield wounding mechanisms. This approach is essential to reproduce not only the severity of the injuries but also the impact of the injury on local and systemic biologic responses needed to participate in the repair.

Current technologies for the repair of segmental bone defects include the use of nonvascularized autologous bone grafts, vascularized autologous bone grafts, allogeneic bone grafts, intercalary prosthetic devices, and bone transport using distraction osteogenesis. Evolving technologies for the repair of segmental bone defects include the use of autologous bone marrow, recombinant osteoinductive proteins, gene therapy, and synthetic small molecules. Materials produced by any of these technologies may be used in conjunction with resorbable or nonresorbable scaffold devices composed of novel biomaterials.

A typical example of a battlefield injury is illustrated by a soldier who has sustained a high-velocity gunshot wound resulting in a grade IIIB open distal, one third tibial fracture with segmental loss of bone. Because of the need to perform extensive débridement of injured tissue, more extensive débridement than would be required after a low-velocity injury, knowledge of the extent of bone and soft-tissue loss becomes critical. Multiple irrigation and débridement procedures, inclusive of multiple antibiotic bead placement exchanges, result in a segmental skeletal defect of substantial size (Figure 12). Evolving technologies that may enhance the repair of this kind of defect include the use

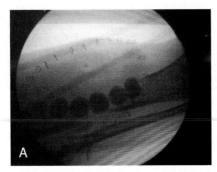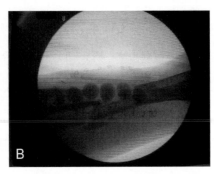

**Figure 12** AP (**A**) and lateral (**B**) radiographs of a 32-year-old man who sustained a high-velocity gunshot wound resulting in a type IIIB open distal, one third tibial fracture with a segmental defect. The patient was treated with multiple irrigation and débridement procedures as well as antibiotic bead placements and exchanges. The segmental defect measures approximately 6 cm in length. (Courtesy of David Casey, MD.)

of autologous bone marrow in conjunction with a structural delivery vehicle such as a hydroxyapatite implant or recombinant bone morphogenetic protein-2.[63,64]

Preclinical data from a canine study suggest that large segmental defects can be bridged with the use of hydroxyapatite material impregnated with culture-expanded bone marrow mesenchymal stem cells.[63] The bone marrow mesenchymal stem cells not only differentiate into osteoblasts, which produce bone to heal the defect, but also secrete paracrine signals that recruit other progenitor cells in the local tissue environment, which may participate in the healing process (Figure 13). A recent report by Hernigou and associates[65] suggests that the yield of bone-forming cells from a bone marrow aspirate may be increased by techniques aimed at harvesting marrow on the endosteal surface of the ilium and by making multiple aspirations of small quantities to reduce dilution of the cellular concentration with peripheral blood. An alternate treatment approach, the use of a recombinant growth factor, is supported by two recent studies showing a reduction in the number of secondary interventions required af-

ter definitive treatment of an open tibial fracture with the implantation of recombinant bone morphogenetic protein-2.[64,66] This osteoinductive protein promotes healing by inducing a mitogenic effect in undifferentiated stem cells and promoting angiogenesis.

A future technology for the repair of segmental bone defects may be the use of gene therapy that involves expression of an osteogenic gene or a combination of genes. Recent studies have shown that skeletal muscle-derived cells, when transduced to express an osteogenic gene (such as bone morphogenetic protein-4) and an angiogenic gene (such as vascular endothelial growth factor), have a synergistic effect on bone formation.[67,68] Studies using direct percutaneous gene delivery have shown enhancement in the healing of segmental bone defects and may lead to technologies that obviate the need for ex vivo transduction of cells or other delivery vectors.[69] Because recombinant growth factors have very short biologic half-lives, are difficult to retain at the site of local application, and require large doses to produce effects, gene therapy may have several advantages. By delivering complementary

DNA rather than the proteins themselves, it is possible to achieve a sustained, local presence of the growth factor at efficacious concentrations with minimal exposure of nontargeted sites.

The devastation produced by some battlefield wounding mechanisms often leads to such extensive loss of bone and soft tissue that the only treatment option is amputation. However, evolving therapies are directed toward the complete restoration of an anatomic part, such as a portion of a limb or joint. Several experiments, using synthetic scaffolds composed of copolymers of polyglycolic and poly-L-lactic acid, or hydroxyapatite, in combination with autologous periosteum or cells, have been used to reconstruct small bones, such as the phalanges of the hand.[70,71] When used in conjunction with well-planned plastic surgical reconstructive protocols involving cutaneous and myocutaneous flaps, actual digits have been reconstructed after civilian injuries.[71]

High cost is one limitation in the development of such therapies. Methods for the development of sophisticated biomaterials, recombinant proteins, or gene therapy mechanisms involve expensive raw materials, time-intensive experimentation, and substantial manpower. The ability to develop synthetic small molecules and proteins using advanced methodologies, such as combinatorial chemistry, may be possible at much lower costs. This would undoubtedly enhance scientific discovery and development and would accelerate the pace at which new and advanced therapies could positively impact the care of injured military personnel.

## Soft-Tissue Coverage of Massive Wounds

Because of improvements in body

armor that protect both the head and the trunk, soldiers are surviving massive blast injuries that would otherwise be fatal; however, the resulting mutilating upper and lower extremity traumatic injuries require bone and soft-tissue reconstruction. Great progress was made in extremity reconstruction during the era of World War II, especially the development of reconstructive hand surgery. To date, almost 1,000 patients have required amputations as a result of the wars in Iraq and Afghanistan. Military efforts have focused on functional rehabilitation of the amputee with improved prostheses, more rapid integration back into the military system, and peer-to-peer work groups that help the injured service member's recovery.

Some of the newer concepts in soft-tissue reconstruction involve preserving amputation levels, either with emergency fillet free flaps from the nonsalvageable injured body part, such as at the shoulder, elbow, or knee, and the use of conventional free-tissue transfer procedures to resurface and provide soft-tissue augmentation to joints, such as the elbow or the knee that have been stripped of soft tissue. If such areas could not be covered, the ultimate amputation levels would be higher.[72]

The need for immediate amputation in the combat theater to save lives, stop hemorrhaging, and control contamination is still a time-honored principle. Even in the combat theater, the amputated extremity should be considered as a source for different structures that can be used for reconstruction.[73] These structures include skin that can be harvested for further reconstruction or coverage immediately after the extremity is amputated; and vessels and nerve, and bone that can be used

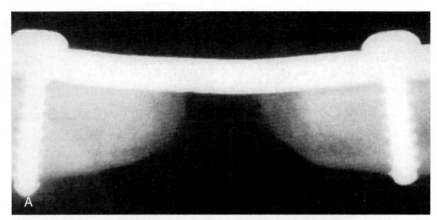
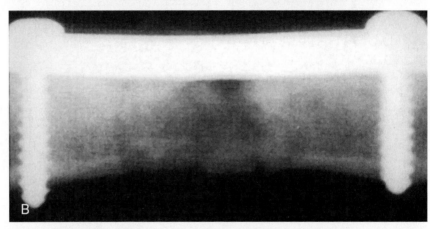
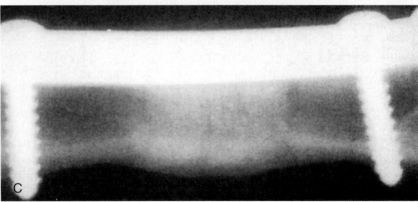

**Figure 13**   **A,** Radiograph of a 21-mm-long osteoperiosteal canine femoral defect that had been left untreated for 16 weeks. Little or no new bone formation is observed, and nonunion has occurred. **B,** Radiograph of the same defect treated with a hydroxyapatite ceramic cylinder that had not been loaded with mesenchymal stem cells. After 16 weeks, union has occurred at the host bone-implant interface, but bone formation has not occurred throughout the entire implant, and callus has not formed around the implant. **C,** Radiograph of the same defect treated with a hydroxyapatite ceramic cylinder that was loaded with mesenchymal stem cells. Union occurred at the host bone-implant interface, bone appears to have formed throughout the implant, and a substantial callus has formed around the implant. (Reprinted with permission from Bruder SP, Kraus KH, Goldberg VM, Kadiyala S: The effect of implants loaded with autologous mesenchymal stem cells on the healing of canine segmental bone defects. *J Bone Joint Surg Am* 1998;80:985-996.).

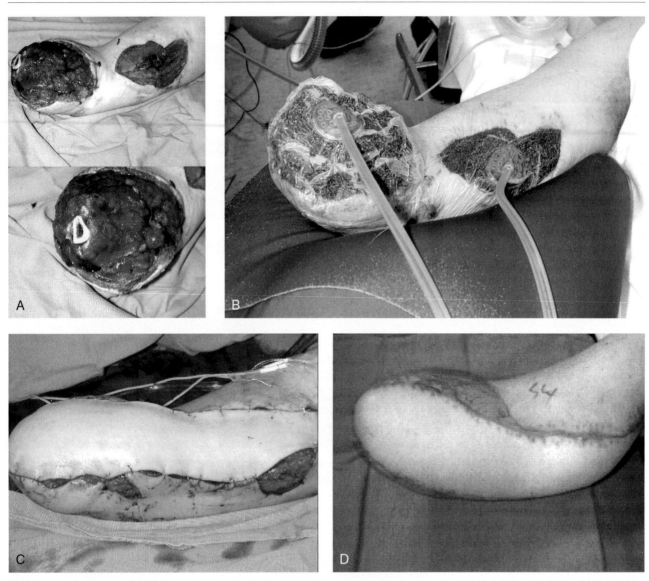

**Figure 14**  A 33-year-old marine was ambushed in Fallujah, Iraq, and sustained severe injuries from a rocket-propelled grenade. **A,** Because of a major vascular injury, his forearm was amputated, but his elbow remained in jeopardy because of soft-tissue coverage concerns. **B,** The patient was initially treated with a wound vacuum-assisted closure device. **C,** The elbow joint was salvaged with a free latissimus flap, and the brachial artery was reconstructed with a vein graft for flap inflow. **D,** The flap underwent one debulking. The patient now uses a conventional prosthesis, has excellent elbow function, no pain, and has returned to work.

for intercalary defects, cancellous, or as osteoarticular grafts.

For example, a 33-year-old Marine was injured by a rocket-propelled grenade in Fallujah, Iraq, causing a near-complete amputation of his forearm that required below-elbow amputation. The patient was subsequently evacuated to the United States for reconstruction that included a brachial artery interposition graft and a free latissimus dorsi flap that was used to provide coverage of the elbow amputation level and salvage function in his below-elbow amputation. The patient is now functional with a lower-elbow prosthesis and has a greater degree of function than would have been possible if the arm had been amputated above the elbow (Figure 14).

## Perforator Flaps

Another new dimension in soft-tissue reconstruction is the use of perforator flaps. The new workhorse for cutaneous coverage is the anterolateral thigh flap, which is based on the lateral femoral circumflex arterial system, particularly the descending branches of the lateral femoral circumflex artery. The advantages of this flap are that large surface areas of skin and subcutaneous tissue can be provided. The muscle-sparing dissection of this free flap is advantageous because no muscles are harvested and a large surface area can be obtained for coverage of other extremity soft-tissue deficiencies. The patient also can be supine while the flap is harvested, which is in contrast to the conventional scapula flaps that require lateral positioning of the patient. The flap is quite versatile and can be taken as an adipofascial flap only. In military personnel, who usually have a fairly thin body habitus, the donor site can be closed primarily.[74] Perforator flaps have been used worldwide during the past decade for a variety of reconstructions and represent an advance in the evolution of free-tissue transfer. Newer techniques rely on perforator flaps only and do not require the harvesting of a major muscle.

### Fasciocutaneous Flaps

Soft-tissue injuries that occur in the combat theater, particularly in the civilian population, and especially lower extremity injuries are challenging for military surgeons to treat. Because they cannot be transported from the area, injured civilians do not have access to reconstructive microsurgery in locations such as LRMC or in medical centers in the United States.

As limb-sparing surgery, fasciocutaneous flaps such as the sural flap have enabled military physicians to provide coverage around the distal third of the leg, in anatomic areas that traditionally would have been closed with free-tissue transfer.[75] The sural flap is used to treat the distal third of the extremity and is based on the perforating vessels of the peroneal artery distally and the neurocutaneous territories, specifically the sural nerve and the vascular

pedicle that accompanies it. The sural flap is a distally based flap with a large surface area that can be used without the need for an operating microscope and relies on soft-tissue principles of harvesting a free flap. Loupe magnification must be available, and the surgeon must be familiar with the regional anatomy to assure that this flap can be viable after harvest. It can be harvested as a fasciocutaneous flap or a fasciosubcutaneous turndown flap, depending on the needs of the patient and the defect.[76] The outflow of the flap can be augmented by venous supercharging, which is the procedure of coapting the proximal lesser saphenous vein to the more distal veins in the foot with loupe magnification and the possible use of 6-0 or 7-0 sutures.

### Other Techniques

Other developments in soft-tissue reconstruction include microsurgical free-tissue transfer for craniofacial defects and soft-tissue and bone composite flaps (that include bone and skin), such as the osteocutaneous fibula transfer that can be used for the reconstruction of the maxilla or mandible. These techniques have been used in the civilian population for the last decade and can readily be applied to wounded military personnel with soft-tissue and bone deficiencies.

Developments in soft-tissue reconstructive surgery continue to evolve to meet the needs of severely injured patients. These techniques are effective, reliable, and can advance the care and recovery of those who sustain major war wounds.

## Battlefield Musculoskeletal Infections

The exigencies of wartime have been a driving factor in improvements in the surgical treatment of

orthopaedic trauma.[77] These improvements also include the prevention and treatment of wound infections that can be attributed to advances in transport, antibiotic development and selection, surgical technique, and aseptic practices. In Iraq and Afghanistan, military medical personnel have provided rapid and highly advanced care aimed at fighting infection; however, research is still needed to prevent opportunistic infections in extremity wounds, particularly those caused by multidrug-resistant organisms.

### Historic Perspective

During the Civil War, amputation was the only prophylaxis against extremity infection. Contrary to some reports, anesthesia (in the form of ether or chloroform) was available to Union forces and was used routinely during surgical procedures. However, because of the perpetual shortage of water, surgeons often would go days without cleaning their hands or surgical instruments, and gangrene was common. Even with these limitations, it is estimated that approximately 75% of amputees survived the Civil War; the importance of sanitary practices in preventing infection was demonstrated to an entire generation of physicians. The Civil War also saw advances in moving wounded personnel more quickly from the battlefield, as the army adopted faster and more stable four-wheeled carts operated under the supervision of an Army Medical Corps.[78,79] Advances in transporting the wounded have continued to play a major role in the successful treatment of orthopaedic infections.

The battlefields of World War I were farmlands fertilized with manure. This environment provided ideal conditions for infection with tetanus bacilli. By this time, surgical practice had evolved and the primary protocol for contaminated wounds was delayed primary closure; prophylactic amputation became much less common.[80] In addition, major advances in triage and ambulance transport, and the more widespread employment of nurses, led to more rapid treatment of infected wounds.[81,82] The mortality rate for lower extremity wounds was 7.7%, and 4.1% for upper extremity wounds. The major cause of death during World War I was not battlefield trauma or wound infection but influenza, which was controlled only after millions of people died in a worldwide pandemic.[77]

The widespread use of antibiotics was the most important development in the treatment of infection during World War II. The American war effort that led to the mass production of planes, bullets, shells, tanks, and aircraft carriers also produced penicillin on a prodigious scale. Penicillin was used to treat wound infection, pneumonia, meningitis, gonorrhea, and syphilis. During World War II the nature of the common wound had changed— approximately 80% of injuries were caused by bombs and mortar and shell fire, not bullets.[78] By this time, delayed primary wound closure was no longer the standard treatment; rather, clinical appearance dictated whether the wound was considered ready for closure. Surgeons also used more aggressive débridement to treat infections. The increased use of antibiotics is considered the primary factor in the marked decrease in the mortality rate in World War II compared with that of World War I, with a mortality rate of 2.1% for lower extremity wounds and 1.1% for upper extremity wounds.[77]

The Korea Conflict and Vietnam War demonstrate the tremendous advances in transport and treatment that are the hallmarks of the current military system. Helicopter evacuation was first used in Korea and was predominantly used in Vietnam. Surgical hospitals were increasingly mobile. By 1970, the overall "died-of-wounds" rate fell to 2.5%. In Korea, and to a greater extent Vietnam, a broader spectrum of antimicrobial agents were used;[83] however, one of the authors reports present complications of increasingly resistant bacteria in war wounds.

In Iraq and Afghanistan, tremendous improvements in military medicine and survivorship have again emphasized the importance of preventing postoperative wound infections. In Iraq, advances in body armor, combined with the enemy's use of IEDs, have led to a decrease in lower extremity and torso wounds and an increase in the number of survivors with head, neck, and upper extremity wounds.[84] Broad-spectrum antibiotics, meticulous débridement, and delayed wound closure when the wound appears clean are protocols used to fight contamination and treat soft-tissue injuries. Treatment is provided by a relatively small number of surgeons. Although troop numbers in Iraq have ranged from 130,000 to 150,000 at any one time, 120 surgeons are on active duty (this includes 10 to 15 orthopaedic surgeons). Army Forward Surgical Teams move swiftly behind the combat lines and rapidly establish mobile hospitals.[85,86]

Although methicillin-resistant *Staphylococcus aureus* and vancomycin-resistant *Enterococci* are of perpetual concern in orthopaedic wounds, other resistant strains have been detected in injuries treated in the United States. The most serious pathogens are multidrug-resistant *Pseudomonas aeruginosa* and *Klebsiella pneumoniae*[87] (HC Yun et al, Brook Army Medical Center, Fort Sam Houston, TX, unpublished data, 2005). A recent survey of type III tibial fractures in soldiers injured in Iraq and Afghanistan, conducted by Brooke Army Medical Center, showed that the most frequently identified initial pathogens were *Acinetobacter baumannii-calcoaceticus* complex, *Enterobacter* spp., and *P aeruginosa*. The infections studied were predominantly caused by gram-negative organisms (33 of 42). Recurrent infections subsequent to surgical débridement, however, were predominately caused by staphylococci (67%); these infections caused delayed union or amputation.[88]

*A baumannii-calcoaceticus* is an aerobic, gram-negative bacillus commonly isolated from the hospital environment and hospitalized patients and is resistant to a broad range of antimicrobial agents. It is an increasingly common cause of infection in personnel returning from overseas conflicts after being cared for in deployed military hospitals.[89-92] Although the source of this pathogen has not been determined, data support the role of acquisition after injury during treatment in health care facilities rather than from inoculation at the time of injury from environmental soil contamination or preinjury skin colonization. Studies have shown that multidrug-resistant *Acinetobacter* is a common cause of nosocomial infection in burn patients, and patients with the infection had more severe burns and comorbidities, with longer lengths of hospitalization. Statistical analysis, however, has shown that *Acinetobacter* infection does not independently affect mortality.[91,93] Infectious outbreaks with *Acinetobacter* have oc-

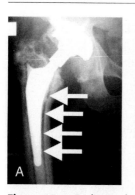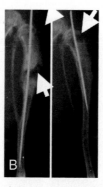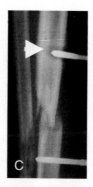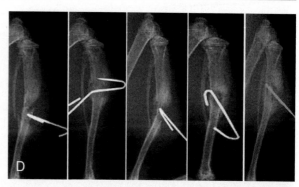

**Figure 15** Radiographs showing intramedullary versus transcortical implant-associated osteomyelitis. The radiographs show the differences between the osteolytic lesions (*arrows*) around an intramedullary implant in a patient (**A**) and in two different experimental mice (**B**) compared with a transcortical implant in a patient (**C**) and five different experimental mice (**D**).

curred in a variety of settings and geographic locations, including in those injured in earthquakes and tsunamis; hospital-acquired infections in Turkey, Brazil, and Baltimore; patients with ventilator-assisted pneumonias in Lebanon; and in ICUs in Kuwait.[94-99]

The principles of antibiotic prophylaxis are the same in the military hospital as in the civilian setting; a single dose of antibiotic administered within 1 hour of a surgical wound is sufficient prophylaxis against infection. Administration of more than one antibiotic for more than 24 hours does not offer additional protection against sepsis, organ failure, and death but rather increases the probability of antibiotic-resistant infections.[100,101] Immediate prophylaxis is generally not possible for patients with open fractures that occur in the field; however, with improvements in battlefield training and techniques, it may be possible to treat injured military personnel with prophylactic antibiotics within 1 hour of injury. Antibiotics with broad coverage aimed at multidrug-resistant pathogens such as *Acinetobacter* are probably not needed at the time of injury; however, more studies are needed to confirm this

hypothesis and provide the tools and knowledge to reduce the infection rate and successfully treat multidrug-resistant organisms. Specific research initiatives should focus on using both new and old drugs in new applications and settings, such as medics administering prophylaxis at time of injury; establishing animal and human trials of new and old drugs in a wound model; early identification of organisms through DNA analysis; and improved infection control practices. The collection of demographic data pinpointing the number and type of infections in orthopaedic wounds, the surgical treatment given, the antibiotic used, and other relevant information would enable researchers to recommend optimal antibiotic and surgical protocols aimed at the prevention of wound infection.

## A Quantitative Murine Transtibial Model of Implant-Associated Osteomyelitis

A major reason for the limited progress in developing novel antibiotic treatments and vaccines for bone infections is the absence of a highly quantitative animal model of osteomyelitis that can be used to evaluate in vivo bacterial growth, in

vivo bacterial load, host immunity, vascularity, and osteolysis. The over-emphasis on the clinical relevance of these animal models, at the expense of scientific rigor in terms of precision, accuracy, and reproducibility of the outcome measures is one explanation for the delayed development of such models.[102-107]

Orthopaedic implant-associated osteomyelitis occurs with the use of intramedullary devices (such as joint prostheses) and transcortical implants (such as external fixation devices) (Figure 15). Although the infection rate of fixation devices is 2.5 times greater, and has an incidence of more than 8 times that of total joint prostheses, it is not considered to be as serious because the revision surgery is simpler to perform.[108] Most instances of an infected transcortical implant can be resolved with a single surgical procedure to relocate the pin; the abscess is treated independently. Two revision procedures are needed to treat most patients with an infected prosthesis.[108] From the standpoint of clinical significance, investigators have focused primarily on models of implant-associated osteomyelitis that involve an intramedullary device with gram-positive *S*

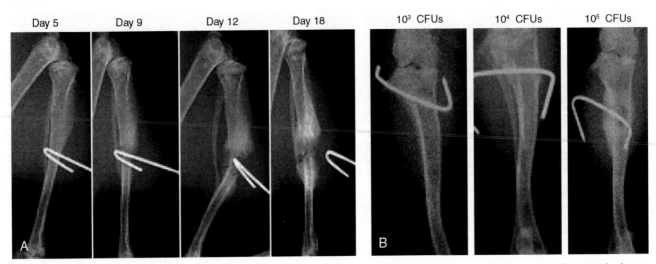

**Figure 16**  Kinetics and inoculum requirements in the transcortical pin model of implant-associated osteomyelitis. **A,** The kinetics of radiographic osteolysis and fracture in the model were evaluated by serial radiographs on days 5, 9, 12, and 18 following implantation of a transcortical pin coated with $10^6$ colony-forming units (CFUs) of UAMS-1 *S aureus*. **B,** To determine the inoculum needed to induce chronic osteomyelitis, the indicated dose of bacteria ($10^3$, $10^4$, and $10^5$ CFUs) were coated onto the pin before implantation, and radiographs were taken on day 9. The data are representative of five mice per group and demonstrate that radiographic evidence of osteolysis around the infected pin can only be seen in mice given $10^4$ and $10^5$ CFUs.

*aureus*.[102-107] Unfortunately, this approach has important limitations, most notably the inability to generate reproducible (temporal and spatial) lesions. Even when guided by the location of a fracture, radiographs confirmed the random location of the lytic lesions, which were distributed between the epiphysis, metaphysis, and diaphysis. In contrast, studies in mice have shown that implantation of an infected transcortical pin always produces lesions adjacent to the pin, and never results in chronic osteomyelitis in other regions of the tibia or hematogenous spreading.

Based on the early success with this murine transtibial model of implant-associated osteomyelitis, time-course and dose-response studies were performed to evaluate the reproducibility of the model (Figure 16). Preliminary results regarding the time course of osteomyelitis indicate that reproducible osteolysis adjacent to the pin is evident by day 9, frac-

tures occur within 3 weeks, and the model closely resembles clinical osteomyelitis around an external fixation pin. The dose-response studies indicate that inoculation with at least $1 \times 10^4$ colony-forming units (CFUs) of UAMS-1 *S aureus* is required to establish chronic osteomyelitis. This osteomyelitis was never observed in negative controls including (1) uncoated pins, (2) pins coated with heat-killed UAMS-1 *S aureus*, and (3) pins coated with $5 \times 10^8$ CFUs of nonpathogenic *Escherichia coli*.[109]

Recently, there has been an emergence of *A baumannii-calcoaceticus* osteomyelitis in military personnel with battlefield injuries that occurred while serving in the Middle East.[110,111] These gram-negative bacteria have shown multidrug resistance against the commercially available antibiotic-impregnated (vancomycin, gentamycin, tobramycin) bone void fillers and coated implants. However, clinical studies have shown sensitivity to

colistin and imipenem.[110,111] Currently, the murine transtibial model on osteomyelitis with isolates of *A baumannii-calcoaceticus* from soldiers is being used to investigate gentamycin- and colistin-impregnated beads that are effective against both gram-positive and gram-negative bacteria.

## Summary

In the *New England Journal of Medicine*, Atul Gwande of the Harvard School of Public Health writes, "The nation's military surgical teams are under tremendous pressure, but they have performed remarkably in this war. They have transformed the strategy for the treatment of war casualties. They have saved the lives of an unprecedented 90% of the soldiers wounded in battle. And they have done so under extraordinarily difficult conditions and with heroic personal sacrifices."[85] This markedly improved survival of service personnel who have been wounded in action has resulted in greater orthopaedic reconstructive challenges than encountered in previous conflicts. Although the treatment of musculoskeletal war wounds pose some of the most difficult treatment challenges faced by military orthopaedic surgeons, techniques of optimal care continue to evolve.[112] Because many of the injured are young, physically fit men and women with long life expectancies, it is hoped that new research will provide enhanced opportunities for orthopaedic surgeons to restore optimal function to these wounded service members.

## References

1. US Department of Defense Website. DefenseLINK US Casualty Status. Available at: http://www.defenselink. mil/news/casualty.pdf. Accessed April 5, 2007.

2. Covey DC: Combat orthopaedics: A view from the trenches. *J Am Acad Orthop Surg* 2006;14:S10-S17.

3. Frykberg ER: Medical management of disasters and mass casualties from terrorist bombings: How can we cope? *J Trauma* 2002;53:201-212.

4. Rand: Infrastructure, Safety, and Environment Website. RAND MIPT Terrorism Incident Database Project. Available at: http://www.rand.org/ise/ projects/terrorismdatabase. Accessed March 12, 2007.

5. Kluger Y: Bomb explosions in acts of terrorism: Detonation, wound ballistics, triage and medical concerns. *Isr Med Assoc J* 2003;5:235-240.

6. Mallonee S, Shariat S, Stennies G, et al: Physical injuries and fatalities resulting from the Oklahoma City bombing. *JAMA* 1996;276:382-387.

7. The CBC Website. The Halifax Explosion. Available at: http://www.cbc. ca/halifaxexplosion. Accessed June 15, 2005.

8. National Archives of Canada Website: Tragedy on the home front: Halifax

explosion-6 December, 1917. Available at: http://www.collectionscanada. ca/education/firstworldwar/0518020 2/0518020203_e.html. National Archives of Canada, RG 24, series D-1-a, vol. 5634, file 37-25-1, part 1. Accessed July 11, 2007.

9. Howell P: The Explosion Website: Available at: http://www.chron.com/ content/chronicle/metropolitan/ txcity/index.html.

10. Ciraulo DL, Frykberg ER, Feliciano DV, et al: A survey assessment of the level of preparedness for domestic terrorism and mass casualty incidents among Eastern Association for the Surgery of Trauma Members. *J Trauma* 2004;56:1033-1041.

11. Stuhmiller JH, Phillips Y, Richmond D: The physics and mechanisms of primary blast injury, in Bellamy R, Zajtchuk R (eds): *Textbook of Military Medicine: Conventional Warfare: Ballistic, Blast and Burn Injuries*. Washington, DC, US Government Printing Office, 1991, pp 241-270.

12. Hull JB: Blast: Injury patterns and their recording. *J Audiov Media Med* 1992;15:121-127.

13. Mayorga MA: The pathology of primary blast overpressure injury. *Toxicology* 1997;121:17-28.

14. Leibovici D, Gofrit ON, Stein M, et al: Blast injuries: Bus versus open-air bombings: A comparative study of injuries in survivors of open-air versus confined-space explosions. *J Trauma* 1996;41:1030-1035.

15. Katz E, Ofek B, Adler J, et al: Primary blast injury after a bomb explosion in a civilian bus. *Ann Surg* 1988;209: 484-488.

16. Gans L, Kennedy T: Management of unique clinical entities in disaster medicine. *Emerg Med Clin North Am* 1996;14:301-326.

17. Caseby NG, Porter MF: Blast injuries to the lungs: Clinical presentation, management and course. *Injury* 1976; 8:1-12.

18. Maynard RL, Cooper GJ, Scott R: Mechanism of injury in bomb blasts and explosions, in Westby S (ed):

*Trauma: Pathogenesis and Treatment*. London, England, Heinemann, 1988, pp 30-41.

19. Coppel DL: Blast injury of the lungs. *Br J Surg* 1976;63:735-737.

20. Jönsson A, Arvebo E, Schantz B: Intrathoracic pressure variations in an anthropomorphic dummy exposed to air blast, blunt impact, and missiles. *J Trauma* 1988;28(suppl 1):S131-S135.

21. Irwin RJ, Lerner MR, Bealer JF, Brackett DJ, Tuggle DW: Cardiopulmonary physiology of primary blast injury. *J Trauma* 1997;43:650-655.

22. Stuhmiller JH: Biological response to blast overpressure: A summary of modeling. *Toxicology* 1997;121:91-103.

23. Harmon JW, Sampson JA, Graeber GM, et al: Readily available serum markers fail to aid in diagnosis of blast injury. *J Trauma* 1988;28:S153-S159.

24. Hull JB, Cooper GJ: Pattern and mechanism of traumatic amputation by explosive blast. *J Trauma* 1996;40: S198-S205.

25. Leibner ED, Weil Y, Gross E, et al: A broken bone without a fracture: Traumatic foreign bone implantation resulting from a mass casualty bombing. *J Trauma* 2005;58:388-390.

26. Boehm TM, James JJ: The medical response to the La Belle Disco bombing in Berlin 1986. *Mil Med* 1988;153: 235-238.

27. Ciraulo DL, Frykberg ER: The surgeon and acts of civilian terrorism: Blast injuries. *J Am Coll Surg* 2006; 203:942-950.

28. Department of Defense Website. DoD Personnel and Procurement Statistics. Directorate for Information and Reports. Available at: http:// siadapp.dmdc.osd.mil. Accessed July 11, 2007.

29. The Physics Behind Air Bags and Crumple Zones. Available at: www. k12.nf.ns/gc/Science/Physics3204/ Projects2003/SlotA/ProjectA2/ link20.htm. Accessed July 11, 2007.

30. Smith RM, Giannoudis PV: Trauma and the immune response. *J R Soc*

*Med* 1998;91:417-420.

31. Bone LB, Johnson KD, Weigelt J, Scheinberg R: Early versus delayed stabilization of femoral fractures: A prospective randomized study. *J Bone Joint Surg Am* 1989;71:336-340.

32. Baker SP, O'Neill B, Haddon W, et al: The injury severity score: A method for describing patients with multiple injuries and evaluation of emergency care. *J Trauma* 1974;14: 187-196.

33. *Surface Ship Survivability: Naval War Publication.* Washington, DC, Department of Defense, 1996, pp 20-31.

34. Rotondo MF, Schwab CW, McGonigal MD, et al: Damage control: An approach for improved survival in exsanguinating penetrating abdominal trauma. *J Trauma* 1993;35:375-382.

35. Eiseman B, Moore EE, Meldrum DR, Raeburn C: Feasibility of damage control surgery in combat casualties. *Arch Surg* 2000;135:1323-1327.

36. Giannoudis PV: Surgical priorities in damage control in polytrauma. *J Bone Joint Surg Br* 2003;85:478-483.

37. Pape HC, Giannoudis P, Krettek C: The timing of fracture treatment in polytrauma patients: Relevance of damage control orthopaedic surgery. *Am J Surg* 2002;183:622-629.

38. Scalea TM, Boswell SA, Scott JD, Mitchell KA, Kramer ME, Pollack AN: External fixation as a bridge to intramedullary nailing for patients with multiple injuries and with femur fractures: Damage control orthopaedics. *J Trauma* 2000;48:613-623.

39. Pape HC, Grimme K, Van Griensven M, et al: EPOFF Study Group: Impact of intramedullary instrumentation versus damage control for femoral fractures on immunoinflammatory parameters: Prospective randomized analysis by the EPOFF Study Group. *J Trauma* 2003;55:7-13.

40. Lee JC, Peitzman AB: Damage-control laparotomy. *Curr Opin Crit Care* 2006;12:346-350.

41. Chambers LW, Green DJ, Sample K, et al: Tactical surgical intervention with temporary shunting of peripheral vascular trauma sustained during Operation Iraqi Freedom: One unit's experience. *J Trauma* 2006;61: 824-830.

42. Alam HB, Burris D, DaCorta JA: Hemorrhage control in the battlefield: Role of new hemostatic agents. *Mil Med* 2005;170:63-69.

43. Alam HB, Chen Z, Jaskille A, et al: Application of a zeolite hemostatic agent achieves 100% survival in a lethal model of complex groin injury in swine. *J Trauma* 2004;56:974-983.

44. Pusateri AE, McCarthy SJ, Gregory KW, et al: The effect of a chitosan-based hemostatic dressing on blood loss and survival in a model of severe venous hemorrhage and hepatic injury in swine. *J Trauma* 2003;54: 177-182.

45. Pusateri AE, Delgado AV, Dick EJ, Martinez RS, Holcomb JB, Ryan KL: Application of a granular mineral-based hemostatic agent (QuikClot) to reduce blood loss after grade V liver injury in swine. *J Trauma* 2004;57: 555-562.

46. Bickell WH, Wall MJ, Pepe PE, et al: Immediate versus delayed fluid resuscitation for hypotensive patients with penetrating torso injuries. *N Engl J Med* 1994;331:1105-1109.

47. Sondeen JL, Coppes VG, Holcomb JB: Blood pressure at which rebleeding occurs after resuscitation in swine with aortic injury. *J Trauma* 2003;54: S110-S117.

48. Kauvar DS, Holcomb JB, Norris GC, Hess JR: Fresh whole blood transfusion: A controversial military practice. *J Trauma* 2006;61:181-184.

49. Grissom TE, Farmer JC: The provision of sophisticated critical care beyond the hospital: Lessons from physiology and military experiences that apply to civil disaster medical response. *Crit Care Med* 2005;33: S13-S21.

50. Bagg MR, Covey DC, Powell ET: Levels of medical care in the global war on terrorism. *J Am Acad Orthop Surg* 2006;14:S7-S9.

51. Venturi ML, Attinger CE, Meshabi AN, et al: Mechanisms and clinical applications of the vacuum-assisted closure (VAC) device. *Am J Clin Dermatol* 2005;6:185-194.

52. Stannard JP, Robinson JT, Anderson ER, et al: Negative pressure wound therapy to treat hematomas and surgical incisions following high energy trauma. *J Trauma* 2006;60:1301-1306.

53. Herscovici D, Sanders RW, Scaduto JM, et al: Vacuum-assisted wound closure (VAC therapy) for the management of patients with high energy soft tissue injuries. *J Orthop Trauma* 2003;17:683-688.

54. Miller Q, Bird E, Bird K, et al: Effect of subatmospheric pressure on the acute healing wound. *Curr Surg* 2004; 61:204-208.

55. Argenta LC, Morykwas MJ: Vacuum-assisted closure: A new method for wound control and treatment: clinical experience. *Ann Plast Surg* 1997;38: 563-577.

56. DeFranzo AJ, Argenta LC, Marks MW, et al: The use of vacuum-assisted closure therapy for the treatment of lower-extremity wounds with exposed bone. *Plast Reconstr Surg* 2001;108:1184-1191.

57. Joseph E, Hamori CA, Bergman S, et al: A prospective randomized trial of vacuum-assisted closure versus standard therapy of chronic nonhealing wounds. *Wounds* 2000;12:60-67.

58. Kirby JP, Fantus RJ, Ward S, et al: Novel uses of a negative-pressure wound care system. *J Trauma* 2002; 53:117-121.

59. Leininger BE, Rasmussen TE, Smith DL, Jenkins DH, Coppola C: Experience with wound vac and delayed primary closure of contaminated soft tissue injuries in Iraq. *J Trauma* 2006;61: 1207-1211.

60. Scurr JH, Machin SJ, Bailey-King S, Mackie IJ, McDonald S, Smith PD: Frequency and prevention of symptom-less deep venous thrombosis in long haul flights: A randomized trial. *Lancet* 2001;357:1485-1489.

61. United States Transportation Command (USTRANSCOM)/Global Patient Movement Requirement Center (GPMRC) data, provided by United States Central Command (CENTCOM), From: https://www.transcom.smil.mil/getfiles/j3/tccc_update/tccc_update.ppt.

62. Fackler ML: Wound ballistics: A review of common misconceptions. *JAMA* 1988;259:2730-2736.

63. Bruder SP, Kraus KH, Goldberg VM, Kadiyala S: The effect of implants loaded with autologous mesenchymal stem cells on the healing of canine segmental bone defects. *J Bone Joint Surg Am* 1998;80:985-996.

64. Govender S, Csimma C, Genant HK, et al: Recombinant human bone morphogenetic protein-2 for treatment of open tibial fractures: A prospective, controlled, randomized study of four hundred patients. *J Bone Joint Surg Am* 2002;84:2123-2134.

65. Hernigou P, Poignard A, Beaujean F, Rouard H: Percutaneous autologous bone-marrow grafting for nonunions: Influence of the number and concentration of progenitor cells. *J Bone Joint Surg Am* 2005;87:1430-1437.

66. Swiontkowski MF, Aro HT, Donnell S, et al: Recombinant human bone morphogenetic protein-2 in open tibial fractures: A subgroup analysis of data combined from two prospective randomized studies. *J Bone Joint Surg Am* 2006;88:1258-1265.

67. Peng H, Wright V, Usas A, et al: Synergistic enhancement of bone formation and healing by stem cell-expressed VEGF and bone morphogenetic protein-4. *J Clin Invest* 2002;110:751-759.

68. Liu TS, Weiss KR, Fu FH, Huard J: Gene therapy and tissue engineering in orthopaedic surgery. *Instr Course Lect* 2006;55:597-611.

69. Betz OB, Betz VM, Nazarian A, et al: Direct percutaneous gene delivery to enhance healing of bone defects. *J Bone Joint Surg Am* 2006;88:355-365.

70. Isogai N, Landis W, Kim TH, Gerstenfeld LC, Upton J, Vacanti JP: Formation of phalanges and small joints by tissue-engineering. *J Bone Joint Surg Am* 1999;81:306-316.

71. Vacanti CA, Bonassar LJ, Vacanti MP, Shufflebarger J: Replacement of an avulsed phalanx with tissue-engineered bone. *N Engl J Med* 2001;344:1511-1514.

72. Kuntscher MV, Erdmann D, Homann HH, Steinau H, Levin SL, Germann G: The concept of Fillet flaps: Classification, indications, and analysis of their clinical value. *Plast Reconstr Surg* 2001;108:885-896.

73. Levin LS, Aponte RL: The use of spare parts in surgery of the hand. *Atlas Hand Clinics (Saunders)* 1998;3:235-251.

74. Wang HT, Fletcher JW, Erdmann DE, Levin LS: Use of the anterolateral thigh free flap for upper extremity reconstruction. *J Hand Surg Am* 2005;30:859-864.

75. Touam C, Rostoucher P, Bhatia A, Oberlin C: Comparative study of two series of distally based fasciocutaneous flaps for coverage of the lower one-fourth of the leg, the ankle, and the foot. *Plast Reconstr Surg* 2001;107:383-392.

76. Bocchi A, Merelli S, Morellini A, et al: Reverse fasciosubcutaneous flap versus distally pedicled sural island flap: two elective methods for distal-third leg reconstruction. *Ann Plast Surg* 2000;45:284-291.

77. Dougherty PJ, Carter PR, Seligson D, Benson DR, Purvis JM: Orthopaedic surgery advances resulting from World War II. *J Bone Joint Surg Am* 2004;86:176-181.

78. Colihan J: Military medicine, in *American Heritage*. New York, NY, Forbes, 1984, vol 35, pp 65-77.

79. Blaisdell FW: Medical advances during the Civil War. *Arch Surg* 1988;123:1045-1050.

80. Helling TS, Daon E: In Flanders fields: the Great War, Antoine Depage, and the resurgence of debridement. *Ann Surg* 1998;228:173-181.

81. Holder VL: From handmaiden to right hand: World War I and advancements in medicine. *AORN J* 2004;80:911-923.

82. Hardaway RM: Wound shock: A history of its study and treatment by military surgeons. *Mil Med* 2004;169:265-269.

83. Kovaric JJ, Matsumoto T, Dobek AS, Hamit HF: Bacterial flora of one hundred and twelve combat wounds. *Mil Med* 1968;133:622-624.

84. Lin DL, Kirk KL, Murphy KP, McHale KA, Doukas WC: Evaluation of orthopaedic injuries in Operation Enduring Freedom. *J Orthop Trauma* 2004;18:S48-S53.

85. Gawande A: Casualties of war: Military care for the wounded from Iraq and Afghanistan. *N Engl J Med* 2004;351:2471-2475.

86. Murray CK, Reynolds JC, Schroeder JM, Harrison MB, Evans OM, Hospenthal DR: Spectrum of care provided at an echelon II medical unit during Operation Iraqi Freedom. *Mil Med* 2005;170:516-520.

87. Murray CK, Roop SA, Hospenthal DR, et al: Bacteriology of war wounds at the time of injury. *Mil Med* 2006;171:826-829.

88. Johnson EN, Burns TC, Hayda RA, Hospenthal DR, Murray CK: Infectious complications of open type III tibial fractures among combat casualties. *Clin Infect Dis* 2007;45:409-415.

89. Centers for Disease Control and Prevention (CDC): Acinetobacter baumannii infections among patients at military medical facilities treating injured U.S. service members, 2002-2004. *MMWR Morb Mortal Wkly Rep* 2004;53:1063-1066.

90. Allen DM, Hartman BJ: Acinetobacter species, in Mandell GL, Bennett JE, Dolin R (eds): *Mandell, Douglas, and Bennett's Principles and Practice of Infectious Diseases*. Philadelphia, PA, Churchill Livingstone, 2000, vol 2, pp 2339-2344.

91. Davis KA, Moran KA, McAllister CK, Gray PJ: Multidrug-resistant Acinetobacter extremity infections in sol-

diers. *Emerg Infect Dis* 2005;11:1218-1224.

92. Murray CK, Hospenthal DR: Treatment of multidrug resistant Acinetobacter. *Curr Opin Infect Dis* 2005;18:502-506.

93. Albrecht MC, Griffith ME, Murray CK, et al: Impact of Acinetobacter infection on the mortality of burn patients. *J Am Coll Surg* 2006;203:546-550.

94. Oncul O, Keskin O, Acar HV, et al: Hospital-acquired infections following the 1999 Marmara earthquake. *J Hosp Infect* 2002;51:47-51.

95. Kanafani ZA, Kara L, Hayek S, Kanj SS: Ventilator-associated pneumonia at a tertiary-care center in a developing country: Incidence, microbiology, and susceptibility patterns of isolated microorganisms. *Infect Control Hosp Epidemiol* 2003;24:864-869.

96. Rotimi VO, al-Sweih NA, Feteih J: The prevalence and antibiotic susceptibility pattern of gram-negative bacterial isolates in two ICUs in Saudi Arabia and Kuwait. *Diagn Microbiol Infect Dis* 1998;30:53-59.

97. Garzoni C, Emonet S, Legout L, et al: Atypical infections in tsunami survivors. *Emerg Infect Dis* 2005;11:1591-1593.

98. Levin AS, Mendes CM, Sinto SI, et al: An outbreak of multiresistant Acinetobacter baumanii in a university hospital in Sao Paulo, Brazil. *Infect Control Hosp Epidemiol* 1996;17:366-368.

99. Lortholary O, Fagon JY, Buu Hoi A, Mahieu G, Gutmann L: Colonization by Acinetobacter baumanii in intensive-care-unit patients. *Infect Control Hosp Epidemiol* 1998;19:188-190.

100. Velmahos GC, Jindal A, Chan L, et al: Prophylactic antibiotics after severe trauma: More is not better. *Int Surg* 2001;86:176-183.

101. Velmahos GC, Toutouzas KG, Sarkisyan G, et al: Severe trauma is not an excuse for prolonged antibiotic prophylaxis. *Arch Surg* 2002;137:537-541.

102. Daum RS, Davis WH, Farris KB, Campeau RJ, Mulvihill DM, Shane SM: A model of Staphylococcus aureus bacteremia, septic arthritis, and osteomyelitis in chickens. *J Orthop Res* 1990;8:804-813.

103. Rissing JP, Buxton TB, Weinstein RS, Shockley RK: Model of experimental chronic osteomyelitis in rats. *Infect Immun* 1985;47:581-586.

104. Passl R, Muller C, Zielinski CC, Eibl MM: A model of experimental post-traumatic osteomyelitis in guinea pigs. *J Trauma* 1984;24:323-326.

105. Worlock P, Slack R, Harvey L, Mawhinney R: An experimental model of post-traumatic osteomyelitis in rabbits. *Br J Exp Pathol* 1988;69:235-244.

106. Varshney AC, Singh H, Gupta RS, Singh SP: Experimental model of staphylococcal osteomyelitis in dogs. *Indian J Exp Biol* 1989;27:816-819.

107. Kaarsemaker S, Walenkamp GH, vd Bogaard AE: New model for chronic osteomyelitis with Staphylococcus aureus in sheep. *Clin Orthop Relat Res* 1997;339:246-252.

108. Darouiche RO: Treatment of infections associated with surgical implants. *N Engl J Med* 2004;350:1422-1429.

109. Li D, Gromov K, Awad H, O'Keefe RJ, Drissi H, Schwarz EM: Anti-catabolic therapy exacerbates osteomyelitis without altering humoral immunity. *J Bone Miner Res* 2006;21:S37.

110. Davis KA, Moran KA, McAllister CK, Gray PJ: Multidrug-resistant Acinetobacter extremity infections in soldiers. *Emerg Infect Dis* 2005;11:1218-1224.

111. Murray CK, Hospenthal DR: Treatment of multidrug resistant Acinetobacter. *Curr Opin Infect Dis* 2005;186:502-506.

112. Covey DC: Blast and fragment injuries of the musculoskeletal system. *J Bone Joint Surg Am* 2002;84:1221-1234.

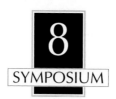
# From Iraq Back to Iraq: Modern Combat Orthopaedic Care

*COL Roman A. Hayda, MD, MC, USA

CDR Michael T. Mazurek, MD, MC, USN

Col Elisha T. Powell IV, MD, MC, USAF

Col Mark W. Richardson, MD, MC, USAF

LTC H. Michael Frisch, MD, MC, USA

LTC Romney C. Andersen, MD, MC, USA

COL James R. Ficke, MD, MC, USA

## Abstract

*War wounds are often large and complex, with high degrees of contamination and tissue loss differing significantly from typical civilian injuries. Infection has been a common complication driving the tenets of care, even in the antibiotic age. Fractures were historically treated with casting or traction because of the risk of infection with internal fixation. However, current civilian fracture care has evolved significantly with extensive use of internal and external fixation with early mobilization and other adjuncts to restore function earlier and more completely. Whether the application of modern techniques and implants can better restore function in patients with these severe injuries is currently being evaluated.*

**Instr Course Lect 2008;57:87-99.**

War by its very nature is associated with severe injuries and death, posing challenges to those who provide medical care. Wars have accelerated medical advances out of necessity. Concepts that form the framework of modern trauma care such as triage, evacuation, and helicopter transport evolved during military conflicts. Surgical advances such as vascular repair, plastic reconstruction, and intramedullary nailing also originated in caring for the complex wounds encountered in war, along with the concepts of wound débridement and use of cleansing solutions.[1] The current global war on terrorism, encompassing Operation Enduring Freedom in Afghanistan and Operation Iraqi Freedom in Iraq, has been no exception in its capacity to produce serious injury and push the envelope of surgical care.

Statistics from 2006 show that there have been approximately 24,000 war-related injuries and 2,600 combat deaths from the fighting in Afghanistan and Iraq over a 4-year period.[2] This translates to a survival rate of more than 90%, which compares favorably with the 70% to 75% survival rates seen during World War II and the Vietnam War. Further analysis shows that the increased survival rate stems from a reduction in battlefield mortality from approximately 20% to 7.5%.[2] Several factors contribute to the enhanced rate of survival. Improved body armor and helmets better protect against high-velocity munitions. Training of medical personnel, the use of tourniquets, and advanced methods of hemorrhage control and resuscitation all play a role in improving battlefield survivability.

*★COL Roman A. Hayda, MD or the department with which he is affiliated has received research or institutional support from Stryker, Synthes, Medtronic, and Smith & Nephew.*

*Disclaimer:* The opinions or assertions contained herein are the private views of the authors and are not to be construed as official or reflecting the views of the Department of Defense or the US government. The authors are employees of the US government.

Blast munitions currently are the predominant mechanism of injury on the battlefield, causing approximately 80% of injuries sustained during combat.[3] Munitions such as improvised devices, mortars, artillery rounds, and rocket-propelled grenades are powerful devices capable of producing these severe injuries. Gunshots are associated with fewer than 20% of injuries, whereas crashes of wheeled and tracked vehicles and helicopters cause the remainder of injuries.

Enhanced survival translates to definitive care of complex injuries. An interim analysis revealed that 54% of those with war injuries have extremity wounds, with 26% of all patients with war injuries sustaining fractures.[3] These fractures are usually complex, and more than 82% are open fractures.[4] These injuries frequently involve the loss of all levels of tissue, including skin, muscle, nerve, vessels, bone, and even significant articular surface area, creating reconstructive challenges regardless of the technology and techniques available. Ongoing studies will assess the successes and challenges faced in restoring function to patients with these injuries.

The care of injuries sustained during war differs from that of civilian trauma in two aspects: (1) As stated earlier, war injuries are typically high-energy, penetrating injuries associated with contamination and tissue loss. (2) The battlefield environment requires levels (or echelons) of care, placing critical life- and limb-saving resources near the battlefield with definitive care taking place in fixed facilities away from the battle zone.

There are five levels in the current matrix of providing care. Level I takes place directly on the battlefield, where the soldier buddy or combat medic provides the critical first step in treatment. This first aid involves triage, bandaging, splinting, hemorrhage control with tourniquets and advanced hemostatic dressings, antibiotics, and low-volume fluid resuscitation. Depending on the type of injury and the tactical situation, the injured individual is evacuated by ground or helicopter to facilities providing level II or III care. Level II is usually an aid station with medical personnel, physician assistants, and physicians. A spartan surgical capability, such as the Army's Forward Surgical Team (20 personnel) or the Navy's Forward Resuscitative Surgical System, may also be in place to provide the best forward life- and limb-saving surgical care. These units are highly mobile to allow proximity to the battlefield. However, supplies and holding capacity are extremely limited. Level III consists of the combat support or combat theater hospital. This medical and surgical facility is more robust and consequently less mobile, and specialists may be available to perform more complex care. At this level, patients are prepared for transport from the combat theater. Level IV is currently represented by Landstuhl Regional Medical Center. The injured arrive by airplane, often within several days of injury. Here they are further evaluated and transported back to the United States for definitive care at a level V facility. Patients with the most complex injuries currently are treated at Walter Reed Army Medical Center, Bethesda Naval Hospital, Brooke Army Medical Center, and San Diego Naval Hospital. (More information on levels of casualty care is also available in chapter 7.) A more detailed account of care rendered at each level follows.

## Battlefield Care

Improved care of those who are wounded during combat has been directly impacted by hemorrhage control, damage control surgery (DCS), damage control orthopaedics (DCO), and the ability to rapidly evacuate patients to higher levels of care. The ability to provide the highest level of care on the battlefield has translated to increased rates of survival on the battlefield.

### Hemorrhage Control

Battlefield injuries with hemorrhage are divided into two categories: compressible and noncompressible. (More information on hemorrhage control is available in chapter 7.) Compressible hemorrhage can be controlled by mechanical means, such as direct pressure or a tourniquet, typically involving the extremity. According to data obtained during the Vietnam War, approximately 40% of soldiers who died on the battlefield as a result of exsanguination had a source of hemorrhage that was believed to have been controllable in the field.[5,6] Lakstein and associates[7] reported on a 4-year experience of the Israeli Defense Force, studying the effectiveness of tourniquets in preventing fatal limb exsanguinations on the battlefield. There were 550 battle injuries over this time period; most of these injuries (78%) were caused by blasts, and 91 tourniquets were applied. None of the 125 fatalities resulted from limb exsanguinations, and there were only 7 neurologic complications, which did not correlate with the longest tourniquet times. The authors of this study concluded that tourniquets are a safe and effective means of compressible hemorrhage control.

The US Army Institute of Surgical Research investigated the effectiveness of seven different self-applied tourniquets for battlefield use. Twenty healthy volunteers ap-

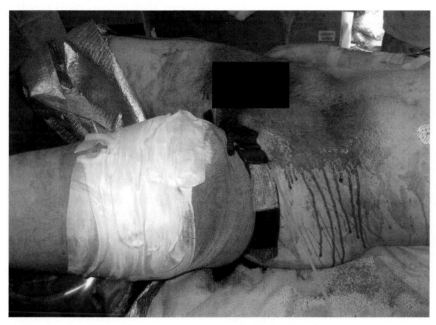

**Figure 1**   Combat application tourniquet and pressure bandage.

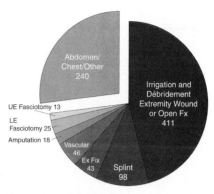

**Figure 2**   Breakdown of trauma cases at a level II facility in Al Anbar Province during Operation Iraqi Freedom II. UE, upper extremity; LE, lower extremity; Fx, fracture; Ex Fix, external fixation.

plied the tourniquets, with the goal being loss of a distal Doppler signal. Only three commercially available designs were found to obliterate Doppler flow in both the upper and lower extremity; all used either pneumatic compression or a windlass strap[8] (Figure 1). As a result, these tourniquets are currently issued to individual service members on the battlefield.

Noncompressible hemorrhage, often involving a major vessel in the groin or axilla, cannot be controlled by mechanical means. For noncompressible hemorrhage, hemostatic dressings have been developed for use on the battlefield. QuikClot (Z-Medica, Wallingford, CT) and Hemcon (HemCon Medical Technologies, Portland, OR) are currently used by US forces on the battlefield. QuikClot is derived from a biologically inert material (zeolite) that absorbs water and causes an exothermic reaction. It has been tested in a porcine model with both simulated groin wounds and grade V liver lac-

erations, demonstrating effective hemorrhage control and no mortality from exsanguination.[9-11] HemCon, derived from a natural polymer in shellfish, controls hemorrhage by adhering to the underlying tissue. It has been tested in grade V liver lacerations and severe extremity wounds and has demonstrated effectiveness in preventing exsanguinations from noncompressible hemorrhage in this model.[11-13]

## Forward Surgical Care

The earliest level of surgical capability on the battlefield is at the second level of care, where military medical units provide life- and limb-saving care as close as possible to the point of injury. These facilities, usually occupying native buildings, do not provide a sterile environment and are suited for emergency surgical stabilization and resuscitation of wounded soldiers rather than for definitive care. Forward surgical care units provide DCS and DCO.[14-16] Data obtained at a level II

facility outside Fallujah, Iraq during Operation Iraqi Freedom II (February 2004 to February 2005) show that approximately 25% of the surgeries performed there were for thoracic or abdominal trauma using damage control techniques (D Covey, MD and associates, Bravo Surgical Company Camp, Fallujah, Iraq, personal communication, 2005) (Figure 2). See chapter 7 for more information on battlefield surgery, DCS, and DCO.

## Resuscitation

Most of the trauma seen on the battlefield is penetrating and associated with significant hemorrhage. Therefore, the focus of stabilization on the battlefield is prevention of the lethal triad, a cascade of events in which the patient becomes cold (core body temperature less than 35°C) because of open body cavities and generous administration of fluids, acidotic because of hypovolemia and lactate overproduction, and then experiences coagulopathy.[17] Hypotensive resuscitation (rebleeding after clot formation at certain levels of arterial pressure)[18] and the administration of fresh whole blood are techniques

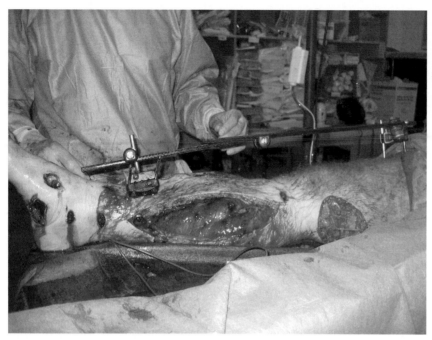

**Figure 3**   External fixation in the field.

used on the battlefield to prevent ongoing hemorrhage, metabolic derangements, and dilutional coagulopathy. See chapter 7 for more information on these techniques. After stabilization, the patient can be moved to facilities providing more advanced levels of care.

From DCS was born the concept of DCO.[19-21] The goal of DCO is to limit the physiologic insult to patients in extremis with the following strategy: hemorrhage control, débridement of contaminated and devitalized tissue, provisional stabilization (traction, splintage, or external fixation), and restoration of distal blood flow when necessary, all while maintaining the greatest number of options for definitive care (Figure 3). As the wounds are débrided and stabilized and surgical hemostasis is obtained, the extremity is evaluated for perfusion. If perfusion of the extremity does not occur because of arterial injury or a lack of outflow because of a major venous transection, the preferred

technique at this level is to place a temporary vascular shunt (a silicone tube to bypass a missing segment of a blood vessel). This technique, which can be performed by nonspecialists, rapidly restores blood flow, limits blood loss and physiologic insult, and does not require immediate transport to a facility with full vascular reconstruction capability. Recent data from a care center in Iraq demonstrated 100% patient survival with 27 temporary vascular shunts placed. Six shunts lost patency because of clot formation, and there were three ultimate amputations not related to failure of revascularization.[22]

After adequate resuscitation and stabilization with improved hemorrhage control, DCS, and DCO techniques are accomplished, patients are rapidly transported to a higher level of care.

## Aeromedical Evacuation

Following initial surgical stabilization and resuscitation, injured and ill pa-

tients are transported from the combat zone to definitive care in fixed facilities. The average time for patients to be transported to Germany and subsequently to the United States is approximately 3 days.[23] This is a great improvement from the Vietnam War, during which the average time from injury to US hospitalization was 45 days. The US military has transitioned from large hospitals located in the rear of the combat theater to smaller, more capable hospitals in the combat zone. These hospitals are located closer to the site of initial injury and are staffed by personnel with the most advanced trauma skills and latest technology. The combined effect of DCS with lighter, leaner, and life-saving trauma hospitals drives the need for rapid medical evacuation of critically ill patients across all levels of care. Injured patients are provided essential care in the combat theater, with definitive care of their complex injuries taking place in facilities in the United States. These patients require close monitoring and at times ongoing resuscitation during transport to higher levels of surgical care, providing a challenge to the care providers.

### En-Route Care

DCS is often performed by forward surgical teams in relatively austere environments (level II). These stabilized patients require rapid evacuation by rotary-wing aircraft to level III care at a combat support hospital or combat theater hospital. Transport times are generally short, usually much less than 2 hours.

This concept of care has been formalized by the US Navy with the development of the En-Route Care (ERC) Team. This two-person team consists of a critical care or emergency department-trained nurse and a medical technician. Recently, training courses for ERC nurses have been developed by the US Navy at Camp Lejeune, North Carolina. The US Army also performs this ERC mission but has no formalized ERC program at the time of this writing.

The goal of ERC is to provide uninterrupted resuscitation in critically ill ventilated patients. Results from the 1st Marine Expeditionary Force from March 2003 to August 2006 were 401 evacuees in 360 missions, with 16% requiring ERC. The mean injury severity score was 17 (range, 4 to 57), with 100% of evacuees arriving safely to the next level of care (HR Bohman, MD, personal communication, February 2007).

### Critical Care Air Transport Team

The transport of critically ill patients from level III (combat theater hospital) to level IV (Landstuhl Regional Medical Center, Germany) facilities and from level IV to V (a medical center in the United States) is the responsibility of the Air Force Critical Care Air Transport Team (CCATT). The team consists of a CCATT-trained physician, a critical care nurse, and a respiratory therapist. In addition to medical training focused on care of the critically ill surgical patient, flight physiology is a critical component of the team's training.

This team works closely with the aircraft crew chief when preparing a critically ill patient for transport. These patients are the last on the aircraft and the first to deplane. Because most air missions involve cargo or personnel transport aircraft reconfigured for patient care, issues such as patient positioning, equipment location, oxygen, and power demands are discussed with the crew chief and resolved with a team effort. Typical missions last 8 hours but at times take longer to arrive at the next level of care.[24]

The understanding of aeromedical transport requires the realization that the flight environment complicates the ability to assess the patient because of cramped space, low light, and limited patient access and has its particular physiologic stresses. Teams learn to optimize therapeutic interventions before placing the patient in the aircraft. Additionally, the stresses of flight take a toll on both the patient and caregivers. These stresses include decreased barometric pressure, decreased partial pressure of oxygen, decreased humidity, temperature fluctuations, noise, vibration, fatigue, and sometimes motion sickness. Decreased barometric pressure during flight produces potentially problematic gas expansion in the patient's hollow viscous organs. In addition, acceleration and deceleration during takeoff and landing may elevate intracranial pressures in neurosurgical patients.[25] CCATT members are trained to handle the stresses of flight both for themselves and their patients to ensure safe arrival at the next level of care. For more information on aero-evacuation of wounded patients, see chapter 7.

### Special Medical Augmentation Response Teams

The US Army Institute of Surgical Research at Brooke Army Medical Center provides expert burn care and also sends specialized burn flight teams to transport patients to the burn center. The four-person burn flight team consists of a burn critical care physician, a critical care registered nurse from the burn center, a licensed practical nurse, and a medical technician. The team carries approximately 800 lb of gear, including specialized equipment such as patient warmers, pressure cycle ventilators, bronchoscopes, and

items for burn wound care.[26] The burn flight team provides critical specialized care both before and during flight in terms of surgery, ventilation, and resuscitation to safely transport these very ill patients, successfully delivering patients with multisystem injury and burns, even those with burns involving greater than 90% of their body surface area.

Military trauma care of the wounded soldier has changed from stable patient care to critical patient care—moving sicker patients sooner rather than holding them in hospitals near or in the battlefield area. Unpublished data from the US Transportation Command Global Patient Movement Requirement Centers show that from October 2001 to December 2006 the aeromedical system has been used to transport 39,452 patients. Specialized teams have been created to transport severely ill patients after DCS. Recognizing the challenges of the aeromedical transport environment requires that surgeons perform meticulous and effective DCS to deliver a patient who is optimally stabilized for transport and ready to receive definitive care.

### Reconstruction of Complex Injuries: Successes and Challenges

On return to the United States, the most severely injured patients are treated at military medical centers across the country. On admission, a thorough head-to-toe evaluation of the extremities and axial skeleton takes place, with particular attention paid to assessing wounds and neurovascular status. Imaging studies are obtained of known injuries and suspected injuries. This is often the first opportunity for a detailed examination given the austere conditions on the battlefield and the necessity for rapid transport. Isolated injuries are the exception rather than the rule, with each patient having an average of three open wounds; 26% of open wounds are associated with a fracture, and 82% of fractures are open.[3] Once all injuries are identified, reconstructive plans are made in a multidisciplinary approach involving orthopaedic surgery to include the subspecialties of trauma, foot and ankle, hand surgery, plastic surgery, general surgery, and vascular surgery.

Wounds are frequently colonized with bacteria and require serial exploration, débridement, and irrigation to prepare for definitive stabilization. Most wounds undergo 4 to 5 serial débridements before definitive fixation, with some complex injuries and infections requiring more than 30 procedures (AT Groth, MD, Paradise Island, Bahamas, unpublished data presented at the Southern Orthopaedic Association annual meeting, 2006). Open wounds are often treated with vacuum-assisted closure dressings that provide soft-tissue edema reduction and wound granulation and potentially reduce bacterial burden.

Definitive fracture reduction and stabilization is achieved by several methods, including intramedullary rods, plate and screw fixation, multiplanar external fixation, or, in rare instances, casting. Soft-tissue coverage is achieved by several methods as well, including local or free tissue transfer, acute shortening with planned lengthening, and delayed primary closure or healing by secondary intention with the assistance of negative-pressure wound therapy.

Each of the medical centers treating a large percentage of injured patients has institutional review board–approved protocols to record patient injuries and document their care. Prospective and retrospective studies are underway to characterize these injuries and obtain outcome data on their eventual function and patients' satisfaction.

## Subtrochanteric Fracture

The constellation of injuries seen in military medical centers differs from those seen in civilian orthopaedic trauma, both in the types of fractures encountered and devastation to the soft tissues. An example of this is the open subtrochanteric fracture, an injury that is seldom seen in civilian orthopaedic trauma. A study described more than 40 open subtrochanteric femur fractures and reported that 56% were Gustilo-Anderson type IIIA fractures and 44% were type IIIB or IIIC. Types IIIB or IIIC have been associated with a 75% rate of deep infection and osteomyelitis. Nonetheless, intramedullary nailing was performed in 78% of patients. Thirty percent of infected patients required hardware removal to eradicate the infection, and no patient to date has required an amputation (AT Groth, MD, Paradise Island, Bahamas, unpublished data presented at the Southern Orthopaedic Association annual meeting, 2006).

## Tibia Fracture

A review of the combined data from the major medical centers has identified more than 300 tibia fractures.[27] In one series, 68% of fractures involving the tibia shaft were either type IIIB or IIIC (R Beer, MD, personal communication, 2006) (Figure 4). In this series, 10% of fractures were treated with intramedullary nailing, 83% with multiplanar external fixation, and 7% with plate fixation. A follow-up study of a cohort treated with tibial nailing initially revealed a 9.1% infection rate; however, as follow-up continued, that rate has risen to 18.2% (AP LaCap, MD, Honolulu HI, unpublished data presented at the Society of Military Orthopaedic Surgeons annual meeting, 2006). In another study of patients with open tibia fractures who were treated with multiplanar external fixation, there were no deep infections; however, 11% of the patients had pin tract infections (AP LaCap, MD, Honolulu HI, unpublished data presented at the Society of Military Orthopaedic Surgeons annual meeting, 2006). In a retrospective study of 32 patients with open tibia fractures treated with bone morphogenetic protein, there were only two nonunions; 88% of the fractures had radiographic union, and, most importantly, there was an infection rate of only 3% (TR Kuklo, MD, Ottawa, Canada, unpublished data presented at the Orthopaedic Trauma Association meeting, 2005).

## Segmental Radius Fracture

Reviewing the databases from major medical centers identified 10 radius fractures in which segmental bone loss had occurred. Most were treated with an autograft; however, one was treated with a free fibula graft and another with an allograft. One study reported healing in 100% of these fractures (CL Ledford, MD, unpublished data presented at the Spring Medical Surgical Behavioral Science Conference, Willingen, Germany, 2006). However, function is related to the soft-tissue injuries associated with the fracture. Segmental nerve injuries and heterotopic ossification had poorer outcomes.

## Open Elbow Fractures

Although open elbow injuries are not uncommon in civilian practice, the mix of fractures sustained during combat could be classified with higher grades of severity. One study reported that 56% of open elbow fractures were grade IIIB or IIIC, which indicates the severe nature of these injuries. In that study, 90% were treated with open reduction and internal fixation, 7% were treated by external fixation, and 7% underwent amputation. In this series, function was related to the soft-tissue injury and heterotopic ossification (K Walick, MD, Vail, CO, unpublished data presented at the Society of Military Orthopaedic Surgeons annual meeting, 2004).

## Knee Extensor Mechanism Injury

Another unique injury occurring in war is open extensor mechanism injury to the knee. Twenty of these injuries have been documented. According to a study by Andersen,[27] 60% of these fractures are grade IIIB; this level of severity results from the relatively small quantity of muscle around the knee joint. This study has not identified any reconstructed grade IIIC injuries because there is a high likelihood that such an injury would lead to amputation, primarily in the combat theater. Thirty-five percent of these injuries involved the quadriceps tendon, 41%, the patella; 65%, the patellar ligament; and 24%, the tibial tubercle. Associated fractures of the distal femur occurred in 64% of the injuries, and proximal tibia fractures were present in 59% of the patients. Reconstruction was performed in 47% of the patients, knee fusion in 29%, and transfemoral amputation in 35%. Complications in these patients were common, and outcomes tend to be related to the amount of soft-tissue damage and associated fractures. Patients with isolated soft-tissue injuries to the patellar ligament or quadriceps tendon fared much better than those with fracture involvement.

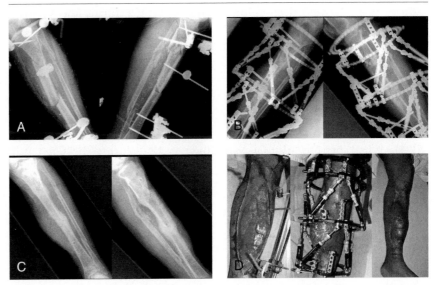

**Figure 4**    Radiographs and photographs of the lower leg of a 33-year-old soldier with a complex gradeIII B/C tibia fracture. Other injuries included an ipsilateral calcaneus fracture, and a contralateral traumatic below-knee amputation. In the combat theater, he underwent débridement, stabilization with external fixation, and vascular reconstruction (**A** and **D**). Following serial débridements, he underwent free flap coverage, bifocal multiplanar external fixation frame stabilization, and bone morphogenetic protein grafting of both sites (**B** and **D**). The hospital course was complicated by two flap infections, which were treated with débridement. He currently ambulates with a cane. **A,** Grade IIIC open tibia fracture in transportation frame. **B,** Bifocal multiplanar external fixator. **C,** Healed grade IIIB/C tibia fracture. **D,** Clinical photographs of (left to right) initial wounds, multiplanar external fixator, and healed tibia.

Significant burns are present in 5% of the treated service members (RA Hayda, MD, San Antonio, TX, unpublished data presented at the 10th Annual Trauma Symposium, 2004). Most have fractures associated with them; care of these fractures is dictated by the injury to the soft tissue. Care of the burn patient is labor intensive, and poorer outcomes are to be expected both in reconstructive surgery and amputation surgery. Wound healing complications, infection, and contractures challenge the recovery of these patients.

## Complications

Heterotopic ossification was reported in 31% of long-bone fractures in one study (S Ahmed, MD,

Phoenix, AZ, unpublished data presented at the Orthopaedic Trauma Association annual meeting, 2006). The incidence was highly correlated with hip and femur fractures as well as higher injury severity scores. Heterotopic ossification correlated negatively with grade I open fractures and tibia fractures. There was no increased incidence of burns, head injury, or vacuum-assisted closure use, although the number of patients in these subsets limits statistical analysis. Interestingly, the resected heterotopic bone demonstrated positive cultures without the patient manifesting any signs of infection.

Infection continues to be common in patients with open fractures resulting from war injuries. In a review,

60% of wounds were deep-culture positive at the time of presentation at the definitive care facility despite serial débridements and antibiotic treatment along the evacuation chain (RA Hayda, MD, San Antonio, TX, unpublished data presented at the 10th Annual Trauma Symposium, 2004). When present, *Pseudomonas* and *Klebsiella* have been exceedingly difficult to eradicate, requiring large resections. *Acinetobacter* is ubiquitous in the battlefield theater. Some of these infections are multidrug-resistant and lead to chronic infection, in which the long-term consequences are unknown. A prospective study showed that wound dehiscence highly correlates to procalcitonin levels and other cytokines in the exudate rather than wound culture or other systemic inflammatory markers (JA Forsberg, MD, Phoenix, AZ, unpublished data presented at the Academic Surgical Congress, 2007).

These examples demonstrate that reconstruction of these complex injuries is demanding and lengthy, requiring patience and persistence on the part of the surgeon, rehabilitation team, and patient. Novel solutions are often required, using the full spectrum of reconstructive techniques. When successful, excellent functional recovery may be achieved. However, certain injuries, particularly periarticular injuries, leave significant functional deficits and result in elective amputation in certain instances. Ongoing detailed analysis of long-term functional outcomes will guide optimal treatment guidelines.

## Amputation Surgery

The destructive nature of war injuries has historically led to amputation. The concept of "Centers of Excellence" for amputee care, which started during World Wars I and II and continued during the Vietnam War, has continued with the Armed Forces Amputee Patient Care Program; its three centers are in Washington, DC; San Antonio, TX; and San Diego, CA.[28-30] Historically, the percentage of amputations in patients with battle injuries has been as high as 12% during the Civil War, decreasing to 3.4% during the Vietnam War, and is presently 2.3%. As of February 2007, the total number of amputees from the conflicts in Iraq and Afghanistan is 553 among all military services. There have been 336 unilateral lower extremity amputations, 113 unilateral upper extremity amputations, 99 double amputees, and 5 triple amputees, with a total of 662 lost limbs.[31] Approximately 40% of amputees have additional fractures, significant soft-tissue injuries, or infections.

Wounds sustained on the battlefield can be severe and may require amputation. However, survival from such injuries may be enhanced with body armor and modern methods of resuscitation. In past conflicts, circular amputation above the zone of injury followed by skin traction was practiced.[32] For wounds healed by secondary intention, myodesis was not performed initially, and more than 90% required later scar revision and closure.[33] Gel liners now can be used instead of a glued stockinette, but frequent painful dressing changes are still required. The infection rate remains low, and the rate of healing is high, but so is the revision rate. Most importantly, although skin traction works, this method confines a patient to bed, resulting in deconditioning, weight gain, and isolation from other patients, delaying rehabilitation.[34]

At the start of the current global war on terrorism, a consensus panel of civilian and military experts developed the concept of open length-preserving amputation. This approach entails (1) excision of devitalized tissue and contaminants; (2) maintenance of all viable tissue to include bone, muscle, and skin for possible use in closure; (3) frequent débridement, leaving the wounds open; (4) selective fracture stabilization to preserve length; and (5) creative myodesis and skin closure to maintain maximal length at the definitive care facility in the United States.[34] Circular amputations are avoided to preserve length.

Open length-preserving amputations treated without skin traction, much like that in circular amputations, lead to soft-tissue retraction, complicating closure. The principles of skin traction can be applied to open length-preserving amputations by using vacuum-assisted closure and vessel loop skin traction (Figure 5, *A* and *B*). This method has several advantages over standard skin traction: decreased edema, maintenance of drainage, containment and isolation of the wound, support of viable muscle and skin flaps, and patient mobility. Maintaining all viable tissue for later use in creative myodesis and closure facilitates length preservation, joint preservation, and prosthetic fitting (Figure 5, *C*). Sometimes length and joint preservation involves fixation of concomitant fractures, which has been used successfully in these patients.

Although proper surgical technique is important, outcome is determined more by an aggressive and comprehensive rehabilitation program. The amputee care program is dependent on a coordinated multidisciplinary team approach to provide the highest quality of care. The amputee care program concentrates on rehabilitation, not just surgery. The rehabilitation of the amputee may take more than 1 year, as the amputee progresses through the phases of therapy to attain maximal functional recovery, and it is not defined by using a specific component or device.[34]

The four phases of physical therapy for amputees are protective healing, preprosthetic training, prosthetic training, and return to duty and progressive activities. Sports and recreation programs are critical to rehabilitation on physical, cognitive, and psychologic levels.

Crucial to the success of the amputee care program is ensuring that the amputee is not isolated and is able to benefit from the experience of the group. Peer visitors are key members of the team and crucial to success, and their presence is consistently highly rated by patients. All peer visitors are trained in the Amputee Coalition of America Peer Visitor Training program. Peer visitors often take patients out for their first meals, socialize with them, and can discuss long-term life challenges.

In past conflicts, amputees were routinely medically separated from the military without regard to their functional outcome. Unfortunately, this practice often had the underlying effect of giving the initial impression that the amputee was not capable of returning to previous levels of duty. Return to duty is now determined by function, not condition. As of February 2007, the total number of amputees who have returned to duty during the current conflicts is 30, with 7 of those having been redeployed to the combat theater.

Advances in prosthetics and prosthetic suspension also have facilitated the ability to maintain effective function with levels previously considered short or nonfunctional, in particular the short transtibial amputation. If the extensor mechanism

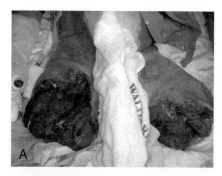
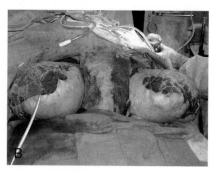
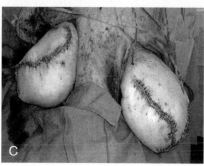

**Figure 5**  **A,** Example of bilateral high transfemoral amputation wounds. **B,** Vacuum-assisted closure vessel loop traction. **C,** Atypical closure without further shortening.

can be maintained, the knee joint should be preserved regardless of absolute length. Vacuum suspension of a microprocessor knee has also facilitated ambulation for patients with hip disarticulations.

The debate between the merits of the Ertl and Burgess transtibial amputations continues. The Ertl amputation is advocated as having a better end-bearing stump, but in the few patients who have undergone bilateral transtibial amputations with an Ertl on one side and a Burgess on the other, there has not been a difference in prosthetic fitting or rehabilitation. Currently, fibular instability is accepted as the primary indication for an Ertl amputation. Outcomes studies are currently underway to compare the two objectively. Many transtibial amputees also develop what has been termed as "auto Ertl," an unplanned synostosis from heterotopic ossification after a Burgess transtibial amputation.[35,36]

Heterotopic ossification has become one of the greatest challenges

in extremity injuries and amputations occurring during war. Although it has been sparsely reported as far back as the Civil War, heterotopic ossification was not identified as a treatment challenge in previous conflicts. Heterotopic ossification is often asymptomatic, but it can result in pain, skin breakdown, and difficulty in wearing a prosthesis. There is a clear correlation between blast injuries and amputations within the zone of injury[37] (Table 1). The exact etiology remains unknown but is believed to be multifactorial and is the focus of ongoing research.

Symptomatic heterotopic ossification can usually be treated with prosthetic modification, but those cases that require excision present multiple challenges. Areas previously skin-grafted may be adherent to the underlying heterotopic ossification, necessitating excision and alternative methods of closure and coverage. Excision also leaves a large cavitary dead space that is prone to the formation of a seroma or a hematoma and infec-

**Table 1**
**Heterotopic Ossification Distribution in Amputees**

| Heterotopic Ossification Amount | Mild | Moderate/Severe |
|---|---|---|
| All amputations (213) | 63% | 34% |
| **Blast injury** | | |
| Amputation in zone of injury (147) | 55% | 45% |
| Amputation above injury (40) | 13% | 3% |
| **Nonblast injury** | | |
| Amputation in zone of injury (20) | 30% | 25% |
| Amputation above injury (6) | 0% | 0% |

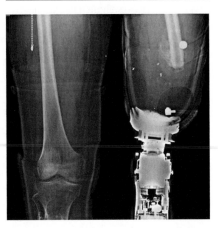

**Figure 6** Limb prosthesis malalignment after adductor myodesis failure demonstrated in a standing radiograph.

tion. Local tissues do not rotate easily into the void, and tissue transfers may be necessary. Care must be taken both preoperatively and intraoperatively because neurovascular structures may be encompassed by heterotopic ossification.

Another challenge is myodesis failure, which can result in pain, bone prominence, and limb prosthesis malalignment (Figure 6). Myodesis failure has been associated with inflammatory reactions to fiber wire, fiber wire eroding through bone, and subclinical infections (AW Mack, MD, Honolulu, HI, presented at the Society of Military Orthopaedic Surgeons annual meeting, 2005).

The Military Extremity Trauma Amputation and Limb Salvage Study (METALS) that is currently underway is a multicenter outcomes study comparing amputee and limb-salvage outcomes and is modeled after the Lower Extremity Assessment Project (LEAP). The METALS study will also include upper extremity injuries. In comparison with the LEAP study, military amputees in the METALS study may be more functional but also require more surgeries and have more complications. To facilitate data collection, some modifications to the Orthopaedic Trauma Association classification have been made, such as adding "X" as a type for amputations. A detailed database, the Military Or-

thopaedic Trauma Registry, will capture the injury demographics and detail the levels of tissue loss and treatment parameters.

## Future Directions
### Far Forward Casualty Care
Substantial progress has been made with respect to the development of a theaterwide trauma system. Much like the community-based trauma systems currently found in most large metropolitan centers in the United States, a system using high-volume, centralized expertise in handling severe injuries is now in place in Iraq and Afghanistan. Although the distances covered by traditional medical evacuation helicopters are significant, and far forward surgery has been battle tested and proven in active military operations, the current system is saving lives effectively. The development of centralized oversight through a theaterwide communications network has provided a timely feedback loop for further process improvement.

### Forward Echelon Surgery
Wound excision and débridement principles are effective but remain subjective with some variation in application. The future in this area rests with the widespread education and dissemination of information to maximize effectiveness and minimize variation. To this end, the Ex-

tremity War Injuries Symposium in January 2007 convened to initiate formal clinical treatment principles and then publish consensus-based protocols in a variety of formats. A growing body of experience, including higher evidence-level studies, is available and will need to be expanded to support formal guidelines. Currently, the American Academy of Orthopaedic Surgeons and the Orthopaedic Trauma Association have collaborated extensively with surgeons in the US Army, Navy, and Air Force with extensive combat and trauma experience to develop, record, and disseminate these principles.

### Evacuation
The previous section describing the current status of evacuation from the combat theater to definitive care facilities in the United States demonstrates the rapid transport of injured military personnel to appropriate care facilities and the potential for improved wound care, closure, and limb reconstruction. With CCATT, wounded patients can be sent from a forward facility to the highest level intensive care units in

the United States within 2 days. This has opened a completely new arena with respect to immediate perioperative analgesia, the potential for in-flight negative-pressure wound therapy management, and an investigation of the impact of altitude on the progression of zones of injury. Current flight testing of airworthy pain pumps and negative-pressure dressings is underway. See chapter 7 for more information on negative-pressure wound management.

### Limb Salvage

Advances in limb stabilization, free tissue transfer, and bone graft substitutes, as well as development of osteoinductive materials to facilitate management of massive segmental bone and soft-tissue loss, are being used to improve rates of limb salvage. In spite of often devastating injuries, return to function is possible. Future study to ascertain predictors of best practices and decision making in limb salvage versus amputation is needed. The METALS project is a step toward this end. This area may well be one of the most significant toward translation of military experience to civilian injury care.

### Amputee Care

The concept of establishing centers of excellence in limb-loss management is not new. The effort currently lies in an advancement of prosthetic design, high return to duty rate relative to all previous conflicts, and maintenance of the lowest possible amputation level. As previously discussed, this practice has led to new challenges involving heterotopic ossification, soft-tissue coverage, and advanced rehabilitation. Future development of prosthetic design is driven by the patient's culture of expectation; many patients

find they can run, climb, drive, and meet many of their previous physical goals. Additionally, existing outcomes measures demonstrate a "ceiling effect," whereby a disproportionate percentage of patients reach maximal outcomes and therefore may actually be doing better than these measures are capable of recording.

An exciting glimpse into the future for amputee rehabilitation can be observed at the Army's new Center for the Intrepid, a 65,000 square foot advanced facility in San Antonio, alongside Brooke Army Medical Center. The Center for the Intrepid was a gift through work by the Fisher Foundation and over 600,000 donations. This center, caring for limb-salvage, burn, and limb-loss patients from the military, has the goal of providing the most advanced rehabilitation and comprehensive care available. This outpatient facility includes rehabilitation and surgical experts and a comprehensive care team to maximize functional outcome. The facility houses an elaborate motion performance laboratory, a virtual reality computer-aided rehabilitation environment, driving simulator, firearm simulator, daily living skills apartment, and aquatics system. The center, which opened in January 2007, promises to become one of the world's foremost rehabilitation facilities.

## Research

The future direction for the care of injured military personnel depends on the accurate and objective collection of the multitude of lessons learned in recent military conflicts. Previous wars have led to advances in surgical care, and the Iraq and Afghanistan conflicts should be no exception. The potential for a prospective, longitudinal study is enormous

and should not to be ignored. In January 2006, collaborators in the first Extremity War Injury Symposium developed a list of research priorities. Congress provided substantial funding through the Orthopaedic Trauma Research Program, and the first panel, in July 2006, approved funding of 14 proposals within the priority areas (Table 2). These projects include military and civilian investigators from all aspects of clinical, translational, and industrial research. Several projects are now underway, and the second Extremity War Injury Symposium confirmed the need for continued investigation and the development of clinical practice principles.

One of the primary areas of interest identified in the initial Extremity War Injury Symposium was the development of a reliable trauma registry, specifically including extremity injuries and details specific to these injuries. The Institute of Surgical Research is working to include a comprehensive registry of all extremity injuries sustained to date, and for all future injuries, based on existing classification standards. This Military Orthopaedic Trauma Registry is intended to allow long-term data collection and access to information as required by researchers. Similar to the Joint Theater Trauma Registry, this will also be accessible through data-sharing agreements and available for investigations.

### Amputee Research

Research into the optimal management of patients with limb loss will focus on developing adaptive prostheses and improving the evaluation of outcomes. As technology and prosthetic manufacturing improves, so must the tools used for patient assessment. To this end, congressionally-mandated amputee research will focus on outcomes measures, pain

**Table 2**
**Orthopaedic Trauma Research Program (OTRP)**

| OTRP Priorities 2006 | OTRP-Funded Proposals 2006 |
|---|---|
| Data collection systems/registry | Mechanisms of heterotopic ossification |
| Timing of treatment | Prevention/treatment of heterotopic ossification |
| Techniques of débridement | Improved outcomes of high-energy contaminated wounds |
| Patient transportation issues | Development of an anti-infective acute wound care gel |
| Wound coverage | Cellular therapy to obtain rapid bone formation |
| Antibiotic treatment | Controlled delivery of growth factors for segmental defects |
| Management of segmental bone defects | Adipose-derived stem cells for the treatment of large bone defects |
| Development of an animal model of complex blast injury | Bone formation in infected segmental defects with bone morphogenetic proteins |
| Amputee issues | Modification of animal osteomyelitis model to simulate war extremity wounds |
| Heterotopic ossification | Expanded options with antibiotic bone cement |
| | Serum markers: predictors of war wound infections |
| | Three studies of *Acinetobacter*-related osteomyelitis |

management, prevention, and treatment of complications such as heterotopic ossification, infections, and limb-socket interface adaptability. The future may see integration of prostheses directly to the patient, or reinnervation of specific muscles to improve myoelectric function. The actual development of these high technology prostheses, in a manner that makes them affordable and widely accessible, is required if long-term use is to be ensured.

## Summary

Injuries sustained in combat are severe and complex, often involving all levels of tissue loss. The care of these injuries has required the selective use of new techniques and technologies to obtain maximal recovery for injured patients. The unprecedented survival rate is related to protective measures and implementation of sophisticated treatment methods on the battlefield applied by highly trained medical personnel. In the combat the-

ater, hemorrhage control, DCS, thorough débridement, and temporary stabilization prepare patients for transport. Definitive care of complex injuries and amputations in stateside facilities use the most current techniques applied by a multidisciplinary team. This process is often lengthy but attempts to restore maximal function despite the complexity of the injury. Through the professional and dedicated service of all those involved in the treatment process, soldiers are afforded optimal opportunity to continue military service if they desire.

Comprehensive research of broad topics, as well as specific injury patterns and treatment algorithms, largely lacking in previous conflicts, will provide information critical to improving the care of injured soldiers. This information is likely to improve the care of complex injuries seen in the civilian sector, whether they result from disasters, terrorist acts, high-energy vehicle crashes, or industrial accidents. Through the continued col-

laboration of the military and civilian sectors, medical and surgical advances can be made for the benefit of all.

## References

1. Noe A: Extremity injury in war: A brief history. *J Am Acad Orthop Surg* 2006;14:S1-S6.

2. Department of Defense Website. Statistical Information Analysis Division, DoD Personnel and Procurement Statistics. Available at: http://siadapp.dmdc.osd.mil/personnel/CASUALTY/castop.htm. Accessed October 17, 2007.

3. Owens BD, Kragh JF Jr, Wenke JC, Macaitis J, Wade CE, Holcomb JB: Combat wounds in Operation Iraqi Freedom and Operation Enduring Freedom. *J Trauma*, in press.

4. Owens BD, Kragh JF Jr, Macaitis J, Svoboda SJ, Wenke JC: Characterization of extremity wounds in Operation Iraqi Freedom and Operation Enduring Freedom. *J Orthop Trauma* 2007;21:254-257.

5. *Joint Technical Coordinating Group for Mutations Effective Evaluation of Wound Data and Munitions Effectiveness in Vietnam (WDMEV), Vol I of III: Final report, December 1970.* Alexandria, VA, Defense Technical Information Center (AD879516), 1970.

6. Alam HB, Burris D, DaCorta JA, Rhee P: Hemorrhage control in the battlefield: Role of new hemostatic agents. *Mil Med* 2005;170:63-69.

7. Lakstein D, Blumenfeld A, Sokolov T, et al: Tourniquets for hemorrhage control on the battlefield: A 4-year accumulated experience. *J Trauma* 2003;54(suppl 5):S221-S225.

8. Walters TJ, Wenke JC, Kauvar DS, McManus JG, Holcomb JB, Baer DG: Effectiveness of self-applied tourniquets in human volunteers. *Prehosp Emerg Care* 2005;9:416-422.

9. Alam HB, Chen Z, Jaskille A, et al: Application of a zeolite hemostatic agent achieves 100% survival in a lethal model of complex groin injury in

swine. *J Trauma* 2004;56:974-983.

10. Pusateri AE, Delgado AV, Dick EJ, Martinez RS, Holcomb JB, Ryan KL: Application of a granular mineral-based hemostatic agent (QuikClot) to reduce blood loss after grade V liver injury in swine. *J Trauma* 2004;57: 555-562.

11. Acheson EM, Kheirabadi BS, Deguzman R, Dick EJ Jr, Holcomb JB: Comparison of hemorrhage control agents applied to lethal extremity arterial hemorrhages in swine. *J Trauma* 2005;59:865-874.

12. Kheirabadi BS, Acheson EM, Deguzman R, et al: Hemostatic efficacy of two advanced dressings in an aortic hemorrhage model in swine. *J Trauma* 2005;59:25-34.

13. Pusateri AE, McCarthy SJ, Gregory KW, et al: The effect of a chitosan-based hemostatic dressing on blood loss and survival in a model of severe venous hemorrhage and hepatic injury in swine. *J Trauma* 2003;54: 177-182.

14. *Surface Ship Survivability: Naval War Publication.* Washington DC, Department of Defense, 1996, vol 3, pp 20-31.

15. Rotondo MF, Schwab CW, McGonigal MD, et al: Damage control: An approach for improved survival in exsanguinating penetrating abdominal trauma. *J Trauma* 1993;35:375-382.

16. Eiseman B, Moore EE, Meldrum DR, Raeburn C: Feasibility of damage control surgery in combat casualties. *Arch Surg* 2000;135:1323-1327.

17. Lee JC, Peitzman AB: Damage-control laparotomy. *Curr Opin Crit Care* 2006;12:346-350.

18. Bickell WH, Wall MJ, Pepe PE, et al: Immediate versus delayed fluid resuscitation for hypotensive patients with penetrating torso injuries. *N Engl J Med* 1994;331:1105-1109.

19. Giannoudis PV: Surgical priorities in damage control in polytrauma. *J Bone Joint Surg Br* 2003;85:478-483.

20. Pape HC, Giannoudis P, Krettek C: The timing of fracture treatment in polytrauma patients: Relevance of damage control orthopaedic surgery. *Am J Surg* 2002;183:622-629.

21. Scalea TM, Boswell SA, Scott JD, Mitchell KA, Kramer ME, Pollack AN: External fixation as a bridge to intramedullary nailing for patients with multiple injuries and with femur fractures: Damage control orthopaedics. *J Trauma* 2000;48:613-623.

22. Chambers LW, Green DJ, Sample K, et al: Tactical surgical intervention with temporary shunting of peripheral vascular trauma sustained during Operation Iraqi Freedom: One unit's experience. *J Trauma* 2006;61: 824-830.

23. Bagg MR, Covey DC, Powell ET: Levels of medical care in the global war on terrorism. *J Am Acad Orthop Surg* 2006;14(suppl 10):S7-S9.

24. Grissom TE, Farmer JC: The provision of sophisticated critical care beyond the hospital: Lessons from physiology and military experiences that apply to civil disaster medical response. *Crit Care Med* 2005;33: S13-S21.

25. Air Force e-Publishing Website. Air Force Instruction 41-307: Aeromedical Evacuation Patient Considerations and Standards of Care. August 20, 2003. Available at: www.e-publishing.af.mil. Accessed December 2007.

26. Cancio LC, Horvath EE, Barillo DJ, et al: Burn support for Operation Iraqi Freedom and related operations, 2003 to 2004. *J Burn Care Rehabil* 2005;26:151-161.

27. Andersen R: From Iraq: Back to Iraq: Modern combat orthopaedic care: Reconstruction of complex injuries. Success and challenges. *74th Annual Meeting Proceedings.* Rosemont, IL, American Academy of Orthopaedic Surgeons, 2007, pp 319-323.

28. Bowker JH, Pritham CH: The history of amputations and prosthetics, in Smith DG, Michael JW, Bowker JH (eds): *Atlas of Amputations and Limb Deficiencies,* ed 3. Rosemont, IL, American Academy of Orthopaedic Surgeons, 2004, pp 3-20.

29. Peterson LT: Amputations, in Mullins WS, Cleveland M, Shands AR Jr (eds): *Surgery in World War II: Orthopaedic Surgery in the Zone of the Interior.* Washington, DC, Office of the Surgeon General, Department of the Army, 1970, pp 849-1014.

30. Mayfield GW, Brown PW: Vietnam War amputees and rehabilitation of the combat-wounded amputee, in Burkhalter WE (ed): *Surgery in Vietnam: Orthopedic Surgery.* Washington, DC, US Government Printing Office, 1994, pp 131-153,189-207.

31. Potter BK, Scoville CR: Amputation is not isolated: An overview of the US Army Amputee Patient Care Program and associated amputee injuries. *J Am Acad Orthop Surg* 2006;14:S188-S190.

32. Dougherty PJ: Wartime amputee care, in Smith DG, Michael JW, Bowker JH (eds): *Atlas of Amputations and Limb Deficiencies,* ed 3. Rosemont, IL, American Academy of Orthopaedic Surgeons, 2004, pp 77-97.

33. Hampton OP: Amputations, in Coates JB, Cleveland M (eds): *Surgery in World War II: Orthopaedic Surgery in the Mediterranean Theater of Operations.* Washington, DC, Office of the Surgeon General, Department of the Army, 1957, pp 245-270.

34. Gajewski D, Granville RR: The United States Armed Forces Amputee Patient Care Program. *J Am Acad Orthop Surg* 2006;14:S183-S187.

35. Dougherty PJ: Transtibial amputees from the Vietnam War: Twenty-eight-year follow-up. *J Bone Joint Surg Am* 2001;83:383-389.

36. Bowker JK: Transtibial amputation: Surgical management, in Smith DG, Michael JW, Bowker JH (eds): *Atlas of Amputation and Limb Deficiencies,* ed 3. Rosemont, IL, American Academy of Orthopaedic Surgeons, 2004, pp 481-501.

37. Potter BK, Burns TC, LaCap AP, Granville RR, Gajewski DA: Heterotopic ossification following traumatic and combat-related amputations. *J Bone Joint Surg Am* 2007;89:476-486.

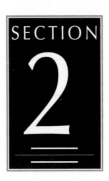

# SECTION 2

# Shoulder

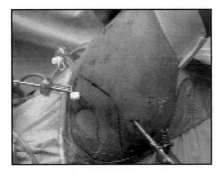

# What Went Wrong and What to Do About It: Pitfalls in the Treatment of Shoulder Impingement

*W. Ben Kibler, MD
Aaron Sciascia, MS, ATC

## Abstract

*Shoulder impingement is a commonly treated disorder; however, the absence of a clear understanding of pathophysiology and causation can create variability in treatment. Pitfalls that can impede optimal patient outcomes can occur in the areas of diagnosis, treatment, and rehabilitation. Diagnostic pitfalls include failing to identify some of the multiple extrinsic diagnoses as well as the intrinsic subacromial pathology in patients with symptoms of impingement. Surgical pitfalls include not addressing the entire pathology and doing an incomplete or excessive decompression. Rehabilitation pitfalls include prescribing the wrong exercises at the wrong time and omitting steps in the rehabilitation process. Every patient who presents for primary treatment of impingement or secondary treatment following failed treatment should have a thorough evaluation of all intrinsic and extrinsic factors that can contribute to the symptoms of shoulder impingement.*

**Instr Course Lect 2008;57:103-112.**

Impingement is the most commonly diagnosed disorder around the shoulder, and subacromial decompression is the most commonly performed surgical procedure around the shoulder.[1] Since Neer's description of impingement, clinical examination, diagnostic tests, radiologic evaluations, surgical treatment techniques, and rehabilitation protocols have been identified to treat this clinical disorder.[2,3] Despite this breadth of experience, the outcomes of treatment are not uniformly satisfactory. There is still not a clear understanding of the etiology, most efficacious evaluation techniques, and definitive treatment for the syndrome characterized by impingement symptoms.[4] Because definitive knowledge is not available, the treating physician must be aware of and must try to avoid pitfalls in the diagnosis, treatment, and rehabilitation of patients with shoulder impingement.

## Pitfalls in Diagnosis

Patients who initially present with shoulder impingement or those in whom initial treatment has failed require a detailed evaluation and diagnosis to guide subsequent treatment. An incomplete diagnosis is a frequent pitfall in failed treatment.

### History

The patient's history is vital for detecting mechanisms of injury and guiding the physical examination. Failure to obtain a history of previous injuries or treatments will limit understanding of the present pathophysiology. The age and occupation of the patient, as well as commonly required motions and tasks, can direct the evaluation toward certain diagnoses.

### Clinical Examination

A large number of clinical tests can be used to define impingement. Almost all of these tests are directed toward identifying causative factors within the subacromial space. Tests for the Neer and Hawkins impingement signs have relatively high sensitivity but low specificity.[3] Another diagnostic test involves anesthetic

*W. Ben Kibler, MD or the department with which he is affiliated has received research or institutional support from Alignmed, holds stock or stock options in AlignMed, and is a consultant or employee for AlignMed.

**Table 1**
**Clinical Diagnosis Associated With Impingement Syndrome and Resultant Biomechanical Effect**

| Diagnosis | Factor | Effect |
|---|---|---|
| Subacromial factors<br>  Os acromiale<br>  Bone spurs<br>  Thickened coracoacromial ligament<br>  Calcific enthesopathy<br>  Synovitis/bursitis | Intrinsic | Alters static dimensions of subacromial space |
| Acromioclavicular joint injury<br>  Arthrosis<br>  Bone spurs<br>  Instability<br>  High grade acromioclavicular separation | Intrinsic<br>Extrinsic | Alters static dimensions<br>Alters scapulohumeral rhythm |
| Rotator cuff injury<br>  Tear<br>  Tendinopathy | Extrinsic | Superior humeral head translation |
| Labral injury | Extrinsic | Superior humeral head translation |
| Biceps tendinopathy | Extrinsic | Impingement |
| Instability | Extrinsic | Alters scapulohumeral rhythm |
| Inflexibility<br>  GIRD<br>  Pectoralis minor | Extrinsic | Alters scapulohumeral rhythm |
| Scapular dyskinesis | Extrinsic | Alters scapulohumeral rhythm |
| Neurologic | Extrinsic | Neurologic |

GIRD = glenohumeral internal rotation

injection into the subacromial space, which anesthetizes the space and reduces pain but does not indicate the mechanisms of pain generation. Radiologic evaluations include plain radiographs, with an emphasis on the supraspinatus outlet view; however, morphologic acromial shape is not associated with the presence of symptoms and has not been identified as a predictor of impingement. The primary pitfall of commonly used clinical tests is that they individually do not provide a complete diagnosis. The grouping of clinical and radiologic findings may provide a more accurate description of a patient's impingement syndrome.[5,6]

Most current studies of shoulder impingement show that intrinsic factors in the subacromial space, and multiple other factors, including abnormal humeral translation, scapular position and motion, alterations in muscle activation balance and patterns, and glenohumeral pathology, all can be involved in the clinical disorder.[5-10] The subacromial space should be conceptualized not as a static space with rigid boundaries but as a dynamic space with dimensions that are affected by many extrinsic factors. The intrinsic factors may create impingement by causing disease within the space. The extrinsic factors can create impingement by altering scapulohumeral rhythm, the coupled motion that maintains congruency between the parts of the humerus and all parts of the scapula during dynamic motion. Because the diagnosis is the basis that determines treatment and rehabilitation plans, the evaluation of a patient with impingement should include all of the possible intrinsic and extrinsic causative factors. An incomplete diagnosis, which does not include other factors or concomitant pathology, is a pitfall that can lead to incomplete treatment.

At least nine specific diagnoses may be associated with symptoms related to impingement syndrome. Each diagnosis is associated with an intrinsic or extrinsic factor that may affect the static or dynamic dimensions of the subacromial space or create pain (Table 1).

Os acromiale, subacromial bone spurs, a thickened coracoacromial ligament with calcific enthesopathy, and/or hypertrophic synovitis have been shown to alter the static dimensions of the space. Acromioclavicular joint arthrosis with bone spurs and instability also will decrease the static dimensions. High-grade acromioclavicular separations alter the strut function of the clavicle on the scapula and allow scapular protraction and decreased dynamic acromial elevation when the arm is elevated. This alteration in scapulohumeral rhythm creates impingement.

Rotator cuff impairment, along the entire spectrum ranging from muscle weakness to tendinopathy to a complete tear, alters the function of the rotator cuff as a compressor cuff and humeral head depressor and allows superior translation of the humeral head during motion.[11,12] This dynamic alteration of the subacromial space can create impingement.

Among the effects of superior labral injury is a change in shoulder capsular stiffness, with increased humeral head translation.[13] This diagnosis also is associated with other diagnoses, including rotator cuff injury and glenohumeral internal rotation deficit (GIRD), which create altered humeral head motion, and scapular dyskinesis, which creates altered acromial motion.[11,14-16] These alterations in scapulohumeral rhythm also affect the subacromial space.

Rotator interval lesions, which include biceps tendinopathy and upper subscapularis lesions, can create impingement-like pain at the anterior acromial edge. Studies have shown that the biceps and rotator interval are the structures that are mechanically impinged in forward flexion and horizontal adduction of the arm.[17]

Glenohumeral instability is characterized by excessive humeral head translation. Microtraumatic instability has been described as being part of the instability/impingement continuum in which impingement disorders frequently occur.[18]

Muscle inflexibility and capsular stiffness can alter scapulohumeral rhythm or create pain. Pectoralis minor tightness is common in patients with impingement and creates altered scapular tilt and acromial elevation.[19] GIRD, a combination of acquired capsular stiffness and acquired muscle stiffness, allows superior humeral head translation in external rotation and internal rotation and creates scapular protraction in arm follow-through.[20-24] It is not uncommon for early stages of adhesive capsulitis to create rotator interval pain similar to impingement or to create altered humeral head translation because of capsular stiffness.

Scapular dyskinesis is associated with impingement by altering the scapular position at rest and on dynamic motion.[25] Scapular dyskinesis is characterized by loss of acromial upward rotation, excessive scapular internal rotation, and excessive scapular anterior tilt.[6,9,15] These positions create scapular protraction, which decreases the subacromial space and decreases demonstrated rotator cuff strength.[16,26,27] Activation se-quencing patterns and the strength of the muscles that stabilize the scapula are altered in patients with impingement and scapular dyskinesis.[5,7]

Cervical radiculopathy or brachial plexus neuropathies can create pain or muscle weakness that cause the symptoms of impingement. C5-C6 radiculopathy with referred pain or suprascapular neuropathy with rotator cuff weakness may be the sole cause of the pain or may be a comorbid factor.

## Pitfalls in Surgical Treatment

The failure to make a complete diagnosis and thereby not treating all of the pathology is one major pitfall leading to unsuccessful surgery. Superior labral and rotator interval lesions are often untreated. In instances of failed treatment, it is important to assess the patient for these pathologies.

Other pitfalls are related to the actual techniques of impingement surgery. The goal of surgery is to create a flat acromial undersurface extending from the acromioclavicular joint to the anterolateral corner of the acromion.[3] Multiple studies have shown that this type of subacromial decompression can be efficacious using an open or arthroscopic approach.[28,29] The technical pitfalls are associated with inadequate or excessive decompression.

Inadequate decompression may be related to inadequate excision of bone or soft tissue. Inadequate removal of the anterolateral acromion is the most common pitfall, but a failure to remove the calcific enthesopathy in the coracoacromial ligament also occurs. Most studies show that coplaning of the inferior clavicular spur does not compromise surgical results and should be considered a routine procedure when a spur is present.[30] Inadequate soft-tissue resection is usually related to incomplete débridement of the superficial bursa. This tissue is a potent source of pain with increased levels of mediators of inflammation, and it should be completely removed.[31] Other pitfalls in soft-tissue surgery include not removing the acromial attachment of the coracoacromial ligament and the occasionally occurring lateral soft-tissue band over the rotator cuff. These causes of failed treatment can be avoided by adequate resection of the tissue.

Excessive decompression relates to resection of too much bone on the acromion or the clavicle on the undersurface of the acromion. Studies recommend removal of 2 to 4 mm of bone, based on an average acromial thickness of 6.5 to 8.0 mm.[32] More than 5 mm of resected bone can lead to an increased risk of acromial fracture and superior humeral head migration.[33] Unlike in instances of inadequate decompression, treatment options following excessive decompression are limited. Fractures can be treated, but superior humeral head migration is difficult to control. This pitfall can be avoided by careful preoperative planning and attention to details such as the site of resection and the depth of bone.

Excessive resection at the acromioclavicular joint is a major pitfall in treating impingement. Distal clavicle excision is frequently done as part of subacromial decompression or as a separate procedure. Resection of as much as 1.0 to 1.5 cm of the distal clavicle has occasionally been advocated. This amount of resection may damage the biomechanics of the acromioclavicular joint. Studies have shown increased shear loads on the acromioclavicular joint when more than 5 mm of distal clavicle has been resected, that resection of more than 8 mm disrupts the attachments of the superior acromioclavicular ligaments and increases translation, and that a 1-cm resection increases acromioclavicular anterior/posterior motion from 1.2 to 8.3 mm.[34,35] Loss of the acromioclavicular ligament attachment sites removes the major restraints to anterior/posterior acromioclavicular joint stability and creates a rotary instability of the scapula in relation to the clavicle around the intact coracoclavicular ligaments. This abnormal translation produces scapular dyskinesis and increasing impingement. This pitfall is difficult to correct. Bone grafting to increase clavicular length has not been successful, and complete ligamentous restoration, either by repair or reconstruction, is not successful because of the shortened clavicle. Scapular retraction by bracing, taping, or exercise is helpful in reducing symptoms.

## Pitfalls in Nonsurgical Treatment and Rehabilitation

The basis of nonsurgical treatment and rehabilitation in impingement is to reestablish normal coupled scapulohumeral rhythm.[36] Restoration of the muscle activation sequences and strength as well as soft-tissue flexibility will optimize humeral head kinematics, maintain three-dimensional scapular motion, and maximize subacromial space height.[21,37] These dynamic factors will decrease the symptoms of impingement.

The most common pitfall is failure to recognize that these deficits exist. Pectoralis minor tightness, which is present in most patients with impingement, is often overlooked.[19] GIRD often is present and can be identified when properly evaluated. Evaluation of scapular dyskinesis is accomplished by observation of static position and dynamic motions.[24] Inadequate treatment can be reversed by recognizing and addressing those deficits in an adequate rehabilitation program.

Pitfalls in rehabilitation include not addressing critical deficits or using unphysiologic progressions. Rehabilitation includes treating the patient's symptoms and also the associated physiologic and biomechanical factors, such as pectoralis minor tightness, GIRD, muscle weakness or imbalance, and scapular dyskinesis.

The emphasis of rehabilitation for impingement should start proximally and end distally.[36,38] Proximal control of core stability leads to control of three-dimensional scapular motion.[39] The goal of this phase of rehabilitation is to achieve the position of optimal scapular function—posterior tilt, external rotation, and upward elevation. The serratus anterior functions most importantly as an external rotator of the scapula, and the lower trapezius acts as a stabilizer of the acquired scapular position. Maximal rotator cuff strength is achieved from a stabilized, retracted scapula.[26,27] After scapular control is achieved, rehabilitation of the rotator cuff should be implemented with an emphasis on closed chain, humeral head cocontraction exercises.[40-42] An increase in impingement pain when doing open chain rotator cuff exercises indicates the wrong emphasis at the wrong stage of the rehabilitation protocol.

## Evaluation and Treatment of the Patient With Prior Failed Treatment

### History

The evaluation of a patient who had unsuccessful treatment for impingement should begin with a detailed assessment of the history of the injury and previous treatment. The history of the original mechanism of injury or appearance of symptoms and subsequent limitations can sometimes provide clues to the origin of the impingement symptoms. A history of trauma such as a fall or sudden forced flexion or extension can indicate a rotator cuff injury, an acromioclavicular joint injury, or a labral tear as comorbid factors. Repetitive overhead activities in work or recreational activities may indicate a labral injury. Pain with repetitive horizontal adduction suggests biceps or acromioclavicular joint injury. Medial scapular border pain and/or crepitus indicates scapular involvement in the symptoms.

The specific details of nonsurgical treatment should be determined. It is important to know the exact composition of the rehabilitation program. Programs that emphasize modalities (ultrasound, iontophoresis, ice/heat, electrical stimulation) have not been shown to be efficacious; most of the evidence is preclinical and can be controversial.[43] Programs that emphasize rotator cuff strengthening, especially those using open chain tubing exercises as the starting point, will often create impingement symptoms.[26,44] If injections have been administered in the patient's treatment, the type of medicine used and the number, location, and short- and long-term effects should be established. The type and effect of other medications, such as anti-inflammatory drugs or supplements, as well as other nonsurgical treatments (acupuncture or massage), should be documented.

It is helpful to review the clinical notes regarding any surgical procedure and the patient's postoperative course. The nature of the surgery, the approach, the surgical findings, the techniques used, the early postoperative management, and the

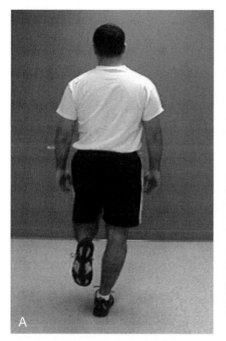
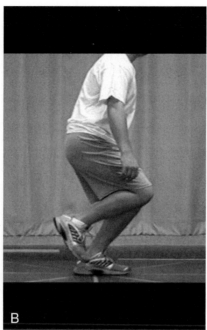

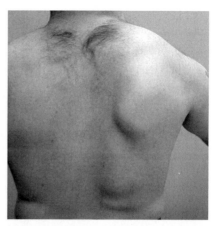

**Figure 2**    Type II scapular dyskinesis with prominence of the entire medial border is shown.

**Figure 1**    **A,** Single leg stance. The patient is asked to stand on one leg with no other cues. A positive Trendelenburg sign indicates gluteus medius weakness. **B,** Single leg squat. The patient is asked to flex the knee 45° in a squat maneuver, and then return to an upright stance. Forward or lateral trunk tilt or rotation of the trunk around the leg indicates a loss of dynamic control.

early and subsequent functional outcomes can all provide clues to the nature of the failed treatment.

### Physical Examination

A thorough physical examination should be done to accurately evaluate the kinetic chain, scapular, and shoulder factors that may have contributed to failed impingement treatment. Kinetic chain factors may be evaluated by screening methods. Hip and trunk stability can be assessed using the single leg stance and single leg squat maneuvers[36,39] (Figure 1). Any deficits found during the screening examination should be evaluated in more depth.

Scapular factors are common in failed impingement treatment and can be assessed by a detailed evaluation. The goals of the physical examination of the scapula are to establish the presence or absence of scapular dyskinesis and to use dynamic maneuvers to assess the effect of correction of dyskinesis on impingement symptoms.

The patient's resting posture should be checked for side-to-side asymmetry and for evidence of inferior medial or medial border prominence (Figure 2). Marking the superior and inferior medial borders may help ascertain the position of the scapula.

To evaluate dynamic scapular motion, the patient raises and lowers the arms three to five times. This process usually reveals any weakness in the muscles and displays the dyskinetic patterns. If necessary, the patient may raise and lower the arms up to 10 times or may hold 3- to 5-lb weights during the evaluation, which will further highlight the scapular dyskinesis. Alteration in medial border motion in any plane,

singly or in combination, is recorded as "present" or "absent." The clinically observed evaluation has a correlation of 0.84 with biomechanically determined abnormalities in symptomatic patients (B. Kibler, MD, unpublished data, Dana Point, CA, 2003).

Dynamic maneuvers that may relieve impingement symptoms include the scapular assistance test and the scapular retraction test.[27,45,46] In the scapular assistance test, the examiner applies gentle pressure to assist scapular upward rotation and posterior tilt as the patient raises his arm (Figure 3). A positive result occurs when the painful symptoms of impingement are relieved and the arc of motion is increased.[45] In the scapular retraction test, the examiner stabilizes the scapula in a retracted position (Figure 4). A positive result is an increase in supraspinatus strength (determined by manual muscle testing).[27] A positive scapular assistance test or scapular retraction test shows that scapular dyskinesis is directly involved in producing the impingement symptoms and indicates the need for inclusion of early scapular rehabilita-

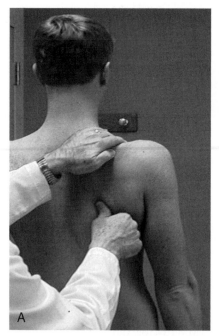

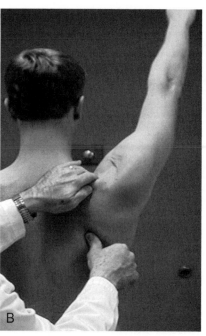

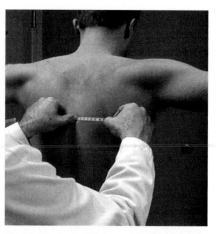

**Figure 5** Lateral scapular slide. Bilateral measurements are taken from the tip of the medial scapular border to the nearest spinous process. A 1.5 cm side-to-side asymmetry is considered abnormal. The arms should not be higher than 90° abducted but should be in maximal internal rotation. This position requires activation of all the scapular stabilizers.

**Figure 3** The scapular assistance test. **A,** The position of the examiner's hands in preparation for the arm elevation is shown. **B,** As the patient elevates the arm, the examiner applies gentle pressure to assist scapular upward rotation and posterior tilt. A positive test results in increased arm motion and decreased symptoms of impingement.

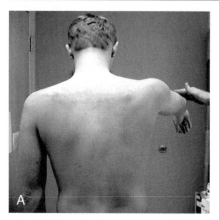

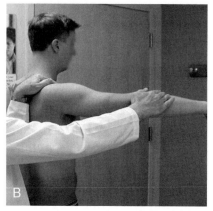

**Figure 4** The scapular retraction test. **A,** A manual muscle examination is used to estimate relative supraspinatus strength and weakness with the patient maintaining a "normal" posture. Note that this patient has type III scapular dyskinesis with superior medial border prominence. **B,** The examiner stabilizes the scapula in a neutral, slightly retracted position and then repeats the manual muscle examination. A positive test results in an increase in demonstrated supraspinatus strength.

tion exercises to improve scapular control. **(DVD 9.1)**

The lateral scapular slide is a semidynamic measurement of scapular control (Figure 5). Bilateral measurements of the distance between the inferior medial scapular tip and the spine are done with the arms in 80° and 90° of abduction and maximally internally rotated. Side-to-side asymmetries greater than 1.5 cm have a 0.84 correlation with biomechanically determined excessive scapular internal rotation.[47]

Evaluation of the shoulder should include assessment of flexibility, strength, and anatomic injury. GIRD should be evaluated by stabilizing the scapula, placing the arm in 90° of abduction in the scapular plane, and rotating the arm (Figure 6). The arm should be rotated until there is tightness in the motion and/ or when the scapula begins to move forward in a windup fashion.[20] Bilateral measurements should be obtained, and treatment should begin if the side-to-side difference in measurements is greater than 25°, or the absolute measurement on the asymptomatic side is less than 25°.[20]

Palpation of the pectoralis minor and the short head of the biceps when the arm and scapula are externally rotated can assess coracoid-based inflexibility because both

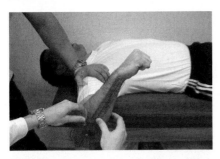

**Figure 6** GIRD is measured by stabilizing the scapula and internally rotating the glenohumeral joint to a feeling of tightness against the rotation.

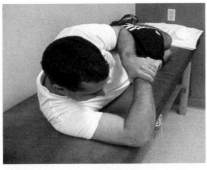

**Figure 7** The sleeper stretch is used to increase glenohumeral internal rotation. The patient stabilizes the scapula by lying on his side, then places the arm into maximal internal rotation.

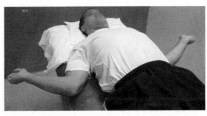

**Figure 8** The open book stretch increases pectoralis minor and biceps short head flexibility. A rolled towel or other support is placed between the scapulae, and the arms are placed in external rotation and horizontal abduction. The arms should have less than 90° abduction to minimize thoracic outlet symptoms.

muscles run off the coracoid tip. The tight muscle will usually be tender to palpation, even if it is not producing overt symptoms during use.

Other shoulder factors can be assessed by standard physical examination techniques for internal derangements of glenohumeral and acromioclavicular joints. Tests should evaluate rotator cuff strength and integrity, glenohumeral instability, superior labral tears, biceps tendinopathy, and acromioclavicular joint arthrosis or instability. All of these pathologic deficits have been associated with symptoms of impingement.

### Imaging
A review of imaging studies related to prior treatments is helpful to evaluate the original disorder and any subsequent treatment alterations. Acromioclavicular or subacromial spurs and rotator cuff or labral injury are common findings both before and after treatment.

The need for new imaging studies should be based on the patient's history and physical examination. Plain radiographs should include AP, lateral, axillary, and outlet views to adequately assess the subacromial space and its boundaries. CT is par-

ticularly helpful in evaluating the acromioclavicular joint pathology. MRI should be used to evaluate soft-tissue injury. In many instances, contrast arthrography is helpful in assessing for labral and biceps injury.

### Treatment
Treatment for previously unsuccessfully treated impingement is guided by the findings from the physical examination and imaging. An understanding of the multiple factors involved in the symptoms of impingement can elucidate the pitfalls that may have hindered prior treatment and can help in the selection of the proper surgical or nonsurgical treatment and in planning a functional rehabilitation program.

Surgical treatment should restore anatomic integrity to the structures that influence the content and boundaries of the subacromial space and allow normal scapulohumeral rhythm. Treatment should include acromial spurs, distal clavicle spurs, acromioclavicular joint arthrosis or instability, rotator cuff pathology, superior labral injury, biceps pathology, or instability.

Postoperative and nonsurgical treatment are related to restoration of nor-

mal scapulohumeral rhythm, which begins with establishing trunk and core stability and using triplanar exercises, including lunges and balance exercises.[39]

A rehabilitation program for a patient with impingement symptoms and scapular dyskinesis should begin with restoration of flexibility. Sleeper stretches are excellent for improving GIRD (Figure 7), and open book stretches (Figure 8) can improve coracoid-based inflexibility. General flexibility exercises for the trunk also should be included. Flexibility exercises should be continued as muscle rehabilitation begins.

Periscapular muscles often are very weak in patients with impingement because of disuse and inhibition of use resulting from pain. Early strengthening should not be done by isolating these weak muscles but rather by taking advantage of the facilitation of periscapular activation by the synergistic proximal trunk and hip muscle activations. Because these exercises are done in a closed chain fashion, they do not place excessive loads on the impinged or injured distal structures.[48] Exercise sets should integrate hip and trunk extension and scapular retraction movements (lawn

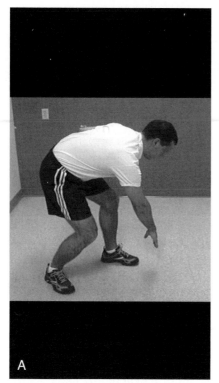
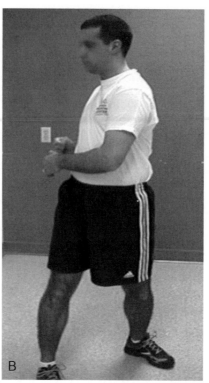
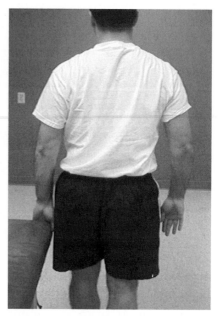

**Figure 9**  The lawn mower pull involves some degree of knee and trunk flexion and rotation. **A,** The starting position can vary based on soreness or restrictions on motion resulting from pain or surgery. In the immediate postoperative period, the starting position can be the arm in a sling. **B,** The ending position is shown. The knee and trunk are extended, and the scapula is retracted so that the elbow ends up in the "back pocket" position.

**Figure 10**  The low row exercise involves hip and trunk extension, scapular retraction, and arm extension against resistance. The resistance can begin as an isometric (as is shown in this photograph) and may progress to isotonic exercises using bands. The low row exercise involves arm positions and motions that do not create impingement and creates scapular positions that activate the serratus anterior as a scapular external rotator. This exercise is ideal for the early stages of rehabilitation.

mower pulls) close to, then farther away from the body (Figure 9), and should integrate trunk extension, scapular retraction, and arm extension exercises (low row exercises) (Figure 10).

In a recent study, low row and lawn mower exercises were shown to be effective in activating key scapular muscles (serratus anterior and lower trapezius) in task-specific patterns at clinically significant moderate levels of intensity (25% to 30% maximal voluntary isometric contraction), which is consistent with physiologic activation. (B. Kibler, MD, Florence, Italy, presented at the International Society for Knee Arthroscopy and Sports Medicine meeting, 2007.) These characteris-

tics suggest that the exercises may be used in the early and middle phases of comprehensive shoulder rehabilitation protocols to establish a stable base for glenohumeral function.

Rotator cuff activation is crucial in maintaining the integrity of the subacromial space; however, maximal rotator cuff activation can occur only off a stabilized scapular base.[26,49] Demonstrated rotator cuff strength may be increased as much as 24% when the scapula is stabilized and retracted.[27] Therefore, the emphasis on rotator cuff rehabilitation in patients with impingement should occur later in the rehabilitation protocol, after proximal stability has been established. Rehabilitation should emphasize cocontraction of the muscles in force

couples and integrated scapular stabilization-humeral head depression exercises. Rotator cuff exercises may progress from the closed to open chain position, from the horizontal to the vertical to the diagonal direction, and from slow to fast speed. Each type of progression increases rotator cuff muscle activation.[40]

## Summary

There are many possible pitfalls in the treatment of patients with symptoms of impingement. The diagnosis of impingement has been considered a simple process and most pitfalls were assumed to be associated with surgical technique. However, pitfalls also may be encountered in the diagnostic process because several diagnoses can be associated with impingement, and each must be carefully evaluated before treatment is initiated. Proper surgical or nonsurgical treatment is crucial for restoration of the anatomy surrounding the subacromial space. Integrated, properly phased rehabilitation is needed to restore normal muscle and joint flexibility, muscle strength and activation patterns, and motions that allow coupled scapulohumeral rhythm. Proper recognition of the complexity of diagnosing and treating impingement will avoid pitfalls and achieve better treatment outcomes in patients who initially present with impingement symptoms and in those with prior failed treatments.

## References

1. van der Windt DA, Koes BW, de Jong BA, Bouter LM: Shoulder disorders in general practice: Incidence, patient characteristics, and management. *Ann Rheum Dis* 1995;54: 959-964.

2. Neer CS: Anterior acromioplasty for the chronic impingement syndrome in the shoulder: A preliminary report. *J Bone Joint Surg Am* 1972;54:41-50.

3. Goldberg SS, Bigliani LU: Shoulder impingement revisited: Advanced concepts of pathomechanics and treatment. *Instr Course Lect* 2006;55: 17-27.

4. Stephens SR, Warren RF, Payne LZ, Wickiewicz TL, Altchek DW: Arthroscopic acromioplasty: A 6-to-10-year follow-up. *Arthroscopy* 1998;14: 382-388.

5. Cools AM, Witvrouw E, DeClercq G: Scapular muscle recruitment pattern: Trapezius muscle latency in overhead athletes with and without impingement symptoms. *Am J Sports Med* 2003;31:542-549.

6. Ludewig PM, Cook TM: Alterations in shoulder kinematics and associated muscle activity in people with symptoms of shoulder impingement. *Phys Ther* 2000;80:276-291.

7. Cools AM, Witvrouw EE, Mattieu NN: Isokinetic scapular muscle performance in overhead athletes with and without impingement symptoms. *J Athl Train* 2005;40:104-110.

8. Kebaetse M, McClure PW, Pratt NA: Thoracic position effect on shoulder range of motion, strength, and three-dimensional scapular kinematics. *Arch Phys Med Rehabil* 1999;80:945-950.

9. Michener LA, McClure PW, Karduna AR: Anatomical and biomechanical mechanisms of subacromial impingement syndrome. *Clin Biomech (Bristol, Avon)* 2003;18:369-379.

10. McClure PW, Bialker J, Neff N, Williams G, Karduna AR: Shoulder function and 3-dimensional kinematics in people with shoulder impingement syndrome before and after a 6-week exercise program. *Phys Ther* 2004;84: 832-848.

11. Deutsch A, Altchek DW, Schwartz E, Otis JC, Warren RF: Radiologic measurement of superior displacement of the humeral head in the impingement syndrome. *J Shoulder Elbow Surg* 1996;5:186-193.

12. Paletta GA, Warner JP, Warren RF: Shoulder kinematics with two-plane x-ray evaluation in patients with anterior instability or rotator cuff tears. *J Shoulder Elbow Surg* 1997;6:516-527.

13. Pagnani MJ, Deng XH, Warren RF, Torzilli PA, Altchek DW: Effect of lesions of the superior portion of the glenoid labrum on glenohumeral translation. *J Bone Joint Surg Am* 1995; 77:1003-1010.

14. Grossman MG, Tibone JE, McGarry MH: A cadaveric model of the shoulder: A possible etiology of superior labrum anterior-to-posterior lesions. *J Bone Joint Surg Am* 2005;87:824-831.

15. Lukasiewicz AC, McClure P, Michener L: Comparison of three dimensional scapular position and orientation between subjects with and without shoulder impingement. *J Orthop Sports Phys Ther* 1999;29: 574-586.

16. Solem-Bertoft E, Thuomas KA, Westerberg CE: The influence of scapular retraction and protraction on the width of the subacromial space: An MRI study. *Clin Orthop Relat Res* 1993;296:99-103.

17. Flatow EL, Soslowsky LJ, Ticker JB: Excursion of the rotator cuff under the acromion: patterns of subacromial contact. *Am J Sports Med* 1994;22: 779-788.

18. Reddy AS, Mohr KJ, Pink M, Jobe FW: Electromyographic analysis of the deltoid and rotator cuff muscles in persons with subacromial impingement. *J Shoulder Elbow Surg* 2000;9: 519-523.

19. Borstad JD, Ludewig PM: The effect of long versus short pectoralis minor resting length on scapular kinematics. *J Orthop Sports Phys Ther* 2005;35: 227-238.

20. Burkhart SS, Morgan CD, Kibler WB: The disabled throwing shoulder: Spectrum of pathology: Part I. Pathoanatomy and biomechanics. *Arthroscopy* 2003;19:404-420.

21. Tyler TF, Nicholas SJ: Quantification of posterior capsule tightness and motion loss in patients with shoulder impingement. *Am J Sports Med* 2000; 28:668-673.

22. Proske U, Morgan DL: Muscle damage from eccentric exercise: Mechanism, mechanical signs, adaptation and clinical applications. *J Physiol* 2001;537:333-345.

23. Harryman DT, Sidles JA, Clark JM: Translation of the humeral head on the glenoid with passive glenohumeral motions. *J Bone Joint Surg Am* 1990;72:1334-1343.

24. Kibler WB, Uhl TL, Maddux JW, Brooks PV, Zeller B, McMullen J: Qualitative clinical evaluation of scapular dysfunction: A reliability study. *J Shoulder Elbow Surg* 2002;11: 550-556.

25. Warner JP, Micheli L, Arslenian L:

Scapulothoracic motion in normal shoulders and shoulders with glenohumeral instability and impingement syndrome. *Clin Orthop Relat Res* 1992; 285:199-215.

26. Smith J, Dietrich CT, Kotajarvi BR, Kaufman KR: The effect of scapular protraction on isometric shoulder rotation strength in normal subjects. *J Shoulder Elbow Surg* 2006;15: 339-343.

27. Kibler WB, Sciascia AD, Dome DC: Evaluation of apparent and absolute supraspinatus strength in patients with shoulder injury using the scapular retraction test. *Am J Sports Med* 2006;34:1643-1647.

28. Husby T, Haugstvedt JR, Brandt M, Holm I, Steen H: Open versus arthroscopic subacromial decompression: A prospective, randomized study of 34 patients followed for 8 years. *Acta Orthop Scand* 2003;74: 408-414.

29. Spangehl MJ, Hawkins RJ, McCormack RG, Loomer RL: Arthroscopic versus open acromioplasty: A prospective, randomized, blinded study. *J Shoulder Elbow Surg* 2002;11: 101-107.

30. Barber FA: Coplaning of the acromioclavicular joint. *Arthroscopy* 2001; 17:913-917.

31. Gotoh M, Hamada K, Yamakawa H, Inoue A, Fukuda H: Increased substance P in subacromial bursa and shoulder pain in rotator cuff diseases. *J Orthop Res* 1998;16:618-621.

32. Nicholson GP, Goodman DA, Flatow EL, Bigliani LU: The acromion: Morphologic condition and age-related changes: A study of 420 scapulas. *J Shoulder Elbow Surg* 1996;5:1-11.

33. Flatow EL, Colman WW, Kalkar R, et al: The effect of anterior acromioplasty on rotator cuff contact: An experimental and computer simulation. *J Shoulder Elbow Surg* 1995;4:553-554.

34. Costic RS, Jari R, Rodosky MW, Debski RE: Joint compression alters the kinematics and loading patterns of the intact and capsule-transected AC joint. *J Orthop Res* 2003;21:379-385.

35. Sahara W, Sugamoto K, Murai M, Tanaka H, Yoshikawa H: 3D kinematic analysis of the acromioclavicular joint during arm abduction using vertically open MRI. *J Orthop Res* 2006;24:1823-1831.

36. Kibler WB, McMullen J, Uhl TL: Shoulder rehabilitation strategies, guidelines, and practice. *Oper Tech Sports Med* 2000;8:258-267.

37. Kamkar A, Irrgang JJ, Whitney SL: Nonoperative management of secondary shoulder impingement syndrome. *J Orthop Sports Phys Ther* 1993; 17:212-224.

38. Kibler WB, McMullen J: Scapular dyskinesis and its relation to shoulder pain. *J Am Acad Orthop Surg* 2003; 11:142-151.

39. Kibler WB, Press J, Sciascia A: The role of core stability in athletic function. *Sports Med* 2006;36:189-198.

40. Wise MB, Uhl TL, Mattacola CG, Nitz AJ, Kibler WB: Shoulder musculature activation during supported and unsupported active range of motion upper extremity exercises. *J Shoulder Elbow Surg* 2004;13: 614-620.

41. Hinterwimmer S, von Eisenhart-Rothe RV, Siebert M, et al: Influence of adducting and abducting muscle forces on the subacromial space

width. *Med Sci Sports Exerc* 2003;35: 2055-2059.

42. Graichen H, Hinterwimmer S, von Eisenhart-Rothe R, Vogl T, Englmeier KH, Eckstein F: Effect of abducting and adducting muscle activity on glenohumeral translation, scapular kinematics and subacromial space width in vivo. *J Biomech* 2005; 38:755-760.

43. Sharma P, Maffulli N: Tendon injury and tendinopathy: Healing and repair. *J Bone Joint Surg Am* 2005;87: 187-202.

44. Thigpen CA, Padua DA, Morgan N, Kreps C, Karas SG: Scapular kinematics during supraspinatus rehabilitation exercise. *Am J Sports Med* 2006; 34:644-652.

45. Kibler WB: The role of the scapula in athletic shoulder function. *Am J Sports Med* 1998;26:325-337.

46. Rabin A, Irrgang JJ, Fitzgerald GK, Eubanks A: The intertester reliability of the scapular assistance test. *J Orthop Sports Phys Ther* 2006;36:653-660.

47. Schwellnus MP: The repeatability of clinical and laboratory tests to measure scapular position and movement during arm abduction. *Int J Sports Med* 2003;4:1-10.

48. Kibler WB, Livingston B: Closed chain rehabilitation for upper and lower extremities. *J Am Acad Orthop Surg* 2001;9:412-421.

49. Smith J, Kotajarvi BR, Padgett DJ, Eischen JJ: Effect of scapular protraction and retraction on isometric shoulder elevation strength. *Arch Phys Med Rehabil* 2002;83:367-370.

# Complications in Arthroscopic Anterior Shoulder Stabilization: Pearls and Pitfalls

*Robert A. Arciero, MD

Jeffrey T. Spang, MD

## Abstract

*Arthroscopic treatment of anterior glenohumeral instability has become increasingly common. As longer-term follow-up studies become available, certain trends dictating the success or failure of arthroscopic stabilization are becoming more evident. Bone defects are important predictors of clinical failure, and the recognition of bone loss and other pathoanatomic variables can help determine which patients will benefit from arthroscopic stabilization for anterior glenohumeral instability. Arthroscopic techniques for anterior shoulder instability must mirror the focus of open methods on retensioning the inferior glenohumeral ligament and restoring the anatomy of the anterior capsulolabral complex. Arthroscopic stabilization for anterior glenohumeral instability has achieved results comparable to those of open stabilization methods in properly selected patients.*

*Advantages of arthroscopic treatment of shoulder instability include lower morbidity, decreased pain, the ability to treat other pathologies, and improved cosmesis. As arthroscopic treatment of recurrent shoulder instability becomes more commonplace, it is crucial to review the factors that influence the success or failure of arthroscopic instability procedures and to understand the guidelines for patient selection, surgical pearls and pitfalls, and adjunctive technical details designed to optimize results.*

**Instr Course Lect 2008;57:113-124.**

Successful arthroscopic stabilization of anterior glenohumeral instability begins with careful patient selection based on a thorough history and physical examination. Results of the history and physical examination should identify patients with the diagnosis of traumatic anterior instability and should rule out patients with other instability disorders such as multidirectional instability, posterior instability, and other labral pathologies. Although arthroscopic techniques are evolving to treat other forms of instability, the most extensive and favorable outcomes with arthroscopic stabilization have been achieved in the treatment of anterior instability.

## Patient Selection

### History

The patient's activity level and expectations are important components of the initial history. The demands the patient will place on any surgical reconstruction must be taken into account in surgical planning. Previous treatment of instability, whether surgical or nonsurgical, will provide important background information. A detailed review of instability episodes is needed to assess the magnitude of the injury. Several important questions that can help identify patients with traumatic anterior instability are shown in Table 1. These questions are used to gauge the severity of the instability, confirm the diagnosis of traumatic anterior instability, and discover any complicating factors such as bone loss.

### Physical Examination

An initial physical examination should include observation as well as motion and strength testing. An examiner may compare the injured and contralateral sides to evaluate muscle atrophy, scapular kinetics, and the resting position of the shoulder. Active and passive range of

*Robert A. Arciero, MD or the department with which he is affiliated has received research or institutional support from Arthrex Smith & Nephew and Mitek.*

## Table 1
### Key Questions for Identifying Patients With Traumatic Anterior Instability

| Question | Value |
| --- | --- |
| What was the initial mechanism of injury? | Quantifies energy required for initial dislocation; greater energy suggests a greater likelihood of associated lesions (glenoid fracture, capsular tear) |
| What was the arm position at the time of injury? | Allows imaging and physical examination to be directed at locations of suspected pathology; abduction/external rotation would indicate a mechanism consistent with anterior instability |
| Did the shoulder dislocate? Was a reduction required? | Need for reduction indicates a mechanism of injury sufficient to cause capsulolabral disruption |
| Were radiographs taken at the time of the initial event? | Early radiographs may show bone or rim avulsion and can verify the direction of dislocation |
| What was the length of disability following the event? | Delayed return to functional activities or persistent disability may indicate more extensive capsulolabral disruption |
| How many episodes of disability have occurred since the index event? Were they dislocations? Subluxations? Were reductions required? | Multiple episodes increase concern for bony defects or concomitant damage and indicate the level of laxity |
| Are there arm positions/activities that you avoid? | Allows assessment of current functional status; permits identification of direction of instability |
| What activities would you like to resume? | Categorizes patient in terms of functional postoperative requirements |

motion should be evaluated, along with a thorough strength examination designed to include the rotator cuff musculature and the deltoid. Neurologic status should be checked, in particular the sensory and motor functions of the axillary nerve. Generalized ligamentous laxity must be determined because it will reflect increased capsular redundancy and may change the selected surgical approach. Asymmetric motion or strength deficits should be categorized and may represent chronic changes or posttraumatic loss of function. Careful motor evaluation should indicate rotator cuff pathology caused by injury. Provocative tests must be used to confirm and quantify the degree of instability.

Vital tests include apprehension testing to determine the amount of abduction and external rotation re-

quired to reproduce symptoms of instability. A relocation maneuver can be performed by applying a posteriorly directed force on the proximal humerus in a supine patient with the arm in abduction and external rotation; the test is positive if the force reduces the feeling of instability. A seated or supine load-and-shift maneuver must be performed to quantify the instability. It is important to note any painful crepitus that results from an anterior or posterior shift. The sulcus/rotator interval should be examined in both internal and external rotation in the adducted arm and must be compared with the contralateral side for appropriate interpretation. The posterior jerk test may be used and, if positive, indicates posterior instability. Recent variations of this test have been used to detect a posterior labral component of anteroinferior instability.[1]

## Imaging

Appropriate imaging studies are a vital component of preoperative assessment. Imaging is necessary to evaluate bone loss because large bone defects of the glenoid and humeral head adversely affect the outcome of arthroscopic stabilization.[2,3] A standard AP view and an AP view of the glenohumeral joint are combined with an axillary view for initial evaluation before the physical examination. Additional specialized radiographs can be obtained in the office setting. Modified axillary views, such as a West Point view, can be helpful in estimating glenoid bone loss.[4] A Stryker notch view can be used to examine and quantify a Hill-Sachs lesion. Unless these views confirm normal anatomy, additional imaging may be warranted.

MRI can be a helpful adjunct in the evaluation of a patient with traumatic instability. The acknowledged superiority of MRI for soft-tissue visualization can assist in preoperative planning and in detecting unusual variants in pathology associated with anterior instability. The addition of intra-articular contrast can improve the ability of MRI to show rotator cuff pathology, humeral avulsion of the glenohumeral ligaments (HAGL), capsular tears, and classic Bankart lesions. Recognizing additional soft-tissue pathology, such as rotator cuff tears, capsular rents, superior labrum anterior and posterior lesions, and extension of the Bankart lesion posteriorly, can lead to improved outcomes if all pathologies are treated.[5,6] In an acute injury (less than 1 week after dislocation), contrast need not be added because the blood and fluid associated with the initial injury are sufficient to provide image enhancement. Although MRI is helpful in viewing bone edema, information from MRI scans may cause an underestimation of bone lesions and should not be substituted for CT scanning for the quantification of bone defects of the glenoid or humeral head (Figure 1).

CT is the most accurate method of evaluating bone injuries of the glenoid or the humerus. Recent software advances have made three-dimensional imaging possible for both glenoid fossa and humeral head lesions, allowing more accurate measurements of bone loss (Figure 2). Multiple studies have shown that the most common reason for failure of arthroscopic stabilization procedures is bone loss.[2,3,7] Bone defects on the glenoid or the humeral head can significantly increase failure rates. Accurate assessment of these injuries is of paramount importance because failure to adequately evaluate bony defects will compromise the results of arthroscopic stabilization.

The indications for preoperative CT scanning are continuing to expand. CT scanning must be considered if the patient reports instability at low abduction angles or has marked apprehension at low abduction/external rotation during provocative testing. A patient with a dislocation produced by severe trauma that required manual reduction and that is followed by unprovoked instability and spontaneous reduction should have a CT scan for the evaluation of possible bone loss. Patients who have multiple dislocations requiring reductions also should be considered for a scan. A CT scan is needed if the frequency of the instability episodes is increasing or the amount of trauma required to cause an instability episode is decreasing. It has been the authors' experience that dislocation while asleep indicates extensive capsulolabral injury or bone loss. If

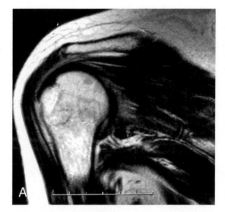
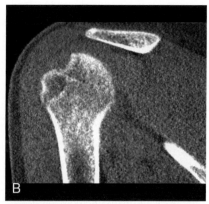

**Figure 1**    MRI (**A**) and CT scan (**B**) of a Hill-Sachs lesion show that MRI can underrepresent bone defects.

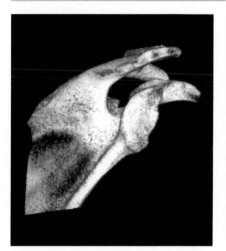
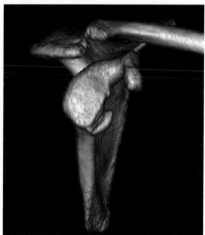

**Figure 2**    CT scan showing anterior bone loss of the glenoid.

**Figure 3**    Three-dimensional CT scan showing an osseous Bankart lesion.

bone injury is detected on any of the initial radiographic examinations, a CT scan is needed to accurately assess the damage. CT should be routinely used when revision arthroscopic surgery is contemplated.

Glenoid deficiency and loss of the glenoid surface reduce the concavity of the glenoid and decrease the arc length of the glenoid.[8-11] Several methods have been described for estimating the extent of glenoid bone loss.[12,13] Sugaya and associates[13] used a three-dimensional CT scan of the glenoid face (Figure 3). To determine the percentage of the defect, the area of bone loss is divided by

the area of a circle based on the inferior glenoid and the quotient is then multiplied by 100%.

Although techniques have been developed for measuring bone loss arthroscopically, it would be optimal to know the extent of the glenoid damage before attempting a stabilization procedure.[14,15] Arthroscopic measurement of glenoid bone loss is accomplished by passing a measuring probe from posterior to anterior while crossing the bare area of the glenoid. The distance from the posterior rim of the glenoid to the bare area is compared with the distance from the anterior rim of the glenoid

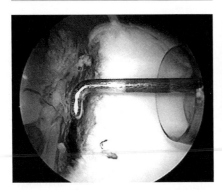

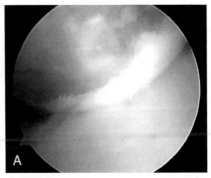

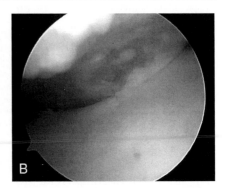

**Figure 4** Arthroscopic measuring of bone loss. In this right shoulder viewed from the posterosuperior portal, a probe is placed from the posterior portal with the hook over the anterior edge of the glenoid. The first laser marking is over the "bare spot." The distance from the anterior hook to the bare spot is divided by the distance from the bare spot to the posterior edge; the quotient represents the amount of anterior glenoid bone loss.

**Figure 5** Arthroscopic view of the left shoulder viewed from the posterior showing a Hill-Sachs lesion engaging on the glenoid rim. **A,** The Hill-Sachs lesion is perched adjacent to the glenoid rim. **B,** With the humeral head dislocated, the Hill-Sachs lesion is engaged or locked on the glenoid rim.

to the bare area to determine the extent of the bone loss (Figure 4). Clinical retrospective studies have reported increased rates of instability recurrence based on glenoid loss ranging from 20% to 30%.[2,7,16] It is critical to accurately quantify bone loss on the glenoid side with a CT scan to avoid arthroscopic surgery on a patient who would be better treated with an open, bone-restoring procedure.

Common options to restore the missing anterior rim include bone grafting procedures using the iliac crest and transfer of the coracoid process.[17-21] For coracoid transfer, either the tip of the coracoid (Bristow) or the entire coracoid (Latarjet) is transferred to the rim of the glenoid to buttress the humerus.[22,23] Multiple studies have confirmed the long-term success of both iliac crest bone grafting and coracoid transfer in restoring stability.[19-21,24-26]

Significant humeral head defects (Hill-Sachs lesions) occur after an-terior dislocation and can compromise the results of arthroscopic procedures. A small Hill-Sachs lesion may be well tolerated, but a large lesion or a lesion combined with anterior glenoid bone loss must be treated.[17] The alignment of the Hill-Sachs lesion also is important. So-called engaging Hill-Sachs lesions run parallel to the face of the glenoid in the abducted, externally rotated position.[7] The humeral head subluxates as the anterior rim of the glenoid sinks, or engages into the defect (Figure 5). Reconstruction of any glenoid bone loss may be enough to lengthen the arc of rotation and eliminate the Hill-Sachs lesion as a cause of recurrent instability.[9] Large defects of the humeral head (20% to 30%) may still require open intervention.[17] Estimation of the size of the defect remains difficult, but CT scanning with three-dimensional reconstruction can help evaluate the defect and plan appropriate reconstruction.

## Surgical Treatment

Although multiple options for the treatment of significant Hill-Sachs lesions have been described, few clinical studies are available for review. Surgical techniques for the humerus include the use of allograft plugs, elevation with bone grafting of the lesion, matched size articular allograft, and rotational humeral osteotomy.[27-30]

### Indications for Arthroscopic Treatment

Patients with traumatic, recurrent anterior shoulder instability are excellent candidates for an arthroscopic instability procedure. A thorough history and physical examination should confirm anteroinferior laxity and the presence of adequate bone stock to support an arthroscopic repair. Patients with bone loss of less than 20% and glenoid rim fractures that retain a sizable fragment also are suitable candidates. Throwing athletes with instability pathology may benefit from an arthroscopic procedure to limit overtightening of capsular tissues.

### Contraindications for Arthroscopic Treatment

The most important contraindication for arthroscopic treatment is the presence of significant bone loss. As noted previously, glenoid bone loss of 20% or more will increase failure rates dramatically. The presence of the "inverted pear" on an

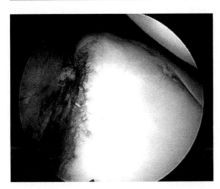

**Figure 6**    The presence of the "inverted pear" on an arthroscopic view indicates significant glenoid bone loss.

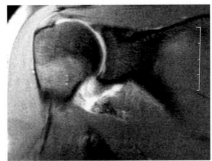

**Figure 7**    MRI scan of HAGL lesion.

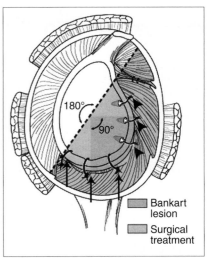

**Figure 8**    Illustration of surgical reconstruction with a 180° focus. Plication sutures (*arrows*), suture anchors (*arrowheads*), and rotator interval closure are shown. (Reproduced with permission from Bicos J, Mazzocca AD, Arciero RA: Anterior instability of the shoulder, in Schepsis AA, Busconi BD (eds): *Orthopaedic Surgery Essentials: Sports Medicine*. Philadelphia, PA, Lippincott Williams & Wilkins, 2005, p 222.)

arthroscopic view also indicates significant bone loss (Figure 6). Significant humeral head bone loss (25% to 30%) also precludes arthroscopic intervention. Soft-tissue injuries associated with anterior dislocation also may rule out arthroscopic repair. Injury to the subscapularis and the humeral insertions of the glenohumeral ligaments and severe capsular damage have all been reported with shoulder dislocations.

HAGL is a rare but important pathoanatomic variant that can occur in patients with traumatic anterior instability. An MRI scan with contrast should show the pathologic lesion, which is estimated to occur in 2% to 9% of traumatic dislocations[31-33] (Figure 7). Although some authors have reported arthroscopic repair of a HAGL lesion, most recommend open repair.[17,34,35] A mini-open approach has been described that avoids violation of the subscapularis tendon.[36] In most patients, the location of the humeral ligament insertion precludes arthroscopic repair.

Capsular deficiency also may be encountered in this patient population. It usually is associated with multiple surgical procedures but may be present in patients with no prior surgeries.[37] Aggressive thermal capsulorrhaphy may result in a severely attenuated capsule.[38] This rare complication should be treated with a revision procedure designed to reconstruct the anteroinferior structures. Allograft can be used, although Millett and associates[17] reported the use of autograft tissue in three patients.

### Controversial Indications

Arthroscopic treatment of traumatic anterior shoulder instability in collision athletes remains a controversial topic. Recent articles describing modern suture anchor techniques have shown similar redislocation rates in collision athletes and noncollision athletes.[39,40] Burkhart and De Beer[7] reported on a large group of patients that included many rugby players. Collision athletes without bone loss did not have a higher dislocation recurrence rate compared with other patients in the study. Other reported studies do show higher rates of postoperative dislocation for collision athletes when compared with historic outcomes for arthroscopic instability surgery, but some authors have attributed this increased rate of failure to the activity rather than the surgical technique.[41,42] One study that directly compared open and arthroscopic techniques did find a higher failure rate for the arthroscopic group.[42] Historic reports of failure rates for open stabilization procedures in contact athletes vary between 3% and 15%.[43,44] Arthroscopic instability procedures for collision athletes without bone loss should result in failure rates that are similar to those reported for traditional open instability surgery.

### Surgical Pearls and Pitfalls

The important anteroinferior capsulolabral complex must be considered when surgical treatment is required[45] (Figure 8). The basis for arthroscopic instability procedures is the reestablishment of normal glenoid labral anatomy and retensioning of the inferior glenohumeral ligament (IGHL) in a manner that mirrors open procedures. Instability surgery should be concentrated an-

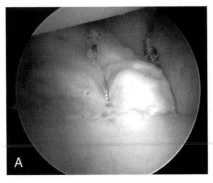
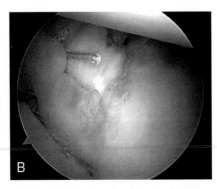

**Figure 9** Completed repair of the labral complex with restored soft-tissue bumper. **A,** Completed capsulolabral repair in a right shoulder viewed from the posterior. **B,** Completed repair viewed from the anterosuperior portal.

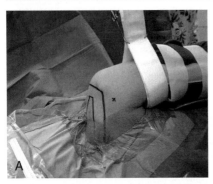
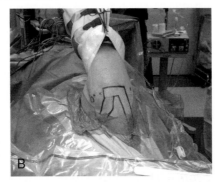

**Figure 10** **A,** View of posterior portal placement in the right shoulder. **B,** Right shoulder viewed from superior to show optimal portal placement—anterosuperior and anteroinferior portals to the left and posterior portal on the right.

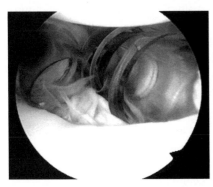
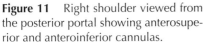
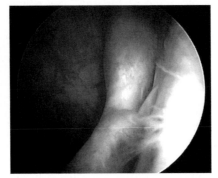

**Figure 11** Right shoulder viewed from the posterior portal showing anterosuperior and anteroinferior cannulas.

**Figure 12** Medially healed IGHL complex.

wise approach to arthroscopic instability surgery can eliminate many of these potential pitfalls.

At the conclusion of surgery, the anteroinferior capsulolabral complex should resemble a soft-tissue buttress on the face of the glenoid, and the capsule should be appropriately tensioned (Figure 9). A typical Bankart lesion extends to the inferior (6 o'clock) position on the glenoid, making access to this area critical. The surgeon must have the ability to place instruments deep into the inferior recess of the shoulder capsule and must place anchors down to at least the 5 o'clock position.[45]

For arthroscopic instability surgery, the authors prefer placing the patient in the lateral position with longitudinal traction. After positioning is complete, proper portal placement enhances access while minimizing iatrogenic trauma to the articular surfaces and facilitates instrumentation in the inferior aspect of the joint (Figure 10). The posterior portal should be placed in line with the glenoid to allow the angle of the arthroscope to parallel the glenoid face. After the posterior portal is established, a 7-mm anterosuperior cannula should be placed high in the rotator interval and an 8.25-mm anteroinferior cannula should be placed just above the subscapularis. Care must be taken to leave an adequate distance (at least 3 cm) between the two cannulas to eliminate instrument crowding. Outside-in needle localization is used to ensure that these cannulas will allow instrumentation of the inferior pouch (Figure 11). The anteroinferior capsulolabral complex then must be adequately mobilized. Often the labrum is healed medially along the scapular neck (Figure 12). The capsulolabral release is considered adequate when the muscular fibers of

teroinferiorly and should reestablish the anatomy and function of the IGHL. Common pitfalls in arthroscopic instability surgery include poor cannula placement limiting exposure in the joint, failure to

properly mobilize the Bankart lesion off the medial glenoid, failure to retension the IGHL, failure to begin the repair at the 6 o'clock position, failure to correct concomitant capsular redundancy, and too few fixation points on the glenoid. A step-the subscapularis are visible under the labrum (Figure 13). Placing the arthroscope in the anterosuperior position can improve viewing of the soft-tissue release and glenoid bone preparation. Positioning tips to improve instrument access to the inferior shoulder include placement of a "bump" into the axilla to lateralize the humeral head and improve visualization (Figure 14). For final preparation, the glenoid must be roughened with a burr or meniscal rasp to encourage soft-tissue healing.

After adequate mobilization is obtained, multiple options exist for retensioning the IGHL. Almost all techniques require shuttling of permanent nonabsorbable sutures housed within the anchor through the capsule and labrum. Suture hooks, penetrators, and other shuttling devices are used to transfer the nonabsorbable suture through the capsule and labrum. The authors use a commercial shuttling hook and 0 Polydioxanone (Ethicon, Somerville, NJ) for this purpose. If the arthroscope is posterior, a traction stitch may be placed inferiorly and brought out of the anterosuperior portal, enabling a more inferior grasp of tissue for the anchor stitch.[46] In the authors' preferred technique, the arthroscope is placed in the anterosuperior portal to better visualize the extent of the shift. A suture-passing instrument can be placed in the anteroinferior cannula for the initial suture pass, but the authors prefer placement of the initial suture pass through the posterior cannula. This technique improves access to the apex of the capsulolabral release, allowing a very inferior primary stitch with excellent visualization (Figure 15).

Suture anchors should be placed 1 to 2 mm onto the articular face of the glenoid and 5 to 10 mm cephalad to

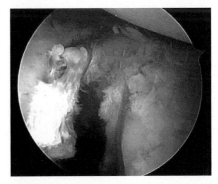

**Figure 13**   Adequate capsulolabral release with muscle fibers visible.

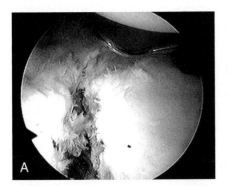
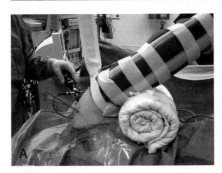
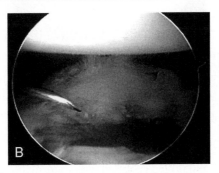
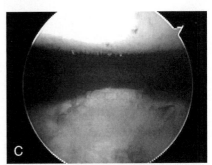

**Figure 14**   **A,** Placement of bump in axilla to improve exposure. View of the inferior joint before the bump is placed (**B**) and after the bump is placed (**C**).

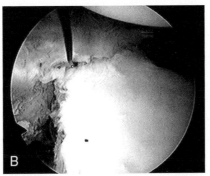
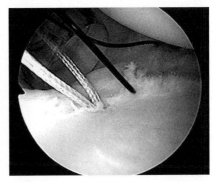

**Figure 15**   Inferior aspect of the right glenohumeral joint. **A,** Suture hook/passing instrument is brought into the joint from the posterior portal. Note access to the IGHL complex near the 6 o'clock position. **B,** Capsule and labrum are pierced with device inferiorly and the suture is being passed.

**Figure 16**   The suture anchor is placed cephalad to the shuttle stitch to achieve the superior tissue shift needed to retension the IGHL and re-create normal labral buttress.

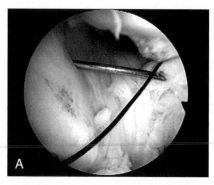
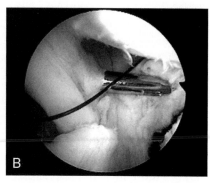

**Figure 17** Needle localization (**A**) and trocar insertion (**B**) for percutaneous transsubscapular anchor placement on the inferior glenoid.

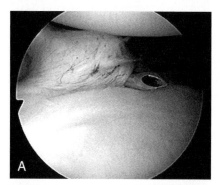
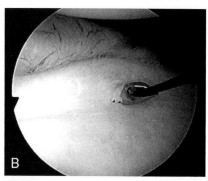

**Figure 18** The right shoulder viewed from the anterosuperior portal showing the capsular plication technique. **A,** Suture hook coming from anteroinferior portal and piercing the anteroinferior capsule (usually 1 cm lateral to the labrum). **B,** After taking a pinch of capsule, the labrum is pierced in a more cephalad position to tension the capsule/ligament.

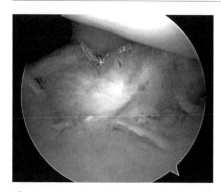

**Figure 19** Completed mattress stitch with both suture limbs on the tissue side.

the shuttle stitch to achieve the superior tissue shift required to retension the IGHL while recreating the normal labral buttress (Figure 16). The capsulolabral complex must be moved onto the face of the glenoid

and pulled cephalad with each anchor to complete the repair. If inferior anchor placement remains difficult despite well-placed anterior cannulas, a transsubscapular anchor can be placed. A stab incision is created using needle localization, and the anchor is inserted percutaneously to ensure correct placement on the inferior glenoid (Figure 17).

Capsular tensioning and labral repair can be combined with a combination stitch (pinch-tuck technique), in which a curved suture-passer pierces the capsule 5 to 10 mm lateral to the labrum, exits the capsule, then reenters at the lateral edge of the labrum to emerge at the articular margin (Figure 18). A

monofilament suture can be used to shuttle a nonabsorbable suture housed in the anchor. The process of shuttle suture/anchor placement should be repeated until normal anatomy is restored. Recently, some authors have recommended at least four anchor points to ensure adequate stabilization of the labral complex.[2,47] It may be necessary to move the arthroscope back to the posterior portal for placement of the most anterior cephalad anchor.

## Adjunctive Techniques

Other techniques are valuable when associated pathology is encountered along with a Bankart lesion. A mattress suture technique can be used with a degenerative or atrophic labrum or poor quality capsular tissue. To create a mattress suture, a second soft-tissue pass is made just superior to an anchor stitch that has already been completed. For this stitch, both limbs of the anchor exit on the soft-tissue side; tying an arthroscopic knot creates a mattress stitch that enhances tissue gathering (Figure 19).

Occasionally a labral injury extends posteriorly past the 6 o'clock position and involves a tear of the posterior labrum. Posterior access often is required to place anchors in the correct position. A percutaneous technique for anchor placement can be used, with needle localization to ensure a correct path (Figure 20). Alternatively, a posteroinferior portal can be created, again using needle localization to ensure appropriate access. This portal typically is 1 to 3 cm more lateral than a routine posterior portal on the shoulder when viewed externally (Figure 21). Even in the absence of labral pathology, the posterior capsule may be patulous and loose. Several authors have recommended routine placement of

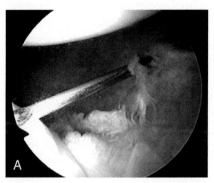
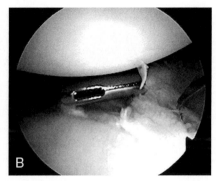
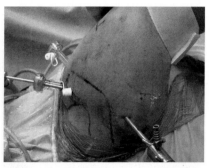

**Figure 20** Needle localization (**A**) and trocar insertion (**B**) for posterolateral percutaneous anchor placement.

**Figure 21** Outside view of posterolateral portal location indicated by 18-gauge spinal needle. (Reproduced with permission from Bottoni CR, Franks BR, Moore JH, DeBerardino TM, Taylor DC, Arciero RA: Operative stabilization of posterior shoulder instability. *Am J Sports Med* 2005;33:998.)

posteroinferior plication sutures to improve results.[48,49] Capsular plication stitches can be placed using the "pinch-tuck" technique to tighten the posteroinferior portion of the IGHL and restore the proper tension to the IGHL complex (Figure 22).

The rotator interval can be closed to provide additional stability for the repair. Many techniques have been described in the literature, but all are designed to reestablish interval integrity and increase stability.[34,50] The superior border of the medial glenohumeral ligament or subscapularis can be grasped with a suture-passing device from the anterosuperior portal. The superior glenohumeral/coracohumeral complex is then pierced with a tissue penetrator to grasp the stitch. Multiple stitches can be placed to increase the closure. A biomechanical study has confirmed that rotator interval closure decreases external rotation and anterior translation.[51] Although the indications for rotator interval closure have not been well established, current recommendations include a sulcus sign greater than 1 cm of inferior translation (1+ sulcus) that does not correct with external rotation or correspond to the uninjured side, laxity with a clear posterior

component, and a collision athlete in whom stability is more important than motion.[41,52]

Capsular tearing may be associated with a traumatic anterior shoulder dislocation. Reported rates of complete capsular tears found at the time of arthroscopy range from 1.5% to 40%.[53,54] A recent retrospective report of 303 shoulders showed a 4% frequency of complete capsular tears.[55] In this study, all tears were treated arthroscopically with capsular repair and only one recurrence was reported (Figure 23). Failure to correct a full-thickness capsular tear may lead to insufficiency of the IGHL complex, even if the labral ligament complex is reduced to the glenoid.

Patients also may present with a glenoid rim fracture, the so-called osseous Bankart lesion (Figure 24). The outcomes of patients with glenoid rim fragments can be contrasted with the outcomes of patients with anterior glenoid bone loss. Boileau and associates[2] reported that patients with rim fractures had outcomes that were not significantly different from those of patients without bony injury. These results compare favorably with results reported by Sugaya and associates[56] for the treatment of patients with chronic instability who re-

tained an osseous fragment in the Bankart lesion. An earlier study of patients with acute bony Bankart injuries also reported excellent clinical results.[5] The reported success of arthroscopic osseous Bankart repair makes it a viable option if the retained bone fragment can be included in the repair.

Rotator cuff pathology should be considered in patients older than 40 years with anterior shoulder dislocations, especially those with recurrent symptoms.[57] A careful physical examination and MRI of soft tissue should alert the examiner to the concomitant pathology. Although subscapularis repairs are reportedly less successful than supraspinatus repairs in patients with instability, patients can expect good pain relief with a minimal decrease in function.[58] Other rotator cuff pathology should be treated at the time of the index procedure for instability.

### Complications
Complications have not been widely reported with arthroscopic shoulder instability surgery and have mainly focused on recurrence of instability

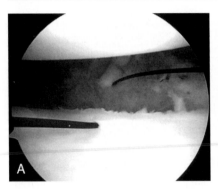
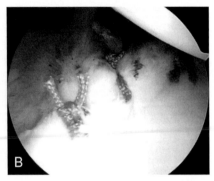

**Figure 22** Capsular plication shuttle stitch placement **(A)** and final repair of the IGHL complex **(B)**.

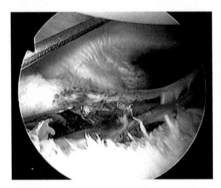

**Figure 23** Anterior capsular tear.

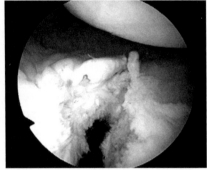

**Figure 24** Arthroscopic view of the osseous Bankart lesion.

as an evaluation end point. Large, recent clinical trials have reported recurrent instability rates (both subluxation and dislocation) ranging from 4% to 15%.[2,16,48,49] Each study noted the high prevalence of bone loss in patients who experienced recurrent episodes of instability. All the studies reported minimal to no significant loss of range of motion and high rates of patient satisfaction.

One well-known complication of intra-articular anchor placement is protrusion of the anchor into the joint surface. In 2004, Rhee and associates[59] reported a case study of five patients with severe arthropathy after protruding anchors were confirmed. Although such protrusions have been reported for open procedures, arthroscopic procedures require extra care to ensure proper anchor placement.[60] Proper portal

creation allows easier instrumentation and anchor placement. Although the literature has many reports of the hazards of incorrectly placed metallic anchors, bioabsorbable anchors also have been implicated in a small case study of severe osteolysis.[61] The authors postulated that micromotion induces the loss of stability in a knotless anchor construct, leading to pullout of the anchors and chondrolysis. Occasional synovitis and foreign body reactions have been reported, but large clinical trials have not shown bioabsorbable anchors to be a consistent complication.[62-64]

## Summary

Arthroscopic stabilization for recurrent anterior instability is rapidly becoming a well-accepted technique.

The surgeon must have a high index of suspicion for significant bone loss because this is an almost universal contraindication for arthroscopic repair, even in the hands of recognized experts. In the past 5 years, outcomes from arthroscopic stabilization using modern techniques are equivalent to those of open methods. The arthroscopic technique is demanding and requires meticulous attention to detail. Proper placement of anchors, placement of instrumentation inferiorly in the detached capsulolabral complex, and secure knot-tying are prerequisites for reestablishing the normal labral anatomy and insuring retensioning of the IGHL. The surgeon should possess the skills required to accommodate variations in pathoanatomy, such as a chronically medialized labrum, atrophic or attenuated labrum, labral tears that extend posteriorly, and excessive capsular laxity.

## References

1. Kim SH, Park JS, Jeong WK, Shin SK: The Kim test: A novel test for posteroinferior labral lesion of the shoulder: A comparison to the jerk test. *Am J Sports Med* 2005;33:1188-1192.

2. Boileau P, Villalba M, Hery JY, Balg F, Ahrens P, Neyton L: Risk factors for recurrence of shoulder instability after arthroscopic Bankart repair. *J Bone Joint Surg Am* 2006;88:1755-1763.

3. Tauber M, Resch H, Forstner R, Raffl M, Schauer J: Reasons for failure after surgical repair of anterior shoulder instability. *J Shoulder Elbow Surg* 2004;13:279-285.

4. Itoi E, Lee SB, Amrami KK, Wenger DE, An KN: Quantitative assessment of classic anteroinferior bony Bankart lesions by radiography and computed tomography. *Am J Sports Med* 2003;31:112-118.

5. Porcellini G, Paladini P, Campi F, Paganelli M: Shoulder instability and related rotator cuff tears: Arthroscopic findings and treatment in patients aged 40 to 60 years. *Arthroscopy* 2006;22:270-276.

6. Rhee YG, Ha JH, Park KJ: Clinical outcome of anterior shoulder instability with capsular midsubstance tear: A comparison of isolated midsubstance tear and midsubstance tear with Bankart lesion. *J Shoulder Elbow Surg* 2006;15:586-590.

7. Burkhart SS, De Beer JF: Traumatic glenohumeral bone defects and their relationship to failure of arthroscopic Bankart repairs: Significance of the inverted-pear glenoid and the humeral engaging Hill-Sachs lesion. *Arthroscopy* 2000;16:677-694.

8. Itoi E, Lee SB, Berglund LJ, Berge LL, An KN: The effect of a glenoid defect on anteroinferior stability of the shoulder after Bankart repair: A cadaveric study. *J Bone Joint Surg Am* 2000;82:35-46.

9. Burkhart SS, Danaceau SM: Articular arc length mismatch as a cause of failed bankart repair. *Arthroscopy* 2000;16:740-744.

10. Bigliani LU, Newton PM, Steinmann SP, Connor PM, McLlveen SJ: Glenoid rim lesions associated with recurrent anterior dislocation of the shoulder. *Am J Sports Med* 1998;26:41-45.

11. Lazarus MD, Sidles JA, Harryman DT II, Matsen FA III: Effect of a chondral-labral defect on glenoid concavity and glenohumeral stability: A cadaveric model. *J Bone Joint Surg Am* 1996;78:94-102.

12. Gerber C, Nyffeler RW: Classification of glenohumeral joint instability. *Clin Orthop Relat Res* 2002;400:65-76.

13. Sugaya H, Moriishi J, Dohi M, Kon Y, Tsuchiya A: Glenoid rim morphology in recurrent anterior glenohumeral instability. *J Bone Joint Surg Am* 2003;85-A:878-884.

14. Burkhart SS, Debeer JF, Tehrany AM, Parten PM: Quantifying glenoid bone loss arthroscopically in shoulder insta-bility. *Arthroscopy* 2002;18:488-491.

15. Lo IK, Parten PM, Burkhart SS: The inverted pear glenoid: An indicator of significant glenoid bone loss. *Arthroscopy* 2004;20:169-174.

16. Kim SH, Ha KI, Cho YB, Ryu BD, Oh I: Arthroscopic anterior stabilization of the shoulder: Two to six-year follow-up. *J Bone Joint Surg Am* 2003;85:1511-1518.

17. Millett PJ, Clavert P, Warner JJ: Open operative treatment for anterior shoulder instability: When and why? *J Bone Joint Surg Am* 2005;87:419-432.

18. Chen AL, Hunt SA, Hawkins RJ, Zuckerman JD: Management of bone loss associated with recurrent anterior glenohumeral instability. *Am J Sports Med* 2005;33:912-925.

19. Bodey WN, Denham RA: A free bone block operation for recurrent anterior dislocation of the shoulder joint. *Injury* 1983;15:184-188.

20. Haaker RG, Eickhoff U, Klammer HL: Intraarticular autogenous bone grafting in recurrent shoulder dislocations. *Mil Med* 1993;158:164-169.

21. Warner JJ, Gill TJ, O'Hollerhan JD, Pathare N, Millett PJ: Anatomical glenoid reconstruction for recurrent anterior glenohumeral instability with glenoid deficiency using an autogenous tricortical iliac crest bone graft. *Am J Sports Med* 2006;34:205-212.

22. Latarjet M: Technic of coracoid preglenoid arthroereisis in the treatment of recurrent dislocation of the shoulder. *Lyon Chir* 1958;54:604-607.

23. Helfet AJ: Coracoid transplantation for recurring dislocation of the shoulder. *J Bone Joint Surg Br* 1958;40-B:198-202.

24. Schroder DT, Provencher MT, Mologne TS, Muldoon MP, Cox JS: The modified Bristow procedure for anterior shoulder instability: 26-year outcomes in Naval Academy midshipmen. *Am J Sports Med* 2006;34:778-786.

25. Hovelius L, Sandstrom B, Sundgren K, Saebo M: One hundred eighteen Bristow-Latarjet repairs for recurrent anterior dislocation of the shoulder prospectively followed for fifteen years: Study I. Clinical results. *J Shoulder Elbow Surg* 2004;13:509-516.

26. Allain J, Goutallier D, Glorion C: Long-term results of the Latarjet procedure for the treatment of anterior instability of the shoulder. *J Bone Joint Surg Am* 1998;80:841-852.

27. Chapovsky F, Kelly JD: Osteochondral allograft transplantation for treatment of glenohumeral instability. *Arthroscopy* 2005;21:1007.

28. Re P, Gallo RA, Richmond JC: Transhumeral head plasty for large Hill-Sachs lesions. *Arthroscopy* 2006;22:798.

29. Yagishita K, Thomas BJ: Use of allograft for large Hill-Sachs lesion associated with anterior glenohumeral dislocation: A case report. *Injury* 2002;33:791-794.

30. Weber BG, Simpson LA, Hardegger F: Rotational humeral osteotomy for recurrent anterior dislocation of the shoulder associated with a large Hill-Sachs lesion. *J Bone Joint Surg Am* 1984;66:1443-1450.

31. Bokor DJ, Conboy VB, Olson C: Anterior instability of the glenohumeral joint with humeral avulsion of the glenohumeral ligament: A review of 41 cases. *J Bone Joint Surg Br* 1999;81:93-96.

32. Taylor DC, Arciero RA: Pathologic changes associated with shoulder dislocations: Arthroscopic and physical examination findings in first-time, traumatic anterior dislocations. *Am J Sports Med* 1997;25:306-311.

33. Wolf EM, Cheng JC, Dickson K: Humeral avulsion of glenohumeral ligaments as a cause of anterior shoulder instability. *Arthroscopy* 1995;11:600-607.

34. Spang JT, Karas SG: The HAGL lesion: An arthroscopic technique for repair of humeral avulsion of the glenohumeral ligaments. *Arthroscopy* 2005;21:498-502.

35. Richards DP, Burkhart SS: Arthroscopic humeral avulsion of the gleno-

humeral ligaments (HAGL) repair. *Arthroscopy* 2004;20(suppl 2):134-141.

36. Arciero RA, Mazzocca AD: Mini-open repair technique of HAGL (humeral avulsion of the glenohumeral ligament) lesion. *Arthroscopy* 2005;21:1152.

37. Warner JJ, Venegas AA, Lehtinen JT, Macy JJ: Management of capsular deficiency of the shoulder: A report of three cases. *J Bone Joint Surg Am* 2002;84-A:1668-1671.

38. Park HB, Yokota A, Gill HS, El Rassi G, McFarland EG: Revision surgery for failed thermal capsulorrhaphy. *Am J Sports Med* 2005;33:1321-1326.

39. Ide J, Maeda S, Takagi K: Arthroscopic Bankart repair using suture anchors in athletes: Patient selection and postoperative sports activity. *Am J Sports Med* 2004;32:1899-1905.

40. Bacilla P, Field LD, Savoie FH: Arthroscopic Bankart repair in a high demand patient population. *Arthroscopy* 1997;13:51-60.

41. Mazzocca AD, Brown FM Jr, Carreira DS, Hayden J, Romeo AA: Arthroscopic anterior shoulder stabilization of collision and contact athletes. *Am J Sports Med* 2005;33:52-60.

42. Cho NS, Hwang JC, Rhee YG: Arthroscopic stabilization in anterior shoulder instability: Collision athletes versus noncollision athletes. *Arthroscopy* 2006;22:947-953.

43. Pagnani MJ, Dome DC: Surgical treatment of traumatic anterior shoulder instability in American football players. *J Bone Joint Surg Am* 2002;84-A:711-715.

44. Uhorchak JM, Arciero RA, Huggard D, Taylor DC: Recurrent shoulder instability after open reconstruction in athletes involved in collision and contact sports. *Am J Sports Med* 2000; 28:794-799.

45. Cole BJ, Millett PJ, Romeo AA, et al: Arthroscopic treatment of anterior glenohumeral instability: Indications and techniques. *Instr Course Lect* 2004; 53:545-558.

46. Boileau P, Ahrens P: The TOTS (temporary outside traction suture): A new technique to allow easy suture placement and improve capsular shift in arthroscopic bankart repair. *Arthroscopy* 2003;19:672-677.

47. Kim SH, Ha KI, Kim YM: Arthroscopic revision Bankart repair: A prospective outcome study. *Arthroscopy* 2002;18:469-482.

48. Westerheide KJ, Dopirak RM, Snyder SJ: Arthroscopic anterior stabilization and posterior capsular plication for anterior glenohumeral instability: A report of 71 cases. *Arthroscopy* 2006;22:539-547.

49. Carreira DS, Mazzocca AD, Oryhon J, Brown FM, Hayden JK, Romeo AA: A prospective outcome evaluation of arthroscopic Bankart repairs: Minimum 2-year follow-up. *Am J Sports Med* 2006;34:771-777.

50. Almazan A, Ruiz M, Cruz F, Perez FX, Ibarra C: Simple arthroscopic technique for rotator interval closure. *Arthroscopy* 2006;22:230.

51. Plausinis D, Bravman JT, Heywood C, Kummer FJ, Kwon YW, Jazrawi LM: Arthroscopic rotator interval closure: Effect of sutures on glenohumeral motion and anterior-posterior translation. *Am J Sports Med* 2006;34: 1656-1661.

52. Stokes DA, Savoie FH, Field LD, Ramsey JR: Arthroscopic repair of anterior glenohumeral instability and rotator interval lesions. *Orthop Clin North Am* 2003;34:529-538.

53. Ogawa K, Yoshida A: Extensive shoulder capsule tearing as a main cause of recurrent anterior shoulder dislocation. *J Shoulder Elbow Surg* 1997;6:1-5.

54. Kuriyama S, Fujimaki E, Katagiri T, Uemura S: Anterior dislocation of the shoulder joint sustained through skiing: Arthrographic findings and prognosis. *Am J Sports Med* 1984;12:339-346.

55. Mizuno N, Yoneda M, Hayashida K, Nakagawa S, Mae T, Izawa K: Recurrent anterior shoulder dislocation caused by a midsubstance complete capsular tear. *J Bone Joint Surg Am* 2005;87:2717-2723.

56. Sugaya H, Moriishi J, Kanisawa I, Tsuchiya A: Arthroscopic osseous Bankart repair for chronic recurrent traumatic anterior glenohumeral instability. *J Bone Joint Surg Am* 2005;87: 1752-1760.

57. Neviaser RJ, Neviaser TJ, Neviaser JS: Concurrent rupture of the rotator cuff and anterior dislocation of the shoulder in the older patient. *J Bone Joint Surg Am* 1988;70:1308-1311.

58. Gerber C, Krushell RJ: Isolated rupture of the tendon of the subscapularis muscle: Clinical features in 16 cases. *J Bone Joint Surg Br* 1991;73: 389-394.

59. Rhee YG, Lee DH, Chun IH, Bae SC: Glenohumeral arthropathy after arthroscopic anterior shoulder stabilization. *Arthroscopy* 2004;20:402-406.

60. Kaar TK, Schenck RC Jr, Wirth MA, Rockwood CA Jr: Complications of metallic suture anchors in shoulder surgery: A report of 8 cases. *Arthroscopy* 2001;17:31-37.

61. Athwal GS, Shridharani SM, O'Driscoll SW: Osteolysis and arthropathy of the shoulder after use of bioabsorbable knotless suture anchors: A report of four cases. *J Bone Joint Surg Am* 2006;88:1840-1845.

62. Burkart A, Imhoff AB, Roscher E: Foreign-body reaction to the bioabsorbable suretac device. *Arthroscopy* 2000;16:91-95.

63. Bostman O, Partio E, Hirvensalo E, Rokkanen P: Foreign-body reactions to polyglycolide screws: Observations in 24/216 malleolar fracture cases. *Acta Orthop Scand* 1992;63:173-176.

64. Barber FA, Snyder SJ, Abrams JS, Fanelli GC, Savoie FH: Arthroscopic Bankart reconstruction with a bioabsorbable anchor. *J Shoulder Elbow Surg* 2003;12:535-538.

# Arthroscopic Anterior Shoulder Instability Repair: Techniques, Pearls, Pitfalls, and Complications

Cordelia W. Carter, MD
Chris Moros, BS
Christopher S. Ahmad, MD
William N. Levine, MD

## Abstract

*Initial attempts to replicate the success of open anterior shoulder instability procedures using arthroscopic procedures were associated with unacceptably high failure rates. The resultant focus on identifying clear surgical indications and improving both arthroscopic technique and instrumentation has culminated in arthroscopic success rates approaching those of established open procedures. Current experience shows that with careful patient selection, strict adherence to proper surgical technique, and the avoidance of common surgical errors, excellent clinical results can be achieved with arthroscopic instability repair.*

**Instr Course Lect 2008;57:125-132.**

When surgical shoulder stabilization is indicated, satisfactory outcomes usually can be achieved regardless of the type of procedure used. Satisfactory outcomes require adherence to the following surgical tenets: anatomic repair of the detached anteroinferior labrum, restoration of proper tension to the inferior glenohumeral ligament complex, capsular plication as needed to eliminate residual capsular laxity, and assessment of the sufficiency of the rotator interval with plication of this region as indicated.

## Indications

As arthroscopic techniques have evolved, the clinical results of arthroscopic shoulder instability repair have approached those of traditional open procedures.[1-3] Advantages of arthroscopic instability surgery include improved ability to identify and treat concomitant intra-articular pathology, less soft-tissue dissection (for example, division of the subscapularis muscle), less intraoperative blood loss, decreased surgical time, a shorter hospital stay, less postoperative pain, easier functional recovery, maximal preservation of joint motion (such as external rotation), and improved cosmesis.[4]

It is critical to identify patients who are not candidates for arthroscopic shoulder stabilization. Contraindications to arthroscopic stabilization include factors such as significant bone deficiency either on the glenoid (inverted pear deformity) or an "engaging" Hill-Sachs deformity of the humeral head.[5] Careful review of preoperative radiographs is critical to success; however, when in doubt, CT scans should be obtained to appropriately evaluate possible bone deficiencies. Other contraindications include humeral avulsion of the glenohumeral ligament (HAGL) lesions, capsular insufficiency associated with previous revision surgeries, and patients with voluntary dislocations. **(DVD 11.1)**

## Surgical Technique

### Anesthesia, Examination Under Anesthesia, and Positioning

Regional interscalene anesthesia is routinely used by the authors. To improve patient flow and efficiency, the block is administered outside the operating room in a regional anesthesia area. The patient is then taken to the operating room where an examination under anesthesia (EUA) is performed. EUA of both shoulders with the patient supine allows the examiner to assess the degree and direction of glenohumeral laxity when involuntary guarding is eliminated, and to make a direct comparison between the symptomatic and asymptomatic shoulder joints. Most importantly, EUA confirms the preoperative diagnosis established based on a careful patient history and physical and radiographic evaluations.

Following EUA, the patient is positioned in either the lateral decu-

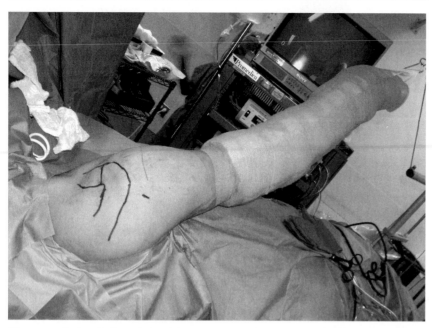

**Figure 1** Patient in lateral decubitus position with traction applied.

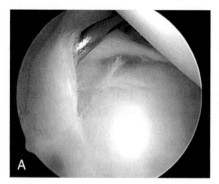

**Figure 2** Arthroscopic view of superior labrum anterior and posterior tear (**A**) found in addition to anterior labral tear (**B**).

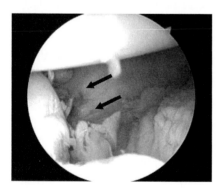

**Figure 3** Arthroscopic view of an anterior labrum periosteal sleeve avulsion, which is best identified from an anterosuperior viewing portal. Arrows indicate medial capsulolabral complex.

capsule and labrum (anterior, posterior, superior, inferior). The use of this position may be desirable in patients requiring capsular plication. The authors prefer the lateral decubitus position for most patients with shoulder instability (Figure 1). (**DVD 11.2**)

### Diagnostic Arthroscopy and Portal Placement

Following the preparation and sterile draping of the patient, a standard posterior portal is established in the anatomic "soft spot," approximately 2 cm inferior and 1 cm medial to the posterolateral edge of the acromion. Systematic diagnostic arthroscopy is performed to evaluate the glenohumeral joint. Diagnostic arthroscopy includes both direct visualization and manual probing to evaluate the biceps anchor and the intra-articular portion of the tendon of the long head of the biceps brachii. This evaluation is followed by a similar inspection of the entire circumference of the glenoid labrum starting from the 12 o'clock position and proceeding 360° around the clock face. Next, the glenoid is examined for evidence of injury, osseous deficiency, or osteochondral wear. The rotator cuff, the rotator interval, and the glenohumeral ligaments are then evaluated with the arm held in various degrees of abduction and external rotation to best assess the degree and direction of pathologic laxity. The presence of the "drive-through" sign (passage of the arthroscope from posterior to anterior at the midhumeral level, indicating significant capsular laxity) is then assessed.[6] It cannot be overemphasized that completion of thorough diagnostic arthroscopy is critical to identifying concomitant intra-articular pathology such as superior labrum anterior and posterior lesions (Figure 2), anterior labrum periosteal

bitus or beach chair position. Successful stabilization can be performed in either position, and arguments can be made to support the use of either position. For example, conversion to an open approach is easier from the beach chair position, which may be relevant when operating on patients with HAGL lesions or severe bony deficiency of the glenoid in whom conversion to an open approach is anticipated. Alternatively, the lateral decubitus position has significant advantages, including enhanced visualization of and access to the entire

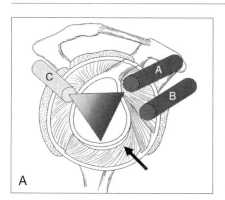
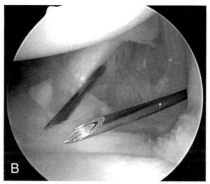
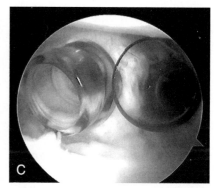

**Figure 4**    **A,** Illustration showing anterosuperior cannula (A) high in the rotator interval and anteroinferior cannula (B) just above the rolled edge of the subscapularis viewed from a posterior cannula (C). **B,** Arthroscopic view showing two spinal needles indicating placement for each anterior cannula. **C,** Anterior cannulas in position.

sleeve avulsion injuries (Figure 3), HAGL injuries, rotator cuff pathology, the size of Hill-Sachs lesions, and the presence and degree of anterior glenoid deficiency. This evaluation is important in planning a comprehensive surgical repair.[7-9]

After initial diagnostic arthroscopy, an anterosuperior portal is made using an outside-in technique with a spinal needle. This portal should be placed high in the rotator interval, superior and lateral to the palpable coracoid process, so that it pierces the rotator interval capsule and enters the joint at the level of the biceps anchor at an insertion angle of approximately 90° to the arthroscope (Figure 4). Too-medial placement of this portal may compromise access to the glenoid. Portal dilators may be used to facilitate cannula placement and minimize the potential for articular cartilage damage while placing cannulas in the joint. A disposable threaded cannula is then inserted through the portal. Use of a cannula enables swift passage of arthroscopic instrumentation into and out of the glenohumeral joint, facilitates arthroscopic knot tying, and creates a seal in the joint, thereby minimizing fluid extravasation into the adjacent soft tis-

sues. Use of a threaded cannula prevents inadvertent back-out of the cannula from the glenohumeral joint. The camera is then placed in the anterior cannula to further evaluate the posterior and inferior capsule and the medial glenoid.

Next, an anteroinferior portal is made, taking care to leave a generous distance (at least 3 cm) between the anterosuperior and anteroinferior cannulas; in this manner, the working space available for passage of arthroscopic instruments is maximized (Figure 4). The anteroinferior portal should be placed just above the superior rolled edge of the subscapularis. Proper lateral placement of this cannula is critical to facilitate placement of suture anchors in the desired orientation on the anteroinferior glenoid.

## Capsulolabral Mobilization and Glenoid Preparation

Before inserting the implants, the capsulolabral complex must be mobilized from its nonanatomic position on the glenoid neck. This mobilization is achieved by positioning the arthroscope in the posterior portal and placing a rasp, periosteal elevator, electrocautery device, or arthroscopic shaver through the working antero-

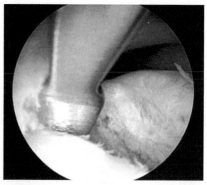

**Figure 5**    Arthroscopic view of the labral-ligamentous complex being mobilized from its scarred nonanatomic position.

inferior portal (Figure 5). Using one or a combination of these instruments, the scarred capsulolabral complex is systematically mobilized from the glenoid neck inferiorly to the 6 o'clock position until it is freely mobile and can be shifted onto the glenoid rim with ease. Capsular mobility is assessed using a soft-tissue grasper to pull the tissue from inferior to superior and also onto the glenoid rim. Attainment of satisfactory tissue mobility occasionally may require release beyond the 6 o'clock position. In this situation, the axillary nerve must be protected. Next, a motorized burr or arthroscopic shaver is used to prepare the glenoid;

the guiding concept is that gentle decortication of the anteroinferior glenoid to expose bleeding bone that extends medially onto the glenoid neck and inferiorly to the 6 o'clock position of the glenoid will enhance subsequent healing of the repaired labrum (Figure 6). **(DVD 11.3)**

### Suture Anchor Placement and Suture Passage

Technical goals for suture anchor placement and suture passage are to place suture anchors directly onto the edge of the articular surface of the glenoid and to pass sutures through the capsulolabral complex, thereby re-creating an anatomic reconstruction (Figures 7 and 8). Improper insertion of suture anchors

medially along the scapular neck increases the risk of recurrent instability. Anchor placement proceeds inferiorly to superiorly, with placement of the first suture anchor through the anteroinferior cannula at the 5:30 position on the glenoid (for a right shoulder). It is essential that anchors be precisely placed with respect to the insertion angle (approximately 45° to the plane of the glenoid) and position (on the glenoid rim). If insertion of the suture anchor at the desired position is impossible to achieve through the anteroinferior cannula, a percutaneous technique can be used to place the most inferiorly positioned anchor (Figure 9). A toothed, cannulated drill guide is used to maintain the

desired position on the glenoid rim during drilling of the anchor hole and insertion of the implant. Following insertion, the anchor is checked to ensure that it is seated in bone, stable to manual tensioning of the sutures, not proud on the glenoid surface, and that the sutures slide easily; these factors are associated with risk for both failure of the stabilization procedure and subsequent osteochondral injury.

At this stage in the repair, either a direct or shuttle technique of suture passing can be used. In the direct technique, both suture limbs are taken out of the anterosuperior cannula using a suture-grasping device; a tissue-penetrating/suture-grasping instrument is then inserted into the anteroinferior cannula and through the capsulolabral tissue at a site approximately 5 to 10 mm inferior to the suture anchor. The suture limb that is closer to the labral tissue is retrieved within the instrument and then withdrawn through the tissue to exit via the anteroinferior portal. This limb will become the post of the arthroscopic knot. Proper identification of the post (the suture limb that traverses the tissue) will ensure that the arthroscopic knot sits in its desired position away from the articular cartilage. Next, the second suture limb is retrieved through

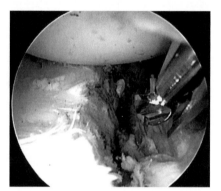

**Figure 6**   A small, round burr, or aggressive shaver or rasp is used to decorticate/abrade the scapular neck to enhance healing of the repaired labral-ligamentous complex.

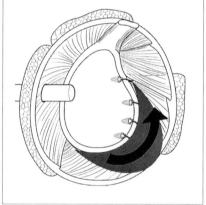

**Figure 7**   Illustration showing the inferior to superior shift of the capsule.

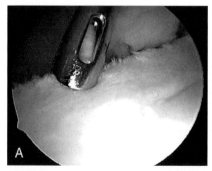 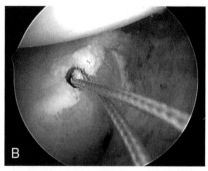

**Figure 8**   **A,** Proper positioning of the suture anchors onto the glenoid rim ensures an anatomic restoration of the labral-ligamentous complex. **B,** Anterosuperior viewing portal shows appropriate placement of the anchors.

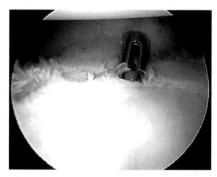

**Figure 9**   Drill guide for suture anchor introduced percutaneously to achieve low 6 o'clock position.

the anteroinferior cannula, and an arthroscopic knot is tied. The knot is tied with an effort to reduce the labrum onto the glenoid face and shift the tissue superiorly. A grasper introduced via the anterosuperior portal may be used to shift the capsule and labrum superiorly during knot tying (Figure 10).

A potential complication of using a direct suture-retrieving device is the risk for articular cartilage injury while maneuvering the device to retrieve the suture. In addition, it is difficult to penetrate tissue inferior to the anchor and then to maneuver the instrument to the sutures to be shuttled. To avoid these complications, a suture shuttle technique can be used quite effectively. With this technique, one suture limb is brought through the anterosuperior cannula and one is left in the anteroinferior cannula. A shuttling device or lasso is passed through the anteroinferior cannula or is passed percutaneously into the capsulolabral tissue inferior to the anchor (Figure 11); the shuttle suture is then retrieved through the anterosuperior cannula. Outside the cannula, the suture shuttle is loaded with the waiting suture limb and both are pulled simultaneously into the joint, through the capsuloligamentous tissue, and out through the anteroinferior cannula. Once shuttling of the suture limb is complete, an arthroscopic knot is tied, as described previously.

After successful placement of the first suture anchor at the 5:30 position, additional anchors are placed into the glenoid in an inferior to superior direction, until three or four anchors (distributed from the 6 o'clock to 3 o'clock positions on the glenoid face) have been inserted (Figure 12). The quality of this repair is assessed using the arthroscopic probe. With the demonstra-

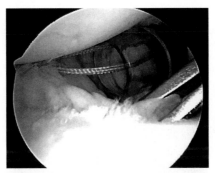

**Figure 10**    A suture lasso is passed from the anteroinferior cannula through the detached anteroinferior labral-ligamentous complex for repair; arthroscopic view from the posterior viewing portal, right shoulder.

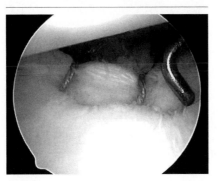

**Figure 12**    Arthroscopic view of the final repair of the labral-ligamentous complex viewed from posterior portal.

tion of residual capsular laxity following anatomic repair of the anteroinferior capsuloligamentous structures, additional stabilization techniques are used. **(DVD 11.4)**

### Capsular Plication

Persistent laxity in the inferior and posterior capsule following arthroscopic Bankart repair can be corrected by suture plication with absorbable or nonabsorbable sutures (Figure 13). With this technique, the capsule is first abraded with an arthroscopic shaver or rasp. Next, a suture-passing device is used to penetrate the redundant capsule approximately 1 cm from the labrum and then to penetrate the labrum itself. If the labrum is deficient, a suture

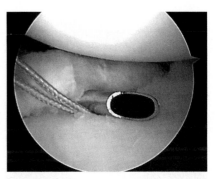

**Figure 11**    Grasper introduced via the anterior-superior cannula is used to shift the tissue superiorly during knot tying.

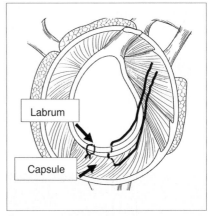

**Figure 13**    Capsular plication sutures are placed in shoulders that have pathologic capsular redundancy as determined by preoperative and intraoperative findings.

anchor should be placed to prevent the suture from pulling out of the labrum (Figure 14). Sutures are passed and tied according to the methods described previously. Two or three plication sutures can be placed, beginning inferiorly then progressing posteroinferiorly, from approximately the 6 o'clock position to the 8 o'clock position. After the inferior capsular plication is complete, the quality of the tissue repair is again evaluated with the arthroscopic probe.

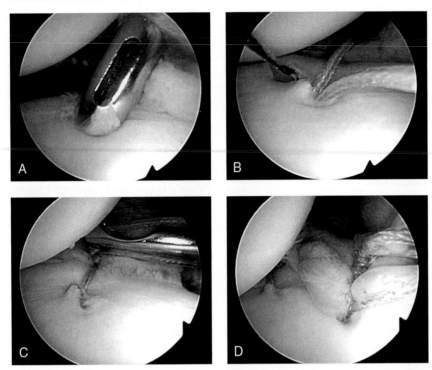

**Figure 14** **A,** Percutaneous portal made for suture anchor placement where the cannula did not allow appropriate angle and direction. **B,** Anchor placed adjacent to the labrum and suture-passer is placed through capsule and labrum. **C,** Knot tying reduces the capsule to the labrum. **D,** Completed capsular plication.

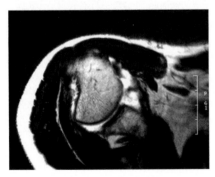

**Figure 15** Two previous arthroscopic anterior instability repairs failed in a right-handed 28-year-old man. Prerevision MRI scan shows significant glenoid bone loss. A Latarjet (coracoid bone transfer) procedure restored stability to his shoulder.

### Rotator Interval Closure

The indications for rotator interval closure are evolving. The rotator interval is primarily responsible for providing stability against posterior and inferior translation of the hu-meral head in the adducted and externally rotated shoulder. Therefore, it is rarely necessary to perform rotator interval closure in routine anterior instability repairs. However, rotator interval closure should be performed in patients with posterior and/or multidirectional instability. Various techniques of interval closure have been described.[10-15] Regardless of the technique used, it is important to place the arm in slight external rotation to avoid postoperative loss of motion secondary to capsular overtightening.

### Pearls of Arthroscopic Instability Repair

Table 1 summarizes the pearls of arthroscopic anterior shoulder instability repair.

### Pitfalls

Preoperative pitfalls of arthroscopic anterior shoulder instability repair include failure to elicit a history of voluntary dislocation; failure to recognize multidirectional instability based on the patient's history and/or physical examination; failure to identify humeral-engaging, Hill-Sachs lesions or HAGL lesions; failure to recognize the surgeon's technical limitations; and failure to identify glenoid deficiency precluding adequate stabilization (> 25%) (Figure 15). Intraoperative pitfalls include poor portal placement resulting in an undesirable anchor insertion angle, or cannulas too close together; incomplete diagnostic arthroscopy resulting in failure to recognize concomitant pathology; inadequate capsulolabral mobilization; inadequate glenoid preparation; improper anchor placement such as articular penetration or placement medially along the scapular neck; poor suture management; failure to recognize loose or proud suture anchors; use of too few suture anchors; unloading of suture anchors; use of thermal energy; and failure to restore proper capsular tension (recurrence versus stiffness).

### Thermal Capsulorrhaphy

Thermal capsulorrhaphy was initially greeted with enthusiasm when it was introduced in the mid 1990s as a novel treatment for shoulder instability attributable to capsular laxity. When used alone or in conjunction with other procedures, the primary concept of thermal capsulorrhaphy was that heat applied to lax shoulder tissues would result in collagen denaturation, tissue shrinkage, and would ultimately improve joint stability. Despite a lack of evidence in the literature to support the efficacy of thermal capsulorrhaphy, it gained widespread acceptance. Over time, however, clinical investigators have been unable to demonstrate the maintenance of shoulder stability, with one study reporting unsatisfactory results in 37% of patients.[16] More worrisome are reports of potentially devastating complications associated with the use of thermal energy, including chondrolysis, capsular necrosis, axillary nerve injury, adhesive capsulitis, and capsular disruption.[17,18] As a result of these reports, thermal capsulorrhaphy has been largely abandoned as a adjunctive surgical technique.[16,19]

## Summary

Arthroscopic shoulder instability repair has evolved over the past 15 years; the results of this procedure now rival those of open instability repair. Attention to detail, appropriate patient selection, meticulous surgical technique, and avoidance of pitfalls have led to successful outcomes in most patients.

## References

1. Carreira DS, Mazzocca AD, Oryhon J, Brown FM, Hayden JK, Romeo AA: A prospective outcome evaluation of arthroscopic Bankart repairs: Minimum 2-year follow-up. *Am J Sports Med* 2006;34:771-777.

2. Kim SH, Ha KI, Cho YB, Ryu BD, Oh I: Arthroscopic anterior stabilization of the shoulder: Two- to six-year follow-up. *J Bone Joint Surg Am* 2003; 85:1511-1518.

3. Mazzocca AD, Brown FM Jr, Carreira DS, Hayden J, Romeo AA: Arthroscopic anterior shoulder stabilization of collision and contact athletes. *Am J Sports Med* 2005;33:52-60.

4. Coughlin L, Rubinovich M, Johansson J, White B, Greenspoon J: Arthroscopic staple capsulorrhaphy for anterior shoulder instability. *Am J Sports Med* 1992;20:253-256.

5. Burkhart SS, De Beer JF: Traumatic glenohumeral bone defects and their relationship to failure of arthroscopic Bankart repairs: Significance of the inverted-pear glenoid and the humeral engaging Hill-Sachs lesion. *Arthroscopy* 2000;16:677-694.

6. Blevins FT: Rotator cuff pathology in athletes. *Sports Med* 1997;24:205-220.

7. Neviaser TJ: The anterior labroligamentous periosteal sleeve avulsion lesion: A cause of anterior instability of the shoulder. *Arthroscopy* 1993;9: 17-21.

8. Wolf EM, Cheng JC, Dickson K: Humeral avulsion of glenohumeral ligaments as a cause of anterior shoulder instability. *Arthroscopy* 1995;11:600-607.

9. Bach BR, Warren RF, Fronek J: Disruption of the lateral capsule of the shoulder: A cause of recurrent dislocation. *J Bone Joint Surg Br* 1988;70: 274-276.

10. Almazan A, Ruiz M, Cruz F, Perez FX, Ibarra C: Simple arthroscopic

## Table 1
### Pearls of Arthroscopic Anterior Shoulder Instability Repair

| | |
|---|---|
| Patient evaluation | Perform a thorough preoperative evaluation to determine if a patient is not a candidate for arthroscopic repair (such as those with significant glenoid bone loss and/or Hill-Sachs lesions). If doubt exists, CT should be used to rule out bone deficiencies. Diagnostic arthroscopy should be used to assess the magnitude of glenoid deficiency. |
| Patient positioning | Both the beach chair and lateral decubitus positions are acceptable. The lateral decubitus position allows greater access to the entire capsule and labrum. |
| Portal placement | If placement of the cannula does not allow access to the inferior glenoid for suture placement, create a percutaneous adjuvant portal that penetrates the subscapularis. This portal needs to be large enough only for the drill guide and blunt obturator. |
| Capsulolabral mobilization | Always view from the anterosuperior portal to ensure appropriate mobilization of the labral-ligamentous complex. |
| Glenoid preparation | Glenoid/scapular neck decortication/abrasion is necessary to enhance healing of the labral-ligamentous complex to anatomic position. |
| Suture anchor placement | The anchors should be placed onto the glenoid articular cartilage surface (not on the medial scapular neck) to avoid nonanatomic repairs and resulting recurrent instability. |
| Suture passage | Several suture-passing instruments with varying angles should be available. |
| Final repair | Always view the repair from the anterosuperior portal to ensure appropriate restoration of the labral-ligamentous complex. |
| Capsular plication | When necessary (such as in cases with a redundant capsule or multidirectional component), capsular plication should be added to routine anterior instability repair. If the labrum is intact, the capsule can be plicated directly to the intact labrum. Care should be taken to ensure that when tying these plication sutures the labrum does not pull away from the glenoid. If this occurs, suture anchors should be placed into the glenoid and then a capsular plication with the suture anchor sutures should be performed. In situations with a torn labrum, routine capsular plication is performed with suture anchor sutures. |
| Rotational interval closure | This type of closure is not routinely necessary for anterior instability surgery but should be considered if there is pathologic sulcus sign (no diminution of sulcus sign with external rotation, adduction, and longitudinal pull of the humerus) and in patients with posterior and multidirectional instability. |

technique for rotator interval closure. *Arthroscopy* 2006;22:230.

11. Cole BJ: Arthroscopic shoulder stabilization with suture anchors: Technique, technology and pitfalls. *Clin Orthop Relat Res* 2001;390: 17-30.

12. Gartsman GM, Hammerman S: Arthroscopic rotator interval repair in glenohumeral instability: Description of an operative technique. *Arthroscopy* 1999;15:330-332.

13. Lewicky YM: Simplified arthroscopic rotator interval capsule closure: An alternative technique. *Arthroscopy* 2005; 21:1276.

14. Treacy SH, Savoie FH: Rotator interval capsule closure: An arthroscopic technique. *Arthroscopy* 1997;13:103-106.

15. Taverna E, Battistella F: Arthroscopic rotator interval repair: The three-step all-inside technique. *Arthroscopy* 2004;20:105-109.

16. D'Alessandro DF, Fleischli JE, Connor PM: Prospective evaluation of thermal capsulorrhaphy for shoulder instability: indications and results: Two- to five-year follow-up. *Am J Sports Med* 2004;32:21-33.

17. Levine WN, Clark AM Jr, D'Alessandro DF, Yamaguchi K: Chondrolysis following arthroscopic thermal capsulorrhaphy to treat shoulder instability: A report of two cases. *J Bone Joint Surg Am* 2005;87: 616-621.

18. Rath E: Capsular disruption as a complication of thermal alteration of the glenohumeral capsule. *Arthroscopy* 2001;17:E10.

19. Levine WN, Bigliani LU, Ahmad CS: Thermal capsulorrhaphy. *Orthopedics* 2004;27:823-826.

# Posterior and Multidirectional Instability of the Shoulder: Challenges Associated With Diagnosis and Management

Matthew T. Provencher, MD, LCDR, MC, USNR
*Anthony A. Romeo, MD

## Abstract

*The diagnosis and treatment of posterior and multidirectional instability of the shoulder remain challenging because of complexities in the classification and etiology of the condition and the physical examination of a patient with suspected posterior and multidirectional instability. With an improved understanding of pertinent clinical symptoms and physical examination findings, a successful strategy for nonsurgical and surgical management can be developed. It is essential to understand the biomechanics of repair procedures, relevant pathoanatomy, and techniques of surgical management to optimize surgical success. Arthroscopic techniques have allowed improved diagnosis and treatment of this condition.*

**Instr Course Lect 2008;57:133-152.**

The diagnosis and management of posterior and multidirectional instability of the shoulder continues to be challenging. Although recent biomechanical and clinical studies have advanced understanding of the pathophysiology of shoulder instability, its relative infrequency makes treatment decisions difficult. However, an improved understanding of clinical symptoms and physical examination findings in patients with posterior and multidirectional instability has led to more appropriate patient selection for surgical intervention. Although improved implants and arthroscopic techniques have produced more reliable results in these patients, attaining an accurate history and diagnosis and accounting for intraoperative pathology are prerequisites for a successful outcome.

True posterior and multidirectional instability may be easily overlooked because the presentation can be confusing, and often patients are referred with diagnoses other than shoulder instability.[1-4] Although the results of surgical treatment of posterior and multidirectional instability have improved, they are not as reliable as those of surgical treatment of anterior instability of the shoulder.

Although posterior instability and multidirectional instability are two separate but often overlapping entities, the principles of diagnosis, management, and inherent complexity are similar.

## Challenges Associated With Shoulder Instability Classification Systems

The first challenge is to identify and classify patients with recurrent shoulder instability. Variations in the definitions of posterior instability and multidirectional instability make extrapolation of biomechanical and clinical results difficult.[5] Multidirectional instability has been defined as symptomatic involuntary shoulder laxity in more than one direction (anterior, posterior, inferior).[3] However, one of the major difficulties in classifying multidirectional instability is determining the presence and direction of true symptomatic instability. It is

*Anthony A. Romeo, MD is a consultant or employee for Arthrex.*

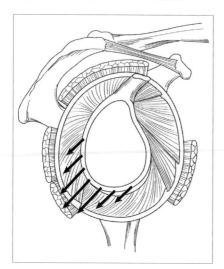

**Figure 1** The predominant direction of posterior instability is in the posteroinferior direction (*arrows*), corresponding to positions on the face of the glenoid between 7 o'clock and 7:30. Posterior instability should be distinguished from bidirectional instability, which is multidirectional instability with a symptomatic sulcus component. The posterior and anterior bands of the inferior glenohumeral ligament are seen in the inferior quadrants of the shoulder.

| Table 1 |
| --- |
| **Challenges of Posterior and Multidirectional Instability Classification: Key Points** |
| Classic anterior and posterior instability are unidirectional (anteroinferior or posteroinferior). |
| Bidirectional instability has a symptomatic sulcus component and is thus considered multidirectional instability. |
| Multiple classifications exist to describe instability (based on etiology, chronicity, and volitional control), making accurate diagnoses difficult. |
| Careful attention to a patient's history and physical examination findings are essential to identify true posterior and multidirectional instability. |

critical to differentiate instability from laxity, a normal physiologic finding of asymptomatic translation of the shoulder joint that is necessary for normal shoulder kinematics. In contrast, instability represents a pathologic condition of increased glenohumeral translation that causes pain or reproduces symptoms of instability.[2,3,5-9] Shoulders that are unstable in two or three directions always have a component of inferior instability. However, the presence of a sulcus sign or inferior laxity should not be considered a factor in multidirectional instability unless it reproduces instability symptoms or there are other intraoperative findings to suggest that the inferior component is pathologic.[2,3,5,10-16]

Multidirectional instability should not be confused with unidirectional anteroinferior or posteroinferior instability of the shoulder. True bidirectional instability or multidirectional instability has a clearly symptomatic sulcus component.[2,3,5,9] Pain and weakness distinguish pathologic instability from normal laxity and it is critical to establish this finding with physical examination.[1-3,6,9,10,12,13,17-21]

McFarland and associates[5] identified significant variabilities in the definition, classification, and diagnosis of multidirectional instability of the shoulder, which leads to an overestimation of the number of patients with that condition. The difficulties in classification are numerous—differentiating a symptomatic sulcus sign from normal sulcus laxity, determining the differences in bidirectional (anterior-inferior with symptomatic sulcus) and unidirectional anterior (in an anteroinferior direction) or posterior (in a posteroinferior direction) instability (Figure 1), and the incorrect interpretation of the ability to subluxate the shoulder over the glenoid rim as diagnostic of instability.[2,3,5]

Patient evaluation should clearly delineate the direction of instability (unidirectional, bidirectional, or more than two directions), the presence of a symptomatic sulcus,[5,17] chronicity of the injury, and should include intraarticular findings to support the diagnosis along with a description of the criteria used to document the instability (such as office setting, under anesthesia, and grading system used).[3,5,22-26] In addition, other important factors for classification are etiology (atraumatic, traumatic, cumulative microtrauma), amount of symptomatic translation, and volitional control (voluntary and involuntary instability). Key points to remember on the challenges of classifying posterior and multidirectional instability of the shoulder are summarized in Table 1.

## Biomechanical Considerations in Posterior and Multidirectional Instability

Recent improvements in understanding the biomechanics and pathophysiology of posterior and multidirectional instability have led to better clinical diagnoses, recognition of pathology, and surgical techniques. Several anatomic findings and biomechanical studies have helped to clarify the role of dynamic and static stabilizers of the glenohumeral joint, with particular attention to the version of the glenoid, the labral and capsular conditions, and dynamic function of the muscular stabilizers.

### Dynamic Stabilizers

During normal active motion, the humeral head is properly oriented and compressed into the glenoid by the dynamic contribution of the rotator cuff muscles and the long head of the biceps tendon.[27-32] Turkel and associates[30] and other investigators identified the subscapularis as the primary stabilizer preventing posterior translation, but all of the rotator cuff muscles have been shown to be important in providing concavity-compression of the shoulder joint.[25,27-36] Dynamic inferior stability of the shoulder joint is maintained by the supraspinatus and, some believe, the long head of the biceps.[31,37] The infraspinatus and teres minor serve as posterior compressors, which underscores the fact that nearly all of the shoulder girdle muscles that cross the glenohumeral joint function to maintain a stable glenohumeral joint.[28,34] If the force of rotator cuff contraction is diminished, significant increases in anterior, posterior, and inferior displacement are seen.[38] The importance of the dynamic stabilizers in shoulder instability cannot be overemphasized, especially when treating a shoulder with instability in more than one direction.

### Static Stabilizers

The bony anatomy and capsulolabral ligamentous complex are the primary static stabilizers of the glenohumeral joint.[8,27,28,30,34,39] The posterior band of the inferior glenohumeral ligament (IGHL) complex is the most important posterior ligamentous stabilizer during internal rotation and forward flexion because this places the posterior band of the IGHL in an anteroposterior orientation, providing resistance to posterior subluxation.[31] The coracohumeral ligament and the posterior capsule also limit posterior translation when the arm is forward flexed, adducted, and internally rotated.[31,40-42] The attachment site of the IGHL usually can be seen arthroscopically and ranges from the 2 o'clock to 4 o'clock position (mean, 3 o'clock) for the anterior band and the 7 o'clock to 9 o'clock position for the posterior band. The architecture of the capsule and ligaments allows the complex movements of the

shoulder joint, with a reciprocal load-sharing principle within the capsule.[43] If the anterosuperior capsule is under tension, there is an obligate simultaneous laxity in the posteroinferior capsule and vice versa.[34,44] This principle is known as the "circle concept" of glenohumeral instability—to have shoulder instability, both sides of the capsular mechanism are disrupted to some extent—although this principle remains controversial.[33,45,46]

The posterior band of the IGHL is an important capsular thickening; however, the posterior capsule is quite different from the anterior capsule.[47] The anterior capsule and anterior IGHL are thicker and biomechanically different from the posterior capsule and posterior IGHL.[47] Despite these differences, the posterior capsule is important in maintaining the stability of the shoulder because posterior instability results only after significant posterior capsular stretch, injury, and subsequent redundancy.[21,28,46] Stretch of the capsule beyond the initial resting length has been implicated as a cause of posterior and multidirectional instability and is present even without a labral tear.[30,34,48] Weber and Caspari,[46] in a biomechanical cadaver study evaluating the restraints to posterior dislocation, reported posterior damage to the capsule (100% of the time) and labrum (70% of the time). However, they noted no injury to the rotator interval (anterosuperior) structures after posterior dislocation, which challenges the circle concept of shoulder stability.

Inferior stability is an important aspect of multidirectional instability that can be easily overlooked. The extent of inferior capsulolabral injury is probably underrecognized and deserves special attention when evaluating a patient with suspected shoulder instability because failure to adequately treat the inferior component

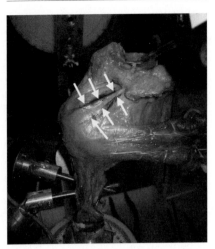

**Figure 2** Cadaveric dissection of the static anterosuperior structures of the glenohumeral joint. The coracohumeral ligament is contained within the rotator interval (*outlined with arrows*), and serves to maintain inferior stability of the adducted shoulder.

of instability may result in recurrence.[2,37] The IGHL complex is important in inferior stability because it provides as much stability as the dynamic contribution of the supraspinatus.[37] The coracohumeral ligament contained within the rotator interval capsule helps prevent inferior subluxation in external rotation[28,37,42,49,50] (Figure 2). Other rotator interval capsular structures (superior glenohumeral ligament, capsule, and long head of the biceps) also are important in maintaining inferior stability, although their relative contributions are not well defined.[28,37,42,49-51] Bony anatomy, the labrum, and scapular inclination also are important for inferior stability.[52,53]

Although the posterior labrum provides resistance to translation, it is less of a factor than the anterior labrum in anterior instability because the posterior labrum is only loosely attached to the surrounding capsule, with less ligamentous reinforce-

**Table 2**
**Biomechanical and Anatomic Considerations in Shoulder Instability: Key Points**

Shoulder and rotator cuff musculature provide important concavity-compression. All muscles contribute to dynamic stability, especially the supraspinatus (inferior stability) and subscapularis (posterior stability).

The bony anatomy, the glenohumeral ligaments, the fibrous labrum, and negative intra-articular pressure provide static stability.

The posterior band of the inferior glenohumeral ligament is a thick, robust structure, important in flexion and internal rotation.

The posterior capsular properties are much different from those of the anterior capsule.

Posterior instability may be associated with posterior glenoid bone loss and loss of posterior chondrolabral containment.

Inferior (multidirectional) instability is associated with an incompetent inferior capsular and potentially incompetent rotator interval structures.

ment.[21,47,54] Thus, the mere presence of a reverse Bankart lesion does not necessarily lead to recurrent posterior instability. However, a loss of chondrolabral containment (both an increase in bony retroversion and loss of posteroinferior labral height) has been found in patients with clinically documented posterior instability.[55] The labrum has been shown to influence glenohumeral stability by increasing the concavity-compression mechanism of the humeral head in the glenoid socket.[32,34,56] The principle of chondrolabral containment also is important in maintaining stability of the shoulder given the shallow depth of the bony glenoid, which is augmented by the fibrous ring of the glenoid labrum.[32,56,57]

### Other Factors Affecting Stability of the Shoulder

Abnormal glenoid shape, such as retroversion or flatness, is believed to affect the humeral head position in patients with atraumatic shoulder instability.[36,58] Posterior instability may result in or be a consequence of excessive glenoid or humeral retroversion, glenoid hypoplasia, or loss of chondrolabral containment.[17,20,32,34,36,55,59-69] However, it is not known if glenoid bony changes, such as retroversion, precede the development of posterior instability.

A normal, negative intra-articular pressure at rest also is important to stability of the shoulder joint, although the pressure fluctuates with load and humeral position.[32,70-73] If the ability to maintain negative pressure is compromised (effusion, hematoma, repetitive trauma, and loss of capsular constraint), the humeral head will more easily subluxate and assume a more inferior position with the arm at the side.[72,73] Key points to remember concerning biomechanical and anatomic factors in shoulder instability are summarized in Table 2.

### Etiology and Pathophysiology

The etiology of instability is challenging to identify; however, three broad categories have been defined: instability that is clearly traumatic, instability that is caused by cumulative microtrauma, and instability that is purely atraumatic.[2,3,9,13,14,16,20-22,25,26,40,62,64,74]

The development of recurrent instability may not be caused by an isolated traumatic occurrence but rather may be a spectrum or continuum of instability. For example, purely unidirectional instability, after continued use and reinjury, may progress to bidirectional (or multidirectional) instability. Along this spectrum, there is recurrent capsu-

lar and labral injury, further compromising the static restraints. With a subsequent loss of static restraints, the dynamic contribution becomes less effective in maintaining concavity-compression of the glenohumeral joint.[31,34,56]

Patients with traumatic posterior instability usually can recall an injury that immediately preceded their symptoms. Such an injury may predispose the patient to recurrent episodes of posterior instability. Unlike the high propensity for recurrent anterior instability after an initial anterior dislocation, recurrent posterior instability following an initial posterior dislocation is not a common cause of recurrent instability. Multidirectional instability remains less well defined.

Multidirectional instability may occur atraumatically in an individual with ligamentous laxity of the shoulder; the onset of pain and a sensation of instability develop gradually. Initially, symptoms are present only with higher-demand activities or provocative positions, including a flexed, internally rotated arm, which causes posterior or inferior subluxation (multidirectional instability). Progression of symptoms may lead to instability during activities of daily living.

The most frequent etiology of recurrent posterior and multidirectional instability is repetitive microtrauma, usually in patients who participate in sports activities that involve repetitive loading of the shoulder in front of the body. These activities include baseball, softball, kayaking, volleyball, rowing, swimming, and football (blocking lineman position), all of which place the shoulder in a flexed and internally rotated position, which predisposes the posterior band of the IGHL to injury.[61,62,64,75-80] These activities repetitively injure the posterior and inferior capsulolabral complex and contribute to a loss of glenoid-labral continuity.[55,81] Neer and Foster[2] reported that approximately 50% of patients in their studies had subjected their shoulders to repetitive injury.

Labral tears in posterior and multidirectional instability may occur after overt trauma or develop after cumulative microtrauma. Tears of the labrum are important to identify because patients with labral pathology have shown uniformly good results with surgical treatment.[75,76,78,82] In the cumulative microtrauma model, an accumulation of shearing forces caused by persistent shoulder subluxation or microtrauma leads to a loss of chondrolabral containment, with subsequent development of posterior labral marginal cracks or partial avulsions of the glenoid labrum, termed a Kim lesion (an incomplete avulsion of the posterior labrum)[81] (Figure 3).

It is important to remember that the etiology of posterior and multidirectional instability is atraumatic (usually resulting from an underlying ligamentous condition), traumatic (overt event), or, most commonly, results from cumulative microtrauma. Sports and activities that repetitively load the capsulolabral complex cause injury, such as capsular stretch and various forms of labral pathology. It is challenging to identify the etiology so that treatment can be tailored to the specific cause and to understand the specific pathology that accompanies each etiology.

## Voluntary Versus Involuntary Instability

It is important to determine the presence of a voluntary, willful instability because patients with voluntary instability respond poorly to surgical treatment. Voluntary instability (especially with a posterior component) is of two types—volun-

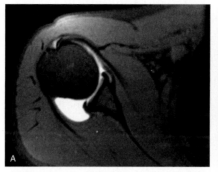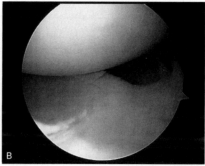

**Figure 3** **A,** Magnetic resonance arthrography of a Kim lesion of the posterior-inferior labrum. Contrast between the posterior labrum and the glenoid signifies an incomplete tear of the posterior labrum and is important to recognize in patients with posterior shoulder instability. **B,** Arthroscopic view of a Kim lesion seen in the posteroinferior quadrant of the shoulder, highlighting the marginal crack and incomplete stripping but loss of chondrolabral containment caused by this injury.

tary positional and voluntary muscular.[21,62,64,76] Patients with voluntary positional instability demonstrate subluxation in the provocative position (flexion, adduction, and internal rotation), whereas voluntary muscular instability occurs with the arm in an adducted (nonpositional-dependent) position. Patients with voluntary positional instability who can positionally reproduce their instability should not be excluded from surgical treatment.[26,61,62,64,74] The positional control is unique to posterior instability because of the volitional control offered by the posterior muscle girdle. Voluntary positional subluxation of the shoulder in posterior instability results more from positional control than from a volitional desire for secondary gain, and reflects the underlying pathophysiology of capsulolabral injury within the glenohumeral joint in up to 80% of patients.[61,62,74] Although voluntary instability in the anterior direction may be associated with an underlying psychiatric diagnosis, this usually is not the situation with multidirectional or posterior instability.[20,21,62,80] The ability of an athlete to voluntarily posteriorly

subluxate the shoulder in the provocative position should not be regarded as predictive of decreased surgical success.

## Clinical Presentation

Patients with posterior and multidirectional instability often present with multiple nonspecific reports of pain, decreased athletic performance, and loss of strength.[26,61,62,64,66,74-76,82-92] Pain associated with posterior instability often is described as generalized throughout the shoulder or at the posterior aspect of the shoulder. Pain caused by subluxation may be associated with rotator cuff tendinitis secondary to excessive stretching of these structures. Apprehension is uncommon in patients with posterior subluxation and should alert the physician that the shoulder may be subluxating anteriorly.[21,25,62]

The primary direction of instability can be determined by identifying the provocative position that reproduces instability symptoms. As instability progresses, patients may learn certain maneuvers that will subluxate their shoulders, as well as other maneuvers that will reduce a posteriorly subluxated shoulder.[62]

The diagnosis of posterior and multidirectional instability may be difficult because it can masquerade as or coincide with other shoulder conditions. Patients may have multiple, nonspecific reports of shoulder pain, discomfort, and weakness, and may have been seen by several other health care providers.[9,20,62,64,74] If no clear diagnosis of other shoulder conditions can be easily made (such as a superior labrum anterior and posterior lesion, rotator cuff tear, or biceps tendinitis), and the clinical history suggests a possible etiology for instability, posterior instability or multidirectional instability should be considered.

Patients with posterior instability also may have an element of multidirectional instability, and those with multidirectional instability may report multiple nonspecific symptoms of shoulder pain, paresthesias, and difficulties carrying weight at the side (such as a gallon of milk) or may report neuritic or radicular-type symptoms that mimic thoracic outlet syndrome.[3,16,62,93] Subluxation events during sleep may be common. Correlation of symptoms with the position of the arm is important to ensure that the correct diagnosis is made and that surgical treatment is customized to the symptomatic areas of instability.

Posterior instability or multidirectional instability should be suspected in a young patient with multiple nonspecific reports of shoulder pain, weakness, or paresthesias; activity-related pain is more common than symptoms of instability. These patients may have been evaluated, had surgery for an incorrect diagnosis, or may be referred from other health care providers with other diagnoses. It is important to identify provocative arm positions and the athletic activity that cause the shoulder symptoms.

## Physical Examination

A comprehensive physical examination is one of the most important aspects in the evaluation of a patient with suspected posterior and multidirectional instability of the shoulder. Both shoulders should be examined, observing any obvious dislocation, asymmetry, abnormal motion, muscle atrophy, swelling, and scapular winging and tracking. Wide scars may suggest a collagen disorder.[12] Scapulothoracic dyskinesis should be carefully evaluated.[94] The asymptomatic shoulder may be examined first to gain patient confidence and relaxation.[18,40,64] Radiographic and magnetic resonance arthrography findings have been described, but the mainstay of diagnosis remains symptoms of posterior instability or multidirectional instability that are identified by shoulder examination in the office. The diagnosis can be confirmed by examination under anesthesia.[95]

Range-of-motion testing in patients with posterior instability usually is normal and symmetric, although an increase in external rotation and mild loss of internal rotation may be observed.[77,80,96] These patients also have tenderness to palpation at the posterior glenohumeral joint line.[62,96] Altered scapulothoracic motion resulting from asymmetric scapular winging is common.[96,97]

Provocative maneuvers help determine the direction and degree of instability. The posterior apprehension or stress test may reproduce the specific shoulder symptoms; however, apprehension usually is not demonstrated by patients who have posterior instability.[10,62,77,96] Additional posterior instability tests include the jerk test, the posterior stress test, the Kim test, and the load and shift test.[10,31,40,48,98,99] Patients with a painful jerk test show a higher

failure rate with nonsurgical treatment than those who do not have this finding.[99] Asymmetrical or increased shoulder laxity in an asymptomatic athlete does not necessarily indicate glenohumeral instability. The precise method of surgical treatment should be decided only after the magnitude of translation and other clinical examination findings are correlated with the patient's symptoms.

Excessive inferior translation of the humerus on the glenoid often is associated with posterior subluxation and may indicate bidirectional instability or multidirectional instability if the inferior sulcus test reproduces the patient's symptoms[2,17,62,100] (Figure 4). To perform the test, the examiner directs a force inferiorly on the humerus with the shoulder in neutral to 20° of abduction and observes the distance between the anterior margin of the acromion and the superior humeral head.[17,49] A positive test is indicated by reproduction of pain and symptoms of instability with approximately 1 cm or more inferior translation. Inferior instability also may be demonstrated with the arm in 90° of abduction by applying a downward force on the proximal humerus to cause inferior displacement.[20,62] When assessing the amount of inferior humeral head translation, the patient's reaction to the test provides more important information than the actual amount of translation.

Multidirectional instability is associated with apprehension during range-of-motion testing, and patients have tenderness along the medial angle of the scapula and anterior rotator cuff.[12] Internal rotation strength also is decreased up to 30% in patients with multidirectional instability, which emphasizes the dynamic muscular dysfunction in this condition.[97] Anterior impingement also may be present in multidirectional instability because of increased excursion of the humeral head into the cuff tendons.[62] A careful and thorough physical examination remains the diagnostic method of choice. Serial office visits and repeat examinations are particularly useful to confirm the diagnosis.

Generalized ligamentous laxity has been associated with glenohumeral instability. Hyperextension of the elbows of more than 5°, the ability to touch the thumb to the ipsilateral forearm, hyperextension of the metacarpophalangeal joints more than 90° (Figure 5), and touching the palm of each hand to the floor while keeping the knees extended all are indicative of generalized ligamentous laxity.[2,6,95] This laxity has been documented in 40% to 75% of patients who had surgery for multidirectional instability and has been associated with decreased surgical success rates.[2,3,17,19] Key points to remember concerning the physical examination for shoulder instability are summarized in Table 3.

## Electromyography Findings

There are several abnormal electromyography findings in patients with multidirectional instability. The shoulder musculature, including the deltoid, supraspinatus, and infraspinatus, have atypical patterns of activity, suggesting that neuromuscular control is a contributing factor to the etiology of multidirectional instability.[101,102] There also is a more prominent spinal stretch reflex in multidirectional instability, which alters the motor control of rotator cuff muscles and diminishes the ability of the upper limbs to perform proprioceptive tasks in space.[103,104] The dynamic centering

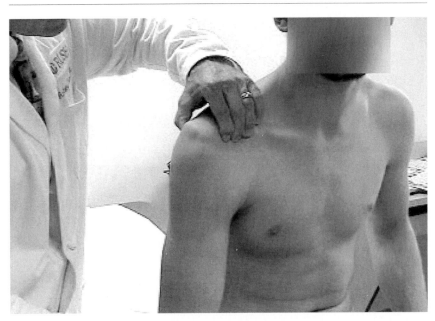

**Figure 4**   Sulcus examination performed in the office shows a 1+ to 2+ inferior translation below the lateral edge of the acromion. It is important to determine if the sulcus finding is symptomatic and reproduces the patient's symptoms.

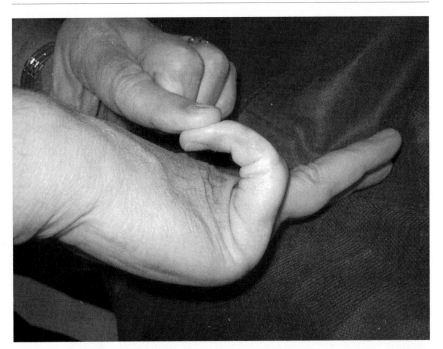

**Figure 5**   Metacarpophalangeal joint hyperextension is demonstrated in a patient with an underlying collagen disorder. The generalized ligamentous examination is an important part of the instability evaluation.

capability of the glenohumeral joint also is altered because the humeral head is translated posteriorly in patients with multidirectional instability.[105] Electromyography findings in multidirectional instability support the concept of targeted muscle strengthening exercises.[101-104]

## Radiographic Evaluation and Other Imaging Studies

Patients who experience a traumatic posterior dislocation may have a reverse Hill-Sachs lesion, which is an impaction fracture of the anterosuperior humerus; however, this rarely occurs and radiographs usually are normal. Although radiographs are usually normal in posterior instability and multidirectional instability, they should still be obtained, especially an axillary lateral view to assess for potential dislocation, subluxation, and bony injury. The axillary view indicates the direction and degree of displacement of the humeral head relative to the glenoid; the presence and size of humeral head compression fractures characteristically found at the level of the lesser trochanter; posterior glenoid rim defects such as fractures, erosions, or calcifications; fractures of the humeral tuberosities; calcification of the capsule or the tendons; and formation of osteophytes.[21,77,80,96] Glenoid hypoplasia also can be identified on a standard radiograph by a shallow or irregular glenoid fossa, prominent coracoid process, enlarged acromion, distal clavicle abnormalities, hypoplasia of the upper ribs, and flattening of the humeral head.[69] In multidirectional instability, the AP radiograph may show inferior subluxation of the humerus in the glenoid. CT is excellent for assessing glenoid hypoplasia, glenoid bone loss, and glenoid retroversion (Figure 6).

MRI and magnetic resonance arthrography offer additional information about the posterior and inferior capsulolabral structures, the rotator interval, the biceps labral anchor, and rotator cuff and are the authors' choice of imaging modalities (Figure 7). Magnetic resonance arthrography is the most sensitive and

---

**Table 3**
**Physical Examination of a Patient With Suspected Posterior and Multidirectional Instability: Key Points**

Provocative examination maneuvers demonstrate posterior (unidirectional posterior instability) and potentially inferior instability.

The posterior loading and Kim test may be positive for pain alone (subluxation is not as commonly seen as in anterior instability testing)

Documentation of a symptomatic inferior sulcus examination is paramount to the diagnosis of multidirectional instability.

Patients with posterior instability who have a symptomatic inferior sulcus are better classified as having multidirectional instability.

Hyperlaxity signs should be documented because these patients may have an underlying collagen disorder that decreases the efficacy of soft-tissue procedures.

---

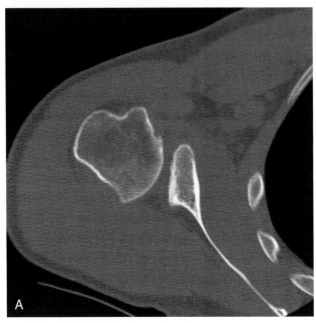 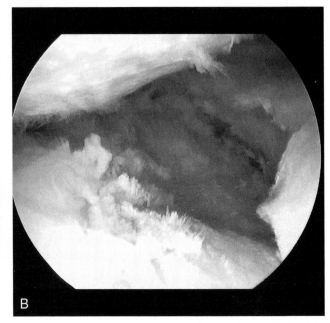

**Figure 6**  A patient with recurrent posterior instability and severe posterior glenoid bone loss secondary to traumatic injury shown on CT scan (**A**) and arthroscopic view of the posteroinferior quadrant of the glenohumeral joint from the anterosuperior portal (**B**).

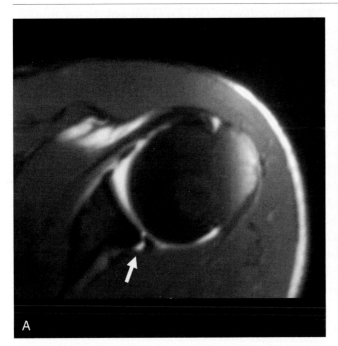
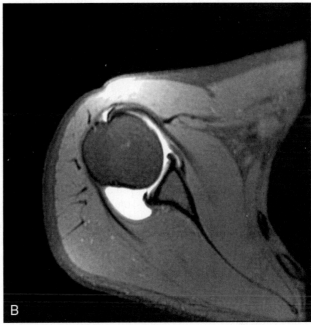

**Figure 7** **A,** Magnetic resonance arthrogram showing a posterior labral tear (*arrow*). **B,** Arthrogram of a patient with multidirectional instability and without labral tears shows a patulous posteroinferior capsule corresponding to examination findings of excessive laxity and instability.

specific imaging modality to assess labral pathology, capsular tears and condition (size), and associated pathology. Arthrography findings of a Kim lesion[81] include a loss of posterior labral height, with incomplete extrusion of contrast into the posterior chondrolabral junction.

## Treatment Decisions
### Nonsurgical Treatment
Determining the optimal approach for the management of posterior instability or multidirectional instability is a challenge; however, certain characteristics are associated with successful nonsurgical treatment. Rehabilitative treatment remains the initial treatment of choice.[2-4,65,77,90,106,107] Diminished pain and improved stability have been reported in approximately two thirds of patients with recurrent posterior instability treated with a strengthening program.[58,77,90,96,107] In particular, patients with generalized ligamentous laxity and instability

caused by repetitive microtrauma are likely to respond to an aggressive exercise program, whereas patients with a history of a traumatic event or cumulative microtrauma are less likely to respond to nonsurgical treatment.[25,77,107,108] Burkhead and associates[107] reported that 16% of patients who had a traumatic subluxation had good or excellent results from an exercise program, compared with 89% of those who had atraumatic subluxation. Tibone and Bradley[80] reported that 70% of athletes with posterior instability had improvement in symptoms after 6 months of rehabilitation; results were subjective. Shoulder orthoses to increase scapular inclination have been tested in a strengthening program, with failure noted in only 3 of 46 patients with multidirectional instability.[109] However, a recent study by Misamore and associates[89] showed a relatively poor response to nonsurgical treatment of multidirectional insta-

bility in young athletic patients followed for 7 to 10 years.

Patients with both posterior instability and multidirectional instability (especially) demonstrate altered dynamic shoulder muscular kinematics. Targeted nonsurgical therapy and muscle strengthening along with proprioception training can improve symptoms of instability. A minimum of 6 months of therapy is a reasonable first-line treatment, although young patients with overt, traumatic posterior and multidirectional instability respond less favorably to such treatment.

### Surgical Treatment
Many challenges are associated with the surgical management of posterior and multidirectional instability. Surgical stabilization should be considered only in patients with limited function of the involved shoulder because of pain or instability who are psychologically stable and in whom

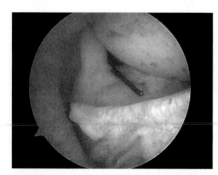

**Figure 8** Arthroscopic view (sky box view) of a patulous posteroinferior capsule without a labral tear in a patient with multidirectional instability of the shoulder. As the arthroscope is slowly retracted to the edge of the posterior capsule, nearly the entire posterior glenoid from the 12 o'clock to 6 o'clock position is visualized, signifying an excessively lax posteroinferior capsule in this patient.

an adequate trial of conservative therapy has failed.[2,19,25,77,96,108] Open bone procedures include bone blocks, glenoid osteotomy, and rotational osteotomy of the proximal humerus.[4,54,100,110-117] Open soft-tissue procedures for posterior instability and multidirectional instability include capsular shifts, subscapularis tendon transfer, posterior capsular plication and infraspinatus advancement, reverse Putti-Platt plication, reverse Bankart repair, Boyd-Sisk procedure, and biceps tendon transposition.[2,10,17,19,48,58,63,67-69,87,118-124] The results of open procedures for posterior instability and multidirectional instability have been mixed, with 40% to 91% deemed successful. Open treatment of multidirectional instability has served as the gold standard, especially when inferior capsular pathology is corrected.[2,10,17,19,63,68,87,90,119] The results of open treatment of posterior instability have not been as good, probably because of the larger surgical dissection and biomechanical properties of the posteroinferior capsule and

labrum that are different from those of the anterior aspect of the shoulder.[20,62,100,125,126] Hawkins and associates[62] reported an overall recurrence rate of 50% after three different open posterior procedures.

The advent of less invasive, advanced arthroscopic techniques has made arthroscopy a viable treatment for the surgical management of posterior and multidirectional instability in patients without significant bone loss or fracture. The advantages of arthroscopic treatment include less surgical dissection and an increased ability to treat concomitant pathology and access the posterior capsulolabral complex. However, the success of arthroscopic treatment is predicated on the success of reproducing open surgical techniques with arthroscopic means. Because of the increased technical demands of these arthroscopic procedures, several areas are particularly challenging to treat surgically in patients with posterior and multidirectional instability.

### Labral Tears Versus Intact Labrum

Patients with multidirectional instability and even posterior instability may have an intact labrum; however, the pathology is within an excessively lax capsule, especially in the posterior and inferior quadrants of the shoulder. The capsular laxity present in multidirectional instability also is noted in posterior instability and may exist with or without tears of the glenoid labrum.[2,10,17,22,62,75,78,119,126,127] This is immediately apparent when the arthroscope is placed in the posterior portal and the entire glenoid is seen as the tip of the arthroscope is pulled back to the edge of the capsule. Termed a "sky box" view and caused by excessive laxity of the posteroinferior capsular pouch, this is almost always correlated to the direction of symptomatic instability[126] (Figure 8).

This excessive pouch size must be surgically corrected.

Large circumferential tears of the glenoid labrum, termed the triple labral lesion, have been described.[128] The finding of a circumferential labral tear does not automatically imply multidirectional instability or posterior instability because some patients with circumferential 360° labral tears have clinical findings of multidirectional instability (Figure 9). Good results have been reported when extensive labral injuries are repaired with seven or eight anchors.

### Capsulolabral Anchor Repair Versus Capsular Plication

A capsular plication is a surgical technique that imbricates and decreases the size of the shoulder capsule with a suture (absorbable or nonabsorbable), using as the fixation point an intact glenoid labrum[7] (Figure 10). This technique is in contrast to a capsulolabral repair with anchors, which uses the glenoid as the fixation point (Figure 11). The indications for an anchor repair rather than a capsular plication (sutures only into the capsule and intact labrum) are not well defined; however, it is generally believed that capsular plication is sufficient if the posteroinferior glenoid labrum is completely intact. Although the labrum has been shown to be a solid fixation point, concerns about shear stress, small labral tear propagation, an unrecognized Kim lesion, and suture breakage make anchor fixation preferable because it remains the strongest and most predictable repair construct.[81,129]

### Surgical Capsular Plication and the Safety of Plicating the Inferior Capsule Complex

The determination of how much capsular plication is necessary in posterior and multidirectional instability remains a challenge. The pri-

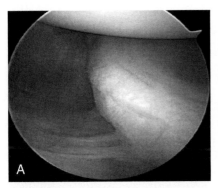 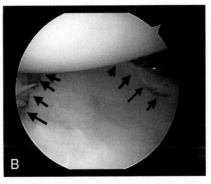 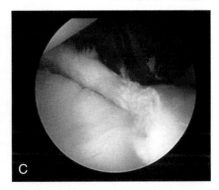

**Figure 9** **A,** Arthroscopic view of the posteroinferior capsule and ligaments in a patient with multidirectional instability caused by symptomatic and excessive capsular laxity without a labral tear. **B,** Arthroscopic view of a circumferential labral tear and capsular injury in a patient with multidirectional instability. A complete 360° labral tear is shown (*arrows*). **C,** Arthroscopic view of a posterior labral tear in a semiprofessional football lineman with posterior instability caused by a traumatic blocking injury.

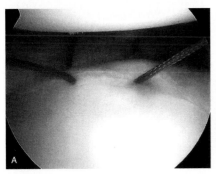 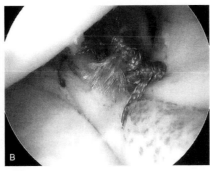 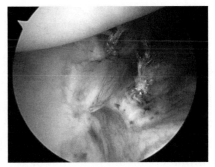

**Figure 10** **A,** Example of capsulolabral plication of the posteroinferior aspect of the glenohumeral joint. **B,** The labrum, rather than glenoid bone anchors, is used as the anchor point.

**Figure 11** Example of a capsulolabral repair with suture anchors in a patient with posterior instability of the shoulder.

mary direction of instability, translation of examination findings under anesthesia (compared with the contralateral limb), and capsular injury will determine the overall amount and location of capsular plication. Although there is no universally accepted amount, a 1-cm plication is believed to provide good stability.[130,131] Plications are done to imbricate areas of the glenohumeral joint that have evidence of excessive capsular laxity corresponding to the primary direction of clinical instability. The important areas of plication include the posteroinferior and inferior aspects of the capsule. Generally, three to five plication sutures, an-

chored either to the labrum or a glenoid anchor, are sufficient. However, it should be kept in mind that capsular plications are not without consequence and result in a predictable time-zero rotational loss.[132] An isolated posteroinferior plication of 1 cm results in 9° of internal rotation loss (at 0° abduction) and 11° loss of abduction, whereas a 1-cm plication of the entire posterior capsule results in a 15° loss of abduction and a 21° loss of internal rotation under similar conditions. The amount of capsular plication remains one of the most challenging aspects in the treatment of posterior and multidirectional instability; further clinical

study into this area is necessary to better define volume change and surgical outcomes.

Injury to the axillary nerve must be avoided during capsular plication. The location of the axillary nerve during arthroscopic capsular plication has been well defined, and the distance from the capsule to the nerve varies with patient positioning. Placing the arm in abduction and external rotation with perpendicular traction increases the zone of safety during arthroscopic plication.[133] An anteroinferior 1-cm plication has been shown to be 12.5 mm away from the axillary nerve; this distance is increased

### Table 4
### Surgical Treatment of Posterior and Multidirectional Instability: Key Points

Posterior and multidirectional instability associated with labral tears is etiologically different from that in patients without labral tears. Those with traumatic labral tears that are repaired tend to have better overall outcomes compared with those with a pure capsular injury.

Both plication (repair directly to labrum) and anchor repair (fixation to glenoid bone) have been described to correct instability pathology.

Capsular plication results in a predictable loss in rotation; a balance must be maintained between sufficient repair and overconstraint.

The axillary nerve is closest to the glenoid from the 5 o'clock to 6 o'clock position (12 to 15 mm), with an increasing distance in the posterior quadrant. Thermal and plication injuries to the nerve have been described.

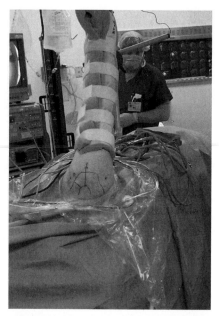

**Figure 12** Lateral decubitus position in the operating room. The arm is abducted 60° to 65° and flexed 10° to 15°. Approximately 10 lb of in-line traction are used.

(24.1 mm) with plications in the posteroinferior quadrant of the shoulder.[134] The closest point between the glenoid rim and the axillary nerve is 12.4 mm at the 6 o'clock position.[135] Because of the close proximity of the axillary nerve to the capsule, thermal devices have been implicated in axillary nerve injury, resulting in deltoid dysfunction, loss of sensation, and a burning-type dysesthesia.[136-138]

### Biomechanical Evaluation of Stabilization Procedures

The biomechanics of posterior and multidirectional repair procedures have been investigated, although most of these have used thermal devices.[56,59,139-141] The use of thermal devices for the primary treatment of instability is no longer advocated because of unacceptable failure rates and irreversible capsular damage.[136-138,142] Capsular and labral repair procedures have been shown to restore chondrolabral containment, which restores stability of the joint after injury.[34,56,130,139,141] Biomechanical time-zero findings are important to understanding repair strength and success; however, clinical correlation has yet to be fully determined.

### Surgical Treatment: Key Points

Although surgical treatment of pa-

tients with posterior and multidirectional instability is challenging, it is appropriate in a select population of patents. Key points to remember concerning surgical treatment are summarized in Table 4.

### Arthroscopic Surgical Techniques

Both the beach chair and lateral decubitus positions have been advocated for the arthroscopic treatment of posterior and multidirectional instability. Although both techniques are effective, it has been clinically shown that the lateral decubitus position more effectively opens up the inferior and posterior quadrants of the shoulder and allows for ease of access to these areas with well-placed arthroscopic portals.[7,143] To improve access in the lateral decubitus position, the arm is abducted 65° and flexed approximately 15° by means of an overhead traction sleeve. An axillary traction device (direct superior traction) or pillow bump placed into the axilla further opens up the posteroinferior area of the shoulder (Figure 12).

An additional challenge is obtaining correct portal placement to allow repair of all quadrants of the shoulder, but accessing pathology in the posteroinferior aspect of the shoulder is paramount. Following a diagnostic arthroscopic examination from a standard posterior portal, an

anterosuperior portal is made in the superior aspect of the rotator interval, entering the joint laterally under the biceps tendon to allow good glenoid trajectory. To access the posterior structures, the arthroscope is then placed into the anterosuperior portal. Accessory posterior portals can then be made to facilitate repair, instrumentation, or anchor placement. Under the guidance of an 18-gauge spinal needle, an accessory posterolateral portal enters the joint inferiorly, approximately 1 cm anterior and 2 cm lateral to the original arthroscopic posterior portal.[144-146] (Figure 13, A). A clear 8.25-mm cannula is inserted to accommodate the instruments that will work in the posterior and posteroinferior aspects of the shoulder (Figure 13, B).

For repair of a posterior labral tear, preparation of the chondrolabral junction may be more easily accomplished with an elevator instrument

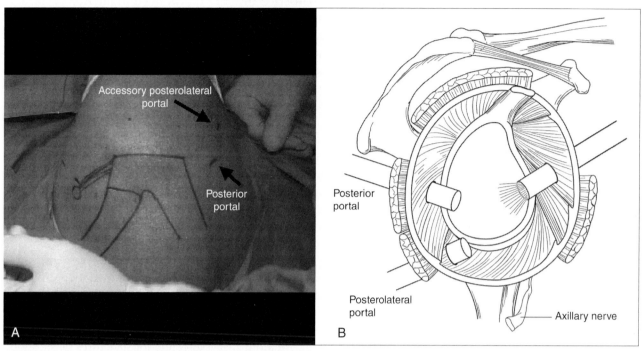

**Figure 13** Arthroscopic portal placement is used to gain access to the posterior and posteroinferior areas of the glenohumeral joint. The accessory posterolateral portal is placed approximately 2 cm lateral and 1 cm anterior to the standard posterior portal **(A)**. This allows posterolateral entry into the inferior aspect of the glenohumeral joint **(B)**. An 8.25-mm cannula may be placed to accommodate all capsulolabral repair instrumentation.

inserted from the anterior portal rather than preparing the labrum from a posterior or accessory posterior portal (Figure 14). The trajectory from the anterior portal allows the labrum to be easily elevated off the glenoid without traumatic injury, similar to the way a pancake is elevated off a hot griddle. During the preparation, the labrum should be meticulously probed, and if a crack or tear is seen or palpated, the labrum should be completely taken down and an anchor repair performed.

The sequence of repair is dictated by the primary direction of instability and the extent of capsulolabral pathology. Because the shoulder volume is diminished after each capsulolabral repair, each successive repair becomes increasingly difficult because of the diminished working space. Generally, the inferior and posteroinferior pa-

thology is treated first, followed by any remaining anterior areas or superior labrum anterior and posterior injuries. With the arthroscope in the anterosuperior portal, the inferior and posterior repairs are sequentially done in a superior direction from the accessory posterolateral and posterior portals.

When using arthroscopic techniques it is important to remember that although both beach chair and lateral decubitus positions have been described, the lateral decubitus position allows ease of access to the posteroinferior quadrant of the shoulder. Posterior labral preparation at the chondrolabral junction is facilitated with an elevator device inserted from an anterior portal (rather than posterior). An accessory posterolateral portal allows access to the posterior and inferior areas of the shoulder.

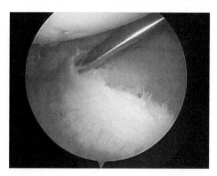

**Figure 14** Arthroscopic view shows elevation of the labrum from the anterosuperior portal. Using the elevator device from the anterior portal facilitates labral and glenoid separation of the posterior, posteroinferior, and inferior aspects of the glenohumeral joint.

## Results of Arthroscopic Treatment

Although the results of arthroscopic treatment of posterior and multidirectional instability continue to improve, overall results have not been as encouraging as those achieved after treatment of unidirectional anterior instability.[75,76,78,82,88,92,126,147] This is the result of patient selection (especially for multidirectional instability), the inherent biomechanical differences of the posteroinferior capsulolabral complex, and unrecognized pathology. Overall, recent results of arthroscopic treatment are encouraging, although longer-term studies are needed to truly assess the arthroscopic efficacy of these procedures.[75,76,78,82,92] Because of the relative infrequency of the condition, studies with more than 40 patients are rare, which makes clinical interpretation somewhat difficult.

## Postoperative Rehabilitation and Return-to-Sport Decision Making

Postoperatively, patients are immobilized in a 30° abduction pillow in neutral rotation for 4 to 6 weeks. During this period, patients are allowed to perform passive pendulum exercises, gentle passive scaption, and active elbow and wrist motion. Active motion of the glenohumeral joint is started at 4 to 6 weeks, depending on the magnitude of injury and repair. Internal rotation and adduction are restricted for a total of 6 weeks (posterior instability treatment). At the 4- to 6-week point, patients increase range of motion and subsequently begin a strengthening program of the rotator cuff and scapular stabilizing musculature. At the 6-month point, patients are allowed unrestricted return to full activities, with a sports-specific training program.

It is important to remember that postoperative rehabilitation should be based on the individual pathology, the direction of primary instability, and the surgical treatment used.

## Deciding When Closure of the Rotator Interval Should Be Performed

The role of the rotator interval in posterior and multidirectional instability of the shoulder is frequently discussed, and surgical treatment of this area is suggested as an adjunct to the primary repair. Closure of the rotator interval has been frequently touted as a useful adjunct in both multidirectional instability and posterior instability; however, arthroscopic closure of the rotator interval may not be as biomechanically robust as its open counterpart. Many surgeons do not close the rotator interval in patients with posterior instability and multidirectional instability and have obtained satisfactory results without the potential loss of external rotation that has been described biomechanically.[76,78,88,92,126,148-154] The basis for treatment of lesions of the rotator interval was initially investigated by Ovesen and Nielsen,[50] Ikeda,[155,156] Harryman and associates,[42] and others[37,51,157] who showed that the rotator interval is an important structure in both posterior and inferior stability of the shoulder joint. Harryman and associates[42] also determined that posterior and inferior stability of the shoulder was improved after open, medial-to-lateral imbrication of the rotator interval structures. The potential problem is that these results of open rotator interval closure have been extrapolated to a procedure that is generally performed arthroscopically—a superior to inferior imbrication of the interval structures. The arthroscopic closure imbricates different structures than those described by Harryman and associates,[42] shifting the middle glenohumeral ligament to the superior rotator interval capsule (superior glenohumeral ligament), and does not necessarily imbricate the coracohumeral ligament, which has been

shown to be an inferior stabilizer of the glenohumeral joint. Recent biomechanical evidence has suggested that arthroscopic rotator interval closure is not beneficial to improve posterior and inferior shoulder stability.[151,152,154]

The circle concept is the essential basis for routine rotator interval closure—that a posterior instability event cannot occur without concomitant injury to the anterosuperior structures of the shoulder (the rotator interval complex).[45] However, the circle concept of injury to the anterosuperior structures has not been uniformly demonstrated; in a biomechanical posterior dislocation model, Weber and Caspari[46] documented no injury to the anterosuperior structures of the shoulder. It remains a challenge to determine when to close the rotator interval of the shoulder because plication in this area also decreases external rotation at the side, with questionable clinical benefit. Rotator interval closure may be indicated in patients with a symptomatic, excessively lax inferior capsular component and a sulcus sign that does not obliterate in external rotation (suggesting loss of integrity of the rotator interval capsule).[50,155] If rotator interval closure is done, the arm should be externally rotated 30° to 45° to minimize loss of motion after repair. There is no clear evidence that arthroscopic rotator interval closure adds to stability of the shoulder in patients with posterior and multidirectional instability; however, in selected patients with excessive laxity, it may be a useful adjunct to adequate capsulolabral repair.[85,86]

The role of the rotator interval (composed of the coracohumeral ligament, superior glenohumeral ligament, long head of the biceps, and capsule) in posterior and multidirectional instability remains controversial. In a cadaveric model, open closure of the rotator interval has been shown to improve inferior and posterior stability (medial to lateral closure).[42] Arthroscopic closure of the rotator interval (superior to inferior closure) is less predictable in affecting biomechanical function; it may be useful in instances of excessive laxity after repair and in instances of the persistence of a sulcus sign in external rotation, although this is highly debatable.[152]

## Summary

Posterior and multidirectional instability of the shoulder presents diagnostic and clinical challenges. Once recognized, a variety of open and arthroscopic surgical procedures have been advocated. Because of the relative infrequency of the condition, there have been only a few reports in the literature. The overall results of surgical treatment of posterior and multidirectional instability are not equivalent to those of anterior instability treatment. An understanding of the pathoanatomy, careful patient selection, and adherence to techniques designed to address the pathology are critical to optimizing patient outcomes. As arthroscopic stabilization procedures and techniques are refined, improved results are hoped for when addressing this complex disorder.

## References

1. Foster CR: Multidirectional instability of the shoulder in the athlete. *Clin Sports Med* 1983;2:355-368.

2. Neer CS, Foster CR: Inferior capsular shift for involuntary inferior and multidirectional instability of the shoulder. *J Bone Joint Surg Am* 1980; 62:897-908.

3. Neer CS II: Involuntary inferior and

multidirectional instability of the shoulder: Etiology, recognition, and treatment. *Instr Course Lect* 1985;34: 232-238.

4. Rowe C, Yee L: A posterior approach to the shoulder joint. *J Bone Joint Surg Am* 1944;26:580-594.

5. McFarland EG, Kim TK, Park HB, Neira CA, Gutierrez MI: The effect of variation in definition on the diagnosis of multidirectional instability of the shoulder. *J Bone Joint Surg Am* 2003;85:2138-2144.

6. Cofield RH, Irving JF: Evaluation and classification of shoulder instability: With special reference to examination under anesthesia. *Clin Orthop Relat Res* 1987;223:32-43.

7. Hewitt M, Getelman MH, Snyder SJ: Arthroscopic management of multidirectional instability: Pancapsular plication. *Orthop Clin North Am* 2003; 34:549-557.

8. Lintner SA, Levy A, Kenter K, Speer KP: Glenohumeral translation in the asymptomatic athlete's shoulder and its relationship to other clinically measurable anthropometric variables. *Am J Sports Med* 1996;24:716-720.

9. Lo IK, Bishop JY, Miniaci A, Flatow EL: Multidirectional instability: Surgical decision making. *Instr Course Lect* 2004;53:565-572.

10. Bigliani LU, Pollock RG, McIlveen SJ, Endrizzi DP, Flatow EL: Shift of the posteroinferior aspect of the capsule for recurrent posterior glenohumeral instability. *J Bone Joint Surg Am* 1995;77:1011-1020.

11. Bigliani LU, Kelkar R, Flatow EL, Pollock RG, Mow VC: Glenohumeral stability: Biomechanical properties of passive and active stabilizers. *Clin Orthop Relat Res* 1996;330:13-30.

12. An YH, Friedman RJ: Multidirectional instability of the glenohumeral joint. *Orthop Clin North Am* 2000;31: 275-285.

13. Arendt EA: Multidirectional shoulder instability. *Orthopedics* 1988;11:113-120.

14. Flatow EL, Warner JI: Instability of

the shoulder: Complex problems and failed repairs. Part I: Relevant biomechanics, multidirectional instability, and severe glenoid loss. *Instr Course Lect* 1998;47:97-112.

15. Levine WN, Prickett WD, Prymka M, Yamaguchi K: Treatment of the athlete with multidirectional shoulder instability. *Orthop Clin North Am* 2001;32:475-484.

16. Mallon WJ, Speer KP: Multidirectional instability: Current concepts. *J Shoulder Elbow Surg* 1995;4:54-64.

17. Altchek DW, Warren RF, Skyhar MJ, Ortiz G: T-plasty modification of the Bankart procedure for multidirectional instability of the anterior and inferior types. *J Bone Joint Surg Am* 1991;73:105-112.

18. Bahk M, Keyurapan E, Tasaki A, Sauers EL, McFarland EG: Laxity testing of the shoulder: A review. *Am J Sports Med* 2007;35:131-144.

19. Cooper RA, Brems JJ: The inferior capsular-shift procedure for multidirectional instability of the shoulder. *J Bone Joint Surg Am* 1992;74:1516-1521.

20. Hawkins RJ, Belle RM: Posterior instability of the shoulder. *Instr Course Lect* 1989;38:211-215.

21. Hawkins RJ, McCormack RG: Posterior shoulder instability. *Orthopedics* 1988;11:101-107.

22. Antoniou J, Harryman DT: Posterior instability. *Orthop Clin North Am* 2001;32:463-473.

23. Paxinos A, Walton J, Tzannes A, Callanan M, Hayes K, Murrell GA: Advances in the management of traumatic anterior and atraumatic multidirectional shoulder instability. *Sports Med* 2001;31:819-828.

24. Schenk TJ, Brems JJ: Multidirectional instability of the shoulder: Pathophysiology, diagnosis, and management. *J Am Acad Orthop Surg* 1998;6:65-72.

25. Schwartz E, Warren RF, O'Brien SJ, Fronek J: Posterior shoulder instability. *Orthop Clin North Am* 1987;18: 409-419.

26. Steinmann SP: Posterior shoulder instability. *Arthroscopy* 2003;19(suppl 1): 102-105.

27. Ovesen J, Nielsen S: Anterior and posterior shoulder instability: A cadaver study. *Acta Orthop Scand* 1986; 57:324-327.

28. Ovesen J, Nielsen S: Posterior instability of the shoulder: A cadaver study. *Acta Orthop Scand* 1986;57: 436-439.

29. Saha AK: Mechanics of elevation of glenohumeral joint: Its application in rehabilitation of flail shoulder in upper brachial plexus injuries and poliomyelitis and in replacement of the upper humerus by prosthesis. *Acta Orthop Scand* 1973;44:668-678.

30. Turkel SJ, Panio MW, Marshall JL, Girgis FG: Stabilizing mechanisms preventing anterior dislocation of the glenohumeral joint. *J Bone Joint Surg Am* 1981;63:1208-1217.

31. Blasier RB, Soslowsky LJ, Malicky DM, Palmer ML: Posterior glenohumeral subluxation: Active and passive stabilization in a biomechanical model. *J Bone Joint Surg Am* 1997;79: 433-440.

32. Lippitt S, Matsen F: Mechanisms of glenohumeral joint stability. *Clin Orthop Relat Res* 1993;291:20-28.

33. Blasier RB, Goldberg RE, Rothman ED: Anterior shoulder stability: Contributions of rotator cuff forces and the capsular ligaments in a cadaver model. *J Shoulder Elbow Surg* 1992;1: 140-150.

34. Matsen FA III, Chebli C, Lippitt S: Principles for the evaluation and management of shoulder instability. *J Bone Joint Surg Am* 2006;88:648-659.

35. Naggar L, Morrey BF, An KN: Major capsuloligamentous constraints to posterior instability of the shoulder. *J Shoulder Elbow Surg* 1991;4:S43.

36. Inui H, Sugamoto K, Miyamoto T, et al: Glenoid shape in atraumatic posterior instability of the shoulder. *Clin Orthop Relat Res* 2002;403:87-92.

37. Soslowsky LJ, Malicky DM, Blasier RB: Active and passive factors in inferior glenohumeral stabilization: A biomechanical model. *J Shoulder Elbow Surg* 1997;6:371-379.

38. Wuelker N, Korell M, Thren K: Dynamic glenohumeral joint stability. *J Shoulder Elbow Surg* 1998;7:43-52.

39. O'Brien SJ, Neves MC, Arnoczky SP, et al: The anatomy and histology of the inferior glenohumeral ligament complex of the shoulder. *Am J Sports Med* 1990;18:449-456.

40. Gerber C, Ganz R: Clinical assessment of instability of the shoulder with special reference to anterior and posterior drawer tests. *J Bone Joint Surg Br* 1984;66:551-556.

41. Harryman DT, Sidles JA, Clark JM, McQuade KJ, Gibb TD, Matsen FA: Translation of the humeral head on the glenoid with passive glenohumeral motion. *J Bone Joint Surg Am* 1990;72:1334-1343.

42. Harryman DT II, Sidles JA, Harris SL, Matsen FA III: The role of the rotator interval capsule in passive motion and stability of the shoulder. *J Bone Joint Surg Am* 1992;74:53-66.

43. Wang VM, Flatow EL: Pathomechanics of acquired shoulder instability: A basic science perspective. *J Shoulder Elbow Surg* 2005;14(suppl S):2S-11S.

44. Curl LA, Warren RF: Glenohumeral joint stability: Selective cutting studies on the static capsular restraints. *Clin Orthop Relat Res* 1996;330:54-65.

45. Bowen MK, Warren RF: Ligamentous control of shoulder stability based on selective cutting and static translation experiments. *Clin Sports Med* 1991;10:757-782.

46. Weber SC, Caspari RB: A biomechanical evaluation of the restraints to posterior shoulder dislocation. *Arthroscopy* 1989;5:115-121.

47. Bey MJ, Hunter SA, Kilambi N, Butler DL, Lindenfeld TN: Structural and mechanical properties of the glenohumeral joint posterior capsule. *J Shoulder Elbow Surg* 2005;14:201-206.

48. Pollock RG, Bigliani LU: Recurrent posterior shoulder instability: Diagnosis and treatment. *Clin Orthop Relat Res* 1993;291:85-96.

49. Helmig P, Sojbjerg JO, Kjaersgaard-Andersen P, Nielsen S, Ovesen J: Distal humeral migration as a component of multidirectional shoulder instability. *Clin Orthop Relat Res* 1990; 252:139-143.

50. Ovesen J, Nielsen S: Experimental distal subluxation in the glenohumeral joint. *Arch Orthop Trauma Surg* 1985;104:78-81.

51. Warner JJ, Deng X-H, Warren RF, Torzilli PA: Static capsuloligamentous restraints to superior-inferior translation of the glenohumeral joint. *Am J Sports Med* 1992;20:675-685.

52. Halder AM, Kuhl SG, Zobitz ME, Larson D, An KN: Effects of the glenoid labrum and glenohumeral abduction on stability of the shoulder joint through concavity-compression: An in vitro study. *J Bone Joint Surg Am* 2001;83:1062-1069.

53. Itoi E, Motzkin NE, Morrey BF, An KN: Scapular inclination and inferior stability of the shoulder. *J Shoulder Elbow Surg* 1992;1:131-139.

54. Hawkins RJ, Janda DH: Posterior instability of the glenohumeral joint: A technique of repair. *Am J Sports Med* 1996;24:275-278.

55. Kim SH, Noh KC, Park JS, Ryu BD, Oh I: Loss of chondrolabral containment of the glenohumeral joint in atraumatic posteroinferior multidirectional instability. *J Bone Joint Surg Am* 2005;87:92-98.

56. Lazarus MD, Sidles JA, Harryman DT II, Matsen FA III: Effect of a chondral-labral defect on glenoid concavity and glenohumeral stability: A cadaveric model. *J Bone Joint Surg Am* 1996;78:94-102.

57. Howell SM, Galinat BJ: The glenoid-labral socket: A constrained articular surface. *Clin Orthop Relat Res* 1989; 243:122-125.

58. Hurley JA, Anderson TE, Dear W, Andrish JT, Bergfeld JA, Weiker GA: Posterior shoulder instability: Surgical versus conservative results with evaluation of glenoid version. *Am J*

*Sports Med* 1992;20:396-400.

59. Metcalf MH, Duckworth DG, Lee SB, et al: Posteroinferior glenoplasty can change glenoid shape and increase the mechanical stability of the shoulder. *J Shoulder Elbow Surg* 1999; 8:205-213.

60. Weishaupt D, Zanetti M, Nyffeler RW, Gerber C, Hodler J: Posterior glenoid rim deficiency in recurrent (atraumatic) posterior shoulder instability. *Skeletal Radiol* 2000;29:204-210.

61. Abrams JS: Arthroscopic repair of posterior instability and reverse humeral glenohumeral ligament avulsion lesions. *Orthop Clin North Am* 2003;34:475-483.

62. Hawkins RJ, Koppert G, Johnston G: Recurrent posterior instability (subluxation) of the shoulder. *J Bone Joint Surg Am* 1984;66:169-174.

63. Krishnan SG, Hawkins RJ, Horan MP, Dean M, Kim YK: A soft tissue attempt to stabilize the multiply operated glenohumeral joint with multidirectional instability. *Clin Orthop Relat Res* 2004;429:256-261.

64. Millett PJ, Clavert P, Hatch GF III, Warner JJ: Recurrent posterior shoulder instability. *J Am Acad Orthop Surg* 2006;14:464-476.

65. Millett PJ, Clavert P, Warner JJ: Arthroscopic management of anterior, posterior, and multidirectional shoulder instability: Pearls and pitfalls. *Arthroscopy* 2003;19(suppl 1):86-93.

66. Norwood LA, Terry GC: Shoulder posterior subluxation. *Am J Sports Med* 1984;12:25-30.

67. Rhee YG, Lee DH, Lim CT: Posterior capsulolabral reconstruction in posterior shoulder instability: Deltoid saving. *J Shoulder Elbow Surg* 2005;14: 355-360.

68. van Tankeren E, de Waal Malefijt MC, van Loon CJ: Open capsular shift for multi directional shoulder instability. *Arch Orthop Trauma Surg* 2002;122: 447-450.

69. Wirth MA, Groh GI, Rockwood CA: Capsulorrhaphy through an anterior approach for the treatment of atrau-

matic posterior glenohumeral instability with multidirectional laxity of the shoulder. *J Bone Joint Surg Am* 1998;80:1570-1578.

70. Hashimoto T, Suzuki K, Nobuhara K: Dynamic analysis of intraarticular pressure in the glenohumeral joint. *J Shoulder Elbow Surg* 1995;4:209-218.

71. Hurschler C, Wulker N, Mendila M: The effect of negative intraarticular pressure and rotator cuff force on glenohumeral translation during simulated active elevation. *Clin Biomech (Bristol, Avon)* 2000;15:306-314.

72. Inokuchi W, Sanderhoff Olsen B, Sojbjerg JO, Sneppen O: The relation between the position of the glenohumeral joint and the intraarticular pressure: An experimental study. *J Shoulder Elbow Surg* 1997;6:144-149.

73. Itoi E, Motzkin NE, Browne AO, Hoffmeyer P, Morrey BF, An KN: Intraarticular pressure of the shoulder. *Arthroscopy* 1993;9:406-413.

74. Robinson CM, Aderinto J: Recurrent posterior shoulder instability. *J Bone Joint Surg Am* 2005;87:883-892.

75. Bottoni CR, Franks BR, Moore JH, DeBerardino TM, Taylor DC, Arciero RA: Operative stabilization of posterior shoulder instability. *Am J Sports Med* 2005;33:996-1002.

76. Bradley JP, Baker CL III, Kline AJ, Armfield DR, Chhabra A: Arthroscopic capsulolabral reconstruction for posterior instability of the shoulder: A prospective study of 100 shoulders. *Am J Sports Med* 2006;34:1061-1071.

77. Fronek J, Warren RF, Bowen M: Posterior subluxation of the glenohumeral joint. *J Bone Joint Surg Am* 1989; 71:205-216.

78. Provencher M, Bell S, Menzel K, Mologne T. Arthroscopic treatment of posterior shoulder instability: Results in 33 patients. *Am J Sports Med* 2005;33:1463-1471.

79. Tibone J, Ting A: Capsulorrhaphy with a staple for recurrent posterior subluxation of the shoulder. *J Bone Joint Surg Am* 1990;72:999-1002.

80. Tibone JE, Bradley JP: The treatment of posterior subluxation in athletes. *Clin Orthop Relat Res* 1993;291: 124-137.

81. Kim SH, Ha KI, Yoo JC, Noh KC: Kim's lesion: An incomplete and concealed avulsion of the posteroinferior labrum in posterior or multidirectional posteroinferior instability of the shoulder. *Arthroscopy* 2004;20: 712-720.

82. Kim SH, Ha KI, Park JH, et al: Arthroscopic posterior labral repair and capsular shift for traumatic unidirectional recurrent posterior subluxation of the shoulder. *J Bone Joint Surg Am* 2003;85:1479-1487.

83. Fuchs B, Jost B, Gerber C: Posterior-Inferior capsular shift for the treatment of recurrent, voluntary posterior subluxation of the shoulder. *J Bone Joint Surg Am* 2000;82:16-25.

84. Gartsman GM, Roddey TS, Hammerman SM: Arthroscopic treatment of bidirectional glenohumeral instability: Two- to five-year follow-up. *J Shoulder Elbow Surg* 2001;10:28-36.

85. Gartsman GM, Roddey TS, Hammerman SM: Arthroscopic treatment of multidirectional glenohumeral instability: 2- to 5-year follow-up. *Arthroscopy* 2001;17:236-243.

86. Kim SH, Kim HK, Sun JI, Park JS, Oh I: Arthroscopic capsulolabroplasty for posteroinferior multidirectional instability of the shoulder. *Am J Sports Med* 2004;32:594-607.

87. Lebar RD, Alexander AH: Multidirectional shoulder instability: Clinical results of inferior capsular shift in an active-duty population. *Am J Sports Med* 1992;20:193-198.

88. McIntyre LF, Caspari RB, Savoie FH: The arthroscopic treatment of posterior shoulder instability: Two-year results of a multiple suture technique. *Arthroscopy* 1997;13:426-432.

89. Misamore GW, Sallay PI, Didelot W: A longitudinal study of patients with multidirectional instability of the shoulder with seven- to ten-year follow-up. *J Shoulder Elbow Surg* 2005;14:466-470.

90. Pollock RG, Owens JM, Flatow EL, Bigliani LU: Operative results of the inferior capsular shift procedure for multidirectional instability of the shoulder. *J Bone Joint Surg Am* 2000; 82:919-928.

91. Vidal L, Bradley JP: Management of posterior shoulder instability in the athlete. *Curr Opin Orthop* 2006;17: 164-171.

92. Williams RJ III, Strickland S, Cohen M, Altchek DW, Warren RF: Arthroscopic repair for traumatic posterior shoulder instability. *Am J Sports Med* 2003;31:203-209.

93. Leffert RD, Gumley G: The relationship between dead arm syndrome and thoracic outlet syndrome. *Clin Orthop Relat Res* 1987;223:20-31.

94. Kibler WB: The role of the scapula in athletic shoulder function. *Am J Sports Med* 1998;26:325-337.

95. Cofield RH, Nessler JP, Weinstabl R: Diagnosis of shoulder instability by examination under anesthesia. *Clin Orthop Relat Res* 1993;291:45-53.

96. Petersen SA: Posterior shoulder instability. *Orthop Clin North Am* 2000;31: 263-274.

97. Warner JJ, Micheli LJ, Arslanian LE, Kennedy J, Kennedy R: Patterns of flexibility, laxity, and strength in normal shoulders and shoulders with instability and impingement. *Am J Sports Med* 1990;18:366-375.

98. Kim SH, Park JC, Park JS, Oh I: Painful jerk test: A predictor of success in nonoperative treatment of posteroinferior instability of the shoulder. *Am J Sports Med* 2004;32: 1849-1855.

99. Kim SH, Park JS, Jeong WK, Shin SK: The Kim test: A novel test for posteroinferior labral lesion of the shoulder: A comparison to the jerk test. *Am J Sports Med* 2005;33:1188-1192.

100. Hawkins RH: Glenoid osteotomy for recurrent posterior subluxation of the shoulder: Assessment by computed axial tomography. *J Shoulder Elbow Surg* 1996;5:393-400.

101. Morris AD, Kemp GJ, Frostick SP: Shoulder electromyography in multidirectional instability. *J Shoulder Elbow Surg* 2004;13:24-29.

102. Barden JM, Balyk R, Raso VJ, Moreau M, Bagnall K: Atypical shoulder muscle activation in multidirectional instability. *Clin Neurophysiol* 2005;116:1846-1857.

103. Auge WK II, Morrison DS: Assessment of the infraspinatus spinal stretch reflex in the normal, athletic, and multidirectionally unstable shoulder. *Am J Sports Med* 2000;28: 206-213.

104. Barden JM, Balyk R, Raso VJ, Moreau M, Bagnall K: Dynamic upper limb proprioception in multidirectional shoulder instability. *Clin Orthop Relat Res* 2004;420:181-189.

105. Inui H, Sugamoto K, Miyamoto T, et al: Three-dimensional relationship of the glenohumeral joint in the elevated position in shoulders with multidirectional instability. *J Shoulder Elbow Surg* 2002;11:510-515.

106. Beasley L, Faryniarz DA, Hannafin JA: Multidirectional instability of the shoulder in the female athlete. *Clin Sports Med* 2000;19:331-349.

107. Burkhead WZ, Rockwood CA: Treatment of instability of the shoulder with an exercise program. *J Bone Joint Surg Am* 1992;74:890-896.

108. Kiss J, Damrel D, Mackie A, Neumann L, Wallace WA: Non-operative treatment of multidirectional shoulder instability. *Int Orthop* 2001;24:354-357.

109. Ide J, Maeda S, Yamaga M, Morisawa K, Takagi K: Shoulder-strengthening exercise with an orthosis for multidirectional shoulder instability: Quantitative evaluation of rotational shoulder strength before and after the exercise program. *J Shoulder Elbow Surg* 2003;12:342-345.

110. Arciero RA, Mazzocca AD: Posterior acromial bone block augmentation for the treatment of posterior glenoid bone loss associated with recurrent posterior shoulder instability. *Tech Shoulder Elbow Surg* 2006;7:210-217.

111. Gosens T, van Biezen FC, Verhaar JA: The bone block procedure in recurrent posterior shoulder instability. *Acta Orthop Belg* 2001;67: 116-120.

112. Bessems JH, Vegter J: Glenoplasty for recurrent posterior shoulder instability: Good results in 13 cases followed for 1-16 years. *Acta Orthop Scand* 1995; 66:535-537.

113. Gerber C, Ganz R, Vinh TS: Glenoplasty for recurrent posterior shoulder instability: An anatomic reappraisal. *Clin Orthop Relat Res* 1987; 216:70-79.

114. Graichen H, Koydl P, Zichner L: Effectiveness of glenoid osteotomy in atraumatic posterior instability of the shoulder associated with excessive retroversion and flatness of the glenoid. *Int Orthop* 1999;23:95-99.

115. Boyd HB, Sisk TD: Recurrent posterior dislocation of the shoulder. *J Bone Joint Surg Am* 1972;54:779-786.

116. Chaudhuri GK, Sengupta A, Saha AK: Rotation osteotomy of the shaft of the humerus for recurrent dislocation of the shoulder: Anterior and posterior. *Acta Orthop Scand* 1974;45: 193-198.

117. Surin V, Blader S, Markhede G, Sundholm K: Rotational osteotomy of the humerus for posterior instability of the shoulder. *J Bone Joint Surg Am* 1990;72:181-186.

118. Caprise PA Jr, Sekiya JK: Open and arthroscopic treatment of multidirectional instability of the shoulder. *Arthroscopy* 2006;22:1126-1131.

119. Choi CH, Ogilvie-Harris DJ: Inferior capsular shift operation for multidirectional instability of the shoulder in players of contact sports. *Br J Sports Med* 2002;36:290-294.

120. Dreese JC, D'Alessandro DF: Posterior capsulorrhaphy through an infraspinatus split for posterior instability. *Tech Shoulder Elbow Surg* 2005;6: 199-207.

121. Massoud SN, Levy O, Copeland SA: Inferior capsular shift for multidirectional instability following failed laser-assisted capsular shrinkage. *J Shoulder Elbow Surg* 2002;11:305-308.

122. Misamore GW, Facibene WA: Posterior capsulorrhaphy for the treatment of traumatic recurrent posterior subluxations of the shoulder in athletes. *J Shoulder Elbow Surg* 2000;9:403-408.

123. Papendick LW, Savoie FH III: Anatomy-specific repair techniques for posterior shoulder instability. *J South Orthop Assoc* 1995;4:169-176.

124. Thomas SC, Matsen FA III: An approach to the repair of avulsion of the glenohumeral ligaments in the management of traumatic anterior glenohumeral instability. *J Bone Joint Surg Am* 1989;71:506-513.

125. Tibone JE, Prietto C, Jobe FW, et al: Staple capsulorrhaphy for recurrent posterior shoulder dislocation. *Am J Sports Med* 1981;9:135-139.

126. Wolf EM, Eakin CL: Arthroscopic capsular plication for posterior shoulder instability. *Arthroscopy* 1998;14: 153-163.

127. Kim SH, Noh KC, Park JS, Ryu BD, Oh I: Loss of chondrolabral containment of the glenohumeral joint in atraumatic posteroinferior multidirectional instability. *J Bone Joint Surg Am* 2005;87:92-98.

128. Lo IK, Burkhart SS: Triple labral lesions: Pathology and surgical repair technique: Report of seven cases. *Arthroscopy* 2005;21:186-193.

129. Provencher MT, Verma N, Obopilwe E, Rincon LM, Tracy J, Romeo AA, Mazzocca A: A biomechanical analysis of capsular plication versus anchor repair of the shoulder: Can the labrum be used as a suture anchor? *Arthroscopy* 2007, in press.

130. Metcalf MH, Pon JD, Harryman DT II, Loutzenheiser T, Sidles JA: Capsulolabral augmentation increases glenohumeral stability in the cadaver shoulder. *J Shoulder Elbow Surg* 2001; 10:532-538.

131. Schneider DJ, Tibone JE, McGarry MH, Grossman MG, Veneziani S, Lee TQ: Biomechanical evaluation after five and ten millimeter anterior glenohumeral capsulorrhaphy using a novel shoulder model of increased laxity. *J Shoulder Elbow Surg* 2005;14: 318-323.

132. Gerber C, Werner C, Macy J, Jacob H, Nyffeler R: Effect of selective capsulorrhaphy on the passive range of motion of the glenohumeral joint. *J Bone Joint Surg Am* 2003;85:48-55.

133. Uno A, Bain GI, Mehta JA: Arthroscopic relationship of the axillary nerve to the shoulder joint capsule: An anatomic study. *J Shoulder Elbow Surg* 1999;8:226-230.

134. Eakin CL, Dvirnak P, Miller CM, Hawkins RJ: The relationship of the axillary nerve to arthroscopically placed capsulolabral sutures: An anatomic study. *Am J Sports Med* 1998;26: 505-509.

135. Price MR, Tillett ED, Acland RD, Nettleton GS: Determining the relationship of the axillary nerve to the shoulder joint capsule from an arthroscopic perspective. *J Bone Joint Surg Am* 2004;86:2135-2142.

136. Greis PE, Burks RT, Schickendantz MS, Sandmeier R: Axillary nerve injury after thermal capsular shrinkage of the shoulder. *J Shoulder Elbow Surg* 2001;10:231-235.

137. McCarty EC, Warren RF, Deng XH, Craig EV, Potter H: Temperature along the axillary nerve during radiofrequency-induced thermal capsular shrinkage. *Am J Sports Med* 2004; 32:909-914.

138. Wong KL, Williams GR: Complications of thermal capsulorrhaphy of the shoulder. *J Bone Joint Surg Am* 2001;83(suppl 2 pt 2):151-155.

139. Werner CM, Nyffeler RW, Jacob HA, Gerber C: The effect of capsular tightening on humeral head translations. *J Orthop Res* 2004;22:194-201.

140. Karas SG, Creighton RA, DeMorat GJ: Glenohumeral volume reduction in arthroscopic shoulder reconstruction: A cadaveric analysis of suture plication and thermal capsulorrhaphy. *Arthroscopy* 2004;20:179-184.

141. Remia LF, Ravalin RV, Lemly KS, McGarry MH, Kvitne RS, Lee TQ: Biomechanical evaluation of multidi rectional glenohumeral instability and repair. *Clin Orthop Relat Res* 2003;416: 225-236.

142. Miniaci A, McBirnie J: Thermal capsular shrinkage for treatment of multidirectional instability of the shoulder. *J Bone Joint Surg Am* 2003;85: 2283-2287.

143. Mazzocca AD, Brown FM Jr, Carreira DS, Hayden J, Romeo AA: Arthroscopic anterior shoulder stabilization of collision and contact athletes. *Am J Sports Med* 2005;33:52-60.

144. Difelice GS, Williams RJ III, Cohen MS, Warren RF: The accessory posterior portal for shoulder arthroscopy: Description of technique and cadaveric study. *Arthroscopy* 2001;17:888-891.

145. Goubier JN, Iserin A, Augereau B: The posterolateral portal: A new approach for shoulder arthroscopy. *Arthroscopy* 2001;17:1000-1002.

146. Goubier JN, Iserin A, Duranthon LD, Vandenbussche E, Augereau B: A 4-portal arthroscopic stabilization in posterior shoulder instability. *J Shoulder Elbow Surg* 2003;12: 337-341.

147. Antoniou J, Duckworth DT, Harryman DT II: Capsulolabral augmentation for the management of posteroinferior instability of the shoulder. *J Bone Joint Surg Am* 2000;82:1220-1230.

148. Duncan R, Savoie FH III: Arthroscopic inferior capsular shift for multidirectional instability of the shoulder: A preliminary report. *Arthroscopy* 1993;9:24-27.

149. McIntyre LF, Caspari RB, Savoie FH: The arthroscopic treatment of anterior and multidirectional shoulder instability. *Instr Course Lect* 1996;45:47-56.

150. Treacy SH, Savoie FH III, Field LD: Arthroscopic treatment of multidirectional instability. *J Shoulder Elbow Surg* 1999;8:345-350.

151. Plausinis D, Bravman JT, Heywood C, Kummer FJ, Kwon YW, Jazrawi LM: Arthroscopic rotator interval closure: Effect of sutures on glenohu

meral motion and anterior-posterior translation. *Am J Sports Med* 2006;34: 1656-1661.

152. Provencher MT, Mologne TS, Hongo M, Zhao K, An KN: Arthroscopic versus open rotator interval closure: Biomechanical evaluation of stability and motion. *Arthroscopy* 2007; 23:583-592.

153. Van der Reis W, Wolf E: Arthroscopic rotator cuff interval capsular closure. *Orthopedics* 2001;24:657-661.

154. Yamamoto N, Itoi E, Tuoheti Y, et al: Effect of rotator interval closure on glenohumeral stability and motion: A cadaveric study. *J Shoulder Elbow Surg* 2006;15:750-758.

155. Ikeda H: "Rotator interval" lesion: Part 1. Clinical study. *Nippon Seikeigeka Gakkai Zasshi* 1986;60: 1261-1273.

156. Ikeda H: "Rotator interval" lesion: Part 2. Biomechanical study. *Nippon*

*Seikeigeka Gakkai Zasshi* 1986;60: 1275-1281.

157. Itoi E, Berglund LJ, Grabowski JJ, Naggar L, Morrey BF, An KN: Superior-inferior stability of the shoulder: Role of the coracohumeral ligament and the rotator interval capsule. *Mayo Clin Proc* 1998;73: 508-515.

# Massive Irreparable Tendon Tears of the Rotator Cuff: Salvage Options

Bassem Elhassan, MD

Nathan K. Endres, MD

Laurence D. Higgins, MD

Jon J.P. Warner, MD

## Abstract

*The management of massive, irreparable rotator cuff tears is challenging. Arthroscopic débridement has produced reasonable short-term outcomes in patients who experience good relief from pain and improved range of motion after a subacromial injection with local anesthetic. Arthroscopic débridement with partial repair also has resulted in good outcomes, especially in patients with documented suprascapular nerve traction neurapraxia. Tendon transfer can offer a long-lasting solution in a patient with a weak shoulder who still has the ability to raise the shoulder past the horizontal position. Shoulder replacement with the use of a reverse prosthesis has emerged as a viable option in patients with pseudoparalysis with or without osteoarthritis of the glenohumeral joint.*

**Instr Course Lect 2008;57:153-166.**

A massive rotator cuff tear was defined by Cofield as a tear with a diameter of 5 cm or more.[1] Gerber defined this condition as a tendon tear involving two or more tendons after débridement.[2] The latter definition is more functional than a definition based on a simple measurement of the length of the tear because an exact measurement of the extent of the tendon tear can be made only after the degenerated rim of the tendon tissue has been débrided. The length of the tendon tear is then measured in centimeters with the arm at the side; the involved tendons are also noted.

## General Considerations

Tauro[3] suggested that the size of the tear should not only represent the anteroposterior dimension but also should include the mediolateral dimension. He proposed an index (square centimeters) of tear dimension created by multiplying the anteroposterior dimension by the mediolateral dimension.[3] Although knowledge of all the dimensions of a rotator cuff tear after débridement allows a more quantitative measure of tear size, the determination of an index of tear size does not provide additional significant data because tendon tears are rarely rectangular. The mediolateral distance also changes with arm position. The dimension of the tear as a percentage of the humeral head may have more prognostic value because of significant variations in patient size.[4]

A massive tear does not necessarily mean an irreparable tear, and an irreparable rotator cuff tear can be defined as one in which the quality of the tendon tissue is so poor that primary direct tendon-to-bone repair is not possible with the arm adducted at the side after débridement of avascular tissue.[5] Acute massive tears may be much larger than 5 cm in diameter but may have good quality tendon that is elastic and easily repaired to its anatomic insertion. Conversely, a chronic small tear may have friable, inelastic, thin tendon tissue that is impossible to mobilize and repair.[6,7] Other important indicators of an irreparable tear include static superior subluxation of the humeral head with an acromiohumeral distance of less than 5 mm, MRI scans showing severe atrophy of rotator cuff muscles, and advanced fatty degeneration of the muscles.[8,9]

Another factor that has recently been shown to be important when considering if a tendon tear will be reparable is the patient's history of cigarette smoking.[10] Tendon tears in patients who are chronic smokers are larger than tears in control groups of nonsmokers, and the quality of the tissue and its potential to heal are also reduced.

Massive rotator cuff tears usually are of two different configurations: the more common posterosuperior configuration that involves the supraspinatus and infraspinatus, and the less common anterosuperior configuration that involves the subscapularis and the supraspinatus.[11] Complete disruption of the supraspinatus, infraspinatus, and subscapularis is rare and is usually associated with a chronic tendon tear that is irreparable.

Most literature reviews report on posterosuperior tears, which make up 10% to 20% of all tendon tears. Neer and associates[12] reported 145 massive posterosuperior tears in 340 rotator cuff tears treated over a 13-year period. Bigliani and associates[13] reported 61 such tears over 6 years. Ellman and associates[14] reported 9 massive tears in 50 rotator cuff tears over 12 years, and Harryman and associates[15] reported 28 of 100 over 5 years. Warner and associates[16] reported their 5-year experience with 53 massive tears in 213 rotator cuff tears (20%) undergoing surgical repair.

Anterosuperior rotator cuff tears have been reported less frequently.[5] Warner and associates[16] reported 19 such tears in 407 rotator cuff tears (5%) treated surgically over a 6-year period. Among 105 tears reported by Harryman and associates,[15] 22 involved the anterosuperior cuff. Kruz and associates[17] reported treating 18 anterosuperior tears over a 5-year period. A recent review reported 73 isolated ruptures of the subscapularis or combined ruptures of the subscapularis and supraspinatus in 1,345 patients treated with rotator cuff repair.[18]

Despite the fact that massive rotator cuff tears are more challenging to treat, most can be repaired or reconstructed with good outcomes.[9,11] Based on the experience of the senior authors and others, fewer than 5% of all rotator cuff tears remain irreparable, not only because of their size but also because of the quality of the tendon tissue.[14,19]

## Treatment Options for Irreparable Tendon Tears

Few surgical options exist for an irreparable rotator cuff tear. Simple débridement through an arthroscopic or open technique has been suggested by some authors who believe that this approach can provide good pain relief and a possibility of functional improvement.[19-22] These techniques are indicated primarily for elderly patients who have pain and low physical demands. Although shoulder strength does not improve in these patients, function usually is enhanced because of relief from pain caused by mechanical impingement. The ideal patient for this approach is older than 60 years, has preoperative active flexion of at least 120° (after subacromial anesthetic injection), and has at least 80% of normal external rotation strength. In patients with poor preoperative function, this procedure cannot guarantee durable pain relief or recovery of function.

Reported outcomes of such treatment are variable. Apoil and Augereau[23] reported poor long-term results after open subacromial débridement and resection of the coracoacromial ligament. In contrast, Rockwood and associates[5] reported decreased pain and improvement of function and strength in 83% of patients after acromioplasty, decompression, and tear débridement, with no deterioration over time. Gartsman[24] reported results that were inferior to those reported by Rockwood and associates.[5] In the study by Gartsman, open débridement and subacromial decompression led to decreased pain and improved function; however, strength decreased. Other studies have reported good results in biomechanically compensated, irreparable tears after arthroscopic acromioplasty.[21,22] Significant reduction in pain but no improvement in strength or function has been reported after arthroscopic débridement.[25,26] However, Zvijac and associates[27] reported deterioration of function and strength over time, especially in patients with massive tears treated with arthroscopic débridement and subacromial decompression. Kempf and associates[28] reported no significant improvement in the overall Constant score in patients with massive tears after arthroscopic débridement and long-term postoperative rehabilitation.

Other suggested treatment options have included the use of synthetic fabrics or tendon allografts to patch massive, irreparable rotator cuff tears. These techniques have demonstrated fair to poor clinical effectiveness. Moore and associates[29] reported on 32 patients who had allograft reconstruction of irreparable rotator cuff tears over a 14-year period. MRI scans of 15 patients at a mean follow-up of 31 months showed radiographic failure of the allograft rotator cuff reconstruction in all patients. Iannotti and associates[30] also showed that the use of porcine small intestinal mucosa to augment massive rotator cuff tears did not improve the rate of tendon healing or clinical outcome scores.

Tendon transfers around the shoulder have become an established method for the management of massive, irreparable rotator cuff tears in selected patients.[15,20] Local tendon transfers include the use of the subscapularis or teres minor tendons to cover a large defect in the superior portion of the rotator cuff.[31,32] Most of these approaches have been abandoned because their efficacy could not be validated.[33] Some patients may have worse function after local transfers, possibly because of weakening of the remaining anteroposterior force couple.

Isolated teres major transfer to reconstruct an irreparable infraspinatus tear has been reported, but this repair is not favored because the tendon is short and bulky.[14,20,34] Others have recommended transfer of the trapezius tendon, but results have not been reproducible.[35] Some European surgeons have recommended the use of the anterior deltoid for reconstruction of massive cuff tears; however, this technique has not been independently validated.[36]

Transfer of the latissimus dorsi to reconstruct massive tears in the rotator cuff was originally proposed and reported by Gerber and associates.[20] This transfer provides a strong, vascularized tendon, which may close the cuff defect and act as a humeral head depressor. In practice, it probably improves function by restoring lost external rotation rather than active depression of the humeral head. It is now considered a viable option for treatment of irreparable posterosuperior cuff tears in certain patients. Longer follow-up studies have confirmed initial reports of the value of this treatment.[16,37-40] The subscapularis tendon and deltoid origin must be intact for the transfer to provide benefit. The patient also must have only moderate weakness about the shoulder and not pseudoparalysis. In the latter situation, the patient has profound weakness and can barely lift the arm from the side.

The pectoralis major tendon transfer has been described for patients with irreparable anterosuperior rotator cuff tears.[11,17,41] Its loca-

tion and line of action make this transfer feasible for treatment of irreparable subscapularis tears; however, the pectoralis major tendon transfer cannot recenter a humeral head that is statically subluxated anteriorly and superiorly. This transfer is best suited for an isolated, irreparable subscapularis tendon tear, not a combined subscapularis-supraspinatus tendon tear.[17]

When a patient has profound shoulder weakness with the appearance of a pseudoparalytic shoulder, isolated tendon transfer is not effective in restoring function. Shoulder fusion is rarely an option because patients with such dysfunction are usually older and may have bilateral disease. Shoulder fusion is not well tolerated by these patients. However, in the rare instance of a young patient with multiple failed surgeries, a fusion may be considered.[42]

Hemiarthroplasty has been proposed for patients with limited functional goals. This treatment may be reasonable for a patient with an irreparable massive posterosuperior tendon tear in which the subscapularis remains intact and the humeral head is not subluxated anterosuperiorly.[43]

In patients with massive rotator cuff tears, profound weakness, and superior and/or anterior subluxation of the humeral head, reverse or inverse shoulder arthroplasty is an effective short-term to midterm treatment approach.[44-46] Improved outcomes have been reported when using a reverse shoulder prosthesis along with a tendon transfer to restore weak external rotation.[47-49]

## Pathomechanical Considerations

The extrinsic and intrinsic muscles around the glenohumeral joint work in synergy to maintain balanced force

couples in all planes. The deltoid and inferior parts of the rotator cuff maintain the coronal force couple, whereas the subscapularis and infraspinatus/teres minor maintain the transverse force couple. Each of the four rotator cuff muscles has a force potential based on the individual physiologic cross-sectional areas.[4,24,50,51] A perpendicular line drawn from the line of action of a muscle to the center of rotation determines the leverage of the muscle.[52] The functional contribution is determined for each muscle by multiplying the force potential of the muscle by its leverage. The percentage of physiologic cross-sectional area of the subscapularis muscle is 52%, the supraspinatus 15%, and infraspinatus (and teres minor) 33%.[53] The average moment arm of the subscapularis is 2.3 cm; supraspinatus, 2.0 cm; and infraspinatus (and teres minor), 2.2 cm. Thus, the rotational contribution of the subscapularis is 52%, the supraspinatus 14%, and the infraspinatus (and teres minor) 32%. This demonstrates the primary importance of the anterior and posterior components in shoulder joint rotation.[52]

During simple scapular plane abduction, the tendon excursion of the rotator cuff muscles is minimal compared with that of the deltoid muscle (deltoid, 6.5 cm; supraspinatus, 3.8 cm; infraspinatus, 3.5 cm; and subscapularis, 0.4 cm). The rotator cuff muscles function more as stabilizers than as prime movers, providing a fixed fulcrum for concentric rotation of the humeral head on the glenoid.[54,55] During abduction, the deltoid creates a relative upward shearing moment that must be resisted by a force couple produced by the rotator cuff muscles.[50] A rotator cuff tear involving the supraspinatus in combination with either the infraspinatus or the subscapularis will lead to disruption of this force couple and may eventually lead to loss of a stable fulcrum for glenohumeral joint motion.[56,57]

Although some studies have shown that the long head of the biceps may resist superior and anterior translation of the humeral head on the glenoid, its role as an active stabilizer and head depressor in patients with a massive rotator cuff tear has not been proven.[58,59] Because the long head of the biceps is often enlarged and hypertrophied in patients with massive rotator cuff tears, it has been suggested that it substitutes for a deficient rotator cuff.[60] Recent electromyographic studies have shown that the long head of the biceps is electrically inactive in patients with a massive rotator cuff tear who attempt abduction, so it probably is not an active humeral head depressor.[28,59] Walch and associates[61] provided compelling evidence that the long head of the biceps acts as a significant pain generator, and that biceps tenotomy provides significant pain relief in patients with irreparable massive rotator cuff tears.

Several studies have shown good motion and concentric rotation of the glenohumeral joint in patients with massive rotator cuff tears.[21,22,62] Complete loss of containment usually results from extension of the tear inferior to the equator into the subscapularis or the infraspinatus and teres minor.[2,8,38] However, the existence of an extended tear is not always associated with poor function, because many patients have poor function even with a small rotator cuff tear.[1,5,13] It is not known why symptoms and function manifest differently in patients with rotator cuff tears of varying sizes.

Fatty infiltration of atrophic rotator cuff muscles has been proposed as a major factor influencing the reparability and outcome of massive rotator cuff tears.[38,39,63] Warner and associates[64] studied patients with massive rotator cuff tears of similar size and found a correlation between the MRI appearance of atrophy and fatty degeneration and overall shoulder biomechanics and function. They believed that it was possible to identify factors that would help predict poor outcomes in patients with massive rotator cuff tears. These factors include profound weakness of external rotation, superior displacement of the humeral head, and MRI scans showing atrophy and fatty replacement of the muscles. If a true AP radiograph of the shoulder with the arm in neutral rotation shows that the acromiohumeral interval is less than 5 mm, and if MRI shows advanced muscular atrophy and fatty degeneration, surgical repair is unlikely to result in restoration of function and strength.[65]

A decrease in muscle compliance has been documented in chronic cuff tears and may preclude direct repair to bone.[66] With chronic tears, the pennation angle between the individual muscle fibers decreases, the length of the muscle fiber shortens, and increased amounts of fat fill the space between the muscle fibers.[67] Warner and associates[16] found a correlation between the degree of change in muscle fat on preoperative MRI scans and the tendon quality observed intraoperatively. It was found that the more advanced the fatty infiltration of muscle, the more friable and stiff the tendon, and the lower the rate of success of tendon-to-bone repair.

The coracoacromial ligament is another anatomic structure that is believed to play a secondary static role in preventing anterosuperior migration of the humeral head when rotator cuff containment function is lost.[58] This ligament must be preserved because it acts as the last barrier to unchecked anterosuperior translation of the humeral head. Routine acromioplasty in this situation should be avoided because it can destabilize the coracoacromial ligament.[68]

## Tendon Transfer for Irreparable Cuff Tears

For irreparable posterosuperior tears, latissimus dorsi transfer is a good treatment option. Studies have reported 80% good to excellent results that remained stable over a 10-year period.[2,20,51] This type of transfer is not recommended in patients with an irreparable subscapularis tear. Miniaci and Macleod[37] reported 80% satisfactory results after failed rotator cuff repair. Warner and Parsons[38] reported 70% overall patient satisfaction; however, they had a 30% rupture rate and significantly worse outcomes were reported in patients who had latissimus dorsi transfer as a salvage procedure after failed rotator cuff repair. Iannotti and associates[69] reported 64% satisfactory results and suggested that gender, preoperative shoulder function, and general strength may influence the outcome. Female patients with generalized muscle weakness and poor shoulder function are more likely to have a poor clinical outcome.

For an irreparable anterosuperior tear, pectoralis major transfer has been described.[70] Wirth and Rockwood[41] reported satisfactory results in 10 of 13 patients, and Resch and associates[71] reported good to excellent results in 9 of 12 patients. Less predictable results were found in the evaluation of 10 patients who had complex shoulder disorders and required pectoralis major transfer for subscapularis insufficiency after failed surgery.[35] The authors of another study reported satisfactory results in 24 of 30 pectoralis transfers (80%) and noted that outcomes were better in patients who had isolated irreparable subscapularis tears.[70] In patients with associated irreparable supraspinatus tears, the results were less favorable.

This approach has been modified for anterosuperior irreparable tears by combining pectoralis major and teres major transfers. This modification is based on the rationale that when these two muscles are transferred together, a better vector is achieved to replace the deficient subscapularis muscle (Figure 1). In several patients, the humeral head was recentered, and the patient's function was improved. However, too few of these procedures have been performed for comparison with isolated pectoralis major transfer.

### Indications for Tendon Transfer

An ideal candidate for a tendon transfer has mild to moderate shoulder weakness without subluxation of the humeral head. For an irreparable posterosuperior rotator cuff tear, a latissimus tendon transfer is performed when the subscapularis tendon and the deltoid are intact.[2,8] Other important factors are patient related and include no current use of tobacco and a willingness to comply with a protracted postoperative program to train the transferred tendon. Specific contraindications to latissimus transfer include arthritis, loss of the subscapularis tendon, deltoid insufficiency, and stiffness.[11,32,38]

### Technical Considerations
#### Débridement

For massive tears, no differences in outcome have been reported between open and arthroscopic débridement. Some authors believe that after subacromial decompression, débridement of the cuff itself is not necessary.[63] Additional procedures on the biceps tendon are controversial. Some authors recommend its preservation, whereas others recommend tenotomy.[5,28] Preservation of the coraco-

acromial arch is a key to success with either tendon transfer or débridement. Loss of the arch will lead to failure of either intervention.

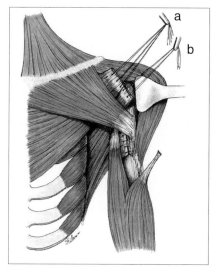

**Figure 1** Drawing showing a combined transfer of the sternal head of the pectoralis major (a) and teres major (b). (Reproduced with permission from Higgins L, Warner JJP: Massive tears of posterior superior rotator cuff, in Warner JJP, Iannotti J, Flatow E (eds): *Complex and Revision Problems in Shoulder Surgery*. Philadelphia, PA, Lippincott Williams & Wilkins, 2005.)

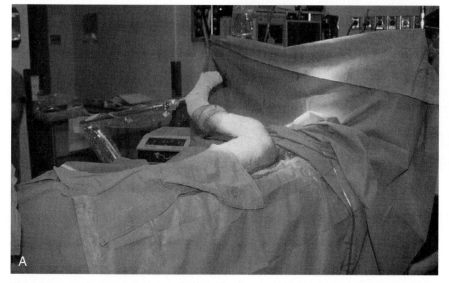
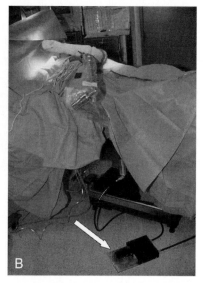

**Figure 2** **A,** Photograph shows the benefit of using a hydraulic arm holder. **B,** The arrow points to the foot pedal for the hydraulic arm control. (Reproduced with permission from Higgins L, Warner JJP: Massive tears of posterior superior rotator cuff, in Warner JJP, Iannotti J, Flatow E (eds): *Complex and Revision Problems in Shoulder Surgery*. Philadelphia, PA, Lippincott Williams & Wilkins, 2005, p 149.)

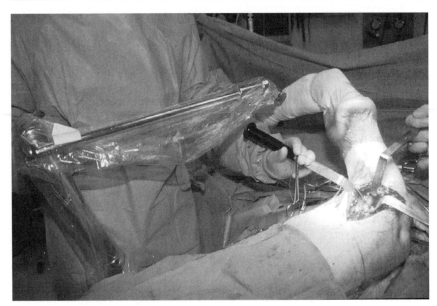

**Figure 3**    The hydraulic arm holder is useful for keeping the shoulder in abduction and internal rotation during latissimus dorsi harvesting. (Reproduced with permission from Higgins L, Warner JJP: Massive tears of posterior superior rotator cuff, in Warner JJP, Iannotti J, Flatow E (eds): *Complex and Revision Problems in Shoulder Surgery*. Philadelphia, PA, Lippincott Williams & Wilkins, 2005, p 149.)

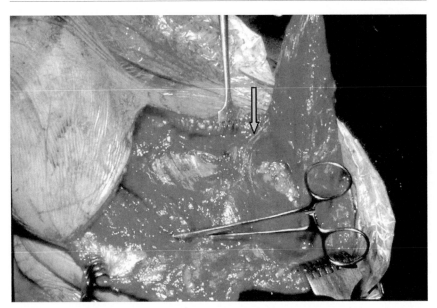

**Figure 4**    The latissimus dorsi tendon is detached from its insertion and dissected in a retrograde fashion to its neurovascular pedicle (*arrow*). (Reproduced with permission from Higgins L, Warner JJP: Massive tears of posterior superior rotator cuff, in Warner JJP, Iannotti J, Flatow E (eds): *Complex and Revision Problems in Shoulder Surgery*. Philadelphia, PA, Lippincott Williams & Wilkins, 2005, p 150.)

### Latissimus Dorsi Transfer

A latissimus dorsi transfer can be done with the patient either seated or in the lateral decubitus position. Gerber and others originally described the lateral decubitus position but have modified their approach to allow for a seated position that is more familiar to most surgeons performing rotator cuff repair.[2,8] The seated position works well for most patients; however, exposure and harvesting of the latissimus dorsi are difficult in an obese patient. For these patients, the lateral decubitus position is recommended.

The use of a hydraulic arm holder is helpful to reproducibly position the arm (Figure 2). An incision is first made along the latissimus dorsi muscle and curved underneath the axilla. The arm is placed in a position of abduction and internal rotation (Figure 3). The latissimus dorsi muscle is dissected from the teres major and isolated to its insertion on the humerus. The latissimus dorsi tendon is then detached from its insertion and dissected in a retrograde fashion to its neurovascular pedicle (Figure 4). The muscle attachments to the surrounding chest wall are released, and the muscle is freed over the inferior border of the scapula. This process usually provides sufficient length for the transfer. The interval underneath the deltoid is then developed, and the tendon is transferred over the greater tuberosity. The tendon is fixed along the greater tuberosity while the arm is maintained in abduction and external rotation to set tendon tension so that active external rotation can be achieved by the transfer (Figure 5). If some rotator cuff remains, it can be repaired or sewn into the tendon transfer. After closure of all incisions, the arm is positioned in an orthotic device to maintain abduction and external rotation (Figure 6).

### Postoperative Care

Postoperative treatment can be divided into four phases. Phase I includes the first 6 weeks after surgery, during which time the patient re-

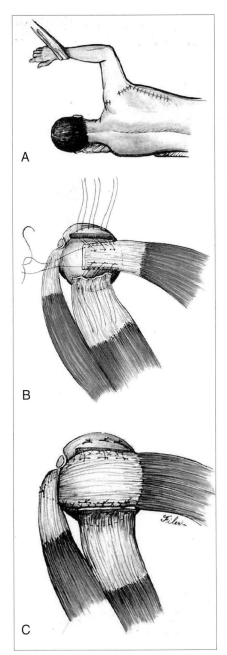

**Figure 5**    While the arm is maintained in abduction and external rotation (**A**) the latissimus dorsi tendon is fixed along the greater tuberosity to set tendon tension so that active external rotation can be achieved by the transfer (**B** and **C**). (Reproduced with permission from Higgins L, Warner JJP: Massive tears of posterior superior rotator cuff, in Warner JJP, Iannotti J, Flatow E (eds): *Complex and Revision Problems in Shoulder Surgery*. Philadelphia, PA, Lippincott Williams & Wilkins, 2005, p 151.)

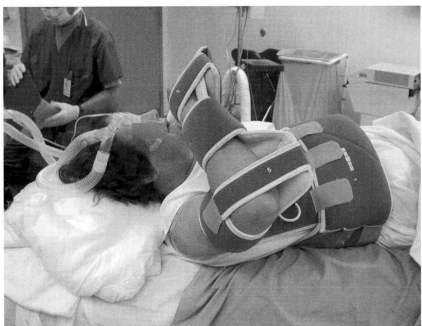

**Figure 6**    After skin closure and dressing application, the arm is positioned in an orthotic device to maintain abduction and external rotation. (Reproduced with permission from Higgins L, Warner JJP: Massive tears of posterior superior rotator cuff, in Warner JJP, Iannotti J, Flatow E (eds): *Complex and Revision Problems in Shoulder Surgery*. Philadelphia, PA, Lippincott Williams & Wilkins, 2005, p 152.)

mains in the abduction orthosis except for passive therapy when the shoulder is moved into abduction and external rotation but not into adduction or internal rotation. This passive motion ensures that the graft does not scar in its transferred position.

In phase II, the orthosis is removed and the patient is permitted to use the arm for active range of motion for all activities of daily living; however, no lifting is permitted. Active assisted motion and passive motion continue. This phase lasts for an additional 6 weeks.

During phase III, the patient is taught to activate the tendon transfer by means of biofeedback training. This phase begins 12 weeks after surgery. A biofeedback unit with cutaneous electrodes gives the patient feedback about latissimus dorsi muscle activity. The patient is then instructed in two methods (the J

maneuver and the adduction external rotation maneuver) that activate the latissimus dorsi as an elevator and external rotator of the arm.

In the J maneuver, the patient's arm is held by the therapist in approximately 90° of abduction. The patient is then instructed to pull downward and across the body to make the latissimus dorsi contract. As the therapist resists this movement, the patient is asked to try to flex the shoulder once the arm crosses the midline. In this manner, the patient learns to maintain latissimus dorsi contraction while attempting to flex the arm. The hand traces the letter J, and the biofeedback unit helps the patient maintain muscle activity. The patient can use the contralateral arm to assist in this maneuver.

In the adduction external rotation maneuver, the patient's arm is abducted approximately 30° away from the body, and the patient is instructed to forcefully adduct the arm while the therapist resists this adduction with a hand above the patient's elbow. This action causes the latissimus dorsi to contract. The patient is then asked to simultaneously externally rotate the shoulder. The therapist may help the patient with external rotation. By observing muscle activity with the biofeedback device, the patient can train the latissimus dorsi to become an active external rotator (Figure 7).

Phase IV of treatment begins after 16 weeks and consists of strengthening exercises.

### Pectoralis Major Transfer

For an irreparable subscapularis tendon tear, a transfer of the sternal head of the pectoralis major is recommended.[32] The sternal head of the pectoralis major is routed underneath the clavicular head, which acts as a fulcrum for the sternal head when both contract (Figure 8). This helps in guiding the axis of pull of the pectoralis major to be more in line with the vector of the subscapularis. Other authors have described transfer of a portion of the pectoralis major underneath the conjoined tendon;[71,72] however, Gerber and associates[39] did not observe any advantage in their patients using this

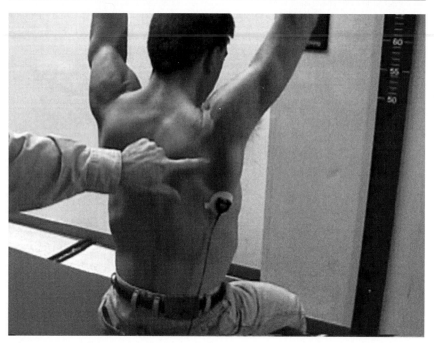

**Figure 7** Biofeedback is used to train the patient to use the transferred latissimus dorsi. (Reproduced with permission from Higgins L, Warner JJP: Massive tears of posterior superior rotator cuff, in Warner JJP, Iannotti J, Flatow E (eds): *Complex and Revision Problems in Shoulder Surgery*. Philadelphia, PA, Lippincott Williams & Wilkins, 2005, p 151.)

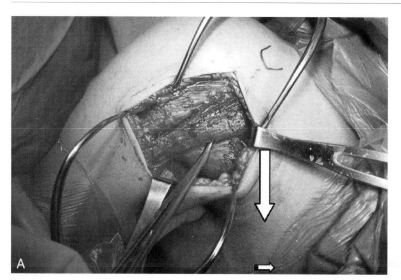
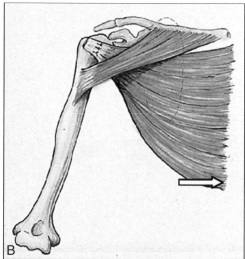

**Figure 8** **A,** Intraoperative photograph showing a clamp placed between the clavicular head (*large arrow*) and sternal head (*small arrow*) of the pectoralis major. **B,** Diagram showing transfer of the sternal head of the pectoralis major under the clavicular head with fixation on the lesser tuberosity of the humerus (*arrow*). (Reproduced with permission from Warner JJP, Iannotti J, Flatow E (eds): *Complex and Revision Problems in Shoulder Surgery*. Philadelphia, PA, Lippincott Williams & Wilkins, 2005, p 41.)

method compared with direct transfer of the pectoralis major.

In rare instances, the subscapularis tendon may be chronically deficient and anterior subluxation of the humeral head may occur. This condition is very difficult to treat. In this situation, the addition of a teres major transfer may help recenter the humeral head on the glenoid. The teres major tendon is located underneath the latissimus dorsi, which is detached and repaired after mobilizing the teres major. The teres major is transferred to the lower portion of the lesser tuberosity, and the pectoralis major is transferred to the upper portion of the lesser tuberosity (Figure 1). In the setting of revision surgery, when there is significant scar formation, the senior author has found a modified Latarjet procedure to be helpful in providing stability by recentering the humeral head.

## Reverse Shoulder Prosthesis

Standard total shoulder arthroplasty as a treatment for rotator cuff tear arthropathy (RCTA) has been largely abandoned because of unsatisfactory clinical results related to altered biomechanics.[73-75] In the absence of a functioning rotator cuff, the glenoid component is exposed to excessive shear forces produced by the deltoid. This "rocking-horse" phenomenon leads to early failure secondary to glenoid loosening.[76]

The role of hemiarthroplasty is still debated. Hemiarthroplasty may provide pain relief; however, active motion usually is not improved because functional mechanics are not restored. Results may deteriorate with time because of progressive glenoid erosion. Published rates of persistent postoperative pain range from 6% to 53%, with active elevation ranging from 86° to 120°.[77-79] Some patients with irreparable tears

have significant pain but maintain reasonably good function because of an intact anteroposterior force couple across the joint and compensatory scapulothoracic mechanics. In these patients, hemiarthroplasty may be the initial procedure of choice if nonsurgical treatment or arthroscopic débridement fails to provide satisfactory pain relief.

Because of the disappointing results with conventional arthroplasty, reverse (or inverse) total shoulder arthroplasty (RTSA) has gained attention as an alternative treatment option for patients with RCTA. The shoulder mechanics in the patients are often so poor that they appear to have pseudoparalysis of the affected extremity. Typically this pseudoparalysis is associated with static superior subluxation of the humerus on plain radiographs (Figure 9).

Neer first introduced the concept of constrained arthroplasty for the treatment of RCTA in the 1970s. However, early designs generally were associated with poor clinical results and were not widely accepted.[80-84] The early designs usually failed because the axis of rotation of the joint was moved lateral to its normal position. This altered position increased the force of the lever arm across the glenoid during elevation, which usually resulted in failure caused by pullout of the glenoid component.

In 1985, a new prosthesis design addressed the perceived shortcomings of the earlier prostheses. The basic biomechanical goal of the new design was to medialize the center of rotation to decrease shear forces and also increase the deltoid lever arm, thus producing more efficient arm elevation. Practically, this goal was achieved by affixing a hemisphere with no neck (glenosphere) to a baseplate on the glenoid. It has been

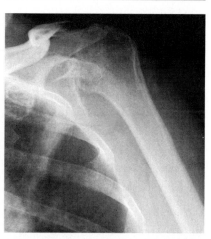

**Figure 9** In patients with significant shoulder weakness that creates the appearance of pseudoparalysis of the affected extremity, the radiographs of the shoulder typically show static superior subluxation of the humerus.

shown that by medializing the center of rotation by 10 mm, deltoid torque (primarily the middle deltoid with some contribution from the anterior and posterior deltoid) increases 20% to 60%. Lowering the center of rotation by 10 mm also increases deltoid torque by 30% to 60%. The large diameter of the glenosphere (36 or 42 mm) offered greater stability and a larger arc of motion than the smaller components used in earlier designs.[46]

In 1987, the initial results of the new prosthesis were presented.[85] The Delta III (DePuy International, Leeds, UK), a modification of the original prosthesis, has been used in France since 1991 and recently received Food and Drug Administration approval in the United States. Other models, including the Anatomic Inverse (Zimmer, Warsaw, IN) and the Reverse Shoulder Prosthesis (Encore Medical, Austin, TX), have recently become available.

Preoperative patient evaluation should consist of the usual focused

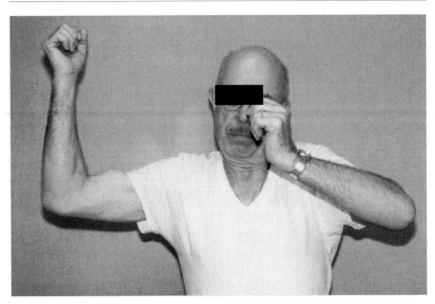

**Figure 10**    A patient with a massive rotator cuff tear and positive hornblower's sign that indicates severe external rotation weakness.

physical examination and appropriate radiographic and laboratory studies. Of particular importance is the establishment of normal deltoid function as well as teres minor function. The external rotation lag and hornblower's signs (Figure 10) are helpful in assessing the status of the posterior cuff (infraspinatus and teres minor).[86,87] This assessment is important because the clinical results of RTSA are worse when there is significant dysfunction of the posterior cuff, specifically teres minor.[88] In some patients, a tendon transfer can be combined with RTSA to improve external rotation.[47-49]

If the patient has an existing prosthesis in place that is being converted to a RTSA, markers of inflammation (erythrocyte sedimentation rate and C-reactive protein) should be obtained preoperatively. If there is a suspicion of infection, aspiration can be done using image guidance. Imaging studies generally consist of true AP and axillary radiographs and a CT scan to evaluate alignment, glenoid bone stock, and

fatty infiltration of the rotator cuff muscle bellies. MRI also can be used to assess fatty infiltration, but its use is not mandatory.

Complete details of the surgical procedure for insertion of a reverse prosthesis are described elsewhere.[73] Two surgical approaches can be used. The deltopectoral approach usually is the most familiar to surgeons and is best suited to revision surgery; however, it is associated with a higher incidence of instability. The superior approach is a good option in primary surgery and is associated with a lower incidence of instability but also a higher incidence of inferior scapular notching. Repair of the subscapularis tendon after placement of a reverse prosthesis is controversial. Because the humerus and center of rotation are effectively lowered with this procedure, it often is impossible to repair the subscapularis back to its insertion.

The early clinical results of using the reverse prosthesis for the treatment of RCTA are promising; however, most of the studies are small, and follow-up is limited.[74,80,89-92] Re-

cently, larger studies with longer follow-up periods have been published.[44-46,93,94]

In 2004, the authors of a multicenter study from Europe reported the results of 80 prostheses in 77 patients with a minimum 2-year follow up (mean, 44.5 months).[46] The mean patient age at the time of surgery was 72.8 years. The average Constant score improved from 22.6 to 65.6, with active elevation improving from 73° to 138°. Clinical results were worse in patients with a positive hornblower's sign preoperatively. With surgical failure defined as revision of the prosthesis or failure of the implant, survivorship was 91.3% at 5 years, 74.6% at 7 years, and 29.8% at 8 years. The precipitous decline between years 7 and 8 remains a source of concern; the reasons for the deterioration are not known.

In 2005, Werner and associates[93] evaluated 58 patients (average age, 68 years) with irreparable rotator cuff tears treated with RTSA. Seventeen of the procedures involved primary treatment of rotator cuff insufficiency and 41 were revisions, mainly failed hemiarthroplasty for fracture. Average follow-up was 38 months. The subjective shoulder value increased from 18% to 56%, the Constant score from 29 to 64, and active elevation from 42° to 100°. Patients in the primary group and the revision group showed similar rates of improvement. The overall complication rate was 50%, with hematoma formation the most common complication. The revision rate was 33%.

The authors of another 2005 study reported results on 60 patients with an average age of 71 years and an average follow-up of 33 months. They found significant improvements in the American Shoulder and Elbow Surgeons scores for pain, active flexion, and active abduction. Forty-one of 60 patients rated their result as good or excellent. The complication rate was 17%, with 12% requiring revision surgery.[45]

A 2006 study reported a detailed analysis of a heterogeneous group of 45 patients treated with RTSA.[94] Twenty-one of 45 patients had RCTA. The average age in this subgroup was 77 years. The complication rate in the RCTA group was 5%, compared with 47% in the revision group. Active elevation increased from 55° to 121°, with no change in internal or external rotation. Constant and American Shoulder and Elbow Surgeons scores were higher in the RCTA group.

Despite recent promising results with RTSA, several problems remain unsolved. Instability may be related to undertensioning of the deltoid, medial impingement of the humeral cup on the scapular neck, hematoma formation, or damage to the deltoid. Overtensioning of the deltoid can lead to fracture of the acromion, especially in elderly patients with osteoporosis. These fractures usually can be treated nonsurgically with little consequence to the patient. Scapular notching is another concern. It is believed to be related to impingement of the medial aspect of the polyethylene humeral cup on the inferior scapular neck with the arm adducted. Polyethylene wear has been identified on some retrieved humeral cups, which raises the concern of osteolysis and component loosening. Sirveaux and associates[46] reported inferior scapular notching in 63% of patients. Smaller notches had no effect on clinical outcome, whereas large notches (extending beyond the inferior screw) had a negative effect on clinical outcome. In another study, notching occurred in 46 of 48 patients who had adequate follow-up; however, in contrast to the findings of Sirveaux and associates, notching did not correlate with clinical outcome, regardless of size.[93] Notching was reported in 68% of patients by Boileau and associates,[94] but no glenoid loosening was seen even when notching extended beyond the inferior screw.

As mentioned previously, external rotation is not restored in patients who have a deficient posterior cuff preoperatively. In the study by Boileau and associates,[94] deficiency of the teres minor was associated with lower functional results. Medialization of the center of rotation decreases the amount of posterior deltoid that can be used to compensate for posterior cuff deficiency. Retroversion of the humeral component will increase external rotation, but at the expense of internal rotation. Recently, some surgeons have attempted to improve external rotation by transferring the latissimus major/teres major tendons (the modified L'Episcopo procedure) in patients with profound external rotation lag and the hornblower's sign. This procedure can be done through a deltopectoral approach at the same time as the RTSA or through a separate incision posteriorly.[47-49]

The durability of RTSA over time is still unknown. A recent multicenter study with a minimum 5-year follow-up determined the survival rate of the prosthesis according to the initial indication for surgery.[44] The overall survival rate, with implant replacement as the end point, was 91% at 120 months. Shoulders with RCTA had significantly better results than those with other disorders (95% survival rate at 9 years compared with 77%, respectively); however, progressive deterioration was seen after 6 years. The group with rheumatoid arthritis had the highest revision rate.

As with any arthroplasty, infection remains a major concern. Dealing with an infected RTSA is extremely challenging. After RTSA, there is a large dead space in which a sizable hematoma can form. This potentially can lead to instability and serves as a medium for bacterial growth. Many surgeons routinely place a drain after RTSA.

RTSA has been shown to improve pain and function in patients with RCTA. Recent designs, based on sound biomechanical principles, have demonstrated better results and increased longevity compared with earlier designs. Newer surgical techniques and materials also have contributed to improved success rates. Nonetheless, reported complication and revision rates are still high and long-term outcomes are unknown. For these reasons, candidates for this procedure should be carefully chosen. Patients should be informed of the goals of the procedure and the associated risks. In general, RTSA is reserved for elderly patients with low physical demands.

## Summary

Massive, irreparable rotator cuff tears can be treated with a variety of methods, but the optimal approach tailors treatment to the individual patient. Tendon transfer can result in significant pain relief and improved function in selected patients. RTSA provides significant improvement in pain and function in the short term, but the risk of complication remains high. In some instances, the combination of a reverse prosthesis and tendon transfer can significantly improve patient function. Surgeons should carefully consider different treatment options and should inform their patients of the relative risks as well as the potential for a prolonged recovery after surgery.

# References

1. Cofield RH: Rotator cuff disease of the shoulder. *J Bone Joint Surg Am* 1985;67:974-979.

2. Gerber C: Latissimus dorsi transfer for the treatment of irreparable tears of the rotator cuff. *Clin Orthop Relat Res* 1992;275:152-160.

3. Tauro JC: Arthroscopic repair of large rotator cuff tears using the interval slide technique. *Arthroscopy* 2004;20: 13-21.

4. Thompson WO, Debski RE, Boardman ND III, et al: A biomechanical analysis of rotator cuff deficiency in a cadaveric model. *Am J Sports Med* 1996;24:286-292.

5. Rockwood CA Jr, Williams GR Jr, Burkhead WZ Jr: Debridement of degenerative, irreparable lesions of the rotator cuff. *J Bone Joint Surg Am* 1995; 77:857-866.

6. Gerber C, Fuchs B, Hodler J: The results of repair of massive tears of the rotator cuff. *J Bone Joint Surg Am* 2000; 82:505-515.

7. Hodler J, Fretz CJ, Terrier F, Gerger C: Rotator cuff tears: Correlation of sonographic and surgical findings. *Radiology* 1988;169:791-794.

8. Gerber C, Hersche O: Tendon transfers for the treatment of irreparable rotator cuff defects. *Orthop Clin North Am* 1997;28:195-203.

9. Goutallier D, Postel JM, Bernageau J, Lavau L, Voisin MC: Fatty infiltration of disrupted rotator cuff muscles. *Rev Rhum Engl Ed* 1995;62:415-422.

10. Galatz LM, Silva MJ, Rothermich SY, Zaegel MA, Havlioglu N, Thomopoulos S: Nicotine delays tendon-to-bone healing in a rat shoulder model. *J Bone Joint Surg Am* 2006;88: 2027-2034.

11. Warner JP, Gerber C: Treatment of massive rotator cuff tears: Posterior-superior and anterior-superior, in Iannotti JP (ed): *The Rotator Cuff: Current Concepts and Complex Problems*. Rosemont, IL, American Academy of Orthopaedic Surgeons, 1998, pp 59-94.

12. Neer CS II (ed): *Shoulder Reconstruction*. Philadelphia, PA, WB Saunders, 1990, pp 41-142.

13. Bigliani LU, Cordasco FA, McIlveen SJ, Musso ES: Operative repairs of massive rotator cuff tears: Long-term results. *J Shoulder Elbow Surg* 1992;1: 120-130.

14. Ellman H, Hanker G, Bayer M: Repair of the rotator cuff: End-result study of factors influencing reconstruction. *J Bone Joint Surg Am* 1986; 68:1136-1144.

15. Harryman DT II, Mack LA, Wang KY, Jackins SE, Richardson ML, Matsen FA III: Repairs of the rotator cuff: Correlation of functional results with integrity of the cuff. *J Bone Joint Surg Am* 1991;73:982-989.

16. Warner JJ, Higgins L, Parsons IM IV, Dowdy P: Diagnosis and treatment of anterosuperior rotator cuff tears. *J Shoulder Elbow Surg* 2001;10:37-46.

17. Kreuz PC, Remiger A, Erggelet C, Hinterwimmer S, Niemeyer P, Gachter A: Isolated and combined tears of the subscapularis tendon. *Am J Sports Med* 2005;33:1831-1837.

18. Flury MP, John M, Goldhahn J, Schwyzer HK, Simmen BR: Rupture of the subscapularis tendon (isolated or in combination with supraspinatus tear): When is a repair indicated? *J Shoulder Elbow Surg* 2006;15: 659-664.

19. Rokito AS, Cuomo F, Gallagher MA, Zuckerman JD: Long-term functional outcome of repair of large and massive chronic tears of the rotator cuff. *J Bone Joint Surg Am* 1999;81:991-997.

20. Gerber C, Vinh TS, Hertel R, Hess CW: Latissimus dorsi transfer for the treatment of massive tears of the rotator cuff: A preliminary report. *Clin Orthop Relat Res* 1988;232:51-61.

21. Burkhart SS: A stepwise approach to arthroscopic rotator cuff repair based on biomechanical principles. *Arthroscopy* 2000;16:82-90.

22. Burkhart SS: Reconciling the paradox of rotator cuff repair versus debridement: A unified biomechanical rationale for the treatment of rotator cuff tears. *Arthroscopy* 1994;10:4-19.

23. Apoil A, Augereau B: Anterior-superior arthrolysis of the shoulder for rotator cuff degenerative lesions, in Post M, Morrey B, Hawkins R (eds): *Surgery of the Shoulder*. St Louis, MO, Mosby-Year Book, 1990, pp 267-270.

24. Gartsman GM: Massive, irreparable tears of the rotator cuff: Results of operative debridement and subacromial decompression. *J Bone Joint Surg Am* 1997;79:715-721.

25. Ellman H: Arthroscopic subacromial decompression: Analysis of one- to three-year results. *Arthroscopy* 1987;3: 173-181.

26. Ellman H, Kay SP, Wirth M: Arthroscopic treatment of full-thickness rotator cuff tears: 2- to 7-year follow-up study. *Arthroscopy* 1993;9:195-200.

27. Zvijac JE, Levy HJ, Lemak LJ: Arthroscopic subacromial decompression in the treatment of full thickness rotator cuff tears: A 3- to 6-year follow-up. *Arthroscopy* 1994;10: 518-523.

28. Kempf JF, Gleyze P, Bonnomet F, et al: A multicenter study of 210 rotator cuff tears treated by arthroscopic acromioplasty. *Arthroscopy* 1999;15: 56-66.

29. Moore DR, Cain EL, Schwartz ML, Clancy WG Jr: Allograft reconstruction for massive, irreparable rotator cuff tears. *Am J Sports Med* 2006;34: 392-396.

30. Iannotti JP, Codsi MJ, Kwon YW, Ciccone J, Brems JJ: Porcine small intestine submucosa augmentation of surgical repair of chronic two-tendon rotator cuff tears: A randomized, controlled trial. *J Bone Joint Surg Am* 2006; 88:1238-1244.

31. Ozaki J, Fujimoto S, Masuhara K, Tamai S, Yoshimoto S: Reconstruction of chronic massive rotator cuff tears with synthetic materials. *Clin Orthop Relat Res* 1986;202:173-183.

32. Neviaser JS, Neviaser RJ, Neviaser TJ: The repair of chronic massive ruptures of the rotator cuff of the shoulder by use of freeze-dried rotator cuff. *J Bone Joint Surg Am* 1978;60:681-684.

33. Karas SE, Giachello TL: Subscapularis transfer for reconstruction of

massive tears of the rotator cuff. *J Bone Joint Surg Am* 1996;78:239-245.

34. Cofield RH: Subscapular muscle transposition for repair of chronic rotator cuff tears. *Surg Gynecol Obstet* 1982;154:667-672.

35. Warner JJ: Management of massive irreparable rotator cuff tears: The role of tendon transfer. *Instr Course Lect* 2001;50:63-71.

36. Handelberg FW: Treatment options in full thickness rotator cuff tears. *Acta Orthop Belg* 2001;67:110-115.

37. Miniaci A, Macleod M: Transfer of the latissimus dorsi muscle after failed repair of a massive tear of the rotator cuff: A two to five-year review. *J Bone Joint Surg Am* 1999;81:1120-1127.

38. Warner JJ, Parsons IM IV: Latissimus dorsi tendon transfer: A comparative analysis of primary and salvage reconstruction of massive, irreparable rotator cuff tears. *J Shoulder Elbow Surg* 2001;10:514-521.

39. Gerber C, Mauieira G, Espinosa N: Latissimus dorsi transfer for the treatment of irreparable rotator cuff tears. *J Bone Joint Surg Am* 2006;88:113-120.

40. Guettler JH, Basamania CJ: Muscle transfers involving the shoulder. *J Surg Orthop Adv* 2006;15:27-37.

41. Wirth MA, Rockwood CA Jr: Operative treatment of irreparable rupture of the subscapularis. *J Bone Joint Surg Am* 1997;79:722-731.

42. Safran O, Iannotti JP: Arthrodesis of the shoulder. *J Am Acad Orthop Surg* 2006;14:145-153.

43. Sanchez-Sotelo J, Cofield RH, Rowland CM: Shoulder hemiarthroplasty for glenohumeral arthritis associated with severe rotator cuff deficiency. *J Bone Joint Surg Am* 2001;83: 1814-1822.

44. Guery J, Favard L, Sirveaus F, Oudet D, Mole D, Wach G: Reverse total shoulder arthroplasty: Survivorship analysis of eighty replacements followed for five to ten years. *J Bone Joint Surg Am* 2006;88:1742-1747.

45. Frankle M, Siegal S, Pupellp D, Saleem A, Mighell M, Vasey M: The Reverse Shoulder Prosthesis for glenohumeral arthritis associated with severe rotator cuff deficiency: A minimum two-year follow-up study of sixty patients. *J Bone Joint Surg Am* 2005;87:1697-1707.

46. Sirveaux F, Favard L, Oudet D, Huquet D, Walch G, Mole D: Grammont inverted total shoulder arthroplasty in the treatment of glenohumeral osteoarthritis with massive rupture of the cuff: Results of a multicentre study of 80 shoulders. *J Bone Joint Surg Br* 2004;86:388-395.

47. Boileau P, Chuinard C, Trojani C: Modified latissimus dorsi and teres major transfer for external rotation deficit of the shoulder: As an isolated procedure or with a reverse arthroplasty, in *Nice Shoulder Course-Arthroscopy and Arthroplasty*. Montpellier, France, Sauramps Medical, 2006, pp 335-346.

48. Gerber C, Pennington SD, Lingenfelter EJ, Sukthankar A: Reverse Delta-III shoulder replacement combined with latissimus dorsi transfer. *J Bone Joint Surg Am* 2007;89:940-947.

49. Habermeyer P, Magosch P, Rudolph T, Lichtenberg S, Liem D: Transfer of the tendon of latissimus dorsi for the treatment of massive tears of the rotator cuff: A new single-incision technique. *J Bone Joint Surg Br* 2006; 88-B:208-212.

50. Lehtinen JT, Tingart MJ, Apreleva M, et al: Practical assessment of rotator cuff muscle volume using MRI. *Acta Orthop Scand* 2003;74:722-730.

51. McMahon PJ, Debski RE, Thompson WO, Warner JJ, Fu FH, Woo SL: Shoulder muscle forces and tendon excursions during glenohumeral abduction in the scapular plane. *J Shoulder Elbow Surg* 1995;4:199-208.

52. Tingart MJ, Apreleva M, Letinen JT, Capell B, Palmer WE, Warner JJ: Magnetic resonance imaging in quantitative analysis of rotator cuff muscle volume. *Clin Orthop Relat Res* 2003; 415:104-110.

53. Bassett RW, Cofield RH: Acute tears of the rotator cuff: The timing of sur-gical repair. *Clin Orthop Relat Res* 1983;175:18-24.

54. Keating JF, Waterworth P, Shaw-Dunn J, Crossan J: Acute tears of the rotator cuff: The timing of surgical repair. *J Bone Joint Surg Br* 1993;75: 137-140.

55. Inman VT, Saunder JB, Abbott LC: Observations of the function of the shoulder joint. *Clin Orthop Relat Res* 1996;330:3-12.

56. Poppen NK, Walker PS: Forces at the glenohumeral joint in abduction. *Clin Orthop Relat Res* 1978;135:165-170.

57. Watson M: Major ruptures of the rotator cuff: The results of surgical repair in 89 patients. *J Bone Joint Surg Br* 1985;67:618-624.

58. Neer CS, Satterlee CC, Dalsery RM: On the value of the coracohumeral ligament release. *Orthop Trans* 1989; 13:235-241.

59. Yamaguchi K, Riew KD, Galatz LM, Syme JA, Neviaser RJ: Biceps activity during shoulder motion: An electromyographic analysis. *Clin Orthop Relat Res* 1997;336:122-129.

60. Weiner DS, Macnab I: Superior migration of the humeral head: A radiological aid in the diagnosis of tears of the rotator cuff. *J Bone Joint Surg Br* 1970;52:524-527.

61. Walch G, Boileau P, Noel E, Leotard JP, Dejour H: Surgical treatment of painful shoulders caused by lesions of the rotator cuff and biceps, treatment as a function of lesions: Reflections on the Neer's concept. *Rev Rhum Mal Osteoartic* 1991;58:247-257.

62. Burkhart SS: Arthroscopic debridement and decompression for selected rotator cuff tears: Clinical results, pathomechanics, and patient selection based on biomechanical parameters. *Orthop Clin North Am* 1993;24: 111-123.

63. Neviaser RJ, Neviaser TJ, Neviaser JS: Concurrent rupture of the rotator cuff and anterior dislocation of the shoulder in the older patient. *J Bone Joint Surg Am* 1988;70:1308-1311.

64. Warner JP, Waskowitz R, Marks PH, et al: Function in patients with mas-

sive rotator cuff tear with attention to muscle atrophy. *60th Annual Meeting Proceedings.* Rosemont, IL, American Academy of Orthopaedic Surgeons, 1993, pp 18-20.

65. Nove-Josserand L, Levigne C, Noel E, et al: The acromio-humeral interval: A study of the factors influencing its height. *Rev Chir Orthop Reparatrice Appar Mot* 1996;82:379-382.

66. Hersche O, Gerber C: Passive tension in the supraspinatus musculotendinous unit after long-standing rupture of its tendon: A preliminary report. *J Shoulder Elbow Surg* 1998;7: 393-396.

67. Meyer DC, Hoppeler H, con Rechenberg B, Gerber C: A pathomechanical concept explains muscle loss and fatty muscular changes following surgical tendon release. *J Orthop Res* 2004;22:1004-1007.

68. Arntz CT, Matsen FA, Jackins S: Surgical management of complex irreparable rotator cuff deficiency. *J Arthroplasty* 1991;6:363-370.

69. Iannotti JP, Hennigan S, Herzog R, et al: Latissimus dorsi tendon transfer for irreparable posterosuperior rotator cuff tears: Factors affecting outcome. *J Bone Joint Surg Am* 2006;88:342-348.

70. Jost B, Puskas GJ, Lustenberger A, Gerber C: Outcome of pectoralis major transfer for the treatment of irreparable subscapularis tears. *J Bone Joint Surg Am* 2003;85:1944-1951.

71. Resch H, Povacz P, Ritter E, Matschi W: Transfer of the pectoralis major muscle for the treatment of irreparable rupture of the subscapularis tendon. *J Bone Joint Surg Am* 2000;82: 372-382.

72. Galatz LM, Connor PM, Calfee RO, Hsu JC, Yamaguchi K: Pectoralis major transfer for anterior-superior subluxation in massive rotator cuff insufficiency. *J Shoulder Elbow Surg* 2003; 12:1-5.

73. Boileau P, Watkinson DJ, Hatzidakis AM: Grammont reverse prosthesis: Design, rationale and biomechanics. *J Shoulder Elbow Surg* 2005;14: 147S-161S.

74. Boulahia A, Edwards TB, Walch G, Baratta RV: Early results of a reverse design prosthesis in the treatment of arthritis of the shoulder in elderly patients with a large rotator cuff tear. *Orthopedics* 2002;25:129-133.

75. Nyffeler RW, Werner CM, Gerber C: Biomechanical relevance of glenoid component positioning in the reverse Delta III total shoulder prosthesis. *J Shoulder Elbow Surg* 2005;14: 524-528.

76. Franklin JL, Barrett WP, Jackins SE, Matsen FA III: Glenoid loosening in total shoulder arthroplasty: Association with rotator cuff tear deficiency. *J Arthroplasty* 1988;3:39-46.

77. Field LD, Dines DM, Zabinski SJ, Warren RF: Hemiarthroplasty of the shoulder for rotator cuff tear arthropathy. *J Shoulder Elbow Surg* 1997;6:18-23.

78. Williams GR Jr, Rockwood CA Jr: Hemiarthroplasty in rotator cuff-deficient shoulders. *J Shoulder Elbow Surg* 1996;5:362-367.

79. Zuckerman JD, Scott AJ, Gallagher MA: Hemiarthroplasty for cuff tear arthropathy. *J Shoulder Elbow Surg* 2000;9:169-172.

80. Brostrom LA, Wallensten R, Olsson E, Anderson D: The Kessel prosthesis in total shoulder arthroplasty: A five year experience. *Clin Orthop Relat Res* 1992;277:155-160.

81. Coughlin MJ, Morris JM, West WF: The semiconstrained total shoulder arthroplasty. *J Bone Joint Surg Am* 1979;61:574-581.

82. Lettin AW, Copeland SA, Scales JT: The Stanmore total shoulder replacement. *J Bone Joint Surg Br* 1982;64: 47-51.

83. Post M, Haskell SS, Jablon M: Total shoulder replacement with a constrained prosthesis. *J Bone Joint Surg Am* 1980;62:327-335.

84. Sirveaux F, Molé D, Boileau P: The reversed prosthesis, in Warner JP, Iannotti JP, Flatow EL (eds): *Complex and Revision Problems in Shoulder Surgery*, ed 2. New York, NY, Lippincott Williams and Wilkins, 2005, pp 497-513.

85. Grammont P, Trouilloud P, Laffay J, Deries X: Etude et réalisation d'une nouvelle prosthèse d'épaule. *Rhumatologie* 1987;39:407-418.

86. Hertel R, Ballmer FT, Lambert SM, Gerber C: Lag signs in the diagnosis of rotator cuff rupture. *J Shoulder Elbow Surg* 1996;5:307-313.

87. Walch G, Boulahia A, Calderone S, Robinson AHN: The dropping and hornblower's signs in evaluation of rotator cuff tears. *J Bone Joint Surg Br* 1998;80:624-628.

88. Simovitch RW, Helmy N, Zumstein MA, Gerber C: Impact of fatty infiltration of the teres minor muscle on the outcome of reverse total shoulder arthroplasty. *J Bone Joint Surg Am* 2007;89:934-939.

89. De Buttet M, Boucho Y, Capon D, Delfosse J: Grammont shoulder arthroplasty for osteoarthritis with massive rotator cuff tears: Reports of 71 cases. *J Shoulder Elbow Surg* 1997; 6:197.

90. Grammont PM, Baulot E: Delta shoulder prosthesis for rotator cuff rupture. *Orthopedics* 1993;16:65-68.

91. Jacobs R, DeBeer P, De Smet L: Treatment of rotator cuff tear arthropathy with a reversed delta shoulder prosthesis. *Acta Orthop Belg* 2001; 67:344-347.

92. Rittmeister M, Kerschbaumer F: Grammont reverse total shoulder arthroplasty in patients with rheumatoid arthritis and nonreconstructible rotator cuff lesions. *J Shoulder Elbow Surg* 2001;10:17-22.

93. Werner CM, Steinmann PA, Gilbart M, Gerber C: Treatment of painful pseudoparesis due to irreparable rotator cuff dysfunction with the Delta III reverse-ball-and-socket total shoulder prosthesis. *J Bone Joint Surg Am* 2005; 87:1476-1486.

94. Boileau P, Watkinson D, Hatzidakis AM, Hovorka I: The Grammont reverse shoulder prosthesis: Results in cuff tear arthritis, fracture sequelae, and revision arthroplasty. *J Shoulder Elbow Surg* 2006;15:527-540.

# The Reverse Total Shoulder Arthroplasty

*Frederick A. Matsen III, MD
*Pascal Boileau, MD
*Gilles Walch, MD
*Christian Gerber, MD
Ryan T. Bicknell, MD, MSc

## Abstract

*A reverse total shoulder arthroplasty is a prosthesis that should be used in patients who have specific contraindications to the more conventional total shoulder prosthetic replacements. The patient and surgeon should understand that this reconstruction is technically more difficult and is associated with more complications than conventional shoulder reconstructions. The reverse total shoulder arthroplasty has been used in Europe more than in North America, and the experience in Europe is guiding its use in North America. An understanding of the mechanics of the reverse total shoulder arthroplasty and the technical details of its implantation will help in understanding its role in shoulder reconstruction.*

**Instr Course Lect 2008;57:167-174.**

A reverse total shoulder arthroplasty is a procedure considered for patients whose shoulder problem cannot be effectively managed with a conventional total shoulder replacement. The reverse total shoulder prosthesis is based on a concept introduced by Professor Paul Grammont, in which a convex articular surface is fixed to the glenoid and a concave articular surface is fixed to the proximal part of the humerus[1] (Figure 1). This prosthesis addresses some of the limitations of conven-

tional arthroplasty. To understand the role of the reverse total shoulder arthroplasty, one must first understand the limitations of conventional arthroplasty.

## Limitations of Conventional Arthroplasty

A conventional or anatomic shoulder arthroplasty is the replacement of damaged joint surfaces with prosthetic components that approximate the normal joint surfaces and are stabilized by mechanisms similar to

those stabilizing a native glenohumeral joint. In performing a conventional arthroplasty, the surgeon is faced with several limitations.

### Limited Ability to Manage Glenohumeral Translation

The normal glenohumeral joint consists of a small, shallow, concave glenoid with a compliant rim for articulation and a spherical humeral head. The small articular surface and minimal constraint of the glenoid allow a large range of rotational motion before the humeral neck abuts on the glenoid rim. They also allow small physiologic translations of the humeral head on the glenoid in response to loads that are applied tangential to the glenoid joint surface. Translation also occurs at the extremes of glenohumeral motion, permitting a greater range of motion than would be possible if the humeral head did not translate.

Although the compliant rim of the normal glenoid enables full surface contact during small humeral translations, this attribute is not replicated by the much less compliant polyethylene joint surface of a con-

*Frederick A. Matsen III, MD or the department with which he is affiliated has received research or institutional support from DePuy. Pascal Boileau, MD and Gilles Walch, MD or the departments with which they are affiliated have received royalties from Tornier. Christian Gerber, MD or the department with which he is affiliated has received royalties from Zimmer.*

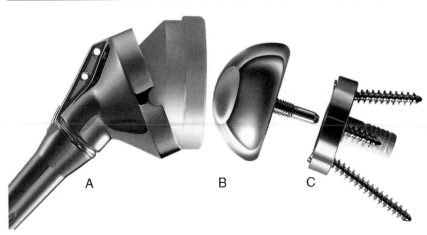

**Figure 1**    A reverse total shoulder prosthesis. **A,** The humeral stem and metaphysis, and polyethylene humeral concavity insert. **B,** The glenosphere. **C,** The metaglene. (Courtesy of DePuy Orthopaedics, Inc.)

ventional shoulder arthroplasty. If the prosthetic glenoid surface conforms exactly to the humeral head (that is, if each has the same radius of curvature), no translation can occur without loading of the polyethylene glenoid rim. Rim loading is associated with markedly diminished contact area, increased contact pressure (load per unit contact area), and cold flow of the rim. Rim loading also challenges glenoid component fixation through the so-called rocking-horse mechanism. A prosthetic glenoid surface that does not conform exactly to the humeral head (that is, it has a radius of curvature that is larger than that of the humeral head) allows translation but also diminishes contact area, increases local contact pressure, and increases the risk of polyethylene failure.

### Limited Fixation of the Glenoid Component to Bone

The normal glenoid joint surface is well fixed to the subjacent glenoid bone. This fixation is critical for the management of tangential humeral loads that are directed off-center to the glenoid center line. In conven-

tional arthroplasty, the polyethylene glenoid surface can be fixed to the bone with bone cement or with screws and tissue ingrowth through a metal back. With the repeated application of off-center loads, bone-cement fixation is at risk of failing as a result of cement fatigue and bone resorption. Although metal backs can be secured to bone, the fixation of the polyethylene to the metal back is also at risk of failing.

### Limited Intrinsic Stability

The normal glenohumeral joint is stabilized by the concavity compression mechanism, in which the joint forces compress the humeral head into the glenoid fossa. These compressive forces are caused by the combined action of muscular and capsuloligamentous restraints. A loss of any of the normal osseous, capsuloligamentous, or muscular constraints leads to glenohumeral instability and a loss of normal shoulder function. Anterior instability results from defects in the subscapularis, anterior aspect of the capsule, glenoid labrum, anterior glenoid bone, rotator cuff, or posterior humeral articular surface. Pos-

terior instability results from glenoid dysplasia; posterior glenoid erosion or fracture; and defects in the posterior aspect of the labrum, posterior aspect of the capsule, posterior aspect of the rotator cuff, or anterior humeral articular surface. Superior instability results from loss of the compression and spacer effect of the normal supraspinatus. Upward displacement of the humerus slackens the deltoid so that it is less effective in humeral elevation. If the deltoid cannot compensate for this slack, the humerus cannot be elevated, a situation known as pseudoparalysis. The coracoacromial arch serves as a backstop limiting upward translation of the humeral head with rotator cuff deficiency. Deficiency of the coracoacromial arch from wear, fracture, or surgical acromioplasty can allow the humeral head to slip out from underneath it, a condition known as anterosuperior escape, which compounds the pseudoparalysis.

Conventional arthroplasty can be used in some patients with arthritis and glenohumeral instability. When arthritis is coupled with instability resulting from deficiencies of the humeral head, the full articular surface can be restored by a humeral component. When the glenoid is deficient, its contour can be restored by a glenoid prosthesis as long as the bone beneath it offers sufficient support. When arthritis is coupled with instability resulting from acute reparable rotator cuff tears, stability may be restored by cuff repair in association with conventional shoulder arthroplasty. When arthritis is coupled with instability resulting from excessive capsular laxity, capsular tightening or the use of a larger humeral head component may restore the capsular tension needed for stability. When the cuff is deficient and the upwardly displaced humeral head is stabilized by an intact coracoacromial arch and the deltoid has not been slackened to the point where it is unable to raise the arm, a conventional or extended articular surface humeral hemiarthroplasty may enhance shoulder comfort and function.

Conventional arthroplasty usually cannot be used to manage instability resulting from unreconstructible soft-tissue or osseous deficiencies, such as severe posterior glenoid bone deficiency. If the posterior aspect of the capsule and rotator cuff have been lost as a result of trauma or previous surgery, conventional arthroplasty cannot restore posterior stability. Similarly, in the presence of anterosuperior escape and pseudoparalysis of the shoulder, resurfacing of the humeral head and glenoid cannot restore shoulder stability or deltoid function.

### Limited Ability to Compensate for Deltoid Dysfunction

Conventional shoulder arthroplasty can only minimally modify the tension and moment arm of the deltoid. Deltoid tension can be adjusted by raising and lowering the humeral component, but such changes may adversely affect the alignment of the humeral and glenoid articular surfaces. With a conventional arthroplasty, the center of rotation of the humeral head cannot be medialized to increase the deltoid moment arm.

### Limitations of Any Type of Shoulder Reconstruction

Conventional shoulder and reverse shoulder arthroplasty are limited by the same factors that limit any surgical reconstruction. Shoulders with skin, vascular, lymphatic, or osseous deficiency may be at excessive risk when treated with reconstructive surgery.[1] Patients who have fragile bone or general medical, emotional, motivational, or social health issues usually are not candidates for any type of shoulder arthroplasty. Deltoid deficiency, limited scapular mobility, and infection usually preclude effective reconstruction.[2]

## Features of the Reverse Total Shoulder Arthroplasty
### Glenohumeral Translation

In a reverse total shoulder arthroplasty, the deep, conforming concavity of the humeral articular surface does not permit glenohumeral translation. Although this constraint reduces the range of motion before contact occurs between the humeral and glenoid elements, it eliminates the possibility of rim loading and the resulting problems of cold flow of the rim polyethylene and the creation of eccentric forces that can contribute to component loosening. Full surface contact is maintained during the allowed range of the articulation.[3-6]

### Fixation of the Glenoid Component

In a reverse total shoulder arthroplasty, a metal "metaglene," or base plate, is fixed to a prepared glenoid with locking and nonlocking screws along with a press-fit hydroxyapatite-coated central peg. No bone cement is used. The spherically convex glenoid articular surface, the "glenosphere," is fitted to the metaglene and held in position with a Morse taper and screw. The glenoid component does not have a polyethylene element, therefore avoiding the challenges associated with securing a polyethylene surface to a metal-backed glenoid fixation system. The geometry of the glenoid prosthesis medializes the center of rotation of the glenoid prosthesis on the osseous surface of the glenoid, so that eccentrically applied loads have a small lever arm, reducing the moments that challenge glenoid fixation.

### Intrinsic Stability

One of the measures of the intrinsic stability of an articulation is the balance stability angle, that is, the maximal angle that the net joint reaction force can form with the concavity before dislocation occurs. In most conventional shoulder arthroplasty systems, the net humeral joint-reaction force must be directed within 30° or less of the glenoid center line to avoid dislocation. In reverse total shoulder arthroplasty, the glenosphere is stabilized in the humeral socket as long as the net joint-reaction force exerted by the glenoid convexity is within 45° of the center of the humeral articular concavity. Because the center line of the humeral concavity forms an angle of 155° with the long axis of the humeral shaft, the joint is stable against forces applied to it by the deltoid, although these forces may be parallel to the surface of the osseous glenoid. This high degree of intrinsic stability frees the reverse total shoulder prosthesis from dependence on soft-tissue constraints and the coracoacromial arch for stability. It can also provide stability when there is glenoid osseous deficiency, as long as there is sufficient bone stock for glenoid fixation.

### Compensation for Deltoid Dysfunction

In contrast with conventional arthroplasty, reverse arthroplasty provides the opportunity to restore tension to the deltoid by moving the deltoid insertion distally and provides an increased deltoid lever arm by increasing the perpendicular distance from the center of rotation (on the osseous surface of the glenoid

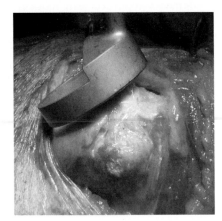

**Figure 2**  The humeral resection guide is inserted into the humeral canal and placed in 0° of retroversion.

bone) to the deltoid muscle. Finally, the intrinsic stability of the reverse total shoulder prosthesis allows for humeral elevation by the lateral deltoid even in the presence of an anterior deltoid defect that may have resulted from injury or previous surgery.

## Possible Applications of Reverse Total Shoulder Arthroplasty

Reverse total shoulder arthroplasty is considered when rehabilitation has not satisfactorily addressed, and conventional surgical reconstruction methods cannot satisfactorily manage, shoulder pain and loss of function. Because of the magnitude and potential risks of the reverse shoulder arthroplasty, nonsurgical means of improving the patient's quality of life merit a dedicated trial before surgery. The patient should be treated initially with a specific exercise program and analgesics before any surgery is considered.

The reverse total shoulder arthroplasty may be considered for the management of a patient with refractory rotator cuff tear arthropathy, especially with anterosuperior

escape and pseudoparalysis; a failed prosthetic reconstruction with superior, anterior, or posterior instability; or a failed reconstruction for a traumatic injury with pseudoparalysis and instability. As is the case with any major surgical procedure, the surgeon must consider the adequacy of the skin, bone, and deltoid muscle. When the procedure is being done as a revision of a previous operation, consideration must be given to the possibility of occult infection with organisms such as *Pseudomonas acnes* or *Staphylococcus epidermidis*. The surgeon needs to assess the patient's physical, emotional, and social situation to determine if those factors favor a successful outcome. Finally, the surgeon needs to be confident of his or her ability to manage the complex intraoperative decision making and any complications that may arise with this procedure.

## One Technique for Reverse Total Shoulder Arthroplasty

There are now several different reverse total shoulder arthroplasty systems and many variations on the technique. The following is an example of a reverse total shoulder arthroplasty technique involving the Delta Reverse Shoulder Prosthesis (DePuy, Warsaw, IN). It is beyond the scope of this chapter to present each of these methods and perhaps too soon to understand their relative advantages and disadvantages. The presentation of this example provides the opportunity to describe some of the key principles and technical aspects of the procedure.

Preoperative planning is critical. The surgeon must consider the osseous anatomy, the reconstructibility of the soft tissues, and the alterations resulting from previous injury and surgery. An anteroposterior radiograph made in the plane of

the scapula and a transparent glenoid template are used to estimate the most inferior position of the glenoid that will result in the inferior screw being contained in the thick bone of the scapular axillary border. An anteroposterior humeral radiograph is used to estimate the size and fit of the diaphyseal and metaphyseal humeral components.

Although the deltopectoral approach may be associated with an increased prevalence of instability, it is often used because it is familiar, safe, and versatile. Any adhesions are lysed and bursal tissue is removed while the deltoid, the acromion, and any residual rotator cuff tissue are protected. The rotator cuff tear is examined to verify that it cannot be repaired, and, if it cannot, useless tendon tissue is resected. The glenohumeral joint is opened by incising the subscapularis and capsule from their insertion on the lesser tuberosity. The surgeon should preserve as much length of the subscapularis as possible. The inferior aspect of the capsule is released from the humerus, and the axillary nerve is identified. The subscapularis is dissected so that it is freed circumferentially. It will be repaired to the humerus later.

The humeral head is removed first to expose the glenoid. Final preparation of the humerus is deferred until the glenoid prosthesis is in place. The humeral resection guide stem is inserted into the medullary canal (Figure 2), and the humeral head is resected in 0° of retroversion. When the arm is pulled distally, the plane of the humeral cut should pass just below the inferior aspect of the glenoid face.

Secure fixation of the all-metal glenoid component to the bone of the glenoid is one of the unique features of the reverse total shoulder arthroplasty. This secure fixation depends on proper preparation of the bone, positioning of the component, and screw placement. The surgeon should be sure to identify and protect the axillary nerve. First, the capsule is dissected from the anterior aspect of the glenoid down to and around the inferior pole so that the superior aspect of the axillary border of the scapula can be palpated and seen. The origin of the long head of the triceps is released as necessary. All abnormal glenoid anatomy is identified. The surgeon should note the amount of overhang of the inferior aspect of the glenoid with respect to the axillary border of the scapula. The labrum and cartilage are removed from the glenoid. A point is marked 13 mm anterior to the posterior rim of the glenoid and 19 mm superior to the inferior glenoid rim, and a guidewire is drilled into the glenoid at this point (Figure 3). The metaglene is placed over this guidewire (with the peg laterally) to verify the appropriateness of this center point. If the metaglene rim is flush with the extrapolated axillary border, the metaglene is removed and the central hole is drilled with a step drill. The glenoid is reamed conservatively, with removal of only enough bone to make the surface relatively flat, and the surgeon makes sure that the reamer handle remains perpendicular to the face of the glenoid. Bone graft harvested from the humeral head is added to any defects in the osseous glenoid, and the metaglene peg is inserted into the central peg hole.

The anterior and posterior aspects of the axillary border of the scapula are palpated, and the metaglene is rotated so that the inferior hole is centered over the axillary border. With a drill guide, the hole is drilled for the inferior locking screw.

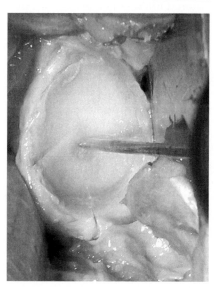

**Figure 3** A guidewire is drilled 13 mm anterior to the posterior glenoid lip and 19 mm superior to the inferior glenoid lip.

(The inferior locking screw makes a 16° angle with the central peg.) The surgeon should check frequently to ensure that the drill is in bone by pushing on the drill while it is not rotating. A 2-mm drill bit is used unless the bone is unusually hard. At least 36 mm of intraosseous drilling is recommended. If this is not achieved, the rotation of the metaglene with respect to the axillary border of the scapula should be reexamined. Once an adequate hole has been made, the inferior locking screw is inserted. A similar technique is used to drill the hole for and insert the superior locking screw. Then the hole for the anterior nonlocking screw is drilled and the screw is inserted into the best bone available, with the orientation guided by palpation of the anterior aspect of the glenoid neck. The posterior nonlocking screw is then inserted, again in the best bone accessible. A trial glenosphere is inserted into the metaglene and the inferior aspect of the glenoid is inspected,

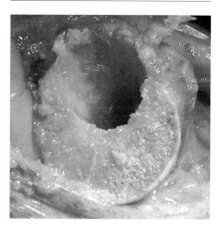

**Figure 4** Humeral reaming is stopped when cortical contact is first achieved.

with removal of bone that may abut against the humeral polyethylene component. Any axillary glenoid bone is resected as necessary. The adequacy of the bone resection can be verified by placing a trial polyethylene component over the glenosphere and making sure that it can be adducted fully, while recalling that the humeral cup makes a 155° angle with the humeral shaft.

The final preparation of the humerus must preserve humeral bone stock while optimizing the height, version, and fixation of the humeral component. The humeral canal is prepared by inserting progressively larger reamers until cortical contact is first achieved (Figure 4). The trial stem is inserted with the metaphyseal reamer guide in 0° of retroversion, and the metaphysis is reamed until bone purchase is achieved.

The trial humeral component is assembled and is inserted in 0° of retroversion. A 3-mm trial plastic cup is used, and the joint is reduced. The surgeon checks for medial abutment of the polyethylene against the axillary border of the glenoid, for stability, and for range of motion. There should be less than 2 mm of distraction when distal traction is applied to the arm. If

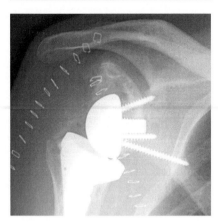

**Figure 5**  AP radiograph showing a low position of the glenoid component and the inferior screw in the thick bone of the axillary border of the scapula.

the joint cannot be reduced, the surgeon should consider lowering the humeral component by sequentially resecting small amounts of humeral bone.

The glenosphere should be inserted before the humeral component. The glenosphere is inserted into the metaglene, with the surgeon making sure that there is no soft tissue interposed between them, that the glenosphere is aligned to avoid cross-threading, and that it is fully seated.

Positioning of the humeral component and selection of the humeral polyethylene cup are the definitive steps for adjusting deltoid tension. The definitive humeral component is securely assembled with a strong crescent wrench on the stem and the component inserter on the metaphysis. The humeral medullary canal is brushed and irrigated. A cement restrictor is inserted 13 mm distal to the lateral aspect of the humeral cut. Six drill holes and number-2 nonabsorbable sutures are placed in the anterior neck cut for later attachment of the subscapularis. The assembled humeral component is cemented in 0° of retroversion without the polyethylene

insert. Different heights of polyethylene liners, starting with 3 mm, are tried to discover the height that allows reduction of the shoulder but less than 2 mm of distraction with traction. The surgeon checks again for abutment of polyethylene against the lateral aspect of the glenoid inferiorly with the patient's arm adducted. Finally, the surgeon places the definitive polyethylene component, making sure that it is inserted straight. The subscapularis is repaired to the humerus with the sutures that had been previously placed at the anterior neck cut. A postoperative radiograph is recommended (Figure 5).

This is a major operation for individuals who are usually older and less robust than those treated with conventional arthroplasty; thus, rehabilitation is gentle and gradual. The arm is rested in a sling for 36 hours. Hand-gripping exercises are started immediately. Hand-to-mouth exercises are started after 36 hours, and physical activity is limited to gentle activities of daily living, with a lifting limit of 1 lb (0.45 kg) until 6 weeks after the surgery. Activities are progressed from that point, with the range of motion limited to 0° of external rotation and 90° of elevation for 3 months.

## Results of Reverse Total Shoulder Arthroplasty

A retrospective study including all reverse shoulder prostheses implanted over a 10-year period at three shoulder centers was conducted in France. Of the original group of 457 patients, 242 (53%) had a rotator cuff lesion: 149 had cuff tear arthropathy, 48 had a massive cuff tear, and 45 had failed rotator cuff surgery. Ninety-nine patients (22%) had a revision of a previous prosthesis; 60 (13%) had fracture-related complications; 26 (6%) had osteoarthritis; and 2% each had rheumatoid arthritis, a tumor, or another

condition. Three hundred eighty-nine shoulders (85%) were available for follow-up more than 2 years postoperatively. The average age at the time of follow-up was 75.6 years (range, 22 to 92 years). The average duration of follow-up was 43.5 months (range, 24 to 142 months).

Significant improvement was noted in the mean Constant scores for pain (from 3.5 points preoperatively to 12.1 points at the time of follow-up), activity (from 5.8 to 15.1 points), mobility (from 12.1 to 24.5 points), and strength (from 1.3 to 6.1 points; $P < 0.0001$). Active elevation improved, but active internal and external rotation did not. The operations for the treatment of cuff tear arthropathy had the best results, whereas the revision procedures had the worst outcomes. A young age, preoperative stiffness, teres minor deficiency, tuberosity nonunion, and pain rather than loss of function as the preoperative symptom tended to be associated with inferior results. The deltopectoral approach tended to result in greater active elevation but also a greater risk of instability. Survivorship to the end points of revision and loosening was better for patients with rotator cuff problems than for those with a failed prior hemiarthroplasty. The functional results were noted to deteriorate progressively after 6 years in the group treated for a cuff tear, after 5 years in the group treated with a revision of a prior hemiarthroplasty, after 3 years in the group with osteoarthritis, and after 1 year in the group managed with a revision of a total shoulder arthroplasty.

## Complications of Reverse Total Shoulder Arthroplasty

Reverse total shoulder arthroplasty is a new, unconventional approach for the treatment of a variety of difficult shoulder conditions in older individuals. Thus, it is not surprising that it would be associated with frequent and substantial complications. Indeed, complication rates as high as 60% with revision rates as high as 50% have been reported.[2] Complications are more frequent and more serious when reverse total shoulder arthroplasty is used to revise a failed prior arthroplasty.

Humeral cortical perforations, shaft fractures, or tuberosity fractures may occur during surgery. Intraoperative humeral fractures are most commonly associated with revision of a prior humeral arthroplasty, with a rate as high as one in four. Prevention requires careful removal of the prosthesis and respect for the thin bone that is often encountered in candidates for reverse shoulder arthroplasty. These fractures can often be treated at the time of the surgery with a longer stem and cerclage wires or tension band wire fixation. The surgeon performing a reverse total shoulder arthroplasty must be prepared and equipped for these eventualities. Furthermore, humeral fractures may increase the risk of subsequent humeral loosening.

Intraoperative glenoid fracture may involve the rim, major portions of the glenoid surface, or the glenoid neck. These fractures occur during glenoid reaming or during tightening of glenoid screws. Prevention requires respect for the osteopenic bone of older patients and gentle reaming of the glenoid by hand. Rim fractures can often be stabilized by the metaglene. If fixation is questionable, placement of the humeral component can be delayed until fracture consolidation is achieved. If the central peg of the metaglene cannot be secured to intact bone, a staged reconstruction with bone graft should be considered.

Postoperative hematomas are common and may be prevented by careful hemostasis, the use of drains, and delaying motion of the shoulder for several days after the surgery. Large hematomas may require surgical drainage.

A humeral shaft fracture is another relatively common postoperative complication. These fractures usually are the result of a fall or too abrupt passive elevation or rotation of the arm. They often occur at the tip of the prosthesis, probably because of the abrupt transition between the stiff cemented segment of the humerus containing the prosthesis and the osteopenic bone distal to it. Treatment may include bracing, additional fixation, or revision to a longer component.

Loosening of the humeral component is uncommon and usually is associated with a fracture or infection. Unscrewing of the junction between the metaphyseal and diaphyseal portions of the humeral component can be avoided by vigorous tightening at the time of the surgery and by maintaining tuberosity support for the metaphysis.

Loosening of the glenoid component results when the component is insecurely anchored, because of either glenoid bone deficiency or suboptimal positioning, or it occurs secondary to trauma in which the force on the arm is transmitted directly to the glenoid fixation. The risk of glenoid loosening can be minimized by ensuring that (1) the glenoid component is positioned low on the glenoid bone so that upwardly directed forces on the glenosphere can be resisted by compression of the superior aspect of the metaglene against solid glenoid bone and (2) the fixation screws are securely anchored in the best scapular bone available. Secure anchoring is particularly important for the inferior screw, which must resist pull-out when inferiorly directed loads are applied to the glenosphere.

Infection is a relatively frequent and serious complication of reverse total shoulder arthroplasty. Contributing causes include hematoma formation, revision of a previous arthroplasty, the magnitude of the surgery, and the compromised general health of some patients. Infection with persistent low-virulence organisms, such as *Propionibacterium acnes* and *Staphylococcus epidermidis,* are particularly prevalent in patients treated with revision arthroplasty. Prevention is optimized by obtaining culture specimens in a thorough fashion at the time of the revision surgery and maintaining the cultures for several weeks to allow growth of these slow-growing organisms. Once a specific organism is identified, culture-specific treatment should be employed. The inclusion of appropriate antibiotics in the cement is recommended.

Dislocation is a relatively common complication, especially after the revision of a previous arthroplasty, when the osseous and soft-tissue anatomy has been distorted by prior trauma, when components are malpositioned, or when the humeral component levers against glenoid bone. Instability can be prevented by careful intraoperative examination to ensure full motion, proper version, absence of abutment, and no separation (pistoning) of the components when traction is applied to the humerus, combined with repairs of the subscapularis and other soft tissues. If there is any question about intrinsic stability, delaying shoulder motion for 6 weeks after the surgery may allow healing of the soft-tissue envelope around the reconstruction. If the components have been properly positioned with adequate soft-tissue tension and without medial glenohumeral abutment in adduction, an early postoperative dislocation may be managed with closed reduction and immobilization with the arm at the side in a sling. If instability results from component malpositioning, osseous abutment, or inadequate soft-tissue tension, revision surgery may be required.

Fractures of the acromion occur commonly as a result of a preexisting acromial lesion, overtensioning of the deltoid, or osseous fatigue from loading of an osteopenic acromion. Distal acromial fractures with inferior angulation usually require only the treatment of symptoms. However, fractures of the scapular spine may cause clinically relevant pain and loss of function. Anteroposterior, axillary, and scapular Y radiographs as well as CT scans may be used to evaluate patients with unexpected pain or poor function after a reverse total shoulder arthroplasty. Internal fixation should be considered for such patients, despite the difficulties presented by poor bone and substantial loads.

Neurologic injuries include axillary nerve damage from surgical dissection or traction injuries from excessive tension resulting from lengthening of the arm. These injuries are most common in revisions with difficult surgical exposures.

## Socioeconomic Considerations

Reverse total shoulder prostheses and the support for their application tend to be expensive. Being that this prosthesis is generally recommended for individuals 65 years of age and older, the cost of its implantation may substantially exceed a medical center's reimbursement from Medicare and other insurance programs. However, there are many individuals whose comfort, function, and quality of life are compromised by severe rotator cuff lesions and failed surgical reconstructions who could potentially benefit from this procedure. Finally, the substantial risks of the procedure create the need for informed consent and assessment of the total context in which the patient will live after this reconstruction.

## Summary

Reverse total shoulder arthroplasty is a powerful and technically demanding tool for managing shoulder conditions in relatively older, less active patients who previously had no solution for these problems. It is tempting to expand its application to an increasing number of conditions in younger and more active individuals, such as irreparable rotator cuff tears, severe proximal humeral fractures, and complex instability patterns. This temptation needs to be balanced by an awareness of the complications, cost, and potential for deteriorating function with time after this method of reconstruction.

## References

1. Grammont PM, Baulot E: Delta shoulder prosthesis for rotator cuff rupture. *Orthopedics* 1993;16:65-68.

2. Bohsali KI, Wirth MA, Rockwood CA Jr: Complications of total shoulder arthroplasty. *J Bone Joint Surg Am* 2006;88:2279-2292.

3. Guery J, Favard L, Sirveaux F, Oudet D, Mole D, Walch G: Reverse total shoulder arthroplasty: Survivorship analysis of eighty replacements followed for five to ten years. *J Bone Joint Surg Am* 2006;88:1742-1747.

4. Werner CM, Steinmann PA, Gilbart M, Gerber C: Treatment of painful pseudoparesis due to irreparable rotator cuff dysfunction with the Delta III reverse ball-and-socket total shoulder prosthesis. *J Bone Joint Surg Am* 2005; 87:1476-1486.

5. Frankle M, Levy JC, Pupello D, et al: The reverse shoulder prosthesis for glenohumeral arthritis associated with severe rotator cuff deficiency. *J Bone Joint Surg Am* 2006;88(suppl 1 Pt 2):178-190.

6. Boileau P, Watkinson D, Hatzidakis AM, Hovorka I: Neer Award 2005: The Grammont reverse shoulder prosthesis: Results in cuff tear arthritis, fracture sequelae, and revision arthroplasty. *J Shoulder Elbow Surg* 2006;15:527-540.

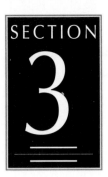
# Elbow and Wrist

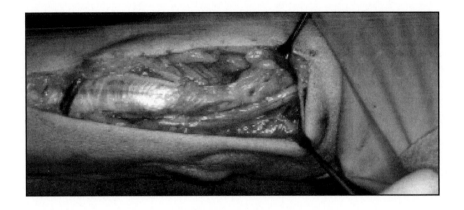

# Median and Radial Nerve Compression About the Elbow

Peter Tsai, MD

David R. Steinberg, MD

## Abstract

*It is important for physicians who treat upper extremity disorders to understand motor palsy or pain syndromes caused by compression of the median and radial nerves about the elbow and forearm. Patients with anterior interosseous nerve syndrome may report hand weakness, whereas those with pronator syndrome may present with pain and paresthesia that can be confused with carpal tunnel syndrome. Patients with posterior interosseous nerve syndrome report hand weakness, whereas those with radial tunnel syndrome report pain in the lateral elbow and forearm, which may be confused with lateral epicondylitis. Because each syndrome has overlapping symptoms, serial examinations are needed to determine the correct diagnosis.*

**Instr Course Lect 2008;57:177-185.**

Cubital tunnel syndrome is the most well-recognized compression/traction neuropathy occurring around the elbow. Compression of the median and radial nerves about the elbow and forearm are less often encountered yet must be understood by any physician who treats upper extremity pathology.

Nontraumatic compression of the median and radial nerves at the elbow may each present in one of two forms: as a motor palsy or as a pain syndrome. Patients with anterior interosseous nerve syndrome present with hand weakness, whereas patients with pronator syndrome report pain and paresthesias that can be easily confused with carpal tunnel syndrome. Patients with posterior interosseous nerve syndrome present with hand weakness, whereas patients with radial tunnel syndrome report lateral elbow and fore-

arm pain that can be easily confused with lateral epicondylitis. A discussion of each condition will include information on presentation, evaluation, the approach to management, and the results of treatment, with particular emphasis on controversial issues, such as differential diagnosis, surgical indications, and surgical approaches.

## Median Nerve
### Anatomy

The median nerve is formed distal to the axilla from portions of the medial and lateral cords of the brachial plexus, composed of fibers from C6, C7, C8, and T1. The lateral cord provides mostly sensory axons from C6 and C7, with the medial cord contributing the bulk of motor input through C8 and T1. The terminal divisions of the medial and lateral cords coalesce in a Y

shape to become the median nerve, which then courses lateral and superficial to the brachial artery. The median nerve is parallel and anterior to the medial intermuscular septum. At the middle of the brachium, the median nerve crosses over the brachial artery to lie just medial to the artery. The nerve and artery pass under the lacertus fibrosus (bicipital aponeurosis) and enter the antecubital region medial to the biceps tendon and anterior to the brachialis (Figure 1, *A*). The median nerve then passes beneath the humeral (superficial) head of the pronator teres and subsequently passes between the humeroulnar and radial portions of the flexor digitorum superficialis, under the proximal arch of this muscle belly (Figure 1, *B*). The nerve courses further down the forearm under cover of the flexor digitorum superficialis and lies over the flexor digitorum profundus along the lateral side of this muscle.

The last major branch of the median nerve in the forearm is the anterior interosseous nerve. It departs from the median nerve approximately 4 cm distal to the medial epicondyle of the humerus, passing under fibrous tissue originating from either the flexor digitorum superficialis or its pronator teres. It runs along the interosseous membrane between the flexor digitorum pro-

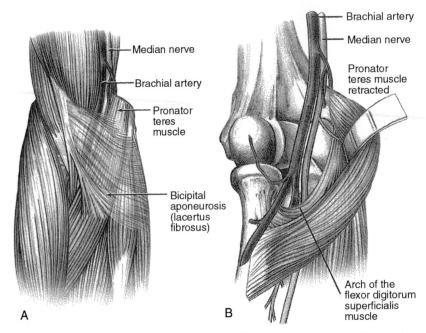

**Figure 1** Illustrations depicting proximal median nerve anatomy. **A,** The median nerve and the brachial artery are covered by the pronator teres and the lacertus fibrosus. **B,** After reflection of the humeral head of the pronator teres muscle and the bicipital aponeurosis, the median nerve can be visualized proximally. It disappears beneath the flexor digitorum superficialis arch. (Adapted with permission from Berger RA, Weiss APC (eds): *Hand Surgery.* Philadelphia, PA, Lippincott Williams and Wilkins, 2004, p 898.)

fundus and flexor pollicis longus, and finally terminates in the distal part of the forearm, deep to the pronator quadratus, innervating the flexor digitorum profundus, flexor pollicis longus, and pronator quadratus muscles along the way. Anatomic dissections have demonstrated the innervation of the flexor pollicis longus and flexor digitorum profundus through multiple nerve branches along the medial and lateral edges of these muscles, respectively.[1,2] The autonomous zone of sensory innervation for the median nerve includes the palmar surfaces of the index and long fingers and their dorsal aspects past the level of the distal interphalangeal joint.

When considering the normal anatomy of the median and anterior interosseous nerves, the potential anomalous structures and innervation patterns of the upper extremity must be kept in mind. The presence of a Martin-Gruber anastomosis in the forearm may change the clinical presentation of pronator syndrome. Additionally, anatomic variations as the anterior interosseous nerve courses distally in the antebrachium may affect sites of compression of the nerve. In the study by Beaton and Anson,[3] the nerve passed between the deep and superficial heads of the pronator teres in 82% of the limbs, deep to the ulnar head in 7%, and through the superficial head of the pronator teres in 2%; in the remaining 9%, the deep head was absent. Additionally, there have been descriptions of the nerve passing anterior to the superficial head. Underneath the deep head of the pro-

natorteres, Gantzer's muscle (the accessory head of the flexor pollicis longus) may be found. In a recent investigation, al-Qattan[4] found the muscle in 52% of 25 specimens; the muscle arose from the medial epicondyle in approximately 85% of the specimens in which it was present and from the medial epicondyle and coronoid in the remaining 15%. A supracondyloid process of the distal part of the humerus (present in approximately 1% of individuals of European descent) may indicate the presence of the ligament of Struthers, which can cause compression of the median nerve as it passes through the foramen formed by the fibrous band.[5]

Compression of the median nerve at the elbow can present in one of two forms: anterior interosseous nerve syndrome and pronator syndrome. Anterior interosseous nerve syndrome presents as a motor palsy, whereas pronator syndrome is associated with pain and paresthesias that can be easily confused with carpal tunnel syndrome. Although anterior interosseous nerve palsy may occur after fracture or surgery about the elbow, only nontraumatic anterior interosseous nerve syndrome will be discussed in this chapter.

### Anterior Interosseous Nerve Syndrome

The earliest reports of anterior interosseous nerve syndrome appeared in a 1948 report by Parsonage and Turner[6] that described anterior interosseous nerve palsy associated with paralytic lesions about the shoulder. Subsequently, Kiloh and Nevin[7] reported cases of spontaneous neuritis of the anterior interosseous nerve with isolated paralysis of the flexor pollicis longus and median-innervated flexor digitorum profundus. Although Parsonage and Turner had described this lesion years earlier, they had not believed that it was anatomically possible to have an isolated lesion of the anterior interosseous nerve.

Sites of isolated anterior interosseous nerve compression include the fibrous arch of the flexor digitorum superficialis and the pronator teres, under which the nerve travels early in its course. A patient who has anterior interosseous nerve syndrome will report weakness of pinch, which can affect activities such as writing and picking up small objects. A careful history may reveal an antecedent episode of spontaneous forearm pain followed by progressive weakness in the hand. Repetitive elbow flexion or forearm pronation have been proposed as dynamic causes of compression of the anterior interosseous nerve in the proximal part of the forearm. A history of transient shoulder pain (often following an immunization or viral illness) preceding the development of upper extremity weakness or paresthesias should alert one to the possibility of brachial neuritis (Parsonage-Turner syndrome). Although a variety of cutaneous and motor nerves can be affected, anterior interosseous nerve palsy has been described in a high percentage of patients with brachial neuritis. These cases need to be differentiated from those presumably occurring at the elbow because the treatment will be very different.

Anterior interosseous nerve syndrome leads to an inability to flex the interphalangeal joint of the thumb and the distal interphalangeal joint of the index finger (and occasionally the long finger) because of weakness of the flexor pollicis longus and the radial half of the flexor digitorum profundus. Although the pronator quadratus is also involved, the patient will not be aware of this involvement because of intact function of the pronator teres. During examination, the contribution of the pronator teres can be partially eliminated by testing the strength of resisted pronation with the elbow maximally flexed. The flexor pollicis longus and flexor digitorum profundus of the index finger are examined by asking the patient to make an "OK sign" by firmly opposing the tips of the thumb and index finger. A patient who has anterior interosseous nerve palsy will compensate with a key, or lateral, pinch using the thumb adductor and the first dorsal interosseous muscle (which are innervated by the ulnar nerve).

## Pronator Syndrome

The symptoms and signs of pronator syndrome overlap those of carpal tunnel syndrome. Both conditions are associated with pain and paresthesias in the radial three and one-half digits, with the symptoms often being worse with certain activities. Patients with either of these conditions may have a tender nerve over both the wrist and the proximal part of the forearm, although the Tinel sign is most prominent at the main site of compression, which can include a ligament of Struthers originating from a supracondylar process, the pronator teres, the lacertus fibrosus, and the fibrous arcade of the flexor digitorum superficialis. There are, however, some features that may help to differentiate the two diagnoses. Painful symptoms that awaken the patient from sleep are much more common in association with carpal tunnel syndrome. A careful examination of a patient who has pronator syndrome may reveal decreased sensibility in the palm over the thenar eminence (innervat-ed by the palmar cutaneous branch, which branches from the median nerve proximal to the carpal tunnel). The Phalen maneuver will be negative. Provocative testing for pronator syndrome stresses structures that potentially can compress the median nerve. If symptoms are reproduced during resisted forearm pronation or resisted elbow flexion/supination, one should suspect the pronator teres or the lacertus fibrosus, respectively. Resisted grasp (the "middle finger flexion test") is less helpful because the result could be positive in association with either condition: contraction of the flexor digitorum superficialis muscle belly may compress the nerve proximally, and finger flexion may draw prominent lumbrical muscle bellies into the carpal canal and cause distal nerve compression.[8]

## Evaluation of the Median Nerve

Standard radiographs of the elbow will aid in the diagnosis of structural anomalies such as a supracondylar process.[5] MRIs are rarely needed unless a mass is suspected. Electrodiagnostic studies can be helpful for the evaluation of anterior interosseous nerve palsy but usually reveal normal findings in cases of pronator syndrome.

## Treatment and Outcomes

Patients with pronator syndrome or anterior interosseous nerve syndrome should be managed with a trial of nonsurgical treatment, which should include the avoidance of provocative activities that involve repetitive elbow flexion, forearm pronation, or forceful gripping. A posterior elbow splint may reinforce the importance of resting the extremity. Oral nonsteroidal anti-inflammatory medications may be helpful, particularly in patients with pronator syndrome.

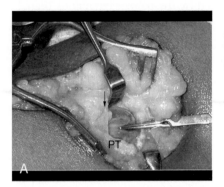 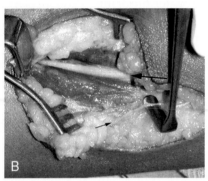

**Figure 2** Decompression of the proximal aspect of the median nerve. **A,** The lacertus fibrosus has already been transected, and the pronator teres (PT) has been retracted. The median nerve (under the curved Jacobson clamp) runs under the fibrous arch of the flexor digitorum superficialis (*arrow*). **B,** With transection of the flexor digitorum superficialis arch, the median nerve is decompressed (*large arrow*). Note the proximity of the medial antebrachial cutaneous nerve (*small arrow*).

It has been reported that 50% to 70% of patients with pronator syndrome may respond to conservative therapy.[9,10] Patients who do not respond to such therapy are candidates for surgical decompression, which has been associated with a success rate of approximately 90%.[11,12] The indications for surgical decompression in patients with anterior interosseous nerve syndrome are more controversial. Recommendations in the literature have been empirical or anecdotal, based mainly on small retrospective series. The authors of those studies have recommended surgical decompression if no motor recovery is detected after 8 to 12 weeks. Improvement has been documented anywhere from 4 weeks to 2 years after surgical release.[13,14] To further complicate the matter, a few reports have described series of patients with anterior interosseous nerve syndrome who recovered function without surgical intervention; spontaneous resolution occurred between 3 and 24 months after the onset of symptoms.[15,16]

During surgery, the nerve is decompressed from proximal to distal. The surgeon should begin the decompression proximal to the an-

tecubital crease to easily identify the median nerve and explore this region for a ligament of Struthers. If present, the ligament and the supracondylar process should be removed. Decompression in the forearm includes release of the lacertus fibrosus and the proximal fibrous edge of the flexor digitorum superficialis arch (Figure 2). The superficial head of the pronator teres should be mobilized; if still causing compression, it may be released with a stepcut at the distal tendon and then repaired in a lengthened position.[17] The surgeon should also explore the region for the presence of anomalies such as Gantzer's muscle, an accessory muscle of the flexor pollicis longus arising from the medial epicondyle and occasionally the coronoid.[18] The arm is immobilized in a well-padded posterior splint with the elbow at 90° and the forearm in neutral rotation. The splint is discontinued and motion is allowed approximately 1 week after surgery.

## Radial Nerve

### Anatomy

The radial nerve is the terminal branch of the posterior cord and is

actually the largest terminal branch of the brachial plexus. It is composed of C5 through C8 nerve roots and lies posterior to the axillary artery. As the nerve travels distally, it falls further posteriorly and passes through the triangular space to enter the posterior aspect of the brachium. It then runs along the anterior aspect of the long head of the triceps, leaving this area and coursing along the posterior aspect of the humerus in the spiral groove to lie on the lateral aspect of the humerus under the brachioradialis and on top of the brachialis. As the nerve courses distally, it is under the cover of the extensor carpi radialis longus and brevis, with the joint capsule and capitellum of the humerus lying posterior to the nerve at this point. This region, from the joint capsule to the proximal supinator, was originally referred to as the "radial tunnel" by Roles and Maudsley,[19] who began decompressing the radial nerve as a part of the treatment of recalcitrant lateral epicondylitis. The radial nerve divides into its two terminal branches, the sensory branch and the posterior interosseous nerve. The superficial sensory branch takes off from the radial nerve proximal to the radial tunnel and travels distally on the undersurface of the brachioradialis. The posterior interosseous nerve crosses the elbow joint and lies in adipose tissue anterior to the radiocapitellar joint capsule. The first potential structures causing nerve compression in the radial tunnel, tethering fibrous bands that arise between the brachioradialis and the joint capsule, can be found at the level of the radial head (Figure 3). The next anatomic area of possible compression includes the branches of the radial recurrent artery that are believed to cause increased pressure on the pos-

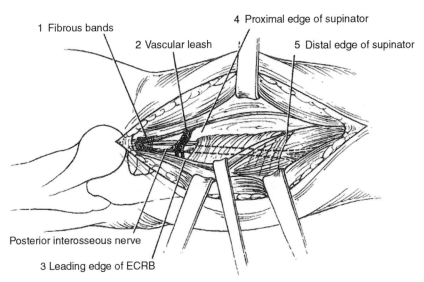

Figure 3   Five possible anatomic sites of compression of the posterior interosseous nerve within the radial tunnel. ECRB = extensor carpi radialis brevis. (Reproduced with permission from Gelberman RH (ed): *Surgical Nerve Repair and Reconstruction*. Philadelphia, PA, JB Lippincott, 1991, p 1007.)

In illustration labels:

1 Fibrous bands
2 Vascular leash
4 Proximal edge of supinator
5 Distal edge of supinator
Posterior interosseous nerve
3 Leading edge of ECRB

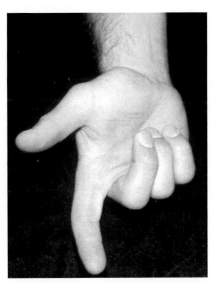

Figure 4   Photograph of the hand and wrist of a patient with a partial posterior interosseous nerve palsy. The patient presented with loss of extensor digitorum communis function but with preservation of index finger and thumb extension.

terior interosseous nerve. As the nerve courses distally, it lies underneath the extensor carpi radialis brevis, which can itself cause compression of the nerve under its tendinous edge. The nerve travels between the superficial and deep heads of the supinator after passing under the arcade of Frohse. Interestingly, this proximal fibrous arcade of the superficial head of the supinator does not appear to be present in the human fetus but develops at some point later in life in approximately 30% of individuals (with the rest having a membranous leading edge of the supinator).[20] In a minority of patients, the nerve also may be compressed under the distal edge of the supinator.

Before the nerve enters the supinator, it sends branches to the extensor carpi radialis brevis and supinator muscles. As it runs under the cover of the distal supinator, it branches into two parts; the superficial portion innervates the extensor carpi ulnaris, extensor digitorum communis, and extensor digiti minimi; and the deep branch serves the abductor pollicis longus, extensor pollicis brevis, extensor pollicis longus, and extensor indicis proprius. The bifurcated nerve then continues into the posterior aspect of the forearm, deep to the extensor digitorum communis and superficial to the outcropper muscles, to terminate as an articular branch to the radiocarpal joint.

Compression of the radial nerve at the elbow can present in one of two forms: posterior interosseous nerve syndrome and radial tunnel syndrome. Patients with posterior interosseous nerve syndrome present with a motor palsy, whereas patients with radial tunnel syndrome report lateral elbow and forearm pain that can easily be confused with lateral epicondylitis. Both posterior interosseous nerve syndrome and radial tunnel syndrome have the same sites of compression; these sites can be recalled by the mnemonic FREAS, which stands for fibrous bands about the radiocapitellar joint, radial recurrent branches, extensor carpi radialis brevis, arcade of Frohse, and, finally, the distal edge of the supinator.

## Posterior Interosseous Nerve Syndrome

A patient who has posterior interosseous nerve syndrome may present with a transient episode of forearm pain followed by progressive weakness of the digital extensors as well as the extensor carpi ulnaris. Posterior interosseous nerve palsy, while usually complete, occasionally involves only some of the extensor muscles (Figure 4). Muscles of the mobile wad are spared because they

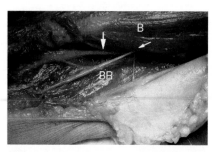

**Figure 5** Photograph showing the close proximity of the lateral antebrachial cutaneous nerve (*small arrow*) and the radial nerve (*large arrow*). The more superficial lateral antebrachial cutaneous nerve exits between the biceps (B) and the brachioradialis (BR), whereas the radial nerve lies in the plane between the brachialis and the brachioradialis.

are innervated more proximally. If the brachioradialis or the radial wrist extensors (the extensor carpi radialis brevis and extensor carpi radialis longus) are also weak, the examiner should suspect more proximal compression by, for example, the lateral head of the triceps or a humeral exostosis. Posterior interosseous nerve syndrome may occur idiopathically or be caused by compression of the posterior interosseous nerve by masses such as ganglia. In the rheumatoid arthritis population, the examiner should palpate for rheumatoid nodules, radiocapitellar synovitis, or a subluxated radial head.

The examiner should not assume that a patient with rheumatoid arthritis who presents with a loss of digital extension necessarily has posterior interosseous nerve palsy. Other diagnoses to be considered in the differential include extensor tendon rupture (usually at the level of the distal part of the ulna), sagittal band rupture, or inflammatory involvement of the metacarpophalangeal joints leading to palmar-ulnar subluxation. Extensor tendon rupture is characterized by loss of the tenode-

sis effect (compensatory digital extension during passive wrist flexion). When the sagittal band ruptures, the extensor tendon usually subluxates ulnarly between the metacarpal heads. Passive extension of the finger allows the extensor mechanism to centralize over the metacarpophalangeal joint, and the patient is then able to actively maintain extension (but not initiate digital extension).

### Radial Tunnel Syndrome

Radial tunnel syndrome also is caused by compression of the posterior interosseous nerve in the proximal part of the forearm. The factors that cause radial tunnel syndrome to develop in some patients and posterior interosseous nerve syndrome to develop in others are not well understood. Radial tunnel syndrome is characterized by proximal dorsal forearm pain. Some patients may have weakness secondary to the pain, although actual motor involvement is rare. Symptoms may occur at night or may be aggravated with repetitive activities such as forearm rotation, elbow extension, and maximum wrist flexion-extension.

The symptoms of radial tunnel syndrome overlap those of the much more prevalent lateral epicondylitis (tennis elbow); a careful history and examination are required to differentiate the two. In fact, 5% of patients with tennis elbow also have radial tunnel syndrome.[21] Conversely, 50% of patients with radial tunnel syndrome may have concomitant lateral epicondylitis.[22] This may be caused by involvement of the extensor carpi radialis brevis in both conditions or to the fact that the superficial belly of the supinator produces some tension of the common extensor.[23] The possibility of radial tunnel

syndrome should always be considered in patients with resistant lateral epicondylitis.[19] The most common finding is tenderness over the mobile wad rather than over the lateral epicondyle. The diagnosis is strengthened with positive provocative maneuvers, including resisted supination with the elbow extended. The middle finger extension test, heralded in some texts as pathognomonic for radial tunnel syndrome, has not been found to be useful in our experience because it is often positive in patients with lateral epicondylitis (because of stressful contraction of the extensor carpi radialis brevis). A small group of patients may present with point tenderness over the dorsal aspect of the middle part of the forearm, distal and ulnar to the mobile wad; these patients represent the 5% of cases in which the posterior interosseous nerve is compressed under the distal edge of the supinator. Because of the absence of objective findings associated with radial tunnel syndrome, the physical examination should be repeated on more than one occasion and the findings should be compared with those for the contralateral extremity.

Another rare cause of lateral elbow/proximal forearm pain that may be confused with radial tunnel syndrome is compression of the lateral antebrachial cutaneous nerve, first described in 1982 by Bassett and Nunley.[24] This condition is caused by compression of the lateral edge of the biceps tendon and may be aggravated by active elbow flexion and supination or maximum forearm pronation. The diagnostic dilemma exists because of the close proximity of the lateral antebrachial cutaneous nerve and the radial nerve in the antecubital region (Figure 5).

## Evaluation of the Radial Nerve

Differential lidocaine injections may be helpful for distinguishing among lateral epicondylitis, radial tunnel syndrome, and lateral antebrachial cutaneous nerve compression. Electrodiagnostic studies may be positive for patients with posterior interosseous nerve syndrome and those with lateral antebrachial cutaneous nerve pathology but are usually normal for patients with radial tunnel syndrome. Imaging studies may be helpful if a mass around the elbow or the proximal part of the forearm is suspected.

## Treatment and Outcomes

Most patients with posterior interosseous nerve syndrome and radial tunnel syndrome initially should be treated nonsurgically with the avoidance of provocative activities, immobilization in a wrist or elbow splint, and use of oral nonsteroidal anti-inflammatory medications.

Surgical decompression should be considered for patients with a clear diagnosis of radial tunnel syndrome after 3 months of failed conservative treatment. For patients with posterior interosseous nerve syndrome, surgical indications include progressive weakness, late presentation with severe weakness and atrophy, or the absence of improvement after 4 to 12 weeks of conservative treatment.

The surgical approach to the radial nerve in the forearm may vary depending on the comfort of the surgeon with the procedure and with his or her knowledge of the offending anatomic structures. At least four approaches have been described; however, not all approaches allow equal access to all potential points of compression. The brachioradialis-splitting approach is most direct, but it involves

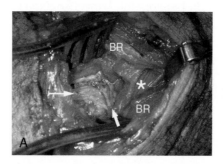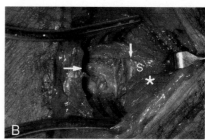

**Figure 6** Decompression of the posterior interosseous nerve with the brachioradialis-splitting approach (the elbow is to the left, and the distal part of the forearm is to the right). **A,** Dissection through the brachioradialis (BR) reveals the posterior interosseous nerve (*large arrow*) running under the radial recurrent vessels (*small arrow*) and the oblique fibers of the extensor carpi radialis brevis (*asterisk*). **B,** Deeper dissection reveals the posterior interosseous nerve (*large arrow*) running under the fibrous arch (*small arrow*) of the supinator (S), which lies deep to the extensor carpi radialis brevis (*asterisk*).

blunt dissection through muscle and requires careful placement of the incision.[25] The relatively bloodless interval between the brachioradialis and the extensor carpi radialis longus requires a more extensive incision, but it can be combined with the surgical approach used for the treatment of lateral epicondylitis.[26] A dorsal approach, commonly used for the treatment of proximal radial diaphyseal fractures, provides better access to the distal edge of the supinator but provides poorer visualization of the posterior interosseous nerve more proximally and associated potential compressive structures.[27] An anterior approach may be useful for exposure of the anterior aspect of the joint and masses, but it requires a deeper dissection and provides poor visualization of the distal edge of the supinator.[28,29]

Regardless of approach, one key to successful decompression of the radial nerve is the identification of both the extensor carpi radialis brevis and the proximal edge of the supinator. If the surgeon believes that the decompression is finished after releasing the first muscle en-

countered, the arcade of Frohse may have been missed. One should realize that the extensor carpi radialis brevis passes over the posterior interosseous nerve obliquely, whereas fibers of the supinator run at right angles to the nerve (Figure 6).

After satisfactory release and wound closure, the arm is immobilized in a well-padded posterior splint with the elbow at 90° and the forearm in neutral rotation. The splint is discontinued and motion is allowed approximately 1 week after surgery.

Good to excellent recovery of function after the surgical treatment of posterior interosseous nerve syndrome may be expected in as many as 90% of patients.[30] Results of radial tunnel surgery are much more variable. Good to excellent relief of symptoms have been reported in 51% to 92% of patients.[31-33] This wide range of satisfactory outcomes may be the result of numerous factors, including the more subjective nature of the diagnosis, with poor localization of pain, a more chronic presentation leading to permanent changes within the nerve, or a more frequent association with workers' compensation claims.

## Summary

The less common nerve compression syndromes about the elbow require a high level of suspicion and, in some patients, may be confidently diagnosed only after serial examinations. Each syndrome has a series of overlapping conditions that must be considered in the differential diagnosis. Most patients with pronator syndrome will respond to nonsurgical management. The role of surgery for the treatment of anterior interosseous nerve syndrome is controversial, particularly in light of the fact that the condition may actually be caused by more proximal nerve pathology. Most patients with posterior interosseous nerve syndrome will recover good to excellent function after surgical release. The results of decompression in patients with radial tunnel syndrome can be equally gratifying with adherence to careful patient-selection criteria.

## References

1. Canovas F, Mouilleron P, Bonnel F: Biometry of the muscular branches of the median nerve to the forearm. *Clin Anat* 1998;11:239-245.

2. Spinner M: The anterior interosseous-nerve syndrome, with special attention to its variations. *J Bone Joint Surg Am* 1970;52:84-94.

3. Beaton LB, Anson BJ: The relation of the median nerve to the pronator teres muscle. *Anat Rec* 1939;75:23-26.

4. al-Qattan MM: Gantzer's muscle: An anatomical study of the accessory head of the flexor pollicis longus muscle. *J Hand Surg Br* 1996;21:269-270.

5. Barnard LB, McCoy SM: The supracondyloid process of the humerus. *J Bone Joint Surg Am* 1946;28:845-850.

6. Parsonage MJ, Turner JWA: Neuralgic amyotrophy: The shoulder-girdle syndrome. *Lancet* 1948;251:973-978.

7. Kiloh LG, Nevin S: Isolated neuritis of the anterior interosseous nerve. *BMJ* 1952;1:850-851.

8. Cobb TK, An KN, Cooney WP, Berger RA: Lumbrical muscle incursion into the carpal tunnel during finger flexion. *J Hand Surg Br* 1994;19:434-438.

9. Morris HH, Peters BH: Pronator syndrome: Clinical and electrophysiological features in seven cases. *J Neurol Neurosurg Psychiatry* 1976;39:461-464.

10. Johnson RK, Spinner M, Shrewsbury MM: Median nerve entrapment syndrome in the proximal forearm. *J Hand Surg Am* 1979;4:48-51.

11. Tsai TM, Syed SA: A transverse skin incision approach for decompression of pronator teres syndrome. *J Hand Surg Br* 1994;19:40-42.

12. Hartz CR, Linscheid RL, Gramse RR, Daube JR: The pronator teres syndrome: Compressive neuropathy of the median nerve. *J Bone Joint Surg Am* 1981;63:885-890.

13. Schantz K, Riegels-Nielsen P: The anterior interosseous nerve syndrome. *J Hand Surg Br* 1992;17:510-512.

14. Sood MK, Burke FD: Anterior interosseous nerve palsy: A review of 16 cases. *J Hand Surg Br* 1997;22:64-68.

15. Miller-Breslow A, Terrono A, Millender LH: Nonoperative treatment of anterior interosseous nerve paralysis. *J Hand Surg Am* 1990;15:493-496.

16. Goulding PJ, Schady W: Favourable outcome in non-traumatic anterior interosseous nerve lesions. *J Neurol* 1993;240:83-86.

17. Mackinnon SE, Novak CB: Compression neuropathies, in Green DP, Hotchkiss RN, Pedersen WC, Wolfe SW (eds): *Green's Operative Hand Surgery*, ed 5. Philadelphia, PA, Elsevier, 2005, pp 999-1046.

18. Dellon AL, Mackinnon SE: Musculoaponeurotic variations along the course of the median nerve in the proximal forearm. *J Hand Surg Br* 1987;12:359-363.

19. Roles NC, Maudsley RH: Radial tunnel syndrome: Resistant tennis elbow as a nerve entrapment. *J Bone Joint Surg Br* 1972;54:499-508.

20. Spinner M: The arcade of Frohse and its relationship to posterior interosseous nerve paralysis. *J Bone Joint Surg Br* 1968;50:809-812.

21. Werner CO: Lateral elbow pain and posterior interosseous nerve entrapment. *Acta Orthop Scand Suppl* 1979;174:1-62.

22. Kalb K, Gruber P, Landsleitner B: Compression syndrome of the radial nerve in the area of the supinator groove: Experiences with 110 patients. *Handchir Mikrochir Plast Chir* 1999;31:303-310.

23. Erak S, Day R, Wang A: The role of supinator in the pathogenesis of chronic lateral elbow pain: A biomechanical study. *J Hand Surg Br* 2004;29:461-464.

24. Bassett FH III, Nunley JA: Compression of the musculocutaneous nerve at the elbow. *J Bone Joint Surg Am* 1982;64:1050-1052.

25. Lister GD: Radial tunnel syndrome, in Gelberman RH (ed): *Operative Nerve Repair and Reconstruction*. Philadelphia, PA, JB Lippincott, 1991, pp 1023-1037.

26. Hall HC, Mackinnon SE, Gilbert RW: An approach to the posterior interosseous nerve. *Plast Reconstr Surg* 1984;74:435-437.

27. Thompson JE: Anatomical methods of approach in operations on the long bones of the extremities. *Ann Surg* 1918;68:309-329.

28. Henry AK: *Extensile Exposure Applied to Limb Surgery*, ed 2. Baltimore, MD, Williams and Wilkins, 1957.

29. Eversmann WW Jr: Entrapment and compression neuropathies, in Green DP (ed): *Operative Hand Surgery*, ed 3. New York, NY, Churchill Livingstone, 1993, pp 1341-1385.

30. Hashizume H, Nishida K, Nanba Y, Shigeyama Y, Inowe H, Morito Y: Non-traumatic paralysis of the posterior interosseous nerve. *J Bone Joint Surg Br* 1996;78:771-776.

31. Ritts GD, Wood MB, Linscheid RL: Radial tunnel syndrome: A ten-year surgical experience. *Clin Orthop Relat Res* 1987;219:201-205.

32. Lawrence T, Mobbs P, Fortems Y, Stanley JK: Radial tunnel syndrome: A retrospective review of 30 decom

pressions of the radial nerve. *J Hand Surg Br* 1995;20:454-459.

33. Jebson PJ, Engber WD: Radial tunnel syndrome: Long-term results of surgical decompression. *J Hand Surg Am* 1997;22:889-896.

# Compression of the Ulnar Nerve at the Elbow: Cubital Tunnel Syndrome

Harris Gellman, MD

## Abstract

*Although cubital tunnel syndrome has been described as the most common entrapment of the ulnar nerve, there is still considerable difficulty identifying the exact location of the pathologic compression of the nerve and deciding on the correct surgical or nonsurgical treatment. The most commonly recommended surgical techniques include simple (in situ) decompression, decompression with medial epicondylectomy, anterior subcutaneous transposition, and anterior submuscular transposition of the ulnar nerve at the elbow. It is important to understand the pitfalls and possible complications of these commonly used treatments.*

**Instr Course Lect 2008;57:187-197.**

Cubital tunnel syndrome has been described as the most common entrapment of the ulnar nerve.[1] As early as 1878, Panas[2] reported the association of slowly progressive ulnar nerve palsy with compression of the ulnar nerve at the elbow. Feindel and Stratford[3] proposed the term cubital tunnel to specifically describe that area where nerve compression occurs distal to the medial epicondyle. They described the anatomy of the cubital tunnel as the area beginning immediately proximal to and ending immediately distal to the medial epicondyle. Despite this attempt at specificity, the most difficult aspect of the treatment algorithm is identifying the exact location of pathologic compression of the nerve. After the diagnosis has been made, there is debate concerning the appropriate treatment of the compressive neuropathy of the ulnar nerve at the elbow. Simple (in situ) decompression, decompression with medial epicondylectomy, anterior subcutaneous transposition, and anterior submuscular transposition are the most commonly recommended surgical techniques, with proponents arguing in favor of their chosen technique.[4-12] None of these techniques is applicable to every patient.

## Anatomy

The cubital tunnel is a restrictive area immediately distal to the medial epicondyle, the roof of which is formed by the aponeurosis over the flexor carpi ulnaris (FCU) origin spanning the olecranon and medial epicondyle; the floor is formed by the medial ligaments of the elbow joint. Within the cubital tunnel, the ulnar nerve lies beneath the fascial arcade between the deep and the superficial heads of the FCU and is anterior to the flexor digitorum profundus (Figure 1).

Proximally, the ulnar nerve sends off an articular branch before innervating the FCU and the ulnar head of the flexor digitorum profundus muscle. Compression of the ulnar nerve commonly occurs at the fascial origin between the ulnar and humeral heads of the FCU, immediately distal to the medial epicondyle at the area known as Osborne's ligament. In addition to being the most common site of ulnar nerve compression, it is the second most common site of peripheral nerve entrapment. Other sources of compression include the arcade of Struthers; the medial head of the triceps; the aponeurosis of the FCU; synovial hypertrophy of the elbow (as found in rheumatoid disease); and the presence of tumors (ganglia or lipomata), aberrant muscles (anconeus epitrochlearis), cubitus valgus, and bone spurs.

Nerve subluxation that occurs during elbow flexion often results in pain with elbow flexion/extension or throwing activities. Cubital tunnel syndrome also has been reported after surgery (for example, cardiac or shoulder surgery) and has been associated with the use of a blood pressure cuff or a tourniquet, or can result from patient positioning; many of these patients report a preexisting neuropathy.[13]

## Pathophysiology

The ulnar nerve is subject to compression, traction, and friction with

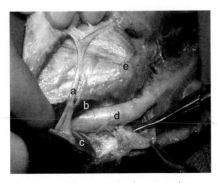

**Figure 1** Photograph showing the cubital tunnel anatomy including the medial antebrachial cutaneous nerve (a), superficial head of the flexor carpi ulnaris (b), deep head of the flexor carpi ulnaris (c), ulnar nerve (d), and medial epicondyle (e).

normal elbow motion. The cubital tunnel normally narrows during elbow flexion as Osborne's ligament stretches and becomes taut, and the medial collateral ligament bulges beneath the nerve.[3,12] The cross-sectional contour of the tunnel changes from an oval during elbow extension to a flattened ellipse during elbow flexion.[14] Iba and associates[15] reported increased pressure during elbow flexion 1 to 2 cm distal to the proximal edge of the cubital tunnel retinaculum.

Osborne's ligament stretches 5 mm for every 45° of elbow flexion, elongating up to 40% from full extension to full flexion.[12] As the elbow is flexed, the arcuate ligament elongates, decreasing the canal volume by 55%; pressure within the tunnel increases sevenfold, rising to more than twentyfold when contraction of the FCU is added.[16] Gelberman and associates[17] reported that during elbow motion from full extension to 135° of flexion, the mean cross-sectional area of the three regions of the cubital tunnel (medial epicondyle, deep to the tunnel aponeurosis, deep to the flexor carpi ulnaris muscle) decreased by

30%, 39%, and 41%, and the mean area of the ulnar nerve decreased by 33%, 50%, and 34%, respectively. These changes were significant in all three regions of the cubital tunnel ($P < 0.05$). The greatest changes occurred in the region beneath the aponeurosis of the cubital tunnel with the elbow at 135° of flexion. The mean intraneural pressure within the cubital tunnel was significantly greater than the mean extraneural pressure when the elbow was flexed 90°, 100°, 110°, and 130°. With the elbow flexed 130°, the mean intraneural pressure was 45% greater than the mean extraneural pressure. Similarly, with the elbow flexed 120° or more, the mean intraneural pressure 4 cm proximal to the cubital tunnel was significantly greater than the mean extraneural pressure (15.6 ± 5 mm Hg at 120° flexion versus 9.3 ± 4.8 mm Hg at extension; an increase of approximately 63%).

Motion and traction of the nerve occurs both proximal and distal to the medial epicondyle as a result of elbow flexion. Normal excursion of the ulnar nerve is as great as 10 mm proximal to the medial epicondyle and 6 mm distal to the epicondyle.[18] The combined motion of the wrist, fingers, elbow, and shoulder results in 21.9 mm of ulnar nerve excursion at the elbow. The nerve itself elongates 4.7 mm with elbow flexion, increasing to 8 mm with abduction and external rotation of the shoulder. Wright and associates[19] found that an average strain of 29% occurred at the elbow with elbow flexion, and another study reported the largest increase in strain during shoulder abduction.[20] Strain may be a factor associated with a tension neuropathy and may be a factor in the development of cubital tunnel syndrome.

## Signs and Symptoms: Diagnosis

Numbness in the ulnar nerve distribution of the hand is the most common finding in patients with cubital tunnel syndrome, varying in severity depending on the degree and the duration of nerve compression. The sensory deficits usually include the radial and ulnar sides of the small finger and the ulnar half of the ring finger, although normal variations in sensory distribution of the ulnar nerve may extend the numbness to the entire ring finger. Patients often report pain at the medial aspect of the elbow, which radiates into the proximal forearm, as well as weakness of intrinsic muscles and grip strength. In severe instances, significant wasting of the intrinsic musculature, especially the first dorsal interosseous muscle, also may occur.

Tinel sign often is positive at the elbow with an exacerbation of symptoms during compression (or percussion) of the nerve near the origin of the FCU. The elbow flexion test is a provocative test analogous to Phalen's maneuver for carpal tunnel syndrome. In the elbow flexion test, the elbow is maintained in full flexion, with the wrist extended for 1 minute. The test is considered positive when paresthesias or numbness occurs in the ulnar nerve distribution; however, the test has been reported to be more sensitive than specific, and false positive results have been reported in 10% of individuals with normal function.[21] Care must be taken to differentiate this condition from nerve entrapment at the wrist (ulnar nerve compression in Guyon's canal), generalized peripheral neuropathy, thoracic outlet syndrome, cervical nerve root disorders, and focal dystonia.

## Electrodiagnostic Studies

The number of patients who report ulnar neuritis at the elbow far exceeds the number who will ultimately require surgical decompression. Therefore, electrodiagnostic studies should be reserved until the patient is considered a surgical candidate. Most patients will respond to a 4- to 6-week period of work modification, the use of splints when typing, correction of elbow position when typing to one of a less acute angle (45° rather than 90°), and the use of nonsteroidal anti-inflammatory medications. If no improvement occurs after a reasonable period of conservative treatment, nerve conduction velocity (NCV) studies should be performed as part of the preoperative evaluation.

Entrapment neuropathies are typically localized by finding evidence of abnormal conduction (usually slowing conduction); temporal dispersion and/or conduction block in the nerve may also occur, although less frequently. Typically, motor conduction velocities greater than 47 m/s and sensory conduction velocities greater than 54 m/s are considered normal levels. Occasionally, patients with the classic signs and symptoms of nerve compression have normal conduction velocities across the 10-cm elbow segment.[9] Use of an "inching" technique, in which the nerve is studied in three 2-cm segments, allows increased and more accurate detection of focal sites of compression. Miller[22] showed that prolongation of latency in elbow segment 3, which is 2 cm distal to the medial epicondyle, localizes the area of compression to the cubital tunnel in the area of the FCU. When evaluating segmental conduction velocities (reported in m/s), a delay greater than 0.40 m/s is considered abnormal.[23]

## Treatment

Since the original description of the condition, debate has continued concerning the most appropriate treatment for cubital tunnel syndrome. Simple (in situ) decompression, anterior subcutaneous transposition, anterior submuscular transposition, and decompression with medial epicondylectomy are the most commonly recommended procedures.[4-12] Modified in situ decompression is also used for a select group of patients.

### Nonsurgical Treatment

Indications for nonsurgical treatment include mild, intermittent symptoms with a normal or slightly abnormal NCV study. The patient should have normal two-point sensory testing, with no evidence of atrophy of the ulnar-innervated musculature. Nonsurgical treatment consists of eliminating all sources of external and dynamic compression of the nerve at the elbow.

The patient should be cautioned to avoid triceps strengthening exercises and minimize elbow positioning with greater than 45° of flexion. Typists and keyboard operators should elevate their chairs and lower their keyboards to help maintain the elbow at approximately 45° of flexion. Protecting the ulnar nerve from prolonged elbow flexion during sleep is important, whether or not the patient is experiencing paresthesias at night or on awakening. Night splints should immobilize the elbow in 40° to 60° of flexion, ensuring that no straps cross the ulnar nerve at the cubital tunnel.[24]

Conservative treatment has been shown to be effective. Eisen and Danon[25] reported spontaneous recovery in 90% of patients with subjective symptoms, normal sensory examination, and NCV greater than 47 m/s (mild abnormality). Dimond and Lister[26] reported an 86% improvement in patients with cubital tunnel syndrome treated with long arm splints compared with 58% for those treated surgically.

### Simple In Situ Decompression

In situ decompression has been recommended for patients with mild compression.[5,27-32] Although there have been many arguments both for and against simple in situ decompression, the primary difficulty has been identifying which patients will respond best to this technique.[30,33]

A longitudinal incision is made immediately anterior to the medial epicondyle. The ulnar nerve is exposed by opening the cubital tunnel and following the nerve proximally to the level of the tourniquet and distally into the FCU muscle. The medial intermuscular septum is released from its attachment to the medial epicondyle, and the FCU muscle fascia is released for approximately 4 cm distally into the muscle. The deep fascia over the nerve is released to open the distal area of compression. The nerve is followed from proximal to distal to ensure that no additional areas of compression remain. One key point to remember for in situ decompression is that the nerve itself is not released from the fascial attachments deep to the nerve and is, therefore, not mobilized. This step helps to prevent later subluxation of the nerve, which may result in painful snapping of the nerve over the medial epicondyle (Figure 2).

### Anterior Subcutaneous Transposition

In anterior subcutaneous transposition, a longitudinal incision is made immediately anterior to the medial epicondyle. The ulnar nerve is

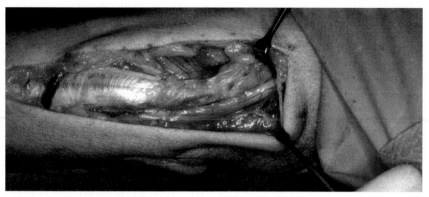

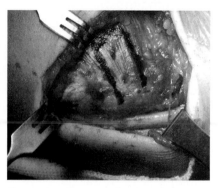

**Figure 2**  Photograph shows in situ decompression. Anterior subluxation of the ulnar nerve is shown after complete in situ ulnar nerve release.

**Figure 3**  Photograph shows the creation of a fascial flap using the anterior subcutaneous transposition procedure.

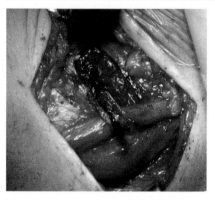

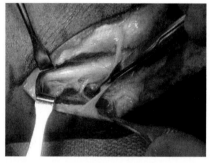

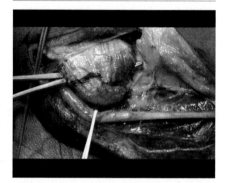

**Figure 4**  Using the anterior subcutaneous transposition procedure, the ulnar nerve is held in place and prevented from subluxation by the fascial flap.

**Figure 5**  Using the anterior submuscular transposition procedure, the nerve is released through the cubital tunnel and into the flexor carpi ulnaris. The medial antebrachial branches are identified and protected.

**Figure 6**  Using the anterior submuscular transposition procedure, the flexor pronator origin is released from the medial epicondyle distal to the insertion of the ulnar collateral ligament.

exposed by opening the cubital tunnel and by following the nerve proximally to the level of the tourniquet and distally into the FCU muscle. It is important to fully mobilize the nerve 4 to 5 cm proximal to the epicondyle and 4 to 5 cm distal to the medial epicondyle into the FCU. The medial intermuscular septum is released from its attachment to the medial epicondyle and a portion is excised. This step prevents kinking of the nerve during anterior transposition because this area is a potential iatrogenic point of nerve compression after surgery. A pocket is created from fascia or subcutaneous fat to avoid the complication of subluxation of the nerve back into the

cubital groove (Figure 3). The nerve should lie anteriorly under the fascial flap without enduring tension or compression (Figure 4).

## Anterior Submuscular Transposition

Learmonth[34] first described submuscular transposition in 1942. The theoretic advantage of this procedure is that all areas of nerve compression are released during the procedure, which permits the nerve to lie in an unscarred anatomic plane. Deep to the flexor-pronator origin, the nerve is held in an intermuscular interval with a good vascular bed, protecting the nerve from external compressive forces. This aspect

makes this technique appropriate for throwing athletes because of the increased need to protect the nerve from trauma. The nerve lies in a relatively straight line and is therefore less subject to tension. The procedure is technically more demanding, and care is required to prevent the creation of new sites of constriction from scarring around the nerve (Figures 5 through 8).

## Medial Epicondylectomy

Medial epicondylectomy for the treatment of cubital tunnel syndrome removes two potential impinging structures: the proximal FCU arcade and the pulley effect of the medial epicondyle. Removing the medial epicondyle pulley allows gentle anterior movement of the nerve with flexion and avoids devascularization and kinking.

The elbow is flexed and the upper extremity is abducted and externally rotated on the hand table. After incision, care is taken to prevent damage to the medial antebrachial cutaneous nerve during dissection. The ulnar nerve is exposed by incising the cubital tunnel roof. The nerve is released proximally and distally, and the medial intermuscular septum is released from its attachment to the medial epicondyle. The nerve is released at approximately 4 cm into the FCU. The nerve is then protected, and a subperiosteal dissection of the flexor-pronator origin is done to expose the medial epicondyle (Figure 9). An oscillating saw or osteotome is then used to remove approximately 1 to 1.5 cm of bone (Figure 10). Removing a larger portion of bone presents the risk of destabilizing the elbow by releasing all or part of the medial collateral ligament. It is advisable to reattach the muscle origin with the elbow in extension to minimize the postoperative risk of elbow flexion contracture.[34,35]

### Modified In Situ Decompression

Many reports discuss treatment options for failed surgical management of cubital tunnel syndrome.[1,36-38] Because of variations in pathology that are found at the time of surgical exploration, it is usually necessary to vary surgical technique to suit the physical needs and body habitus of the patient.[4,12,14,39] Whereas in situ decompression has been recommended for patients with mild compression,[5,27-33] a modification of in situ decompression is an excellent choice for a select group of patients with compression isolated to the

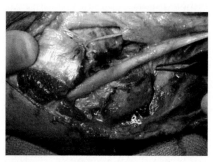

**Figure 7** The ulnar nerve is transposed anterior to the medial epicondyle, deep to the flexor-pronator origin during the anterior submuscular transposition procedure.

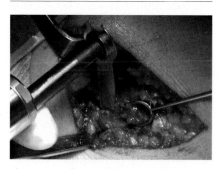

**Figure 9** The medial epicondyle is exposed subperiosteally during medial epicondylectomy. Approximately 1 to 1.5 cm of medial epicondyle is removed, using an oscillating saw or an osteotome. The nerve is carefully protected behind a retractor throughout the procedure.

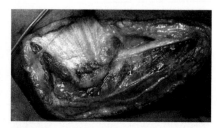

**Figure 8** Using the anterior submuscular transposition procedure, the flexor-pronator origin is repaired, ensuring that the nerve is not compressed or restricted by a suture.

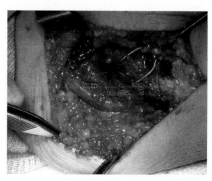

**Figure 10** With the medial epicondylectomy procedure, the bone is smoothed and the periosteum repaired before wound closure. The elbow is taken through flexion and extension to ensure that the nerve can roll freely, without kinking or snapping over the residual medial epicondyle.

aponeurosis and fascial band at the origin of the FCU distal to the medial epicondyle. It is quick, easy, and requires minimal dissection and little disturbance to the nerve.

In an attempt to more accurately determine the exact site or sites of nerve compression, Miller[22] and others evaluated patients (over a 22-month period) with symptoms of ulnar nerve compression of the cubital tunnel using a modified electrodiagnostic testing technique.[25,33,40] Motor and sensory conduction velocities were first performed in a standard fashion, evaluating the ulnar nerve both across the elbow and from below the elbow to the wrist. A

standard distance of 10 cm across the elbow, with the elbow flexed 90°, was used.[22] With surface electrodes placed over the abductor digiti quinti muscle, compound muscle action potential was recorded, and sensory responses were then recorded from the small finger using surface electrodes separated by 2 cm. Patients were again evaluated using an inching technique, in which the stimulator was moved along the nerve in several steps to detect focal sites of compression. The nerves were studied in three 2-cm segments: segment 1, proximal to the medial epicondyle; segment 2, across the medial epicondyle; and segment 3,

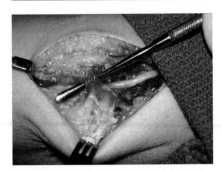

**Figure 11** Using the modified in situ decompression technique, a 1-cm portion of the aponeurosis is left intact to prevent anterior subluxation of the ulnar nerve during elbow flexion. An instrument is placed under the tissue to ensure that the nerve is completely free.

distal to the medial epicondyle. Miller[22] showed that prolongation of latency in segment 3, which is 2-cm distal to the medial epicondyle, localizes the area of compression to the area at the origin of the FCU.

In a study of 59 symptomatic arms (41 patients) for which the standard in situ decompression technique was used, 34 arms were found to have slowing of conduction across the elbow segment.[36] By adding the inching technique, 51 segments were found to have evidence of compression, for a mean of 1.5 compressed segments per nerve; 19 had compression through segment 1, 19 in segment 2, and 14 in segment 3. Seven patients had evidence of compression isolated to segment 3, and surgery was recommended. Of these seven patients, two declined surgery, and five had decompression of the nerve with a modified in situ decompression technique. Twenty of the 34 arms had surgical release of the ulnar nerve. As noted earlier, 5 of these arms had decompression of the nerve with a modified in situ decompression technique; the remaining 15 arms were decompressed by

either medial epicondylectomy or submuscular transposition.

Using the inching technique, of the 25 symptomatic arms initially believed to have normal conduction of the ulnar nerve across the 10-cm elbow segment, 17 were found to have segmental compression of the nerve. A total of 22 segments were compressed. An average of 1.3 segments had slowing of the ulnar nerve across one of the segments at the elbow; 8 had slowing in segment 1, 7 in segment 2, and 7 in segment 3. Four arms only had slowing in segment 3 and were decompressed using the modified in situ technique. An additional four arms were treated by decompression and medial epicondylectomy or by submuscular transposition. Eight of the symptomatic arms had normal NCV studies, both across the elbow and by inching techniques. None of these arms had surgical release.

### Technique Description

The modified in situ decompression technique is advantageous in preventing subluxation of the ulnar nerve over the medial epicondyle after release, which often occurs after in situ decompression.[36] After placing and inflating the tourniquet, an incision approximately 6 cm in length is made anterior to the medial epicondyle, parallel to the ulna with the elbow extended. Care should be taken not to injure the small branches of the medial brachial or the medial antebrachial cutaneous nerves. The medial epicondyle is exposed, allowing identification of the ulnar nerve proximally. The nerve is released proximally through the medial intermuscular septum, and a portion of the medial intermuscular septum is released from its attachment to the medial epicondyle to prevent compression or kinking of the nerve with

elbow flexion. The aponeurosis spanning the interval between the medial epicondyle and the olecranon is identified and isolated but not completely released (Figure 11).

The aponeurotic band converging with the thick fibrous arcade of the FCU muscle is released immediately distal to the medial epicondyle, allowing visualization of the nerve in this area. The muscle is divided distally, splitting the two heads of the FCU to at least the midportion of the proximal third of the forearm and thereby releasing all constricting deep fascial bands within the muscle found compressing the nerve. Care is taken not to damage the branches of the ulnar nerve to the FCU and ulnar half of the flexor profundus. There is commonly a second constricting fascial band deep within the substance of the FCU, located 1 to 2 cm distal to the proximal fibrous arcade; this band also must be released. The nerve is usually found to be flattened and hyperemic within this area.

Attention is then directed to the unreleased portion of nerve at the medial epicondyle. The nerve is carefully dissected free from the overlying aponeurosis (which is now approximately 1 to 1.5 cm in length), and the aponeurosis is dissected free from any surrounding tissue, which may be adherent and may be causing restriction of this area during elbow flexion. The nerve portion within the region of the cubital tunnel should now be fully visualized. The nerve is carefully examined to ensure that no compression of the nerve under the remaining portion of aponeurosis or roof remains. After release, no constriction of the nerve under the ligament should exist; the nerve should be free in both extension and flexion (Figure 12). The surgeon should check to ensure that the nerve does not subluxate over the medial epicondyle with full elbow flexion and that the nerve remains free.

When evidence of continued nerve compression or nerve subluxation over the medial epicondyle during passive elbow flexion is seen, use of this procedure is not appropriate. Childress[41] reported that, in 12% of asymptomatic individuals, the ulnar nerve moved onto the tip of the medial epicondyle when the elbow was flexed to or beyond 90°, and the nerve completely passed across and anterior to the epicondyle in 4% of that group. Eversman[42] noted that the incidence of subluxation after surgery can be decreased by limiting decompression to an area distal to a line drawn from the medial epicondyle to the olecranon. If the nerve is seen to subluxate, the remainder of the cubital tunnel is released, and a medial epicondylectomy, anterior transposition, or submuscular transposition is performed.

### Postoperative Management

Postoperatively, a long arm bulky dressing with plaster splint is used for 1 week, after which the patient is seen for a wound check and a dressing change. The long arm splint is discarded, and a cock-up volar wrist splint is used for an additional 1 to 2 weeks for comfort and to assist in healing the tissues at the elbow. Gentle elbow range-of-motion exercises are started at the first postoperative visit; strengthening exercises are not started for at least 3 weeks after surgery.

### Discussion

A high level of correlation was found between the clinical findings at the time of surgery and the findings of electrodiagnostic studies in those patients who underwent surgical decompression.[36] The addition of inching conduction studies of the ulnar nerve across the elbow aids in

preoperative evaluation and planning. At surgery, each patient was found to have a dense aponeurosis at the FCU origin, tightly constricting the nerve when the elbow was flexed to 90°. At release, the portion of the nerve segment that passed under the fibrous aponeurosis was constricted and hyperemic. None of the nerves subluxated at surgery. Postoperatively, all nine patients treated by modified in situ decompression had resolution of their pain, and eight of the nine had resolution of their paresthesias. One patient who had severe compression at surgery and marked slowing of nerve conduction (23 m/s) preoperatively had continued paresthesias for 6 months, which then resolved. This patient had severe intrinsic atrophy and abnormal two-point discrimination, which did not improve after nerve release. The eight remaining patients had normal two-point discrimination, both preoperatively and postoperatively. At an average follow-up of 18 months, none of the patients had worsening or a recurrence of their symptoms. The only patient in this group in whom electrodiagnostic studies were repeated after surgery also was the patient who showed poor response to decompression. Although this patient remained symptomatic when the electrodiagnostic studies were repeated at 3 months postoperatively, NCV improved but not to normal levels.

## Comparison of Techniques

A literature review on the surgical treatment of cubital tunnel syndrome shows that no single procedure is superior.[4,5,7-9,37,43-48] Foster and Edshage[45] compared in situ decompression with anterior subcutaneous transposition and found that both procedures provided equally good

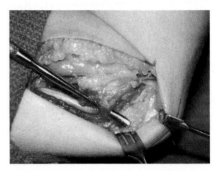

**Figure 12** During the modified in situ decompression technique, a probe is placed and the elbow is passively flexed to ensure that the nerve remains uncompressed and does not subluxate throughout all positions of elbow flexion.

results in relief of pain and dysesthesias. Transposition resulted in a greater incidence of complete relief from paresthesias than did in situ decompression (53% versus 36%, respectively), complete resolution of weakness (50% versus 35%, respectively), and complete resolution of muscle atrophy (43% versus 0%, respectively), although the differences between the results were not statistically significant.

Dellon[5] reported that 13 of 15 patients (90%) described as having minimal nerve compression obtained excellent results with any surgical procedure; however, simple decompression was rarely successful in patients with moderate compression. The modified in situ technique also worked best in those patients with abnormal electrodiagnostic studies defined by the inching technique but with normal or only mildly abnormal NCVs across the 10-cm elbow segment.

Manske and associates[49] reported relief of pain and dysesthesias in 22 of 27 patients (80%) treated with simple decompression. In 25 of the patients, the ulnar nerve was narrowed and hyperemic with adhesions. Of the five failed treatments with simple decompression, four were revised by anterior transposition; three of the four obtained only partial relief of symptoms.

Macnicol[28] found anterior transposition superior to simple decompression when adhesion of the nerve was present in the posterior condylar groove or when no abnormality of the nerve could be identified. For patients with little or no muscle involvement, Chan and associates[44] reported that 82% improved after simple decompression and anterior transposition; however, a higher percentage of full recovery was seen in those treated by simple decompression. Conversely, Heithoff[30] argued against transposition of the nerve, citing high complexity, numerous complications, and damage resulting from devascularization of the ulnar nerve. Other studies that compared in situ decompression with subcutaneous or submuscular transposition also have reported no statistically significant differences in outcome.[43]

Proponents of medial epicondylectomy have reported good to excellent results in several studies. Hicks and Toby[51] found that a strain of 5.3% of the ulnar nerve preoperatively only decreased to 4.3% after in situ decompression, whereas adding medial epicondylectomy resulted in a strain of –0.54%. They concluded that in situ decompression alone did not relieve the strain of the ulnar nerve at the elbow; however, by adding medial epicondylectomy, nerve strain was completely eliminated. Tomaino and associates[52] reported excellent relief of symptoms in a group of 16 patients (18 elbows) with electrodiagnostic-negative cubital tunnel syndrome treated with in situ release and medial epicondylectomy. In their meta-analysis on treatment of cubital tunnel syndrome, Mowlavi and associates[53] reported that medial epicondylectomy was the most successful surgical treatment for patients with minimal symptoms, but it produced the poorest results in patients with severe symptoms. Amako and associates[54] compared partial medial epicondylectomy (> 40% of the width of the medial epicondyle, which is approximately 10 mm from the tip of the epicondyle) in 14 patients with minimal medial epicondylectomy (< 20% of the width of the medial epicondyle, approximately 5 mm from the tip of the epicondyle) in 18 patients with ulnar nerve decompression for the treatment of cubital tunnel syndrome. Both groups had significant improvement in motor conduction velocity following medial epicondylectomy, with no significant difference in the improvement of motor conduction velocity between the two groups, although valgus instability of the elbow was significantly greater in the partial epicondylectomy group. They concluded that the combination of minimal medial epicondylectomy with ulnar nerve decompression is an effective treatment of cubital tunnel syndrome, and a larger excision of the medial epicondyle during this procedure should be avoided.

The most common complication after in situ decompression is failure to relieve symptoms, most often resulting from nerve compression at another level.[55] The addition of inching studies during electrodiagnostic testing adds diagnostic accuracy, thereby minimizing the risk of missing a second area of nerve compression. In one study, only 34 of 59 symptomatic arms had electrical evidence of nerve compression. By adding inching techniques, nerve compression was confirmed in an additional 17 arms, increasing the accuracy of the electrodiagnostic testing from 57.6% (34 of 59 arms) to 86% (51 of 59 arms).[36]

Modified in situ decompression is not indicated in all patients with compression of the ulnar nerve in the region of the cubital tunnel. It is recommended only for those patients with NCV studies that document slowing in the segment of the nerve as it passes into and through the proximal FCU muscle, distal to the medial epicondyle.[31,32,36] This method should be reserved for patients with mild abnormalities in nerve conduction, a nerve that does not subluxate with elbow flexion, and normal osseous anatomy. In patients undergoing this procedure, findings from the physical examination should correlate with other findings that provide the clinical picture; for example, a positive Tinel's sign or tenderness of the nerve at the insertion of the nerve into the FCU that has been identified from the physical examination should also be evident from clinical studies.

Advantages of the modified in situ technique include the ability to release the area of compression with minimal disturbance of the vascular supply to the nerve. Subluxation of the nerve, frequently seen after simple release, can lead to recurrence of symptoms as a result of repeated contusion of the nerve as it snaps over the medial epicondyle. By leaving a noncompressing portion of the aponeurosis intact, subluxation of the nerve is avoided. This is a safe and simple technique with minimal postoperative morbidity and quicker recovery than with other methods.

It is important, however, to be aware of the limitations of the technique. It is only recommended for a limited select group of patients and is not recommended for patients with preoperative evidence of subluxation of the ulnar nerve, radiographic evidence of osteophytes within the cubital tunnel or under the medial epicondyle, or those with rheumatoid arthritis with synovitis of the elbow joint causing extrinsic compression on the nerve. In situ decompression also would be contraindicated in patients with cubitus valgus as a cause of nerve palsy. In patients with any of these contraindications, one of the other described methods is preferred.

## Complications and Treatment Failure of Ulnar Nerve Surgery at the Elbow

Cubital tunnel surgery has an average 20% overall rate of failure, which can be defined as failure to relieve symptoms, with up to 35% of patients having residual symptoms at the surgical site after undergoing surgery.[56] Failed surgeries can be attributed to inaccurate diagnosis (nerve compression at another level), inadequate decompression, creation of iatrogenic compression, iatrogenic nerve injury, diabetes, peripheral neuropathy, scar formation, or nerve subluxation. Kinking of the ulnar nerve has been seen at reoperation for persistent cubital tunnel syndrome.[37]

Failure to completely release compression at the cubital tunnel or deep flexor origin is the most common cause for failed decompression. Rogers and associates[57] and others have reported incomplete release as the factor that is responsible for continued symptoms in 57% of their patients.[58] Iatrogenic compression of the nerve can occur at the medial intermuscular septum, with anterior transposition as a result of inadequate proximal and distal mobilization of the nerve, as well as kinking of the nerve over an unreleased septum.

Failures after medial epicondylectomy can result from several causes. The most common findings at reoperation are scarring of transposed nerve anterior to the medial epicondyle. Flexion contracture, which rarely exceeds 30°, can occur after submuscular transposition or medial epicondylectomy, with a reported incidence of up to 10%.[8,37] Flexion contracture usually responds to therapy, active range-of-motion treatment, and dynamic and static splinting. Occasionally, however, patients experience a permanent loss of extension.

Medial epicondylitis also occurs after medial epicondylectomy or submuscular transposition[59] and is typically treated successfully with heat, massage, and corticosteroid injection therapy; the use of a wrist splint to rest the flexor origin also helps to expedite pain relief. Persistent pain at the osteotomy site may be related to the completeness of the ostectomy.[7] Complete ostectomy, partial ostectomy, and minimal ostectomy result in 81%, 67%, and 40% good to excellent results, respectively.

When performing a medial epicondylectomy, or during submuscular transposition, nonunion of the epicondyle may occur. The ulnar collateral ligament lies below the common flexor origin, and medial elbow instability may occur as a result of detachment or division. O'Driscoll and associates[60] described the anatomy of the anterior medial collateral ligament as exclusively originating from the medial epicondyle and having no attachment to the condyle.

Flexor origin avulsion can be avoided by using subperiosteal dissection during medial epicondylectomy, with use of a wrist splint to protect the flexor-pronator origin for 3 to 6 weeks postoperatively after submuscular transposition.

Cutaneous neuromas are a common cause of continued pain after cubital tunnel surgery. The medial antebrachial cutaneous nerve may be injured or transected during exposure of the ulnar nerve. Careful dissection at the time of the original surgery is key to preventing nerve injury. Injury to the medial antebrachial cutaneous nerve has been reported in as many as 90% of patients who have persistent pain following cubital tunnel surgery. One to three branches course from the midbrachium to the medial epicondyle, olecranon, and posterior forearm. MacKinnon and associates[61] reported that injury to one of these three branches is the most common cause of sensitive elbow after cubital tunnel surgery.[26,57] Lowe and associates[62] showed that the posterior branch of the medial antebrachial cutaneous nerve courses in proximity to the cubital tunnel and is particularly prone to injury during ulnar nerve release at the elbow. Because of the potential for iatrogenic division of small branches of the medial antebrachial cutaneous nerve, Tomaino and associates[52] recommended formal neurolysis to facilitate exposure of the branches at the time of ulnar nerve surgery.

Revision surgery may be successful for relief of pain and paresthesias.[57] Indications for reoperation include significant pain (neuroma, nerve pain), progressive motor or sensory loss, and unimproved neurologic deficit with either no clinical improvement or worsening results on electrodiagnostic studies. Although nerve decompression in spite of normal NCV studies and electromyography has been reported to be successful, it is important to obtain preoperative nerve studies to have a baseline for comparison in patients in whom the outcome is less successful than desired.[52]

Caputo and Watson[63] reported 75% good to excellent results with secondary subcutaneous anterior transposition. Vogel and associates[64] reported that after revision surgery using anterior submuscular transposition, most patients had at least partial pain relief, with an overall satisfaction rate of 78%. Although these results are less favorable than those for the primary procedure, submuscular as well as simple anterior transposition have been reported as useful techniques for revision of failed cubital tunnel syndrome surgery.[57,63] Internal neurolysis has not been shown to improve the results of revision surgery.[64]

## Summary

Proponents of each surgical method used to treat cubital tunnel syndrome argue in favor of their chosen technique. In spite of the numerous options that are available, large numbers of patients have unsuccessful surgical treatments.[1,37,38] It is important to realize that no single technique is applicable to every patient. Because of variations in pathology, it is usually necessary to choose a surgical technique that is suited to the needs and body habitus of the individual patient and the pathology found at the time of surgical exploration.[4,12,14,39]

## References

1. Bednar MS, Blair SJ, Light TR: Complications of the treatment of cubital tunnel syndrome. *Hand Clin* 1994;10: 83-92.

2. Panas P: Sur une cause peu connue de paraysie du nerf cubtal. *Arch gen de Med* 1878;2 (viie serie):5.

3. Feindel W, Stratford J: The role of the cubital tunnel in tardy ulnar palsy. *Can J Surg* 1958;1:287-301.

4. Amadio PC: Anatomic basis for a technique of ulnar nerve transposition. *Surg Radiol Anat* 1986;8:155-161.

5. Dellon AL: Review of treatment results for ulnar nerve entrapment at the elbow. *J Hand Surg Am* 1989;14: 688-700.

6. Folberg CR: Cubital tunnel syndrome: Part II. Treatment. *Orthop Rev* 1994;23:233-241.

7. Heithoff SJ, Millender LH, Nalebuff EA, Petruska AJ Jr: Medial epicondylectomy for the treatment of ulnar nerve compression at the elbow. *J Hand Surg Am* 1990;15:22-29.

8. Janes PC, Mann RJ, Farnworth TK: Submuscular transposition of the ulnar nerve. *Clin Orthop Relat Res* 1989; 238:225-232.

9. Brown WF, Dellon AL, Campbell WW: Electrodiagnosis in the management of focal neuropathies: The "WOG" syndrome. *Muscle Nerve* 1994;17:1336-1342.

10. Kuschner SH: Cubital tunnel syndrome: Treatment by medial epicondylectomy. *Hand Clin* 1996;12: 411-419.

11. Rayan GM: Proximal ulnar nerve compression, cubital tunnel syndrome. *Hand Clin* 1992;8:325-336.

12. Vanderpool DW, Chalmeres J, Lamb DW, Whiston TB: Peripheral compressive lesions of the ulnar nerve. *J Bone Joint Surg Br* 1968;50:792-803.

13. Alvine FG, Schurrer ME: Postoperative ulnar-nerve palsy: Are there predisposing factors? *J Bone Joint Surg Am* 1987;69:255-259.

14. Apfelberg DB, Larson SJ: Dynamic anatomy of the ulnar nerve at the elbow. *Plast Reconstr Surg* 1973;51: 79-81.

15. Iba K, Wada T, Aoki M, et al: Intraoperative measurement of pressure adjacent to the ulnar nerve in patients with cubital tunnel syndrome. *J Hand Surg Am* 2006;31:553-558.

16. Werner CO, Ohlin P, Elmqvist D: Pressures recorded in ulnar neuropathy. *Acta Orthop Scand* 1985;56: 404-406.

17. Gelberman RH, Yamaguchi K, Hollstein SB, et al: Changes in interstitial pressure and cross-sectional area of the cubital tunnel and of the ulnar nerve with flexion of the elbow: An experimental study in human cadavera. *J Bone Joint Surg Am* 1998;80: 492-501.

18. Wilgis EF, Murphy R: The significance of longitudinal excursion in peripheral nerves. *Hand Clin* 1986;2: 761-766.

19. Wright TW, Lowczewski F, Cowin D, et al: Ulnar nerve excursion and strain at the elbow and wrist associated with upper extremity motion. *J Hand Surg Am* 2001;26:655-662.

20. Byl C, Puttlitz C, Byl N: Strain in the median and ulnar nerves during upper-extremity positioning. *J Hand Surg Am* 2002;27:1032-1040.

21. Rayan GM, Jensen C, Duke J: Elbow flexion test in the normal population. *J Hand Surg Am* 1992;17:86-89.

22. Miller RG: The cubital tunnel syndrome: Diagnosis and precise localization. *Ann Neurol* 1979;6:56-59.

23. Felsenthal G, Freed MJ, Kalafut R, Hilton EB: Across-elbow ulnar nerve sensory conduction technique. *Arch Phys Med Rehabil* 1989;70:668-672.

24. Idler RS: General principles of patient evaluation and nonoperative management of cubital tunnel syndrome. *Hand Clin* 1996;12:397-403.

25. Eisen A, Danon J: The mild cubital tunnel syndrome: Its natural history and indications for surgical intervention. *Neurology* 1974;24:608-613.

26. Dimond MI, Lister GD: Cubital tunnel syndrome treated by long-arm splintage. *J Hand Surg Am* 1985;10:432.

27. Lavyne MH, Bell WO: Simple decompression and occasional microsurgical epineurolysis under local anesthesia as treatment for ulnar neuropathy at the elbow. *Neurosurgery* 1982;11:6-11.

28. Macnicol MF: The results of operation for ulnar neuritis. *J Bone Joint Surg Br* 1979;61:159-164.

29. Miller RG, Hummel EE: The cubital tunnel syndrome: Treatment with simple decompression. *Ann Neurol* 1980;7:567-569.

30. Osborne G: Compression neuritis of the ulnar nerve at the elbow. *Hand* 1970;2:10-13.

31. Thomsen PB: Compression neuritis of the ulnar nerve treated with simple decompression. *Acta Orthop Scand* 1977;48:164-167.

32. Wilson DH, Krout R: Surgery of ulnar neuropathy at the elbow: 16 cases treated by decompression without transposition. *J Neurosurg* 1973;38:780-785.

33. Payan J: Electrophysiological localization of ulnar nerve lesions. *J Neurol Neurosurg Psychiatry* 1969;32:208-220.

34. Learmonth JR: A technique for transplanting the ulnar nerve. *Surg Gynecol Obstet* 1942;:792-793.

35. Craven PR, Green DP: Cubital tunnel syndrome: Treatment by medial epicondylectomy. *J Bone Joint Surg Am* 1980;62:986-989.

36. Gellman H, Campion D: Modified in-situ decompression of the ulnar nerve at the elbow. *Hand Clin* 1996;12:405-410.

37. Gabel GT, Amadio PC: Reoperation for failed decompression of the ulnar nerve in the region of the elbow. *J Bone Joint Surg Am* 1990;72:213-219.

38. Kleinman WB: Revision ulnar neuroplasty. *Hand Clin* 1994;10:461-477.

39. Amadio PC, Beckenbaugh RD: Entrapment of the ulnar nerve by the deep flexor-pronator aponeurosis. *J Hand Surg Am* 1986;11:83-87.

40. Eisen A: Early diagnosis of ulnar nerve palsy. *Neurology* 1974;24:256-262.

41. Childress HM: Recurrent ulnar nerve dislocation at the elbow. *Clin Orthop Relat Res* 1975;108:168-173.

42. Eversman WW: Complications of compression or entrapment neuropathies, in Bostwick JA (ed): *Complications in Hand Surgery*. Philadelphia, PA, WB Saunders, 1988, pp 99-115.

43. Adelaar RS, Foster WC, McDowell C: The treatment of cubital tunnel syndrome. *J Hand Surg Am* 1984;9:90-95.

44. Chan RC, Paine KW, Varughese G: Ulnar neuropathy at the elbow: Comparison of simple decompression and anterior transposition. *Neurosurgery* 1980;7:545-550.

45. Foster RJ, Edshage S: Factors related to the outcome of surgically managed compressive ulnar neuropathy at the elbow level. *J Hand Surg Am* 1981;6:181-192.

46. King T: The treatment of traumatic ulnar neuritis: Mobilization of the ulnar nerve at the elbow by removal of the medial epicondyle and adjacent bone. *Aust N Z J Surg* 1950;20:33-42.

47. Kleinman WB: Cubital tunnel syndrome: Anterior transposition as a logical approach to complete nerve decompression. *J Hand Surg Am* 1999;24:886-897.

48. King T, Morgan FP: Late results of removing the medial humeral epicondyle for traumatic ulnar neuritis. *J Bone Joint Surg Br* 1959;41:51-55.

49. Manske PR, Johnston R, Pruitt DL, et al: Ulnar nerve decompression at the cubital tunnel. *Clin Orthop Relat Res* 1992;274:231-237.

50. Heithoff SJ: Cubital tunnel syndrome does not require transposition of the ulnar nerve. *J Hand Surg Am* 1999;24:898-905.

51. Hicks D, Toby EB: Ulnar nerve strains at the elbow: The effect of in situ decompression and medial epicondylectomy. *J Hand Surg Am* 2002;27:1026-1031.

52. Tomaino MM, Brach PJ, Vansickle DP: The rationale and efficacy of surgical intervention for electrodiagnostic-negative cubital tunnel syndrome. *J Hand Surg Am* 2001;26:1077-1081.

53. Mowlavi A, Andrews K, Lille S, Verhulst S, Zook EG, Milner S: The management of cubital tunnel syndrome: A meta-analysis of clinical studies. *Plast Reconstr Surg* 2000;106:327-334.

54. Amako M, Nemoto K, Kawaguchi M, et al: Comparison between partial and minimal medial epicondylectomy combined with decompression for the treatment of cubital tunnel syndrome. *J Hand Surg Am* 2000;25:1043-1050.

55. Ferlic DC: Clinical assessment and conservative treatment of cubital tunnel syndrome, in Gelberman RH (ed): *Operative Nerve Repair and Reconstruction*. Philadelphia, PA, JB Lippincott, 1991, pp 1055-1061.

56. Jackson LC, Hotchkiss RN: Cubital tunnel surgery: Complications and treatment failures. *Hand Clin* 1996;12:449-456.

57. Rogers MR, Bergfield TG, Aulicino PL: The failed ulnar nerve transposition: Etiology and treatment. *Clin Orthop Relat Res* 1991;269:193-200.

58. Broudy AS, Leffert RD, Smith RJ: Technical problems with ulnar nerve transposition at the elbow: Findings at reoperation. *J Hand Surg Am* 1978;3:85-89.

59. Goldberg BJ, Light TR, Blair SJ: Ulnar neuropathy at the elbow: Results of medial epicondylectomy. *J Hand Surg Am* 1989;14:182-188.

60. O'Driscoll SW, Jaloszynski R, Morrey BF, et al: Origin of the medial ulnar collateral ligament. *J Hand Surg Am* 1992;17:164-168.

61. Mackinnon SE, Dellon AL, Hudson AR: A primate model for chronic nerve compression. *J Reconstr Microsurg* 1985;1:185-192.

62. Lowe JB, Maggi SP, Mackinnon SE: The position of crossing branches of the medial antebrachial nerve during surgery in humans. *Plast Reconstr Surg* 2004;114:692-696.

63. Caputo AE, Watson HK: Subcutaneous anterior transposition of the ulnar nerve for failed decompression of cubital tunnel syndrome. *J. Hand Surg Am* 2000;25:544-551.

64. Vogel RB, Nossaman BC, Rayan GM: Revision anterior submuscular transposition of the ulnar nerve for failed subcutaneous transposition. *Br J Plast Surg* 2004;57:311-316.

# Controversies in Carpal Tunnel Syndrome

Michael J. Botte, MD

## Abstract

*Compression of the median nerve at the wrist (carpal tunnel syndrome) is the most common compression neuropathy of the upper extremity. Surgical decompression has become one of the most frequently performed peripheral nerve procedures. Despite the popularity of the procedure, and the volume of clinical and basic science information available, differences of opinion exist as to diagnosis and management. This review discusses several of these controversies and presents both recent and historical data that have led to some of these disagreements.*

**Instr Course Lect 2008;57:199-212.**

Compression of the median nerve at the wrist (carpal tunnel syndrome [CTS]) was described by Paget in 1854 and Putnam in 1880.[1] Surgical decompression was suggested by Marie and Foix in 1913.[2] CTS was discussed further by Learmonth,[3] Cannon and Love,[4] and Phalen and associates[5-9] and has since become the most frequently recognized upper extremity nerve compression syndrome. Surgical decompression has become one of the most common and successful extremity procedures.[10-16] Despite its incidence and the volume of clinical and basic science information available, CTS generates controversy and questions regarding aspects of its diagnosis and management. Several of these questions form the basis for this discussion. Each question is sequentially addressed, with objective discussion based on data available from clinical and basic science investigations.

## What Are the Best Indicators for Evaluating CTS?

CTS remains primarily a clinical diagnosis, based on history and physi-

cal examination.[11-15] Patients' complaints are well recognized and include the classic pain or tenderness in the carpal tunnel area and the associated paresthesias or pain that radiates to the hand in the median nerve distribution (palmar thumb, index, long, and radial ring finger). There is often an associated feeling of weakness or clumsiness of the hand, with patients frequently dropping objects. Symptoms can be perceived as worse at night and are usually exacerbated with repetitive wrist motion. Additionally, placement of the wrist in a position of fixed or exaggerated flexion or extension often exacerbates symptoms. As nerve compression increases or becomes chronic, weakness and atrophy of the thenar muscles become more evident.

Physical examination includes inspection (for thenar atrophy), palpation of the carpal canal for tenderness, evaluation of sensibility and motor function, and the use of provocative tests.[11-31] Described methods of sensibility assessment have included evaluation by

Semmes-Weinstein monofilament measurements, vibrometry threshold evaluation, static two-point discrimination, and moving two-point discrimination. Early studies by Szabo, Gelberman, and associates have compared the efficacy of different methods[13,17-19]

### Sensibility Evaluation

Szabo[13] has divided sensibility testing into threshold tests (either Semmes-Weinstein monofilament testing or vibrometry evaluation) and innervation density tests (two-point discrimination and moving two-point discrimination). Threshold tests evaluate a single nerve fiber innervating a receptor or group of receptor cells, whereas innervation density tests measure multiple overlapping peripheral receptor fields and the density of the innervation in the region being tested. Innervation density tests may remain apparently normal in a patient with nerve compression as long as a few fibers are conducting normally to their correct cortical end points. The threshold tests, in general, are more consistent and reliable in the diagnosis of CTS. Studies on the clinical indicators of CTS have shown abnormal vibratory thresholds in 87%, abnormal monofilament testing in 83%, and abnormal two-point discrimination in only 22%.[13,17-19] Moving two-point discrimination offers no advantage in the determination of sensory abnormalities in CTS[13,18] (Figure 1).

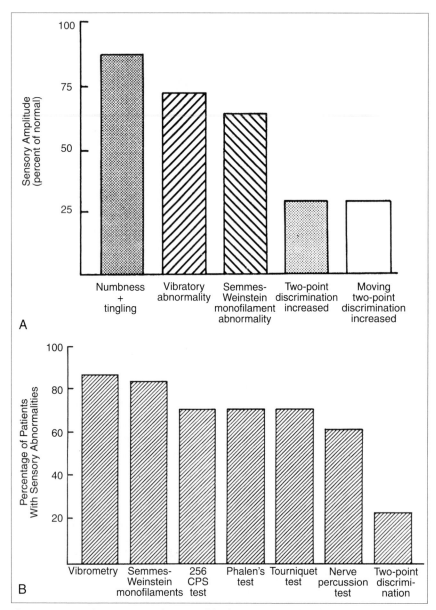

**Figure 1** **A,** Subjective complaints and findings compared with median sensory amplitude as a percentage of normal baseline amplitude (summary of data from 12 subjects tested using an experimentally controlled external compression device. (Reproduced with permission from Gelberman RH, Szabo RM, Williamson RV, Dimick MP: Sensibility testing in peripheral nerve compression syndromes: An experimental study in humans. *J Bone Joint Surg Am* 1983;65:632-638.) **B,** Results of preoperative sensory testing in 20 patients (23 hands) with CTS. The percentage of patients demonstrating a specific sensory abnormality is illustrated by the bar graphs. CPS = Cycles per second tuning fork test. (Reproduced with permission from Szabo RM, Gelberman RH, Dimick MP: Sensibility testing in patients with carpal tunnel syndrome. *J Bone Joint Surg Am* 1984;66:60-64.)

## Motor Evaluation

Motor weakness of the thenar muscles is a relatively late finding in CTS and usually does not occur until there is marked sensory loss. There may be dual innervation of the flexor pollicis brevis by the ulnar nerve as well; therefore, even with complete median nerve dysfunction, some thenar muscle function may remain. The abductor pollicis brevis is usually innervated only by the median nerve (without ulnar nerve contribution), and specific testing with palpation of this muscle may provide useful information.[14,15] Thenar atrophy is usually a late finding and indicates more chronic or severe nerve dysfunction. Isolated thenar atrophy with minimal sensibility loss may indicate specific compression of the recurrent motor branch of the median nerve.

### *Provocative Tests*

Provocative tests for CTS offer important adjuncts to the motor and sensibility evaluation.[11-15,20-32] Provocative tests include the Phalen test (wrist held in flexion for 60 seconds), Tinel sign (percussion of the median nerve at the carpal tunnel to produce paresthesias), the tourniquet test (tourniquet compression in the extremity), the manual forearm compression test,[28] the quantitative provocative diagnostic test using monofilament measurements with the wrist in neutral and in flexion,[29] and evaluation with wrist flexion combined with median nerve compression[30] (Table 1).

Phalen[8] originally found the wrist flexion test to be positive in 74% of patients with CTS. Others have found the Phalen test to be positive in 61% to 88% of patients with CTS and positive in 16% to 20% of normal patients.[20,21,25,29,31]

The Tinel percussion sign has been shown to have variable described sensitivities and specificities. Reported sensitivities have ranged from 14% to 74%, and specificities from 35% to 94%.[5-9,13,20,21,25,28,30] In comparing the Phalen test and Tinel sign, Gellman and associates[20] originally concluded that the Phalen test was the more sensitive and perhaps the more useful, with the Tinel sign less sensitive but more specific. Further studies have shown wide ranges in sensitivity and specificity.[9,13,21,25,28,30] These differences may be caused by variations in examiner technique. Kuschner and associates[21] have concluded that the Tinel sign alone was not useful in the diagnosis of CTS, but when it is combined with the Phalen test, there is a positive predictive value of 88%. The ranges of sensitivities and specificities of the Phalen test and Tinel sign are listed in Table 1.

Tourniquet provocative testing, described by Gilliatt and Wilson,[23] has been shown to have a 40% false positive rate.[13,20] With the newer, more sensitive and specific provocative tests, the tourniquet test no longer has useful clinical application and is mentioned here only for its historical significance.

The median nerve compression test, popularized by Durkan,[28] Williams and associates,[25] and Paley and McMurtry,[24] is performed by the examiner applying direct pressure over the palmar wrist or carpal tunnel for 15 to 120 seconds. The test is considered positive if a patient reports paresthesias in the distribution of the median nerve. Pain or subjective tenderness is not interpreted as a positive test. Reported values for sensitivity of this test have ranged from 23% to 100%, with specificity varying from 29% to 100%. Compression testing using a commercial device has been shown to have a sensitivity of 87% and specificity of 90%.[28]

A provocative test was introduced by Koris and associates[29] that combines the sensitivity of the Semmes-Weinstein monofilament measurements with the specificity of the wrist flexion provocational test. Monofilament measurements in patients with CTS were obtained with the wrist both in the neutral and flexed positions. The sensitivity was 82%, and the specificity was 86%. This combined test is among the most sensitive and specific quantitative clinical tests available.

An additional provocative test was introduced by Tetro and associates[30] that combines wrist flexion with manual median nerve compression. Their results indicate a sensitivity of 82% and a specificity of 99%, which is significantly improved to those of the Phalen or Tinel tests alone. This combined test appears to be the most sensitive and specific provocative test available for the diagnosis of CTS.

## Is There a Role for Ultrasound or MRI in CTS?

Diagnostic ultrasound has recently shown potential in providing data for the diagnosis of CTS. Wiesler and associates[33] have used high-resolution diagnostic ultrasound to demonstrate an increased cross-sectional area of the median nerve in patients with CTS. Bayrak and associates,[34] also using ultrasound, have noted cross-sectional area and morphology changes in patients with CTS. Although these studies are promising, they are preliminary, and the routine use of high-resolution ultrasound has yet to be established.

MRI has been valuable in anatomic studies of the wrist and carpal canal contents.[35-41] MRI has demonstrated anatomic changes in the carpal tunnel with wrist flexion and extension and has led to a better understanding of the dynamic nature of the carpal tunnel shape, cross-sectional area, and volume.[14,37-39] Richman and associates[40] have shown that the anteroposterior diameter of

| Table 1 |
|---|
| **Sensitivity and Specificity of Provocative Tests Used for CTS** |
| Phalen wrist flexion test |
|    Sensitivity 61% to 88% |
|    Specificity 80% to 84% |
| Tinel percussion sign |
|    Sensitivity 14% to 74% |
|    Specificity 35% to 94% |
| Median nerve (manual) compression test |
|    Sensitivity 23% to 100% |
|    Specificity 29% to 100% |
| Quantitative provocative diagnostic test: monofilament measurements with the wrist neutral and in flexion |
|    Sensitivity 82% |
|    Specificity 86% |
| Wrist flexion combined with median nerve compression |
|    Sensitivity 82% |
|    Specificity 99% |

the carpal tunnel increases after transection of the transverse carpal ligament and provide additional rationale for surgical management. From the standpoint of a diagnostic tool, MRI can help identify suspected space-occupying lesions such as benign tumors, proliferative tenosynovitis, anomalous muscles, or the extent of granulomatous infections. However, its routine use in the diagnosis of CTS has not been established.[35-41]

## What Is the Role of Electrodiagnostic Studies?

Electrodiagnostic studies consist of evaluating nerve conduction velocity (NCV) of the median nerve across the carpal tunnel and electromyography (EMG) of the thenar muscles.[42-56] Controversy exists as to the role and validity of electrodiagnostic studies in the routine diagnosis of CTS. Several authors and surgeons emphasize that carpal tunnel is a clinical syndrome,[11-15] and some question the need for electrodiagnostic studies for surgical decision making in CTS.[11,14] However, others note the value of these studies as an adjunct to history and physical examination, and, along with provocative tests, they provide a more complete collection of data for decision making.[13,51-53]

Although generally not used for initial diagnosis, electrodiagnostic studies provide a number of potential benefits. (1) NCV and EMG studies can confirm a suspected CTS diagnosis, if clinical findings are not entirely clear. (2) The studies can give insight as to suspected double-crush syndromes (such as concomitant cervical radiculopathy) or coexisting metabolic conditions (for example, diabetes) that can produce an overlying component of peripheral neuropathy. (3) Complete NCV studies, including measurement of velocity, amplitude, and latency, in addition to EMG studies of the thenar muscles, can help quantitate the severity of nerve compression. (4) NCV and EMG studies can provide a baseline for comparison of a slowly progressive syndrome, if studies are repeated in the future. (5) The studies can provide a baseline for comparison if the response to surgery is less than expected. (6) The studies are often regarded as definitive information or part of the "standard of care" in a medicolegal situation. A surgeon may be criticized if surgical treatment was performed without obtaining electrodiagnostic studies. (7) NCV and EMG studies are often required by insurance companies or workers' compensation evaluators to obtain approval for surgical management. (Unfortunately, workers' compensation boards can delay or not approve surgical management based on a negative electrodiagnostic study, regardless of clinical findings.)

Several studies support and promote electrodiagnostic studies as sensitive and objective tests used to diagnose CTS, with reported sensitivities up to 96.7%.[13,42-45,47-55] Jablecki and associates[45] performed a meta-analysis of electrodiagnostic studies and concluded that these tests are valid, reproducible, highly sensitive, and highly specific. Grundberg,[46] however, studied 292 patients with clinical CTS, and found 11.3% to have normal electrodiagnoistic studies. Others have found that 10% to 15% of patients with clinically evident and surgically relieved CTS had normal electrodiagnostic studies. False positive results can also occur, with abnormal studies obtained from patients without clinical symptoms.[42-56]

Inconsistences (including false positive and false negative results) associated with electrodiagnostic studies can occur from differences in electrodiagnostic standards, which may vary between investigators or institutions. The experience and techniques used by the electrodiagnostician may add additional variability to the quality or reproducibility of the examinations. In general, distal motor latencies of more than 4.5 ms and distal sensory latencies of more than 3.5 ms have been considered abnormal.[13] Asymmetry of conduction between both hands of more than 1 ms for motor conduction or 0.5 ms for sensory conduction time is also considered abnormal.[13] From the motor standpoint, electromyograms with positive waves or fibrillation in the thenar muscles suggest severe and chronic median nerve injury.

Despite the electrodiagnostic findings, CTS remains a clinical diagnosis. Surgical management should not be performed with a normal clinical examination and abnormal electrodiagnostic findings. Conversely, clear clinical symptoms in the face of normal electrodiagnostic findings may still warrant surgical management. Electrodiagnostic studies are valuable adjuncts to the clinical examination but not the definitive determining factor.

## What Are the Outcomes of Corticosteroid Injection?

Corticosteroid injection into the carpal canal was popularized by researchers[57,58] in the 1960s and has since been shown to be a successful adjunct in the management of CTS[57-68] (Figure 2). However, specific indications, optimal patient candidates, and long-term expectations are not always discussed or appreciated. About 80% to 90% of patients show initially improvement following injection. Results gradually deteriorate over time (Figure 2, A), with 50% to 90% eventually undergoing surgical treatment.[59-62,67,68]

Gelberman and associates[60] evaluated patients with CTS who received corticosteroid injection over a 2-year period. Initially, 90% obtained substantial improvement. However, by 24 months, only 8% maintained the improvement. In further examination of the patients and clinical responses, the investigators were able to predict the more optimal candidates for the procedure. Good candidates are, in general, those with milder symptoms and clinical findings. These favorable conditions include symptoms for less than 1 year, numbness that is diffuse and intermittent, normal two-point discrimination, no motor weakness or atrophy, 1- to 2-ms prolongations of distal motor and sensory latencies, and no denervations. When these more optimal candidates were evaluated, 40% were found to be symptom free longer

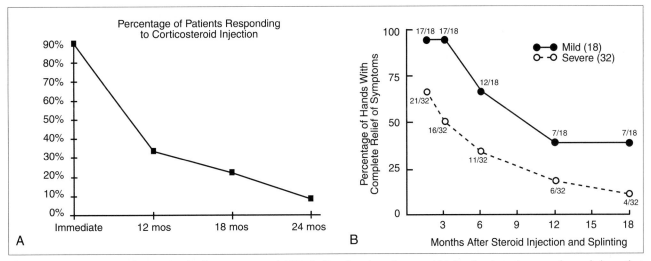

**Figure 2** Corticosteroid injection in the treatment of CTS. **A,** Results of corticosteroid injection into the carpal canal show that the response deteriorates over time. (Courtesy of Clayton A. Peimer, MD.) **B,** Results of corticosteroid injection and splinting in hands with mild versus severe CTS. Patients with the milder symptoms have more sustained relief. (Reproduced with permission from Gelberman R, Aronson D, Weisman M: Carpal-tunnel syndrome: Results of a prospective trial of steroid injection and splinting. *J Bone Joint Surg Am* 1980;62:1181-1184.)

than 1 year after the injection[60] (Figure 2, *B*).

Seror and associates[55] demonstrated initial improvement in the NCVs of patients treated with corticosteroid injection. However, the patients returned to the baseline preinjection level over time.[55] Those with initial milder changes in electrodiagnostic studies had a better response.

Green[62] found that a good response to injection indicated a good response to surgery in 94%. In addition, improvement after injection also confirms the diagnosis.[15]

Recently, Dammers and associates[68] evaluated the effectiveness of different doses of methylprednisolone in CTS in a randomized double-blind trial. They concluded that a single local injection of methylprednisolone using 20, 40, or 60 mg resulted in long-lasting improvement in approximately half the patients. There was slight improvement with a higher (60-mg) dose. A second injection could further re-

duce the number of patients requiring surgery.[68]

Median nerve injury is a potential complication associated with carpal tunnel injection, as initially noted by Phalen in 1966[8] and subsequently reported by others.[63-65,69] So that the procedure can be performed safely, Gelberman and other authors have discussed these procedures in detail[60,63-65] (Figure 3). The needle is inserted midway between the palmaris longus and flexor carpi ulnaris tendons just proximal to the transverse carpal ligament, in line with the flexor digitorum superficialis of the ring finger, and advanced 2 cm while angled 45° distally. The needle is removed and redirected if any paresthesias are encountered during either insertion or injection.[60,63,64]

## How Should CTS Be Managed in Pregnancy?

CTS is a recognized condition that may occur during pregnancy.[11,14,15,70-75] Approximately 20% of pregnant women have occasional symptoms

of CTS, although the reported incidence has been as high as 62%.[73] Bilateral symptoms occur in half of these patients. Positive physical examination findings are less frequent. Despite the number of women developing CTS symptoms, these findings are rarely noted in the patients' charts. Of 10,873 women with 14,574 pregnancies, a diagnosis of CTS was recorded in only 90 of the pregnancies; this is an incidence of only 0.34%.[70]

Symptoms arise most commonly in the third trimester and are associated with generalized edema.[73] Paresthesias are the most common symptom. Most symptoms resolve postpartum. Conservative management using wrist splints is usually adequate. Seven of 50 pregnant women with CTS failed to improve postpartum. Symptoms resolved following carpal tunnel release.[70] Residual mild symptoms usually respond to conservative care. Some patients continue with mild symptoms and require carpal tunnel

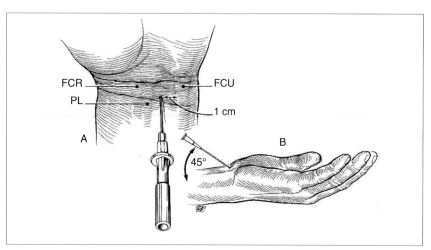

**Figure 3** Technique of carpal tunnel injection. **A,** A 22-gauge needle originally inserted 1 cm proximal to the distal wrist flexion crease through the flexor carpi radialis (FCR) tendon is now inserted just lateral to the ulnar artery for a greater margin of safety. **B,** The needle is angled 45° to 60° distally and advanced 2 cm through the flexor retinaculum, and the solution is injected. PL, palmaris longus; FCU, flexor carpi ulnaris. (Reproduced with permission from Gelberman RH, Rydevik BL, Pess GM, Szabo RM, Lundborg G: Carpal tunnel syndrome: A scientific basis for clinical care. *Orthop Clin North Am* 1988;19:115-124.)

release more than 2 years later. Padua and associates[74] noted that 54% of women with CTS symptoms during pregnancy had symptoms 1 year later. Patients with residual postpartum symptoms justify long-term follow-up.[71,74]

Very few patients have required carpal tunnel release in the third trimester. Relatively few data are available regarding the management of these patients. Local anesthesia should be considered over general anesthesia, and an attempt should be made to minimize systemic medications. The obstetrician and the pediatrician should be involved with all management plans.[11,14,15,70-75]

## Is There a Role for Oral Medications in the Treatment of CTS?

Oral medications used in the treatment of CTS have included nonsteroidal anti-inflammatory drugs (NSAIDs), diuretics, oral steroids, and vitamin $B_6$.[76-83] Although commonly recommended and used, NSAIDs alone have not been adequately evaluated or proven effective in the treatment of CTS. Diuretics have also been used in the treatment of CTS, but in the absence of other conditions, the effectiveness of diuretics for CTS has not been adequately evaluated.

Oral steroids may have a role in the treatment of CTS. Chang and associates[76] performed a prospective, randomized, double-blind placebo-controlled study of patients with CTS. The study compared 4 weeks of oral placebo treatment to tenoxicam (NSAID), trichlormethiazide (diuretic), and prednisolone (20 mg daily for 2 weeks followed by 10 mg daily for 2 weeks). In these patients with clinical and electrodiagnostically established CTS, only the steroid-treated group had a statistically significant improvement in a global symptom scale that rated pain, numbness, paresthesias, weakness, and clumsiness. Patients treated with diuretic or NSAID did not show significant improvement.[15,76]

Subclinical vitamin $B_6$ deficiency was proposed as a possible cause of CTS in the 1980s.[77-80] Ellis and associates[77,78] subsequently reported significant improvement in patients with CTS treated with pyridoxine. This established a treatment rationale for vitamin $B_6$ treatment in CTS. Other investigators were unable to reproduce the findings of Ellis. Subsequent well-controlled studies by Amadio,[81] Stransky and associates,[83] and Spooner and associates[82] failed to show improvement in CTS symptoms with vitamin $B_6$ treatment. Currently, pyridoxine as a treatment of CTS does not seem justified, unless the patient has a known vitamin $B_6$ deficiency. The efficacy of its treatment remains unproven, and routine evaluation of vitamin $B_6$ is probably not warranted in patients with CTS. Unfortunately, vitamin $B_6$ as a treatment of carpal tunnel is still used or advocated occasionally in the literature and frequently by the lay press.

## What Is the Natural History of Untreated CTS?

North and Kaul[14] noted that there are few studies providing insight into untreated CTS. Futami and associates[84] noted that approximately one third of patients had resolution of their symptoms within 5 months without specific treatment. Observation and reassurance may be sufficient for patients who have had a recent onset of mild symptoms or those with very transient symptoms. Conversely, Seror and associates[55] found no improvement in NCV studies of nine patients not treated. Of those treated with various nonsurgical methods, approximately two thirds did not gain sustained improvement. Poor prognostic indicators include symptoms of greater than 6 months duration, the presence of thenar muscle atrophy, and older age groups.[85] Kaplan and associates[86] found that age older than 50 years was a poor prognostic indicator. However, others note that age did not, by itself, affect the ultimate clinical result.[55,87] Age as a factor may be related to the findings that patients older than 70 years who present with CTS may have severe or chronic CTS, but pain may not be as prominent a symptom in elderly patients.[88]

## What Is the Value of or Indication for Neurolysis or Epineurotomy?

For several years, neurolysis or epineurotomy of the median nerve was discussed, recommended, or performed at the time of carpal tunnel release for patients with more severe conditions.[4,89-95] Many had suggested neurolysis for patients who had either refractory or severe symptoms or those with marked atrophy of the thenar muscles. Lister[91] recommended epineurotomy when there was scarring noted of the epineurium and around the fascicles. In the mid-1980s, however, the effectiveness of neurolysis or epineurotomy was questioned. Several authors noted no consistent benefit from neurolysis[95-99] or from epineurotomy.[100-102] Additionally, others have suggested that routine neurolysis may harm the median nerve by either mechanical nerve injury, disruption of the longitudinal vessels that traverse the internal epineurium, or promotion of additional fibrosis.[99,103] Based on

more recent studies, routine use of neurolysis or epineurotomy does not seem warranted.[95-102]

## When Should Tenosynovectomy Be Performed?

Tenosynovectomy at the time of carpal tunnel release has been advocated as a means to "debulk" the carpal tunnel and remove any potential space-occupying tissue that could encroach on the median nerve. In 1989, tenosynovectomy was recommended as the sole surgical treatment of CTS (M. Melvin, MD, Seattle, WA, unpublished data, 1989). A distal forearm incision was used, and the transverse carpal ligament was left intact. In 105 patients, less hand tenderness and a rapid return to work were noted following this procedure. All patients were cured of pain, and all but four had resolution of numbness. These results have not been reproduced. When the transverse carpal ligament is released, routine tenosynovectomy has not been shown to be beneficial and has been associated with an increase in infection[104] and stiffness. As early as 1966, routine flexor tenosynovectomy was discouraged by Phalen.[8] In a prospective randomized study of 88 wrists, Shum and associates[105] noted that there was no benefit from routine tenosynovectomy with open carpal tunnel release.

Tenosynovectomy at the time of release of the transverse carpal ligament is indicated only for invasive, proliferative tenosynovitis, as seen in rheumatoid arthritis or gout, granulomatous infection (from atypical bacterial or fungal infections), or markedly thickened tenosynovium from amyloid deposition in dialysis patients.[11-15]

## What Are the Risks and Benefits of the Different Methods of Decompression (Open Versus Endoscopic Release)?

Perhaps the most currently debated controversy in the treatment of CTS involves the aspects of open carpal release (including limited open techniques) versus endoscopic carpal tunnel release. There are advantages and disadvantages to each method, and each has its advocates.[106-172]

In the 1980s, recommended incisions for carpal tunnel release usually extended proximally to the distal forearm, crossing the wrist crease.[106,107,111,113,114] Some authors advocated extensile exposure for complete nerve decompression or to allow tenosynovectomy as needed. The distal portion of the deep antebrachial fascia was often visualized and incised as well as the transverse carpal ligament. Subsequently, patients often reported a painful incision, especially at the base of the palm. The area of pain, often referred to as "pillar pain," was especially evident when the hand was used to push off with the wrist extended. Scar contracture across the wrist crease was an additional concern. These symptoms related to the incision initially prompted the development of generally shorter incisions. Two newer techniques were developed: (1) the endoscopic carpal tunnel release and (2) the "limited-open" carpal tunnel release.

Endoscopic carpal tunnel release using a single incision was introduced by Okutsu and associates[108] in 1987 and further developed and popularized by Agee and associates,[117,134] Menon,[112,118] Tsai and associates,[120] Murphy,[119] and others[121,125,139,150] (Figure 4). Chow[116] described the double portal technique

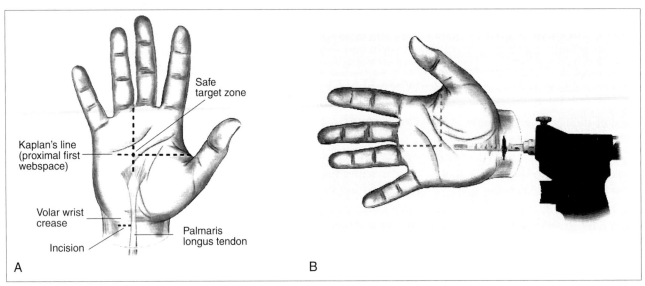

**Figure 4** Single portal endoscopic carpal release as popularized by Agee and associates, showing placement of the incision (**A**) followed by insertion of the Agee endoscopic device (**B**) before transverse carpal ligament division. (Reproduced with permission from Akelman E: Carpal tunnel syndrome, in Berger RA, Weiss AP (eds): *Hand Surgery.* Philadelphia, PA, Lippincott Williams & Wilkins, 2004, pp 867-885.)

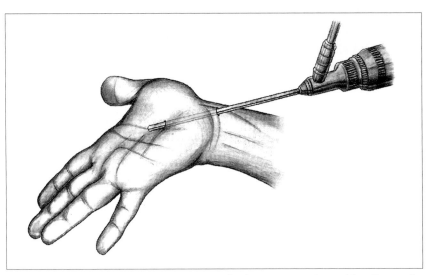

**Figure 5** Double portal endoscopic carpal release as popularized by Chow. The endoscope is placed in the proximal opening of the tube. (Reproduced with permission from Akelman E: Carpal tunnel syndrome, in Berger RA, Weiss AP (eds): *Hand Surgery.* Philadelphia, PA, Lippincott Williams & Wilkins, 2004, pp 867-885.)

(Figure 5). Endoscopic techniques, which required the development of specialized equipment, were shown to be effective, required much smaller incisions, and could avoid incision in the palm over the high-contact area (pillar area).[108-110,116-120,124,125,128]

During development of the endoscopic carpal tunnel release, an additional method was used, using a very limited open incision.[129,130,147,160,162] This method (often referred to as the "mini-open" technique) required special-

ized equipment, used an open but minimal incision, and did not violate the skin of the base of the palm. It was shown to be effective. A popular method, the "SafeGuard" technique, was described by Baratz and Bragdon[129] (Figure 6).

When comparing the traditional open technique of carpal tunnel release to the endoscopic carpal tunnel release to the "mini-open" carpal tunnel release, results and opinions vary. Endoscopic and mini-incision techniques seem to have similar reliability and temporal courses as standard open techniques.[117,119,128,137] Pillar pain may still develop secondary to the transection of the transverse carpal ligament. Some series have been unable to demonstrate any statistically significant difference between patients who undergo open versus mini or endoscopic carpal tunnel release.[132,133] However, most randomized prospective studies support the findings of less midpalmar tenderness and earlier return to work using the endoscopic or mini-open techniques[134,135,138] (Figure 7).

Several authors have brought attention to the potential higher complication rates using endoscopic techniques.[131,165-168] Of particular concern is injury to the ulnar nerve and its branches. In addition, injury to the median nerve, common digital nerves, superficial palmar arch, ulnar artery, and flexor tendon injury have been reported.[131,165-168] Conversely, some recent studies indicate that complications of endoscopic carpal tunnel release are no more frequent than those using open techniques.[161,169]

The benefits of endoscopic and mini-incision techniques decrease with time, and final results seem to be similar to the carpal tunnel release. Investigators have stressed the required learning curve for these techniques, and recent developments have allowed safer procedures. Both endoscopic and mini-open techniques seem to be safe if performed by a surgeon who has become proficient in these techniques. The techniques should probably be avoided by the surgeon who only performs them rarely or sporadically.

## Summary

The two most sensitive and specific provocative tests available for carpal tunnel evaluation are (1) monofilament measurements combined with manual wrist flexion and (2) manual wrist flexion combined with manual compression of the median nerve. Diagnostic ultrasound can be useful for showing changes in nerve morphology in patients with CTS, but its routine use in diagnosis has not been established. MRI evaluation of the carpal tunnel can identify anatomy and abnormal morphology in diseased states, but routine use in diagnosing CTS is not justified. Elec-

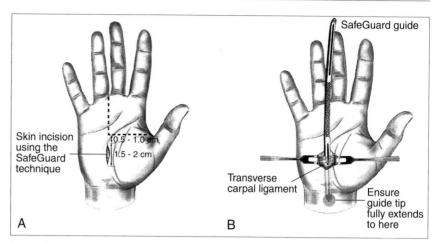

**Figure 6** Limited open carpal tunnel release popularized by Baratz and Bragdon. **A,** Placement of the limited incision. **B,** The SafeGuard guide (KMI, San Diego, CA) facilitates transection of the transverse carpal ligament. (Reproduced with permission from Akelman E: Carpal tunnel syndrome, in Berger RA, Weiss AP (eds): *Hand Surgery.* Philadelphia, PA, Lippincott Williams & Wilkins, 2004, pp 867-885.)

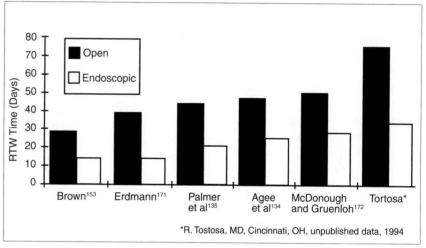

**Figure 7** The results of several studies comparing the return-to-work times (RTW) following carpal tunnel release by open versus endoscopic techniques. (Courtesy of Clayton A. Peimer, MD.)

trodiagnostic studies are valuable adjuncts to the clinical examination, but the final diagnosis of CTS is based primarily on the clinical examination.

Corticosteroid injection into the carpal tunnel can be initially effective, although symptoms often recur within 24 months. Longer-lasting results occur in patients with less severe symptoms. CTS in a pregnant patient will usually resolve in the postpartum period, and surgery is rarely needed. Although NSAIDs, diuretics, vitamin $B_6$, and oral steroids have been used as part of a medical regimen, only oral steroids provide significant improvement. Neurolysis, epineurotomy, or flexor tenosynovectomy should not be used routinely to treat CTS but may have a role in specific disease states.

Open carpal release and endoscopic carpal tunnel release are effective surgical treatments. Endoscopic carpal release may provide earlier return to work, but the risks of complications appear to be greater.

## References

1. Putnam J: A series of cases of paresthesia, mainly of the hand, of periodic recurrence, and possibly of vasomotor origin. *Arch Med* 1880;4:147.

2. Marie P, Foix C: Atrophie isolee de l'eminence thenar d' origine nervitique: Role du ligament annulaire anterieur du carpe dans les pathogenie de la lesion. *Rev Neurol* 1913;26:647.

3. Learmonth J: The principle of decompression in the treatment of certain diseases of peripheral nerves. *Surg Clin North Am* 1933;13:905.

4. Cannon B, Love J: Tardy median palsy: Median neuritis amenable to surgery. *Surgery* 1946;20:210-216.

5. Phalen G, Gardner W, LaLonde A: Neuropathy of the median nerve due to compression beneath the transverse carpal ligament. *J Bone Joint Surg Am* 1950;32:109.

6. Phalen G: Spontaneous compression of the median nerve at the wrist. *JAMA* 1951;145:1128.

7. Phalen G, Kendrick J: Compression neuropathy of the median nerve in the carpal tunnel. *JAMA* 1957; 164:524.

8. Phalen GS: The carpal tunnel syndrome: Seventeen years' experience in diagnosis and treatment of six hundred fifty-four hands. *J Bone Joint Surg Am* 1966;48:211-228.

9. Phalen GS: The carpal tunnel syndrome: Clinical evaluation of 598 hands. *Clin Orthop Relat Res* 1972;83: 29-40.

10. Hanrahan LP, Higgins D, Anderson H, Smith M: Wisconsin occupational carpal tunnel syndrome surveillance: The incidence of surgically treated cases. *Wis Med J* 1993;92:685-689.

11. Von Schroeder HP, Botte MJ: Carpal tunnel syndrome. *Hand Clin* 1996;12: 643-655.

12. Botte MJ, von Schroeder HP, Abrams RA, Gellman H: Recurrent carpal tunnel syndrome. *Hand Clin* 1996;12:731-743.

13. Szabo RM: Carpal tunnel syndrome, in Szabo RM (ed): *Nerve Compression Syndromes: Diagnosis and Treatment.* Thorofare, NJ, SLACK, 1989, pp 101-120.

14. North ER, Kaul MP: Compression neuropathies: Median, in Peimer CA (ed): *Surgery of the Hand and Upper Extremity.* New York, NY, McGraw-Hill, 1996, pp 1307-1336.

15. Akelman E: Carpal tunnel syndrome, in Berger RA, Weiss APC (eds): *Hand Surgery.* Philadelphia, PA, Lippincott Williams & Wilkins, 2004, pp 867-885.

16. Gelberman RH, North ER: Carpal tunnel release, in Gelberman RH (ed): *Operative Nerve Repair and Reconstruction.* Philadelphia, PA, JB Lippincott, 1991, pp 899-912.

17. Gelberman RH, Szabo RM, Williamson RV, Dimick MP: Sensibility testing in peripheral nerve compression syndromes: An experimental study in humans. *J Bone Joint Surg Am* 1983;65: 632-638.

18. Szabo RM, Gelberman RH, Dimick MP: Sensibility testing in patients with carpal tunnel syndrome. *J Bone Joint Surg Am* 1984;66:60-64.

19. Szabo RM, Gelberman RH, Williamson RV, Dellon AL, Yaru NC, Dimick MP: Vibratory sensory testing in acute peripheral nerve compression. *J Hand Surg Am* 1984;9: 104-109.

20. Gellman H, Gelberman RH, Tan AM, Botte MJ: Carpal tunnel syndrome: An evaluation of the provocative diagnostic tests. *J Bone Joint Surg Am* 1986;68:735-737.

21. Kuschner SH, Ebramzadeh E, Johnson D, et al: Tinel's sign and Phalen's test in carpal tunnel syndrome. *Orthopedics* 1992;15:1297-1302.

22. De Smet L: Value of some clinical provocative tests in carpal tunnel syndrome: Do we need electrophysiology and can we predict the outcome? *Hand Clin* 2003;19:387-391.

23. Gilliatt R, Wilson T: A pneumatic tourniquet test in the carpal tunnel syndrome. *Lancet* 1953;265:595-597.

24. Paley D, McMurtry R: Median nerve compression test in carpal tunnel syndrome diagnosis reproduces sign and symptoms in affected wrist. *Orthop Rev* 1985;14:411.

25. Williams TM, MacKinnon SE, Novak CB, et al: Verification of the pressure provocative test in carpal tunnel syndrome. *Ann Plast Surg* 1992;29:8-11.

26. Palumbo CF, Szabo RM: Examination of patients for carpal tunnel syndrome sensibility, provocative, and motor testing. *Hand Clin* 2002;18: 269-277.

27. Dellon AL: Management of peripheral nerve problems in the upper and lower extremity using a quantitative sensory testing. *Hand Clin* 1999;15: 697-715.

28. Durkan JA: A new diagnostic test for carpal tunnel syndrome. *J Bone Joint Surg Am* 1991;73:535-538.

29. Koris M, Gelberman RH, Duncan K, Boublick M, Smith B: Carpal tunnel syndrome: Evaluation of a quantitative prevocational diagnostic test. *Clin Orthop Relat Res* 1990;251:157-161.

30. Tetro AM, Evanoff BA, Hollstien SB, Gelberman RH: A new provocative test for carpal tunnel syndrome: Assessment of wrist flexion and nerve compression. *J Bone Joint Surg Br* 1998;80:493-498.

31. Seror P: Phalen's test in the diagnosis of carpal tunnel syndrome. *J Hand Surg Br* 1988;13:383-385.

32. Seror P: Tinel's sign in the diagnosis of carpal tunnel syndrome. *J Hand Surg Br* 1987;12:364-365.

33. Wiesler ER, Chloros GD, Cartwright MS, et al: The use of diagnostic ultrasound in carpal tunnel syndrome. *J Hand Surg Am* 2006;31:726-732.

34. Bayrak IK, Bayrak AO, Tilki HE, Nural MS, Sunter T: Ultrasonography in carpal tunnel syndrome: Comparison with electrophysiological stage and motor unit number estimate. *Muscle Nerve* 2007;35:344-348.

35. Jarvik JG, Kliot M, Maravilla KR: MR nerve imaging of the wrist and hand. *Hand Clin* 2000;16:13-24.

36. Zeiss J, Skie M, Ebraheim N, et al: Anatomic relations between the median nerve and flexor tendon in the carpal tunnel: MR evaluation in normal volunteers. *AJR Am J Roentgenol* 1989;153:533-536.

37. Garcia-Elias M, Sanchez-Freijo J, Salo J, et al: Dynamic changes of the transverse carpal arch during flexion-extension of the wrist: Effects of sectioning the transverse carpal ligament. *J Hand Surg Am* 1992;17:1017-1019.

38. Yoshioka S, Okuda Y, Tamai K, et al: Changes in carpal tunnel shape during wrist joint motion: MRI evaluation of normal volunteers. *J Hand Surg Br* 1993;18:620-623.

39. Skie M, Zeiss J, Ebraheim N, et al: Carpal tunnel changes and median nerve compression during wrist flexion and extension seen by magnetic resonance imaging. *J Hand Surg Am* 1990;15:934-939.

40. Richman JA, Gelberman RH, Rydevik BL, et al: Carpal tunnel syndrome: Morphologic changes after release of the transverse carpal ligament. *J Hand Surg Am* 1989;14:852-857.

41. Siegel S, White LM, Brahme S: Magnetic resonance imaging of the musculoskeletal system: Part 5. The wrist. *Clin Orthop Relat Res* 1996;332:281-300.

42. Kopell HP, Goodgold J: Clinical and electrodiagnostic features of carpal tunnel syndrome. *Arch Phys Med Rehabil* 1968;49:371-375.

43. Ghavanini MR, Haghijhat M: Carpal tunnel syndrome: Reappraisal of five clinical tests. *Electromyogr Clin Neurophysiol* 1998;38:437-441.

44. Aulisa L, Tamburrelli F, Padua R, et al: Carpal tunnel syndrome: Indication for surgical treatment based on electrophysiologic study. *J Hand Surg Am* 1998;23:687-691.

45. Jablecki CK, Andary MT, So YT, Wilkins DE, Williams FH: Literature review of the usefulness of nerve conduction studies and electromyography for the evaluation of patients with carpal tunnel syndrome. *Muscle Nerve* 1993;16:1392-1414.

46. Grundberg AB: Carpal tunnel decompression in spite of normal electromyography. *J Hand Surg Am* 1983;8:348-349.

47. Braun RM, Jackson WJ: Electrical studies as a prognostic factor in the surgical treatment of carpal tunnel syndrome. *J Hand Surg Am* 1994;19:893-900.

48. Concannon MJ, Gainor B, Petroski GF, Puckett CL: The predictive value of electrodiagnostic studies in carpal tunnel syndrome. *Plast Reconstr Surg* 1997;100:1452-1458.

49. Glowacki KA, Breen CJ, Sachar K, Weiss AP: Electrodiagnostic testing and carpal tunnel release outcome. *J Hand Surg Am* 1996;21:117-121.

50. Choi SJ, Ahn DS: Correlation of clinical history and electrodiagnostic abnormalities with outcome after surgery for carpal tunnel syndrome. *Plast Reconstr Surg* 1998;102:2374-2380.

51. Hilburn JW: General principles and use of electrodiagnostic studies in carpal and cubital tunnel syndromes: With special attention to pitfalls and interpretation. *Hand Clin* 1996;12:205-221.

52. Kilmer DD, Davis BA: Electrodiagnosis in carpal tunnel syndrome. *Hand Clin* 2002;18:243-255.

53. Harris CM, Tanner E, Goldstein MN, Pettee DS: The surgical treatment of the carpal-tunnel syndrome correlated with preoperative nerve-conduction studies. *J Bone Joint Surg Am* 1979;61:93-98.

54. Prakash KM, Fook-Chong S, Leoh TH, et al: Sensitivities of sensory nerve conduction study parameters in carpal tunnel syndrome. *J Clin Neurophysiol* 2006;23:565-567.

55. Seror P, Bectarte M, Mortier J: Carpal tunnel syndrome: Electrophysiological aspects of treated and untreated cases. *Rev Chir Orthop Reparatrice Appar Mot* 1988;74:466-472.

56. Goodwill CJ: The carpal tunnel syndrome: Long-term follow-up showing relation of latency measurements to response to treatment. *Ann Phys Med* 1965;10:12-21.

57. Foster JB: Hydrocortisone and the carpal tunnel syndrome. *Lancet* 1960;1:454-456.

58. Goodman HV, Foster JB: Effect of local corticosteroid injection on median nerve conduction in carpal tunnel syndrome. *Ann Phys Med* 1962;6:287-294.

59. Wood MR: Hydrocortisone injections for carpal tunnel syndrome. *Hand* 1980;12:62-64.

60. Gelberman RH, Aronson D, Weisman MH: Carpal-tunnel syndrome: Results of a prospective trial of steroid injection and splinting. *J Bone Joint Surg Am* 1980;62:1181-1184.

61. Girlanda P, Datola R, Venuto C, et al: Local steroid treatment in idiopathic carpal tunnel syndrome: Short- and long-term efficacy. *J Neurol* 1993;240:187-190.

62. Green DP: Diagnostic and therapeutic value of carpal tunnel injection. *J Hand Surg Am* 1984;9:850.

63. Gelberman RH, Rydevik BL, Pess GM, Szabo RM, Lundborg G: Carpal tunnel syndrome: A scientific basis for clinical care. *Orthop Clin North Am* 1988;19:115-124.

64. Frederick HA, Carter PR, Littler JW: Injection injuries to the median and ulnar nerves at the wrist. *J Hand Surg Am* 1992;17:645-647.

65. Kay NR, Marshall PD: A safe, reliable method of carpal tunnel injection. *J Hand Surg Am* 1992;17:1160-1161.

66. Weiss AP, Sachar K, Gendreau M: Conservative management of carpal tunnel syndrome: A reexamination of steroid injection and splinting. *J Hand Surg Am* 1994;19:410-415.

67. Dammers JW, Veering MM, Vermuelen M: Injection with methylprednisolone proximal to the carpal tunnel: Randomized double blind trial. *BMJ* 1999;319:884-886.

68. Dammers JW, Roos Y, Veering MM, Vermuelen M: Injection with methylprednisolone in patients with the carpal tunnel syndrome: A randomized double blind trial testing three different doses. *J Neurol* 2006;253:574-577.

69. McConnell JR, Bush D: Intraneural steroid injection as a complication in the management of carpal tunnel syndrome: A report of three cases. *Clin Orthop Relat Res* 1990;250:181-184.

70. Stolp-Smith KA, Pascoe MK, Ogburn PL: Carpal tunnel syndrome in pregnancy: Frequency, severity, and prognosis. *Arch Phys Med Rehabil* 1998;79: 1285-1287.

71. al Qattan MM, Manktelow RT, Bowen CV: Pregnancy-induced carpal tunnel syndrome requiring surgical release longer than 2 years after delivery. *Obstet Gynecol* 1994;84:249-251.

72. Ritchie JR: Orthopedic considerations during pregnancy. *Clin Obstet Gynecol* 2003;46:456-466.

73. Padua L, Aprile I, Caliandro P, et al: Symptoms and neurophysiological picture of carpal tunnel syndrome in pregnancy. *Clin Neurophysiol* 2001; 112:1946-1951.

74. Padua L, Aprile I, Caliandro P, et al: Carpal tunnel syndrome in pregnancy: Multiperspective follow-up of untreated cases. *Neurology* 2002;59: 1643-1646.

75. Weimer LH, Yin J, Lovelace RE, Gooch CL: Serial studies of carpal tunnel syndrome during and after pregnancy. *Muscle Nerve* 2002;25: 914-917.

76. Chang MH, Chang HT, Lee SSJ, et al: Oral drug of choice in carpal tunnel syndrome. *Neurology* 1998;51: 390-393.

77. Ellis J, Folkers K, Watanabe T, et al: Clinical results of a cross-over treatment of pyridoxine and placebo of carpal tunnel syndrome. *Am J Clin Nutr* 1979;32:2040-2046.

78. Ellis JM, Folkers K, Levy M, et al: Response of vitamin B6 deficiency and the carpal tunnel syndrome to pyridoxine. *Proc Natl Acad Sci USA* 1982; 79:7494-7498.

79. Fuhr JE, Farrow A, Nelson H: Vitamin B6 levels in patients with carpal tunnel syndrome. *Arch Surg* 1989;124: 1329-1330.

80. Byers CM, Delisa JA, Frankel DL, Kraft GH: Pyridoxine metabolism in carpal tunnel syndrome with and without peripheral neuropathy. *Arch Phys Med Rehabil* 1984;65:712-716.

81. Amadio PC: Pyridoxine as an adjunct in the treatment of carpal tunnel syndrome. *J Hand Surg Am* 1985;10: 237-241.

82. Spooner GR, Desai HB, Angel JF, Reeder BA, Donat JR: Using pyridoxine to treat carpal tunnel syndrome: Randomized control trial. *Can Fam Physician* 1993;39:2122-2127.

83. Stransky M, Rubin A, Lava N, et al: Treatment of carpal tunnel syndrome with vitamin B6: A double blind study. *South Med J* 1989;82:841.

84. Futami T, Kobayashi A, Wakabayshi N, et al: Natural history of carpal tunnel syndrome. *J Jpn Soc Surg Hand* 1992;9:128-130.

85. Mühlau G, Both R, Kunath H: Carpal tunnel syndrome: Course and prognosis. *J Neurol* 1984;231:83-86.

86. Kaplan SJ, Glickel SZ, Eaton RG: Predictive factors in the non-surgical treatment of carpal tunnel syndrome. *J Hand Surg [Br]* 1990;15:106-108.

87. Fardin P, Negrin P, Carteri A: Clinical and electromyographical considerations on 150 cases of carpal tunnel syndrome. *Acta Neurol Scand* 1979; 73:121.

88. Seror P: Carpal tunnel syndrome in the elderly. *Ann Chir Main Memb Super* 1991;10:217-225.

89. Curtis RM, Eversmann WW Jr: Internal neurolysis as an adjunct to the treatment of the carpal tunnel syndrome. *J Bone Joint Surg Am* 1973;55: 733-740.

90. Eversmann WW Jr, Ritsick JA: Intraoperative changes and motor nerve conduction latency in carpal tunnel syndrome. *J Hand Surg Am* 1978;3: 77-81.

91. Lister G: Compression, in Lister G (ed): *The Hand: Diagnosis and Indications*, ed 3. Edinburgh, Scotland, Churchill Livingstone, 1993, pp 283-322.

92. Cseuz KA, Thomas JE, Lambert EH, Love JG, Lipscomb PR: Long-term results of operation for carpal tunnel syndrome. *Mayo Clin Proc* 1966;41: 232-241.

93. Rietz KA, Onne L: Analysis of sixty-five operative cases of carpal tunnel syndrome. *Acta Chir Scand* 1967;133: 443-447.

94. Mackinnon SE, Dellon AL: Carpal tunnel syndrome, in Mackinnon SE, Dellon AL (eds): *Surgery of the Peripheral Nerve*. New York, NY, Thieme Medical Publishers, 1988, pp 149-169.

95. Lowry WE Jr, Follender AB: Interfascicular neurolysis in the severe carpal tunnel syndrome: A prospective randomized, double blind controlled study. *Clin Orthop Relat Res* 1988;227: 251-254.

96. Holmgren-Larsson H, Leszniewski W, Linden U, et al: Internal neurolysis of ligament division only in carpal tunnel syndrome: Results of a randomized study. *Acta Neurochir (Wien)* 1985;74:118-121.

97. Rhoades CE, Mowery CA, Gelberman RH: Results of internal neurolysis of the median nerve for severe carpal tunnel syndrome. *J Bone Joint Surg Am* 1985;67:253-256.

98. Gelberman RH, Pfeffer GB, Galbraith RT, et al: Results of treatment of severe carpal tunnel syndrome without internal neurolysis of the median nerve. *J Bone Joint Surg Am* 1987;69:896-903.

99. Rydevik B, Lundborg G, Nordborg C: Interneural tissue reactions induced by internal neurolysis. *Scand J Plast Reconstr Surg* 1976;10:3-8.

100. Foulkes GD, Atkinson RE, Beuchel C, Doyle JR, Singer DI: Outcome following epineurotomy and carpal tunnel syndrome: A prospective randomized clinical trial. *J Hand Surg Am* 1994;19:539-547.

101. Blair WF, Goetz DD, Ross MA, Steyers CM, Chang P: Carpal tunnel release with and without epineurotomy: A comparative prospective trial. *J Hand Surg Am* 1996;21:655-661.

102. Leinberry CF, Hamond NL III, Seigfried JW: The role of epineurotomy in the operative treatment of carpal tunnel syndrome. *J Bone Joint Surg Am* 1997;79:555-557.

103. Spinner M: *Injuries to Major Branches of Peripheral Nerves in the Forearm*, ed 2. Philadelphia, PA, WB Saunders, 1978.

104. Hanssen AD, Amadio PC, DeLilva SP, Ilstrup DM: Deep postoperative wound infection after carpal tunnel release. *J Hand Surg Am* 1989;14: 869-873.

105. Shum C, Parisien M, Strauch RJ, Rosenwasser MP: The role of flexor tenosynovectomy in the operative treatment of carpal tunnel syndrome. *J Bone Joint Surg Am* 2002;84:221-225.

106. Burton R, Littler JW: Nontraumatic soft tissue affliction of the hand, in *Current Problems in Surgery*. Chicago, IL, Year Book Medical Publishers, 1975.

107. Jabaley ME: Personal observations on the role of the lumbrical muscles in carpal tunnel syndrome. *J Hand Surg Am* 1978;3:82.

108. Okutsu I, Ninomiya S, Takatori Y, et al: Endoscopic management of carpal tunnel syndrome. *Arthroscopy* 1989;5:11-18.

109. Chow JC: Endoscopic release of the carpal ligament: A new technique for carpal tunnel syndrome. *Arthroscopy* 1989;5:19-24.

110. Chow JC: Endoscopic release of the carpal ligament for carpal tunnel syndrome: 22-month clinical result. *Arthroscopy* 1990;6:288-296.

111. McFarland GB: Entrapment syndromes, in Evarts CM (ed): *Surgery of the Musculoskeletal System*, ed 2. New York, NY, Churchill Livingstone, 1990, pp 961-981.

112. Menon J: Endoscopic release of carpal ligaments. *Arthroscopy* 1991;7:413-414.

113. Beckenbaugh RD: Carpal tunnel syndrome, in Cooney WP, Linscheid RL, Dobyns JH (eds): *The Wrist: Diagnosis and Operative Treatment*. St. Louis, MO, Mosby, 1998, pp 1197-1233.

114. Szabo RM: Entrapment and compression neuropathies, in Green DP, Hotchkiss RN, Pederson WC (eds): *Green's Operative Hand Surgery*, ed 4. New York, NY, Churchill Livingstone, 1999, pp 1404-1447.

115. Okutsu I, Hamanaka I, Tanabe T, Takatori Y, Ninomiya S: Complete endoscopic carpal tunnel decompression. *Am J Orthop* 1996;25:365-368.

116. Chow JC: Endoscopic carpal tunnel release, two-portal technique. *Hand Clin* 1994;10:637-646.

117. Agee JM, McCarroll HR, North ER: Endoscopic carpal tunnel release using the single proximal incision technique. *Hand Clin* 1994;10:647-659.

118. Menon J: Endoscopic carpal tunnel release: Preliminary report. *Arthroscopy* 1994;10:31-38.

119. Murphy MS: Distal one portal carpal tunnel release. *Atlas Hand Clin* 2002:1-7.

120. Tsai TM, Tsuruta T, Syed SA, Kimura H: A new technique for endoscopic carpal tunnel decompression. *J Hand Surg Br* 1995;20:465-469.

121. Mirza MA, King ET, Tanveer S: Palmar uniportal extrabursal endoscopic carpal tunnel release. *Arthroscopy* 1995; 11:82-90.

122. Bozentka DJ, Osterman AL: Complications of endoscopic carpal tunnel release. *Hand Clin* 1995;11:91-95.

123. Steinberg DR, Szabo RM: Anatomy of the median nerve at the wrist: Open carpal tunnel release: Classic. *Hand Clin* 1996;12:259-269.

124. Fischer TJ, Hastings H II: Endoscopic carpal tunnel release: Chow technique. *Hand Clin* 1996;12:285-297.

125. Ruch DS, Poehling GG: Endoscopic carpal tunnel release: The Agee technique. *Hand Clin* 1996;12:299-303.

126. Urbaniak JR, Desai SS: Complications of nonoperative and operative treatment of carpal tunnel syndrome. *Hand Clin* 1996;12:325-335.

127. Szabo RM: Acute carpal tunnel syndrome. *Hand Clin* 1998;14:419-429.

128. Chow JC: Endoscopic release of the carpal ligament for carpal tunnel syndrome: Long-term results using the Chow technique. *Arthroscopy* 1999;15: 417-421.

129. Baratz ME, Bragdon G: Limited open carpal tunnel release using the Safeguard system. *Atlas Hand Clin* 2002: 15-22.

130. Lee WP, Plancher KD, Strickland JW: Carpal tunnel release with a small palmar incision. *Hand Clin* 1996;12: 271-284.

131. Murphy RX Jr, Jennings JF, Wukich DK: Major neurovascular complications of endoscopic carpal tunnel release. *J Hand Surg Am* 1994;19: 114-118.

132. Bande S, DeSmet L, Fabry G: The results of carpal tunnel release: Open versus endoscopic technique. *J Hand Surg Br* 1994;19:14-17.

133. Gibbs KE, Rand W, Ruby LK: Open versus endoscopic carpal tunnel release. *Orthopedics* 1996;19:1025-1028.

134. Agee JM, McCarroll HR Jr, Tortosa RD, et al: Endoscopic release of the carpal tunnel: A randomized prospective multicenter study. *J Hand Surg Am* 1992;17:987-995.

135. Palmer DH, Paulson JC, Lane-Larsen CL, Peulen VK, Olson JD: Endoscopic carpal tunnel release: A comparison of two techniques with open release. *Arthroscopy* 1993;9:498-508.

136. Lewicky RT: Endoscopic carpal tunnel release: The guide tube technique. *Arthroscopy* 1994;10:39-49.

137. Nagle D, Harris G, Foley M: Prospective review of 278 endoscopic carpal tunnel release using the modified Chow technique. *Arthroscopy* 1994;10:259-265.

138. Kerr CD, Gittins ME, Sybert DR: Endoscopic versus open carpal tunnel release: Clinical results. *Arthroscopy* 1994;10:266-269.

139. Berger RA: Endoscopic carpal tunnel release: A current perspective. *Hand Clin* 1994;10:625-636.

140. Cobb TK, Knudson GA, Cooney WP: The use of topographical landmarks to improve the outcome of Agee endoscopic carpal tunnel release. *Arthroscopy* 1995;11:165-172.

141. Nagle DJ, Fischer TJ, Harris GD, et al: A multicenter prospective review of 640 endoscopic carpal tunnel releases using the transbursal and extrabursal Chow techniques. *Arthroscopy* 1996;12:139-143.

142. Jebson PJ, Agee JM: Carpal tunnel syndrome: Unusual contraindications to endoscopic release. *Arthroscopy* 1996;12:749-751.

143. Del Pinal F, Cruz-Camara A, Jado E: Total ulnar nerve transection during endoscopic carpal tunnel release. *Arthroscopy* 1997;13:235-237.

144. Makowiec RL, Nagle DJ, Chow JC: Outcome of first-time endoscopic carpal tunnel release in a teaching environment. *Arthroscopy* 2002;18:27-31.

145. Szabo RM: Open carpal tunnel release is the preferred method of surgical treatment for carpal tunnel syndrome. *J Bone Joint Surg Am* 2002;84:1489.

146. Steinberg DR: Surgical release of the carpal tunnel. *Hand Clin* 2002;18:291-298.

147. Higgins JP, Graham TJ: Carpal tunnel release via limited palmar incision. *Hand Clin* 2002;18:299-306.

148. Nagle DJ: Endoscopic carpal tunnel release. *Hand Clin* 2002;18:307-313.

149. Braun RM, Rechnic M, Fowler E: Complications related to carpal tunnel release. *Hand Clin* 2002;18:347-357.

150. Trumble TE, Diao E, Abrams RA, et al: Single-portal endoscopic carpal tunnel release compared with open release: A prospective randomized trial. *J Bone Joint Surg Am* 2002;84:1107-1115.

151. Ferdinand RD, MacLean JG: Endoscopic versus open carpal tunnel release in bilateral carpal tunnel syndrome: A prospective, randomized, blinded assessment. *J Bone Joint Surg Br* 2002;84:375-379.

152. Wong KC, Hung LK, Ho PC, et al: Carpal tunnel release. A prospective, randomized study of endoscopic versus limited-open methods. *J Bone Joint Surg Br* 2003;85:863-868.

153. Brown LG: Endoscopic compared with open carpal tunnel release. *J Bone Joint Surg Am* 2003;85:964.

154. Kuschner SH: Endoscopic compared with open carpal tunnel release. *J Bone Joint Surg Am* 2003;85:1167.

155. Meals RA: Endoscopic compared with open carpal tunnel release. *J Bone Joint Surg Am* 2003;85:1168-1169.

156. Tuzuner S, Sherman GM, Ozkaynak S, et al: Endoscopic carpal tunnel release: Modification of Menon's technique and data from 191 cases. *Arthroscopy* 2004;20:721-727.

157. Kwok TG, Huang CH, Kao HC: Endoscopic carpal tunnel release using a new median nerve protector. *Arthroscopy* 2004;20:841-847.

158. Nagaoka M, Nagoa S, Matsuzake H: Endoscopic release for carpal tunnel syndrome accompanied by thenar muscle atrophy. *Arthroscopy* 2004;20:848-850.

159. Teoh LC, Tan PL: Endoscopic carpal tunnel release for recurrent carpal tunnel syndrome after previous open release. *Hand Surg* 2004;9:235-239.

160. Cellocco P, Rossi C, Bizzarri F, et al: Mini-open blinded procedure versus limited open techniques for carpal tunnel release: A 30-month follow-up study. *J Hand Surg Am* 2005;30:493-499.

161. Benson LS, Bare AA, Nagle DJ, et al: Complications of endoscopic and open carpal tunnel release. *Arthroscopy* 2006;22:919-924.

162. Alizadeh K, Lahiji F, Phalsaphy M: Safety of carpal tunnel release with a short incision: A cadaver study. *Acta Orthop Belg* 2006;72:415-419.

163. Nagaoka M, Nagao S, Matsuzaki H: Endoscopic carpal tunnel release in the elderly. *Minim Invasive Neurosurg* 2006;49:216-219.

164. Siegmeth AW, Hopkinso-Woolley JA: Standard open decompression in carpal tunnel syndrome compared with a codified open technique preserving the superficial skin nerves: A prospective randomized study. *J Hand Surg Am* 2006;31:1483-1489.

165. Arner M, Hagberg L, Rosen B: Sensory disturbances after two-portal endoscopic carpal tunnel release: A preliminary report. *J Hand Surg Am* 1994;19:548-551.

166. De Smet L, Fabry G: Transection of the motor branch of the ulnar nerve as a complication of tow-portal endoscopic carpal tunnel release: A case report. *J Hand Surg Am* 1995;20:18-19.

167. Stark R: Ulnar nerve transection as a complication of two-portal endoscopic carpal tunnel release. *J Hand Surg Am* 1994;19:522-523.

168. Nath RK, Mackinnon S, Weeks P: Ulnar nerve transection as a complication of two-portal endoscopic carpal tunnel release: A case report. *J Hand Surg Am* 1993;18:896-898.

169. Oertel J, Schroeder H, Gaab M: Dual-portal endoscopic release of the transverse ligament in carpal tunnel syndrome: Results of 411 procedures with special reference to technique, efficacy, and complications. *Neurosurgery* 2006;59:333-340.

170. Brown RA, Gelberman RH, Seiler JG III, et al: Carpal tunnel release: A prospective randomized assessment of open and endoscopic methods. *J Bone Joint Surg Am* 1993;75:1265-1275.

171. Erdmann MW: Endoscopic carpal tunnel decompression. *J Hand Surg Br* 1994;19:5-13.

172. McDonough JW, Gruenloh TJ: A comparison of endoscopic and open carpal tunnel release. *Wis Med J* 1993;92:675-677

# Adult Reconstruction: Hip

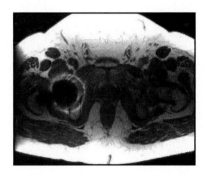

# Minimally Invasive Total Hip Arthroplasty: An Overview of the Results

*Paul J. Duwelius, MD
*Lawrence D. Dorr, MD

## Abstract

*Small-incision total hip arthroplasty (THA) has been shown to be safe and effective in achieving early postoperative improvements in pain and function. The comparative published reports of the two-incision, anterior, and mini-posterior techniques have defined indications for small-incision THAs. The mini-posterior approach appears to be better than the traditional posterior approach for THA in terms of early patient function and acceptance. There may be little difference among the mini-incision techniques when preoperative patient education and postoperative rehabilitation are equivalent.*

*Correct component positioning has been consistently achieved with small-incision procedures, and short-term results are the same as those of traditional THA. The mini-posterior approach also has been shown to have psychological advantages because it allows patients to be more confident about their outcomes. New anesthesia and pain management techniques have also improved early functional results. With time and technical advances such as computer navigation, the use of minimally invasive THA will become more prevalent.*

**Instr Course Lect 2008;57:215-222.**

The focus of minimally invasive surgery (MIS) is to reduce pain in the early postoperative period, which helps to improve immediate function. MIS does not change the basic principles of total hip arthroplasty (THA) and should not affect long-term outcomes. Although the media has been criticized for promoting minimally invasive THA, in reality, it has been popularized by patients because MIS creates a positive psychological experience for the patient.[1] Multiple recent studies suggest that patient satisfaction with MIS is very high.[2-7]

The benefits of MIS compared with traditional surgical approaches in THA have been questioned because there is no conclusive scientific data that confirm physical benefits for patients as measured by traditional scoring instruments.[2,8,9] Because THA done through traditional long incisions has proven results, it is understandable that some surgeons are reluctant to change to small-incision surgery.[10] Much of the skepticism is caused by a misunderstanding of the goals and benefits of MIS, which is simply a new surgical approach and not a new operation. There was skepticism when the posterior approach replaced the trochanteric osteotomy approach to THA; however, trochanteric osteotomy is now no longer used for primary surgery.

Small-incision surgery gives patients more hope that the desired outcomes will be achieved.[7] Patients want pain relief and functional improvement, but true satisfaction with any orthopaedic procedure is not achieved until the patient's psychosocial goals are met.[11-15] Patients want independence and to regain their normal lifestyle.[15,16] MIS gives patients more confidence that they can achieve their goals and expectations. MIS must be shown to be as safe as traditional THA with minimal complications. This chapter will use evidence-based data to establish

*Paul J. Duwelius, MD and Lawrence D. Dorr, MD or the departments with which they are affiliated have received research or institutional support and royalties from Zimmer.

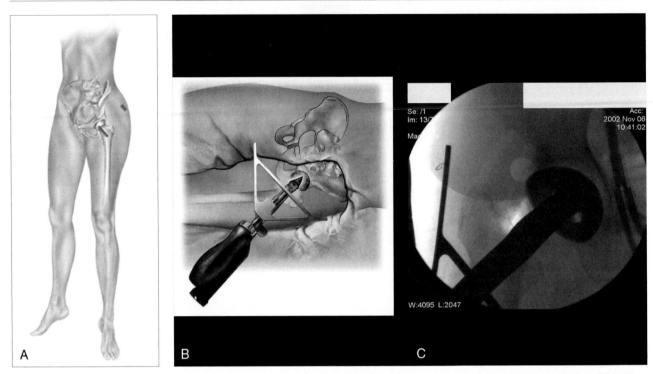

**Figure 1**    **A,** The two-incision surgical technique is performed with the patient supine. **B,** A specialized acetabular insertion guide is used. **C,** Fluoroscopic visualization assists with component insertion.

that small-incision THA is safe, achieves the goal of short-term improvement, and gives patients more confidence that positive outcomes will be realized.

## Technique Guidelines

MIS is more complex than surgery done through a larger incision because at any given moment only part of the surgical field is exposed.[17] The surgeon must be committed to learning the special techniques associated with the greater degree of difficulty of MIS procedures. Correct exposure must be obtained to ensure the safety of MIS. Specialized instrumentation is also needed to allow the surgeon to operate through the soft-tissue windows required by these approaches. Difficulties can be minimized if specialized instruments developed for each technique are used.[2,5,10,17,18] These instruments include lighted retractors, curved acetabular insertion guides, beveled (half-size) acetabular reamers to facilitate insertion and removal and avoid skin and muscle injury, and femoral stem insertion handles to avoid varus stem position and protect muscles.

The common characteristics of all MIS approaches are the need for adequate training and the use of specialized instruments specific to each surgical technique. All MIS techniques cause some soft-tissue injury, but the goal of this type of surgery is to reduce soft-tissue trauma below the level of the skin. The use of specific instrumentation is critical in mobilizing the surgical window to expose the appropriate landmarks and anatomy without unnecessary tissue damage. Trained assistants can facilitate the procedure because of their knowledge on how to use the wound as a mobile window.[17,19-21] If exposure is not sufficient, single-incision techniques allow extension of the incision for improved visualization.

Intraoperative landmarks for some incisions are different from those used in standard surgery because less bone is exposed, and different reference points are necessary. The changes from the normal surgical references are most obvious with the two-incision technique, which is done with the patient supine and with fluoroscopy required for component positioning[2,3,5,20,22,23] (Figure 1). In this technique, the two incisions are made between muscle planes as is the standard anterior incision. The posterior and anterolateral incisions incise muscle during the exposure. No postoperative clinical benefit has been observed in patients in whom there is no muscle cut. All of the incisions allow visualization of the capsule, removal of the femoral head, and retraction of the femur for exposure of the acetabulum.

The benefits of minimally invasive hip surgery include a shorter skin incision and less dissection of the deep hip tissues. For this reason, minimally invasive techniques are described as tissue-sparing procedures. Cadaver studies have shown that retractor damage with the "no muscle cut incisions" is equivalent to damage caused by the posterior mini-incision.[24,25] Although some muscle damage occurs with all small-incision approaches, tissue trauma is less than with standard approaches. For example, with the posterior mini-incision technique, no incision is made into the tensor fascia, the gluteus maximus muscle is split for only 6 cm compared with 10 to 12 cm with a long-incision technique, and neither the gluteus maximus tendon nor the quadratus femoris muscle is released as is done with the long-incision technique[10,26,27] (Figure 2).

Computer navigation can be of great benefit for correct component positioning with the decreased exposure of MIS.[28] Correct numerical inclinations and anteversion are displayed by the software, with adjustments made for the tilt of the pelvis. Many studies have shown improved component placement using computer navigation.[28-33]

## Impact on the Patient

Multiple factors play a role in the success of minimally invasive THA. Patients often have preoperative anxiety that they will not achieve their functional goals and expectations and will be more crippled after surgery than before. The patient's disability may have resulted in anxiety, depression, and a loss of independence.[7,13-15,34] Preoperative patient education is required to allevi-

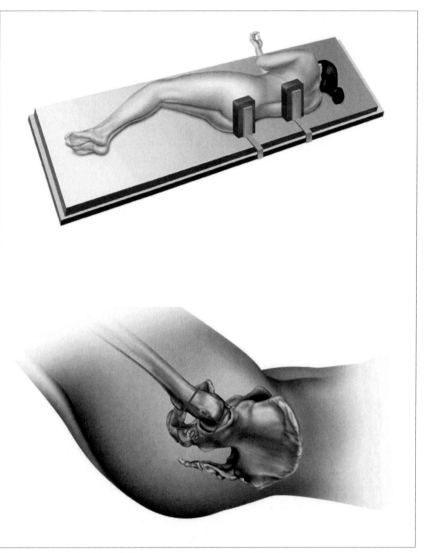

**Figure 2** **A,** The lateral decubitus position is used for the miniposterior approach. **B,** Illustration showing the miniposterior skin incision.

ate this anxiety and instill confidence in the success of the THA.[7,17,21,34-36] Patients should be instructed on the three goals of a successful outcome—pain relief, return of function, and patient satisfaction. Hudak and associates[11,12] defined satisfaction with an orthopaedic operation to mean that the patient does not feel self-conscious about his or her result and has incorporated the treated limb back into the whole-body image.

To patients, minimally invasive

THA means less trauma, which translates to more confidence that they will achieve the envisioned outcome.[7,21] The cosmetic appearance of the wound symbolizes less violation of the patient's body and all of the psychological benefits that accrue from that concept. Preoperatively, the surgeon should determine the patient's most important reasons for undergoing THA (usually mobility and pain relief) and then discuss the patient's goals and expectations. If goals include a small incision and rapid recovery, and this is not realistic for a particular patient, the surgeon must educate the patient on the limitations of achieving those expectations and establish new goals the patient can achieve. Realistic goals are critical for patient satisfaction, and the most satisfied patients are those who exceed their expectations.[12]

Patients identify a small incision with helping them achieve all three components of success (less pain, improved function, satisfaction) as evidenced in the study by Dorr and associates,[7] who reported on a psychological survey of 165 patients, 56 of whom were treated using traditional long posterior incisions and 109 with small posterior mini-incisions. Both preoperatively and at 6 weeks postoperatively, all patients (even those with long incisions) believed that a small incision would enhance all three goals of recovery. At 6 weeks, patients with small incisions had exceeded their expectations, which promoted ultimate satisfaction with their surgery. By 6 months to 1 year after surgery, all patients had achieved their primary goals of pain relief and return of function, and the length of the incision was less important. Despite this, 22 of 56 patients (40%) with a long incision still wished that they had a small incision; therefore, total satisfaction with the outcome was not achieved. The reasons given by these patients suggested that they were self-conscious about aspects of their hip surgery and had not reincorporated their hip into their whole-body image.

## Safety

With any new incisional approach, complications should not be increased and long-term outcomes should not be compromised.[8,10,27]

One frequently cited study reported numerous complications associated with the wound and component position with THA done with a posterior mini-incision; it was suggested that these incisions should not be used.[37] Other studies from multiple centers have shown that MIS does not compromise component position or increase postoperative complications.[4,19,22,30,35,38-45] Randomized prospective studies, such as that of Oganda and associates,[40] have compared a traditional posterior approach to a mini-posterior approach and concluded that both were safe and reproducible because the component positions were the same, complications were the same, and there was no difference in ambulatory ability or length of the hospital stay. Sculco and associates[44] evaluated the benefits of small-incision surgery in a pilot study and concluded that the procedure was safe. These preliminary results were confirmed in a randomized prospective study.[4] In a prospective randomized study by Pour and associates,[45] safe and reproducible results were reported with the anterior mini-incision approach compared with the standard anterior approach. Several retrospective studies have confirmed the safety of minimally invasive THA.[2,5,19,22,30,35,39,43,44,46-48] A follow-up of the patients in the pilot study by Sculco and associates concluded that this technique did not influence the clinical and radiographic results.[4] Floren and Lester[38] reported that 10 years after THA done through a posterior mini-incision there was no compromise to the durability of implant fixation.

In several studies, two-incision MIS had the most complications. Several authors reported a steep learning curve for the two-incision technique. Acceptable learning of

the technique involved more than 10 surgeries, with complications inherent to the technique still occurring after 25 surgeries.[41,49-51] The most prevalent complication was periprosthetic fractures, with a range of occurrence of 1% to 6%. Pagnano and associates,[41] in a randomized comparison of posterior mini-incision and the two-incision techniques, found an increased occurrence of periprosthetic fractures (4%) with the two-incision technique. However, the incidence of fractures reported with the two-incision technique was not greater than that reported by Berend and associates[52,53] with long incisions: 26 of 1,959 fractures (1.3%) with posterior incisions and 32 of 476 (6.3%) with anterior incisions. These data suggest that the two-incision technique is not associated with a clinically significant increased rate of fractures.

Berger and Duwelius[22] reported a 2% frequency of periprosthetic fracture with two-incision THA surgery. A comparison of the results reported by Pagnano and associates[6] and Berger and Duwelius[22] indicates that two distinct differences in technique may have contributed to the differences in fracture rate. Two different femoral stems were used in the studies, and more obese women were included in the study population of Pagnano and associates[6] than in the Berger and Duwelius[22] study. Other than periprosthetic fractures, injury to the lateral femoral cutaneous nerve in 10% to 20% of patients was common to both studies, with resolution of the nerve deficit in most patients.

## Functional Recovery

The goals of MIS are to reduce pain and increase function immediately after THA. Almost all of the studies showed equivalent safety between long and short incisions and showed equivalent functional recovery.[4,30,39,40,43] All of the patients in these studies used the same postoperative physical therapy program. When all patients are treated with an identical program, it is termed a passive therapy program. To determine whether small-incision surgery can allow patients to function better and faster, it is necessary to use an active physical therapy program. An active program is adapted to each individual patient and allows that patient to improve according to his or her capabilities. In a randomized prospective study of THA patients by Dorr and associates,[54] an active rehabilitation program was used. Patients were encouraged to use a single assistive device and be discharged from the hospital within 48 hours. Twenty-nine of 30 patients (97%) with posterior mini-incision THAs were discharged by the second postoperative day compared with 20 of 30 patients (67%) with long incisions ($P = 0.003$). Twenty-six of 30 patients (86.7%) with mini-incisions were discharged from the hospital using only a single assistive device (single cane or crutch) compared with 16 patients (63.3%) with long incisions ($P = 0.005$). Kahn and associates[39] did not randomize their patients but did confirm that patients with mini-posterior incisions were discharged earlier.

A randomized study by Chimento and associates[4] found that patients with posterior mini-incisions had less limp than those with traditional posterior incisions for up to 6 weeks after surgery. DiGioia and associates[30] also reported significantly less limp ($P < 0.05$) and better ability to climb stairs ($P < 0.01$) in those with mini-incisions; these advantages were maintained through the 6-month

postoperative period. Pagnano and associates,[41] in a randomized comparison of posterior mini-incision and two-incision techniques, found that recovery after the posterior mini-incision technique was easier and faster than after the two-incision approach.

The greatest advancement in functional recovery in patients with THA has been the advent of same-day discharge from the hospital. Berger and associates[34] pioneered this rapid return to function by allowing same-day discharge of patients who had two-incision procedures. Study results showed no readmissions, complications, or patient dissatisfaction with going home the same day as surgery. A matched-pairs study of posterior mini-incision and two-incision techniques also suggested that patients treated with the two-incision technique returned to satisfactory function more quickly.[5]

## Associated Techniques, Protocols, and Therapy

Improved anesthetic techniques, pain management protocols, and rapid recovery therapy have been developed in parallel with small-incision surgery. These techniques are as important as the type of incision used for reducing the length of hospitalization and speeding functional recovery.[5,34,35,54,55] Regional anesthesia avoids the nausea, vomiting, and malaise associated with general anesthesia. If narcotics are not used in the epidural or spinal anesthetic, and intravenous narcotics are avoided, there is little postoperative emesis.[55] Regional anesthesia should allow rapid return of the patient's ability to move his or her feet and legs in the recovery room, which comforts both the surgeon and the patient, and allows the patient to be

mobilized from bed within 2 hours of surgery. The type of anesthesia used was less important in the past when parenteral narcotics were used for pain control and patients were not mobilized from bed for 1 to 2 days after surgery. Propofol (Novaplus, Wilmington, DE), when used as an intraoperative sedative, allows the patient to be fully awake immediately after cessation of this intravenous drug.

The use of regional anesthesia and sedation, the effects of which can be rapidly dissipated, has profoundly changed the attitude of patients regarding their recovery in the early postoperative period. The anxiety and dissatisfaction that accompany nausea and vomiting,[7,34,54] as well as the lethargy caused by parenteral narcotics, create a negative perception of the surgical experience for the patient. The patient's surgical experience will influence a decision to have another joint replacement if needed. The patient's positive experience will also influence friends and family members to undergo the procedure if needed. One reason that many patients do not seek treatment for arthritic joints is apprehension regarding the surgery and postoperative recovery.[56]

Another important change has occurred in pain management protocols. Pain is now prevented with a multimodal analgesic protocol that provides protection against pain at the peripheral wound site, the spinal cord transmission site, and the brain. Wound injections provide a high level of pain relief, as was shown in studies by Lombardi and associates[57] and Busch and associates.[58] Pain transmission through the spinal cord (dorsal horn neurons and spinothalamic tract) to the brain is blocked intraoperatively with regional anesthesia. The pain management protocol includes administration of cyclooxygenase-2 (COX-2) inhibitors, pain medication, and an antiemetic 1 hour preoperatively. No intravenous spinal or epidural narcotics are used. In the recovery room, oral pain medications and intravenous ketorolac are used for pain control, with intravenous narcotics administered as needed. For the remainder of the hospitalization, oral pain medications are used, which are adapted to the patient's age and pain tolerance.[55]

Pain can be modified by using COX-2 inhibitors, which block the cyclooxygenase enzymes that are transmitters of pain through the spinal cord to the thalamus. In the brain, pain can be modified in the thalamus by a COX-2 inhibitor and a COX-3 inhibitor (acetaminophen). The response in the brain also can be modified by preoperative education that conditions patients to believe that their pain can be controlled postoperatively and that they should not anticipate having significant pain; this helps with sensitization of the central response.

The effect of this multimodal program, which avoids parenteral narcotics and uses only oral medications, is shown in the study by Maheshwari and associates.[55] When this program was combined with a posterior MIS incision, the average pain scores after administration of the oral medications was 1 on an analog scale of 10. The pain scores before medication were only slightly more than 2. The incidence of emesis was 3.7%. A multimodal program that eliminates parenteral narcotics and uses only oral pain medications, combined with wound injections, is highly effective in controlling the pain of patients with minimally invasive THAs.[5,34,55,57,58]

Another important factor in successful minimally invasive THA is the use of an active physical therapy program. An active physical therapy program promotes progress of the patient based on the capability of the individual patient rather than using a common physical therapy pathway for all patients. An active physical therapy program allows patients to go home on the day of surgery if they can do so. It allows patients to participate in a physical therapy program at home without supervision from a therapist, when the patient will take that responsibility. Patients can initiate a walking program immediately after discharge and can combine that with stretching exercises for flexibility. Results are based on the patient's own pace and level of motivation. This program also has allowed patients to return to work within days after surgery rather than at 3 months as was the traditional time frame.[5,34,35]

## Discussion
It is common sense that small injuries are preferable to larger injuries; therefore, MIS is a less disruptive procedure than traditional THA. MIS may be more difficult and stressful for the surgeon who must learn to work in a smaller surgical field. Surgeons may justify their reluctance to use MIS because of the absence of positive, evidence-based studies confirming the benefits of MIS. Some surgeons believe that the evidence, based on randomized studies, of equivalent safety and functional results achieved by MIS compared with traditional techniques has not been adequate to support change.[4,40,51,54]

MIS is simply a change in surgical incisions and exposure. Previous changes in incisions and exposures have also created disruption but were quickly assimilated into the techniques used by surgeons. The change to the posterior approach for THA avoided trochanteric osteotomy and the complication of nonunion and allowed patients full weight bearing immediately after surgery. Charnley did not embrace this change because it affected his biomechanical theory of leveling moment arms by lateralizing the trochanter. The simplicity of the technique, however, quickly won converts. Hardinge[59] altered the anterior approach by cutting part of the gluteus medius muscle, increasing exposure. Hardinge's approach was adopted by the advocates of the Porous-Coated Anatomic hip prosthesis (Howmedica, Rutherford, NJ) and helped to popularize that device. Some hip surgeons who favored the posterior approach rejected the change because they did not advocate cutting the gluteus medius muscle; however, surgeons who had used the anterior approach favored the simplification of the exposure. MIS, like all new and challenging technologies, will gradually be accepted.

## Summary
Scientific evidence overwhelmingly confirms the safety of THA using small-incision techniques. If component positions do not differ, the durability of the prosthesis will not be altered from that achieved by traditional techniques. Randomized studies have shown that the complication rate for THAs using small and long incisions do not differ. Small-incision THA, using either the posterior or anterior approach, is safe and can reduce pain and improve functional recovery. Active physical therapy programs based on the individual patient's capabilities and motivations will replace passive programs that treat all patients the same. With appropriate education

and good instrumentation, minimally invasive THA can be used successfully by both high- and low-volume surgeons.

## References

1. Klein GR, Parvizi J, Sharkey PF, Rothman RH, Hozack WJ: Minimally invasive total hip arthroplasty: Internet claims made by members of the Hip Society. *Clin Orthop Relat Res* 2005;441:68-70.

2. Berry DJ, Berger RJ, Callaghan JJ, et al: Minimally invasive total hip arthroplasty: Development, early results, and a critical analysis. *J Bone Joint Surg Am* 2003;85:2235-2255.

3. Berger RA: The technique of minimally invasive hip surgery using the two incision approach. *Instr Course Lect* 2004;53:149-155.

4. Chimento GF, Pavone V, Sharrock N, Kahn B, Cahill J, Sculco TP: Minimally invasive total hip arthroplasty: A prospective randomized study. *J Arthroplasty* 2005;20:139-144.

5. Duwelius PJ, Burkhart RL, Hayhurst JO, et al: Comparison of the 2-incision and mini-posterior total hip arthroplasty technique: A retrospective match-pair controlled study *J Arthroplasty* 2007;22:48-56.

6. Pagnano MW, Leone J, Lewallen DG, Hanssen AD: Two-incision THA had modest outcomes and some substantial complications. *Clin Orthop Relat Res* 2005;441:86-90.

7. Dorr LD, Sirianni LE, Thomas D, et al: Psychological reasons for patients preferring minimally invasive total hip arthroplasty. *Clin Orthop Relat Res* 2007;458:94-100.

8. Ranawat CS, Ranawat AS: Minimally invasive total joint arthroplasty: Where are we going? *J Bone Joint Surg Am* 2003;85-A:2070-2071.

9. Woolson ST: In the absence of evidence-Why bother? A literature review of minimally invasive total hip replacement surgery. *Instr Course Lect* 2006;55:189-193.

10. Keener JD, Callaghan JJ, Goetz DD, Pederson D, Sullivan P, Johnston RC: Long-term function after Charnley total hip arthroplasty. *Clin Orthop Relat Res* 2003;417:148-156.

11. Hudak PL, Hogg-Johnson S, Bombardier C, Mckeever PD, Wright JG: Testing a new theory of patient satisfaction with treatment outcome. *Med Care* 2004;42:726-739.

12. Hudak PL, McKeever PD, Wright JG: Understanding the meaning of satisfaction with treatment outcome. *Med Care* 2004;42:718-725.

13. Iversen MD, Daltroy LH, Fossel AH, Katz JN: The prognostic importance of patient preoperative expectations of surgery for lumbar spinal stenosis. *Patient Educ Couns* 1998;34:169-178.

14. Mancuso CA, Salvati EA, Johanson NA, Peterson MGE, Charlson ME: Patients' expectations and satisfaction with total hip arthroplasty. *J Arthroplasty* 1997;12:387-396.

15. Chamberlain K, Petrie K, Azarih R: The role of optimism and sense of coherence in predicting recovery following surgery. *Psychol Health* 1992;7:301-310.

16. Orbell S, Johnston M, Rowley D, Espley A, Davey P: Cognitive representations of illness and functional and affective adjustment following surgery for osteoarthritis. *Soc Sci Med* 1998;47:93-102.

17. Howell JR, Garbuz DS, Duncan CP: Minimally invasive hip replacement: Rationale, applied anatomy, and instrumentation. *Orthop Clin North Am* 2004;35:107-118.

18. Yerasimides JG, Matta JM: Primary total hip arthroplasty with a minimally invasive anterior approach, in *Seminars in Arthroplasty*. Philadelphia, PA, Elsevier, 2005, vol 16, pp 186-190.

19. Hartzband MA: Posterolateral minimal incision for total hip replacement: Technique and early results. *Orthop Clin North Am* 2004;35:119-129.

20. Duwelius PJ: Two-incision minimally invasive total hip arthroplasty: Techniques and results to date. *Instr Course Lectr* 2006;55:215-222.

21. Szendroi M, Sztrinkai G, Vass R, Kiss J: The impact of minimally invasive total hip arthroplasty on the standard procedure. *Int Orthop* 2006;30:167-171.

22. Berger RA, Duwelius PJ: The two-incision minimally invasive total hip arthroplasty: Technique and results. *Orthop Clin North Am* 2004;35:163-171.

23. Berger RA: Total hip arthroplasty using the minimally invasive two incision approach. *Clin Orthop Relat Res* 2003;417:232-241.

24. Mardones R, Pagnano MW, Nemanich JP, Trousdale RT: Muscle damage after total hip arthroplasty done with the two-incision and mini-posterior techniques. *Clin Orthop Relat Res* 2005;441:63-67.

25. Meneghini RM, Pagnano MW, Trousdale RT, Hozack WJ: Muscle damage during MIS total hip arthroplasty: Smith-Peterson versus posterior approach. *Clin Orthop Relat Res* 2006;453:293-298.

26. Inaba Y, Dorr LD, Wan Z, Sirianni L, Boutary M: Operative and patient care techniques for posterior mini-incision total hip arthroplasty. *Clin Orthop Relat Res* 2005;441:104-114.

27. Teet JS, Skinner HB, Khoury L: The effect of the "mini" incision in total hip arthroplasty on component position. *J Arthroplasty* 2006;21:503-507.

28. Murphy SB, Ecker TM, Tannast M: THA performed using conventional and navigated tissue-preserving techniques. *Clin Orthop Relat Res* 2006;453:160-167.

29. DiGioia AM III , Blendea S, Jaramaz B: Computer-assisted orthopaedic surgery: Minimally invasive hip and knee reconstruction. *Orthop Clin North Am* 2004;35:183-189.

30. DiGioia AM III , Plakseychuk AY, Levison TJ, Jaramaz B: Mini-incision technique for total hip arthroplasty with navigation. *J Arthroplasty* 2003;18:123-128.

31. Wixson RL, MacDonald MA: Total hip arthroplasty through a minimal posterior approach using imageless

computer-assisted hip navigation. *J Arthroplasty* 2005;20(suppl 3)51-56.

32. Kalteis T, Handel M, Bathis H, Perlick L, Tingart M, Grifka J: Imageless navigation for insertion of the acetabular component in total hip arthroplasty: Is it as accurate as CT-based navigation? *J Bone Joint Surg Br* 2006;88:163-167.

33. Nogler M, Kessler O, Prassl A, et al: Reduced variability of acetabular cup positioning with use of an imageless navigation system. *Clin Orthop Relat Res* 2004;426:159-163.

34. Berger RA, Jacobs JJ, Meneghini RM, Della Valle C, Paprosky W, Rosenberg AG: Rapid rehabilitation and recovery with minimally invasive total hip arthroplasty. *Clin Orthop Relat Res* 2004;429:239-247.

35. Parvataneni H, Ranawat CS, Ranawat AS, Zikria J, Pate J: Abstract: Modifying the pain response after THR using local periarticular injections. *73rd Annual Meeting Proceedings*. Rosemont, IL, American Academy of Orthopaedic Surgeons, 2006, p 491.

36. Howell JR, Masri BA, Duncan CP: Minimally invasive versus standard incision anterolateral hip replacement: A comparative study. *Orthop Clin North Am* 2004;35:153-162.

37. Woolson ST, Mow CS, Syquia JF, Lannin JV, Schurman DJ: Comparison of primary total hip replacements performed with a standard incision or a mini incision. *J Bone Joint Surg Am* 2004;86:1353-1358.

38. Floren M, Lester DK: Durability of implant fixation after less-invasive total hip arthroplasty. *J Arthroplasty* 2006;21:783-790.

39. Khan RJ, Fick D, Khoo P, Yao F, Nivbrant B, Wood D: Less invasive total hip arthroplasty: Description of a new technique. *J Arthroplasty* 2006;21: 1038-1046.

40. Oganda L, Wilson R, Archbald P, Lawlor M, Humphreys P, O'Brien SA: Minimal incision technique does not improve early postoperative outcomes: A prospective randomized controlled trial. *J Bone Joint Surg Am* 2005;87:699-700.

41. Pagnano MW, Trousdale RT, Meneghini RM, Hanssen AD: Patients preferred a mini-posterior THA to a contralateral two-incision THA. *Clin Orthop Relat Res* 2006;453:156-159.

42. Sculco TP: Minimally invasive total hip arthroplasty: In the affirmative. *J Arthroplasty* 2004;19(4, Suppl 1):78-80.

43. Wright JM, Crockett HC, Delgado S, Lyman S, Madsen M, Sculco TP: Mini-incision for total hip arthroplasty: A prospective, controlled investigation with 5-year follow-up evaluation. *J Arthroplasty* 2004;19:538-545.

44. Sculco TP, Jordan LC, Walter WL: Minimally invasive total hip arthroplasty: The Hospital for Special Surgery experience. *Orthop Clin North Am* 2004;35:137-142.

45. Pour AE, Parvizi J, Sharkey PF, Hozack WJ, Rothman RH: Minimally invasive hip arthroplasty: What role does patient preconditioning play? *J Bone Joint Surg Am* 2007;89: 1920-1927.

46. Swanson TV: Early results of 1000 consecutive, posterior, single incision minimally invasive surgery total hip arthroplasties. *J Arthroplasty* 2005;20 (suppl 3):26-32.

47. Waldman BJ: Minimally invasive total hip replacement and perioperative management: Early experience. *J South Orthop Assoc* 2002;11:213-217.

48. Wenz JF, Gurkan L, Jibodh SR: Mini-incision total hip arthroplasty: A comparative assessment of perioperative outcomes. *Orthopedics* 2002;25:1031-1043.

49. Archibeck MJ, White RE Jr: Learning curve for the two-incision total hip replacement. *Clin Orthop Relat Res* 2004;429:232-238.

50. Bal BS, Haltom D, Aleto T, Barrett M: Early complications of primary total hip replacement performed with the two incision technique. *J Bone Joint Surg Am* 2005;87:2432-2438.

51. Porucznik MA: Award-winning study debunks advantages of two-incision THA. *AAOS Now* 2007;1:45.

52. Berend KR, Lombardi AV Jr, Mallory TH, Chonko DJ, Dodds KL, Adams JB: Cerclage wires or cables for the management of intraoperative fracture associated with a cementless, tapered femoral prosthesis: Results at 2 to 16 years. *J Arthroplasty* 2004;19 (suppl 2):17-21.

53. Berend ME, Smith A, Meding JB, Ritter MA, Lynch T, Davis K: Long-term outcome and risk factors of proximal femoral fracture in uncemented and cemented total hip arthroplasty in 2551 hips. *J Arthroplasty* 2006;21 (suppl 2 ):53-59.

54. Dorr LD, Maheswari AV, Long WT, et al: Early pain and functional results comparing minimally invasive to conventional total hip arthroplasty: A prospective, randomized blinded study. *J Bone Joint Surg Am* 2007;89: 1153-1160.

55. Maheshwari AV, Boutary M, Yun AG, Sirianni LE, Dorr LD: Multimodal analgesia without routine parenteral narcotics for total hip arthroplasty. *Clin Orthop Relat Res* 2006;453:231-238.

56. Hawker GA, Wright JG, Coyte PC, et al: Differences between men and women in the rate of use of hip and knee arthroplasty. *N Engl J Med* 2000; 342:1016-1022.

57. Lombardi AV Jr, Berend KR, Mallory TH, Dodds KL, Adams JB: Soft tissue and intra-articular injection of bupivacaine, epinephrine, and morphine has a beneficial effect after total knee arthroplasty. *Clin Orthop Relat Res* 2004;428:125-130.

58. Busch CA, Shore BJ, Vhandri FR, et al: Efficacy of periarticular multimodal drug injection in total knee arthroplasty: A randomized trial. *J Bone Joint Surg Am* 2006;88:959-963.

59. Hardinge K: The direct lateral approach to the hip. *J Bone Joint Surg Br* 1982;64:17-19.

# Muscle Damage in Minimally Invasive Total Hip Arthroplasty: MRI Evidence That It Is Not Significant

B. Sonny Bal, MD, MBA
Jason A. Lowe, MD
Alan E. Hillard, MD

## Abstract

*The prevalence of damage to the musculature surrounding the hip joint was assessed in a random selection of patients who had a unilateral primary total hip replacement with either the two-incision minimally invasive technique, the standard posterolateral approach, or the direct lateral approach. The musculature of the operated hip was compared with that of the normal contralateral side using MRI with a special metal subtraction protocol that allowed visualization of the muscles and tendons while minimizing metal artifacts. All patients had undergone total hip arthroplasty at least 18 months before the investigation. The data show that the standard posterolateral and direct lateral approaches are associated with an increased incidence of postoperative alterations in the hip muscles after total hip arthroplasty, when compared with two-incision minimally invasive hip replacement. The results from this study suggest that the two-incision technique for total hip replacement may have muscle-sparing advantages over other standard approaches.*

**Instr Course Lect 2008;57:223-229.**

Minimally invasive hip replacement is attractive to patients and surgeons alike because less invasive surgery done with smaller incisions can achieve improved cosmetic outcomes and an earlier return to function.[1-3] Some authors have reported excellent short-term outcomes with minimally invasive hip replacement, whether performed as a modification of a standard posterolateral or direct lateral approach to the hip joint[4,5] or by using an entirely new technique to access the hip joint.[6,7] Specifically, total hip arthroplasty (THA) performed with two small incisions was introduced as a

revolutionary new procedure in 2002, with very early discharge from the hospital and virtually no complications after surgery in selected patients.[7,8]

However, the excellent outcomes of minimally invasive hip replacement have not always been reproducible. Minimally invasive THA using the posterolateral approach has been associated with an increased risk of complications, even in the hands of experienced surgeons.[9] Others have been unable to demonstrate any benefit of minimally invasive hip replacement over the standard surgical approaches.[10-12]

The outcomes of two-incision minimally invasive hip replacement have also been inconsistent. Some investigators have reported an increased risk of complications and repeat surgery with two-incision minimally invasive hip replacement, citing the difficulty in surgical exposure, increased surgical times, and technical challenges inherent in performing minimally invasive hip replacement with unfamiliar surgical approaches and short incisions.[13,14]

In a recent study of two-incision minimally invasive hip replacement in 89 patients, there was an increased risk of complications, such as femoral fracture, femoral nerve palsy, thigh numbness, repeat surgery, and inconsistent implant positioning, especially early in the learning curve.[13] Complications declined sharply with surgeon experience, and the procedure subsequently had consistent and predictable outcomes.[15] The reasons for continuing with two-incision minimally invasive hip replacement included patient demand, faster recovery (in patients who did not have complications) in comparison with conventional THA, easier positioning and surgery in the supine patient position, and the preservation of mus-

## Table 1
**Demographic and Radiographic Data After Modified Two-Incision Minimally Invasive Hip Replacement Without Intraoperative Fluoroscopy**

| Patient Demographic Data | |
| --- | --- |
| Patients/hips | 102/102 |
| Mean age in years (range) | 60.6 (37-88) |
| Number of males (%) | 61 (59.8%) |
| Mean body mass index (range) | 31.1 (18.3-60.8) |
| Diagnosis of hip disease | |
| Osteoarthritis | 89 |
| Osteonecrosis | 7 |
| Rheumatoid arthritis | 3 |
| Other | 3 |
| Operated hip | |
| Number of right hips (%) | 56 (64.9%) |
| Mean intraoperative blood loss (range) | 335 mL (60-1,300 mL) |
| Mean surgical time (range) | 77 min (66-127 min) |
| Mean hospital stay (range) | 2.4 days (2-6 days) |
| **Radiographic Data** | |
| Incomplete radiolucent lines between cup and pelvis | 2 |
| Complete radiolucent line between cup and pelvis | 0 |
| Mean cup abduction angle in degrees (range) | 43.8 (39.7-48.5) |
| Limb-length discrepancy (mm) | 1.7 (–1.3 to 3.7) |

cles and tendons during component insertion.

The two-incision minimally invasive hip replacement procedure was modified from its original description to include slightly longer incisions, improved surgeon visualization of bony anatomy, a femoral stem that did not require canal reaming, and the elimination of intraoperative fluoroscopy.[13,15] As a result of these technique modifications, and with increased surgeon experience, the clinical and radiographic outcomes of 102 consecutive patients who underwent two-incision minimally invasive hip replacement immediately following the 89 patients reported earlier[13] had outcomes that were comparable to the excellent results of THA using other techniques.[16] These data are summarized in Table 1; no patient underwent repeat surgery or demonstrated the complications that were encountered earlier.

When two-incision minimally invasive hip replacement is performed appropriately, excellent outcomes in terms of early recovery of independent ambulation and patient satisfaction are possible, in part because of the preservation of muscles and tendons. However, visible damage to 15% to 17% of the surface of the gluteus medius and gluteus minimus muscles has been reported following two-incision minimally invasive hip replacement.[17] These observations were based on inspection of the muscles after the procedure was performed on cadavers, using a previously described method to measure muscle damage during reamed intramedullary nailing.[18]

The prevalence of damage to the hip musculature was investigated in a random selection of patients from the first 89 patients who underwent consecutive two-incision minimally invasive hip replacement,[13] and ex-

amining the operated hip joints using MRI with a special metal subtraction protocol that allowed visualization of the muscles and tendons, while minimizing metal artifacts. For comparison, historical control groups were used—one group consisting of patients who had undergone primary THA with the standard posterolateral approach and another group consisting of patients who had undergone primary THA with the direct lateral approach. Both control groups had previously undergone primary THA before the advent of the two-incision method.

## Methods

The 32 patients who were enrolled in this investigation were distributed as follows: two-incision minimally invasive hip replacement ($n = 17$), standard posterolateral approach ($n = 8$), and standard direct lateral approach ($n = 7$). All patients who underwent THA with the posterolateral approach had repair of the posterior hip capsule and short external rotators.[19] In the direct lateral group, a modification of the Hardinge approach[20] was used, by elevating approximately 30% to 50% of the anterior gluteus medius and vastus lateralis subperiosteally to expose the hip joint. All patients had undergone unilateral THA at least 18 months before the study and had recovered without complications. No patient demonstrated a limp or used support for ambulation at the time of the investigation. Each patient underwent MRI of the operated hip and contralateral nonoperated hip following approval by the Institutional Review Board.

MRI of the pelvis was done with a 1.5-T MRI system (Signa Horizon, GE Healthcare, Milwaukee, WI). The standard pelvis protocol for patients with THA is T1 (spin echo

[SE], 5 mm thickness; echo time [TE], 9 ms; repetition time [TR], 816 ms; 512 × 512) and T2 (SE, 5 mm thickness; TE, 103 ms; TR, 4,566 ms; 512 × 512) axial, and coronal T1 (SE, 5 mm thickness, TE, 9.93 ms; TR, 516 ms; 512 × 512) and short T1 inversion recovery (STIR) (IR, 140 ms; TE, 38.3 ms; TR, 5,600 ms; 512 × 512). A send-receive phased-array body coil was used at a field of view of 38 cm for the T1-weighted images and 38 cm for the STIR-weighted images. Axial imaging was done with a field of view of 38 cm (software version 8.3, Horizon CX, GE Healthcare). The examinations were evaluated on diagnostic monitors using the Dynamic Imaging Integrad PACS system (Dynamic Imaging, Allendale, NJ), and all study interpretations were done by an independent board-certified musculoskeletal diagnostic radiologist who was blinded to the surgical procedure.

An SE T1 technique was selected to evaluate postoperative injury to the surrounding soft tissues of the hip. The T1 technique is an accepted means of evaluating for fatty changes in muscles. The patient was positioned along the long axis of the hip arthroplasty and imaged only in the frequency-encoding direction so that metal artifacts could be directed away from the surrounding musculature. The receiver bandwidth was maximized to increase the amplitude of the frequency-encoding gradients. Misregistration artifacts are inversely proportional to the applied frequency-encoding gradient strength. The trade-off is a decrease in signal-to-noise ratio. The high-image 512 × 512 matrix improved the signal-to-noise ratio. These changes did not decrease the diagnostic quality of the scan to evaluate for fatty atrophy in the surrounding musculature.

STIR coronal imaging was also done as a way of suppressing the fat signal to evaluate for other pathology around the hip. This technique is particularly effective for fluid changes around the hip. Residual edema in the surrounding musculature, marrow edema, lymphoceles, abscesses, or other fluid-containing structures or abnormalities related to the postsurgical procedure can be evaluated on this heavily T2-weighted sequence. An additional T2 axial conventional SE sequence was also used to increase reader confidence but did not yield any additional information.

The surrounding soft tissues on the operated side were compared with those of the nonoperated side for muscle tear, atrophy, tendon disruption, and abnormal fluid collections. Muscle atrophy was graded as follows: grade 0, normal; grade 1, minimal decrease in muscle size (≤ 30% compared with the opposite hip) with fatty replacement; grade 2, 30% to 70% of muscle involvement with fatty changes as judged on the T1-weighted images, with corresponding decreased muscle mass; and grade 3, more than 70% fatty replacement with the muscle unit measuring 20% or less of that of the contralateral hip. This grading system was used to measure the postoperative appearance of each of the following muscles: tensor fascia lata, gluteus maximus, gluteus medius, gluteus minimus, piriformis, iliopsoas, sartorius, quadratus femoris, and rectus femoris.

## Results

No complications occurred in this study because of the MRI protocol previously described, and all patients completed the study. Two hips in the two-incision group showed minimal atrophic changes (grade 1) in the glu-

teus minimus muscle; one of these two hips also had similar changes in the gluteus medius muscle. Another hip in the two-incision group showed similar changes in the gluteus maximus muscle (Figure 1). The remaining hips in the two-incision group had normal-appearing hip muscles (grade 0) on MRI that were similar in appearance to the contralateral, nonoperated side (Figure 2). All hips in the standard posterolateral group showed atrophic changes (≥ grade 2) in one or more of the following muscles: gluteus medius, gluteus maximus, tensor fascia lata, piriformis, and quadratus femoris (Figure 3). Similarly, all hips in the direct lateral group showed atrophy (≥ grade 2) in one or more of the following muscles: gluteus medius, gluteus maximus, gluteus minimus, and tensor fascia lata muscles (Figure 4). Complete tendon disruption was not found in any hip in this study. The changes in hip musculature following primary THA after each of the three surgical approaches are summarized in Table 2.

## Discussion

Postoperative MRI of a metal THA is not usually done because of the metallic susceptibility artifact that makes evaluation of both the prosthesis and the surrounding soft tissues unrewarding.[21] The artifacts include diffusion-related signal loss, inhomogeneous or paradoxical tissue-selective signal suppression, misregistration, and intravoxel dephasing, with the latter predominating. The artifacts resulting from a metal prosthesis are accentuated by a gradient-refocused echo technique; thus, when imaging is done, conventional SE parameters are used.

For this investigation, an attempt was made to minimize the inherent artifacts generated by the metal hip

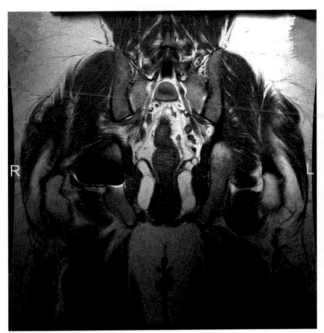

**Figure 1**   Coronal MRI scan showing minimal changes to the gluteus maximus following two-incision minimally invasive hip replacement.

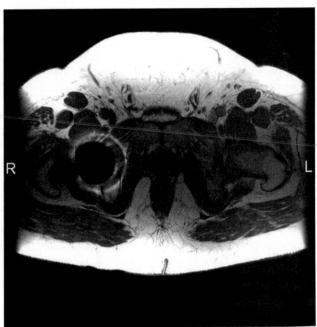

**Figure 2**   Axial MRI scan showing no atrophy of hip musculature following two-incision minimally invasive hip replacement.

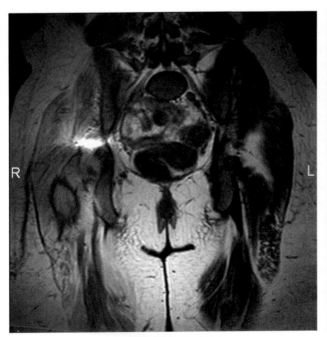

**Figure 3**   Coronal MRI scan showing atrophy in right gluteus musculature following THA with the posterolateral approach.

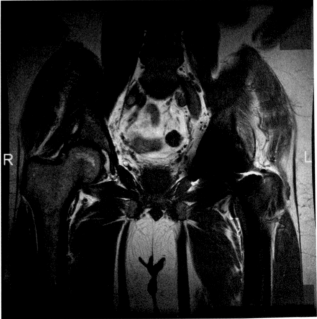

**Figure 4**   Coronal MRI scan showing atrophy in left gluteus medius muscle following THA with the direct lateral approach.

prosthesis by using SE techniques with a 180° refocused radiofrequency pulse. This recovers transverse signal loss caused by inhomogeneities within the static magnetic field. Field inhomogeneities caused by large metal objects also cause local hydrogen-spin dephasing in adjacent, randomly diffusing water molecules. This process is accentuated by a long TE sequence. Fast SE, another technique, also was not used because of misregistration artifacts. For SE techniques, this type of misregistration can be seen in the frequency-encoding direction, and the magnitude is related to the magnitude of the metallic inhomogeneity.[22]

This investigation showed that the standard posterolateral and direct lateral approaches were associated with more postoperative alterations in the hip muscles after THA, when compared with two-incision minimally invasive hip replacement. The pattern of muscle alterations is consistent with the anatomic rationale of the respective surgical approaches. The posterolateral approach typically includes splitting the gluteus maximus muscle fibers, division of the short external rotators, traction on the gluteus medius muscle as the femur is retracted anteriorly, and repair of the short external rotators at the end of the procedure. During the direct lateral surgical approach or its various modifications, the gluteus maximus muscle fibers are split, followed by division and elevation of the gluteus medius and minimus tendons from the greater trochanter, with or without a split in the proximal part of the vastus lateralis muscle. Anterior retraction of the divided abductors permits hip exposure, and the longitudinal split in the musculature is stitched together at the conclusion of the operation.

## Table 2
**Postoperative Hip Muscle Alterations Detected on MRI**

| | Muscle Changes[*] | | | |
|---|---|---|---|---|
| | Grade 0 | Grade 1 | Grade 2 | Grade 3 |
| Two-incision | 14 | 3 | 0 | 0 |
| Posterolateral | 0 | 0 | 3 | 5 |
| Direct lateral | 0 | 0 | 5 | 2 |

[*]Grade 0 = normal (like contralateral side); grade 1 = < 30% decrease in muscle size; grade 2 = 30% to 70% fatty replacement of muscle; grade 3 = > 70% fatty replacement of muscle.

In two-incision minimally invasive hip replacement, the plane of dissection is between the abductors and the sartorius superficially and between the abductors and the rectus femoris muscles in the deep plane.[23] Femoral component insertion is achieved by developing a plane posterior to the abductors and entering the femoral canal close to the insertion of the piriformis tendon. At least in theory, two-incision minimally invasive hip replacement can be performed without disrupting any muscle or tendon origin, thereby making it a true muscle-sparing technique.

Several explanations exist to reconcile the findings of other authors who have found muscle damage to the abductors in cadavers undergoing two-incision minimally invasive hip replacement[14,17] with the findings of this study. First, the method of measuring muscle damage by physical inspection following cadaver surgery may yield different results than evaluating subtle muscle changes in living subjects on MRI scans done many months after surgery. The two techniques of determining muscle alterations have not been compared side by side, and their correlation is unknown. Second, subtle variations in surgical technique could produce different degrees of muscle trauma. Specifically, during two-incision minimally invasive hip replacement, instru-

ments and implants are inserted blindly with radiographic guidance into the posterior incision.[24] Even slight deviations from the ideal entry point into the femur can produce damage to the adjacent gluteal musculature and piriformis tendon during reaming and nail insertion for femur fractures.[18] Third, inadequate mobilization of the tensor fascia lata during two-incision minimally invasive hip replacement can lead to muscle damage, as retractors are placed directly on this muscle during the procedure.[25] Unless the abductor muscle mass is adequately mobilized by blunt dissection during the anterior dissection and the muscle is protected during retraction, damage to the tensor and abductors can result.

Other investigations have shown that muscle and tendon damage is possible during the Smith-Petersen approach to THA and during femoral canal preparation for a reamed nail.[18,25] Two-incision minimally invasive hip replacement includes both surgical techniques, thereby increasing the potential for muscle injury. In evaluating muscle damage after two-incision minimally invasive hip replacement, the present investigation has significant limitations. These include the small number of patients in each group and the lack of functional outcomes, such as muscle strength grading between the groups of patients to validate the MRI findings. The goals of the study were limited to examining the muscles using an objective method after primary THA with different surgical techniques. Further studies are needed to resolve whether muscle damage is inevitable during two-incision minimally invasive hip replacement or if it can be avoided. Our findings with postoperative MRI following two-incision minimally invasive hip replacement are consistent with the muscle-sparing surgical dissection during the procedure. However, as other authors have observed, the two-incision technique is technically challenging and associated with a steep learning curve.[6,14]

Technique modifications to two-incision minimally invasive hip replacement have resulted in consistent and safe outcomes; these methods have been described previously[15,16] and may help protect the hip muscles against inadvertent injury. Another strategy to avoid muscle damage during blind posterior instrumentation and femoral component insertion during two-incision minimally invasive hip replacement is to avoid the second incision entirely. An evolution of the two-incision minimally invasive hip replacement is the minimally invasive single-incision anterior THA, in which both acetabular and femoral components are inserted through the Smith-Petersen interval,[23] using an orthopaedic table to facilitate exposure.[26,27] The advantage is one less incision and the ability to perform the entire operation under direct vision. The Smith-Petersen approach uses planes between muscles, such that no tendon or muscle detachment is necessary. By avoiding the blind passage of instruments in the posterolateral approach, the concerns relating to muscle damage

with two-incision minimally invasive hip replacement can be addressed, while preserving the benefits of a true muscle-sparing approach for primary THA.

## Summary

In theory, two-incision minimally invasive hip replacement involves surgical exposure that separates muscles along natural planes, instead of dividing tendons or splitting muscle fibers. In practice, given the technical difficulties associated with two-incision minimally invasive hip replacement, muscle damage can occur; this phenomenon has been well described in cadavers. In the present investigation, MRI of the hip muscles following THA demonstrated fewer postoperative alterations following two-incision minimally invasive hip replacement when compared with other standard surgical approaches. These results suggest that despite the muscle damage encountered in cadavers by other authors, hip muscle size and integrity are preserved on MRI scans obtained after two-incision minimally invasive hip replacement.

## References

1. Dorr LD, Maheshwari AV, Long WT, Wan Z, Sirianni LE: Early pain relief and function after posterior minimally invasive and conventional total hip arthroplasty: A prospective, randomized, blinded study. *J Bone Joint Surg Am* 2007;89:1153-1160.

2. Murphy SB, Ecker TM, Tannast M: THA performed using conventional and navigated tissue-preserving techniques. *Clin Orthop Relat Res* 2006; 453:160-167.

3. Khan RJK, Fick D, Khoo P, Yao F, Nivbrant B, Wood D: Less invasive total hip arthroplasty: Description of a new technique. *J Arthroplasty* 2006; 21:1038-1046.

4. Berger RA: Mini-incision total hip replacement using an anterolateral approach: Technique and results. *Orthop Clin North Am* 2004;35:143-151.

5. Sculco TP: Minimally invasive total hip arthroplasty: In the affirmative. *J Arthroplasty* 2004;19(4 suppl 1): 78-80.

6. Duwelius PJ, Burkhart RL, Hayhurst JO, Moller H, Butler JB: Comparison of the 2-incision and mini-incision posterior total hip arthroplasty technique: A retrospective match-pair controlled study. *J Arthroplasty* 2007;22:48-56.

7. Berger RA, Duwelius PJ: The two-incision minimally invasive total hip arthroplasty: Technique and results. *Orthop Clin North Am* 2004;35: 163-172.

8. Berger RA: The technique of minimally invasive total hip arthroplasty using the two-incision approach. *Instr Course Lect* 2004;53:149-155.

9. Woolson ST, Mow CS, Syquia JF, Lannin JV, Schurman DJ: Comparison of primary total hip replacements performed with a standard incision or a mini-incision. *J Bone Joint Surg Am* 2004;86:1353-1358.

10. Kim Y-H: Comparison of primary total hip arthroplasties performed with a minimally invasive technique or a standard technique: A prospective and randomized study. *J Arthroplasty* 2006;21:1092-1098.

11. Asayama I, Kinsey TL, Mahoney OM: Two-year experience using a limited-incision direct lateral approach in total hip arthroplasty. *J Arthroplasty* 2006;21:1083-1091.

12. Ogonda L, Wilson R, Archbold P, et al: A minimal-incision technique in total hip arthroplasty does not improve early postoperative outcomes: A prospective, randomized, controlled trial. *J Bone Joint Surg Am* 2005;87:701-710.

13. Bal BS, Haltom D, Aleto T, Barrett M: Early complications of primary total hip replacement performed with a two-incision minimally invasive technique. *J Bone Joint Surg Am*

2005;87:2432-2438.

14. Pagnano MW, Leone J, Lewallen DG, Hanssen AD: Two-incision THA had modest outcomes and some substantial complications. *Clin Orthop Relat Res* 2005;441:86-90.

15. Bal BS, Haltom D, Aleto T, Barrett M: Early complications of primary total hip replacement performed with a two-incision minimally invasive technique: Surgical technique. *J Bone Joint Surg Am* 2006;88(suppl 1 Pt 2):221-233.

16. Bal BS, Barrett MO, Lowe J: A modified two-incision technique for primary total hip replacement. *Semin Arthroplasty* 2005;16:198-207.

17. Mardones R, Pagnano MW, Nemanich JP, Trousdale RT: The Frank Stinchfield Award: Muscle damage after total hip arthroplasty done with the two-incision and mini-posterior techniques. *Clin Orthop Relat Res* 2005;441:63-67.

18. McConnell T, Tornetta P III, Benson E, Manuel J: Gluteus medius tendon injury during reaming for gamma nail insertion. *Clin Orthop Relat Res* 2003;407:199-202.

19. Su EP, Mahoney CR, Adler RS, Padgett DE, Pellicci PM: Integrity of repaired posterior structures after THA. *Clin Orthop Relat Res* 2006;447:43-47.

20. Hardinge K: The direct lateral approach to the hip. *J Bone Joint Surg Br* 1982;64:17-19.

21. Czerny C, Krestan C, Imhof H, Trattnig S: Magnetic resonance imaging of the postoperative hip. *Top Magn Reson Imaging* 1999;10:214-220.

22. White LM, Buckwalter KA: Technical considerations: CT and MR imaging in the postoperative orthopedic patient. *Semin Musculoskelet Radiol* 2002;6:5-17.

23. Smith-Petersen MN: Approach to and exposure of the hip joint for mold arthroplasty. *J Bone Joint Surg Am* 1949;31:40-46.

24. Berger RA: Total hip arthroplasty using the minimally invasive two-incision approach. *Clin Orthop Relat Res* 2003;417:232-241.

25. Meneghini RM, Pagnano MW, Trousdale RT, Hozack WJ: Muscle damage during MIS total hip arthroplasty: Smith-Petersen versus posterior approach. *Clin Orthop Relat Res* 2006;453:293-298.

26. Matta JM, Shahrdar C, Ferguson T: Single-incision anterior approach for total hip arthroplasty on an orthopaedic table. *Clin Orthop Relat Res* 2005;441:115-124.

27. Matta JM, Ferguson TA: The anterior approach for hip replacement. *Orthopedics* 2005;28:927-928.

# Muscle Damage During Minimally Invasive Total Hip Arthroplasty: Cadaver-Based Evidence That It Is Significant

Sebastien Parratte, MD
*Mark W. Pagnano, MD

## Abstract

*Minimally invasive total hip arthroplasty has generated substantial interest in both patients and surgeons. The concept that smaller incisions and less extensive surgical dissection should lead to less pain and a quicker recovery is inherently appealing. Advocates of minimally invasive total hip arthroplasty have suggested that some minimally invasive total hip approaches can be done without cutting any muscle or tendon. This contention has been carefully examined through a series of comparative cadaver studies, and the authors have determined that it is not possible to routinely perform minimally invasive total hip arthroplasty without causing some measurable degree of muscle damage. Anatomic studies showed that the two-incision approach with fluoroscopy, the posterior mini-incision approach, and the mini-incision Smith-Petersen approach all were associated with measurable muscle damage. The clinical importance of this muscle damage cannot be answered by these cadaver studies.*

**Instr Course Lect 2008;57:231-234.**

Patient expectations toward total hip arthroplasty (THA) have changed over the past three decades; however, Charnley and Ferreiraade's belief that restoration of abductor power is essential in allowing a patient to walk without an assistive device or a Trendelenburg limp remains valid.[1] Numerous standard approaches for THA have been described, and, more recently, several so-called minimally invasive approaches have been developed to preserve abductor power and, more generally, the hip muscles.[2] The fundamental concept of minimally invasive surgery is that less surgical dissection should result in less pain and a quicker recovery. Minimally invasive THA approaches involve smaller skin incisions and theoretically limited deep dissection, but the extent and location of muscle and tendon that is damaged with these approaches has only recently been characterized scientifically.[2] Minimally invasive THA has generated considerable interest among patients, surgeons, and payers, but the scientific data have been limited. Assertions that no muscles or tendons are damaged when using a particular type of minimally invasive THA approach should be scientifically proven before being widely accepted.

## Purpose of the Study

At the authors' institution, a stepwise, logical approach was applied to examining the scientific merits of minimally invasive THA. The first step in this comprehensive approach was the anatomic evaluation of the extent and location of damage to the hip musculature with various surgical approaches. This anatomic evaluation was designed to answer the first fundamental question: is it possible to perform minimally invasive THA without routinely causing some measurable muscle damage during the procedure?

*Mark W. Pagnano, MD or the department with which he is affiliated has received royalties from DePuy and Zimmer.*

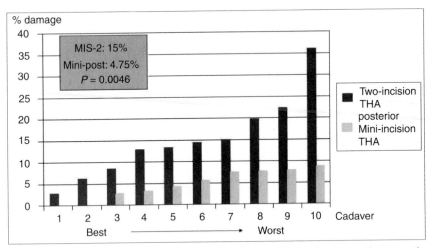

**Figure 1**  Comparison of the percentage of damage of the gluteus medius muscle after minimally invasive two-incision THA and posterior mini-incision THA on 10 cadavers. MIS-2 = minimally invasive two-incision THA, Mini-post = posterior mini-incision THA. (Adapted with permission from Mardones R, Pagnano MW, Nemanich JP, Trousdale RT: Muscle damage after total hip arthroplasty done with the two-incision and mini-posterior techniques. *Clin Orthop Relat Res* 2005;441:63-67.)

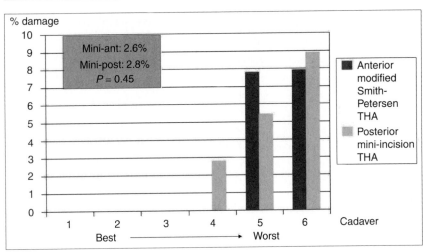

**Figure 2**  Comparison of the percentage of damage of the gluteus medius muscle after minimally invasive modified Smith-Petersen THA and posterior mini-incision THA on six cadavers. Mini-ant = anterior modified Smith-Petersen THA, Mini-post = posterior mini-incision THA. (Adapted with permission from Meneghini RM, Pagnano MW, Trousdale RT, Hozack WJ: Muscle damage during MIS total hip arthroplasty. *Clin Orthop Relat Res* 2006;453:293-298.)

## Materials and Methods

Anatomic studies were designed to compare muscle damage following two-incision minimally invasive THA as described by Berger,[3] the mini-incision anterior Smith-Petersen procedure similar to that described by Matta and associates,[4] and the posterior mini-incision THA procedure described by Berry and associates.[5] A standardized protocol was applied to each study. Fresh frozen cadavers free of hip deformity were used. In these matched-paired studies, the type of minimally invasive THA was randomly assigned to each side of the same cadaver. In each cadaver, the specific minimally invasive THA procedure was done by an experienced surgeon who had extensive clinical experience with the technique. Muscular damage secondary to acetabular and femoral canal preparation and implant insertion was then evaluated by independent surgeons who were not involved in the cadaver surgical procedures. Muscle damage was graded according to a method previously described by McConnell and associates[6] that had been used to evaluate gluteus medius muscle injury during reaming for femoral nail insertion. With this method, damaged muscle was defined as muscle fibers that were cut or torn from their insertion. The average length and width of the damaged area was measured and recorded for each muscle using the different approaches. Gluteus medius and minimus, piriformis, conjoined tendon (superior gemellus, obturator internus, and inferior gemellus), and quadratus muscle damage was quantified using the same method. Additionally, in the Smith-Petersen approach, the tensor fascia latae, the sartorius, and the anterior rectus femoris were evaluated. The surface area of each muscle and tendon insertion was calculated using a product of the width by the length of each muscle and tendon at its insertion on the femur. The percentage of the muscle and tendon disrupted by the procedure was calculated with respect to the muscle and tendon area measured. Muscle damage was compared for each type of procedure.

## Results

The results of these cadaver studies showed that all of the evaluated minimally invasive surgical approaches caused measurable muscle damage.[2,7] The extent and location of damage to particular muscles was related to the type of approach used[2-4,7] (Figures 1 through 3). Substantial damage was observed involving the gluteus minimus and the external rotators after the posterior mini-incision approach.[2,7] A small amount of damage to the gluteus medius also occurred with the posterior mini-incision approach (Figure 4). With the minimally invasive Smith-Petersen approach, damage involved the anterior part of the gluteus medius, the tensor fascia latae, and the external rotators[7] (Figures 5 and 6). The two-incision approach caused measurable damage to the gluteus medius (Figure 7), gluteus minimus, and external rotators.[2] The extent of damage to the abductor muscles was substantially greater for the two-incision approach than for the posterior mini-incision approach.[2]

This comprehensive anatomic approach provides cadaver-based evidence that measurable muscular damage occurs when performing minimally invasive THA, even when using a so-called muscle-sparing approach. In these anatomic studies, the modified direct lateral approach and the modified anterolateral approach were not evaluated.[8-10] However, the modified direct lateral approach requires incision of the gluteus medius, including one third to one half of the muscle and tendon.[8] In the modified anterolateral approach, with the patient in the lateral position or supine, damage to the anterior part of the gluteus medius can be observed following femoral preparation.[1,2,9,10] Specific evaluation of the extent and location of muscle damage after these approaches should be determined by anatomic studies.

## Discussion

The strength of these anatomic cadaver studies is that the extent and location of muscle damage could be measured directly. Such direct mea-

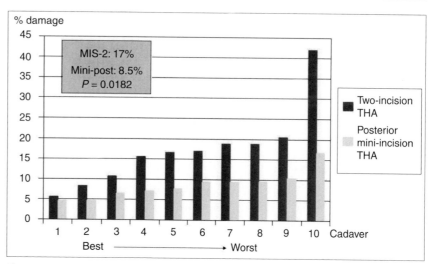

**Figure 3** Comparison of the percentage of damage of the gluteus minimus muscle after minimally invasive two-incision THA or mini-posterior THA on 10 cadavers. MIS-2 = minimally invasive two-incision THA, Mini-post = posterior mini-incision THA. (Adapted with permission from Mardones R, Pagnano MW, Nemanich JP, Trousdale RT: Muscle damage after total hip arthoroplasty done with the two-incision and mini-posterior techniques. *Clin Orthop Relat Res* 2005;441:63-67.)

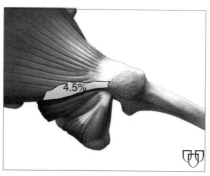

**Figure 4** Schematic representation of the location and amount of damage to the gluteus medius after posterior mini-incision THA. (Reproduced with permission from Mayo Foundation.)

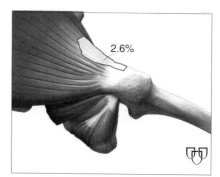

**Figure 5** Schematic representation of the location and amount of damage on the gluteus medius after a minimally invasive modified Smith-Petersen THA. (Reproduced with permission from Mayo Foundation.)

surements are not possible in vivo because the overlying skin and subcutaneous tissue can obscure some damage. However, these cadaver-based studies do have some limitations. The soft tissues and bones in cadaveric specimens behave differently than the same structures in vivo. Such differences can result in underestimating or overestimating the true clinical situation. Also, quantitative measurements of muscle damage do

not necessarily translate into substantial functional differences for patients. Although it seems logical that more muscle damage would cause functional impairment, it may be that some threshold value of damage must be met before clinically important differences in function are observed. Another limitation is that each of these studies relies on the experience of a few surgeons. Because each of the

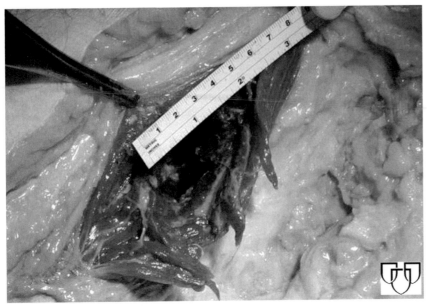

**Figure 6** Damage to the muscle of the tensor fascia latae is clearly visualized and can be measured. (Reproduced with permission from Mayo Foundation.)

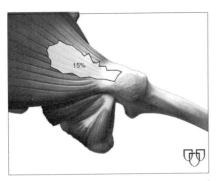

**Figure 7** Schematic representation of the location and amount of damage on the gluteus medius after minimally invasive two-incision THA. (Reproduced with permission from Mayo Foundation.)

surgeons involved in these studies was a fellowship trained, total joint specialist with a high-volume practice, review by other surgeons may result in greater discrepancies in the measured muscle damage. These limitations, however, do not undermine the core finding of these anatomic studies—that measurable muscle damage occurs in most THAs.

## Summary

Despite changes in technique, instrumentation, and implant design, anatomic analysis suggests that it is not possible to routinely perform minimally invasive THA in broad groups of typical patients without causing some measurable muscle damage. By varying the surgical approach, the surgeon can choose which muscle will typically be damaged, but no technique eliminates muscle damage. The clinical impact of this muscle damage cannot be measured by these anatomic cadaver-based studies and should be further evaluated with prospective randomized clinical trials.

## References

1. Charnley J, Ferreiraade S: Transplantation of the greater trochanter in arthroplasty of the hip. *J Bone Joint Surg Br* 1964;46:191-197.

2. Mardones R, Pagnano MW, Nemanich JP, Trousdale RT: Muscle damage after total hip arthroplasty done with the two-incision and mini-posterior techniques. *Clin Orthop Relat Res* 2005;441:63-67.

3. Berger RA: The technique of minimally invasive total hip arthroplasty using the two-incision approach. *Instr Course Lect* 2004;53:149-155.

4. Matta JM, Shahrdar C, Ferguson T: Single-incision anterior approach for total hip arthroplasty on an orthopaedic table. *Clin Orthop Relat Res* 2005;441:115-124.

5. Berry DJ, Berger RA, Callaghan JJ, et al: Minimally invasive total hip arthroplasty: Development, early results, and a critical analysis. *J Bone Joint Surg Am* 2003;85:2235-2246.

6. McConnell T, Tornetta P, Benson E, Manuel J: Gluteus medius tendon injury during reaming for gamma nail insertion. *Clin Orthop Relat Res* 2003;407:199-202.

7. Meneghini RM, Pagnano MW, Trousdale RT, Hozack WJ: Muscle damage during MIS total hip arthroplasty: Smith-Petersen versus posterior approach. *Clin Orthop Relat Res* 2006;453:293-298.

8. Asayama I, Kinsey TL, Mahoney OM: Two-year experience using a limited-incision direct lateral approach in total hip arthroplasty. *J Arthroplasty* 2006;21:1083-1091.

9. Bertin KC, Rottinger H: Anterolateral mini-incision hip replacement surgery: A modified Watson-Jones approach. *Clin Orthop Relat Res* 2004;429:248-255.

10. Jerosch J, Theising C, Fadel ME: Antero-lateral minimal invasive (ALMI) approach for total hip arthroplasty technique and early results. *Arch Orthop Trauma Surg* 2006;126:164-173.

# Surgical Nuances to Minimize Muscle Damage During the Direct Lateral Approach in Minimally Invasive Hip Replacement

*Kenneth Gustke, MD

## Abstract

*Compared with total hip replacements performed using a standard incision direct lateral approach, a minimally invasive direct lateral approach can produce less pain and blood loss without increasing the rate of complications. To minimize the potential for limping after detaching the anterior gluteus medius and the gluteus minimus tendons, special handling of the abductors (which is more difficult because of the limited exposure afforded by the smaller incision) is required. Using special retractors, minimizing overzealous retraction, and achieving strong repair has resulted in no increase in the incidence of limping.*

**Instr Course Lect 2008;57:235-241.**

More patients are interested in having minimally invasive surgery (MIS) for their hip replacement as a result of patient-to-patient conversations, Internet searches, and direct-to-consumer marketing by the orthopaedic implant industry. Patients are attracted by the cosmesis of a smaller incision and the potential for faster rehabilitation.[1-4] However, conventional total hip replacement is a well-established and reproducible procedure providing success rates of more than 90% over 10 years.[5,6] When new approaches and techniques are used, the surgeon is obligated to provide results that are at least equal to those that can be achieved with traditional approaches and techniques. In ideal circumstances, comparison studies will show better results from a new technique than from an older approach, otherwise the new approach will lose favor.

The direct lateral approach for total hip replacement was first introduced in 1982 by Hardinge.[7] It has become a popular approach because of reported lower dislocation rates, which result from the ease of and potentially more accurate acetabular component positioning from the more direct orientation for acetabular preparation, and by not violating the posterior capsule and external rotators.[8-10] The reported disadvantage of the direct lateral approach is the greater incidence of a persistent limp.[8,11,12] This complication can occur because of direct abductor muscle trauma, if the repair of the detached anterior abductors does not heal, or if the superior gluteal nerve is damaged by too proximal splitting of the gluteus medius.[13-16] Anatomic studies have shown the superior gluteal nerve travels in a variable distance from 3 to 8 cm above the tip of the greater trochanter.[13,17,18] Intraoperative care of the detached abductors is needed to prevent the complications that will compromise ultimate patient outcomes.

Operating through a smaller incision provides more limited visualization that can result in a potentially higher complication rate. With the mini-incision direct lateral approach, proper management of the abductors is critical to prevent an increase in the incidence of limp. Special curved retractors are used to

*Kenneth Gustke, MD or the department with which he is affiliated has received research or institutional support and royalties from Zimmer Orthopaedics and is a consultant or employee for Zimmer Orthopaedics.*

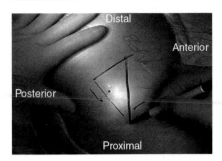

**Figure 1** An incision is made from the anterior vastus ridge to the posterior greater trochanter.

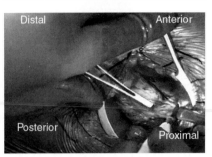

**Figure 2** The mid greater trochanter is incised and carried 1 cm into the gluteus medius proximally and 1 cm into the vastus lateralis fascia distally.

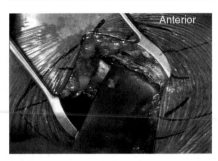

**Figure 3** The anterior gluteal/vastus lateralis flap with a bone sliver is elevated off the anterolateral greater trochanter.

avoid direct damage to the abductors during retraction. Leg positioning and use of the mobile skin window facilitate excellent exposure to the acetabulum and femur, so excessive retraction is not needed; the inadvertent higher proximal splitting of the gluteus medius and damage to the superior gluteal nerve is prevented. A reliable technique for accurate and rigid repair of the anterior gluteus medius and the gluteus minimus tendon is mandatory to prevent postoperative avulsion.

## Surgical Technique

The patient is positioned in the lateral decubitus position, and the operated leg is initially flexed at approximately 30° in neutral abduction and adduction and is neutrally rotated. A sterile bolster is placed between the thighs, and the foot is placed on a Mayo stand. The operating surgeon initially stands on the posterior side of the table, and one assistant stands on the anterior side. The surgeon's use of a head lamp is advantageous. The borders of the greater trochanter are palpated and marked. If the patient is obese and bony landmarks are not obvious, a spinal needle is used to outline the greater trochanter. The vastus tubercle is also palpated and marked. The incision is slightly ob-

lique from the longitudinal direction and extends one finger breadth proximal to the posterosuperior border of the trochanter to one finger breadth posterior to the junction of the anterior greater trochanter and the vastus tubercle line (Figure 1). The incision length varies from 8 to 12 cm depending on the size of the greater trochanter.

The key to the minimally invasive hip technique is the concept of a mobile window. Soft tissue is dissected off the fascia so that the skin can move independent of the fascia. The fascial incision is made less oblique than the skin incision but not truly longitudinal. The gluteus maximus fibers are split longitudinally in the line of their fibers to the superior aspect of the incision. The fascial retractor is inserted. With the leg still in 30° of flexion and neutral abduction and rotation, an incision is made longitudinally over the lateral aspect of the greater trochanter with an electrocautery (Figure 2). The incision is extended about 1.5 cm into the gluteus medius fibers. The thick tendinous portion of the posterior gluteus medius should be left attached to the greater trochanter. The incision is extended approximately 1 cm into the vastus lateralis fascia. Using a wide, curved Lambotte os-

teotome, a sliver of bone approximately 2 cm long, 1 cm wide, and 2 mm deep is elevated off the anterior greater trochanter (Figure 3). Taking a sliver of bone allows for a more reliable bone-to-bone reattachment and demonstrates where to reattach the soft-tissue flap later by reducing the bone sliver into its bone bed.

The foot is removed from the Mayo stand and the hip allowed to externally rotate. The posterior gluteus medius is retracted posteriorly, exposing the gluteus minimus. The gluteus minimus is elevated off the superior joint capsule. The anterior vastus lateralis fascia is dissected off the anterior vastus lateralis muscle until the vastus intermedialis muscle is exposed. Next, the anterior capsule is exposed by elevating the rectus femoris muscle from the capsule anteriorly. There should be a contiguous flap composed of the gluteus minimus tendon, the anterior half of the gluteus medius, and the anterior half of the vastus lateralis fascia. A specially designed lighted anterior acetabular retractor is inserted in the interval between the anterior acetabulum and the iliopsoas tendon. The retractor surface is curved to avoid cutting into the anterior abductor vastus lateralis contiguous flap. A

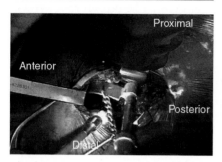

Figure 4    The superior acetabular retractor is inserted.

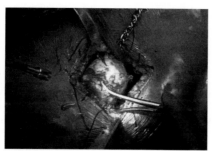

Figure 5    The femoral head is removed.

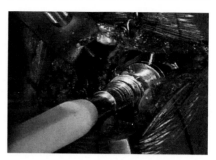

Figure 6    Acetabular reaming. Note the use of a lighted, rounded anterior acetabular retractor.

weight can be attached to the retractor and dangled down into a sterile drape pocket off the side of the table, freeing the assistant's hand. The superior and anterior capsule should be completely exposed. An S-shaped incision is made into the capsule beginning at the acetabulum at the 11 o'clock position for a right hip or the 1 o'clock position for a left hip. The incision extends distally to the greater trochanter and is then carried along the capsular attachment on the intertrochanteric line. The incision is then taken medially through the anterior capsule down to the acetabulum. The anterosuperior capsule is left attached to the acetabulum, with the intent to later repair the superior incision in the capsule.

With the superior capsule and the anterior abductor flap retracted superiorly, a specially designed right or left superior acetabular retractor is then inserted with the long pin at the 12 o'clock position with the handle straight up and down and with the anterior limb of the retractor following the anterior acetabular rim (Figure 4). This retractor holds the capsule out of the way. The retractor handle is removed, but the extension is left attached. The leg is placed back in neutral rotation. A 3.2-mm drill bit is drilled vertically into the greater trochanter parallel to

the extension on the superior acetabular retractor. The distance between the extension and the drill bit is measured and recorded to assist later in decisions about leg length. The extension piece is then removed from the superior acetabular retractor.

The fascial retractor is removed. A large, blunt, bone hook is placed around the femoral neck, and the hip is dislocated anteriorly. The leg is adducted, flexed, and externally rotated, and the lower leg and foot are placed in a sterile drape pocket off the anterior side of the table. With the leg maximally externally rotated, the lesser trochanter is exposed. Using the osteotomy ruler against the proximal lesser trochanter, a mark is made with an electrocautery on the femoral neck at the appropriate level for the femoral neck osteotomy based on preoperative templating. The leg is then rotated back to a position perpendicular to the floor in the sterile drape pocket. The femoral neck osteotomy is made, and the femoral head is then removed (Figure 5).

The leg is removed from the drape pocket and placed on top of the contralateral lower leg. The tip of the posterior acetabular retractor is placed through the posterior capsule, behind the labrum, and hammered into the ischium. A weight can be placed on the retractor and

dangled into a sterile drape pocket off the posterior side of the table. This weight retracts the femur posteriorly. The mobile skin window is moved to provide a straight-on view of the circumferentially exposed acetabulum. At this point, the incision should be directly in line with the center of the acetabulum. The fixed retractors should allow the assistant's hands to be free. The fixed retractors also minimize overzealous retraction, which could unnecessarily extend the split proximally into the gluteus medius. The operating surgeon now moves to the anterior side of the operating table and the assistant to the posterior side. The acetabulum is débrided of soft tissue and osteophytes. For most patients, cutout reamers with sleeves over straight shafts are used to protect the soft tissues (Figure 6). If the patient is very obese, special, angled-handle reamers may be helpful. Reaming begins with a small reamer directed with some anteversion transversely toward the cotyloid notch. The acetabulum is deepened to the proper level to maintain normal offset and obtain adequate lateral cup coverage, as indicated from preoperative planning. Reaming continues at an angle of 40° of abduction and 20° of anteversion until a hemisphere with rim contact is obtained. The shell trial is

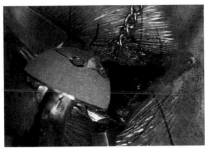

**Figure 7**  The acetabular component is inserted.

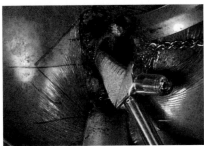

**Figure 8**  Femoral broaching is performed with the femur externally rotated.

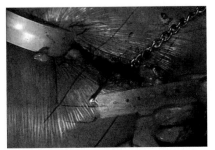

**Figure 9**  The leg length is checked.

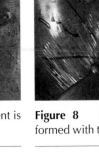

**Figure 10**  The femoral component is inserted.

inserted with the standard shell aligner/positioner to determine fit and stability. Remaining acetabular osteophytes are removed. The shell trial is removed, and the final acetabular implant is impacted into the prepared acetabulum at 40° of abduction and 20° of anteversion (Figure 7). Screws can be inserted if desired. The acetabular insert is then impacted into the shell. Because of the increased stability typical of this surgical approach, standard non-hooded inserts are used.

The operating surgeon moves back to the posterior side of the table and the assistant to the anterior side. The posterior acetabular retractor is removed. The femoral elevator retractor is placed between the posterior greater trochanter and posterior fascia. The leg is adducted and flexed, with the lower leg and foot placed in the anterior drape pocket. A weight is placed on the femoral elevator and allowed to

dangle off the table into the posterior drape pocket. A combination of the force of the assistant's body pushing on the knee and the femoral elevator should bring the proximal femur close to the proximal skin opening.

The leg is maximally externally rotated. Any remaining cortical bone in the lateral neck is removed. The canal finder is inserted to open the intramedullary canal. Successively larger diameter canal reamers are inserted until cortical bone is contacted. This process should confirm the size of the stem determined by the preoperative template. The lower leg is then placed perpendicular to the floor. Femoral broaches are then partially inserted in the appropriate rotation. Part of the way down the canal, the medial broach or broach handle may impinge on the skin edge. If so, the assistant should maximally externally rotate the leg

(Figure 8). The broach rotation will usually be fixed at this point, and the broach can be fully seated without injuring the skin edges. If a collared prosthesis is desired, the calcar is planed with the leg maximally externally rotated. The femoral elevator is removed. A trial neck and head are applied. The hip is reduced and rotated to check for impingement and stability. The extension piece is inserted onto the superior acetabular retractor. A 3.2-mm drill bit is inserted into the previously made hole in the greater trochanter. The bolster is placed between the thighs, and the foot is placed back on the Mayo stand so that the two pins are parallel. Measurement is then made to determine if the leg length is appropriate (Figure 9). The superior acetabular retractor extension is removed. The hip is dislocated, and the trial neck and head are removed. The femoral elevator retractor is again placed between the posterior greater trochanter and posterior fascia. The lower leg and foot are placed into the anterior drape pocket, and the leg is maximally externally rotated. The trial broach is removed.

The porous femoral component is partially inserted into the canal. The implant is inserted following the broached canal (Figure 10). Once the implant is approximately two-thirds seated, the lower leg is placed in neutral rotation perpendicular to the floor, upward pressure is released on the femur by the assistant, and the femoral elevator retractor is removed. The neck of the stem will slide under the anterior skin edge. The femoral component is fully seated in the appropriate rotation. If a cemented stem has been chosen, the canal can be plugged, cleaned, and cement inserted with a cement gun and pressurized. The stem is inserted with its rotation following the broached hole. Once nearly seated, the lower leg can be brought back into neutral rotation or perpendicular to the floor position, and the implant fully seated in the appropriate rotation. Reduction with trial heads may again be performed, or the implant with the previously determined head length can be inserted and the hip reduced. Hip length can again be checked with the superior acetabular retractor extension and drill bit in the femur.

The anterior acetabular and superior acetabular retractors are then removed. The fascial retractor is reinserted. The thigh bolster is placed and the leg extended and externally rotated. The anterior abductor flap is retracted, exposing the anterosuperior capsule flap. The superior limb of the capsular incision is repaired with absorbable suture. The foot is now placed on the Mayo stand with the leg in neutral rotation. The anterior gluteus medius, minimus, vastus lateralis gluteus flap is reduced to its anatomic position using the sliver of bone as a guide. Three no. 5 heavy, nonabsorbable sutures are placed around the bone sliver, then through the greater trochanter anterior to and exiting posterior to the bone sliver bed (Figure 11). The gluteus minimus should still be attached to the anterior flap. To further strengthen the repair, a no. 1 nonabsorbable suture is placed around the gluteus minimus tendon, securing it to the tendinous portion of the gluteus medius (Figure 12). The quality of the repair can be checked by externally rotating the leg. The short incisions in the gluteus medius and vastus lateralis fascia are repaired with no. 1 nonabsorbable sutures. The fascial retractor is removed. The fascia, subcutaneous tissue, and skin are then closed.

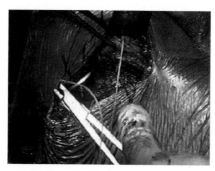

**Figure 11** The sliver of bone in the gluteus medius, minimus, vastus lateralis flap is attached to the bony bed in the greater trochanter.

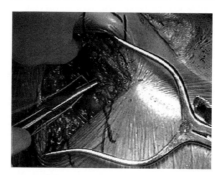

**Figure 12** The gluteus minimus tendon is sutured to the tendinous portion of the gluteus medius.

## Results

The author's first 57 patients undergoing hip replacement with a mini-incision direct lateral approach were compared with a similar set of patients who had hip surgery with a traditional direct lateral approach. Patients were matched for gender, diagnosis, age, body mass index, Charnley type, bone type, and mode of implant fixation. No changes were made in the anesthesia, pain management, or rehabilitation protocols to allow comparison of differences between the surgical approaches. The average incision length with MIS was 11 cm versus 20 cm with the extensile approach. With MIS, the average surgery time was 14 minutes shorter and blood loss was less. The average blood loss during surgery and in the drain collection device was 368 mL for the MIS group compared with 456 mL for the group treated with the standard approach. The average amount of pain (scale, 0 to 10) was less for the MIS patients during the hospital stay but was equal to the other group by 2 weeks after surgery. MIS patients and patients treated with the standard approach had scores of 3.0 versus 3.6 on day 1, 3.0 versus 3.2 on day 2, and 2.6 versus 3.3 on day 3,

respectively. At weeks 2 and 3, MIS patients and those treated with the standard approach had scores of 2.3 versus 2.0; at week 6, scores of 0.9 versus 1.0; at month 3, 0.6 versus 1.0; and at month 6, 0.4 versus 0.5, respectively.

Because of concern about disruption of the abductor repair producing a limp, patients in both groups were restricted to partial weight bearing for 6 weeks and resistive abduction exercises were avoided for 6 weeks. Postoperatively, there was no statistically significant difference in the distance patients in the two groups could walk. On day 1, the patients in the MIS group could walk 36 ft versus 34 ft for the patients treated with the standard approach; on day 2, 101 ft versus 96 ft; on day 3, 169 ft versus 146 ft, respectively. There was no difference in the incidence of limp in either group by 6 months. At 3 months, 67% of the MIS patients had no limp versus 46% of those treated with the standard approach. At 6 months, 74% of patients in each group had no limp, and the remainder had a slight limp. The average length of hospital stay was 3.3 days in both groups; this resulted from no change in the hospital critical care pathways protocols. All patients in both groups had acetabular and femoral component alignments within acceptable ranges. There were no dislocations, infections, or fractures in either group. Eight patients in this study had bilateral total hip replacements, one with the minimally invasive approach and one with the extensile approach. All patients reported less pain; however, patients treated with the minimally invasive approach reported the perception of faster recovery and had a more favorable view of the scar.

## Summary

These data show that minimally invasive total hip replacement using a mini-incision direct lateral approach is better than standard incision total hip replacement. Patients are satisfied with the appearance of the scar, there is less blood loss, and there is less pain during the hospital stay. Most importantly, there is no increase in complications when compared with the standard approach, and implant alignment remains satisfactory; good long-term results can be expected. However, these data do not show any faster rehabilitation rates. All minimally invasive approaches, as well as wide open approaches, can be expected to cause some muscle damage. The mini-incision direct lateral approach is not a muscle-sparing approach because some muscle is still detached. Because the sutured anterior abductor muscles needs time to heal, it is recommended that resistive exercises and range of motion be restricted. Other MIS hip approaches such as the minimally invasive anterolateral Watson-Jones approach, in which no muscle is detached, may allow for faster rehabilitation because postoperative restrictions may not be needed.[19,20] Speed of rehabilitation is also influenced by preopera-

tive patient muscle strength, patient motivation, the type of anesthesia used, and pain management protocols.[21]

The major criticism of the MIS direct lateral approach is that it may increase the potential for limp. Because surgery is more difficult when performed through a smaller incision, the surgeon must be even more careful with management of the abductors. Theoretically, the smaller exposure would require more vigorous retraction for exposure. The use of curved retractors helps to lessen direct trauma to the muscle during retraction. The use of self-retaining retractors after the desired exposure is achieved will decrease the chance that overzealous retraction by assistants will split the gluteus medius too proximally, resulting in damage to the superior gluteal nerve. Removing a sliver of bone with the contiguous flap of the anterior gluteus medius, gluteus minimus tendon, and anterior vastus lateralis fascia will aid with proper placement of the repair and will achieve a stronger repair by resisting pull-through of the sutures. In the author's study, no increased incidence of limping was noted in surgeries with a minimally invasive direct lateral approach compared with those performed with a standard extensile approach. Partial detachment of the abductors is required for exposure using the mini-incision direct lateral approach; however, the use of special techniques will minimize the potential for permanent weakness of the abductors.

## References

1. Wenz JF, Gurkan I, Jibodh SR: Mini-incision total hip arthroplasty: A comparative assessment of perioperative outcomes. *Orthopedics* 2002;25:1031-1043.

2. Berger RA: Mini-incisions: Two for the price of one! *Orthopedics* 2002; 25:472.

3. Wright JM, Crockett HC, Delgado S, Lyman S, Madsen M, Sculco TP: Mini-incision for total hip arthroplasty. *J Arthroplasty* 2004;19:538-545.

4. Goldstein WM, Branson JJ, Berland KA, Gordon AC: Minimal-incision total hip arthroplasty. *J Bone Joint Surg Am* 2003;85(suppl 4):33-38.

5. Engh CA Jr , Culpepper WJ, Engh CA: Long-term results of the anatomic medullary locking prosthesis in total hip arthroplasty. *J Bone Joint Surg Am* 1997;79:177-184.

6. Firestone DE, Callaghan JJ, Liu SS, et al: Total hip arthroplasty with a cemented, polished, collared femoral stem and a cementless acetabular component. *J Bone Joint Surg Am* 2007;89:126-131.

7. Hardinge K: The direct lateral approach to the hip. *J Bone Joint Surg Br* 1982;64:17-19.

8. Ritter MA, Harty LD, Keating ME, Faris PM, Meding JB: A clinical comparison of the anterolateral and posterolateral approaches to the hip. *Clin Orthop Relat Res* 2001;385:95-99.

9. Woo RY, Morrey BF: Dislocations after total hip arthroplasty. *J Bone Joint Surg Am* 1982;64:1295-1306.

10. Mallory TH, Lombardi AV, Fada RA, Herrington SM, Eberle RW: Dislocation after total hip arthroplasty using the anterolateral abductor split approach. *Clin Orthop Relat Res* 1999; 358:166-172.

11. Stephenson PK, Freeman MA: Exposure of the hip using a modified anterolateral approach. *J Arthroplasty* 1991;6:137-145.

12. Frndak PA, Mallory TH, Lombardi AV: Translateral approach to the hip. *Clin Orthop Relat Res* 1993;295: 135-141.

13. Baker AS, Bitounis VC: Abductor function after total hip replacement: An electromyographical and clinical review. *J Bone Joint Surg Br* 1989;71: 47-50.

14. Picado CH, Garcia FL, Marques W Jr: Damage to the superior gluteal nerve after direct lateral approach to the hip. *Clin Orthop Relat Res* 2007;455:209-211.

15. Abitbol JJ, Gendron D, Laurin CA, Beaulieu MA: Gluteal nerve damage following total hip arthroplasty: A prospective analysis. *J Arthroplasty* 1990;5:319-322.

16. Ramesh M, O'Byrne J, McCarthy N, Jarvis A, Mahalingham K, Cashman W: Damage to the superior gluteal nerve after the Hardinge approach to the hip. *J Bone Joint Surg Br* 1996;78:903-906.

17. Jacobs LG, Buxton RA: The course of the superior gluteal nerve in the lateral approach to the hip. *J Bone Joint Surg Am* 1989;71:1239-1243.

18. Foster DE, Hunter JR: The direct lateral approach to the hip for arthroplasty: Advantages and complications. *Orthopedics* 1987;10:274-280.

19. Bertin KC, Rottinger H: Anterolateral mini-incision hip replacement surgery: A modified Watson-Jones approach. *Clin Orthop Relat Res* 2004; 429:248-255.

20. Gustke K: Limited incision muscle-sparing anterolateral Watson-Jones approach for total hip arthroplasty, in O'Conner M (ed): *Limited Incisions for Total Hip Arthroplasty*. Rosemont, IL, American Academy of Orthopaedic Surgeons, 2007, pp 27-36.

21. Dorr L: Single-incision minimally invasive total hip arthroplasty. *J Bone Joint Surg Am* 2003;85:2236-2237.

# Surgical Nuances to Minimize Muscle Damage During the Anterolateral Intermuscular Approach in Minimally Invasive Hip Replacement

Wael Rahman, MD, MSc
Corey J. Richards, MD, MASc, FRCSC
Clive P. Duncan, MD

## Abstract

*Muscle damage that can occur during minimally invasive total hip replacement is an important concern. Minimizing this iatrogenic injury can help achieve the goals of the minimally invasive approach: decreased postoperative pain, decreased blood loss, and faster rehabilitation. Knowledge of particular aspects of minimally invasive anterolateral total hip arthroplasty is important, with focus on the nuances that aid in reducing muscle injury.*

**Instr Course Lect 2008;57:243-247.**

The term minimally invasive surgery (MIS) total hip arthroplasty (THA) is applied to any hip arthroplasty performed through a 10 cm or smaller incision.[1] This modification has been applied to various surgical approaches for THA, including anterior, posterior, lateral, and anterolateral approaches.[2-4] In addition, a two-incision technique was developed using two small incisions.[5] The impetus for the development of the MIS THA was patients' displeasure with the cosmetic appearance of a standard THA incision, as well as a desire for a more rapid recovery and a decreased rate of complications.

The anterolateral intermuscular approach is a surgical approach to the hip initially described by Sayre in 1894 and later modified by Watson-Jones.[6,7] The intermuscular interval is located anterior to the ab-

ductor muscle group and posterior to the tensor fascia lata, sparing the abductor muscles and the posterior capsule and short external rotators. The surgical approach was modified so that it could be used for primary total hip replacements.[8] It was expected that this intermuscular approach would permit rapid rehabilitation and minimize the risk of posterior dislocation.

The orthopaedic literature is deficient in well-designed studies to support the clinical superiority of minimally invasive THA. Most of the available evidence is derived from retrospective cohort studies or personal case series with conflicting results.[9] Cadaveric studies have verified that muscle damage is not minimized with MIS THA, which challenges earlier claims that decreased muscle damage is a benefit of the MIS approach.[10,11]

## Procedure Modifications

Although the application of the label MIS is determined by the length of the skin incision, the philosophy of MIS is to minimize soft-tissue trauma while achieving the excellent long-term outcomes of standard THA approaches. Care must be taken to avoid excessive retraction force, leading to damage to wound edges and underlying muscles, while still obtaining accurate positioning and solid fixation of the THA components. To achieve this goal when performing MIS THA via the anterolateral approach, changes in the surgical process are needed, including modifications in patient selection, preoperative templating, the operating room table, and patient positioning, as well as adopting the use of specialized instruments, precisely locating the incision, and choreographing the movements of the assistant.

### Patient Selection

When selecting patients to undergo MIS THA using the anterolateral approach, it is important to understand the difficulties that can be encountered during the procedure. Particularly relevant to patient selection are adequate posterior retraction of the

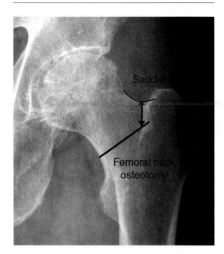

**Figure 1** A measurement is made from the saddle to the level of the femoral neck osteotomy.

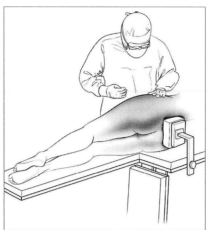

**Figure 2** The operating room table must be modified. (Redrawn from Bertin KC, Rottinger H: Anterolateral mini-incision hip replacement surgery: A modified Watson-Jones approach. *Clin Orthop Relat Res* 2004;429:248-255.)

gluteus medius, proper orientation of the acetabular component during impaction, and adequate adduction of the leg during femoral preparation. Retraction of the gluteus medius is more difficult in heavily muscled patients, resulting in one of two negative outcomes: poor visualization or adequate visualization with unacceptable damage to the gluteus medius muscle. In obese patients, particularly those with increased adipose tissue around the proximal lateral thigh, proper orientation of the acetabular component also can be difficult. The increased depth of the surgical wound can result in an acetabular component that is less anteverted and more vertical than recommended. Patients with body mass indices greater than 30 kg/m² are not ideal candidates, although clinical assessment of the distribution of adipose tissue is important in the decision-making process. Limited hip range of motion can make achieving the desired leg positions difficult. Preparation of the femur can be particularly difficult in this patient population because up to 40° of adduction is required during this

step.[12] As with any MIS THA, the degree and nature of the hip pathology also should be considered. If the procedure is intended to increase the limb length by 2 cm or more (for example, in patients with prior Legg-Calvé-Perthes disease or slipped capital femoral epiphysis), the inherent stability of the intermuscular anterolateral approach can make this goal difficult to achieve. Such patients are not ideal candidates for the procedure and should be warned that limb-length equalization may be incomplete.

### Preoperative Templating

The importance of preoperative planning and templating, with the objective of enabling the surgeon to define anatomic parameters that allow accurate placement of the femoral and acetabular implants, cannot be overemphasized. Optimal femoral and acetabular component fit, the level of femoral neck cut, the prosthetic neck length, and the femoral component offset can be evaluated by preoperative radiographic analy-

sis.[13] The location of the femoral neck osteotomy during standard THA is most commonly referenced off the lesser trochanter. Because of the limited exposure during an anterolateral MIS THA, the lesser trochanter is difficult to visualize. An additional point of reference, the nidus of the superior femoral neck or "saddle," often can be helpful. The distance from this point to the level of the osteotomy, along a line parallel to the shaft of the femur, is measured and recorded (Figure 1).

### Operating Table Modification and Patient Positioning

The patient is positioned on the operating table in the lateral decubitus position with the affected side up and the pelvis firmly secured. A table that allows removal of the distal posterior half of the table is used to permit the significant hip adduction required during femoral preparation (Figure 2). The hip is prepared and draped using contemporary techniques that allow the affected leg to be draped free to facilitate mobilization during the surgical procedure. A draping system with a sterile side bag is used to maintain sterility during preparation of the femur.[8]

### Specialized Instruments

Instrument modifications are required for several steps in the surgical procedure—visualization, acetabular preparation and component insertion, and femoral canal preparation and component insertion. Excellent visualization can be achieved, despite the smaller incision, by using modified retractors. Posterior acetabular retractors with rounded borders, twisted bodies, and long, curved handles provide benefits of decreased edge loading to the retracted soft tissue, uniform distribution of the load applied to the soft tissues, and more

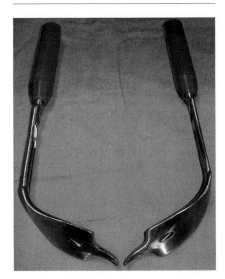

**Figure 3**    Modified posterior acetabular retractors.

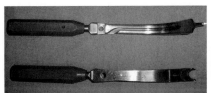

**Figure 4**    Modified femoral retractors.

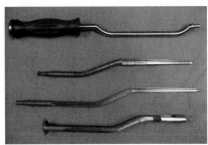

**Figure 6**    Offset femoral instrumentation for canal preparation and component insertion.

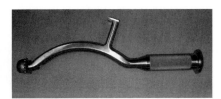

**Figure 5**    Offset acetabular impactor.

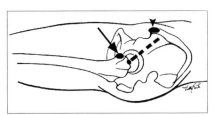

**Figure 7**    Illustration showing the position of the skin incision (*dashed line*). The anterior superior iliac spine (*arrowhead*) and the bunion of the greater trochanter (*arrow*) are shown. (Redrawn from Toms A, Duncan CP: The limited incision, anterolateral, intermuscular technique for total hip arthroplasty. *Instr Course Lect* 2006;55:199-203.)

remote positioning of the assistant's hand to avoid obscuring visualization (Figure 3). The use of flanged retractors is helpful in decreasing the number of retractors required for adequate visibility. The reduced length of the incision inevitably leads to a reduction in light to the surgical field; additional light sources, connected to the retractors, can provide considerable assistance in this respect[14] (Figure 4).

During MIS THA, acetabular reamers and impactors are forced into a more perpendicular and anterior orientation with respect to the sagittal and coronal planes of the patient. If this change in orientation is not recognized and addressed, a vertical and overanteverted acetabular component will result. The use of offset reamers and impactors can help prevent this technical error (Figure 5). Similarly, modified offset instrumentation is available for femoral preparation and component insertion, allowing implantation with the appropriate orientation while avoiding injury to the soft tissue (Figure 6).

## Precise Incision Location
A well-positioned skin incision can greatly improve visualization while minimizing soft-tissue trauma. Two anatomic landmarks must be identified for the anterolateral approach: the anterior superior iliac spine and the "bunion" of the greater trochanter (the inferior prominence of the anterior bulge of the greater trochanter). A line connecting these two points corresponds to the anterior border of the gluteus medius, which can be palpated easily in thin patients. The incision is made parallel and 1 to 2 inches posterior to this line[15] (Figure 7).

## Assistant Choreography
A series of five specific limb positions is used during intermuscular, anterolateral MIS THA. These positions optimize visualization while minimizing tension on the retracted soft tissue during each step of the procedure. The assistant is required to maintain the limb in these positions and ideally should understand

how each position aids visualization and reduces soft-tissue tension.

## Position One
In position one, the hip is abducted 30° with slight external rotation. This position relaxes the gluteus medius and thereby facilitates blunt dissection of the intermuscular plane between the tensor fascia lata and the gluteus medius. Modified Hohmann retractors are placed superior and inferior to the femoral neck overlying the hip capsule. Gentle force is applied to the superolateral retractor to avoid damage to the anterior border of the gluteus medius. The inferomedial retractor must be positioned deep to the iliopsoas to avoid injury to the femoral nerve. At this point in the procedure, the plane between the capsule and the gluteus minimus is developed. It is useful to look for the reflected head of the rectus femoris, which clearly indicates the lip of the acetabulum.[8,15] An inverted T-shaped

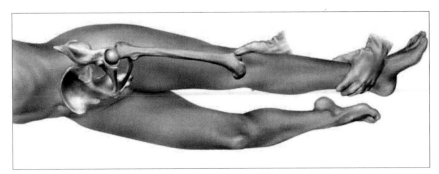

**Figure 8**   In position four (acetabular preparation), the hip is placed in slight external rotation, neutral abduction, and slight flexion. (Reproduced with permission from Zimmer, Inc.)

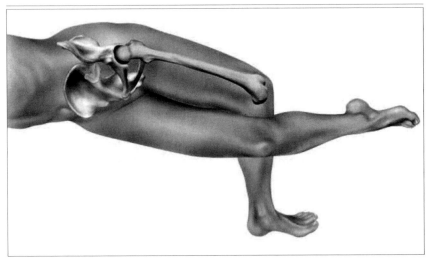

**Figure 9**   In position five (femoral preparation), the hip is in 90° external rotation, 20° hyperextension, and 40° of hip adduction. (Reproduced with permission from Zimmer, Inc.)

capsulotomy is completed by incising the capsule along the anterior aspect of the femoral neck as far as the intertrochanteric line. Both the superior and the inferior capsular flap are then raised, allowing reinsertion of the two Hohmann retractors around the exposed femoral neck. It is important to extend the superior capsular incision as far back as the piriformis fossa while extending the inferior incision laterally and inferiorly as close to the lesser trochanter as possible, to allow adequate mobilization of the femur.[15]

### Position Two
Position two involves maximum hip external rotation, 20° of hip abduction, and placement of the foot in the sterile bag. This position enables visualization of the head-neck junction as far as the base of the greater trochanter. The femoral neck is divided just proximal to the head-neck junction, avoiding damage to the acetabulum by directing the cut angle distally. A Cobb elevator or broad osteotome is placed in the osteotomy site and levered, while the assistant simultaneously forces the limb into external rotation.

### Position Three
In position three, the hip is in 90° of external rotation, the femur is paral-lel to the ground, the tibia is perpendicular to the floor, and the foot is placed in the sterile bag.[15] Retractors are positioned superolateral and inferomedial to the femoral neck, and the definitive osteotomy of the neck is planned. The increased external rotation improves visualization of the femoral neck, allowing for a more accurate osteotomy. The saddle is used as a reference point, as previously discussed, and a second osteotomy is made at a level determined during preoperative templating. The head and neck fragment can be extracted with a threaded Steinmann pin.

### Position Four
In position four, the hip has slight external rotation, neutral abduction, and slight hip flexion (Figure 8). By detensioning the gluteus medius, the femur can be safely retracted posteriorly, allowing visualization of the acetabulum. The acetabulum is then exposed by placing retractors at the 4 o'clock and 8 o'clock positions. If desired, a third retractor can be placed on the anterior acetabular rim. The leg is kept externally rotated during acetabular preparation; traction on the leg may improve exposure. The acetabulum is prepared and the component inserted in the usual manner, using modified instrumentation.[8]

### Position Five
Position five involves 90° of external hip rotation, 20° of hyperextension, and 40° of hip adduction, with the foot and leg placed in the sterile bag (Figure 9). The increased adduction allows more direct access to the femoral canal for preparation and implantation. A modified, flanged elevating retractor is placed posterior and medial to the femoral neck, levering the femur out of the wound. A second modified Hohmann retractor

is used to retract the gluteus medius and minimus. The standard steps in femoral preparation and component insertion, using modified instruments, are then followed.

## Summary

The goal of MIS THA is to reduce soft-tissue trauma, thereby decreasing blood loss and postoperative pain, and allowing earlier patient rehabilitation and more rapid return of function. The MIS anterolateral approach can be used in most patients. However, the ideal candidate is a slender, nonmuscular patient with reasonably good range of motion and minimal deformity. With particular attention to leg positioning during the procedure, the use of modified instrumentation, and a conscious effort for careful retraction, a well-aligned, well-fixed THA can be achieved via the MIS anterolateral approach with minimal soft-tissue trauma.

## References

1. Wright JM, Crockett HC, Delgado S, Lyman S, Madsen M, Sculco TP: Mini-incision for total hip arthroplasty: A prospective, controlled investigation with 5-year follow-up evaluation. *J Arthroplasty* 2004;19: 538-545.

2. Kennon RE, Keggi JM, Wetmore RS, Zatorski LE, Huo MH, Keggi KJ: Total hip arthroplasty through a minimally invasive anterior surgical approach. *J Bone Joint Surg Am* 2003;85-A(suppl 4):39-48.

3. Berry DJ, Berger RA, Callaghan JJ, et al: Minimally invasive total hip arthroplasty: Development, early results, and a critical analysis. *J Bone Joint Surg Am* 2003;85-A:2235-2246.

4. Duncan CP, Toms A, Masri BA: Minimally invasive or limited incision hip replacement: Clarification and classification. *Instr Course Lect* 2006;55:195-197.

5. Berger RA: Total hip arthroplasty using the minimally invasive two-incision approach. *Clin Orthop Relat Res* 2003;417:232-241.

6. Jergesen F, Abbott LC: A comprehensive exposure of the hip joint. *J Bone Joint Surg Am* 1955;37-A:798-808.

7. Watson-Jones R: Fractures of the neck of the femur. *Br J Surg* 1936;23: 787-808.

8. Bertin KC, Rottinger H: Anterolateral mini-incision hip replacement surgery: A modified Watson-Jones approach. *Clin Orthop Relat Res* 2004; 429:248-255.

9. Woolson ST: In the absence of evidence, why bother? A literature review of minimally invasive total hip replacement surgery. *Instr Course Lect* 2006;55:189-193.

10. Mardones R, Pagnano MW, Nemanich JP, Trousdale RT: Muscle damage after total hip arthroplasty done with the two-incision and mini-posterior techniques. *Clin Orthop Relat Res* 2005;441:63-67.

11. Meneghini RM, Pagnano MW, Trousdale RT, Hozack WJ: Muscle damage during MIS total hip arthroplasty: Smith-Petersen versus posterior approach. *Clin Orthop Relat Res* 2006;453:293-298.

12. Sculco TP, Jordan LC, Walter WL: Minimally invasive total hip arthroplasty: The Hospital for Special Surgery experience. *Orthop Clin North Am* 2004;35:137-142.

13. Berger RA: Mini-incision total hip replacement using an anterolateral approach: Technique and results. *Orthop Clin North Am* 2004;35:143-151.

14. Howell JR, Garbuz DS, Duncan CP: Minimally invasive hip replacement: Rationale, applied anatomy, and instrumentation. *Orthop Clin North Am* 2004;35:107-118.

15. Toms A, Duncan CP: The limited incision, anterolateral, intermuscular technique for total hip arthroplasty. *Instr Course Lect* 2006;55:199-203.

# Functional Recovery of Muscles After Minimally Invasive Total Hip Arthroplasty

Samuel R. Ward, PT, PhD
*Richard E. Jones, MD
William T. Long, MD
Debra J. Thomas, MD
*Lawrence D. Dorr, MD

## Abstract

*Whether mini-incision total hip arthroplasty is associated with accelerated postoperative recovery is a subject of considerable controversy. A study was conducted to compare objective outcomes using gait analysis as a measure for recovery of function in patients treated with three different minimally invasive surgical approaches and the traditional posterior approach. Sixty-nine patients underwent instrumented gait analysis at self-selected and fast velocities preoperatively and at 6 weeks and 3 months postoperatively. Four surgical groups were studied—30 treated with posterior mini-incisions, 11 anterolateral, 10 anterior Judet, and 18 traditional posterior long incisions. Overall, gait velocity increased slightly at 6 weeks and significantly at 3 months. However, there were no significant differences between groups for velocity, cadence, stride length, single-limb support time, or double-limb support time at 6 weeks or 3 months postoperatively. These data indicate that patients undergoing total hip arthroplasty with any of these surgical approaches recover muscle function, as measured by gait analysis, to preoperative levels within 6 weeks postoperatively. No advantage was shown with the use of any of the three different small-incision approaches. This finding suggests that the amount of muscle, or the particular muscle cut, does not have a significant effect on the recovery of postoperative gait function.*

**Instr Course Lect 2008;57:249-254.**

Minimally invasive surgery (MIS) for total hip arthroplasty has been described as a reduction in surgical incision size to 10 cm or less and as a muscle-sparing procedure. A number of studies have documented the technical success and safety of various minimally invasive operations performed by experienced surgeons and have found outcomes equivalent to those achieved with the standard incision technique previously used by that surgeon or a group of surgeons.[1-8] Two studies have reported improvements in either postoperative limp or stair-climbing ability in patients who have undergone MIS.[9,10] There are limited objective data comparing the recovery of gait function in patients who have undergone MIS and those who have been treated with a traditional-length incision.[11] Therefore, this study compared the recovery of temporospatial gait characteristics following total hip arthroplasty in each of four surgical groups: those treated with a long posterior traditional incision, posterior mini-incision, anterolateral mini-incision, and anterior Judet MIS performed on a special table. The hypothesis of this study was that patients treated with the small-incision operations would perform better than those treated with the traditional posterior incision with early (6 weeks and 3 months) objective gait-analysis testing. The basis of this hypothesis

*Richard E. Jones, MD is a consultant or employee for Zimmer. Lawrence D. Dorr, MD or the department with which he is affiliated has received research or institutional support and royalties from Zimmer.

**Table 1**
**Patient Demographics (Mean ± Standard Error)**

| | Anterolateral MIS (*n* = 11) | Anterior MIS (*n* = 10) | Posterior Standard (*n* = 18) | Posterior MIS (*n* = 30) |
|---|---|---|---|---|
| Age (years) | 55.0 ± 2.0 | 64.0 ± 2.0 | 61.0 ± 2.0 | 64.0 ± 1.0[†‡] |
| Body mass index | 28.9 ± 1.2 | 27.8 ± 1.1 | 29.8 ± 1.0 | 26.1 ± 0.5[*] |
| Preoperative self-selected velocity (m/min) | 60.6 ± 2.4 | 62.8 ± 3.4 | 56.9 ± 2.1 | 62.8 ± 1.3 |
| Preoperative fast velocity (m/min) | 81.7 ± 5.3 | 70.6 ± 2.6[†§] | 69.9 ± 4.2[†‖] | 80.4 ± 3.9 |

MIS = minimally invasive surgery
·Significantly different from posterior standard ($P = 0.019$)
†Significantly different from anterolateral MIS
‡$P = 0.004$
§$P = 0.016$
‖$P = 0.040$

was that muscle function would improve more quickly and be stronger with small-incision surgery, and this would be reflected in the objective gait analysis.

## Methods

Sixty-nine patients were enrolled in the study at the time of their preoperative clinical visit for total hip arthroplasty. Informed consent was obtained from each patient in accordance with the local ethics committee guidelines. Demographics of age and body mass index, plus the preoperative self-selected and fast gait velocities, are shown in Table 1. Patients in the posterior MIS group were on average 9 years older than the anterolateral MIS group and 9.7 kg lighter than the posterior long-incision surgical group.

The traditional posterior long incision was performed in 18 patients, the posterior mini-incision was performed in 30 patients, the anterolateral mini-incision was done in 11 patients, and the "no muscle cut" anterior Judet MIS using a special traction table was done in 10 patients.[12,13] The participating surgeons' familiarity with the approach used.

Gait analysis was performed at two different walking velocities: a self-selected speed that felt most comfortable and a "fast" gait speed at which patients were asked to walk as rapidly as could be tolerated without discomfort. Patients were allowed to practice each velocity until they were comfortable with the device and the instructions. Three representative trials were obtained for each velocity and averaged for final analysis. Gait data were collected using a battery-operated instrumented device, the IDEEA (MiniSun LLC, Fresno, CA) physical activity monitor with leads taped to the feet and legs that recorded data that were analyzed using computer software (Figure 1). The device was simple and convenient enough to be used in the office hallway. Data were collected at three times: preoperatively, and at 6 weeks and 3 months postoperatively. Stride characteristics that were measured included gait velocity, cadence, stride length, single-limb support time, and double-limb support time. Average values were compared for each patient at each time point (preoperatively, 6 weeks postoperatively, and 3 months postoperatively).

## Statistics

To compare the recovery of these parameters between surgical groups, repeated measures analyses of covariance and post hoc tests with corrections for multiple comparisons were used. Statistical computations were made with SPSS software (SPSS version 11.0, SPSS Inc., Chicago, IL) using a significance threshold of $\alpha = 0.05$. Data are presented as mean ± standard deviation, unless otherwise noted.

## Results

Preliminary data analysis indicated that patient age negatively correlated with self-selected gait velocity at 6 weeks ($r^2 = 0.048$, $P = 0.022$) and at 3 months ($r^2 = 0.113$, $P < 0.001$); likewise, preoperative self-selected gait velocity correlated positively to the 6-week result ($r^2 = 0.280$, $P < 0.001$) and the 3-month result ($r^2 = 0.360$, $P < 0.001$) (Figure 2). Although there were no obvious differences in self-selected or fast preoperative gait velocities between groups, these data indicated that preoperative temporospatial gait parameters should be included in the analyses as covariates. This step simply allows surgical groups to be

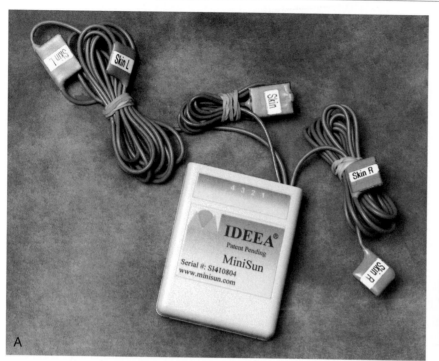

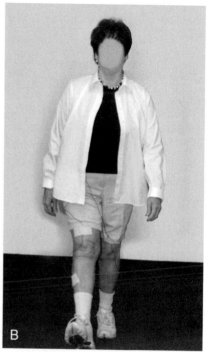

**Figure 1**    **A,** The IDEEA physical activity monitor is a portable device that was used for instrumented gait analysis. Stride characteristic data were collected from this device and analyzed with computer software. **B,** Patient walking in clinic, instrumented with leads attached. No special gait laboratory was necessary.

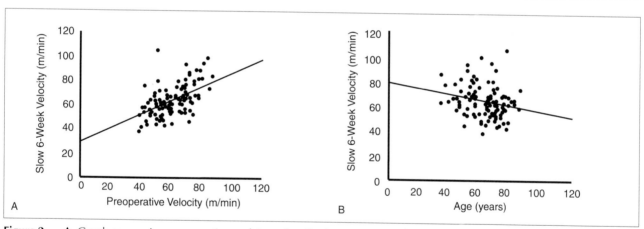

**Figure 2**    **A,** Graph comparing preoperative and 6-week self-selected gait velocity. **B,** Age correlates negatively with 6-week velocity ($r^2 = 0.0.048$, $P = 0.022$) and 3-month velocity ($r^2 = 0.113$, $P = 0.001$).

compared without the confounding effect of preoperative gait velocity.

Self-selected and "fast" gait velocities improved significantly over preoperative values by 3 months (Tables 2 and 3). At the patient's self-selected pace, velocity (in m/min) increased from 60.1 ± 1.42 to 61.5 ± 1.4 at 6 weeks, and to 68.8 ± 1.2 at 3 months ($P < 0.001$), a 5% and 16% improvement, respectively. When patients were asked to walk fast, velocity increased from 77.2 ± 1.5 to 78.3 ± 1.9 at 6 weeks and to 84.9 ± 2.0 at 3 months ($P < 0.05$), a 10% improvement. These improvements were the product of increases in cadence (steps/min) and stride length in all groups.

At 6 weeks and 3 months, there were no significant differences between groups for velocity ($P = 0.243$ and 0.61), cadence ($P = 0.18$ and 0.19), stride length ($P = 0.71$ and

**Table 2**
**Six-Week Temporospatial Gait Characteristics (Mean ± Standard Deviation)**

|  | Anterolateral MIS | Anterior MIS | Posterior Standard | Posterior MIS |
|---|---|---|---|---|
| **Self-selected velocity (m/min)** | 62.30 ± 6.60 | 54.40 ± 9.80 | 61.40 ± 13.00 | 66.50 ± 13.50 |
| Cadence (steps/min) | 99.00 ± 16.00 | 100.00 ± 14.00 | 106.00 ± 20.00 | 108.00 ± 12.00 |
| Stride length (m) | 1.26 ± 0.30 | 1.04 ± 0.11 | 1.16 ± 0.26 | 1.23 ± 0.30 |
| Single support (msec) | 393.50 ± 37.00 | 413.70 ± 32.80 | 393.20 ± 36.60 | 404.20 ± 27.00 |
| Double support (msec) | 139.20 ± 28.40 | 150.00 ± 47.50 | 130.50 ± 58.50 | 129.10 ± 38.90 |
| **Fast velocity (m/min)** | 80.00 ± 8.60 | 72.60 ± 7.10 | 71.80 ± 18.40 | 77.10 ± 14.50 |
| Cadence (steps/min) | 121.00 ± 11.00 | 101.00 ± 14.00 | 117.00 ± 21.00 | 119.00 ± 12.00 |
| Stride length (m) | 1.29 ± 0.14 | 1.10 ± 1.16 | 1.24 ± 0.38 | 1.29 ± 0.20 |
| Single support (msec) | 365.70 ± 31.90 | 393.10 ± 30.00* | 363.60 ± 48.40 | 384.20 ± 31.00† |
| Double support (msec) | 91.60 ± 15.50 | 115.60 ± 35.40 | 110.90 ± 39.30 | 102.50 ± 30.70 |

MIS = minimally invasive surgery
*Significantly different from posterior standard ($P = 0.009$)
†Significantly different from posterior standard ($P = 0.013$).

**Table 3**
**Three-Month Temporospatial Gait Characteristics (Mean ± Standard Deviation)**

|  | Anterolateral MIS | Anterior MIS | Posterior Standard | Posterior MIS |
|---|---|---|---|---|
| **Self-selected velocity (m/min)** | 71.50 ± 7.90 | 63.80 ± 10.80 | 69.10 ± 11.90 | 69.20 ± 11.10 |
| Cadence (steps/min) | 112.00 ± 12.00 | 108.00 ± 11.00 | 116.00 ± 14.00 | 114.00 ± 10.00 |
| Stride length (m) | 1.24 ± 0.10 | 1.16 ± 0.18 | 1.18 ± 0.13 | 1.23 ± 0.19 |
| Single support (msec) | 387.80 ± 32.10 | 396.20 ± 30.30 | 380.10 ± 34.50 | 401.70 ± 28.90* |
| Double support (msec) | 121.10 ± 25.30 | 128.10 ± 34.00 | 124.70 ± 49.90 | 115.80 ± 34.30 |
| **Fast velocity (m/min)** | 91.80 ± 14.80 | 82.70 ± 19.60 | 81.80 ± 19.80 | 82.70 ± 13.80 |
| Cadence (steps/min) | 133.00 ± 16.00 | 119.00 ± 11.00 | 128.00 ± 18.00 | 126.00 ± 10.00 |
| Stride length (m) | 1.36 ± 0.14 | 1.20 ± 00.12 | 1.27 ± 0.18 | 1.33 ± 0.20 |
| Single support (msec) | 348.70 ± 32.90 | 374.90 ± 26.30 | 364.80 ± 38.40 | 380.90 ± 31.60† |
| Double support (msec) | 85.40 ± 15.40 | 102.20 ± 25.30 | 101.80 ± 45.80 | 91.30 ± 30.20 |

MIS = minimally invasive surgery
*Significantly different from posterior standard ($P = 0.003$).
†Significantly different from posterior standard ($P = 0.015$).

0.70), single-limb support time ($P = 0.50$ and 0.40), or double-limb support time ($P = 0.35$ and 0.418). Careful inspection of each time point showed that single-limb support time was significantly shorter in the posterior standard-incision group than the posterior MIS group at 3 months at self-selected gait speeds, and at 6 weeks and 3 months during fast gait (Tables 2 and 3). However, it has been shown that single-limb support time is negatively correlated with gait velocity.[14] This concept makes intuitive sense because as velocity increases, the time one spends in stance declines. When single-limb support time was normalized by walking ve-

locity at the same time point, these differences were no longer apparent, suggesting that the differences were likely caused by small velocity differences between groups at 3 months.

## Discussion

The authors' hypothesis—that patients treated using small incision operations would perform better with objective gait analysis and therefore had better muscle function than did those treated with a posterior long incision—was not proved. Furthermore, the operations that had no muscle cut did not perform better than the small-incision operations that did have muscle cut. The results

showed that the most important predictor of postoperative gait function is preoperative gait function, and age is negatively correlated with gait velocity. As patient age increased, walking velocity declined; this finding is consistent with aging-associated velocity changes in the normal population.[14] The absence of influence of small-incision surgery on the results of gait analysis is an important finding because MIS, particularly the approaches that do not cut muscles, were expected to promote more rapid gait recovery.[1,13,15] However, more rapid recovery is mainly related to how well the patient walked preoperatively and to the patient's age.

The use of a small incision, and whether or not muscle was cut with the approach, seems to have no influence on recovery of gait at 6 weeks and 3 months postoperatively.

The first limitation of this study is that it is underpowered. For the data presented in this report, the study would have required at least 162 patients in each group to reach a power of 80%. To account for this weakness, the authors considered as many confounding factors as possible (age, body mass index, and preoperative gait velocity). The second weakness of this study is that the demographics of the group were not statistically equivalent. However, by correlating postoperative gait function to preoperative gait function for each patient, this difference in demographics did not influence the study results.

Patients' self-selected walking velocity at 6 weeks postoperatively was similar to their preoperative velocity; only by 3 months did they walk 16% faster (on average) than preoperatively. At 3 months, all groups could walk at normal gait velocity when they used their fast walk (normal gait velocity is 80 m/min). These patients achieved the ability to walk at a normal gait velocity with their fast walk more rapidly than did patients the authors had previously studied.[16] These data support early aggressive postoperative mobilization and walking for postoperative therapy.

Although several studies have reported early postoperative recovery with small-incision total hip replacement, such as improvements in postoperative limp and stair-climbing ability,[1,2,9,10] the objective data of this study do not support early improvements in gait. Bennett and associates[11] reported no signifi-

cant improvements in gait with the posterior MIS approach. It has been argued that anterior and posterior MIS approaches have different effects on postoperative recovery; the data presented here do not support these claims. Patients improved even with the anterolateral approach, which divides the gluteus medius muscle. Patients with a "no muscle cut" anterior approach had no better results than any other patients, although with a sufficient patient sample the finding of a better single-limb stance time for these patients than those with the anterolateral approach may be confirmed. The findings of a better single-limb stance time in patients treated with a posterior mini-incision compared with those treated with a posterior long incision approach also might be confirmed with a larger patient sample size. The statistically better single-limb stance time for the direct anterior approach and the posterior mini-incision was not present when corrected for gait velocity.

The absence of significant differences in postoperative gait function between surgical approach groups most likely is explained by muscle physiology and cadaveric muscle-damage studies.[17-19] Repair of muscle damage by elective surgery has already occurred by 6 weeks postoperatively. Muscle undergoes four phases of healing: degeneration, inflammation (these first two occur in the first few days after injury), regeneration, and fibrosis. The regeneration process can peak as early as 2 weeks after injury, and formation of scar tissue begins between the second and third weeks after injury.[17] The regeneration of muscle is directly related to the amount of scar tissue formed, which is related to the amount of damage. The large skeletal muscles, such as those

around the hip, contain up to 1,000 myofibers per single motor unit, compared with muscles with coordinated movements such as extraocular muscles, which have 10 myofibers per motor unit.[17] Large skeletal muscles can sustain more damage before substantial impact on their function. The amount of damage to muscles is essentially the same with all the MIS approaches studied (direct anterior approach, posterior mini approach, and two-incision approach) in the cadaver studies of Mardones and associates[18] and Meneghini and associates.[19] The comparison of muscle damage between the small incisions and the posterior long incision was not studied in the cadaveric model. The healing of bone also influences gait, and bone injury is essentially the same regardless of the surgical approach. Bone healing is dependent on osteon remodeling time, which averages 6 months, with no known factors that can accelerate it.[20,21] The rapid healing of muscle, and the prolonged healing of bone, diminish the influence of the incision size on the physiologic healing of tissues after total hip arthroplasty.

The most influential recovery factor that may be responsible for improved function for patients treated with a small incision may be the patient's mental response to the incision.[22] Psychological studies of patients showed that those treated with either a posterior mini-incision or a posterior long incision believed that the small incision contributed to improved function at 6 weeks postoperatively. Increased confidence in patients who had a small incision could easily affect their daily functional activities and their attitude toward their functional recovery. Improvements in patient education, anesthesia, and pain management also contribute to earlier recovery.[23,24] These effects would not be factors in this study because all patients were treated with similar education and pain management methods.

## Summary

This gait analysis study showed that the muscle injury associated with the four different approaches studied is not clinically important with respect to gait function by 6 weeks postoperatively. This finding suggests that muscle injury may not play a significant role and is not a rate-limiting factor in recovery following total hip replacement. The factors most important for the rapid recovery of patients postoperatively may be their psychological satisfaction with the operation as well as the anesthesia and pain management treatment used.[22,23]

## References

1. Berger RA, Jacobs JJ, Meneghini RM, Della Valle C, Paprosky W, Rosenberg AG: Rapid rehabilitation and recovery with minimally invasive total hip arthroplasty. *Clin Orthop Relat Res* 2004;429:239-247.

2. Berger RA, Duwelius PJ: The two-incision minimally invasive total hip arthroplasty: Technique and results. *Orthop Clin North Am* 2004;35: 163-172.

3. Goldstein WM, Branson JJ, Berland KA, Gordon AC: Minimal-incision total hip arthroplasty. *J Bone Joint Surg Am* 2003;85:33-38.

4. Wenz JF, Gurkan I, Jibodh SR: Mini-incision total hip arthroplasty: A comparative assessment of perioperative outcomes. *Orthopedics* 2002;25:1031-1043.

5. de Beer J, Petruccelli D, Zalzal P, Winemaker MJ: Single-incision, minimally invasive total hip arthroplasty: Length doesn't matter. *J Arthroplasty* 2004;19:945-950.

6. Siguier T, Siguier M, Brumpt B: Mini-incision anterior approach does not increase dislocation rate: A study of 1037 total hip replacements. *Clin Orthop Relat Res* 2004;426:164-173.

7. Berry DJ, Berger RA, Callaghan JJ, et al: Minimally invasive total hip arthroplasty: Development, early results, and a critical analysis. Presented at the Annual Meeting of the American Orthopaedic Association, Charleston, South Carolina, USA, June 14, 2003. *J Bone Joint Surg Am* 2003;85: 2235-2246.

8. Wright JM, Crockett HC, Delgado S, Lyman S, Madsen M, Sculco TP: Mini-incision for total hip arthroplasty: A prospective, controlled investigation with 5-year follow-up evaluation. *J Arthroplasty* 2004;19: 538-545.

9. DiGioia AM, Plakseychuk AY, Levison TJ, Jaramaz B: Mini-incision technique for total hip arthroplasty with navigation. *J Arthroplasty* 2003; 18:123-128.

10. Chung WK, Liu D, Foo LS: Mini-incision total hip replacement: Surgical technique and early results. *J Orthop Surg (Hong Kong)* 2004;12:19-24.

11. Bennett D, Ogonda L, Elliott D, Humphreys L, Beverland DE: Comparison of gait kinematics in patients receiving minimally invasive and traditional hip replacement surgery: A prospective blinded study. *Gait Posture* 2006;23:374-382.

12. Dorr LD: *Hip Arthroplasty: Minimally Invasive Techniques and Computer Navigation.* Philadelphia, PA, Elsevier, 2006.

13. Matta JM, Shahrdar C, Ferguson T: Single-incision anterior approach for total hip arthroplasty on an orthopaedic table. *Clin Orthop Relat Res* 2005;441:115-124.

14. Perry J: *Gait Analysis: Normal and Pathological Function.* Thorofare, NJ, Slack Inc, 1992.

15. Jerosch J, Theising C, Fadel ME: Antero-lateral minimal invasive (ALMI) approach for total hip arthroplasty technique and early results. *Arch Orthop Trauma Surg* 2006;126: 164-173.

16. Long WT, Dorr LD, Healy B, Perry J: Functional recovery of noncemented total hip arthroplasty. *Clin Orthop Relat Res* 1993;288:73-77.

17. Huard J, Li Y, Fu FH: Muscle injuries and repair: Current trends in research. *J Bone Joint Surg Am* 2002;84: 822-832.

18. Mardones R, Pagnano MW, Nemanich JP, Trousdale RT: Muscle damage after total hip arthroplasty done with the two-incision and mini-posterior techniques. *Clin Orthop Relat Res* 2005;441:63-67.

19. Meneghini RM, Pagnano MW, Trousdale RT, Hozack WJ: Muscle damage during MIS total hip arthroplasty. *Clin Orthop Relat Res* 2006;453: 293-298.

20. Kalfas IH: Principles of bone healing. *Neurosurg Focus* 2001;10:E1.

21. Einhorn TA: Enhancement of fracture-healing. *J Bone Joint Surg Am* 1995;77:940-956.

22. Dorr LD, Thomas D, Long WT, Polatin PB, Sirianni LE: Psychologic reasons for patients preferring minimally invasive total hip arthroplasty. *Clin Orthop Relat Res* 2007;458: 94-100.

23. Maheshwari AV, Boutary M, Yun AG, Sirianni LE, Dorr LD: Multimodal analgesia without routine parenteral narcotics for total hip arthroplasty. *Clin Orthop Relat Res* 2006;453: 231-238.

24. Inaba Y, Dorr LD, Wan Z, Sirianni L, Boutary M: Operative and patient care techniques for posterior mini-incision total hip arthroplasty. *Clin Orthop Relat Res* 2005;441:104-114.

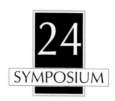

# Hot Topics and Controversies in Arthroplasty: Cementless Femoral Fixation in Elderly Patients

Andrew Dutton, FRCS
*Harry E. Rubash, MD

## Abstract

*Cementless femoral fixation has been established as the gold standard for hip arthroplasty in young patients because of its exceptional longevity. Because older Americans are living longer and staying active, cementless femoral fixation for hip arthroplasty should be considered in all patients who have good bone quality. Numerous studies have shown excellent results using cementless fixation for hip arthroplasty in elderly patients. Histologic analysis, radiographic review, and dual-energy x-ray absorptiometry have shown solid osseointegration for biologic fixation and minimal bone loss. Cementless fixation provides superb functional outcomes with results comparable to those achieved using cemented fixation for hip arthroplasty. Additional advantages of cementless femoral fixation include shorter surgical times and substantial savings in health care costs.*

**Instr Course Lect 2008;57:255-259.**

Total hip arthroplasty (THA) can provide patients with an exceptional quality of life.[1-3] The femoral component may be cemented or cementless. Cementless femoral stems are proximally or fully coated to provide biologic fixation. Despite similar long-term results compared with cemented fixation, cementless femoral fixation provides additional benefits, including decreased morbidity and improved cost-effectiveness. Cementless femoral implants for THAs are an excellent choice for the elderly patient population.

## The Aging Population: Implant Considerations

Elderly individuals are becoming an increasingly large proportion of the US population.[4] In 2000, 12.4% of the US population was older than 65 years. It is estimated that this percentage will increase to 16.3% by 2020. According to data from 2003 from the US Department of Health and Human Services, the life expectancy at birth was 75.3 years for males and 80.1 years for females.[4] At 75 years of age, the mean life expectancy was 10.5 years for males and 12.6 years for females (Table 1). Trends show an increase in life expectancy projections[4] (Table 2).

A study by Ritter and associates[5] compared the life expectancy of patients treated with THA to that of the general population. The 10-year life expectancy rate for women who were treated with THA at age 71 to 80 years was 75%, and 58% for those older than 80 years at the time of THA. In contrast, women in the general population age 71 to 80 years had a 10-year life expectancy rate of 60%, and those older than 80 years had a 10-year life expectancy rate of 27%. This improved life expectancy rate may be due in part to the medical screening of patients prior to THA and to the health status of those who are eligible for the procedure. Because patients undergoing THA have the potential for a long life, it is important that implants used in THA will properly function throughout the patient's lifetime.

## Advantages of Cementless Implants

### Implant Survival

The biologic fixation provided by cementless stems has led to excellent

*Harry Rubash, MD or the department with which he is affiliated has received research or institutional support and royalties from Zimmer.*

long-term implant survival (Table 3). Pieringer and associates[6] retrospectively reviewed the clinical and radiologic results of 80 patients (87 hips) who were older than 80 years at the time of cementless THA. A grit-blasted, titanium alloy femoral stem (Alloclassic SL; Centerpulse, Winterthur, Switzerland) was used in all patients; mean follow-up was 69.3 months. No femoral stems were removed for

aseptic loosening during this period. One intraoperative femoral fracture occurred. Deep infection occurred in two patients, with one patient requiring repeat surgery with a liner and femoral head exchange. Two early postoperative dislocations occurred and were treated successfully with closed reduction. Keisu and associates[7] performed 123 cementless THAs using a plasma-sprayed, titanium alloy femoral stem (Taperloc; Biomet, Warsaw, IN) in patients 80 to 89 years of age. Ninety-two hips (86 patients) had a mean follow-up of 5 years. There were no femoral revisions. One patient who had recurrent dislocations was again treated with closed reduction. Two late periprosthetic fractures occurred; one was treated with open reduction and internal fixation and the other was treated with traction. No perioperative deaths occurred, but the rate of medical complications was 24%. Complications included pulmonary emboli in 6.5% of patients and cardiac abnormalities in 2.4%. McAuley and associates[8] reviewed 159 cementless THAs that used the fully porous-coated Anatomic Medullary Locking femoral

stem (DePuy, Johnson and Johnson, Warsaw, IN) in patients with a mean age of 71 years and a mean follow-up of 8.5 years. One intraoperative, periprosthetic fracture occurred and was treated with cerclage wiring. There was one femoral revision for aseptic loosening at 2.3 years, which was revised successfully to a larger stem. Nine hips dislocated postoperatively, with only one requiring a revision. Two other revisions were needed, one for sepsis and another for an avulsion fracture of the greater trochanter secondary to osteolysis. In another study, Bourne and associates[9] reviewed 307 cementless THAs using a proximally plasma-sprayed, titanium alloy femoral stem (Mallory Head; Biomet Inc, Warsaw, IN) in patients with a mean age of 64 years. With a follow-up period of 10 to 13 years, two femoral revisions were needed; one revision was for a periprosthetic fracture and the other for sepsis. Berend and associates[10] reviewed the outcome of 49 cementless THAs using the Mallory Head femoral component in patients with a mean age of 79 years. With a mean follow-up of 5 years,

## Table 1
### Life Expectancy in the United States in 2003[4]

|        | Male (years) | Female (years) |
|--------|--------------|----------------|
| Birth  | 75.3         | 80.1           |
| Age 65 | 16.8         | 19.8           |
| Age 75 | 10.5         | 12.6           |
| Age 85 | 5.7          | 6.9            |

## Table 2
### Life Expectancy at Birth (Based on Year of Birth)[4]

| Year of Birth | Male | Female |
|---------------|------|--------|
| 1900          | 46.3 | 48.3   |
| 1950          | 65.6 | 71.1   |
| 1990          | 71.8 | 78.8   |
| 2000          | 74.3 | 79.7   |

## Table 3
### Results of Cementless THAs in Elderly Patients

| Study | Patient Age (Years) | Number of Hips | Femoral Stem Type | Follow-up (Years) | Stem Survival | Resurgery (Number and Reason) |
|-------|---------------------|----------------|-------------------|-------------------|---------------|-------------------------------|
| Pieringer et al[6] | > 80 | 87 | Grit-blasted titanium alloy (Alloclassic SL) | Mean 5.8 | 100% | 2 PPFXs 1 Sepsis |
| Keisu et al[7] | 80 to 89 | 92 | Plasma-sprayed titanium tapered (Taperloc) | Mean 5 | 100% | 1 PPFX |
| McAuley et al[8] | Mean 71 | 159 | Fully coated anatomic (Anatomic Medullary Locking) | Mean 8.5 | 98% | 1 Loose 1 Dislocation 1 Sepsis 1 PPFX |
| Bourne et al[9] | Mean 64 | 307 | Plasma-sprayed titanium tapered (Mallory Head) | 10 to 13 | 100% | 1 Sepsis 1 PPFX |
| Berend et al[10] | Mean 79 | 49 | Plasma-sprayed titanium tapered (Mallory Head) | Mean 5 | 100% | 1 Pain |

PPFX = periprosthetic fracture

no femoral revisions for aseptic loosening occurred. One intraoperative femoral fracture was treated with cerclage wiring, and one femoral stem was revised unsuccessfully for unexplained leg (not thigh) pain; intraoperatively, the stem was noted to be well fixed. These studies show excellent results for the survival of cementless femoral components in elderly patients; these results are comparable to the results achieved using cemented femoral implants.

### Preservation of Femoral Bone Stock

The preservation of femoral bone stock is desirable in elderly patients with osteoporosis. The variety of stem geometries and surface coatings available with cementless femoral stems allow biologic fixation in a variety of femoral canal geometries. Grit-blasted, titanium femoral components have shown excellent histologic osseointegration.[11] Marshall and associates[12] radiographically reviewed 200 cementless THAs using plasma-sprayed, titanium alloy femoral stems (Integral, Biomet). Spot welds were seen in 99.3% of the stems, and endosteal bone formation around the tip was noted in 51%. Cortical hypertrophy in zones 2, 3, 5, and 6 was noted in 26%. Akhavan and associates[13] reviewed the results of THA using a cementless stem consisting of a cobalt-chromium core surrounded by polyaryletherketone and titanium mesh (Epoch; Zimmer, Warsaw, IN). Twenty-eight patients were followed for an average of 6.2 years. There was no radiographic evidence of femoral loosening. Although there was a small, initial decrease in bone mass at the proximal zones of 1, 2, 6, and 7 on dual-energy x-ray absorptiometry, bone mass did not decrease significantly over time. Minimal bone loss was noted in the distal zones. There

was one femoral revision for a periprosthetic fracture. Cementless femoral components allow excellent biologic fixation and minimize bone loss.

### Modularity and Geometry of Femoral Stems

Cementless femoral stems also provide the necessary modularity and geometry for fixation in most types of femoral canals. With aging, there is significant remodeling of the femur, which is most pronounced in women.[14] Radiographic analysis of cadaveric femurs revealed an average of 3° of varus remodeling of the femoral neck with aging. At the isthmus, canal expansion averaged 0.092 mm per year. The femoral canal changes from a so-called champagne flute shape to that resembling a stovepipe. Because of these morphologic changes, using a cemented generic femoral component in an elderly woman may compromise the proximal medial cement mantle. To avoid this complication, the stem may be downsized; however, this leads to an excessively thick cement mantle. The option of multiple cementless femoral stem geometries can accommodate the variations in femoral morphology associated with aging.

### Cost Implications

THAs performed in the increasingly larger elderly population have substantial economic implications. From 1990 to 2002, the number of THAs performed has increased by 46%.[15] Health cost assessment and minimization is essential in orthopaedic procedures.[1] Barrack and associates[16] analyzed 50 cases to compare the cost of implanting cemented versus cementless femoral stems. The cases were divided into two groups: uncomplicated, primary, cementless THAs or hybrid THAs. Femoral cementation

involved extra equipment including a canal water pik and brush, canal plug, stem centralizer, and cement. Cemented THAs required longer surgical times (average increase, 20 minutes) that were related to cement insertion and setting. Overall, cementless femoral fixation was approximately 8% less costly than cemented fixation.

### Functional Outcomes

Functional outcomes for cementless THAs in elderly patients have been excellent. Zimmerman and associates[17] compared functional outcomes of cementless versus hybrid THAs in 272 patients older than 65 years. Assessment at 2, 6, and 12 months postoperatively found no differences in pain level, walking speed, and lower extremity function in performing activities of daily living between the two groups. In a study analyzing the clinical results of cementless THAs in patients with an average age of 79 years and an average follow-up of 5 years, 71% of patients were able to walk more than two blocks, 44% did not require an assistive device, 35% required a cane, and 19% used a walker.[10] Jones and associates[18] reviewed the functional outcomes of 454 patients treated with THA. Using the Western Ontario and McMaster Universities Osteoarthritis Index and the Medical Outcomes Society 36-Item Short Form survey, they determined that age was not related to functional outcome. Cementless femoral THA has superb and comparable functional results to cemented THA.

## Complications: Considerations of Cementless Versus Cemented THAs

Cemented femoral fixation has distinct disadvantages compared with cementless fixation. Data from the

Norwegian Arthroplasty Register show that patients with cemented THAs have a significantly increased risk (1.8 times higher) of infection compared with patients with cementless THAs.[19] This finding may be related to bone necrosis secondary to either direct cement toxicity or from heat generated from cement polymerization. Elderly patients are often susceptible to infection because of medical comorbidities.

Elderly patients are more susceptible to cardiopulmonary compromise resulting from the pulmonary emboli related to cemented femoral fixation. Clark and associates[20] evaluated 20 patients age 59 to 83 years who were treated with cemented hemiarthroplasty and monitored with a transesophageal Doppler probe. During cementation, patients had a 33% reduction in cardiac output and a 44% reduction in stroke volume. Hagio and associates[21] evaluated 88 patients treated with a hybrid THA who were monitored with a transesophageal echocardiograph. Severe embolic events (cascade of fine emboli or embolic masses) occurred in 61.5% of patients in the hybrid THA group compared with 5.9% of patients in the group treated with cementless THA. These events were associated with significant decreases in arterial oxygen saturation and systolic blood pressure. Parvizi and associates[22] reviewed the records of 23 patients who died during surgery from cardiorespiratory compromise during THA. These deaths represented 0.06% of THAs performed at the authors' institution. The mean patient age was 80.9 years, and all patients had undergone cemented femoral component fixation. Autopsies were performed in 13 patients. Bone marrow microemboli were found in the lungs of 11 patients,

and methylmethacrylate particles were found in 3 patients.

Hemodynamic changes caused by cementation may be associated with a higher rate of postoperative confusion in elderly patients. Pagnano and associates[23] reviewed the clinical outcome of THAs in 47 patients older than 90 years. Twenty-two patients had 35 medical complications; 9 were caused by transient postoperative confusion. These serious adverse effects of femoral cementation can be particularly problematic in elderly patients with underlying cardiac and pulmonary pathology.

Cemented femoral fixation in THA is associated with prolonged surgical times. The mean surgical time for cementless THA was 120 minutes compared with 140 minutes for cemented THA.[16] The Norwegian Arthroplasty Register noted that surgical times for cementless THAs were on average 15 minutes shorter than for cemented THAs.[19] Smabrekke and associates[24] further analyzed the Register's data and noted that cemented implants with surgical times of less than 51 minutes and more than 90 minutes were associated with an increased risk of revision because of aseptic loosening. Prolonged surgical times (> 150 minutes) were associated with an increased risk of revision because of infection. Because cemented femoral fixation in THA is associated with longer surgical times, operating room and anesthesia costs are increased, as well as the risk of infection.

Another disadvantage of cement fixation is the difficulty encountered in revision surgery. Removing the cement mantle of a femoral stem is challenging and time consuming.[25] Cement removal may necessitate bone damage secondary to procedures such as an extended trochan-

teric osteotomy or the creation of a cortical window.[26,27] Thirteen percent of intraoperative fractures occur during cement removal.[28] The use of specialized instruments to remove cement also carry inherent risks, including the risk of femoral perforation, thermal tissue damage with the use of an ultrasonic device, and increased infection risk secondary to contaminated aerosols from a burr device.[29,30] The preservation of bone stock by avoiding stress shielding can be valuable in the revision setting.

## Summary

The use of cementless femoral prostheses should be considered for THA in all patients with good bone quality. These implants allow biologic fixation with physiologic loading of the bone to minimize stress shielding and have excellent survivorship in elderly patients with all types of bone morphology. With an increasingly large elderly population, cementless femoral prostheses have demonstrated superior cost-effectiveness compared with cemented prostheses. Cementless THA is not associated with the disadvantages of cemented femoral fixation that include cement-related emboli, longer surgical times, increased infection risk, and the difficulties inherent in cement extraction. Cementless femoral implants for THA are an excellent choice for elderly patients.

## References

1. Bozic KJ, Saleh KJ, Rosenberg AG, Rubash HE: Economic evaluation in total hip arthroplasty: Analysis and review of the literature. *J Arthroplasty* 2004;19:180-189.

2. Chang RW, Pelliser JM, Hazen GB: Cost-effectiveness analysis of total hip

arthroplasty for osteoarthritis of the hip. *JAMA* 1996;275:858-865.

3. Brander VA, Malhotra S, Jet J, Heinemann AW, Stulberg DS: Outcome of hip and knee arthroplasty in persons aged 80 years and older. *Clin Orthop Relat Res* 1997;345:67-78.

4. Centers for Disease Control Website. National Center for Health Statistics. Available at: www.cdc.gov/nchs/fastats/lifexpec.html. Accessed March, 2007.

5. Ritter MA, Albohm MJ, Keating M, Faris P, Meding JB: Life expectancy after total hip arthroplasty. *J Arthroplasty* 1998;13:874-875.

6. Pieringer H, Labek G, Auersperg V, Bohler N: Cementless total hip arthroplasty in patients older than 80 years of age. *J Bone Joint Surg Br* 2003;85:641-645.

7. Keisu KS, Orozco F, Sharkey PF, Hozack WJ, Rothman RH: Primary cementless total hip arthroplasty in octogenarians: Two to eleven year follow-up. *J Bone Joint Surg Am* 2001; 83-A:359-363.

8. McAuley JP, Moore KD, Culpepper WJ II, Engh CA: Total hip arthroplasty with porous coated prostheses fixed without cement in patients who are sixty-five years of age and older. *J Bone Joint Surg Am* 1998;80:1648-1655.

9. Bourne RB, Rorabeck CH, Patterson JJ, Guerin J: Tapered titanium cementless total hip replacements: A 10 to 13 year follow-up. *Clin Orthop Relat Res* 2001;393:112-120.

10. Berend KR, Lombardi AV, Mallory TH, Dodds KL, Adams JB: Cementless double-tapered total hip arthroplasty in patients 75 years of age and older. *J Arthroplasty* 2004;19:288-295.

11. Feighan JE, Goldberg VM, Davy D, Parr JA, Stevenson S: The influence of surface-blasting on the incorporation of titanium-alloy implants in a rabbit intramedullary model. *J Bone Joint Surg Am* 1995;77:1380-1395.

12. Marshall AD, Mokris JG, Reitman RD, Dandar A, Mauerhan DR: Cementless titanium tapered-wedge femoral stem: 10-15 year follow-up. *J Arthroplasty* 2004;19:546-552.

13. Akhavan S, Matthiesen MM, Schulte L, et al: Clinical and histologic results related to a low-modulus composite total hip replacement. *J Bone Joint Surg Am* 2006;88:1308-1314.

14. Noble PC, Box GG, Kamaric E, Fink MJ, Alexander JW, Tullos HS: The effect of aging on the shape of the proximal femur. *Clin Orthop Relat Res* 1995;316:31-44.

15. Kurtz S, Mowat F, Ong K, Chan N, Lau E, Halpern M: Prevalence of primary and revision total hip and knee arthroplasty in the United States from 1990 through 2002. *J Bone Joint Surg Am* 2005;87:1487-1497.

16. Barrack RL, Castro F, Guinn S: Cost of implanting a cemented versus cementless femoral stem. *J Arthroplasty* 1996;11:373-376.

17. Zimmerman S, Hawkes WG, Hudson JI, et al: Outcomes of surgical management of total hip replacement in patients aged 65 years and older: Cemented versus cementless femoral component and lateral or anterolateral versus posterior anatomical approach. *J Orthop Res* 2002;20:182-191.

18. Jones CA, Voaklander DC, Johnston DW, Suarez-Almazor ME: The effect of age on pain, function, and quality of life after total hip and knee arthroplasty. *Arch Intern Med* 2001;161:454-460.

19. Engesaeter LB, Espehaug B, Lie SA, Furnes O, Havelin LI: Does cement increase the risk of infection in primary total hip arthroplasty? Revision rates in 56,275 cemented and uncemented primary THAs followed for 0-16 years in the Norwegian Arthroplasty Register. *Acta Orthop* 2006;77:351-358.

20. Clark DI, Ahmed AB, Baxendale BR, Moran CG: Cardiac output during hemiarthroplasty of the hip: A prospective, controlled trial of cemented and uncemented prostheses. *J Bone Joint Surg Br* 2001;83:414-418.

21. Hagio K, Sugano N, Takashina M, Nishii T, Yoshikawa H, Ochi T: Embolic events during total hip arthroplasty: An echocardiographic study. *J Arthroplasty* 2003;18:186-192.

22. Parvizi J, Holiday A, Ereth M, Lewallen DG: Sudden death during primary hip arthroplasty. *Clin Orthop Relat Res* 1999;369:39-48.

23. Pagnano MW, McLamb LA, Trousdale RT: Primary and revision total hip arthroplasty for patients 90 years of age and older. *Mayo Clin Proc* 2003; 78:285-288.

24. Smabrekke A, Epehaug B, Havelin LI, Furnes O: Operating time and survival of primary total hip replacements: An analysis of 31,745 primary cemented and uncemented total hip replacements from local hospitals reported to the Norwegian Arthroplasty Register 1987-2001. *Acta Orthop Scand* 2004;75:524-532.

25. Schurman DJ, Maloney WJ: Segmental cement extraction at revision total hip arthroplasty. *Clin Orthop Relat Res* 1992;285:158-163.

26. Taylor JW, Rorabeck CH: Hip revision arthroplasty: Approach to the femoral side. *Clin Orthop Relat Res* 1999;369:208-222.

27. Paprosky WG, Weeden SH, Bowling JW: Component removal in revision total hip arthroplasty. *Clin Orthop Relat Res* 2001;393:181-193.

28. Meek RM, Garbuz DS, Masri BA, Greidanus NV, Duncan CP: Intraoperative fracture of the femur in revision total hip arthroplasty with a diaphyseal fitting stem. *J Bone Joint Surg Am* 2004;86-A:480-485.

29. Nogler M, Lass-Florl C, Wimmer C, Mayr E, Bach C, Ogon M: Contamination during removal of cement in revision hip arthroplasty: A cadaver study using ultrasonic and high speed cutters. *J Bone Joint Surg Br* 2003;85:436-439.

30. Brooks AT, Nelson CL, Stewart CL, Skinner RA, Siems ML: Effect of an ultrasonic device on temperatures generated in bone and on bone-cement structure. *J Arthroplasty* 1993;8:413-418.

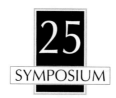

# Cement Fixation of the Femoral Component in Older Patients

*Paul F. Lachiewicz, MD

## Abstract

*Polymethylmethacrylate cement fixation of the femoral component in total hip arthroplasty is still a reasonable option in a select group of patients. Cement fixation is indicated in sedentary patients older than 75 years, certain older patients with rheumatoid arthritis, and patients with femoral neck fractures or conversion surgery. Hips with severe osteopenia or a "stove-pipe" femur (Dorr type C) may also be considered for cement fixation. The cemented femoral component should be fabricated of a cobalt-chromium alloy with a modern geometry and offset. Third-generation cementing techniques should be used to obtain a grade A or B cement mantle. Antibiotic cement may be used in patients at higher risk for infection. The 10-year results of cemented femoral components in these patient populations are excellent.*

**Instr Course Lect 2008;57:261-265.**

The use of polymethylmethacrylate cement for fixation of the femoral component in total hip arthroplasty (THA) has decreased with the successful use of cementless components in a wide variety of patients. However, cement fixation is still indicated for use in a select group of patients. Cement fixation of the femoral component has several distinct advantages. Immediate fixation of the component in the femoral canal is possible even in hips with a large medullary canal. There is no need for "perfect" broach preparation of the femur because cement will fill any gaps. Because postopera-tive thigh pain with full weight-bearing ambulation usually does not occur with cement fixation, more rapid rehabilitation may be possible. In patients at higher risk for infection, antibiotic-impregnated cement can be used.

## Indications

The general indications for the use of cement for femoral component fixation in THA include factors that are related to the patient, the diagnosis, and the femoral bone type. In general, cement is used in older, sedentary or less active patients older than 75 years (Figure 1). In the author's practice, patients in this age group comprise 19% of the primary THAs performed. According to data from the American Academy of Orthopaedic Surgeons, 29% of patients in the United States who had primary THAs in 1999 were in this age group.[1] Although good results with cementless femoral components have been reported in octogenarians,[2] the author generally uses cement for femoral component fixation in patients in this age group. Although cementless fixation has been used, cement fixation is preferred for older patients with rheumatoid arthritis, acute femoral neck fracture (Figure 2), and in patients who require conversion of failed fixation of proximal femoral fractures[3,4] (Figure 3).

Prepackaged tobramycin bone cement (Simplex P with tobramycin, Howmedica, Limerick, Ireland), which may decrease the risk of infection, can be used in patients with a higher risk of infection, including those with rheumatoid arthritis, psoriatic arthritis, and diabetes mellitus. Patients with severe osteopenia of the proximal femur and those with a Dorr type C or "stove-pipe" femur should be considered for cement

*Paul F. Lachiewicz, MD is a consultant or employee of Zimmer.*

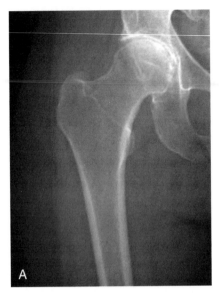
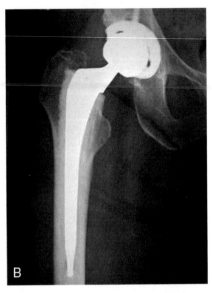

**Figure 1** **A,** Radiograph of the right hip of an 82-year-old woman with medial osteoarthritis. **B,** The postoperative radiograph shows a hybrid THA, cement grade A.

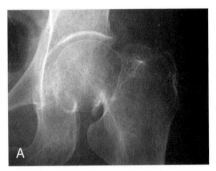
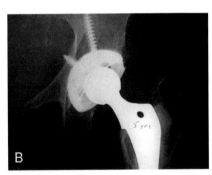

**Figure 2** **A,** Radiograph of a displaced fracture in the left femoral neck in an 81-year-old healthy, active woman. **B,** Postoperative radiograph 5 years after treatment with a hybrid THA.

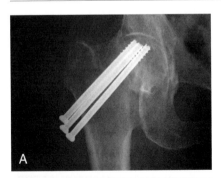
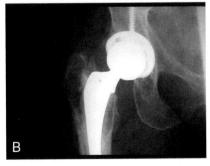

**Figure 3** **A,** AP radiograph of the femur of a 78-year-old woman with failure of fixation of a femoral neck fracture. **B,** Radiograph following conversion to a hybrid THA.

fixation.[5] Another factor that may influence the use of cement fixation is the presence of a contralateral cemented femoral component, which

has provided good patient satisfaction. Patients with concomitant spine arthritis, spinal stenosis, or a psychological disorder such as anxiety or depression, may be considered for cement fixation to avoid possible postoperative activity-related thigh pain.[6] In these groups of patients, it may be difficult to determine the exact cause of residual leg pain if a cementless femoral component is implanted.

## Contraindications

Certain patient groups have a higher risk of early and late failure of cemented femoral components. These groups include patients younger than 65 years, heavy patients (> 90 kg), and patients with high-demand activity levels. It has been noted by the author that, in older male patients, a specific anatomic configuration of the proximal femur may result in a higher failure rate with the use of cemented femoral component fixation. These patients have a narrow (10 to 12 mm) medullary canal with thick cortices, but with a large (medial to lateral) metaphysis and intertrochanteric region. Standard cemented femoral components may fit poorly in patients with these anatomic characteristics and may result in a higher rate of loosening (Figure 4).

Cement fixation should not be routinely used in patients on hemodialysis because of renal failure, bleeding dyscrasia, and bone marrow disorders.[7] In these situations, it may be technically difficult to obtain a good femoral cement mantle because of excessive bleeding. There is some controversy concerning the use of cement fixation in patients with severe cardiopulmonary disease because of the risk of fat embolization with cement pressurization and cardiac arrhythmias caused by systemic cement monomer.[8]

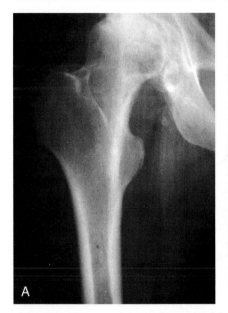

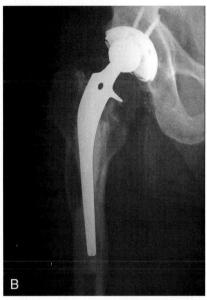

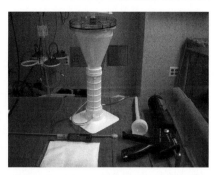

**Figure 5** The equipment needed for implanting a cemented femoral component includes a polyethylene canal plug, cement, vacuum-mixer, syringe, and cement gun.

**Figure 4** **A,** Preoperative radiograph of the femur of an active 60-year-old man with osteoarthritis; the medullary canal is narrow and has thick cortices. **B,** Radiograph 12 years after THA with a cemented femoral component shows loosening and large areas of osteolysis.

## Techniques

Preoperative planning and the use of conventional or digital radiographs to make a template showing the size and offset of the femoral component are recommended. A box with the template-sized component (and a component one size smaller) is placed in a blanket warmer adjacent to the operating room. Some evidence exists that preheating the femoral component improves the cement strength and interface while reducing the time needed for polymerization.[9,10]

Adequate exposure of the hip is recommended for implanting a cemented femoral component; moist sponges are placed on the incision edges. The femoral medullary canal is entered with a canal finder, and broaching is started with a rasp one size smaller than the templated component size. If the smaller rasp fits easily, the rasp that matches the size of the template is placed. If nec-

essary, the rasp is countersunk and a calcar planer is used to shorten the femoral neck. A trial femoral neck and head is placed and the hip is reduced. A thorough check of stability is performed. The author uses a posterior approach and prefers at least 60° of internal rotation stability during trial reduction range of motion. The rasp is then removed and the medullary canal is checked with a metal measuring device for a distal cement centralizer, which is usually 2 mm smaller than the implant. The medullary canal is routinely occluded with a 25-mm polyethylene plastic plug that is placed 1 to 2 cm below the anticipated tip of the prosthesis. Plug stability is checked with a suction tip.

The prosthetic components—stem, head, and distal centralizer—are assembled on the back table. The author does not use a proximal centralizer. Third-generation cementing techniques are recommended.[11,12] The

surgical technician prepares three packages of Simplex-P cement (Stryker Orthopaedics, Mahwah, NJ) using a vacuum mixer-syringe system (Figure 5) while the surgeon irrigates the femoral medullary canal using a long-stem water pik for several minutes. After irrigating the canal with approximately 1.5 L of water, the medullary canal is packed with thrombin-sprayed gauze (vaginal packing) using a long nontoothed forceps. At approximately 6 minutes after the start of cement mixing, a rod is placed into the femoral component extraction hole and a small amount of cement is placed over the distal centralizer and implant tip to prevent distal cement bubbles or voids. The packing is then removed, the canal is suctioned for the final time, and the cement is introduced in a retrograde fashion using the cement gun. The proximal cement is pressurized two to three times manually with two fingers on a rubber dam. The prosthesis is then inserted, holding the femoral head and the extraction-hole rod. Excess cement is removed, preferably with a long-handled knife.[13] After the cement removal, the extraction-hole rod is removed and the prosthesis is manually pushed the final 2 mm into

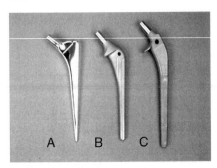

**Figure 6**  Three types of femoral components for cement fixation are shown—polished-tapered (**A**), macrotextured (**B**), proximal precoated (**C**).

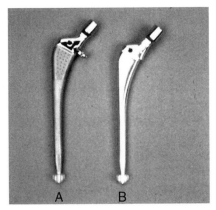

**Figure 7**  Two modern stems for cement fixation with distal centralizer: macrotextured-precoated (**A**) and polished (**B**) are shown.

position. Final packing and cleaning of cement is done with an angled curet. After cement polymerization, the hip is irrigated, the incisional sponges are removed, and the hip reduced. Repair of the posterior capsule and short external rotators is routinely performed. **(DVD 25.1)**

## Results

The femoral component used for cement fixation should be fabricated of a cobalt-chromium alloy with a broad and curved medial surface. A variety of sizes and offsets are available for anatomic reconstruction of the hip. As described, third-

generation cementing techniques should be used to obtain an excellent (grade A or B) cement mantle.[11,12] A wide variety of femoral component surface finishes have been used over the past 15 years including polished, matte finish, macrotextured, and precoated with a film of polymethylmethacrylate (Figure 6).

Longer-term results of several of these different types of femoral components have been reported. The 8- to 12-year follow-up of the first 325 polished, tapered Exeter stems (Stryker Howmedica Osteonics, Mahwah, NJ) showed 100% femoral component survival in a group of patients with a mean age of 67 years.[14] Two studies also have shown a high rate of success at 10-year follow-up for femoral components with a roughened and precoated surface.[15,16] In one study of 75 hips in patients with a mean age of 67 years, there was no femoral loosening at 10 years using a hybrid THA with the Precoat component (Zimmer, Warsaw, IN).[15] Another study reported on the results with a roughened, precoated stem with proximal and distal cement centralizers. In 166 hips in patients with a mean age of 69 years, a cement grade of A or B was achieved in 95% of hips.[16] The 10-year implant survival rate was 95%; only 2.4% of the femoral components were definitely loose. One study, however, reported an early failure rate of 12% at a mean follow-up of 3 years with the use of this precoated femoral component.[17] This study had confounding variables involving the use of highly crystalline polyethylene (Hylamer, DePuy, Warsaw, IN) and ceramic heads in younger patients (mean age, 48 years) with failed implants.

Vail and associates[18] reported on a multicenter, prospective, random-

ized study comparing 226 hybrid THAs in which the femoral component differed only in surface finish (polished Ra 4 microinches versus grit-blasted Ra 80 to 100 microinches. There was no difference in loosening, osteolysis, or radiolucent lines at a mean follow-up of 4.8 years. Another prospective, randomized study comparing a polished (Ra 7 to 12) and a precoated (Ra 70 to 90) femoral component and found no significant difference in the fixation of the components at a mean follow-up of 4 years (PF Lachiewicz, MD, unpublished data, 2003) (Figure 7). However, both of these prospective, randomized studies were underpowered if the difference in the rate of failure was only 2% to 4%. At present, because of implant availability, the author uses a polished femoral component when cement fixation is performed. Over a recent 4-year period, a study of 164 THAs using polished cemented femoral components in patients with a mean age of 75.8 years and a follow-up period of 2 to 5 years found no loosening of the femoral component; only one component was removed to treat a nonunion of a distal periprosthetic fracture (PF Lachiewicz, MD, unpublished data, 2006).

## Summary

Fixation of the femoral component with polymethylmethacrylate cement in THAs is still a valuable treatment and is now used in a select group of patients. Cement fixation should be considered in older, less active patients and in patients with severe osteopenia or Dorr type C femoral canals. The femoral component should be fabricated of a cobalt-chromium alloy; a polished surface finish is recommended. With modern third-generation cementing techniques, a high rate of successful outcomes at 10-year follow-up is achieved using cement fixation of the femoral component.

## References

1. Praemer A, Furner S, Rice DP: *Musculoskeletal Conditions in the United States*, ed 3. Rosemont, IL, American Academy of Orthopaedic Surgeons, 1999, pp 127-138.

2. Keisu KS, Orozco F, Sharke PF, Hozack WJ, Rothman RH, McGuigan FX: Primary cementless total hip arthroplasty in octogenarians: Two to eleven-year follow-up. *J Bone Joint Surg Am* 2001;83-A:359-363.

3. Thomason HC II, Lachiewicz PF: The influence of technique on fixation of primary total hip arthroplasty in patients with rheumatoid arthritis. *J Arthroplasty* 2001;16:628-634.

4. Macaulay W, Pagnotto MR, Iorio R, Mont MA, Saleh KJ: Displaced femoral neck fractures in the elderly: Hemiarthroplasty versus total hip arthroplasty. *J Am Acad Orthop Surg* 2006;14:287-293.

5. Dossick PH, Dorr LD, Gruen T, et al: Techniques for preoperative planning and postoperative evaluation of noncemented hip arthroplasty. *Tech Orthop* 1991;6:1-6.

6. Maloney WJ, Harris WH: Comparison of a hybrid with an uncemented total hip replacement. *J Bone Joint Surg Am* 1990;72:1349-1352.

7. Barrington JW, Lachiewicz PF: Systemic diseases resulting in hip pathology, in Callaghan JJ, Roenberg AG, Rubash HE (eds): *The Adult Hip*, ed 2. Philadelphia, PA, Lippincott, Williams & Wilkins, 2007.

8. Pitto RP, Koessler M, Kuehle JW: Comparison of fixation of the femoral component without cement and fixation with use of a bone-vacuum cementing technique for the prevention of fat embolism during total hip arthroplasty: A prospective, randomized clinical trial. *J Bone Joint Surg Am* 1999;81:831-843.

9. Iesaka K, Jaffe WL, Kummer FJ: Effects of pre-heating of hip prostheses on the stem-cement interface. *J Bone Joint Surg Am* 2003;85A:421-427.

10. Jafri AA, Green SM, Partington PF, McCaskie AW, Muller SD: Pre-heating of components in cemented total hip arthroplasty. *J Bone Joint Surg Br* 2004;86:1214-1219.

11. Barrack RL, Mulroy RD, Harris WH: Improved cementing techniques and femoral component loosening in your patients with hip arthroplasties: A 12-year radiographic review. *J Bone Joint Surg Br* 1992;74:385-389.

12. Oishi CS, Walker RH, Colwell CW Jr: The femoral component in total hip arthroplasty: Six to eight-year follow-up of one hundred consecutive patients after use of a third-generation cementing technique. *J Bone Joint Surg Am* 1994;76:1130-1136.

13. Kamineni S, An KN, Morrey BF: Methods of removing excess bone cement. *Orthopaedics* 2007;30:12-16.

14. Williams HD, Browne G, Gie GA, Ling RS, Timperly AJ, Wendover NA: The Exeter universal cemented femoral component at 8 to 12 years: A study of the first 325 hips. *J Bone Joint Surg Br* 2002;84:324-334.

15. Lachiewicz PF, Messick P: Precoated femoral component in primary hybrid total hip arthroplasty: Results at a mean 10-year follow-up. *J Arthroplasty* 2003;18:1-5.

16. Jarrett SD, Lachiewicz PF: Precoated femoral component with proximal and distal centralizers: Results at 5 to 12 years. *J Arthroplasty* 2005;20:309-315.

17. Sylvain GM, Kassab S, Coutts R, Santore R: Early failure of a roughened surface, precoated femoral component in total hip arthroplasty. *J Arthroplasty* 2001;16:141-148.

18. Vail TP, Goetz P, Tanzer M, Fisher DA, Mohler CG, Callaghan JJ: A prospective randomized trial of cemented femoral components with polished vs grit-blasted surface finish and identical stem geometry. *J Arthroplasty* 2003;18(suppl 1):95-102.

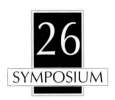

# Hip Resurfacing Arthroplasty: Time to Consider It Again? No

James D. Slover, MD, MS
*Harry E. Rubash, MD

## Abstract

*Total hip arthroplasty (THA) is one of the most successful operations in orthopaedics. A new procedure designed to replace THA, such as hip resurfacing arthroplasty, even for select indications, must offer a definite improvement over the well-established gold standard of treatment. Hip resurfacing does not currently meet this standard. THA is a proven and durable procedure with excellent results and superior short-term implant survival compared with hip resurfacing arthroplasty. Patients treated with hip resurfacing arthroplasty incur unique risks associated with implant malpositioning resulting from the surgeons' steep learning curve, the complex instrumentation involved, and the technical difficulty of the procedure, as well as a risk of femoral neck fracture. Hip resurfacing has limited ability to appropriately restore hip biomechanics and limb length, and concerns for the effects of metal ion and potential revision challenges remain. To date, there is a lack of literature supporting the claim of superior functional outcomes in hip resurfacing compared with THA. Reconsideration of hip resurfacing arthroplasty is unwarranted until appropriate comparative studies can demonstrate a clear benefit to patients.*

**Instr Course Lect 2008;57:267-271.**

Innovation and change are vital to the advancement of the field of orthopaedic surgery. However, total hip arthroplasty (THA) is one of the most successful operations in orthopaedics. Therefore, a new procedure designed to replace THA, even for select patients and indications, should be more than novel; it must provide a definite improvement over the well-established gold standard of treatment. Hip resurfacing arthroplasty does not meet this criterion.

## Total Hip Versus Hip Resurfacing Arthroplasty

Hip resurfacing arthroplasty has recently been advocated as superior to THA for patients younger than 50 years.[1] Proponents of hip resurfacing refer to the higher implant survival rates in younger patients versus the poor THA survival rate in this population and to the preservation of femoral bone stock that this procedure allows. Improved fixation interfaces and alternative bearing surfaces have emerged that contribute to improved outcomes of hip resurfacing in young patients. However, recent results also show improved survival of THAs in this population. Indications for resurfacing are more limited, with studies showing that the outcomes of resurfacing are dependent on preoperative patient characteristics; therefore, hip resurfacing is not as versatile as THA. Patients treated with hip resurfacing incur unique risks that include a significant learning curve for the surgeon, more complex instrumentation, greater exposure resulting from the larger incision and complete capsulectomy required in resurfacing, as well as an increased risk for femoral neck fracture. Also, resurfacing implants require use of metal-on-metal bearing surfaces, which generate cobalt and chromium ions, the long-term

*Harry E. Rubash, MD or the department with which he is affiliated has received research or institutional support and royalties from Zimmer.*

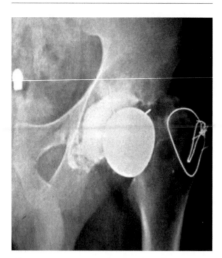

**Figure 1** AP radiograph showing a failed hip resurfacing combined with a thin polyethylene liner. The primary cause of failure was polyethylene wear and osteolysis.

effects of which are currently unknown. Although some studies show improved functional outcomes with hip resurfacing arthroplasty, short-term follow-up periods as well as other factors make the significance of these studies unclear. Therefore, hip resurfacing arthroplasty fails to demonstrate superiority to THA and should not displace this gold standard of treatment.

### Implant Survival Rates in Younger Patients

Recently, despite the outstanding performance of THA, hip resurfacing arthroplasty has been advocated for younger patients because of the historically inferior survival of THAs in this population.[2] Improved fixation interfaces and alternative bearing surfaces have emerged, allowing metal-on-metal resurfacing, which reduces the potential for polyethylene particle-induced osteolysis, a primary cause of failure of past resurfacing implants (Figure 1).[3-5] These developments have led some authors to recommend hip resurfacing in young

patients to preserve femoral bone stock to allow potentially improved patient activity levels and to protect young patients from the possibility of stem breakage from fatigue failure of femoral stems left in place for many years.[4]

More recently, however, the results of THA in young patients have shown improved survival rates with the advent of new surgical techniques, implant designs, and alternative bearing surfaces. Eskelinen and associates[6] reported on the results of 4,661 THAs in patients younger than 55 years treated with circumferential proximally porous-coated cementless stems and found a 10-year survival rate of 99% with aseptic loosening as the end point. Kearns and associates[7] reported on the results of 221 cementless THAs in patients younger than 50 years and found femoral stem survival rates of 99.3%, 98.9%, and 96.8% at 5, 10, and 15 years, respectively. McAuley and associates[8] reviewed the results of 561 extensively porous-coated THAs in patients younger than 50 years and reported a 10-year survival rate of 89% of both femoral and acetabular components. Kerboull and associates[9] reported the results of 287 cemented THAs in patients younger than 50 years and reported a 20-year survival rate of 85.4% for femoral and acetabular components. McLaughlin and Lee[10] reported a 98% bone ingrowth rate and a 2% fibrous ingrowth rate for cementless THAs with no revisions for loosening at 8 to 13 years. These results, which do not include outcomes of new, improved, highly cross-linked, ultra-high molecular weight polyethylene implants, show that THA can be a highly durable procedure, even in a young patient population.

In head-to-head comparisons, the survival rates of THAs have been superior to those of hip resur-

facing arthroplasties. Mont and associates[11] evaluated 30 matched pairs of patients with osteonecrosis treated with THA and hip resurfacing arthroplasty and found a 93% survival of the THAs, with only a 90% survival of the hip resurfacing arthroplasties at 7 years. The Australian Registry, which contains data on more than 4,900 hip resurfacing arthroplasty procedures, also reports superior short-term survival for THA compared with hip resurfacing arthroplasty.[12]

### Revision and Candidate Considerations

The indications for hip resurfacing are also more limited than for THA. The Australian Registry results show significantly higher revision rates for hip resurfacing in women younger than 65 years, with 1.69 to 2.33 revisions per 100 component years compared with 0.54 to 1.04 revisions per 100 component years for men in the same age group.[12] For men younger than 50 years, one of the primary patient groups for which resurfacing is believed to be appropriate, revision rates were also increased, with 1.04 revisions per 100 component years compared with 0.54 to 0.66 revisions per 100 component years for men age 50 to 64 years.[12] Advocates of resurfacing have acknowledged that the outcomes of the procedure are dependent on the preoperative characteristics of the femur.[13] A recent study reviewed the radiographs of 108 patients younger than 50 years presenting for THA to determine if they were candidates for hip resurfacing.[1] Because of morphologic considerations, those with femoral deformities, the presence of large cysts, and head collapse were considered unsuitable for hip resurfacing. Researchers classified 46% as suitable, 43% as unsuitable, and 11% as technically challenging for resurfacing. Hip resurfacing is not as versatile as THA for the treatment of degenerative hip disease in the young patient population.

## Risk Analysis
### Surgery-Related Factors
Patients undergoing a hip resurfacing arthroplasty also incur risks that differ from those incurred with a THA. As a new procedure, hip resurfacing arthroplasty may be associated with a significant learning curve for surgeons, negatively impacting early results.[14] Proponents of hip resurfacing and implant manufacturers have claimed that hip resurfacing is less invasive than THA because of the conservation of femoral bone stock. However, the instrumentation used in resurfacing is more complex and may be less accurate than the instrumentation necessary to perform a successful THA. This difference in instrumentation can lead to component malpositioning, including varus or valgus positioning and notching, placing the patient at further risk for future complications or revision. Hip resurfacing generally requires a larger incision and a complete capsulectomy to mobilize the femoral head for acetabular preparation. The larger exposure may increase the risk for blood loss, nerve palsy, vascular injury, and infection and may lead to increased surgical time, postoperative pain, and poorer cosmesis, which can impact patient satisfaction. In addition, the larger exposure may compromise soft-tissue integrity if revision becomes necessary in the future.

### Femoral Neck Fractures
The increased exposure and dissection necessary for hip resurfacing may also negatively impact the blood supply to the femoral head and neck, placing the patient at increased risk for femoral neck fracture. Performing electrode measurements in the femoral head of patients undergoing hip resurfacing, Steffen and associates[15] showed a 60% drop in oxygen concentration during the surgical approach and an additional 20% drop with component insertion. Little and associates[16] histologically examined the femoral heads from 13 resurfacing revision procedures and found osteonecrosis in 12 of 13 specimens. In the six revisions for fracture, osteonecrosis was seen along the fracture line in all six revisions, whereas a patchy pattern was observed in the six specimens with osteonecrosis and no femoral neck fracture.

The risk of femoral neck fracture in hip resurfacing arthroplasty is significant, ranging from 1.46% to 22%.[14,17] This complication is unique to hip resurfacing when compared with THA. Mont and associates[14] reported a 22% fracture rate in a series of the first 50 hip resurfacing arthroplasties, with a 2% rate in the next series of 50, indicating that a significant learning curve may exist for surgeons. Shimmin and Back[17] reported the findings of an Australian Registry study, which showed a 1.46% overall incidence of femoral neck fracture, with no evidence of a relationship between surgeon experience and the risk of fracture, suggesting the incidence of this complication may persist over time.

### Implications for Femoral Bone Stock
One of the arguments for hip resurfacing is that it preserves femoral neck bone stock. Clearly, femoral neck bone stock is preserved in hip resurfacing, when compared with THA; however, the impact on future revision surgery is unknown. To date, no studies show revisions of hip resurfacing arthroplasties to be technically easier or to have im-

proved outcomes compared with revisions of primary THAs. This fact should be carefully considered given the poorer survival rates of hip resurfacing arthroplasty. An analysis by Loughead and associates[18] found that a larger cup size is needed for hip resurfacing arthroplasty to accommodate the femoral prosthesis, which results in increased removal of acetabular bone stock when compared with conventional THA. The reduced acetabular bone stock could compromise the results of future revision procedures for hip resurfacing arthroplasties, which suggests that hip resurfacing may be a bone-depleting rather than a bone-conserving procedure. Because the acetabular component of a hip resurfacing arthroplasty is nonmodular, it can only accommodate a highly specific femoral implant. Therefore, if a well-fixed hip resurfacing acetabular component must be removed for femoral revision because of this lack of modularity, acetabular bone stock may be further compromised.

### Hip Biomechanics
Hip resurfacing arthroplasty does not restore hip biomechanics as accurately as does THA. In a study of 28 hip resurfacings and 26 THAs, Loughead and associates[19] found a significant decrease in femoral offset in hip resurfacing patients compared with THA patients. The authors also found that hip resurfacing resulted in a statistically significant hip length discrepancy compared with THA, with an average change of 3.6 mm for resurfacing and 0.3 mm for THA.[19] Another study of 40 hip resurfacing arthroplasties showed that resurfacing is incapable of increasing femoral offset, resulting in an offset of 8 mm or less compared with the contralateral hip versus an average offset increase of 9.5 mm in

40 THAs, which resulted in an off-set equal to or greater than the offset of the contralateral hip.[20] The authors also found that hip resurfacing was capable of lengthening limbs by a maximum of 1 cm.[20]

### Metal Ion Formation

Another important factor to consider is the issue of metal ion formation. Current hip resurfacing arthroplasty implants require the use of a metal-on-metal bearing surface, which has been shown to generate cobalt and chromium ions in vivo in both THA and resurfacing procedures.[21,22] The long-term impact of these ions remains unknown, but significant concerns for carcinogenesis as well as renal and liver toxicity exist.[21,23,24] In patients with metal-on-metal bearing arthroplasties, a lymphocyte-dominated immunologic response, which leads to persistent or early recurrence of pain, joint effusions, and the formation of radiolucent lines around the implant, also have been shown.[24] The level of lymphocyte reactivity increases linearly with respect to the level of metal ions.[25] Even when a metal-on-metal THA is selected, the patient's exposure to ions is lower than that in a hip resurfacing arthroplasty, likely because of the smaller diameter of the bearing surface.[22] THA also presents the opportunity to use alternative bearing surfaces to metal-on-metal, with good results in younger patients.[26] Although the long-term impact of metal ion release in vivo is unknown, concerns regarding biologic effects remain, making this an important consideration for patients and surgeons.

### Functional Outcomes

An additional argument for hip resurfacing arthroplasty has been the assertion that the procedure is associated with improved functional outcomes. THA has been one of the most successful operations in orthopaedics in improving patient function. Patients have reported that these improvements are highly valued, assigning the procedure an average utility value of 0.87 (scale 0-1) using a time trade-off utility measurement score.[27] Select studies, including one prospective randomized controlled study, have suggested hip resurfacing arthroplasty patients have higher activity levels postoperatively than THA patients.[28,29] This randomized study evaluated 210 patients who were followed for 1 year postoperatively.[28] There was no difference in Western Ontario McMaster Osteoarthritis Index scores between the two groups, but the resurfacing group had an average University of California at Los Angeles activity score of 7.1, compared with 6.3 for the THA group. A study by Pollard and associates[30] retrospectively compared 54 hybrid THAs with 54 resurfacings and found no difference in functional outcomes scores. The resurfacing group did have an average University of California at Los Angeles activity score of 9 compared with 7 for the THA patients.[30] However, the short-term follow-up and the magnitude of the activity score difference make the significance of these studies unclear. In fact, most studies examining the functional outcomes of hip resurfacing arthroplasty have been plagued by patient selection issues, lack of randomization, and lack of blinded assessment, rendering it impossible at this time to directly attribute any differences to the specific procedure or implant. Further randomized clinical trials with longer follow-up that compare the functional results of these two procedures are needed to establish superior outcomes of either procedure.

### Summary

THA is a proven durable procedure with excellent results and superior short-term survival compared with hip resurfacing arthroplasty. The unique risks of hip resurfacing arthroplasty, including the surgeon's steep learning curve, technical difficulty, and the risk of femoral neck fracture, in addition to the concerns for metal ion effects, the potential revision challenges, and the lack of evidence in the literature to support the claim of superior functional outcomes, render the expected outcomes less reliable than those of THA. THA should remain the gold standard of treatment; reconsideration of hip resurfacing arthroplasty is unwarranted until appropriate comparative studies can prove a clear benefit to patients.

## References

1. Eastaugh-Waring SJ, Seenath S, Learmonth DS, Learmonth ID: The practical limitations of resurfacing hip arthroplasty. *J Arthroplasty* 2006;21: 18-22.

2. Dorr LD, Luckett M, Conaty JP: Total hip arthroplasties in patients younger than 45 years: A nine- to ten-year follow-up study. *Clin Orthop Relat Res* 1990;260:215-219.

3. Schmalzried TP, Fowble VA, Ure KJ, Amstutz HC: Metal-on-metal surface replacement of the hip: Technique, fixation, and early results. *Clin Orthop Relat Res* 1996;329:S106-S114.

4. Schmalzried TP: The optimal metal-metal arthroplasty is still a total hip arthroplasty: In opposition. *J Arthroplasty* 2006;21( suppl 1)77-79.

5. Howie DW, Campbell D, McGee M, Cornish BL: Wagner resurfacing hip arthroplasty: The results of one hundred consecutive arthroplasties after eight to ten years. *J Bone Joint Surg Am* 1990;72:708-714.

6. Eskelinen A, Remes V, Helenius I, Pulkkinen P, Nevalainen J, Paavolainen P: Total hip arthroplasty for primary osteoarthrosis in younger patients in the Finnish arthroplasty register: 4,661 primary replacements followed for 0-22 years. *Acta Orthop* 2005;76:28-41.

7. Kearns SR, Jamal B, Rorabeck CH, Bourne RB: Factors affecting survival of uncemented total hip arthroplasty in patients 50 years or younger. *Clin Orthop Relat Res* 2006;453:103-109.

8. McAuley JP, Szuszczewicz ES, Young A, Engh CA Sr: Total hip arthroplasty in patients 50 years and younger. *Clin Orthop Relat Res* 2004; 418:119-125.

9. Kerboull L, Hamadouche M, Courpied JP, Kerboull M: Long-term results of Charnley-Kerboull hip arthroplasty in patients younger than 50 years. *Clin Orthop Relat Res* 2004; 418:112-118.

10. McLaughlin JR, Lee KR: Total hip arthroplasty in young patients: Eight- to 13-year results using an uncemented stem. *Clin Orthop Relat Res* 2000;373: 153-163.

11. Mont MA, Rajadhyaksha AD, Hungerford DS: Outcomes of limited femoral resurfacing arthroplasty compared with total hip arthroplasty for osteonecrosis of the femoral head. *J Arthroplasty* 2001;16(suppl 1):134-139.

12. AOA National Joint Replacement Website. Available at: http://www.dmac.adelaide.edu.au/aoanjrr/publications.jsp. Accessed July 25, 2007.

13. Schmalzried TP, Silva M, de la Rosa MA, Choi ES, Fowble VA: Optimizing patient selection and outcomes with total hip resurfacing. *Clin Orthop Relat Res* 2005;441:200-204.

14. Mont MA, Ragland PS, Etienne G, Seyler TM, Schmalzried TP: Hip resurfacing arthroplasty. *J Am Acad Orthop Surg* 2006;14:454-463.

15. Steffen RT, Smith SR, Urban JP, et al: The effect of hip resurfacing on oxygen concentration in the femoral head. *J Bone Joint Surg Br* 2005;87: 1468-1474.

16. Little CP, Ruiz AL, Harding IJ, et al: Osteonecrosis in retrieved femoral heads after failed resurfacing arthroplasty of the hip. *J Bone Joint Surg Br* 2005;87:320-323.

17. Shimmin AJ, Back D: Femoral neck fractures following Birmingham hip resurfacing: A national review of 50 cases. *J Bone Joint Surg Br* 2005;87: 463-464.

18. Loughead JM, Starks I, Chesney D, Matthews JN, McCaskie AW, Holland JP: Removal of acetabular bone in resurfacing arthroplasty of the hip: A comparison with hybrid total hip arthroplasty. *J Bone Joint Surg Br* 2006; 88:31-34.

19. Loughead JM, Chesney D, Holland JP, McCaskie AW: Comparison of offset in Birmingham hip resurfacing and hybrid total hip arthroplasty. *J Bone Joint Surg Br* 2005;87:163-166.

20. Silva M, Lee KH, Heisel C, Dela Rosa MA, Schmalzried TP: The biomechanical results of total hip resurfacing arthroplasty. *J Bone Joint Surg Am* 2004;86-A:40-46.

21. Brodner W, Bitzan P, Meisinger V, Kaider A, Gottsauner-Wolf F, Kotz R: Serum cobalt levels after metal-on-metal total hip arthroplasty. *J Bone Joint Surg Am* 2003;85-A:2168-2173.

22. Clarke MT, Lee PT, Arora A, Villar RN: Levels of metal ions after small- and large-diameter metal-on-metal hip arthroplasty. *J Bone Joint Surg Br* 2003;85:913-917.

23. Tharani R, Dorey FJ, Schmalzried TP: The risk of cancer following total hip or knee arthroplasty. *J Bone Joint Surg Am* 2001;83-A:774-780.

24. Willert HG, Buchhorn GH, Fayyazi A, et al: Metal-on-metal bearings and hypersensitivity in patients with artificial hip joints: A clinical and histomorphological study. *J Bone Joint Surg Am* 2005;87:28-36.

25. Hallab NJ, Anderson S, Caicedo M, Skipor A, Campbell P, Jacobs JJ: Immune responses correlate with serum-metal in metal-on-metal hip arthroplasty. *J Arthroplasty* 2004;19 (suppl 3):88-93.

26. Murphy SB, Ecker TM, Tannast M: Two- to 9-year clinical results of alumina ceramic-on-ceramic THA. *Clin Orthop Relat Res* 2006;453:97-102.

27. Laupacis A, Bourne R, Rorabeck C, et al: The effect of elective total hip replacement on health-related quality of life. *J Bone Joint Surg Am* 1993;75: 1619-1626.

28. Vendittoli PA, Lavigne M, Roy AG, Lusignan D: A prospective randomized clinical trial comparing metal-on-metal total hip arthroplasty and metal-on-metal total hip resurfacing in patients less than 60 years old. *Hip Int* 2006;16:S73-S81.

29. Vail TP, Mina CA, Yergler JD, Pietrobon R: Metal-on-metal hip resurfacing compares favorably with THA at 2-years' follow-up. *Clin Orthop Relat Res* 2006;453:123-131.

30. Pollard TC, Baker RP, Eastaugh-Waring SJ, Bannister GC: Treatment of the young active patient with osteoarthritis of the hip: A five- to seven-year comparison of hybrid total hip arthroplasty and metal-on-metal resurfacing. *J Bone Joint Surg Br* 2006;88:592-600.

# Digital Templating in Total Hip Arthroplasty

LCDR David R. Whiddon, MD
*James V. Bono, MD

## Abstract

*Preoperative templating for total hip arthroplasty requires precision and accuracy. The current method of acetate overlays is subject to errors in magnification. Digital radiography permits the use of software programs that calculate the x-ray magnification with precision and then adjust the templates to match the exact magnification. A reproducible set of steps is described that allows a surgeon to preoperatively template in the digital environment.*

**Instr Course Lect 2008;57:273-279.**

Total hip arthroplasty is widely considered to be one of the most successful orthopaedic procedures in terms of improved patient quality of life and cost-effectiveness.[1,2] It is performed at both specialized centers and in small community hospitals throughout the world. Surgeons must precisely place implants to optimize the biomechanical and biologic function of the joint. By using a digital templating algorithm, the surgeon is offered a stepwise method to determine which size prosthesis to use and where to place the prosthesis within the bone to optimize the long-term function of the joint. In the authors' experience, digital templating permits preoperative planning with a level of precision previously unobtainable with acetate overlays. This improvement in planning translates into less intraoperative guesswork with respect to limb-length equalization and restoration of offset.

## Importance of Preoperative Planning

The primary goal in hip replacement surgery is to restore the biomechanics of the hip back to "normal." Preoperative planning is necessary to correct the pathologic state of the hip. Specifically, this means achieving equal limb length and the appropriate offset following surgery. Many patients with arthritic conditions of the hip have a limb-length discrepancy. This may be caused by erosion of the cartilage of the hip joint or deformity leading to the arthritic condition (such as Legg-Calve-Perthes disease). In most instances, several millimeters of limb shortening will occur. Thus, the goal of surgery is to restore the limb back to its original length, which will restore the original biomechanics of the joint.[3] Determining the exact amount of limb-length discrepancy is necessary to achieve limb-length equality and to avoid overlengthening or shortening of the leg.

Femoral offset is the measurement of the distance from the center of rotation of the hip joint to the longitudinal axis of the femoral shaft. This measurement determines the moment arm of the abductor muscles. The amount of offset determines how hard the muscles have to work; the greater the offset the greater the moment arm, given that the same force is applied. It is important to appropriately restore the offset for the hip to function properly. For example, if a hip prosthesis is placed with an insufficient offset, the hip muscles will have to generate increased force, leading to discomfort and easy fatigability. The extra force applied to the joint can be harmful over the long term, leading to premature

*James V. Bono, MD or the department with which he is affiliated has received royalties from Sectra and is a consultant or employee for Sectra.

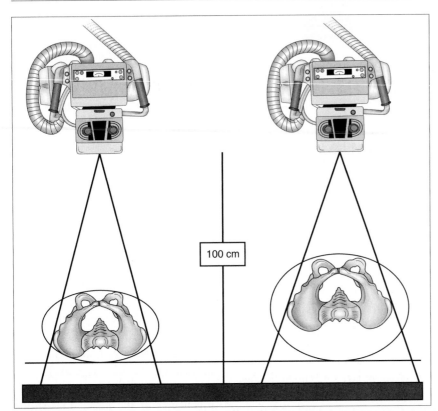

**Figure 1** Illustration showing the effect of bone-to-plate distance on overall magnification. As the distance between the bone and the x-ray plate increases (depicted on the right half of the illustration), the shadow of the bone on the cassette becomes larger.

wear and loosening.[4] Insufficient offset also can create joint laxity, leading to dislocation.[5,6]

Cementless femoral components rely on intimate contact with host bone for stability and long-term survival. An undersized implant is susceptible to early loosening because the component will not be well supported within the bone. Conversely, the desire to achieve a stable fit with an oversized implant may result in fracture of the bone. Increased accuracy in preoperative planning is important to avoid these complications.

## Advances in Digital Radiography

There are numerous advantages in the conversion to digital radiography. Digital images are archived in a readily accessible format that is easily manipulated and transferred among clinicians. Images are seldom lost because they are stored and backed up electronically. There also are potential cost savings associated with the cessation of film processing and printing of radiographs. The images can be printed, if necessary, but are usually viewed on a computer monitor. As digital radiography becomes more widely implemented, orthopaedic surgeons will be required to adapt their practices to this technology. Digital preoperative planning enables the surgeon to select from a library of templates and to electronically overlay them on an image. The surgeon can then perform the necessary measurements critical to the templating and preop-

erative planning process in a digital environment. The preoperative planning process is fast, precise, and cost-efficient, and it provides a permanent, archived record of the templating process.[7]

One important point that must not be overlooked is that high-quality radiographs are a prerequisite in the templating process. Radiographs should be obtained with the patient supine with the legs internally rotated 15° to 20°. This position is intended to place the femoral necks parallel to the cassette, maximizing the offset. The x-ray beam should be centered just below the pubic symphysis to obtain a "low" AP pelvis radiograph. This view permits sufficient visualization of the proximal femur to template the femoral component.

All radiographs must be magnified because of the distance between the bone and the radiographic cassette. The farther away the bone is from the cassette for a given tube-to-cassette distance, the more magnified the bone will appear on the radiograph (Figure 1). This means that the magnification needed for the radiograph of an obese patient will be more than that needed for a slender patient. Conventional radiographs are obtained with a magnification factor that varies. The acetate overlays provided by prosthesis vendors typically come with a fixed 15% or 20% magnification factor. Thus, they cannot be adjusted to the many variations that may occur as a result of body habitus.

One additional problem unique to digital radiography is that the printed images can be rescaled to fit the radiographic film with margins. Rescaling may occur automatically in the printing software and may not represent the true magnification of the osseous structures. Therefore, caution is advised when templating with acetate overlays on printed digital images. The use of radiographic size markers is encouraged to mitigate potential errors. Most manufacturers provide a type of magnification marker that consists of two ball bearings embedded 10 cm apart in plastic. This marker provides an easy calculation of magnification because the actual measurement will correspond with the percentage of magnification. Alternatives to this marker include the use of a sphere of known diameter (for example, a prosthetic head ball) or a coin[8] (Figure 2).

## Digital Templating Algorithm

There are several steps involved in using the digital templating algorithm.

### Step One

The magnification of the radiograph must be determined. To calculate the magnification factor, it is necessary to have a marker of known size at the level of the hip joint. The ideal circumstance occurs when the patient has a contralateral hip arthroplasty and the femoral head size is known and easily measured. With the more widespread use of hard-on-hard bearings, this is sometimes difficult. Otherwise, a radiographic marker of known dimension is placed externally at the level of the hip joint. It may be taped to the skin of the patient at the level of the greater trochanter or placed between the thighs at the same level as the greater trochanter. The software calibrates the image and the templates are scaled to the correct magnification factor. All subsequent steps are based on measurements that have been corrected for magnification (Figure 3).

### Step Two

The orientation of the pelvic axis is determined by drawing a line between the acetabular teardrops

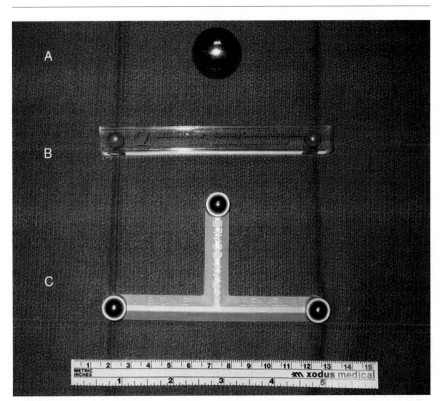

**Figure 2**    Three different templating markers are pictured. **A,** A 25-mm radiopaque marker is small enough to be placed between the thighs. **B** and **C,** Examples of markers provided by prosthetic manufacturers that allow determination of magnification by measuring the distance between the metallic spheres at each end (100 mm).

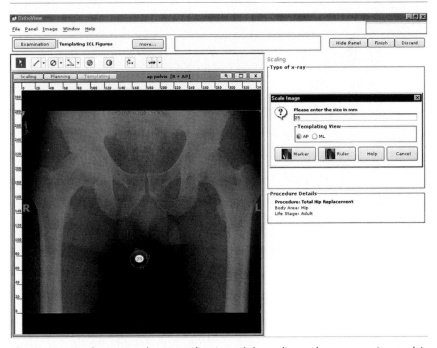

**Figure 3**    To determine the magnification of the radiograph, a measuring tool is applied to the radiograph. The known dimension of the object is input, and the software will adjust all subsequent measurements to this value of magnification.

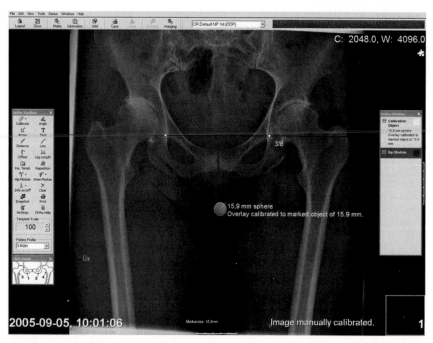

**Figure 4**  The pelvic axis is determined by a line placed between the acetabular teardrops.

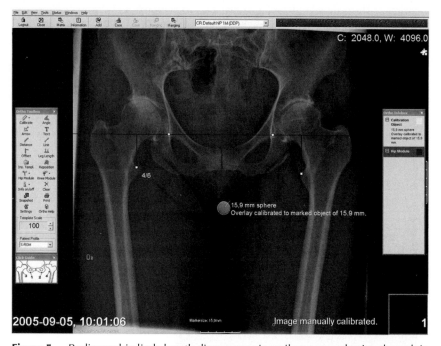

**Figure 5**  Radiographic limb-length discrepancy is easily measured using the pelvic axis and the top of the lesser trochanter.

(Figure 4). The pelvic axis provides the fixed pelvic landmark from which leg length and cup abduction are determined. The acetabular tear-drop is preferable because it is re-producible and closest to the hip center of rotation. Other landmarks can be used, including the ischial tu-berosity, obturator foramen, or greater sciatic notch.

### Step Three

It is necessary to determine whether a limb-length discrepancy is present. A perpendicular line is drawn from the pelvic axis to identical fixed points on the right and left femur. Many landmarks, including the greater and lesser trochanter, can be used. Most commonly, the top of the lesser trochanter is selected be-cause this landmark is easy to identi-fy radiographically and intraopera-tively (Figure 5). The radiographic limb-length discrepancy is corre-lated with the clinical measurement of limb lengths using blocks during preoperative evaluation.

In some patients, a fixed pelvic obliquity exists and correction of clinical limb-length inequality may be undesirable. Often, restoration of normal motion to the hip will cor-rect the obliquity. Seated shoot-through AP pelvic radiographs may be obtained to determine the flexi-bility of the deformity.

### Step Four

The new center of rotation of the hip joint is determined. The digital acetabular component template is placed at a 45° angle to the pelvic axis. The medial border of the pros-thesis is placed between the inner and outer walls of the pelvis, and the template size is chosen that best fills the existing acetabulum without re-moving excessive bone from the weight-bearing dome of the acetab-ulum (Figure 6).

### Step Five

The size of the femur is determined. The proximal metaphysis and proxi-mal diaphysis are measured to deter-mine the closest fit based on the type of component used. Each software program performs this step slightly differently, with wizards available to assist in optimizing the fit and fill (Figure 7). The software then recommends a size of component to fit within the measured dimensions of the femur (Figure 8).

### Step Six

The recommended size of the femoral component is then positioned within the bone so that the center of rotation of the femur overlays the center of rotation of the acetabular component. This may require using a higher offset stem or a different neck-shaft angle implant. If the limb is to be lengthened, the center of rotation of the femoral component is raised the desired distance proximal to the center of rotation of the acetabulum. This adjustment may necessitate using a larger femoral component to maintain proximal metaphyseal fill (Figure 9).

### Step Seven

The level of the femoral neck resection is determined. The length of the femoral neck resection necessary to place the femoral component in position according to step six is measured (proximal to the lesser trochanter or distal to the greater trochanter). This measurement will be corrected for magnification and should be reproducible intraoperatively. Other intraoperative measurements such as the distance between the lesser trochanter and the center of rotation of the head can be measured and recorded at this time (Figure 10).

### Digital Templating Software

Several companies now offer digital templating software, either as part of a digital radiography solution or as a stand-alone product. All major pros-

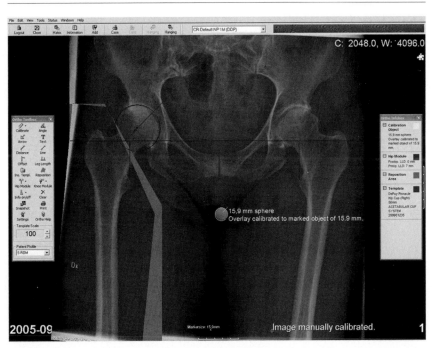

**Figure 6**    The femoral head is outlined; this will determine the center of rotation of the hip and will suggest a cup size. The acetabular component will be placed between the inner and outer walls of the acetabulum.

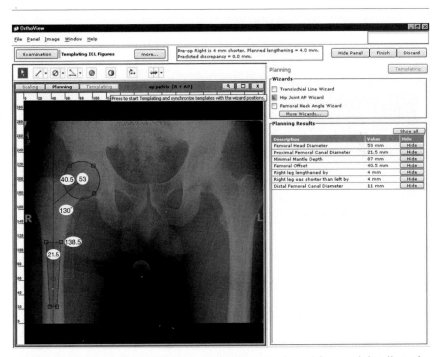

**Figure 7**    The femoral canal is measured at the metaphyseal flare and distally in the diaphysis. This will align the femoral component within the canal and determine the size of the femoral component.

thesis manufacturers now provide template information to software manufacturers; this has enabled most companies to offer a digital templating solution that can provide each surgeon with the necessary implant spe-

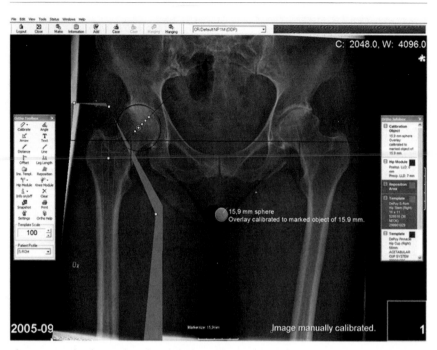

**Figure 8** The femoral and acetabular components are provisionally placed within the bone before fine-tuning component placement.

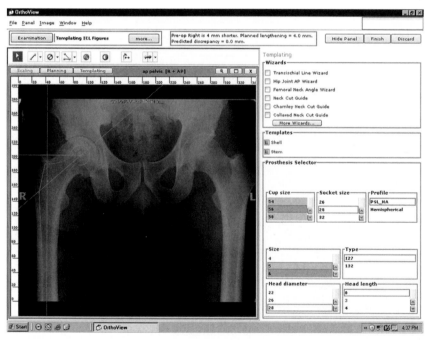

**Figure 9** The high offset femoral component is chosen to reproduce offset and the center of the head is 4 mm proximal to the center of rotation of the cup, thus perfectly restoring limb-length equality.

cific templates to successfully plan surgery. Integration with a picture archiving and communication system allows the record of the templating session to be appended to the digital radiograph jacket of the patient.

The unique features of each software program are beyond the scope of this chapter. Each program provides wizards to simplify the sizing of components and to optimize placement and biomechanics. The seven-step digital templating algorithm previously outlined can be applied to most of the current digital templating programs.

## Discussion

Shortly after the introduction of digital radiography at the New England Baptist Hospital, the senior author (JV Bono, MD) began implementation of this digital templating algorithm; more than 500 total hip arthroplasties have been digitally templated. In 2006, digital templating software was introduced to the arthroplasty fellows and remaining staff. Digital templating is now possible for all primary and revision hip arthroplasties performed at the New England Baptist Hospital. The number of printed films has been reduced and the department is nearing its goal of a filmless radiology department.

Preoperative digitally templated plans were compared with acetate overlay plans in 51 primary total hip arthroplasties (Whiddon and associates, unpublished data, 2006). Comparisons were made between the preoperatively templated cup and stem and the actual cup and stem sizes implanted at surgery. All templating was performed by arthroplasty fellows who participated in the surgery. A high level of correlation was found between the digital preoperative plan and the actual components used during surgery. Specifically, 90% of the stems implanted were within one size of the digital preoperative plan and 82% were within one size of the acetate overlay plan. On the acetabular side,

78% of cups were within one size of the digital preoperative plan and 67% of the cups were within one size of the acetate overlay plan. In another recent study, a randomized trial was conducted to compare digital and analog templating. The use of digital templating resulted in the correct prediction of the component within one size in 84% of the cementless cups and 58% of the cementless stems.[9] These results compared favorably with acetate overlay templating that correctly predicted within one size in 67% of cups and 56% of stems; the only significant difference occurred with size prediction in the cementless cups.

Although these studies have verified the ability of digital templating to accurately predict component sizes preoperatively, a clear benefit in long-term joint function or outcome has not yet been shown. The cost of digital templating software from one vendor is approximately $8,000 for a single user license. Minimizing complications associated with an oversized or undersized implant will likely result in long-term benefits; however, the true benefit to improved long-term outcomes will be realized when proper anatomic and biomechanical relationships are restored.

## Summary

In a short period of time, digital radiography has changed the landscape of orthopaedic surgery. The tools now available for digital templating enable more accurate and precise templating than ever before. The seven steps outlined in this chapter enable the surgeon to preoperatively determine the appropriate cup size, stem size, neck length, and head size, as well as the necessary amount of osseous resection needed to reestablish the proper

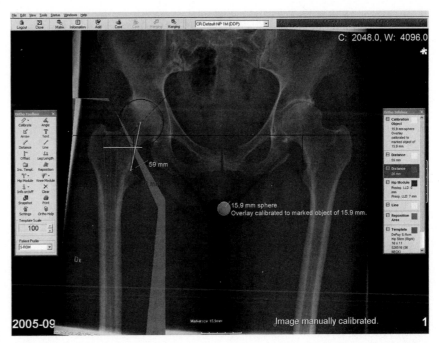

**Figure 10**  The final preoperative plan is shown. Measurements are recorded that will be obtained intraoperatively.

limb length and femoral offset. The only remaining step is to reproduce the plan in the operating room.

## References

1. Kawasaki M, Hasegawa Y, Sakano S, et al: Quality of life after several treatments for osteoarthritis of the hip. *J Orthop Sci* 2003;8:32-35.

2. Garellick G, Malchau H, Herberts P, Hansson E, Axelsson H, Hansson T: Life expectancy and cost utility after total hip replacement. *Clin Orthop Relat Res* 1998;346:141-151.

3. Noble P: Biomechanics of revision hip replacement, in Bono J, McCarthy J, Thornhill T, Bierbaum B, Turner R (eds): *Revision Total Hip Arthroplasty*. New York, NY, Springer, 1999, pp 135-141.

4. Sakalkale DP, Sharkey PF, Eng K, Hozack WJ, Rothman RH: Effect of femoral component offset on polyethylene wear in total hip arthroplasty. *Clin Orthop Relat Res* 2001;388: 125-134.

5. Mahoney CR, Pellicci PM: Complications in primary total hip arthroplasty: Avoidance and management of dislocations. *Instr Course Lect* 2003;52: 247-255.

6. McCabe J, Pellicci P, Salvati E: Dislocation following total hip arthroplasty, in Bono J, McCarthy J, Thornhill T, Bierbaum B, Turner R, (eds): *Revision Total Hip Arthroplasty*. New York, NY, Springer, 1999, pp 391-400.

7. Bono JV: Digital templating in total hip arthroplasty. *J Bone Joint Surg Am* 2004;86(suppl 2):118-122.

8. Conn KS, Clarke MT, Hallett JP: A simple guide to determine the magnification of radiographs and to improve the accuracy of preoperative planning. *J Bone Joint Surg Br* 2002;84: 269-272.

9. The B, Verdonschot N, van Horn JR, van Ooijen PM, Diercks RL: Digital versus analogue preoperative planning of total hip arthroplasties: A randomized clinical trial of 210 total hip arthroplasties. *J Arthroplasty* 2007;22: 866-870.

# Adult Reconstruction: Knee

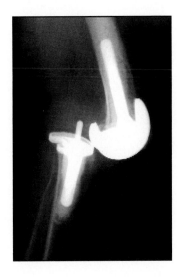

# Extensor Mechanism Complications After Total Knee Arthroplasty

Jay Patel, MD

Michael D. Ries, MD

Kevin J. Bozic, MD, MBA

## Abstract

*Extensor mechanism complications after total knee arthroplasty are relatively uncommon but potentially devastating. The etiology of these complications, which includes patellofemoral instability, periprosthetic patellar fracture, and disruptions of the quadriceps tendon and patellar ligament, has become better defined in recent years, with a subsequent decrease in the incidence, primarily resulting from changes in surgical technique and component design. In addition to addressing the patient's specific failure mechanism, the treatment of extensor mechanism complications after total knee arthroplasty may include nonsurgical management, primary repair, or reconstruction with autogenous, allogeneic, or synthetic tissue. Prevention of these complications, the foremost goal, is achieved through identification of patient and procedure risk factors, meticulous surgical technique, including vigilance during exposure and retractor placement, and a high index of suspicion both during and after the procedure.*

**Instr Course Lect 2008;57:283-294.**

The incidence of extensor mechanism complications after total knee arthroplasty (TKA) is 1% to 10%.[1-8] These complications are a common basis for revision TKA, accounting for as much as 12% of revisions in some studies.[9] A recent multicenter prospective analysis, based on patients from the North American Knee Arthroplasty Revision study, reported that patients who undergo revision TKA secondary to extensor mechanism complications have less favorable outcomes than patients who undergo revision for other reasons.[8] In one such example, patients who have a revision TKA for patellofemoral complications are 23% more likely to need further surgery and have a

higher risk of reoperation than patients requiring revision TKA for aseptic loosening.[10] As the number of TKA procedures increases with the aging US population, the number of revision TKA procedures secondary to extensor mechanism complications is likely to similarly increase. Improvements in patient selection, surgical technique, and prosthetic design have all contributed to a reduction in the current extensor mechanism complication rate, thereby helping to improve patient outcomes.

Extensor mechanism complications after TKA include patellofemoral instability, patellar fracture, and soft-tissue disruptions (patellar ligament avulsions and quadriceps ten-

don rupture). In addition to focusing on the type of failure, both nonsurgical and surgical treatments are tailored to the individual characteristics of the patient, including the underlying diagnosis or comorbidities (particularly infection, rheumatoid arthritis, history of malnutrition, or immunosuppression), bone quality, soft-tissue vascularity, and anticipated activity level or biomechanical demands on the knee.

## Patellofemoral Instability

Patellofemoral instability after TKA is a common disorder, with an incidence of 1% to 12%.[11] This category of complication, the etiology of which is characterized by issues related to both component design and surgical technique, includes patellar subluxation, dislocation, component wear, loosening, failure, and patellar fracture. Surgeons can minimize patellofemoral instability—among the most common of the extensor mechanism complications after TKA—by understanding the various etiologies, careful surgical planning, and meticulous intraoperative technique and evaluation.

Evaluation of the patient with patellofemoral instability after TKA begins with a careful history and physical examination, specifically addressing issues related to pain and functional impairment. Patients commonly report anterior knee pain, difficulty with stair climbing, patellar dislocation, and a painful, audible "clunk." On physical examination, the surgeon may observe an increased Q angle (> 15° in men and 20° in women) and a positive apprehension test. Radiographic examination includes plain radiographs of the knee, with sunrise views to evaluate patellar tilt or subluxation and full-length radiographs, which sometimes are required to accurately measure the Q angle. Femoral and tibial component rotation can be evaluated using a CT scan.[12]

### Causes

Prosthetic design can contribute to patellofemoral stability through a variety of factors, including the depth and orientation of the trochlear groove, patellar component geometry, and conformity of the patellofemoral joint. Studies have shown that the valgus angle of the trochlear groove in the coronal plane can differentially affect the medial and lateral shear forces on the patella at different points of flexion. The design rationale underlying the valgus angle of the trochlear groove, which is between 5° and 7° in most prosthetic designs, is described as one aligning patellar tracking with the extensor mechanism forces; A 0° trochlear groove has been shown to create greater lateral patellofemoral shear forces than a 7° trochlear groove.[13] The depth of the trochlear groove must be balanced to not only maximize patellofemoral stability but also to minimize patellofemoral contact forces. A shallow trochlear groove without a lateral flange can cause instability. Although a deep constrained trochlear groove with a lateral flange addresses this complication by improving stability, it also increases contact forces, which can result in wear,

loosening, and patellar component fracture.[14-16] Patellofemoral complications also have been associated with a femoral component that has a narrow anterior flange and an abrupt anterior to distal transition with a smaller radius of curvature.[17]

Evolution of the design of the patellar component has been primarily based on its role in component failure, such as loosening, fracture, and instability. Design parameters for patellar components can include varying dome shapes, such as a central symmetric dome, an offset dome, an anatomic dome, and a modified sombrero-shaped dome that has a dome-shaped central projection surrounded by a peripheral flat region.[11] Use of the modified sombrero-shaped dome has been reported to result in decreased component tilting and decreased shear forces compared with the central symmetric dome.[18]

Patellar clunk syndrome has been described as a form of patellofemoral instability in posterior cruciate ligament-substituting designs of TKA. The syndrome is characterized by the development of a fibrous nodule on the deep aspect of the quadriceps tendon that falls into the intercondylar notch of the femoral component during knee flexion. The clunk represents movement of the scar tissue out of the intercondylar region during knee extension. To reduce such soft-tissue impingement complications, modified femoral component designs were created that included deepening and elongating the femoral trochlea.[2]

Although prosthetic design can contribute to patellofemoral instability, errors in surgical technique are often implicated as the primary reason for these complications, with component malpositioning, described extensively in the literature, identified as a

significant source of these errors.[12,19-31] As the rotational alignment of the femoral component is a critical factor in determining patellofemoral tracking, several intraoperative landmarks have been described to assess femoral component rotation, including the surgical epicondylar axis, the anteroposterior axis (Whiteside's line), and the posterior condylar axis (Figure 1). Studies have shown the surgical epicondylar axis to be the most accurate landmark for establishing femoral component rotation,[29] whereas rotational alignment of the tibial component remains controversial. Various landmarks including the medial and lateral malleoli, second ray of the foot, tibial tubercle, tibial crest, femoral epicondylar axis, and the flexion gap have been described to align the tibia. Berger and associates[12] recommend that the tibial component be 18° internally rotated relative to the line connecting the geometric center of the tibial plateau to the tibial tubercle. They also describe the importance of combined (femoral and tibial) rotational alignment on patellofemoral tracking: between 1° and 4° of combined internal rotation of the femoral and tibial components correlated with lateral tracking, 3° and 8° with patellar subluxation, and 7° and 17° with early patellar dislocation or late patellar prosthesis failure.[12] Although consensus exists that the femoral component should be aligned with the surgical epicondylar axis, the complication of rotational alignment continues to be an issue. Computer navigation systems, developed to reduce error associated with visualizing alignment axes, show promise in improving alignment but are limited by the variability in the identification of landmarks.[32-34] In a prospective randomized trial comparing computer navigation with conventional techniques, navigation was shown to im-

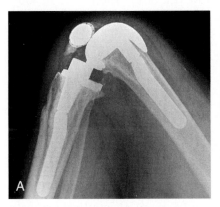
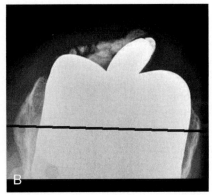
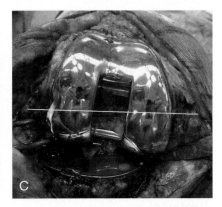

**Figure 1** A 64-year-old man presenting with patellar instability after revision TKA was treated with extensor mechanism realignment and patellar revision without femoral or tibial component revision. His symptoms were not improved. **A,** A lateral radiograph shows recurrent lateral patellar subluxation and tilt. **B,** Patellar radiograph shows lateral tilt and subluxation of the patellar component. A line between the medial and lateral epicondyles suggests that the femoral component is internally rotated. **C,** Intraoperative view showing internal rotation of the femoral component relative to the surgical epicondylar axis (*white line*).

prove frontal plane and sagittal plane alignment but did not improve rotational alignment.[35]

Patellar component positioning also affects patellofemoral tracking in TKA. Medial placement of the patellar component decreases the Q angle and reduces the lateral forces on the patella, whereas central or lateral patellar positioning worsens lateral tracking of the patella.[13,16] Medializing the patellar component also has been shown to decrease the need for lateral release, although the ultimate positioning of the patellar component depends on intraoperative tracking with the components in place.[36] One exception to medializing the patella is in the case of a large patella where a greater than 1.5-cm lateral overhang exists, causing the lateral aspect of the patella to track over the lateral condyle and resulting in anterior knee pain. In this situation, central placement of the patella is acceptable.[37] Alternatively, the exposed lateral facet can be resected after the patellar component is cemented into position.

Soft-tissue balancing is important to optimize patellofemoral stability. In patients with a valgus knee and preoperative patellar maltracking, a lateral retinacular release may often be necessary. An inadequate lateral release, and similarly, failure of the medial retinaculum repair, may result in continued lateral tracking and subluxation. These errors can be avoided by iteratively checking patellar tracking after adjustment of components and soft-tissue balancing. Debate exists as to whether a lateral retinacular release is needed to correct patellar tilt during the primary TKA; some physicians contend that a lateral release to treat patellar tilt will not change outcomes.[38] A vastus-splitting surgical approach has been used as an alternative to the medial parapatellar approach to preserve the extensor mechanism. In a randomized, prospective trial, use of the vastus-splitting approach led to a decreased need for lateral retinacular release without impairing quadriceps function.[39]

Overstuffing the patellofemoral joint should be avoided because it destabilizes the patella. If the patellar height is increased as a result of underresection of the patella or because of a prominent anterior flange of the femoral component, increased tension is applied to the medial and lateral retinaculum. Because of the Q angle, the tension is partially relieved by lateral subluxation of the patella. Overstuffing can be avoided with appropriate resection of the patella, leaving 12 mm of bone to reduce fracture risk.[40] The femoral component also must be appropriately sized—too large a component can cause overstuffing, whereas too small a component can result in notching of the anterior femoral cortex.

Postoperative patellar tilting and subluxation may also result from abnormal tibiofemoral kinematics. "Paradoxical motion" has been observed after a TKA in which the tibia is anteriorly subluxated relative to the femur during knee extension, and the femur moves anteriorly during knee flexion.[41] If, during flexion, the tibia rotates externally relative to the femur, the tibial tubercle is lateralized, resulting in lateral patellar tilt and translation.[42]

Intraoperative assessment of patellofemoral stability is crucial to prevent these complications. Various techniques exist to check maltracking, including applying manual pressure to the lateral aspect of the patella, using a towel clip or stitch to temporarily close the medial arthrotomy, or using nothing ("no thumbs") to secure the medial patella. Release of the tourniquet before intraoperative assessment is recommended because the tourniquet itself can cause maltracking by trapping, therefore limiting excursion of the extensor mechanism.[43]

### Treatment

Treatment of patellofemoral instability after TKA depends on the specific etiology of the condition. Nonsurgical management, including physical therapy to strengthen the vastus medialis obliquus, is often recommended but is rarely successful.[2] In instances of component malpositioning, revision surgery is indicated. If component positioning is correct, a lateral retinacular release may be necessary to address patellofemoral maltracking; however, patients who undergo a lateral release have a higher incidence of patellar fracture and wound complications. Although an attempt should be made to preserve the superior lateral geniculate artery, the patellar fracture rate is not necessarily increased when the artery is sacrificed.[44] Using technetium Tc 99m bone scans, Ritter and associates[45] showed that patients with sacrifice of the superior lateral geniculate artery returned to normal function at 1-year follow-up. Other complications of lateral release include osteonecrosis, infection, and a more painful postoperative course.

Prior to current understanding of component malpositioning, proximal realignment was used to treat symptomatic patellar subluxation that could not be treated with a lateral release. The technique involves advancement of the vastus medialis obliquus and medial placation.[46]

Whiteside[47] was an early proponent of distal realignment characterized by medialization of the tibial tubercle to reduce the Q angle. These techniques, although major advances of their time, do not resolve maltracking complications associated with femoral or tibial component malpositioning. Current consensus recommends implant revision for complications associated with component malalignment.[48]

## Patellar Fracture

The prevalence of patellar fracture after TKA is 0.2% to 21% in resurfaced patellas, whereas the rate of fracture in unresurfaced patellas is 0.05%.[49-52] In a large retrospective review of more than 12,000 TKAs at the Mayo Clinic, the prevalence of patellar fractures was 0.68%. Men have a higher prevalence of patellar fractures compared with women (1.01% versus 0.40%).[53]

### Causes

The etiology of patellar fractures after TKA can be attributed to patient factors, implant design, and surgical technique.[54] Increased fracture risk has been noted in patients with rheumatoid arthritis, osteoporosis, previous surgery, and obesity, with trauma accounting for approximately 15% of fractures.[4,53,55,56] Higher patellofemoral and extensor mechanism forces have been associated with patellar fractures. An example of this is the higher fracture risk men have compared with women, which is believed to be a result of men's increased activity level and body weight.[52] Patients with higher activity levels have greater knee flexion and greater patellofemoral contact forces.[53] Similarly, a sudden contracture of the quadriceps can lead to patella fracture.[57]

The design of the patellar component may also contribute to frac-

ture risk or to maltracking. In some studies, components with a large central peg have been reported to have a higher fracture risk, whereas those with smaller pegs have higher rates of loosening.[1] Patellar components with a large central fixation peg have generally been replaced by patellar components with three small peripheral fixation pegs, although the resulting difference in fracture rate is not statistically significant.[58] Biomechanical studies have supported the three-peg component fixation design with the rationale that peripherally located pegs have better fixation against shear stresses.

Prior to the current all-polyethylene three-peg component fixation designs, metal-backed, cementless patellar components were evaluated. The design rationale was that the metal backing reduced bending forces on the polyethylene and, therefore, would result in more uniform load distribution.[3] This design was quickly shown to have higher failure rates than cemented polyethylene components.[56,59] The mechanisms of failure included dissociation of the metal from bone, dissociation of the polyethylene from the metal backing, polyethylene wear, and fracture, potentially allowing exposed metal to cause further damage to the femoral components. In response to these failures, surgeons returned to all-polyethylene cemented designs.

Surgical technique can affect the vascular supply of the patella, and can lead to an increased risk for osteonecrosis (Figure 2). During a medial parapatellar approach, the medial superior and inferior genicular arteries, lateral inferior genicular artery, and descending genicular artery can be compromised, and a lateral release may sacrifice the lateral superior genicular artery.[60] Thermal necrosis may occur during resection, with vascular

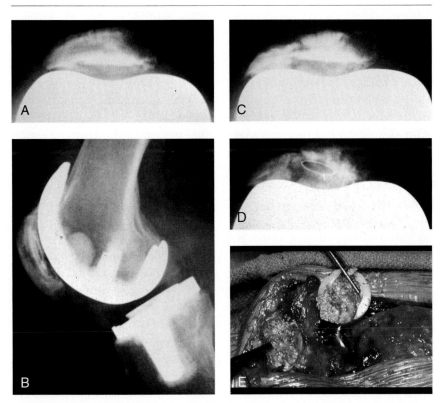

**Figure 2**    **A,** Patellar radiograph after TKA in a patient with a history of renal failure. A lateral retinacular release was required. **B,** Lateral radiograph of the knee showing a normal-appearing patella. **C,** Patellar radiograph 1 year after TKA shows sclerosis consistent with osteonecrosis and fragmentation of the lateral patellar facet. **D,** Patellar radiograph 18 months after TKA shows further fragmentation of the patella, which resulted in extensor mechanism disruption. **E,** Intraoperative view of the loose patella and disrupted extensor mechanism resulting from osteonecrosis.

compromise potentially leading to osteonecrosis, which in turn can cause comminuted fractures of the patella.[50] Controversy remains as to whether sacrificing the lateral superior genicular artery causes higher fracture rates. In some reports, osteonecrosis-related fractures in patients who underwent a lateral retinacular release have been noted.[61] Ritter and associates[45] showed that technetium Tc 99m uptake in the patella is reduced immediately after a lateral release but is restored at 1 year. A later study showed that there is no difference in patella fracture rate by sacrificing the lateral superior genicular artery.[44]

Both overresection and asymmet-

ric resection of the patella can increase fracture risk. A residual thickness of less than 15 mm can lead to significantly increased strain of the patella.[62] Koh and associates[40] reported an increased but statistically insignificant rate of patellar fracture when less than 12 mm of residual bone stock is left. Such underresection of the patella can cause overstuffing of the joint and increase patellofemoral joint forces. Conversely, asymmetric resection, often overresection of the lateral patella, can weaken the patella as well.[63] Component alignment and soft-tissue balancing are as important in preventing patellar fracture as they are in preventing instability. Maltracking

and subluxation of the patella exposes it to greater joint forces and also may lead to patella failure.[12]

### Classification and Treatment

Multiple classification systems have been described for patellar fractures after TKA.[49,53,64,65] Ortiguera and Berry[53] developed a classification system based on a retrospective review of more than 12,000 patients at the Mayo Clinic. Type I fractures have a stable implant and intact extensor mechanism; type II fractures have a disruption of the extensor mechanism; and type III fractures have a loose patellar component. Type III fractures are subclassified into type IIIa with reasonable remaining bone stock ($\geq$ 10 mm) and type IIIb with poor remaining bone stock (< 10 mm).

Type I fractures are most common (49%) and are often asymptomatic, usually detected on routine follow-up radiographs. Type I fractures can be treated nonsurgically with observation or bracing. Only on rare occasions do patients with a symptomatic type I fracture need surgical excision of nonunion fragments. Type II fractures can be treated with open reduction and internal fixation of the patella or by patellectomy, with extensor mechanism repair required in addition to the selected patella procedure. Patients with type II fractures usually have many complications after treatment and often need further surgical treatment. Type IIIa fractures are treated by patelloplasty with component revision or resection, whereas type IIIb fractures are treated by removal of the patellar component with patelloplasty or complete patellectomy. Similar to treatment of patients with type II fractures, surgical treatment for patients with type III fracture is associated with a high rate of complications, with some advocating nonsurgical management of type III fractures because of the high complication rate.[6,53] Complications of patellar fracture after TKA include nonunion, refracture, loss of fixation, extensor mechanism disruption, and infection.

New surgical techniques to manage patellar fractures also have been described. Augmentation with a porous tantalum implant has been used in the revision arthroplasty for deficient patella bone stock.[66] This technique was developed in response to the challenges and complications of bone grafting techniques for deficient patellas.[67,68] Ries and associates[69] reported that the use of porous tantalum augmentation is only successful when at least 50% of the patellar component is covered with host bone stock. The initial limited experience with this implant has shown good clinical success, but more evidence is needed. Allograft reconstruction is another technique that can be used to manage patella fractures. Busfield and Ries[70] recently described the use of whole patellar allograft (patellar ligament, whole patella, quadriceps tendon) for revision TKA in nine knees that had previously undergone patellectomy. The authors did not recommend routine use of this technique because of the high rate of complications (resorption, infection, maltracking), but consider it an option for patients with a severe extensor lag. Others have described success with extensor mechanism allografts, but limited data exist for its specific application to patella fractures.[71,72]

## Soft-Tissue Disruptions of the Extensor Mechanism
### Patellar Tendon Rupture
Patellar tendon rupture after TKA has a prevalence of 0.17% based on a 12-year retrospective study of 8,288 TKAs performed at the Mayo Clinic.[73] Although the etiology of these injuries has not been specifically studied given the low prevalence, the cause of patellar tendon ruptures after TKA is believed to be multifactorial. Patient factors that increase the risk of rupture include prior surgery, systemic disease (such as rheumatoid arthritis, diabetes mellitus, chronic renal insufficiency, obesity), extensor mechanism contractures, osteopenia, and poorly vascularized patellar tendons. Technical reasons for rupture include revision surgery, distal realignment for patellofemoral instability, closed manipulation, or open surgical exposure of a stiff knee.[4,73,74] Excessive lateral patellar retraction or inadequate proximal dissection of the extensor mechanism can put extra strain on the patellar tendon intraoperatively. Acute ruptures can be related to intraoperative or traumatic events, whereas chronic ruptures are often the result of the continual wear of the tendon against the tibial components.[5]

Prevention of patellar tendon rupture is achieved through reducing tension on the tendon during exposure. Patellar subluxation without eversion can be used to reduce tension in some instances, as well as lateral release or rectus snip. Some surgeons advocate reinforcing the insertion of the tendon with a temporary staple or pin. If efforts to reduce tension on the patellar tendon insertion are not successful, extension of the exposure distally, with a tibial tubercle osteotomy, or proximally, with a V-Y turndown, is appropriate to avoid traumatic rupture.[3,75]

### Quadriceps Tendon Rupture
Quadriceps tendon rupture after TKA is also rare. A prevalence of 0.1% was reported in a review of 23,800 primary TKAs done at the Mayo Clinic between 1976 and 2002.[76] In these patients, quadriceps tendon ruptures commonly occurred during walking, rising from a chair, or after falling. Approximately 75% of the patients with ruptures were reported to have underlying systemic risk factors, including steroid use, diabetes mellitus, obesity, and multiple knee surgeries. Lynch and associates[4] noted that a lateral release had been performed in all three cases of quadriceps rupture in their review of 281 TKAs. Poor vascularity of the tendon can be speculated as a reason for this finding.

The Mayo Clinic study found that partial quadriceps tendon tears were best treated nonsurgically.[76] Partial tears were immobilized in extension for 6 to 8 weeks followed by use of a brace for 6 weeks with progressive increase in brace flexion to 90°. Almost all of the patients with complete quadriceps tears were treated surgically but also experienced high complication rates.[76]

### Treatment Options
Primary repair of extensor mechanism disruption without autogenous or allograft soft-tissue augmentation is usually unsuccessful.[4,73] Repair of quadriceps tendon rupture may include direct suture fixation of the tendon with drill holes in the patella, whereas patellar tendon primary repair is accomplished by suture, wire, or staple fixation of the tendon to the bone, or internal fixation of avulsed bone fragments.[77] These repairs are often complicated by infection, rerupture requiring further surgery, and minimal functional improvement for the patient.[76] The high failure rate of primary repair alone is attributed to soft-tissue deficiency and poor vascularity.

Various augmentation techniques involving autogenous tissue, allograft, and synthetic materials have been developed to improve the outcome of

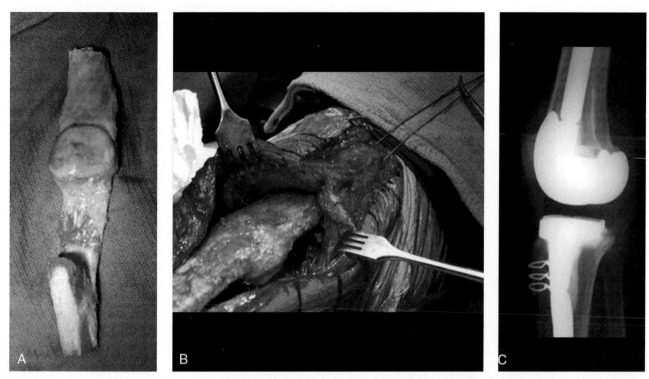

**Figure 3**     **A,** Photograph of a whole patella allograft consisting of the tibial tubercle, patellar ligament, patella, and quadriceps tendon. **B,** The allograft tibial tubercle is fixed into a trough in the host tibia with transverse wires, and the allograft is sutured proximally to the quadriceps tendon. The repair is performed with the knee in full extension, and maximal soft-tissue tension is applied to the soft-tissue repair. **C,** Postoperative lateral radiograph shows the position of the allograft patella and tibial wire fixation. (Reproduced with permission of Burnett RS, Berger RA, Della Valle CJ, et al: Extensor mechanism allograft reconstruction after total knee arthroplasty. *J Bone Joint Surg Am* 2005;87(suppl 1):175-194.)

primary extensor mechanism repair. Cadambi and Engh[74] described using semitendinosus grafts to reconstruct the patellar ligament. In their technique, the semitendinosus distal insertion is left intact. The tendon is passed parallel to the medial aspect of the patellar tendon through a drill hole in the patella and is reattached to itself distally. The authors reported a mean extensor lag of 10° and knee flexion of 79° in their study of seven patients.

Medial gastrocnemius flaps were first described in 1984 for soft-tissue coverage of limb-salvaging tumor resection.[78] Jaureguito and associates[79] later described use of the medial gastrocnemius flap for extensor mechanism disruption after TKA, with the rationale that the flap provides a mus-

cularized vascular bed for improved soft-tissue healing. At a follow-up of 33 months, mean extensor lag was improved from 53° to 24° with this flap. The standard technique includes division of the medial belly of the gastrocnemius at the level of the insertion into the Achilles tendon. The distal end is then transposed anteriorly to cover the tibial tubercle and is sutured to the anterior compartment fascia. The patellar tendon and anterior joint capsule are then attached to the medial aspect of the medial gastrocnemius. In the extended technique, the gastrocnemius is divided more distal to include a tendinous portion of the Achilles tendon. In the situation where a more proximal reconstruction is needed, this tendon is then repaired to the quadriceps ten-

don. The postoperative plan includes immobilization for 6 weeks followed by passive range of motion for 8 weeks, and return to active range of motion. Busfield and associates[80] described using an extended medial gastrocnemius flap as a salvage technique for patients with a failed extensor mechanism allograft or as an alternative for patients with poor soft-tissue coverage, a history of infection, or systemic illness.

Allograft augmentation is often required when autogenous tissues are limited in strength, thickness, and available lengths. In addition, donor site morbidity is a concern, especially in patients who are predisposed to extensor mechanism failure resulting from systemic comorbidities. The extensor mechanism allograft has been

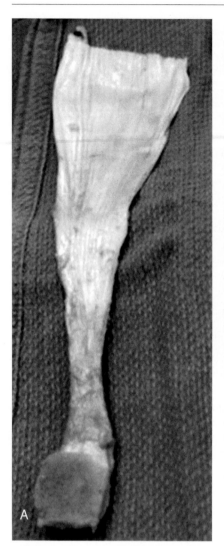

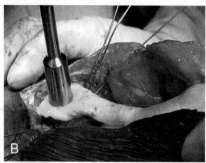

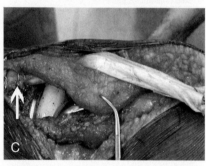

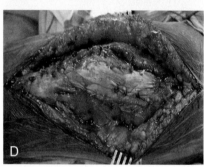

**Figure 4**    **A,** Photograph of Achilles tendon allograft consisting of a calcaneal bone block to be used for tibial fixation. **B,** The calcaneal bone block is impacted into a trough, which has been prepared in the proximal tibia. **C,** Transverse wires (*arrow*) are used to secure the distal allograft bone block, and the tendinous portion is brought proximally to reach the quadriceps tendon. **D,** The allograft tendon is repaired to the quadriceps tendon, and the remaining soft tissue is closed in a side-to-side fashion to seal the arthrotomy and to reinforce the reconstruction. (Reproduced with permission of Burnett RS, Butler RA, Barrack RL: Extensor mechanism allograft reconstruction in TKA at a mean of 56 months. *Clin Orthop Relat Res* 2006;452:159-165.)

extensively described in the literature and is the most common method to repair extensor mechanism deficiencies. The technique was initially described by Emerson and associates[81] in 1990. Their method uses an allograft including the quadriceps tendon, patella, patellar ligament, and tibial tubercle (Figure 3). First, the allograft is prepared by removing facets and fixing the patellar prosthesis. Next, the allograft tibial tubercle is keyed into the tibia, positioned medial of the native tubercle to enhance tracking. The patella is then aligned over the patellar flange of the femoral component, and, with the knee in full tension, the quadriceps tendon is repaired in slight tension, allowing 60° of flexion on the table without excessive tension. The patients were allowed up to 60° of range of motion in the immediate postoperative period. In a study of nine patients treated with this technique for patellar tendon rupture, six patients had no extensor lag, but three had extensor lags between 20° and 40° at an average follow-up of 2 years. Average knee flexion was 105°.[82]

In a modified technique described by Nazarian and Booth,[71] the allograft is tightly tensioned in full extension, the knee is not flexed intraoperatively, most of the allograft patellae are not resurfaced, and the patient is immobilized in extension for 6 weeks. In their study of 36 patients, the mean extensor lag was 1.4° and mean flexion was 98°. Although allograft rupture occurred in 8 patients postoperatively, after repeat allograft repair, 34 of the 36 patients in the study had successful outcomes. Burnett and associates[83,84] reported that outcomes were improved when the allograft is tightly tensioned in extension, as opposed to being minimally tensioned. The mean extensor lag was reduced by tightly tensioning the graft (4° versus 59°), but flexion was not significantly different (104° versus 108°). In a study with a 56-month follow-up, extensor mechanism allografts and Achilles tendon allografts were both found to reduce extensor lag, maintain knee flexion, and improve patient quality of life to a similar extent.[72] However, the allograft patella may resorb over time; Busfield and Ries[70] observed a 38% decrease in the height of the allograft patella in seven patients (nine knees) after an average follow-up of 44 months.

Crossett and associates[85] described using the Achilles tendon allograft for repair of ruptured patellar tendons (Figure 4). In their technique, a primary repair of the patellar tendon is done to maintain proper alignment of the patella. Next, a burr is used to create a window with the dimensions of 2.5 cm long × 1.5 cm wide × 1 cm deep in the tibia, just distal and medial to the insertion of the patellar tendon. A calcaneal bone block is then cut to fit in the window and is fixed with a 4.5-mm screw and reinforced with cerclage wires, when necessary. With the knee in extension, the Achilles tendon is laid over the closed joint capsule and sutured to the extensor mechanism, keeping the tendon taut, without wrinkles. Postoperatively, the knee is kept locked in extension for 4 weeks, at which time range of motion exercises can begin. Full weight bearing is allowed at 3 months. Using this technique in nine patients, the mean extensor lag was decreased from 44° to 3° and range of motion increased from 88° to 107°. Complications included two early failures and proximal patellar migration of 18 mm without functional consequence.

Synthetic ligament augmentation provides an alternative to allografts and autografts. The Leeds-Keio connective tissue prosthesis (L-K CTP, Neoligaments, Leeds, UK) has been used primarily to repair patellar tendon ruptures. It consists of a weave of polyester fibers and functions as scaffold for fibrous ingrowth. Although initial reports of this prosthesis show some promise, the long-term durability of synthetic ligaments has not been established and further data are necessary to determine their role in extensor mechanism reconstruction.[86-89]

## Summary

Extensor mechanism complications after TKA represent a diverse array of clinical scenarios. Treatment modalities for patellofemoral instability, patellar fracture, and soft-tissue disruptions are most effective when tailored to the underlying cause of failure. Although advances are being made in prosthetic design and treatment, outcomes continue to be suboptimal. Careful preoperative planning and meticulous surgical technique are essential in minimizing the incidence of these potentially devastating complications.

## References

1. Brick GW, Scott RD: The patellofemoral component of total knee arthroplasty. *Clin Orthop Relat Res* 1988;231:163-178.

2. Kelly MA: Extensor mechanism complications in total knee arthroplasty. *Instr Course Lect* 2004;53:193-199.

3. Kelly MA: Patellofemoral complications following total knee arthroplasty. *Instr Course Lect* 2001;50:403-407.

4. Lynch AF, Rorabeck CH, Bourne RB: Extensor mechanism complications following total knee arthroplasty. *J Arthroplasty* 1987;2:135-140.

5. Parker DA, Dunbar MJ, Rorabeck CH: Extensor mechanism failure associated with total knee arthroplasty: Prevention and management. *J Am Acad Orthop Surg* 2003;11:238-247.

6. Rand JA: Extensor mechanism complications after total knee arthroplasty. *Instr Course Lect* 2005;54:241-250.

7. Rand JA: Extensor mechanism complications following total knee arthroplasty. *J Knee Surg* 2003;16:224-228.

8. Schoderbek RJ Jr, Brown TE, Mulhall KJ, et al: Extensor mechanism disruption after total knee arthroplasty. *Clin Orthop Relat Res* 2006;446:176-185.

9. Sierra RJ, Cooney WP, Pagnano MW, Trousdale RT, Rand JA: Reoperations after 3200 revision TKAs: Rates, etiology, and lessons learned. *Clin Orthop Relat Res* 2004;425:200-206.

10. Cooney WP, Sierra RJ, Trousdale RT, Pagnano MW: Revision total knees done for extensor problems frequently require reoperation. *Clin Orthop Relat Res* 2005;440:117-121.

11. Eisenhuth SA, Saleh KJ, Cui Q, Clark CR, Brown TE: Patellofemoral instability after total knee arthroplasty. *Clin Orthop Relat Res* 2006;446:149-160.

12. Berger RA, Crossett LS, Jacobs JJ, Rubash HE: Malrotation causing patellofemoral complications after total knee arthroplasty. *Clin Orthop Relat Res* 1998;356:144-153.

13. D'Lima DD, Chen PC, Kester MA, Colwell CW Jr: Impact of patellofemoral design on patellofemoral forces and polyethylene stresses. *J Bone Joint Surg Am* 2003;85-A(suppl 4):85-93.

14. Malo M, Vince KG: The unstable patella after total knee arthroplasty: Etiology, prevention, and management. *J Am Acad Orthop Surg* 2003;11:364-371.

15. Petersilge WJ, Oishi CS, Kaufman KR, Irby SE, Colwell CW Jr: The effect of trochlear design on patellofemoral shear and compressive forces in total knee arthroplasty. *Clin Orthop Relat Res* 1994;309:124-130.

16. Yoshii I, Whiteside LA, Anouchi YS: The effect of patellar button placement and femoral component design on patellar tracking in total knee arthroplasty. *Clin Orthop Relat Res* 1992;275:211-219.

17. Theiss SM, Kitziger KJ, Lotke PS, Lotke PA: Component design affecting patellofemoral complications after total knee arthroplasty. *Clin Orthop Relat Res* 1996;326:183-187.

18. Singerman R, Pagan HD, Peyser AB, Goldberg VM: Effect of femoral component rotation and patellar design on patellar forces. *Clin Orthop Relat Res* 1997;334:345-353.

19. Benjamin J: Component alignment in total knee arthroplasty. *Instr Course Lect* 2006;55:405-412.

20. Lee GC, Cushner FD, Scuderi GR, Insall JN: Optimizing patellofemoral tracking during total knee ar-

throplasty. *J Knee Surg* 2004;17: 144-149.

21. Scuderi GR, Komistek RD, Dennis DA, Insall JN: The impact of femoral component rotational alignment on condylar lift-off. *Clin Orthop Relat Res* 2003;410:148-154.

22. Bankes MJ, Back DL, Cannon SR, Briggs TW: The effect of component malalignment on the clinical and radiological outcome of the Kinemax total knee replacement. *Knee* 2003;10: 55-60.

23. Insall JN, Scuderi GR, Komistek RD, Math K, Dennis DA, Anderson DT: Correlation between condylar lift-off and femoral component alignment. *Clin Orthop Relat Res* 2002;403:143-152.

24. Barrack RL, Schrader T, Bertot AJ, Wolfe MW, Myers L: Component rotation and anterior knee pain after total knee arthroplasty. *Clin Orthop Relat Res* 2001;392:46-55.

25. Matsuda S, Miura H, Nagamine R, Urabe K, Hirata G, Iwamoto Y: Effect of femoral and tibial component position on patellar tracking following total knee arthroplasty: 10-year follow-up of Miller-Galante I knees. *Am J Knee Surg* 2001;14:152-156.

26. Olcott CW, Scott RD: Determining proper femoral component rotational alignment during total knee arthroplasty. *Am J Knee Surg* 2000;13: 166-168.

27. Olcott CW, Scott RD: A comparison of 4 intraoperative methods to determine femoral component rotation during total knee arthroplasty. *J Arthroplasty* 2000;15:22-26.

28. Akagi M, Matsusue Y, Mata T, et al: Effect of rotational alignment on patellar tracking in total knee arthroplasty. *Clin Orthop Relat Res* 1999;366: 155-163.

29. Olcott CW, Scott RD: Femoral component rotation during total knee arthroplasty. *Clin Orthop Relat Res* 1999; 367:39-42.

30. Whiteside LA, Arima J: The anteroposterior axis for femoral rotational alignment in valgus total knee arthro-

plasty. *Clin Orthop Relat Res* 1995;321: 168-172.

31. Berger RA, Rubash HE, Seel MJ, Thompson WH, Crossett LS: Determining the rotational alignment of the femoral component in total knee arthroplasty using the epicondylar axis. *Clin Orthop Relat Res* 1993;286: 40-47.

32. Delp SL, Stulberg SD, Davies B, Picard F, Leitner F: Computer assisted knee replacement. *Clin Orthop Relat Res* 1998;354:49-56.

33. Siston RA, Goodman SB, Patel JJ, Delp SL, Giori NJ: The high variability of tibial rotational alignment in total knee arthroplasty. *Clin Orthop Relat Res* 2006;452:65-69.

34. Siston RA, Patel JJ, Goodman SB, Delp SL, Giori NJ: The variability of femoral rotational alignment in total knee arthroplasty. *J Bone Joint Surg Am* 2005;87:2276-2280.

35. Matziolis G, Krocker D, Weiss U, Tohtz S, Perka C: A prospective, randomized study of computer-assisted and conventional total knee arthroplasty: Three-dimensional evaluation of implant alignment and rotation. *J Bone Joint Surg Am* 2007;89:236-243.

36. Hofmann AA, Tkach TK, Evanich CJ, Camargo MP, Zhang Y: Patellar component medialization in total knee arthroplasty. *J Arthroplasty* 1997;12:155-160.

37. McPherson EJ: Patellar tracking in primary total knee arthroplasty. *Instr Course Lect* 2006;55:439-448.

38. Benjamin J, Chilvers M: Correcting lateral patellar tilt at the time of total knee arthroplasty can result in overuse of lateral release. *J Arthroplasty* 2006;21(6, suppl 2):121-126.

39. Kelly MJ, Rumi MN, Kothari M, et al: Comparison of the vastus-splitting and median parapatellar approaches for primary total knee arthroplasty: A prospective, randomized study. *J Bone Joint Surg Am* 2006; 88:715-720.

40. Koh JS, Yeo SJ, Lee BP, Lo NN, Seow KH, Tan SK: Influence of patellar thickness on results of total knee ar-

throplasty: Does a residual bony patellar thickness of ≤ 12 mm lead to poorer clinical outcome and increased complication rates? *J Arthroplasty* 2002;17:56-61.

41. Dennis DA, Komistek RD, Mahfouz MR, Haas BD, Stiehl JB: Multicenter determination of in vivo kinematics after total knee arthroplasty. *Clin Orthop Relat Res* 2003;416:37-57.

42. Lee KY, Slavinsky JP, Ries MD, Blumenkrantz G, Majumdar S: Magnetic resonance imaging of in vivo kinematics after total knee arthroplasty. *J Magn Reson Imaging* 2005;21: 172-178.

43. Marson BM, Tokish JT: The effect of a tourniquet on intraoperative patellofemoral tracking during total knee arthroplasty. *J Arthroplasty* 1999;14: 197-199.

44. Ritter MA, Pierce MJ, Zhou H, Meding JB, Faris PM, Keating EM: Patellar complications (total knee arthroplasty): Effect of lateral release and thickness. *Clin Orthop Relat Res* 1999; 367:149-157.

45. Ritter MA, Keating EM, Faris PM: Clinical, roentgenographic, and scintigraphic results after interruption of the superior lateral genicular artery during total knee arthroplasty. *Clin Orthop Relat Res* 1989;248:145-151.

46. Merkow RL, Soudry M, Insall JN: Patellar dislocation following total knee replacement. *J Bone Joint Surg Am* 1985;67:1321-1327.

47. Whiteside LA: Distal realignment of the patellar tendon to correct abnormal patellar tracking. *Clin Orthop Relat Res* 1997;344:284-289.

48. Briard JL, Hungerford DS: Patellofemoral instability in total knee arthroplasty. *J Arthroplasty* 1989; 4(suppl):S87-S97.

49. Goldberg VM, Figgie HE III, Inglis AE, et al: Patellar fracture type and prognosis in condylar total knee arthroplasty. *Clin Orthop Relat Res* 1988; 236:115-122.

50. Grace JN, Sim FH: Fracture of the patella after total knee arthroplasty.

*Clin Orthop Relat Res* 1988;230: 168-175.

51. Tria AJ Jr, Harwood DA, Alicea JA, Cody RP: Patellar fractures in posterior stabilized knee arthroplasties. *Clin Orthop Relat Res* 1994;299: 131-138.

52. Windsor RE, Scuderi GR, Insall JN: Patellar fractures in total knee arthroplasty. *J Arthroplasty* 1989;4(suppl): S63-S67.

53. Ortiguera CJ, Berry DJ: Patellar fracture after total knee arthroplasty. *J Bone Joint Surg Am* 2002;84-A:532-540.

54. Burnett RS, Bourne RB: Periprosthetic fractures of the tibia and patella in total knee arthroplasty. *Instr Course Lect* 2004;53:217-235.

55. Goldstein SA, Coale E, Weiss AP, Grossnickle M, Meller B, Matthews LS: Patellar surface strain. *J Orthop Res* 1986;4:372-377.

56. Stulberg SD, Stulberg BN, Hamati Y, Tsao A: Failure mechanisms of metal-backed patellar components. *Clin Orthop Relat Res* 1988;236:88-105.

57. Engh GA, Herzwurm PJ, Parks NL: Treatment of major defects of bone with bulk allografts and stemmed components during total knee arthroplasty. *J Bone Joint Surg Am* 1997;79: 1030-1039.

58. Larson CM, McDowell CM, Lachiewicz PF: One-peg versus three-peg patella component fixation in total knee arthroplasty. *Clin Orthop Relat Res* 2001;392:94-100.

59. Bayley JC, Scott RD, Ewald FC, Holmes GB Jr: Failure of the metal-backed patellar component after total knee replacement. *J Bone Joint Surg Am* 1988;70:668-674.

60. Kayler DE, Lyttle D: Surgical interruption of patellar blood supply by total knee arthroplasty. *Clin Orthop Relat Res* 1988;229:221-227.

61. Holtby RM, Grosso P: Osteonecrosis and resorption of the patella after total knee replacement: A case report. *Clin Orthop Relat Res* 1996;328: 155-158.

62. Reuben JD, McDonald CL, Woodard PL, Hennington LJ: Effect of patella thickness on patella strain following total knee arthroplasty. *J Arthroplasty* 1991;6:251-258.

63. Scott RD, Turoff N, Ewald FC: Stress fracture of the patella following duo-patellar total knee arthroplasty with patellar resurfacing. *Clin Orthop Relat Res* 1982;170:147-151.

64. Hozack WJ, Goll SR, Lotke PA, Rothman RH, Booth RE Jr: The treatment of patellar fractures after total knee arthroplasty. *Clin Orthop Relat Res* 1988; 236:123-127.

65. Keating EM, Haas G, Meding JB: Patella fracture after post total knee replacements. *Clin Orthop Relat Res* 2003;416:93-97.

66. Nasser S, Poggie RA: Revision and salvage patellar arthroplasty using a porous tantalum implant. *J Arthroplasty* 2004;19:562-572.

67. Buechel FF: Patellar tendon bone grafting for patellectomized patients having total knee arthroplasty. *Clin Orthop Relat Res* 1991;271:72-78.

68. Hanssen AD: Bone-grafting for severe patellar bone loss during revision knee arthroplasty. *J Bone Joint Surg Am* 2001;83-A:171-176.

69. Ries MD, Cabalo A, Bozic KJ, Anderson M: Porous tantalum patellar augmentation: The importance of residual bone stock. *Clin Orthop Relat Res* 2006;452:166-170.

70. Busfield BT, Ries MD: Whole patellar allograft for total knee arthroplasty after previous patellectomy. *Clin Orthop Relat Res* 2006;450:145-149.

71. Nazarian DG, Booth RE Jr: Extensor mechanism allografts in total knee arthroplasty. *Clin Orthop Relat Res* 1999; 367:123-129.

72. Burnett RS, Butler RA, Barrack RL: Extensor mechanism allograft reconstruction in TKA at a mean of 56 months. *Clin Orthop Relat Res* 2006;452:159-165.

73. Rand JA, Morrey BF, Bryan RS: Patellar tendon rupture after total knee arthroplasty. *Clin Orthop Relat Res*

1989;244:233-238.

74. Cadambi A, Engh GA: Use of a semi-tendinosus tendon autogenous graft for rupture of the patellar ligament after total knee arthroplasty: A report of seven cases. *J Bone Joint Surg Am* 1992;74:974-979.

75. Scuderi GR, Insall JN, Scott NW: Patellofemoral pain after total knee arthroplasty. *J Am Acad Orthop Surg* 1994;2:239-246.

76. Dobbs RE, Hanssen AD, Lewallen DG, Pagnano MW: Quadriceps tendon rupture after total knee arthroplasty: Prevalence, complications, and outcomes. *J Bone Joint Surg Am* 2005;87:37-45.

77. Abril JC, Alvarez L, Vallejo JC: Patellar tendon avulsion after total knee arthroplasty: A new technique. *J Arthroplasty* 1995;10:275-279.

78. Malawer MM, Price WM: Gastrocnemius transposition flap in conjunction with limb-sparing surgery for primary bone sarcomas around the knee. *Plast Reconstr Surg* 1984;73: 741-750.

79. Jaureguito JW, Dubois CM, Smith SR, Gottlieb LJ, Finn HA: Medial gastrocnemius transposition flap for the treatment of disruption of the extensor mechanism after total knee arthroplasty. *J Bone Joint Surg Am* 1997;79:866-873.

80. Busfield BT, Huffman GR, Nahai F, Hoffman W, Ries MD: Extended medial gastrocnemius rotational flap for treatment of chronic knee extensor mechanism deficiency in patients with and without total knee arthroplasty. *Clin Orthop Relat Res* 2004;428: 190-197.

81. Emerson RH Jr, Head WC, Malinin TI: Reconstruction of patellar tendon rupture after total knee arthroplasty with an extensor mechanism allograft. *Clin Orthop Relat Res* 1990; 260:154-161.

82. Emerson RH Jr, Head WC, Malinin TI: Extensor mechanism reconstruction with an allograft after total knee arthroplasty. *Clin Orthop Relat Res* 1994;303:79-85.

83. Burnett RS, Berger RA, Della Valle CJ, et al: Extensor mechanism allograft reconstruction after total knee arthroplasty. *J Bone Joint Surg Am* 2005;87(suppl 1):175-194.

84. Burnett RS, Berger RA, Paprosky WG, Della Valle CJ, Jacobs JJ, Rosenberg AG: Extensor mechanism allograft reconstruction after total knee arthroplasty: A comparison of two techniques. *J Bone Joint Surg Am* 2004; 86-A:2694-2699.

85. Crossett LS, Sinha RK, Sechriest VF, Rubash HE: Reconstruction of a ruptured patellar tendon with achilles tendon allograft following total knee arthroplasty. *J Bone Joint Surg Am* 2002;84-A:1354-1361.

86. Fujikawa K, Ohtani T, Matsumoto H, Seedhom BB: Reconstruction of the extensor apparatus of the knee with the Leeds-Keio ligament. *J Bone Joint Surg Br* 1994;76:200-203.

87. Fukuta S, Kuge A, Nakamura M: Use of the Leeds-Keio prosthetic ligament for repair of patellar tendon rupture after total knee arthroplasty. *Knee* 2003;10:127-130.

88. Sherief TI, Naguib AM, Sefton GK: Use of Leeds-Keio connective tissue prosthesis (L-K CTP) for reconstruction of deficient extensor mechanism with total knee replacement. *Knee* 2005;12:319-322.

89. Toms AD, Smith A, White SH: Analysis of the Leeds-Keio ligament for extensor mechanism repair: Favourable mechanical and functional outcome. *Knee* 2003;10: 131-134.

# Instability After Total Knee Arthroplasty

Sebastien Parratte, MD
*Mark W. Pagnano, MD

## Abstract

*Instability after total knee arthroplasty is reported to result in implant failure, and substantial instability often requires revision surgery. Successful outcomes can be achieved after revision total knee arthroplasty, particularly if the etiology of the instability is identified before the revision procedure. After careful clinical and radiologic analysis, instability can be classified as extension instability, flexion instability, or genu recurvatum. It is important to understand the causes and recommended treatments of each type of instability.*

**Instr Course Lect 2008;57:295-304.**

Instability after total knee arthroplasty is a cause of failure and a reason for 10% to 22% of revisions.[1-5] Successful outcomes can be obtained in many of these cases, but without identifying the cause of instability, the surgeon risks repeating the mistakes that led to the instability after the initial total knee arthroplasty.[2,3,6] As Vince and associates[6] stated, "the patient's report of instability is not a diagnosis," and particular care should be given to confirming the diagnosis and understanding the causes.

The first step in confirming the diagnosis and understanding the causes is clinical and includes recording an accurate and complete history, including the reason for the original knee replacement, the presence of any preoperative deformity or contracture, previous knee procedures, the specifics of the surgical technique for the knee replacement, the type of prosthesis that was used, the postoperative rehabilitation program, and whether the patient sustained any trauma to the knee after the surgery.[1,2,6] Specific patient-related risk factors are a large surgical correction including an aggressive ligament release, general or regional neuromuscular pathology, hip or foot deformities, and clinical obesity.[6] The postoperative symptoms should be clarified, and a complete physical examination must be performed.[1,2,6] Specific attention should be paid to the knee, with the examiner noting varus-valgus laxity in extension, in 30° of flexion, and in 90° of flexion. Anteroposterior laxity should be tested as well. Laxity in flexion, so-called flexion laxity, is often most evident when an anterior or posterior drawer test is performed with the patient sitting and the knee flexed 90°.[7] Analysis of a complete set of radiographs is necessary and should include measurement of the mechanical and anatomic axes on AP short and full-length weight-bearing radiographs, as well as measurement of implant position on lateral radiographs made with the knee in full extension and in maximum knee flexion.[1,2,6]

After this analysis, the type of instability can be identified. There are three types of instability after a total knee arthroplasty: extension instability, flexion instability, and genu recurvatum. Instability is accentuated by errors in component orientation or overall limb-alignment problems.[1-6] It is important to understand the causes and treatments of each type of instability.

## Extension Instability

Instability in extension may be symmetric or asymmetric. It is usually referred to as extension instability,

*Mark W. Pagnano, MD or the department with which he is affiliated has received royalties from DePuy and Zimmer.*

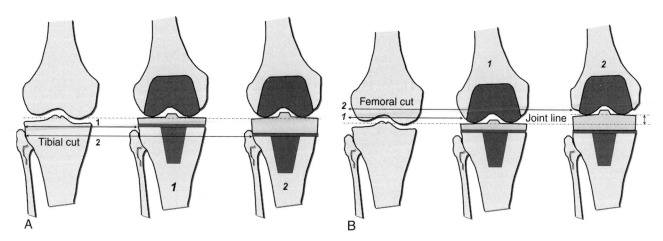

**Figure 1**  **A,** Excessive removal of bone from the proximal part of the tibia affects the space between the femur and tibia equally in knee flexion and knee extension. When the excessive bone removal is recognized during the operation, the potential instability is corrected by using a thicker tibial insert. **B,** Managing excessive bone removal from the distal part of the femur is more challenging. Use of a thicker tibial insert will not solve the problem, as this would elevate the joint line and excessively tighten the flexion space. (Reproduced with permission from Vail TP, Lang JE: Surgical techniques and instrumentation in total knee arthroplasty, in Insall JN, Scott WN (eds): *Surgery of the Knee*, ed 4. Baltimore, MD, Churchill Livingstone, 2006, vol 2, pp 1455-1521.)

and when it is symmetric it is sometimes called "instability due to bone resection."[1,2] Symmetric extension instability occurs when the extension space is not adequately filled by the thicknesses of the components.[8] This may be caused by excessive bone removal from the distal part of the femur or the proximal part of the tibia. Excessive bone removal from the proximal part of the tibia affects the space between the femur and tibia equally in knee flexion and knee extension. When this is recognized during the operation, the potential instability is corrected by using a thicker tibial insert[8] (Figure 1, *A*). A long-term concern is the fixation of the tibial tray, which is more distal than optimal and is in slightly weaker bone.[8]

Managing excessive bone removal from the distal part of the femur is more challenging. A thicker tibial insert will not solve this problem. Using a thicker tibial insert elevates the joint line and excessively tightens the flexion space

(Figure 1, *B*).[2,6,8] Elevating the joint line adversely affects the kinematics of the knee. Depending on the magnitude of the joint line elevation, the symptoms may be only a subtle functional limitation or may be a clinically relevant functional deficit. Marked elevation of the joint line limits knee flexion, adversely affects patellar function, and contributes to so-called midflexion instability, where the knee is stable in extension and 90° of flexion but symmetrically unstable during varus-valgus testing at 30° to 45° of flexion.[2,6,8] Instability caused by overresection of the distal part of the femur is treated by adding distal femoral augments, which are available in most contemporary revision total knee systems.[2,6,8]

Asymmetric extension instability is much more common than symmetric extension instability. It is typically related to a preoperative angular deformity of the knee (Figure 2, *A*) and is caused by persistent or iatrogenic ligamentous asymmetry after the knee is replaced (Fig-

ure 2, *B*).[2,6,8] The most common mistake leading to asymmetric instability is undercorrection of a fixed angular deformity, often out of fear of creating ligamentous instability in the opposite direction.[2,6,8] For instance, concerns about stretching, cutting, or overreleasing the medial collateral ligament in a varus knee can lead to an undercorrection of the varus deformity, leaving the knee still tight on the medial side. This problem is exacerbated if the limb alignment is also left in varus.[2,6,8] Over time, that malalignment and the associated excessive tension on the medial side will stretch out the soft tissues on the lateral side and/or lead to excessive medial polyethylene wear from overload.[2,6,8] In such instances, the varus deformity progressively recurs and the arthroplasty ultimately requires a revision. Laskin and Schob[9] reported four cases of asymmetric extension instability caused by insufficient medial release in a series of 68 total knee arthroplasties done for knees with severe preoperative varus deformity. An appropriate medial release as initially described by Insall and associates[10] should be performed when necessary, with use of a true subperiosteal elevation of the superficial medial collateral ligament from the tibia, with the pes anserinus tendons left intact in most cases (Figure 3). The medial collateral ligament should never be deliberately and improperly stretched by the retractors; instead, the medial collateral ligament should be released with a long soft-tissue sleeve from the proximal part of the tibia.[10]

Undercorrection of a valgus knee will leave the knee still tight laterally with laxity or redundancy in the medial collateral ligament.[1,6,8] Because the medial collateral ligament will not tighten over time, the valgus deformity returns.[1,6,8] Therefore, only minimal laxity of the medial collateral ligament should be accepted when correcting a valgus deformity. To achieve medial and lateral soft-tissue balance, Insall and associates[10] originally advocated a sequential lateral ligamentous release technique.[11] Their original description was of a sequence of releases starting with the lateral collateral ligament and continuing with the popliteus tendon and the lateral head of the gastrocnemius, but they stated that the iliotibial band should be preserved unless a severe external rotation deformity is present.[10,11] Laskin[12] recommended a different release sequence, starting with the iliotibial band and continuing with the popliteus tendon, the lateral collateral ligament, and the lateral head of the gastrocnemius, and, if further correction is needed, advancement of the medial collateral ligament. Both of those techniques, however, lead to overrelease of the lateral ligaments in too many patients.[13] Early

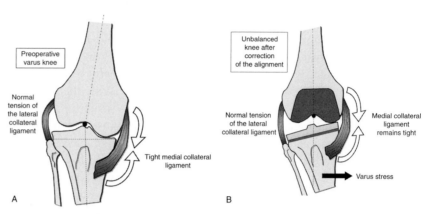

**Figure 2** **A,** An example of a varus knee with a contracted medial collateral ligament that has been incompletely released. **B,** The medial collateral ligament remains tight, and the lateral collateral ligament is subsequently lax. (Reproduced with permission from Vail TP, Lang JE: Surgical techniques and instrumentation in total knee arthroplasty, in Insall JN, Scott WN (eds): *Surgery of the Knee*, ed 4. Baltimore, MD, Churchill Livingstone, 2006, vol 2, pp 1455-1521.)

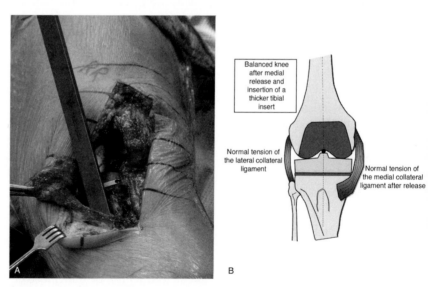

**Figure 3** **A,** The medial release advocated by Insall and associates for treatment of a fixed varus knee deformity involves a true subperiosteal release of the superficial medial collateral ligament from the medial aspect of the tibia. Care is taken to preserve the insertion of the overlying pes anserinus tendons so that the released medial collateral ligament will be held in close contact with the tibia and heal readily. The medial collateral ligament should never be deliberately stretched or pried with retractors. **B,** Satisfactory balance of the knee can be obtained after medial release and insertion of a thicker tibial insert. (Reproduced with permission from Scuderi GR, Insall JN: Fixed varus and valgus deformities, in Lotke PA, Lonner JH (eds): *Master Techniques in Orthopaedic Surgery: Knee Arthroplasty*, ed 2. Philadelphia, PA, Lippincott Williams & Wilkins, 2003, pp 95-109.)

reports of dislocations of posterior stabilized total knee prostheses were almost always related to knees that had a previous preoperative valgus deformity and had undergone one of those types of traditional lateral-sided ligamentous releases.[13] To address this problem, Insall changed his recommendation.[14] He described the "pie crust" or multiple-puncture technique, which has become widely used.[13-15] Clarke and associates[14] used the multiple-puncture technique for a series of 24 valgus knees treated with a posterior stabilized knee prosthesis and reported complete correction without instability. In that series, the mean amount of preoperative valgus was 15° (range, 9° to 30°), and these authors recommended this technique for patients with a fixed valgus deformity of less than 20°.[14] With Insall's pie crust technique, the surgeon fully extends the knee and places a lamina spreader in the extension space. First, a transverse incision is made through the posterolateral aspect of the capsule at the level of the tibial bone cut with a No. 15 surgical blade from just posterior to the lateral collateral ligament to just anterolateral to the popliteus tendon. The popliteus tendon should be carefully protected and not cut. Next, a series of horizontal stab incisions are made with the No. 15 surgical blade (piecrusting) along the lateral side of the knee for any structure that feels tight. The surgeon simply palpates the lateral-sided structures and starts with punctures of the tightest band of tissue. This usually starts with the iliotibial band, but in many knees with a fixed valgus deformity, the lateral collateral ligament itself may also require pie crusting. Specific identification of which structures are being pie crusted is not required, provided that the release is titrated by intermittently checking to determine when a sufficient release has been achieved. On the basis of anatomic and in vivo studies, the depth of the surgical blade should be kept

at less than 5 mm to minimize the risk of a peroneal nerve injury.[13-15] With the aid of lamina spreaders, the lateral side is gently and progressively stretched to effect an in situ lengthening.[13-15] With the pie crust technique, no structure is completely divided; instead, the lateral structures are lengthened in continuity.[13-15] To check for an over-released lateral side, the stability is tested with a trial prosthesis in place. The limb is placed in the "figure-4" position; that is, 90° of knee flexion while the surgeon holds the foot and allows the hip and knee to externally rotate maximally.[14] The knee should be stable in this position; if the post of a posterior stabilized tibial component subluxates from the femoral housing in this position, a thicker or more constrained tibial insert should be used.[14]

In an elderly patient with a valgus deformity of more than 20°, there is a risk of excessive stretching of the peroneal nerve with complete correction.[14,16] Easley and associates[16] reported satisfactory clinical and radiographic results at a mean of almost 8 years after 44 primary constrained condylar knee implants had been used to treat arthritic valgus knees in 37 patients with a mean age of 72 years (range, 60 to 88 years). The deformity can be undercorrected with a varus-valgus constrained condylar implant to compensate for the residual laxity of the medial collateral ligament. According to Easley and associates,[16] this approach has proven successful and is appropriate for an arthritic knee with a substantial valgus deformity in patients approximately 75 years of age with low physical demands.[17] This approach typically is not used in younger, more active patients because of the theoretic concern that a varus-valgus constrained condylar implant

will impart more stresses to the bone-cement interface and lead to a higher rate of revision over time.[16]

Iatrogenic collateral ligament injury may also occur during total knee arthroplasty, most often when the proximal part of the tibia is cut but also during inappropriately vigorous attempts to test varus-valgus stability.[17] The most appropriate treatment of a ligamentous injury is surgical reapproximation of the ligament with Krackow-pattern sutures.[18,19] The repair can be augmented with the hamstring tendons that are left attached distally but freed at the musculotendinous junction with a tendon-stripper.[17] The hamstring tendons are fixed proximally with a ligament washer and screw or are run through a drill hole to the lateral side of the femur and tied over a button or suture post (Figure 4).[17] A constrained condylar implant may be used to add stability.[16,17] This implant essentially acts as an internal splint but clearly is not required in every case of iatrogenic collateral ligament injury. Leopold and associates[17] reported good results with immediate suture repair of an intraoperative avulsion or an intraoperative iatrogenic disruption of the medial collateral ligament without use of a constrained implant and without augmentation. In their series of 600 primary total knee arthroplasties, there were 16 knees (2.7%) in which an intraoperative disruption of the medial collateral ligament was treated with a cruciate-retaining implant combined with direct repair of the medial collateral ligament and bracing for 6 weeks. The results were considered excellent for 13 knees and good for the remaining 3 knees.

## Flexion Instability

Flexion instability is seen most often

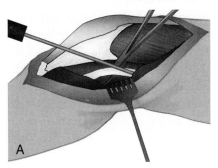
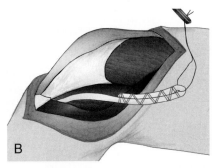
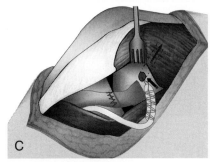

**Figure 4** **A,** In rare cases, the medial collateral ligament may be transected during surgery and require repair. The medial collateral ligament can be augmented with a medial hamstring tendon that is left attached distally but freed with a tendon stripper at the musculotendinous junction. **B,** Preparation of the hamstring tendon. **C,** Proximally, the hamstring tendon can be run through a drill hole to the lateral side of the femur and tied over a button. (Reproduced with permission from Krackow KA, Madanagopal SG: Managing ligament loss, in Lotke PA, Lonner JH (eds): *Master Techniques in Orthopaedic Surgery: Knee Arthroplasty*, ed 2. Philadelphia, PA, Lippincott Williams & Wilkins, 2003, pp 184-186.)

in patients in whom the total knee prosthesis is well aligned axially and well fixed. Historically, this problem has been underdiagnosed in patients with a cruciate-retaining knee implant. The laxity is due to inadequate filling of the flexion space with the implant or disruption of the posterior cruciate ligament. The manifestations of flexion instability range from a vague sense of instability to frank dislocation. This variability depends in part on whether a posterior stabilized or cruciate-retaining implant is in place. Assessment of the knee in 90° of flexion should be part of the routine physical examination of any patient with pain at the site of a total knee arthroplasty, regardless of whether the prosthesis is cruciate retaining, cruciate sacrificing, or cruciate substituting, as this may be the only way to recognize flexion laxity.

Dislocation after a posterior stabilized total knee arthroplasty is a rare but dramatic and disconcerting complication for patient and surgeon alike.[20] Most current posterior stabilized designs have increased the so-called jump distance that is needed for the cam to ride over the post

before dislocating, and dislocation rates are now much lower than 0.5%. However, exceeding the so-called jump distance results in a posterior dislocation of the tibia on the femur, which often requires closed reduction with the patient under anesthesia (Figure 5). Once reduced, the knee typically functions well but is prone to subsequent dislocation. The most common activity that leads to a dislocation is marked knee flexion plus a varus stress (for example, placing the ankle of the surgically treated limb on the contralateral knee to put on a sock or shoe).[20] A posterior stabilized knee prosthesis can resist posterior translation because of the tibial cam, but it does not resist a combination of varus or valgus stress and posterior translation. The standard posterior stabilized knee prosthesis does not provide varus-valgus constraint, and most often a loose flexion gap associated with laxity of a collateral ligament (most often the lateral collateral ligament) is the cause of flexion instability of posterior stabilized knee replacements. At-risk patients include those who had correction of a large valgus deformity, particularly

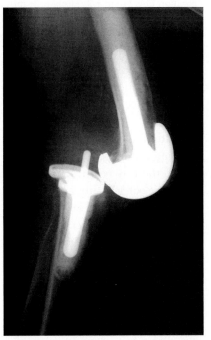

**Figure 5** Dislocation of a posterior stabilized total knee prosthesis. (Reproduced with permission from Insall JN, Clarke HD: Historic development, classification, and characteristics of knee prostheses, in Insall JN, Scott WN (eds): *Surgery of the Knee*, ed 4. Baltimore, MD, Churchill Livingstone, 2006, vol 2, pp 1464-1521.)

if they quickly regained knee flexion with aggressive postoperative rehabilitation.[20] The first episode of dis-

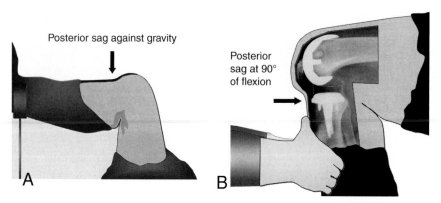

**Figure 6** **A**, Flexion instability is an underrecognized cause of poor results after a cruciate-retaining total knee arthroplasty. Patients with such instability, however, present with a typical constellation of symptoms and a typical constellation of physical findings. Here, a marked posterior sag and posterior drawer are seen. **B**, On the lateral radiograph, the femur can be subluxated posteriorly beyond the anterior lip of the tibial insert. (Reproduced with permission from Pagnano MW, Hanssen AD, Lewallen DA, Stuart MJ: Flexion instability after primary posterior cruciate retaining total knee arthroplasty. *Clin Orthop Relat Res* 1998;356:39-46.)

location should be treated with closed reduction, a trial of bracing, and avoidance of the activity that induced the dislocation. Recurrent dislocation should be addressed by inserting a thicker polyethylene insert (if there is room in the extension space) or by using a constrained condylar implant. The new construct should be checked in the figure-4 position to establish that the instability has been corrected.[20]

A study by Schwab and associates[20] showed that well-aligned and well-fixed posterior stabilized total knee replacements can also be symptomatically unstable in flexion without dislocating. Their patients with this type of instability presented with a typical constellation of symptoms and physical findings, including a sense of instability without frank giving-way, difficulty ascending and descending stairs, and recurrent knee effusions. In many cases, the knee had been aspirated on one or more occasions before the diagnosis of flexion instability was made. The patients had diffuse periretinac-

ular tenderness, especially at the site of tendinous attachments. Examination of the knee in 90° of flexion, particularly with the patient seated and his or her foot planted on the ground, was the most effective way to demonstrate the instability. Excessive anterior translation, especially if it reproduced symptoms, was indicative of flexion instability. In the study by Schwab and associates,[20] 10 of 1,370 revision total knee arthroplasties were done to address symptomatic flexion instability; 8 of these 10 cases of instability were treated successfully with revision of both the femoral and the tibial component, with an emphasis on obtaining balanced flexion and extension gaps. In this group of patients, revision total knee arthroplasty with careful attention to filling the flexion space, usually with a larger femoral component and posterior femoral modular metal augmentation, improved pain relief and stability. With the modular wedges and augments available in contemporary total knee arthroplasty revision sys-

tems, obtaining good balance of the flexion and extension spaces by upsizing the femoral component is consistently possible. The goal in these patients is to have less than 5 mm of anterior translation of the tibia when the knee is tested intraoperatively at 90° of flexion, with the patella reduced in the femoral trochlea.

Flexion instability is an underrecognized cause of poor results after a cruciate-retaining total knee arthroplasty.[7] Typically, this instability occurs in knees in which the prosthesis is well aligned, well fixed, and stable to varus-valgus stress in extension.[7] These patients report a sense of knee instability without giving way, recurrent swelling of the knee, and pain and tenderness about the knee.[7] Usually, physical examination reveals a substantial posterior sag or drawer (best seen with the patient sitting relaxed) (Figure 6), a knee effusion, and multiple areas of soft-tissue tenderness in the retinacular and pes anserinus regions.

In a previous report, two broad groups of causes for flexion instability after posterior cruciate ligament-retaining total knee arthroplasty were identified.[7] One is the creation of an excessive flexion gap by the surgical technical error of undersizing the femoral component or creating an excessive tibial slope. The other is a late failure of the posterior cruciate ligament.[21] A flat tibial liner (in the sagittal plane) offers no inherent resistance to posterior-anterior translation and may contribute to flexion instability. Similarly, posteromedial polyethylene wear functionally increases the flexion space over time and can lead to polyethylene synovitis and flexion instability.

Instability often develops early after a total knee arthroplasty in which the femoral component is undersized in the anteroposterior dimension.[7] Undersizing in the anteroposterior dimension can be detected by comparing a lateral radiograph of the knee made preoperatively with one made after the total knee arthroplasty. If the total knee component is undersized, the posterior condyles of the femur will appear overresected compared with those on the preoperative radiograph. This overresection results in a decrease in the so-called posterior offset of the femur, which contributes to flexion instability and a decrease in the ultimate range of motion of the knee replacement. This undersizing is corrected with revision to a larger femoral component coupled with the use of posterior wedges. An excessive tibial slope can also lead to the total knee prosthesis being well balanced in extension but lax in flexion. Excessive slope also places the posterior cruciate ligament at risk for iatrogenic damage, which often manifests as instability early after the total knee arthroplasty. In these cases, revision total knee arthroplasty with a focus on rebalancing the flexion-extension gaps typically is most reliably achieved by conversion to a posterior stabilized implant design.

Direct iatrogenic injury to the posterior cruciate ligament at the time of the operation may be a cause of flexion instability after a cruciate-retaining total knee arthroplasty.[7] Alternatively, indirect iatrogenic failure of the posterior cruciate ligament can occur when the flexion space is left too tight during the surgery.[7,22] This makes the knee tight in flexion, and some patients will then work aggressively to improve flexion, causing the posterior cruciate ligament to rupture. Those patients can often recall a specific event

when a pop or a snap occurred during vigorous rehabilitation, after which the patient usually had an immediate improvement in the range of motion. This may then be followed by progressive instability. Late instability is also occasionally observed when the posterior cruciate ligament is intrinsically weak secondary to age-related degenerative changes or following the reactivation of inflammatory disease.[23]

Nonsurgical treatment, including quadriceps and hamstring strengthening and local modalities to address tenderness and swelling, is useful for patients with nuisance-type symptoms, but typically it has not been successful when the patient has more marked disability attributable to the flexion instability.[7]

Surgical management with a tibial polyethylene exchange alone is one option, but poor and unpredictable results have been described previously[23] following that isolated procedure. This solution does not address the underlying imbalance between the flexion and extension gaps and is therefore not recommended.[23] A revision to a posterior stabilized total knee arthroplasty is preferred. That procedure allows identification of the cause of instability and addresses it directly so that the knee can be balanced in flexion and extension.[23] At the time of revision, a larger femoral component with posterior augments is often required, and tibial slope, if it is not perpendicular to the long axis of the tibia, should be corrected to closely equalize the flexion and extension spaces. It is important to recognize that the post and cam of the posterior stabilized implant alone is not enough to stabilize these knees, so simply switching to a posterior stabilized prosthesis without carefully balancing the gaps is un-

likely to be successful. In a previous series, 19 of 22 knees that were revised to a posterior stabilized design, with careful intraoperative attention given to balancing the flexion and extension gaps, were satisfactorily improved.[7]

## Recurvatum or Hyperextension Deformity

Recurvatum of the knee after a total knee arthroplasty is difficult to correct. The best management is prevention, and recurvatum seldom develops postoperatively in a knee that does not hyperextend at the end of the procedure, except in patients with a neuromuscular condition or rheumatoid arthritis.[24] Great care should be taken to not accept collateral ligament instability with the implant in place, as this has been associated with increased extension or even hyperextension postoperatively.[25,26]

An existing preoperative recurvatum deformity is challenging to treat. Recurvatum before total knee arthroplasty occurs in less than 1% of patients and is most typically seen in those with neuromuscular disease, particularly poliomyelitis.[25,26] In the absence of neuromuscular disease, recurvatum may be present in knees with a fixed valgus deformity associated with an isolated contracture of the iliotibial band or also associated with cruciate and collateral ligament laxity, as seen in patients with rheumatoid arthritis.[25,26] A patient with marked quadriceps weakness is at particular risk for progressive recurvatum deformity after total knee arthroplasty. Such a patient will continue to force the knee into hyperextension to help to stabilize the limb during the stance phase of gait. For that reason, total knee arthroplasty should be approached with particular caution in patients

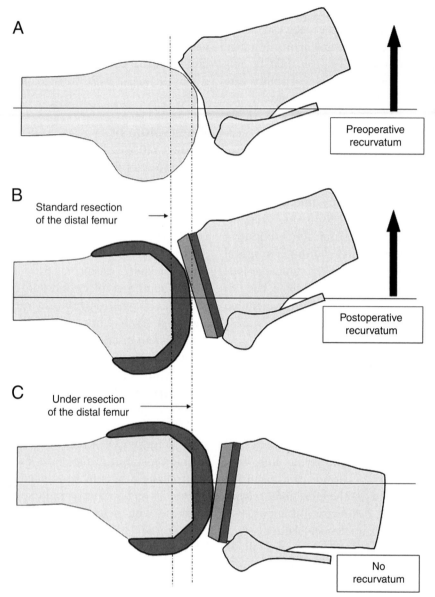

**Figure 7** In patients with marked preoperative hyperextension deformity **(A)** to limit recurvatum **(B)** it may be reasonable to underresect the distal part of the femur and to leave the knee with a slight flexion contracture at the time of the total knee arthroplasty **(C)**. (Reproduced with permission from Insall JN, Clarke HD: Historic development, classification, and characteristics of knee prostheses, in Insall JN, Scott WN (eds): *Surgery of the Knee*, ed 4. Baltimore, MD, Churchill Livingstone, 2006, vol 2, pp 1464-1521.)

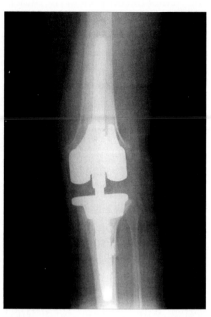

**Figure 8** In knees with marked hyperextension deformity, particularly in the face of quadriceps muscle weakness, a hinged knee design with a hyperextension stop is an implant to consider.

with preoperative recurvatum and quadriceps weakness. Two surgical solutions may be considered for such patients. One is to use a standard prosthesis with a slight under-resection of the distal part of the femur and/or distal femoral augmentation blocks, with the knee left with a slight flexion contracture at the conclusion of the procedure (Figure 7). The other solution, suggested by Krackow and Weiss,[26] is to move the femoral origins of the medial collateral ligament and lateral collateral ligament proximally and posteriorly to re-create the normal tightening action during full extension of the knee. According to Krackow and Weiss,[26] the cam action of the prosthesis with a curved insert combined with transfer of the collateral ligaments prevents recurvatum and avoids the use of a more constrained prosthesis. The principal measure that is necessary is the positioning of one of the attachments of one or both collateral ligaments on the femur to re-create the normal tightening action as full extension of the knee is achieved.

An alternative solution is to use a rotating-hinge total knee prosthesis with an extension stop. This solution is advised particularly for revision of an implant that has already failed. Giori and Lewallen[24] recommended a rotating-hinge prosthesis for knees with less than antigravity quadriceps strength. Hinged total knee arthroplasty implants without a rotating component are seldom used because of the risk of aseptic loosening. However, rotating-hinge prostheses can have a valuable role in cases such as these (Figure 8).

## Summary

Instability after total knee arthroplasty is a condition that often can be avoided by identifying patients who are at risk and by paying close attention to balancing the flexion-extension gaps at the time of the primary total knee arthroplasty. The distal femoral cut will selectively influence the extension space, the posterior femoral cut will selectively influence the extension space, and the tibial cut affects both spaces. The evaluation of an unstable total knee replacement should focus on clear identification of the etiology. In particular, all knees with pain after a total knee arthroplasty should be examined in 90° of flexion to assess for flexion instability, which has historically been underdiagnosed. Surgical treatment is largely aimed at restoring balanced flexion and extension gaps at the time of revision total knee arthroplasty. Selective use of constrained and rotating-hinge total knee arthroplasty designs is appropriate for subgroups of patients with instability.

## References

1. Yercan HS, Ait Si Selmi T, Sugun TS, Neyret P: Tibiofemoral instability in primary total knee replacement: A review. Part 1: Basic principles and classification. *Knee* 2005;12:257-266.

2. Yercan HS, Ait Si Selmi T, Sugun TS, Neyret P: Tibiofemoral instability in primary total knee replacement: A review. Part 2: Diagnosis, patient evaluation, and treatment. *Knee* 2005;12:336-340.

3. Vince KG: Why knees fail. *J Arthroplasty* 2003;18(3 suppl 1):39-44.

4. Callaghan JJ, O'Rourke MR, Saleh KJ: Why knees fail: Lessons learned. *J Arthroplasty* 2004;19(4 suppl 1):31-34.

5. Fehring TK, Valadie AL: Knee instability after total knee arthroplasty. *Clin Orthop Relat Res* 1994;299:157-162.

6. Vince KG, Abdeen A, Sugimori T: The unstable total knee arthroplasty: Causes and cures. *J Arthroplasty* 2006;21(4 suppl 1):44-49.

7. Pagnano MW, Hanssen AD, Lewallen DG, Stuart MJ: Flexion instability after primary posterior cruciate retaining total knee arthroplasty. *Clin Orthop Relat Res* 1998;356:39-46.

8. Brassard MF, Insall JN, Scuderi GR, Faris PM: Complications of total knee arthroplasty, in Scott WN (ed): *Insall & Scott Surgery of the Knee*, ed 4. Philadelphia, PA, Churchill Livingstone/Elsevier, 2006, vol 2, pp 1716-1760.

9. Laskin RS, Schob CJ: Medial capsular recession for severe varus deformities. *J Arthroplasty* 1987;2:313-316.

10. Insall JN, Binazzi R, Soudry M, Mestriner LA: Total knee arthroplasty. *Clin Orthop Relat Res* 1985;192:13-22.

11. Greenwald AS, Black JD, Matejczyk MB, Bryan RS, Insall JN, Wilde AH: Total knee replacement. *Instr Course Lect* 1981;30:301-341.

12. Laskin RS (ed): *Total Knee Replacement*. London, UK, Springer, 1991.

13. Mihalko WM, Krackow KA: Anatomic and biomechanical aspects of pie crusting posterolateral structures for valgus deformity correction in total knee arthroplasty: A cadaveric study. *J Arthroplasty* 2000;15:347-353.

14. Clarke HD, Fuchs R, Scuderi GR, Scott WN, Insall JN: Clinical results in valgus total knee arthroplasty with the "pie crust" technique of lateral soft tissue releases. *J Arthroplasty* 2005;20:1010-1014.

15. Clarke HD, Schwartz JB, Math KR, Scuderi GR: Anatomic risk of peroneal nerve injury with the "pie crust" technique for valgus release in total knee arthroplasty. *J Arthroplasty* 2004;19:40-44.

16. Easley ME, Insall JN, Scuderi GR, Bullek DD: Primary constrained condylar knee arthroplasty for the arthritic valgus knee. *Clin Orthop Relat Res* 2000;380:58-64.

17. Leopold SS, McStay C, Klafeta K, Jacobs JJ, Berger RA, Rosenberg AG: Primary repair of intraoperative disruption of the medical collateral ligament during total knee arthroplasty. *J Bone Joint Surg Am* 2001;83:86-91.

18. Krackow KA, Thomas SC, Jones LC: A new stitch for ligament-tendon fixation: Brief note. *J Bone Joint Surg Am* 1986;68:764-766.

19. Krackow KA, Thomas SC, Jones LC: Ligament-tendon fixation: Analysis of a new stitch and comparison with standard techniques. *Orthopedics* 1988;11:909-917.

20. Schwab JH, Haidukewych GJ, Hanssen AD, Jacofsky DJ, Pagnano MW: Flexion instability without dislocation after posterior stabilized total knees. *Clin Orthop Relat Res* 2005;440:96-100.

21. Waslewski GL, Marson BM, Benjamin JB: Early, incapacitating instability of posterior cruciate ligament-retaining total knee arthroplasty. *J Arthroplasty* 1998;13:763-767.

22. Pagnano MW, Cushner FD, Scott WN: Role of the posterior cruciate ligament in total knee arthroplasty. *J Am Acad Orthop Surg* 1998;6:176-187.

23. Montgomery RL, Goodman SB, Csongradi J: Late rupture of the posterior cruciate ligament after total knee replacement. *Iowa Orthop J* 1993;13:167-170.

24. Giori NJ, Lewallen DG: Total knee arthroplasty in limbs affected by poliomyelitis. *J Bone Joint Surg Am* 2002;84:1157-1161.

25. Meding JB, Keating EM, Ritter MA, Faris PM, Berend ME: Genu recurvatum in total knee replacement. *Clin Orthop Relat Res* 2003;416:64-67.

26. Krackow KA, Weiss AP: Recurvatum deformity complicating performance of total knee arthroplasty: A brief note. *J Bone Joint Surg Am* 1990;72: 268-271.

# Infected Total Knee Arthroplasty: Diagnosis and Treatment

Kevin L. Garvin, MD
Gustavo X. Cordero, MD

## Abstract

*Infection following total knee arthroplasty is a challenging complication for both the patient and the surgeon. Precautions to prevent infection include the use of prophylactic antibiotics, minimized surgical time, and meticulous surgical technique. A patient's risk factors should be thoroughly assessed and medical comorbidities should be treated before surgery.*

*When infection is suspected, prompt evaluation of the patient is necessary. The management of a TKA infection is dictated by the duration of symptoms, suspicion for infection, time since index surgery, the patient's willingness and medical capability for undergoing multiple surgeries, the bacteria's sensitivity to antibiotics, and the surgeon's ability to perform complex surgery. Acute infections are treated with aggressive débridement and parenteral antibiotics. In appropriate circumstances, chronic infections are best treated with two-stage reimplantation, which can reliably eradicate infection, relieve pain, and restore good function.*

**Instr Course Lect 2008;57:305-315.**

The rate of infection after total knee arthroplasty (TKA) has decreased primarily because of the use of prophylactic antibiotics, although other methods also have been reported to lessen the risk of infection.[1] The current infection rate is reported to be 1% to 2% for primary TKAs and 4% to 8% for revision surgeries.[2-7] Although the clinical success of TKA is greater than 90% at 10 years, the number of patients in whom infection develops is projected to increase as more TKAs are performed (Table 1).[8-11] The increased frequency of resistant pathogens further complicates the problem of prosthetic joint infections. The effective treatment of prosthetic joint infec-

tions may require the combined efforts of an orthopaedic surgeon, a plastic surgeon, and an infectious disease specialist. Successful treatment is time consuming and costly, with a delayed diagnosis leading to progressive bone loss, compromise in subsequent salvage attempts, and an increased risk of eventual limb amputation, as well as liability concerns for the surgeon.[12]

## Risk Factors

The risk of infection after TKA is associated with factors related to the surgery, the surgical technique, and the patient's medical status and history (Table 2). A patient with diabetes mellitus has an increased risk of

infection. A retrospective study of 59 TKAs performed in 40 patients with diabetes mellitus found the overall infection rate to be 7%; wound complications occurred in 12% of the TKAs.[13] Yang and associates[14] found the risk of deep joint infection to be 5.5% and wound infection to be 7.3% in a review of 109 TKAs performed in patients with diabetes. A similar increase in the rate of infection occurs in patients with rheumatoid arthritis. In a review of 12,118 primary TKAs, the infection rate at 6 years was 1.7% for patients with a diagnosis of arthrosis compared with 4.4% in those with rheumatoid arthritis ($P = 0.0001$).[2] Multiple studies have confirmed a twofold increase in the risk of developing joint infection following TKA in patients with rheumatoid arthritis.[15,16] In a retrospective review that evaluated the efficacy of eradicating TKA infection according to a study protocol, immunocompromised patients accounted for 83% of unsuccessful treatments and only 43% of successfully treated infections ($P < 0.02$).[17] The immunocompromised group included patients with rheumatoid arthritis, diabetes mellitus, chronic renal insufficiency, and a history of malignant disease. Nutritional status also has been shown to significantly impact postoperative complications. A malnourished

**Table 1**
Projected Number of TKAs and Corresponding Infections

| Year | Primary TKAs | TKA Infections* |
|------|-------------|-----------------|
| 2010 | 663,007 | 9,945 |
| 2020 | 1,520,348 | 22,805 |
| 2030 | 3,481,977 | 52,230 |

*Calculated based on an infection rate of 1.5%

**Table 2**
Risk Factors for Infection Following TKA

Diabetes mellitus
Rheumatoid arthritis
Cancer
Renal insufficiency
Urinary tract infection
Malnutrition
Chemotherapy
Steroid use
Revision surgery
Complex surgery
Organ transplant recipient
Recent dental procedure
Smoking
Obesity
Alcoholism

patient with an albumin level less than 3.5 g/dL has seven times the risk of wound complications and is twice as likely to require prolonged hospitalization following TKA compared with patients with adequate nutritional status.[18,19] A lymphocyte count less than 1,500 cells/mm³ is associated with a fivefold increase in major wound complications.[19]

In a review of 4,171 primary TKAs, patients who had prior knee surgery had a 1.4% risk of joint infection compared with 0.3% in patients without prior surgical intervention (*P* < 0.007).[16] Despite having received adequate treatment, a history of knee sepsis or osteomyelitis before TKA resulted in a 5% infection rate at 5 years in 20 patients.[20] A previous incision around the knee joint is an additional factor that predisposes the skin to necrosis and wound breakdown following TKA.[2,21-23] Prolonged surgical procedures increase the time that the wound is exposed to environmental bacteria and decrease tissue perfusion, thus straining the patient's recuperative capabilities.[1] The use of a hinged prosthesis has been shown to increase the risk of infection, with 10-year rates as high as 15%.[2,24,25] The use of a constrained prosthesis in patients with rheumatoid arthritis has resulted in an increased incidence of hematogenous infection, which is believed to result from the rigid construct producing high interface stress with subsequent pros-

thetic loosening and increased inflammation.[26-28] A thorough patient evaluation before TKA can ensure optimal medical management for immunocompromised patients and patients with risk factors predisposing them to infection, and provide adequate assessment of the postoperative risks for infection.

## Diagnosis
### Presentation
The diagnosis of infection in the acute setting is seldom difficult. Patients often report pain and have physical symptoms suggestive of infection, such as swelling, warmth, erythema, and prolonged drainage. In contrast, the symptoms that are present during an indolent infection are more subtle. Persistent pain following TKA is usually the reason that a patient seeks medical evaluation. Postoperative pain that continues for more than 3 months or the onset of wound drainage should be considered indicative of infection until proven otherwise.[29] Knee pain has been reported in more than 90% of patients with an infected knee replacement.[3,5,23,30-33] Inflammatory processes, such as infection, typically cause pain during rest and will awaken a patient from sleep. Pain from mechanical loosening is generally associated with activity. A decrease in range of motion also should raise suspicion for infection.[32] There are several signs that are rare, but their occurrence is very

specific for infection. Teller and associates[34] found that a fever greater than 99.5°F has a sensitivity of 9% and a specificity of 96% for infection. Joint warmth, erythema, and effusion also have been shown to be highly suggestive of a knee infection, showing a sensitivity of 18% and specificity of 100%.[34] With the exception of pain, the presenting signs of TKA infection lack sensitivity; therefore, a low threshold should be maintained for further evaluation. An algorithm for the evaluation and treatment of TKA infection is shown in Figure 1.

### Patient Evaluation
After completion of a thorough history and physical examination, the evaluation of a patient presenting with a suspected TKA infection involves obtaining serology, joint aspiration, and imaging studies. Erythrocyte sedimentation rate and C-reactive protein are inflammatory markers that may be elevated but correlate poorly with infection.[35] These markers have a high sensitivity and a low specificity, which makes them useful as a screen-

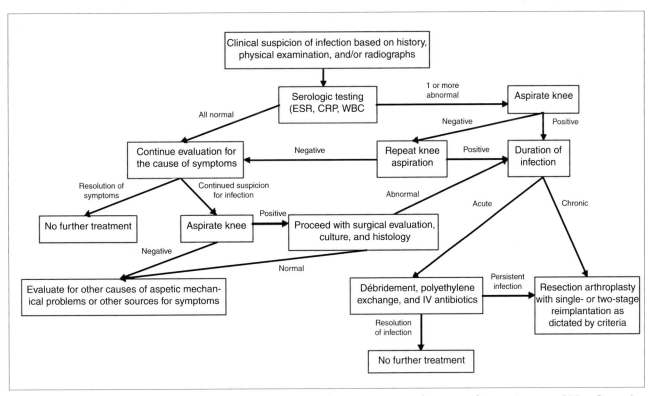

**Figure 1** Algorithm for the diagnosis and treatment of TKA infections. ESR = erythrocyte sedimentation rate; CRP = C-reactive protein; WBC = white blood cell count; IV = intravenous.

ing test for infection when elevated levels are present for more than 3 months following TKA.[1,36] A white blood cell count is usually a less helpful indicator of infection because a fulminant infection usually must be present before the count shows elevation.[5] Infection-specific markers (such as cytokines) and molecular diagnostic tests (such as polymerase chain reaction [PCR] and microarrays) are currently being evaluated for routine use in the diagnosis of prosthetic joint infection.[35-40] PCR is being used to identify the *16S* RNA gene that is conserved in nearly all species of bacteria.[36,41] PCR has a similar sensitivity and specificity as techniques currently used in microbiologic culturing; specific probes are being developed to identify bacteria that are present in orthopaedic infections.[42] The importance of PCR detection of necrotic

bacteria in the absence of clinical infection still remains to be shown.[36]

If any inflammatory marker is elevated in a patient with a suspected TKA infection, a knee aspiration should be obtained under sterile conditions. A fluoroscopically assisted aspiration may be necessary if aspiration is not successful when done on an outpatient basis. To avoid false-negative results, aspiration should be done before administering antibiotics. Bauer and associates[36] reviewed several studies to determine the range of normal leukocyte counts in joint aspirations and found a discrepancy with regard to the level at which a cell count should be considered abnormal. The lack of consistent reporting of units of volume may have further contributed to the discrepancy. The presence of more than 2,500 white

blood cells per milliliter and 60% polymorphonuclear leukocytes can indicate the presence of infection.[43] Windsor and associates[29] found an 82% correlation between the preoperative aspirate and intraoperative culture in 38 infected TKAs. The sensitivity and specificity of a preoperative aspiration in diagnosing infection has been reported as high as 100% in patients with a high clinical suspicion for infection.[35] Aspirations may be less reliable after antibiotics have been administered or when bacteria are tightly bound to the biofilm within the joint.[1] By preoperatively identifying an organism and its sensitivities, appropriate antibiotics can be used in the bone cement during revision surgery.

Imaging studies may be used as an adjunct to serology and aspiration results. Radiographs rarely show changes with acute infection. Periosteal reaction, scattered foci of osteolysis, or generalized bone resorption in the absence of implant wear are nonspecific changes that may occur in prosthetic infections.[5,36] Serial radiographs with early radiolucent lines are strongly indicative of infection. Further imaging studies are rarely needed and are generally not recommended to confirm infection. Scher and associates[44] did not recommend indium-111-labeled leukocyte scintigraphy for evaluation of a loose or painful TKA to determine the presence of infection because it has a sensitivity of 77% and a specificity of 86%. The combined use of technetium TC 99m bone scintigraphy and indium-111-labeled leukocyte scintigraphy also has limited usefulness in the diagnosis of prosthetic infection because of an unacceptably low positive predictive value and high false-positive rate.[34]

### Surgical Evaluation

On occasion, the diagnosis of prosthetic infection is only confirmed at the time of surgery or after a few days when an organism is identified by culture. The diagnosis of TKA infection can be based on a surgeon's experience. Intraoperative frozen sections have been used to assist with the diagnosis of TKA infection. A retrospective review of 33 THA and TKA revisions showed 100% sensitivity and 96% specificity in identifying infection on histopathologic slides when more than five polymorphonuclear leukocytes per high-power field in at least five distinct microscopic fields were observed.[45] In a subsequent study, the histopathologic slides of 64 THA and TKA revisions were reviewed; sensitivity decreased to 25%, and the specificity increased to 98% in identifying infection when more than

10 polymorphonuclear leukocytes were seen per high-power field in the five most cellular areas.[46] The inclusion of multiple sample sites showed an increase in sensitivity from 18.2% to 81% in the diagnosis of prosthetic infection based on frozen sections in 107 total joint revisions.[47] The use of histology in addition to microbiologic evaluation of intraoperative specimens is recommended because microbiologic evaluation alone fails to detect septic loosening in 11% of patients.[48]

Culture of intraoperative tissue and fluid has long been considered the gold standard in diagnosing a prosthetic infection. If the diagnosis is not established before surgery, cultures should be obtained before intraoperative antibiotics are administered. If preoperative antibiotics have been administered, the patient should stop taking antibiotics for 2 to 3 weeks to avoid false-negative cultures.[35,36] Samples from the joint capsule, synovial lining, intramedullary material, granulation tissue, and bone fragments should be sent for culture because it is common for 50% of cultures to be negative in patients with an indolent infection.[5,17] Fungus and acid-fast bacillus cultures also should be obtained because patients may have atypical pathogens. The diagnosis of infection has traditionally been made through isolation of one or more organisms from periprosthetic tissue or fluid samples with the use of conventional microbiologic culture techniques.[36] In a study by Segawa and associates,[17] infection was diagnosed on the basis of multiple positive intraoperative cultures and/or clinically apparent pus in the knee joint. Hanssen and associates[31] based the diagnosis of infection on the identification of the same organism in two or more intraoperative cul-

tures, acute inflammation on histopathologic evaluation, or observation of gross purulence at the time of surgery. Dietz and associates[49] obtained intraoperative cultures from 40 clean, elective orthopaedic procedures without clinical signs of infection and found 58% of the cultures to be positive. Bauer and associates[36] reported that intraoperative culture is a "tarnished" gold standard because it may be falsely negative or falsely positive as reported in multiple studies. In a study by Fehring and McAlister,[47] 4 to 6 of 86 patients with negative cultures were believed to have an underlying infection. Lonner and associates[10] considered 7 of 19 positive cultures to be the result of contamination. Hughes and associates[33] formed criteria for determining hip infection based on multiple factors to minimize the problem of interpreting false-positive cultures. They created a 29-point rating system that accounted for clinical, laboratory, radiographic, bacteriologic, intraoperative, and histopathologic findings. Fifteen or more points were considered diagnostic of deep hip infection. The trend has been to base the final clinical diagnosis on a combination of tests rather than on a single gold standard test.[36] When the culture is negative but other clinical and laboratory tests support the diagnosis of infection, the patient should be treated as having a prosthetic joint infection. The corollary also is true—if just one culture of many is positive and other tests are negative, the positive culture should be interpreted as a false positive.

### Classification

The management of TKA infections is dependent on several factors. The Tsukayama classification system and treatment protocol classifies infec-

**Table 3**
**Classification of Deep Periprosthetic Infection and Treatment**

| | Type I | Type II | Type III | Type IV |
|---|---|---|---|---|
| Timing | Positive intraoperative cultures | Early postoperative infection | Acute hematogenous infection | Late (chronic) infection |
| Definition | Two or more positive cultures at the time of surgery | Infection occurs within the first month after surgery | Hematogenous seeding of a previously well-functioning arthroplasty with acute pain and swelling | Chronic, indolent clinical course; infection present for > 1 month |
| Treatment | Appropriate antibiotics | Attempt at débridement with prosthetic salvage and appropriate intravenous antibiotics | Attempt at débridement with prosthetic salvage and appropriate intravenous antibiotics | Two-stage reimplantation with antibiotic-impregnated spacer and intravenous antibiotics |

tion by type and is based on the time of occurrence of infection from the time of the index procedure.[50] This system is practical and applicable to prosthetic infections (Table 3). Segawa and associates[17] applied this classification system to the treatment of 81 TKA infections. Of 64 infected knees treated by this protocol, 84% were ultimately free of infection and had a functional prosthesis, thus providing support for the usefulness of the classification system.

Acute infections are caused by organisms entering the joint during the index procedure, through hematogenous inoculation, or through a draining wound (Tsukayama type I to III infections).[36] In this system, the presentation of acute infection by definition must occur within 2 to 3 weeks from surgery or within 3 to 4 weeks following the onset of knee pain in a previously well-functioning knee that became hematogenously seeded. Chronic infection presents after 1 month from the index procedure or from the onset of knee pain following hematogenous inoculation (Tsukayama type IV infection). Superficial infection is confirmed at the time of débridement if no inflammation extends into the joint.[17] If extension of inflammation into the joint occurs, the infection is classified as deep.

Deep infections are generally characterized by copious drainage.[1]

## Treatment

The goals of treating an infected TKA are eradicating infection, relieving pain, and providing a stable and functional prosthesis. A successful result is considered clinical eradication of infection at 2 years, and a functional total knee prosthesis.[17] Functionality is defined as minimal pain with ambulation and no visible signs of component loosening on radiographs.

### Antibiotic Therapy Without Surgical Débridement

Antibiotic administration without surgical débridement is rarely indicated because it functions primarily to suppress infection and may select for resistant strains of organisms. A Tsukayama type I infection with two positive intraoperative cultures identified postoperatively after the prosthesis has been placed also would be considered in this category. In this situation, surgical débridement is performed during the index procedure and antibiotics are placed in the cement of the prosthetic joint. Parenteral antibiotics are generally administered for 6 weeks postoperatively to complete the treatment. Long-term suppressive therapy is another treatment

option after parenteral therapy; however, the use of this therapy should be left to the discretion of the treating surgeon after careful evaluation of the risks and benefits.

Suppression of a TKA infection with antibiotics also may be used in patients who refuse surgery or have a medical contraindication to surgery. Goulet[51] proposed using suppressive antibiotics in this group of patients if the organism is sensitive to oral antibiotics, the patient can tolerate the antibiotic therapy, the prosthesis remains well fixed, no signs of systemic sepsis exist, and the patient is compliant. A relative contraindication to suppressive antibiotics is the presence of other joints and artificial implants that may become hematogenously seeded.[7,23] Cultures should be obtained before initiating antibiotic treatment. It is difficult to differentiate between suppression and complete treatment of infection in this situation; therefore, it is recommended that oral antibiotic treatment be continued indefinitely.[51]

### Surgical Débridement With Antibiotic Therapy

Early postoperative wound complication should be treated promptly and aggressively. Superficial infections, characterized by erythema and persistent drainage, that fail to improve after a trial of simple wound manage-

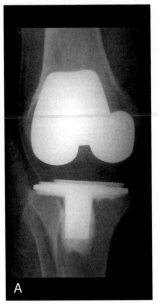 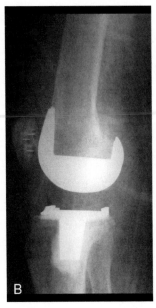 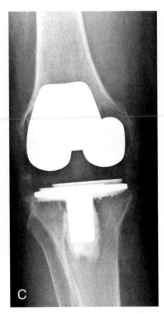 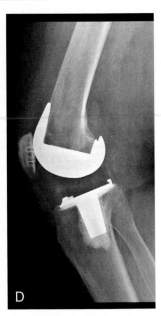

**Figure 2** Four months after TKA, a 76-year-old man reported knee pain and fever for 2 days. Prior to this episode, the patient had been ambulating with a pain-free gait. Physical examination showed a large effusion with overlying erythema. Because the patient reported a recent respiratory infection, hematogenous infection of the TKA was suspected. Preoperative aspiration and intraoperative cultures were positive for *Streptococcus pneumoniae*. AP **(A)** and lateral **(B)** postoperative radiographs after treatment with surgical débridement, polyethylene exchange, and a 6-week course of parenteral antibiotics. AP **(C)** and lateral **(D)** radiographs taken 10 years after the TKA infection show well-fixed components. The patient now ambulates well and without pain.

ment and immobilization will require surgical débridement and a 2-week course of antibiotic therapy.[7,52] Early wound problems result in the extension of superficial infection to deep tissues in one fourth of postoperative wound complications following revision TKA.[2,4] Even with early aggressive treatment, it is possible that these patients may require further extensive surgery. In a retrospective review, 13 patients with TKAs (9 primary and 4 revision TKAs) were treated with surgical débridement of inflammatory tissue that was superficial to the joint, and a 2-week course of antibiotics following persistent drainage or wound dehiscence.[17] At 7.6 years, none of the patients had a recurrence of infection or radiographic findings suggestive of infection.

Deep infection diagnosed within 2 to 3 weeks of surgery or within 3 to 4 weeks following the onset of knee pain in a previously well-functioning knee requires aggressive surgical débridement and parenteral antibiotic therapy[5,17,23,32,53,54] (Figure 2). Surgical débridement with polyethylene exchange permits greater access to the posterior region of the knee, allowing thorough débridement.[17] Débridement is required for removal of biofilm, which has been shown to sequester antibiotics and subsequently increases a bacteria's resistance to antibiotics.[55] Parenteral antibiotics should be continued for 4 to 6 weeks. Mont and associates[56] reviewed 24 acutely infected TKAs treated with serial débridement and parenteral antibiotics for 6 to 12 weeks. Patients were treated with up to three débridements if aspiration at 48 hours postoperatively showed a positive culture, persistently elevated white blood cell count in the fluid (> 100,000 cells), or more than 90% polymorpho-

nuclear leukocytes (regardless of the total count). Antibiotic treatment was extended up to 12 weeks based on findings from knee aspirates obtained at 8 weeks. At 4 years, 100% of 10 early deep postoperative infections and 71% of 14 hematogenous infections treated by this protocol did not have recurrence of infection. The success of treatment also is correlated with the causative pathogen. In a review of 31 patients with acute TKA infections treated with débridement and antibiotics, only 8% of *Staphylococcus aureus* infections were eradicated at 4 years, compared with 56% of *Staphylococcus epidermidis* infections ($P = 0.007$).[57,58]

## Reimplantation of the Prosthetic Joint

Chronic infection in TKA requires complete resection of the prosthesis and cement, aggressive débridement

of soft tissues, and 6 weeks of antibiotic therapy. This is considered the treatment of choice if the pathogen is sensitive to antibiotics, the patient is willing to undergo an extensive treatment course, and the surgeon is willing and qualified to perform the complex surgery. These revisions are complicated by difficult surgical exposure, the potential need for large implants and augmentations, bone and soft-tissue loss, and mechanical difficulties from the absence of ligaments, muscles, and tendons, with the possible need for a constrained prosthesis to help provide joint stability.[7,24,29-31] Soft-tissue defects following revision TKA can generally be successfully treated with a local muscle or musculocutaneous flap.[5,21]

Single- and two-stage reimplantations are rarely indicated without the use of antibiotic therapy. Single-stage reimplantation with antibiotics may be electively performed or occurs by default when a positive intraoperative culture is obtained after revision surgery has been done for presumed aseptic loosening. These patients should be treated with parenteral antibiotics for 6 weeks. In one study, five revision TKAs performed for presumed aseptic loosening were found to have positive intraoperative cultures.[17] Tobramycin-impregnated cement had been used at the time of revision, and parenteral antibiotics were administered for 6 weeks. The infection was successfully eradicated in all five patients at 3.9 years following the revision surgery.

Two-stage reimplantation with antibiotics has become the most common treatment method for chronic TKA infections since it was first described by Insall in 1983.[59,60] The initial treatment involves soft-tissue débridement with removal of the infected prosthesis and cement.

Parenteral antibiotics are then administered for 6 weeks while maintaining a serum bactericidal level of 1:8 or greater. Reimplantation is performed with antibiotic-impregnated cement. Antibiotic administration continues until final cultures from the reimplantation are available, but it is presumed that the joint is sterile.[23] In one study, 38 TKA infections were treated with two-stage reimplantation with a 4-year success rate of 97.4%.[29] Three TKAs were reinfected through a hematogenous source, making the infection rate after two-stage reimplantation 10.4% at 4 years. At 7.5 years, the reimplant survivorship from infection was 91%.[59] Since early success with two-stage reimplantation, only a few modifications have been made to the procedure. Perhaps the most significant change is the use of a static or dynamic cement spacer to act as an antibiotic carrier and maintain soft-tissue tension, which facilitates reimplantation and achieves a better functional recovery.

The success of eradicating infection using two-stage reimplantation has been shown to be greater than 90%.[17,54,59-61] Lonner and associates[62] found a sensitivity of 0% and a specificity of 92% with the use of preoperative aspiration to assess eradication of infection in 34 knees before two-stage reimplantation. Eight knees had recurrence of infection at 4.2 years, none of which were identified by aspiration prior to reimplantation. Hanssen and associates[31] retrospectively reviewed 89 infected TKAs treated by two-stage reimplantation with an average follow-up of 52 months. Recurrent infection developed in 28% of knees treated without antibiotic-impregnated cement and in only 4.7% of knees treated with antibiotic-impregnated cement ($P = 0.0025$).

## Antibiotic-Impregnated Spacers

The advantages of using antibiotic-impregnated cement spacers in patients undergoing two-stage reimplantation are prevention of soft-tissue contraction around the knee and local antibiotic delivery. Dynamic spacers may potentially improve functional recovery by allowing early knee motion and weight bearing. Cement should be placed within the joint space and intramedullary canal before polymerization to provide stability to the débrided ends of the joint. Postoperative knee immobilization provides additional stability. The cement spacer also maintains joint height and prevents contracture of the collateral ligaments. No correlation has been shown between the use of spacer immobilization and loss of motion following reimplantation.[48] A disadvantage to the use of a spacer is its role as a foreign material; dislodgement of the spacer may result in soft-tissue irritation and erosion of healthy bone.

The use of articulating spacers has been advocated to improve range of motion, ease reimplantation, and allow partial weight bearing before reimplantation. Freeman and associates[63] reviewed outcomes of 76 patients who had two-stage reimplantation with interim spacers. Twenty-eight patients were treated with static spacers and 48 with articulating spacers. No significant difference was found between recurrences of infection or Knee Society pain scores; however, the Knee Society functional score was significantly better in the group treated with articulating spacers (65.6) compared with those treated with static spacers (42.5). Improved function and greater soft-tissue compliance with articulating spacers without compromising rates of infection recurrence also has been

**Table 4**
**Comparison of Static and Articulating Spacers**

|  | Static Spacers (Infection Recurrence %) | Articulating Spacers (Infection Recurrence %) | P value of Infection Recurrence | Functional Outcome (Static/Articulating Spacer) | P value of Functional Outcome |
|---|---|---|---|---|---|
| Freeman et al[63] | 28 (18.4) | 48 (9.2) | 0.12 | 42.5/65.6[*] | 0.05 |
| Fehring et al[64] | 25 (12) | 30 (7) | 0.3 | 83/84[†] | 0.83 |
| Emerson et al[65] | 26 (8) | 22 (9) | 0.8 | 94/108[‡] | 0.01 |

[*]Based on Knee Society score
[†]Based on Hospital for Special Surgery rating
[‡]Based on range of motion in degrees

documented in others studies[64,65] (Table 4). Randomized studies are needed to determine if significant improvement in function occurs with articulating spacers compared with static spacers.

In addition to stabilizing the resected joint, antibiotic-impregnated spacers provide local delivery of antibiotics. High-dose antibiotics in spacers (10 to 12 g per cement spacer) are safe and indicated for the treatment of infection. High local concentrations of antibiotics cannot be achieved with the dose used in prophylactic antibiotic-impregnated cement (1 to 2 g per spacer). The decreased mechanical properties of the cement with high-dose antibiotic concentrations are not critical in the short term before definitive reimplantation. Springer and associates[6] treated 34 infected TKAs with resection arthroplasty followed by the administration of both systemic and high-dose local vancomycin and gentamicin. The antibiotic cement spacers contained an average of 10.5 g of vancomycin and 12.5 g of gentamicin per spacer. No clinical evidence of nephrotoxicity or other systemic adverse effects were observed. High-dose clindamycin, vancomycin, and tobramycin have good elution profiles from cement and do not reach breakpoint serum levels.[66] The combination of vanco-

mycin and tobramycin in acrylic bone cement has been shown to improve elution profiles by 103% and 68%, respectively, compared with individual elution profiles.[67] No statistical difference in the rate of infection recurrence has been shown when comparing the treatment of TKA infections with débridement followed by local antibiotics or systemic antibiotics; therefore, combined treatment with both local and systemic antibiotics is recommended.[22] Low-dose antibiotics (1 to 2 g per spacer) do not compromise cement strength and are indicated in high-risk patients at the time of reimplantation surgery. **(DVD 30.1)**

### Resection of the Prosthetic Joint Without Reimplantation

Resection of an infected TKA without reimplantation is indicated for patients who refuse further surgery, patients with resistant pathogens, or those who have insufficient knee tissue for a predictable reconstruction. Despite successful eradication of infection in five patients treated by resection arthroplasty, this procedure should only be considered in severely disabled patients with low functional demands.[5,7,23] Unpredictable pain relief and ambulatory functional difficulties occur after resection arthroplasty, with moderate pain, instability, and requirements

for an ambulatory assistive device in up to 80% of patients.[5,32]

### Arthrodesis

The use of arthrodesis to treat chronic TKA infection has decreased with the increased use of two-stage reimplantation, but it remains a valid option in select patients. Arthrodesis should be considered in patients with extensor mechanism loss, those with resistant bacteria that require toxic doses of antibiotics for adequate therapy, patients with inadequate bone stock or soft tissue for reimplantation, compromised collateral ligaments, and young patients with a high risk of recurrent infection.[7,23,24,68] Wasielewski and associates[54] evaluated patients with 10 chronically infected TKAs. These patients were treated with arthrodesis as the initial treatment secondary to infection with gram-negative organisms, polymicrobial infection, and highly resistant organisms, or the patients had poor soft-tissue coverage or were in poor medical condition. Follow-up at 57 months showed no infection in 100% of patients and good Knee Society scores for pain, but poor Knee Society scores for function. A two-stage arthrodesis with interval parenteral antibiotic therapy also has been shown to eradicate infection in more than 90% of infected knee arthroplasties with poor bone stock.[7,24,30] In a retrospective review of

21 patients who had knee arthrodesis with a modular titanium intramedullary nail, osseous fusion developed in 90% of patients and the overall complication rate was 38%.[69] Despite high rates of pain relief and eradication of infection, patients frequently report an inability to bend the knee, difficulty when transferring from a car or sitting in confined spaces, and an increased energy expenditure with ambulation.[23,30] Arthrodesis in the setting of TKA infections is successful in eradicating infection and alleviating pain but leaves patients with poor function.

### Above-Knee Amputation

An above-knee amputation can be a life-saving procedure in a septic patient with an infected knee prosthesis. Amputation is indicated for resistant pathogens that cannot be controlled despite multiple revisions, inadequate bone stock for subsequent reimplantation or fusion, massive tissue destruction that leaves knee function unsalvageable, or intractable pain. Patients may elect this procedure if multiple attempts at reimplantation have failed.[5,7,12]

## Summary

Infection following TKA is a challenging complication for both the patient and the surgeon. All precautions must be taken to prevent the occurrence of infection, including the use of prophylactic antibiotics, minimized surgical time, and meticulous surgical technique. A patient's risk factors should be thoroughly assessed and medical disorders should be treated before surgery.

The diagnosis of infection requires a high index of suspicion when patients present with knee pain or stiffness, fever, or wound drainage. Prompt evaluation with serology and aspiration can assist with the diagnosis of prosthetic infection, which should be based on a collective interpretation of the data obtained preoperatively and with intraoperative findings including the Gram stain, tissue histology, the presence of gross purulence, the surgeon's impression of the patient's status, and the cultures obtained from fluid and tissue. A single test is not available as the gold standard for making a reliable diagnosis. The treatment of a TKA infection is dictated by the duration of symptoms, suspicion for infection, time since index surgery, the patient's willingness and medical capability of undergoing multiple surgeries, the bacteria's sensitivity to antibiotics, and the surgeon's ability to perform complex surgery. Acute infections require aggressive débridement with parenteral antibiotics. In appropriate circumstances, chronic infections are best treated with a two-stage reimplantation, which can reliably provide eradication of infection, relief of pain, and good function. The use of antibiotic-impregnated spacers in two-stage reimplantation allows for delivery of high-dose local antibiotics, maintenance of soft tissues, and the possibility of improved function with articulating spacers.

## References

1. Gristina AG, Kolkin J: Current concepts review: Total joint replacement and sepsis. *J Bone Joint Surg Am* 1983;65:128-134.

2. Bengtson S, Knutson K: The infected knee arthroplasty: A 6-year follow-up of 357 cases. *Acta Orthop Scand* 1991; 62:301-311.

3. Grogan TJ, Dorey F, Rollins J, Amstutz HC: Deep sepsis following total knee arthroplasty: Ten-year experience at the University of California at Los Angeles Medical Center. *J Bone Joint Surg Am* 1986;68:226-234.

4. Johnson DP, Bannister GC: The outcome of infected arthroplasty of the knee. *J Bone Joint Surg Br* 1986;68: 289-291.

5. Rand JA, Bryan RS, Morrey BF, Westholm F: Management of infected total knee arthroplasty. *Clin Orthop Relat Res* 1986;205:75-85.

6. Springer BD, Lee G, Osmon D, Haidukewych GJ, Hanssen AD, Jacofsky DJ: Systemic safety of high-dose antibiotic-loaded cement spacers after resection of an infected total knee arthroplasty. *Clin Orthop Relat Res* 2004;427:47-51.

7. Windsor RE: Management of total knee arthroplasty infection. *Orthop Clin North Am* 1991;22:531-538.

8. Clayton RA, Amin AK, Gaston MS, Brenkel IJ: Five-year results of the Sigma total knee arthroplasty. *Knee* 2006;13:359-364.

9. Keating EM, Meding JB, Faris PM, Ritter MA: Long-term followup of nonmodular total knee replacements. *Clin Orthop Relat Res* 2002;404:34-39.

10. Lonner JH, Desai P, Dicesare PE, Steiner G, Zuckerman JD: The reliability of analysis of intraoperative frozen sections for identifying active infection during revision hip or knee arthroplasty. *J Bone Joint Surg Am* 1996;78:1553-1558.

11. Kurtz S, Edmund L, Zhao K, Mowat F, Ong K, Halpern M: The future burden of hip and knee revisions: U.S. projections from 2005 to 2030. *73rd Annual Meeting Proceedings.* Rosemont, IL, American Academy of Orthopaedic Surgeons, 2006.

12. Isiklar ZU, Landon GC, Tullos HS: Amputation after failed total knee arthroplasty. *Clin Orthop Relat Res* 1994; 299:173-178.

13. England SP, Stern SH, Insall JN, Windsor RE: Total knee arthroplasty in diabetes mellitus. *Clin Orthop Relat Res* 1990;260:130-134.

14. Yang K, Yeo SJ, Lee BP, Lo NN: Total knee arthroplasty in diabetic pa-

tients: A study of 109 consecutive cases. *J Arthroplasty* 2001;16:102-106.

15. Meding JB, Keating EM, Ritter MA, Faris PM, Berend ME: Long-term followup of posterior-cruciate-retaining TKR in patients with rheumatoid arthritis. *Clin Orthop Relat Res* 2004;428:146-152.

16. Wilson MG, Kelley K, Thornhill TS: Infection as a complication of total knee-replacement arthroplasty: Risk factors and treatment in sixty-seven cases. *J Bone Joint Surg Am* 1990;72:878-883.

17. Segawa H, Tsukayama DT, Kyle RF, Becker DA, Gustilo RB: Infection after total knee arthroplasty: A retrospective study of the treatment of eighty-one infections. *J Bone Joint Surg Am* 1999;81:1434-1445.

18. Del Savio GC, Zelicof SB, Wexler LM, et al: Preoperative nutritional status and outcome of elective total hip replacement. *Clin Orthop Relat Res* 1996;326:153-161.

19. Greene KA, Wilde AH, Stulberg BN: Preoperative nutritional status of total joint patients: Relationship to postoperative wound complications. *J Arthroplasty* 1991;6:321-325.

20. Lee GC, Pagnano MW, Hanssen AD: Total knee arthroplasty after prior bone or joint sepsis about the knee. *Clin Orthop Relat Res* 2002;404:226-231.

21. Bengtson S, Carlsson A, Relander M, Knutson K, Lidgren L: Treatment of the exposed knee prosthesis. *Acta Orthop Scand* 1987;58:662-665.

22. Nelson CL, Evans RP, Blaha JD, Calhoun J, Henry SL, Patzakis MJ: A comparison of gentamicin-impregnated polymethylmethacrylate bead implantation to conventional parenteral antibiotic therapy in infected total hip and knee arthroplasty. *Clin Orthop Relat Res* 1993;295:96-101.

23. Windsor RE, Bono JV: Infected total knee replacements. *J Am Acad Orthop Surg* 1994;2:44-53.

24. Hanssen AD, Trousdale RT, Osmon DR: Patient outcome with reinfec-

tion following reimplantation for the infected total knee arthroplasty. *Clin Orthop Relat Res* 1995;321:55-67.

25. Schoifet SD, Morrey BF: Treatment of infection after total knee arthroplasty by debridement with retention of the components. *J Bone Joint Surg Am* 1990;72:1383-1390.

26. Bengtson S, Blomgren G, Knutson K, Wilgren A, Lidgren L: Hematogenous infection after knee arthroplasty. *Acta Orthop Scand* 1987;58:529-534.

27. Deburge A, Aubriot JH, Genet JP: Current status of a hinge prosthesis (Guepar). *Clin Orthop Relat Res* 1979;145:91-93.

28. Willert HG, Ludwig J, Semlitsch M: Reaction of bone to methacrylate after hip arthroplasty: A long-term gross, light microscopic, and scanning electron microscopic study. *J Bone Joint Surg Am* 1974;56:1368-1382.

29. Windsor RE, Insall JN, Urs WK, Miller DV, Brause BD: Two-stage reimplantation for the salvage of total knee arthroplasty complicated by infection: Further follow-up and refinement of indications. *J Bone Joint Surg Am* 1990;72:272-278.

30. Backe HA Jr, Wolff DA, Windsor RE: Total knee replacement infection after 2-stage reimplantation: Results of subsequent 2-stage reimplantation. *Clin Orthop Relat Res* 1996;331:125-131.

31. Hanssen AD, Rand JA, Osmon DR: Treatment of the infected total knee arthroplasty with insertion of another prosthesis: The effect of antibiotic-impregnated bone cement. *Clin Orthop Relat Res* 1994;309:44-55.

32. Morrey BF, Westholm F, Schoifet S, Rand JA, Bryan RS: Long-term results of various treatment options for infected total knee arthroplasty. *Clin Orthop Relat Res* 1989;248:120-128.

33. Hughes PW, Salvati EA, Wilson PD, Blumenfeld EL: Treatment of subacute sepsis of the hip by antibiotics and joint replacement: Criteria for diagnosis with evaluation of twenty-six cases. *Clin Orthop Relat Res* 1979;141:143-157.

34. Teller RE, Christie MJ, Martin W, Nance EP, Haas DW: Sequential indium-labeled leukocyte and bone scans to diagnose prosthetic joint infection. *Clin Orthop Relat Res* 2000;373:241-247.

35. Duff GP, Lachiewicz PF, Kelley SS: Aspiration of the knee joint before revision arthroplasty. *Clin Orthop Relat Res* 1996;331:132-139.

36. Bauer TW, Parvizi J, Kobayashi N, Krebs V: Diagnosis of periprosthetic infection. *J Bone Joint Surg Am* 2006;88:869-882.

37. Gristina AG: Implant failure and the immuno-incompetent fibro-inflammatory zone. *Clin Orthop Relat Res* 1994;298:106-118.

38. Wozniak W, Wierusz-Kozlowska M, Markuszewski J, Lesniewska K, Wiktorowicz K: Monitoring of IL-6 levels in patients after total hip replacement. *Chir Narzadow Ruchu Ortop Pol* 2004;69:121-124.

39. Di Cesare PE, Chang E, Preston CF, Liu CJ: Serum interleukin-6 as a marker of periprosthetic infection following total hip and knee arthroplasty. *J Bone Joint Surg Am* 2005;87:1921-1927.

40. Deirmengian C, Lonner J, Booth RJ: White blood cell gene expression: A new approach toward the study and diagnosis of infection. *Clin Orthop Relat Res* 2005;440:38-44.

41. Tunney MM, Patrick S, Curran MD, et al: Detection of prosthetic joint biofilm infection using immunological and molecular techniques. *Methods Enzymol* 1999;310:566-576.

42. Kordelle J, Klett R, Stahl U, Hossain H, Schleicher I, Haas H: Infection diagnosis after knee-TEP-implantation. *Z Orthop Ihre Grenzgeb* 2004;142:337-343.

43. Mason JB, Fehring TK, Odum SM, Griffin WL, Nussman DS: The value of white blood cell counts before revision total knee arthroplasty. *J Arthroplasty* 2003;18:1038-1043.

44. Scher DM, Pak K, Lonner JH, Finkel JE, Zuckerman JD, DiCesare PE: The predictive value of indium-111

leukocyte scans in the diagnosis of infected total hip, knee, or resection arthroplasties. *J Arthroplasty* 2000;15: 295-300.

45. Feldman DS, Lonner JH, Desai P, Zuckerman JD: The role of intraoperative frozen sections in revision total joint arthroplasty. *J Bone Joint Surg Am* 1995;77:1807-1813.

46. Della Valle CJ, Bogner E, Desai P, et al: Analysis of frozen sections of intraoperative specimens obtained at the time of reoperation after hip or knee resection arthroplasty for the treatment of infection. *J Bone Joint Surg Am* 1999;81:684-689.

47. Fehring TK, McAlister JA Jr: Frozen histologic section as a guide to sepsis in revision joint arthroplasty. *Clin Orthop Relat Res* 1994;304:229-237.

48. Booth RE Jr, Lotke PA: The results of spacer block technique in revision of infected total knee arthroplasty. *Clin Orthop Relat Res* 1989;248:57-60.

49. Dietz FR, Koontz FP, Found EM, Marsh JL: The importance of positive bacterial cultures of specimens obtained during clean orthopaedic operations. *J Bone Joint Surg Am* 1991;73:1200-1207.

50. Tsukayama DT, Estrada R, Gustilo RB: Infection after total hip arthroplasty: A study of the treatment of one hundred and six infections. *J Bone Joint Surg Am* 1996;78:512-523.

51. Goulet JA, Pellicci PM, Brause BD, Salvati EM: Prolonged suppression of infection in total hip arthroplasty. *J Arthroplasty* 1988;3:109-116.

52. Weiss AP, Krackow KA: Persistent wound drainage after primary total knee arthroplasty. *J Arthroplasty* 1993; 8:285-289.

53. Hanssen AD: Managing the infected knee: As good as it gets. *J Arthroplasty* 2002;17:98-101.

54. Wasielewski RC, Barden RM, Rosenberg AG: Results of different surgical procedures on total knee arthroplasty infections. *J Arthroplasty* 1996;11: 931-938.

55. Ramage G, Tunney MM, Patrick S, Gorman SP, Nixon JR: Formation of Propionibacterium acnes biofilms on orthopaedic biomaterials and their susceptibility to antimicrobials. *Biomaterials* 2003;24:3221-3227.

56. Mont MA, Waldman B, Banerjee C, Pacheco IH, Hungerford DS: Multiple irrigation, debridement, and retention of components in infected total knee arthroplasty. *J Arthroplasty* 1997;12:426-433.

57. Deirmengian C, Greenbaum J, Lotke PA, Booth RE, Lonner JH: Limited success with open debridement and retention of components in the treatment of acute Staphylococcus aureus infections after total knee arthroplasty. *J Arthroplasty* 2003;18:22-26.

58. Deirmengian C, Greenbaum J, Stern J, et al: Open debridement of acute gram-positive infections after total knee arthroplasty. *Clin Orthop Relat Res* 2003;416:129-134.

59. Goldman RT, Scuderi GR, Insall JN: 2-stage reimplantation for infected total knee replacement. *Clin Orthop Relat Res* 1996;331:118-124.

60. Insall JN, Thompson FM, Brause BD: Two-stage reimplantation for the salvage of infected total knee arthroplasty. *J Bone Joint Surg Am* 1983; 65:1087-1098.

61. Haleem AA, Berry DJ, Hanssen AD: Mid-term to long-term followup of two-stage reimplantation for infected total knee arthroplasty. *Clin Orthop Relat Res* 2004;428:35-39.

62. Lonner JH, Siliski JM, Della Valle CD, DiCesare P, Lotke PA: Role of knee aspiration after resection of the infected total knee arthroplasty. *Am J Orthop* 2001;30:305-309.

63. Freeman MS, Fehring TK, Griffin WL, Mason B, Springer BD, Odum SM: Functional improvement of articulating spacers vs. static spacers in infected TKA. *AAHKS 16th Annual Meeting Final Program*. Rosemont, IL, American Association of Hip and Knee Surgeons, 2006, p 63.

64. Fehring TK, Odum S, Calton TF, Mason JB: Articulating versus static spacers in revision total knee arthroplasty for sepsis. *Clin Orthop Relat Res* 2000;380:9-16.

65. Emerson RH, Muncie M, Tarbox TR, Higgins LL: Comparison of a static with a mobile spacer in total knee infection. *Clin Orthop Relat Res* 2002; 404:132-138.

66. Adams K, Couch L, Cierny G, Calhoun J, Mader JT: In vitro and in vivo evaluation of antibiotic diffusion from antibiotic-impregnated polymethylmethacrylate beads. *Clin Orthop Relat Res* 1992;278:244-252.

67. Penner MJ, Masri BA, Duncan CP: Elution characteristics of vancomycin and tobramycin combined in acrylic bone-cement. *J Arthroplasty* 1996;11: 939-944.

68. Bengtson S, Knutson K, Lidgren L: Revision of infected knee arthroplasty. *Acta Orthop Scand* 1986;57: 489-494.

69. Arroyo JS, Garvin KL, Neff JR: Arthrodesis of the knee with a modular titanium intramedullary nail. *J Bone Joint Surg Am* 1997;79:26-35.

# Infection in Primary Total Knee Arthroplasty: Contributing Factors

*William M. Mihalko, MD, PhD
Abhijit Manaswi, MD
Thomas E. Brown, MD
*Javad Parvizi, MD
*Thomas P. Schmalzried, MD
*Khaled J. Saleh, MD

## Abstract

*Infection after a total knee arthroplasty is an infrequent but serious complication that can have devastating consequences. Infection carries a risk of significant morbidity, and the cost of treatment can be a substantial burden to the health care system. Eradication of infection can be very difficult. Prevention of infection remains the ultimate goal. Identification of host risk factors, careful patient selection, and optimization of the wound environment and the operating room remain some of the core fundamental steps that help minimize the overall incidence of infection. Although the exact role of each of these risk factors in a clinical setting can be debatable, a multidisciplinary approach incorporating all known and established methods of infection control can help to minimize the incidence of infection following total knee arthroplasty.*

**Instr Course Lect 2008;57:317-325.**

Infection following total knee arthroplasty (TKA) remains a formidable challenge for both the surgeon and the patient. The overall risk of infection after a primary TKA is approximately 1% to 2%, and the estimated cost for treatment of an infected TKA is well over $60,000.[1]

Any classification method that describes the mechanisms of bacteria entry into the joint (surgical contamination, hematogenous spread, recurrent infection, and infection from direct inoculation) or that is based on the timing of the diagnosis of infection after surgery has limited usefulness in either identifying the specific cause of infection or formulating preventive measures for periprosthetic infections.[2] Classification systems may, however, be helpful in guiding the treatment plan. The high success rate with antibiotic therapy alone that is seen for other bacterial infections has not been achieved in total joint infections. The variable and often unknown mechanism and timing of the seeding of infection, the fewer number of phagocytic cells, and limited delivery of antibiotics to the bone are among some of the unpredictable and limiting factors that lessen the effectiveness of antibiotic therapy for total joint infections. This is why surgeons should consider prevention the best treatment.

Any discussion of preventive measures must acknowledge the critical relationship between the classic epidemiologic triad of bacterium, host, and environment (Figure 1). The risk of a primary infection depends on the number, virulence, and pathogenicity

*William M. Mihalko, MD, PhD has received research or institutional support from Smith & Nephew and is a consultant or employee for Stryker Orthopaedics, Smith & Nephew, and Ethicon. Javad Parvizi, MD and Thomas Schmalzried, MD or the departments with which they are affiliated have received research or institutional support from Stryker Orthopaedics and are consultants or employees for Stryker Orthopaedics. Khaled J. Saleh, MD, MSc or the department with which he is affiliated has received research or institutional support from Stryker Orthopaedics and Smith & Nephew and is a consultant or employee for Stryker Orthopaedics and Smith & Nephew.*

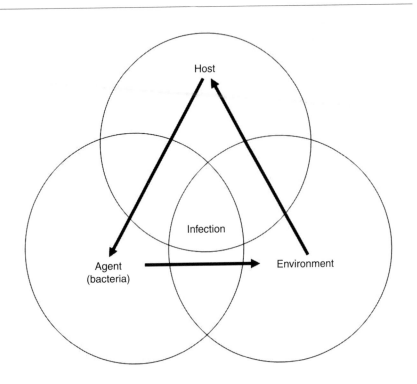

**Figure 1**    The epidemiologic triad relationship.

of the bacteria. In any given wound, the host's ability to mount an inflammatory response to fight these bacteria and the local wound conditions and environment play a major role in the acquisition of an infection. This triad can be affected by several factors, and any imbalance or breach may provide the opportunity for bacteria to initiate the infectious process. Any preventive measures must focus on optimization of the wound environment and the nutritional status of the host, as well as its ability to fight infection and minimize bacterial contamination into the wound. It requires a coordinated effort during the preoperative, surgical, and postoperative time periods.

## Patient-Dependent Factors
### Nutritional Status
Malnutrition adversely affects the following humoral and cell-mediated immune functions: neu-

trophil chemotaxis, bacterial phagocytosis, neutrophil bactericidal function, the delivery of inflammatory cells to infectious foci, and serum complement components.[3-6] A patient's nutritional status can be determined by five factors (1) anthropometric measures, such as muscle mass, triceps skin fold thickness, weight-height ratio, and arm muscle circumference; (2) measurement of cell types—a lymphocyte count less than 1,500/mm³ is associated with increased risk for infection;[5] (3) serum albumin levels—levels less than 3.5 g/dL have been shown to increase wound complications;[3,4] (4) serum transferrin levels, which have been shown to be a very sensitive indicator of wound complications;[3-5] and (5) a recent weight loss of greater than 10% of body mass. These factors also are associated with increased wound complication rates.

The nutritional index of Rainey-MacDonald is a useful screening tool. The formula is (1.2 × serum albumin) + (0.013 × serum transferrin) − 6.43. If the sum is 0 or less, the patient is nutritionally depleted and is thus at a higher risk for sepsis. Jensen and associates[6] reported that 42% of patients undergoing orthopaedic surgery were clinically or subclinically malnourished, and the number of comorbidities that patients possess have been correlated to infections and complications. A prolonged length of hospitalization before the surgical procedure or after the procedure has also been associated with an increased risk of infection.[7]

### Immunologic Status
The ability to fight infection is dictated by the body's ability to mount an inflammatory (white blood cell) and immune (antibody) response, which is aimed at destroying the infecting organism and thus preventing the spread of infection. The mechanisms involved are (1) neutrophil response, (2) humoral immunity, (3) cell-mediated immunity, and (4) the reticuloendothelial system. Any malfunction of these mechanisms, either from congenital or acquired causes, would predispose the host to infection by specific groups of opportunistic pathogens (Table 1). Abnormal neutrophils or humoral and cell-mediated immune deficiencies can lead to infections caused by encapsulated bacteria in infants and elderly subjects, *Pseudomonas* infections in heroin addicts, and *Salmonella* and pneumococcal infections in patients with sickle cell anemia. Diabetes, alcoholism, hematologic malignancy, and cytotoxic therapy are common causes for neutrophil abnormalities. Neutrophil counts less than 55% on a differential or an absolute

**Table 1**
**Conditions Predisposing to Musculoskeletal Infections**

| Congenital | Acquired |
|---|---|
| Hemophilia | Diabetes mellitus |
| Sickle cell disease | Hematologic malignancies |
| Terminal complement deficiencies | Human immunodeficiency virus |
| Leukocyte adhesion deficiency | Uremia |
| Chronic granulomatous disease | Malnutrition |
| | Radiation |
| | Advanced age |
| | Obesity |
| | Vascular disease |
| | Prior infection |
| | Organ transplantation |
| | Collagen vascular disease |

count of $< 1,500/mm^3$ are associated with an increased risk for infections with *Staphylococcus aureus*, gram-negative bacilli, *Aspergillus*, and *Candida*. Immunoglobulin and complement factors play crucial roles in humoral immunity. Splenectomy or hypogammaglobulinemia predispose to infections from encapsulated bacteria such as *Streptococcus pneumoniae*, *Haemophilus influenzae*, and *Neisseria*. Defects in the complement cascade predispose patients to *S aureus* and gram-negative bacillus, whereas hypogammaglobulinemia also predisposes to infections by rare organisms such as *Mycoplasma pneumoniae* and *Ureaplasma urealyticum*.

Cell-mediated immune response is a result of interactions between T lymphocytes and macrophages. Although primary cell-mediated immune deficiencies are rare, secondary cell-mediated immune deficiencies are common. Steroid therapy, malnutrition, lymphoma, systemic lupus erythematosus, immune deficiencies in the elderly, and autoimmune deficiency syndromes can all predispose to fungal, mycobacterial, herpes, and *Pneumocystis carinii* infections.

Anesthetic agents also have an immunosuppressive effect on the patient, and the use of regional anesthesia may result in a slightly lower incidence of infection.[8] Transfusion of homologous blood products has been associated with a slightly lower incidence of postoperative infection compared with autologous blood transfusion (less immunologic modulation of the recipient).[9,10]

## Ectopic Sources of Infection
Many ectopic sources of infection are targeted for discovery during the preoperative work-up of the patient. Dental caries, genitourinary tract infections, pulmonary infections, and skin ulcers are common potential sources for seeding of the primary TKA in the postoperative period. Psoriatic plaques adjacent to the surgical site, thin atrophic skin, abrasions/folliculitis, venous stasis ulcers, toe web-space ulcers, and infected toenails can be associated with a higher rate of infection, and these conditions must be identified and treated appropriately before surgery.[11,12] Recognition of many of these sources involves a thorough history and physical examination before the surgical procedure. The surgeon must remember that other primary care physicians may not realize the importance of these listed sources of bacterial seeding nor may the patient. Therefore, it is the surgeon's obligation to make sure all of these issues are addressed before surgery.

## Surgeon-Dependent Factors
Surgeon-dependent factors are defined as those that can be easily controlled by the surgeon. Specific routines that are developed by the surgeon can help the staff to adhere to many guidelines, which can make a difference in the incidence of postoperative infection rates.

### Skin Preparation
Although it may not be possible to completely disinfect the skin, a significant reduction in the number of pathogens can be achieved before surgery. The skin and hair can be sterilized by applying alcohol, iodine, hexachlorophene, or chlorhexidine, but it is not possible to sterilize the hair follicles and sebaceous glands, which normally harbor bacteria.[13] Hair removal or shaving should be done only in the operating room immediately before surgery to minimize bacterial contamination and reproduction.[14] Skin barriers also help reduce contamination during surgery. Plastic surgical adhesive drapes reduce wound contamination by preventing lateral migration of skin bacteria, but normal recolonization of the skin occurs within 30 minutes, and the microbial counts reach normal levels within 3 hours.[15] However, a plastic drape impregnated with slow-release iodophor effectively eliminates any bacterial colonization on the skin for up to 3 hours.[15] Application of a povidone-iodine solution to the skin margins to reduce the bacterial colony count is a useful method to reduce

contamination. Vigorous scrubbing of the skin on the surgical site should be avoided during preparation of the site because excessive scrubbing may be counterproductive; increased bacterial counts may result from the release of harbored bacteria from follicles and sebaceous glands.

Some of the same issues listed concerning skin preparation of the surgical site are applicable to hand scrubbing by operating room staff and the surgeon. The optimum antiseptic agent and the proper duration for surgical hand scrubbing are not clear, but application of povidone-iodine, waferless alchohol solutions with 0.5% chlorhexidine gluconate, foam alcohol, and a hexachlorophene foam compound all provide excellent bactericidal action.[13,16]

### Prophylactic Antibiotics

Several studies have shown the efficacy of prophylactic antibiotics in reducing infection rates after orthopaedic procedures.[17-21] During the first 24 hours after surgery, the onset of an infection depends on the number of bacteria present. In the first 2 hours, the host defense mechanisms decrease the overall number of bacteria. During the next 4 hours, the number of bacteria remains fairly constant, with the bacteria that are multiplying and those that are being killed by host defenses being approximately equal. The first 6 hours are called the golden period, after which the bacteria multiply exponentially. Antibiotics decrease bacteria multiplication and thus expand the golden period. A good prophylactic antibiotic is one that is safe, bactericidal, and effective against the most common organisms responsible for infection—S aureus, Staphylococcus epidermidis, Escherichia coli, and Proteus. The first-generation cepha-

losporins are nontoxic, inexpensive, and effective against the most potential pathogens in orthopaedic surgery.[18,20] In patients who are allergic to penicillin, vancomycin may be the antibiotic of choice. A maximal dose of antibiotic should be administered 30 to 60 minutes before the skin incision and at least 10 minutes before inflation of the tourniquet. During the procedure, antibiotics should be redosed every 4 hours or whenever the blood loss exceeds 1,000 mL.[22,23] Many studies have shown that 24 hours of antibiotic therapy is just as effective as 48 or 72 hours, and most authorities recommend a single preoperative dose of antibiotics followed by two or three postoperative doses to reduce the possibility of antimicrobial toxicity, and prevent the development of resistant organisms, and reduce unnecessary costs.[24,25]

The role of antibiotic irrigation is still not well established in orthopaedics. However, several studies have shown a decrease in colony counts in wounds and a decrease in infection rates with the use of antibiotic irrigation in general surgical procedures. Triple antibiotic irrigation (neomycin, polymyxin, and bacitracin) is currently one of the most favored solutions in use.[26]

### Local Wound Environment

Careful preoperative assessment and planning are required to minimize the risk of infection in patients with advanced vascular disease, multiple scars from previous surgeries, history of infection, and psoriatic lesions over surgical sites.[2,11,12,27,28] The relatively subcutaneous position of the knee joint makes infection more common than in more deep-seated joints.[29,30] Meticulous closure and good wound care in the postoperative period help in reducing the

overall incidence of infection. Prolonged surgical time also has an impact on the rate of deep prosthetic infection.[2,4]

The well-planned use of preexisting scars around the knee is essential to reduce skin complications; preexisting scars should be excised unless doing so compromises wound closure. All attempts should be made to use the lateralmost previous incision for surgery to optimize the blood supply to the subcutaneous flap. Gentle handling of the tissues, avoiding prolonged use of self-retaining retractors and racks, as well as avoiding the dissection of subcutaneous tissue from underlying fascia, help to prevent devitalization of the subcutaneous tissues. Faulty placement of sutures strangles the tissue and facilitates infection. Meticulous closure of the joint capsule and subcutaneous tissues to avoid dead space and careful homeostasis both help to reduce the incidence of postoperative hematoma formation.

The routine use of drains for TKA is controversial, and many recent studies suggest equivocal results. Good layered closure with epidermal apposition provides early sealing of the wound and minimizes wound drainage. Watertight closure of the joint capsule prevents deep seeding from a superficial infection or stitch abscess. The chemical composition of the suture is an important determinant of infection in the presence of wound infection and contamination. Monofilament absorbable synthetic suture is associated with a lower rate of infection than braided absorbable synthetic suture.[31,32] Although the exact effect of specific physical or chemical properties of implants for total joint arthroplasty are not known, studies suggest that specific biomaterials do influence bacterial adhesion to the implant surface. Coagulase-negative *Staphylococcus* exhibits preferential adhesion to polymers, whereas coagulase-positive *Staphylococcus* adheres more readily to metals.[33] Bacteria alter their metabolic characteristics and antibiotic susceptibility after adhering to biomaterials, and bacteria adherent to methylmethacrylate show very high resistance to antibiotics compared with those that are adherent to metals.[34]

Experimental studies and many clinical trials have found no difference in the infection rates between cementless and cemented implants.[30] Antibiotic-impregnated cement is becoming popular, as it has been shown to lower the incidence of infection, but it is associated with some inherent complications such as weakening of the bone cement, promoting the emergence of resistant organisms, and possible allergic reaction.[35-38] The availability of premixed antibiotics such as tobramycin or gentamicin has led to their use for primary TKA or in patients who have known comorbidities that may increase their chances of infection. However, only long-term studies will reveal whether this practice will decrease infection rates without increasing the rate of aseptic loosening.

## Operating Room Environment
### Clean Air
Airborne bacteria are another source of wound contamination. They are usually gram positive and originate exclusively from the staff in the operating room. Studies have shown that each individual in the operating room sheds 5,000 to 55,000 particles per minute. Interestingly, premenopausal females shed significantly fewer bacteria than males and post-

menopausal females.[39] A conventional operating room may contain as many as 10 to 15 bacteria per cubic foot and as many as 250,000 particles per cubic foot. A laminar airflow system can reduce the number of bacteria by 80%, and a personnel isolator system further reduces the airborne bacterial contamination.[40-43] Clean air is optimally provided by a combination of laminar flow, vertical airflow systems, the use of body exhaust suits, and a room air exchange turnover rate of more than 300 times per hour.[40,42] Body exhaust suits reduce the bacterial counts in the room air, and vertical laminar air-flow systems are more effective than horizontal airway systems.

Ultraviolet light has also been shown to decrease the incidence of wound contamination by reducing the number of airborne bacteria.[44] This concept, although first introduced in 1936, has not been very popular because there is a lack of conclusive evidence about its efficacy and concerns regarding personnel exposure in the operating room. However, ultraviolet light is inexpensive and may be a good alternative to laminar airflow systems.[45,46]

## Methods of Reducing Bacterial Contamination and Optimization of Wound Environment
There are several important practices that help in optimizing the wound and the operating room environment, and their application may help in lowering the incidence of infection. Some of these practices may be obvious, and others have already been mentioned. Sometimes the surgeon may be involved with other duties, such as dictation of operative notes, while these practices are occurring. As one example, it has

been shown that avoiding the use of ward beds in the operating room can affect infection incidence.[12] Similarly, restricting traffic in and out of the operating room also can decrease bacterial counts.[12] Signs and temporary barriers to staff from a main corridor can be put into place so that personnel can enter the operating room only through a substerile corridor or use a phone to call into the room. Identification of personnel who are part of the surgical scrub team and who are bacterial shedders can also aid in decreasing the risk of primary infection.[12] Other actions that may reduce the incidence of bacterial contamination include clamping off of suction tips to avoid continuous airflow through the sucker tip and increased deposition of airborne pathogens on the tip of the sucker. It may be beneficial to change sucker tips every 30 to 45 minutes to help prevent continuous airflow and pathogens on the sucker tip from occurring.[47,48] Letting the scrub technician know that use of a water basin to carry instruments to and from the surgical field is a technique that should be avoided also can help to decrease contamination.[49] The use of impervious gowns and drapes over cloth also has been shown to be helpful.[50] Pulsatile lavage can remove as much as 99% of wound contaminants; this procedure can be added to the surgical regimen to aid in decreasing contamination of the surgical site.[51]

There are also multiple issues that the anesthesiologist can address during the operation that can decrease the risk of surgical site infection. One of these is to ensure the proper timing of prophylactic antibiotic administration. This task is usually the responsibility of the anesthesia team, and they should be educated as to its importance.

The monitoring of the patient's temperature is a concern most orthopaedic surgeons are aware of during trauma procedures but not as focused on during elective procedures. A relationship between patient temperature and risk of surgical site infection in an elective setting has been determined, however. Hypothermia has been shown to cause vasoconstriction; this further reduces the blood supply to the surgical site and makes it more susceptible to infection.[52,53]

Diabetes is a relatively common comorbidity in many patients. Relatively well-controlled diabetes with blood glucose less than 200 mg/dL during the surgical procedure to decrease risk of surgical site infection has been reported.[54]

The number of personnel from the anesthesia team moving in and out of the operating room also should be kept to a minimum. Explaining the importance of this to the anesthesia team as well as posting reminders and barriers as previously noted can be helpful. Ultimately, it takes a multidisciplinary approach to keep all related services involved in patient care in agreement concerning all of these risk factors to minimize the incidence of surgical-site infection in primary TKA.[52-54]

## Postoperative Period

It is important to watch for all risk factors and address the postoperative factors that may contribute to infection. A rapidly expanding hematoma may require timely evacuation and débridement because the pressure on the surrounding tissues may devitalize the adjacent tissues and reduce the influx of antibiotic in the surgical site.[55] A hematoma also provides a prime milieu for bacterial proliferation. Superficial skin necrosis should be treated aggressively, and serous wound drainage should be treated initially with a compressive dressing and prophylactic antibiotic coverage; however, any persistent drainage should be treated in the operating room with open irrigation and débridement.

## Prevention in the Early Postoperative Period: Hematogenous Infection

In the early postoperative period, the hematoma around the surgical wound is susceptible to hematogenous seeding with any episode of bacteremia.[56-58] All intravenous lines and indwelling catheters should be removed as soon as possible. It is advisable to maintain oral antibiotic coverage for any indwelling catheter in the urinary tract. Although it is difficult to document a bacteremic event preceding an infection, it is important to treat remote infections of the urinary tract, respiratory tract, skin, and overt dental infection to prevent any hematogenous seeding.[57,58]

The common risk factors that may also predispose to such infections are rheumatoid arthritis and the use of structural bone grafts.[56,57] The total joint implants are surrounded by an immunocompromised fibroinflammatory zone, wherein the particle debris stimulates the macrophages, leading to superoxide radicals, and a self-perpetuating cytokine-mediated tissue damage cascade is created. This causes a progressive enlargement of the immunocompromised fibroinflammatory zone.[33,59] This condition typically leads to osteolysis, but hematogenous seeding of this immunocompromized zone can occur.[59] Antimicrobial prophylaxis is generally recommended for high-risk patients with a prosthetic joint any time they have a dental procedure or an invasive procedure such as endoscopy, colonoscopy, or cystoscopy, although there is conflicting evidence in the literature and no definitive guidelines are universally agreed on.

## The Future: Self-Protective Smart Implants

In recent years, efforts have been made to coat the surface of the implant with antibiotics or a material with antibacterial properties, such as silver. The antibiotic in the coating or the material on the surface of the implant is believed to prevent bacterial attachment (biofilm formation) and subsequent infection. So far, all the described technologies involve elution of the antibiotics. Biodegradable polymers such as polylactic acid and polyglycolic acid (singly or in combination), collagen, and other carriers have been used to deliver antibiotics. The intrinsic degradation rate of the polymer determines the release kinetics of the antibiotic. Several reports of different antibiotics/polymer systems have recently been described with release rates sufficient to provide prophylaxis against periprosthetic infection. None of these technologies are available for clinical use. One form of coating that contains gentamicin is currently being evaluated in clinical research in Europe. In other technologies, antibiotics are impregnated into a bioactive surface either through formation of a thin, soluble gel film or passive diffusion into other compatible materials such as collagen matrices. Materials such as bioactive glass containing vancomycin have been used to form such a soluble gel film. Using a salt-leaching technique, the thin film acquires a defined porosity that determines the antibiotic release rate.

The thin film/biomaterial interface is less fragile than the biodegradable polymer/metal interface.

Current advances in biomaterials and biotechnology have introduced a new notion of implants with "smart" surfaces. These implants are usually designed to take advantage of molecular knowledge and target specific cellular responses at the cell and molecular level. Advanced surface modifications involve nanoscale chemistry and biomaterial design. Smart implant technology is superior to surface coatings by providing a permanent surface integral to the implant. Using such designs allows for a self-protective surface capable of detecting and responding to infecting organisms, possibly over the life of the implant. In contrast to surface coatings that are susceptible to degradation in the host environment, a smart implant surface is permanent through the application of nanotechnology and has bactericidal effects, without modification or loss of the antibiotic. To create such bactericidal surfaces, organosilane covalent bonds have been used to tether antibiotics and other biofactors to the surface of the implant. During preliminary animal experiments, development of periprosthetic infection was prevented by the organosilane-modified titanium surface. This technology holds great promise for prevention and treatment of periprosthetic infection.

## Summary

All of the variables presented should be carefully considered by the surgeon to optimally decrease infection risk. Obviously, not all topics will be relevant to all patients, but the operating room environment is one all surgeons should be considering to safeguard their patients from acquiring an infected primary TKA. Multi-

ple variables are involved to optimize patient, operating room, and care pathways to minimize the risk of a primary TKA infection.

## References

1. Hebert CK, Williams RE, Levy RS, Barrack RL: Cost of treating an infected total knee replacement. *Clin Orthop Relat Res* 1996;331:140-145.

2. Fitzgerald RH Jr, Nolan DR, Ilstrup DM, et al: Deep wound sepsis following total hip arthroplasty. *J Bone Joint Surg Am* 1977;59:847-855.

3. Dreblow DM, Anderson CF, Moxness K: Nutritional assessment of orthopedic patients. *Mayo Clin Proc* 1981;56:51-54.

4. Gherini S, Vaughn BK, Lombardini AV Jr, Mallory TH: Delayed wound healing and nutritional deficiencies after total hip arthroplasties. *Clin Orthop Relat Res* 1993;293:188-195.

5. Greene KA, Wilde AH, Stulberg BN: Preoperative nutritional status of total joint patients: Relationships to postoperative complications. *J Arthroplasty* 1991;6:321-325.

6. Jensen JE, Jensen TJ, Smith TK, et al: Nutrition in orthopedic surgery. *J Bone Joint Surg Am* 1982;64:1263-1272.

7. Cruse PJ, Foord R: A five year prospective study of 23,649 surgical wounds. *Arch Surg* 1973;107:206-210.

8. Park SK, Brody JI, Wallace HA, et al: Immunosuppressive effect of surgery. *Lancet* 1971;1:53-55.

9. Fernandez MC, Gottlieb M, Monitove JE: Blood transfusion and postoperative infection in orthopedic surgery. *Transfusion* 1992;32:318-322.

10. Murphy P, Heal JM, Blumberg N: Infection or suspected infection after hip replacement surgery with autologous or homologous blood transfusions. *Transfusion* 1991;31:212-217.

11. Maderazo EG, Judson S, Pasternak H: Late infections of total joint prosthesis: A review and recommendations for prevention. *Clin Orthop Relat Res* 1988;229:131-142.

12. Nelson CL: Prevention of sepsis. *Clin Orthop Relat Res* 1987;222:66-72.

13. Gilliam DL, Nelson CL: Comparison of a one-step iodophor skin preparation versus traditional preparation in total joint surgery. *Clin Orthop Relat Res* 1990;250:258-260.

14. Mishriki SF, Law DJW, Jeffery PJ: Factors affecting the incidence of postoperative wound infection. *J Hosp Infect* 1990;16:223-230.

15. Johnston DH, Fairclough JA, Brown J, Hill RA: The rate of skin colonization after surgical preparation: Four methods compared. *Br J Surg* 1987;74:64.

16. Eitzen HE, Ritter MA, French ML, Gioe TJ: A microbiological in-use comparison of surgical hand-washing agents. *J Bone Joint Surg Am* 1979;61:403-406.

17. Doyon F, Evrard J, Mazas F: An assessment of published trials on antibiotic prophylaxis in orthopedic surgery. *Fr J Orthop Surg* 1989;3:49.

18. Gross PA, Barrett TL, Dellinger EP, et al: Quality standard for antimicrobial prophylaxis in surgical procedures. *Clin Infect Dis* 1994;18:421.

19. Heath AF: Antimicrobial prophylaxis for arthroplasty and total joint replacement: Discussion and review of published clinical trials. *Pharmacotherapy* 1991;11:157-163.

20. Hill C, Flamant R, Mazas F, Evrard J: Prophylactic cefazolin versus placebo in total hip replacement: Report of a multicentre double-blind randomised trial. *Lancet* 1981;1:795-796.

21. Nelson CL: The prevention of infection in total joint replacement surgery. *Rev Infect Dis* 1987;9:613-618.

22. Bannister GC, Auchincloss JM, Johnson DP, Newman JH: The timing of tourniquet application in relation to prophylactic antibiotic administration. *J Bone Joint Surg Br* 1988;70:322-324.

23. Burke JF: The effective period of preventive antibiotic action in experi-

mental incisions and dermal lesions. *Surgery* 1961;50:161-168.

24. Heydemann JS, Nelson CL: Short term preventative antibiotics. *Clin Orthop Relat Res* 1986;205:184-187.

25. Maderazo EG, Judson S, Pasternak H: Late infections of total joint prosthesis: A review and recommendations for prevention. *Clin Orthop Relat Res* 1988;229:131-142.

26. Benjamin JB, Volz RG: Efficacy of a topical antibiotic irrigant in decreasing or eliminating bacterial contamination in surgical wounds. *Clin Orthop Relat Res* 1984;184:114-117.

27. Beyer CA, Hanssen TG, Lewallen DG: Pittelkow MR: Primary total knee arthroplasty in patients with psoriasis. *J Bone Joint Surg Br* 1991;73:258-259.

28. Menon TJ, Wroblewski BM: Charnley low friction arthroplasty in patients with psoriasis. *Clin Orthop Relat Res* 1983;176:127-128.

29. Glynn MK, Sheehan JM: An analysis of the causes of deep infection after hip and knee arthroplasties. *Clin Orthop Relat Res* 1983;178:202-206.

30. Hanssen AD, Fitzgerald RH Jr: Infection following cemented and uncemented primary total hip and knee arthroplasty. *American Academy of Orthopaedic Surgeons Fifty-Eighth Annual Meeting Final Program.* Park Ridge, IL, American Academy of Orthopaedic Surgeons, 1991, p 153.

31. Chu CC, Williams DF: Effects of physical configuration and chemical structure of suture material on bacterial adhesion: A possible link to wound infection. *Am J Surg* 1984;147:197-204.

32. Katz S, Izhar M, Mirelman D: Bacterial adherence to surgical sutures: A possible factor in suture induced infection. *Ann Surg* 1981;194:35-41.

33. Gristina AG: Biomaterial centered infections: Microbial adhesion versus tissue intergration. *Science* 1987;237:1588-1595.

34. Naylor PT, Myrvik QN, Gristina A: Antibiotic resistance of biomaterial

adherent coagulase: Negative staphylococci. *Clin Orthop Relat Res* 1990;261:126-133.

35. Josefsson G, Gudmundsson G, Kolmert L, Wijkstriium S: Prophylaxis with systemic antibiotics versus gentamycin bone cement in total hip arthroplasty: A five year survey of 1688 hips. *Clin Orthop Relat Res* 1990;253:173-178.

36. Lynch M, Esser MP, Shelley P, Wroblewski BM: Deep infection in Charnley low friction arthroplasty: Comparision of plain and gentamycin loaded cement. *J Bone Joint Surg Br* 1987;69:355-360.

37. McQueen M, Littlejohn A, Hughes SPF: A comparision of systemic cefuroxime and cefuroxime loaded bone cement in the prevention of early infection after total joint replacement. *Int Orthop* 1987;11:241-243.

38. Robertsson O, Knutson K, Lewold S, et al: The Swedish knee arthroplasty register 1975–1997: An update with special emphasis of 41,223 knees operated on in 1988–1997. *Acta Orthop Scand* 2001;72:503-513.

39. Davies RR, Noble WC: Dispersal of bacteria on desquamated skin. *Lancet* 1962;2:1295-1297.

40. Laurence M: Annotation: Ultra-clean air. *J Bone Joint Surg Br* 1983;65:375-377.

41. Howorth FH: Prevention of airborne infection during surgery. *Lancet* 1985;1:386-388.

42. Lidwell OM, Lowberry EJL, Whyte W, et al: Effect of ultra-clean air in operating rooms on deep sepsis in the joint after total hip or total knee replacement: A randomized study. *Br Med J (Clin Res Ed)* 1982;285:10-14.

43. Salvati EA, Robinson RP, Zeon SM, et al: Infection rates after 3175 total hip and total knee replacements with and without a horizontal unidirectional filtered air flow systems. *J Bone Joint Surg Am* 1982;64:525-535.

44. National Research Council: Report of an ad hoc committee of the committee of trauma, Division of Medical Sciences. Postoperative wound infec-

tions: The influence of ultraviolet radiation of the operating room and various other factors. *Ann Surg* 1964;160:1.

45. Berg M, Bergman BR, Hoborn J: Ultraviolet radiation compared to an ultraclean air enclosure: Comparison of air bacterial counts in operating rooms. *J Bone Joint Surg Br* 1991;73:811-815.

46. Lowell JD, Kundsin RB, Schwartz CM, Pozin D: Ultraviolet radiation and reduction of deep wound infection following hip and knee arthroplasty. *Ann NY Acad Sci* 1980;353:285-293.

47. Greenough CG: An investigation into contamination of operative suction. *J Bone Joint Surg Br* 1986;68:151-153.

48. Meals RA, Knoke L: The surgical suction tip: A contaminated instrument. *J Bone Joint Surg Am* 1978;60:409-410.

49. Baird RA, Nickle FR, Thrupp LD, Rucker S, Hawkins B: Splash basin contamination in orthopedic surgery. *Clin Orthop Relat Res* 1984;187:129-133.

50. Whyte W, Bailey PV, Hamblen DL, Fisher WD, Kelly IG: A bacteriologically occlusive clothing system for use in the operating room. *J Bone Joint Surg Br* 1983;65:502-506.

51. Hamer ML, Robson MC, Kreizek TJ, Southwick WO: Quantitative bacterial analysis of comparative wound irrigations. *Ann Surg* 1975;181:819-822.

52. Dellinger EP: Roles of temperature and oxygenation in prevention of surgical site infection. *Surg Infect (Larchmt)* 2006;7(Suppl 3):S27-S32.

53. Mauermann WJ, Nemergut EC: The anesthesiologist's role in the prevention of surgical site infections. *Anesthesiology* 2006;105:413-421.

54. Sessler DI: Non-pharmacologic prevention of surgical wound infection. *Anesthesiol Clin.* 2006;24:279-297.

55. Nelson CL, Bergfeld JA, Schwartz J, Kolczun M: Antibiotics in human hematoma and wound fluid. *Clin Orthop Relat Res* 1975;108:138-144.

56. Ahlberg A, Carlsson AS, Lindberg L: Hematogenous infection in total joint replacement. *Clin Orthop Relat Res* 1978;137:69-75.

57. Ainscow DAP, Denham RA: The risk of hematogenous infection in total joint replacements. *J Bone Joint Surg Br* 1994;66:580-582.

58. Maniloff G, Greenwald R, Laskin R, Singer C: Delayed post bacteremic prosthetic joint infection. *Clin Orthop Relat Res* 1987;223:194-197.

59. Gristina AG: Implant failure and immuno-incompetent fibro-inflammatory zone. *Clin Orthop Relat Res* 1994;298:106-118.

# Diagnosis and Treatment of the Infected Primary Total Knee Arthroplasty

*William M. Mihalko, MD, PhD
Abhijit Manaswi, MD, MS, FRCS
Quanjun Cui, MD, MS
*Javad Parvizi, MD
*Thomas P. Schmalzried, MD
*Khaled J. Saleh, MD

## Abstract

*A diagnosis of infection in the painful primary total knee replacement is not always a straightforward endeavor. No single, fail-proof diagnostic study for infection exists. Often multiple diagnostic studies that include imaging, blood work, and joint aspiration as well as history and physical examination need to be considered. Infection may not always be determined before surgery, in which case intraoperative frozen sections can help to confirm infection or refute a negative workup. Treatment options vary, depending on the timing in the infection process and the source of the infection and may consist of simpler treatment courses, such as irrigation, débridement, and polyethylene exchange, to more complex treatment courses, such as two-stage revision with an antibiotic spacer to fusion or amputation. The orthopaedic surgeon uses an essential armamentarium of diagnostic and treatment options to determine the presence of infection and tailor the individual treatment of each patient.*

**Instr Course Lect 2008;57:327-339.**

Deep infection after total knee arthroplasty (TKA) represents a significant treatment challenge with the possibility of disastrous consequences. The goal of treatment of a periprosthetic TKA infection is the restoration of a painless, well-functioning joint, with eradication of the infection. The outcome, however, is not always favorable, and the end result could be an arthrodesis, amputation, or a pseudarthrosis. In some instances, the only realistic option is to suppress the infection with continued oral antibiotics while simultaneously retaining the prosthesis. Two-stage resection arthroplasty remains the standard treatment of chronic periprosthetic infections in North America. For each patient, the treatment course should be tailored to the overall prognosis, associated comorbidities, adequacy of local bone stock, availability of soft-tissue coverage (the integrity of the extensor mechanism) for revision surgery, and the functional expectations and wishes of the patient. Preoperative planning is the key to successful outcome, and all attempts should be made to acquire pertinent information before surgery (the prosthesis type, manufacturer, date of placement, revisions, resections, possible surgical complications), as well as any previous diagnostic studies and systemic antibiotic treatment.

## History and Physical Examination

Diagnosis should start with a careful history to identify host factors that may predispose to infection or

*William M. Mihalko, MD, PhD or the department with which he is affiliated, has received research or institutional support from Smith & Nephew and is a consultant or employee for Stryker Orthopaedics, Smith & Nephew, and Ethicon. Javad Parvizi, MD and Thomas Schmalzried, MD or the departments with which they are affiliated have received research or institutional support from Stryker Orthopaedics and are consultants or employees for Stryker Orthopaedics. Khaled J. Saleh, MD, MSc or the department with which he is affiliated has received research or institutional support from Stryker Orthopaedics and Smith & Nephew and is a consultant or employee for Stryker Orthopaedics and Smith and Nephew.

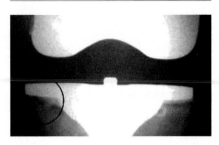

**Figure 1**  AP radiograph shows scalloping under the tibial baseplate and periosteal reaction at the superior aspect of the anterior flange of the femoral component.

complications in wound healing. The physical examination should focus on knee effusion, warmth, erythema, tenderness, painful range of motion, and the presence of nighttime pain, as well as a history of drainage or hematoma after the index procedure. There is usually a complete absence of constitutional symptoms or systemic signs and symptoms of infection.

Because pain is a strong associated factor, infection should be considered in any persistently painful TKA or with the acute onset of pain in a previously well-functioning TKA.[1] The timing of infection can have a significant impact on outcome and is therefore used to guide treatment decisions.

In a patient with a well-functioning, pain-free TKA who experiences sudden onset of acute symptoms, a detailed history should be obtained to determine the presence of hematogenous sources of infection (upper respiratory infection, urinary tract infection, dental procedures, or abscesses). Patients with diabetes should have a complete physical examination of their feet to rule out foot ulcers or secondary skin sources of infection. The history and physical examination remains the initial cornerstone of the workup in

patients with a painful TKA and thus starts the process of determining an infected primary TKA.

## Radiologic Studies
Radiographs must be carefully studied for loosening of the implant, scalloping or bone resorption at the bone-cement interface, cyst formation, periosteal new bone formation, periprosthetic bone resorption, and ectopic bone formation[2-4] (Figure 1). Progressive prosthetic loosening is the most consistent radiographic finding. (Bone destruction is not seen on plain films until an infection has been present for 10 to 21 days, and a lytic lesion is seen only when 30% to 50% of the bony matrix has been destroyed or lost).[2,3] Conventional tomograms and arthrograms have a very limited role in the diagnosis of TKA infection and are largely of historic interest.

## Laboratory Studies
The complete blood count, including the differential count, the erythrocyte sedimentation rate (ESR), and C-reactive protein (CRP) level are obtained during the initial assessment. Because levels can be normal or low in the presence of an infection, the white blood cell (WBC) count is not a reliable indicator of infection; however, the differential usually shows an increase in neutrophils.[1,5] The ESR is elevated in the presence of infection, with peak elevations seen at 3 to 5 days after the onset of infection. Values generally return to normal levels, with eradication of the infection, after 3 weeks of treatment.[6] The ESR is unreliable, however, in patients undergoing steroid therapy or who have anemia/polycythemia, sickle cell disease, or when symptoms are present for less than 48 hours.[6,7] CRP is an acute phase protein that is synthe-

sized in the liver in response to infection. The CRP level rises within 6 hours of the onset of infection, reaching its peak in 2 days after infection and returning to normal levels within 1 week of adequate treatment/eradication.[6,7] The CRP level may return to normal in patients with aseptic loosening but remains elevated in those with septic loosening.[8]

Aspirate from the knee joint should be evaluated for synovial fluid, culture, and antibiotic sensitivity. In patients with septic arthritis, the WBC count is typically greater than $80 \times 10^3$ cells/$\mu$L with more than 75% consisting of neutrophils. In a TKA, however, a leukocyte count of greater than $1.7 \times 10^3$ cells/$\mu$L in the aspirate or a predominance of polymorphonuclear leukocytes of greater than 65% is both sensitive (94% to 97%) and specific (88% to 98%) and is more so when there is clinical evidence of infection.[9-11] When both the CRP and ESR levels are elevated, the probability that a positive aspirate will confirm an infection is approximately 90%.[10] Recent studies suggest that patients with a prosthetic implant having a leukocyte count of less than 2,000/$\mu$L and a differential of less than 50% neutrophils in synovial fluid have a 98% predictive value for the absence of infection.[10] Parvizi and associates[11] also showed that joint aspirations with a cell count of 1,700 cells/$\mu$L or more is predictive of joint infection. This level is far lower than the historic values for septic arthritis of the knee.

In addition to a Gram stain, culture and sensitivity results should be obtained, and, when possible, a bacteriologic culture—the historic gold standard test for infection (however, the bacteriologic culture is positive in approximately only one third of the studies).[12,13] Cultures of superficial wounds or sinus tracts are unreliable and misleading. The preferred specimens are joint aspirate, deep wound biopsy, or bone biopsy (femoral/tibial canal). The tissue culture specimens should be placed in small $CO_2$-filled vacuum containers to reduce exposure to air. For fungal infections, a 10% potassium hydroxide wet mount preparation is helpful for detecting fungal morphology.

The presence of acute inflammation in periprosthetic soft-tissue specimens is specific for infection. Acute inflammation has been described by classifying the number of neutrophils from 1 to 5, 5 to 10, or greater than 10 per 40x high-power field (5 polymorphonuclear leukocytes per high-power field has a sensitivity of 82% to 84% and a specificity of 93% to 96%).[14-17] It is further suggested that multiple samples from suspicious regions be obtained, with areas having the most florid inflammatory cells assessed and at least 10 high-power fields examined to obtain an average count.[15-17]

In a recent study, Parvizi and associates[11] outlined the diagnostic standards for periprosthetic infection as the fulfillment of three of five criteria: (1) a CRP level of greater than 1 mg/dL, (2) an ESR of greater than 30 mm/h, (3) a positive joint aspiration culture, (4) a purulent intraoperative tissue appearance, and (5) a positive intraoperative culture and a defined aseptic failure because prosthetic failure did not meet the criteria for infection described earlier.

## Radionuclide Studies

### Technetium Tc 99m Phosphate
After plain radiographs, this radiographic scan is the one most commonly used for assessing a painful TKA. The uptake of technetium phosphate is primarily a result of os-

teoblastic activity and regional blood flow. After the intravenous injection, the technetium phosphate is distributed to the extracellular compartment, and up to 50% of bony uptake occurs within 1 hour; the kidneys excrete the remaining radioisotope. A three-phase study is then performed, and images are taken in the flow phase, which shows blood flow, similar to a radionuclide angiogram; the immediate or equilibrium phase which shows relative vascular flow and distribution of the radioisotope in the extracellular space; and the delayed phase, which usually occurs 2 to 4 hours after the injection when most of the isotope has been excreted. The three-phase study shows osteoblastic activity and indicates osteomyelitis, tumors, degenerative joint disease, trauma, and postoperative changes. This study can detect osteomyelitis within 48 hours of onset. The sensitivity and positive predictive value is approximately 30% to 38%, and the specificity and negative predictive value is 80% to 89%.[18-20]

### Technetium Tc 99m Sulfur Colloid
A combined study consisting of WBC imaging and complementary bone marrow imaging performed with technetium Tc 99m ([99m]Tc) sulfur colloid is approximately 90% accurate and is especially useful for diagnosing osteomyelitis in situations characterized by altered marrow distribution. The following are limitations in using this study: (1) marrow imaging is not useful when there is no labeled WBC activity in the region of interest; (2) the sulfur colloid image becomes photopenic within approximately 1 week after onset of infection, thus the study is not positive in the acute setting; (3) labeled WBC can accumulate in lymph nodes and can lead to

false image interpretation; and (4) [99m]Tc–sulfur colloid that is improperly prepared or that is more than approximately 2 hours old degrades image quality.

The combined test is used because both WBCs and sulfur colloid accumulate in marrow regardless of the marrow's location, whereas WBCs accumulate during infection, but sulfur colloid does not. The distribution of activity on WBC and marrow images in healthy individuals resembles that in persons with underlying abnormalities; thus, the images are spatially congruent. The exception is osteomyelitis, which stimulates uptake of WBCs and suppresses uptake of sulfur colloid. The WBC-marrow study is positive for infection when activity on the WBC image is seen without corresponding activity on the marrow image; in other words, the images are spatially incongruent. When any other pattern is present, the study is negative for infection. The reported accuracy of combined WBC-marrow imaging has historically been excellent, ranging from 88% to 98%.[21-23]

### Gallium 67 Citrate
This scan is useful for localizing inflammatory lesions. It has direct leukocyte uptake, protein-bound tissue uptake, and perhaps direct bacterial uptake. The specificity of the gallium scan alone is poor but is highly useful in conjunction with [99m]Tc scanning. In regions of acute inflammation, gallium uptake exceeds [99m]Tc uptake, and the sensitivity and specificity of the combined scan are approximately 70% to 90%. A disadvantage of gallium imaging is the slow clearance from the body (up to 72 hours).[19]

### Indium-111-Labeled Leukocytes
In this scan, 50 mL of the patient's blood is obtained, and leukocytes are

separated from the other blood elements and then labeled with indium-111. These labeled leukocytes are then reinjected into the patient, and scans are obtained 24 hours later. The scan is considered positive when the focal accumulation of activity exceeds adjacent normal bony activities. This scan is helpful in the diagnosis of acute infection, but its usefulness in diagnosing chronic infection is doubtful because the inflammatory response is lymphocytic; therefore, the scan result is a cold (negative) scan. The indium-111 scan is sensitive but not specific. Although a negative scan can rule out osteomyelitis, the scan is not helpful for differentiating aseptic from septic loosening in a painful TKA.[24,25] Scher and associates[25] reported that indium-111 leukocyte scans only had 77% sensitivity, 86% specificity, 54% positive predictive value, and 95% negative predictive value when they were used to diagnose infection in 143 patients, 17% of whom had undergone surgery because of a painful joint implant.

### Indium-111-Labeled Monoclonal Immunoglobulin (LeukoScan)

This scan is an alternative to the indium-labeled leukocyte scan. It avoids phlebotomy and radiation to WBCs (risk of malignant transformation). Although still experimental, LeukoScan has better sensitivity, specificity, and diagnostic accuracy than other indium and $^{99m}Tc$ scans and is considered a better diagnostic tool in detecting chronic infection (osteomyelitis) and human immunodeficiency virus.[26,27]

## MRI Scan

With MRI, the classic findings of osteomyelitis are a decrease in the normally high marrow signal on T1-weighted images and a normal or an increased signal on T2-weighted images. The MRI scan is currently considered more sensitive and specific than a bone scan for detecting infection/osteomyelitis. Short tau inversion recovery (STIR) signals have a high negative predictive value of approximately 100% for osteomyelitis. However, the signal changes on MRI are nonspecific, and anything that causes edema or hyperemia (such as fractures, tumors, or inflammation) can produce signal changes that resemble those in osteomyelitis. Although MRI is good for analyzing marrow involvement, it is poor for detecting cortical bone involvement. Gadolinium contrast helps distinguish an abscess from coexisting cellulites and enhances any granulation tissue. The MRI scan is of little help, however, in the early diagnosis of periprosthetic infection because of the artifacts from metallic implants.[28,29]

## Positron Emission Tomography Scan

The 8F-fluorodeoxyglucose positron emission tomography (8F-FDG PET) scan is a promising, highly accurate examination method to detect polyethylene and metal wear-induced chronic inflammation followed by periprosthetic osteolysis.[11] Having a significantly higher sensitivity and specificity than a triple-phase bone scan for differentiating between aseptic loosening and infection, the FDG-PET scan allows reliable prediction of periprosthetic septic inflammatory tissue reactions, and, because of the high sensitivity of this method, a negative PET scan in the setting of a diagnostically unclear situation eliminates the need for revision surgery. In contrast, a positive PET scan gives no clear differentiation regarding the cause of inflammation. In one recent study, the sensitivity/specificity of FDG-PET was 91%/92% (accuracy 91%) compared with 78%/70% (accuracy 74%) for triple-phase bone scans. The authors found a high correlation between FDG-PET investigation and surgical histopathologic findings; however, no significant differences were found regarding cemented and cementless implanted hip arthroplasties.[11]

## Polymerase Chain Reaction Test

The molecular diagnostic tests for the detection of infections are largely experimental. The polymerase chain reaction technique is aimed at the bacterial 16R RNA DNA sequence and holds promise for early detection of infection; however, it currently has a high false-positive rate and is limited in usefulness because live and dead bacteria cannot be differentiated. It is hoped that molecular diagnostic tests that can identify the specific bacteria responsible for producing infection even when prophylactic antibiotics are empirically started will soon become available. However, a recent study aimed to assay the polymerase chain reaction for rapid genomic detection of methicillin resistance in staphylococci (mec-A gene) showed the polymerase chain reaction to be a rapid and reliable approach.[30] In this study, Tarkin and associates[30] validated the feasibility of the molecular approach by using a septic arthritis model consisting of 73 synovial fluid samples inoculated with methicillin-resistant staphylococci and four negative controls. Mec-A polymerase chain reaction was then done on 35 clinical samples from 18 patients obtained at the time of revision arthroplasty. Results of the polymerase chain reaction were compared with cultures. The authors found that mec-A polymerase chain reaction successfully predicted the presence of methicillin-resistant staphylococci in the septic arthritis model. The polymerase chain reaction results were concordant with culture results in 34 of the 35 clinical samples studied. The one discordant result represented a false-positive culture result. The molecular assay was processed in less than 5 hours compared with a processing period of 2 to 3 days for culture. The authors concluded that for the detection of methicillin-resistant staphylococci in periprosthetic infection, the polymerase chain reaction is a rapid and reliable approach.

## Classification of Infection

The classification of infection is based on the timing of the infection process and the clinical presentation. Infection can be classified into four broad categories: types I through IV[31,32] (Table 1).

### Type I: Early Postoperative Infection

An early postoperative infection can be superficial or deep and can occur earlier than 4 weeks after the primary operation. Superficial infections of this type are treated with débridement and a course of antibiotic therapy, whereas deep infections of this type are treated with antibiotic beads, replacement of the polyethylene insert, prosthesis retention, and intravenous antibiotics.

### Type II: Late Chronic Infection

A type II late chronic infection occurs later than 4 weeks after the primary operation and usually presents with worsening pain and loosening of the prosthesis. These infections require a two-stage reconstruction with antibiotic cement spacers.

**Table 1**
**Classification and Treatment of Infected TKA**

| Type | Presentation | Definition | Treatment |
|------|-------------|------------|-----------|
| I | Acute postoperative infection | Acute infection within 4 weeks of surgery | Débridement and prosthetic retention, intravenous antibiotics |
| II | Late chronic infection | Chronic indolent infection 4 weeks after surgery | Two-stage reconstruction |
| III | Acute hematogenous infection | Acute onset of infection in a previously well-functioning joint | Débridement and prosthetic retention, intravenous antibiotics |
| IV | Positive intraoperative culture | Two or more positive intraoperative cultures | A course of appropriate antibiotics |

### Type III: Acute Hematogenous Infection

An acute hematogenous infection is a consequence of bacteremia, which seeds a previously sterile well-functioning prosthetic joint. It requires débridement, replacement of the polyethylene insert, and retention of the prosthesis (provided there is no loosening of the prosthesis), followed by a course of intravenous antibiotics.

### Type IV: Positive Intraoperative Culture With No Clinically Apparent Infection

A type IV infection is characterized by the scenario in which intraoperative cultures are positive, even though no apparent infection exists at the time of revision of a presumed aseptic loosening, and the culture results are positive. This infection type is treated with a course of intravenous antibiotics.

## Surgical Treatment

The usual course of treatment consists of multiple surgeries and a prolonged course of intravenous antibiotics. The extent of the surgical procedure depends on whether the infection is superficial or deep and whether it is acute or chronic. Whereas biofilm formation is more characteristic of chronic infection, early postoperative and acute he-

matogenous infections are less likely to be associated with biofilm formation or prosthetic loosening, and the possibility of cure without prosthetic removal is greater compared with that in instances of indolent infection. Figure 2 shows treatment options.

### Early Superficial Infections

This type of infection is treated with meticulous débridement of the soft tissue, a course of antibiotic therapy, culture of the tissue, and continued draining of fluid. Ideally, débridement includes elliptical excision of the skin margins with inclusion of the subcutaneous fat to the level of the capsule. Any sinus tracts should be curetted and excised prior to primary closure. Proper care should be taken to ensure that there is no extension/breach of the capsule. The wound should be thoroughly washed, preferably with 9 L of pulsatile lavage, and closed over antibiotic-impregnated methylmethacrylate beads. After 2 weeks, the cement beads are removed through a small separate incision, and intravenous antibiotics are continued for an additional 2 weeks. The beads are made by adding vancomycin and tobramycin with methylmethacrylate; the exact combination is a matter of debate. More recently, calcium sulfate beads impregnated with tobramycin have become popular because they are biodegradable.[33]

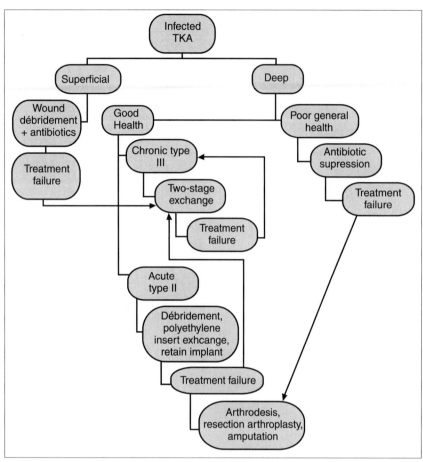

**Figure 2**  Flowchart depicts treatment decision making for infected primary TKA. Treatment should be guided by the patient's health status, functional status, and wishes.

### Early Deep Infection and Acute Hematogenous Infection

The treatment of this type of infection consists of arthrotomy, synovectomy, and débridement of all infected soft tissue. The scar is excised with an elliptical incision, and capsulotomy is done using the previous incision. Gram stains and cultures are taken of the synovial fluid and the synovium. The pseudomembrane is excised with all necrotic tissue. The insert is removed, and all the pseudomembrane and nonviable tissue are removed from the posterior aspect; the gutters also are débrided. The wound is thoroughly irrigated with 9 L of antibiotic solution, and a new polyethylene liner is then inserted. Antibiotic beads are placed in both gutters of the knee, and the arthrotomy is closed. The knee is placed in an immobilizer for 2 weeks, after which range-of-motion therapy is begun. The cement beads are removed at 2 weeks through small incisions. The duration of intravenous antibiotic treatment is generally 6 weeks.[34,35]

### Results of Débridement or Direct Exchange Arthroplasty

In reviewing the literature for this treatment, 30 reports provided outcome data on 530 open débridements, 23 arthroscopic débridements, and 37 one-stage exchange arthroplasties.[36] The average follow-up was 3.95 years, but the range of follow-up was broad (0.02 to 14 years). Successful eradication of infection was reported in 12 of the 23 instances (52.2%) managed by arthroscopic débridement, whereas eradication of infection was reported in 33 of the 37 instances (89.2%) treated by one-stage exchange. Wide variability in associated antibiotic therapy was reported. Factors associated with success included débridement performed less than 4 months after the index procedure, duration of symptoms for less than 4 weeks, antibiotic-sensitive gram-positive organisms, well-fixed components with no radiologic evidence of osteitis, and young, healthy patients. Factors associated with failed débridements included postoperative drainage for more than 2 weeks, sinus tracts present at the time of the débridement, a hinged prosthesis, and an immunocompromised host. Factors associated with successful one-stage exchange included infections by gram-positive organisms, absence of sinus formation, aggressive débridement, using antibiotic-impregnated bone cement for the new prosthesis, and 12 weeks of antibiotic therapy. One-stage exchange arthroplasty failed in 4 of 37 instances; 2 failures occurred in patients with rheumatoid arthritis undergoing corticosteroid therapy. One-stage exchange can be successful with a sensitive organism in a healthy host with prolonged antibiotic therapy. Successful outcomes are more likely when infection is caused by a low virulence organism with a good sensitivity profile, the host is healthy (not immunocompromised), and when there is no sinus tract formation, healthy soft tissue, full débridement, prolonged postoperative antibiotic therapy, and when no bone graft is required. Infection was controlled in only 173 of the 530 infected total knee replacements (32.6%) treated by open débridement and retention of the prosthetic components. Débridement of infected tissue, exchange of the polyethylene insert, and large-volume irrigation followed by prolonged antibiotic therapy can be considered when infection develops within 4 weeks of surgery or after an inciting event (such as dental extraction). The advantages of débridement and retention include limited surgery with preservation of prosthesis and bone stock and faster recovery. The disadvantages of débridement and retention include a serious risk of leaving the infected foreign body in place and inconsistent results, with a failure rate ranging from 14% to 86%.[36]

### Chronic Infection

The two-stage replacement arthroplasty is still the gold standard for chronic infections. The prerequisites for this procedure are adequate bone stock and medical fitness of the patient for multiple surgical procedures. The joint is thoroughly débrided, and all prosthetic components and bone cement are removed.[37] An elliptical incision is made that should include any discharging sinus tracts to excise the scar. Complete excision of the necrotic material and pseudomembrane is performed as deeply as possible. The polyethylene insert is removed first, followed by the removal of femoral, tibial tray, and any remaining cement. At this time, cultures should be obtained from multiple places, including the femoral and tibial canals. The canals should be opened and reamed to remove the pseudomembrane. The two types of antibiotic-impregnated cement spac-

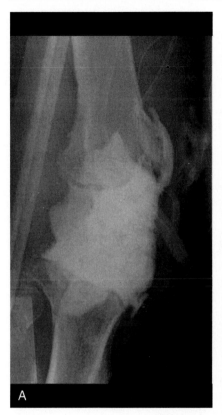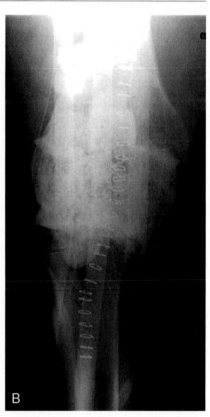

**Figure 3** Lateral **(A)** and AP **(B)** radiographs show a nonarticulating spacer with an intramedullary covered Ilizarov rod for added stability.

ers that are typically referred to in TKA are nonarticulating (block or static) (Figure 3) and articulating (mold or hybrid implant mold combination) (Figure 4). The nonarticulating spacers allow local delivery of a high concentration of antibiotics, and, at the same time, limited function of the joint to maintain joint space for future revision procedures. Disadvantages include limited ability for joint range of motion after surgery, resulting in quadriceps shortening, scar formation, and bone loss, which make surgical exposure more difficult for the final reimplantation of another knee replacement.

Articulating spacers permit more joint motion and can improve function before the second stage of reimplantation. From a technical perspective, improved joint function

and decreased scar formation after resection arthroplasty can facilitate exposure during reimplantation. Better outcomes have been reported with well-molded and properly fitted articulating spacers that restore the soft-tissue tension and allow for a greater degree of joint motion when compared with block-type spacers that may significantly limit joint freedom. Spacers may be commercially made (Figure 5) or custom made in the operating room and may consist entirely of cement, a cement-coated metal composite, or a sterile prosthesis, partially coated with antibiotic-impregnated cement. Favorable results have been reported with each of these types of spacers. **(DVD 32.1)**

Antimicrobials agents are administered 4 to 6 weeks after resection, and

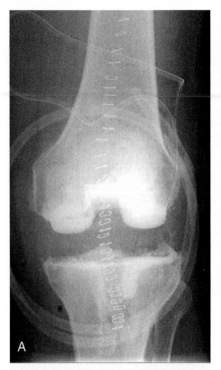 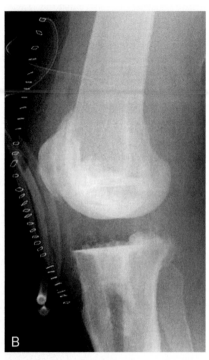

**Figure 4** AP **(A)** and lateral **(B)** radiographs showing an articulating spacer made from a preformed mold, with a polyethylene insert cemented in place.

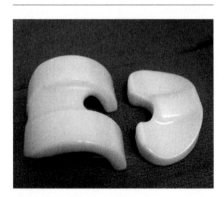

**Figure 5** Photograph of commercial spacers, which are preformed for convenience but are expensive and contain lower doses of antibiotics than that which can be added with a custom mold in the operating room.

the time interval between the two surgical procedures is highly variable.[35,38] No specific scientific protocol has been universally accepted, but confirmation of successful eradication of infection (normal serology and negative aspiration) is required before reim-

plantation. Antimicrobial agents should be stopped for at least 2 weeks before aspiration and serology. The overall success rate of two-stage reimplantation is approximately 87%.[32-35] However, the results with a two-stage early reimplantation (within 2 weeks of removing the infected prosthesis) are as low as 35%, and thus this technique currently is not favored. The delayed reimplantation with more extensive antimicrobial therapy has a success rate of 69% to 92% and, with the additional use of antimicrobial-impregnated cement at revision, success rates of 95% have been reported.[34-39]

### Suppressive Antimicrobial Therapy

This therapy is considered for elderly, frail, or ill patients for whom surgery is not possible or is refused by the patient. This treatment option is likely to be successful when the mi-

croorganism is of low virulence and susceptible to an oral antibiotic, no serious side effect to the antibiotic exists, and the prosthesis is not loose.[39-41] The goal is to provide symptomatic relief, maintain joint function, and prevent systemic spread of infection, rather than the eradication of infection. The long-term cost of such treatment should be discussed with the patient. A success rate of 10% to 25% has been seen, and this rate is improved when the infection is a result of streptococci and coagulase-negative staphylococci, but complications can occur in 8% to 22% of these instances.[42-44]

### Resection Arthroplasty

This procedure is characterized by the removal of all infected components and tissue with no subsequent implantation. The overall success rate for eradication of infection has been reported as between 50% and 89% for TKA infections.[45-48] The limited indications are poor bone and soft tissue, recurrent infections, infection with a multidrug-resistant organism, medical conditions that preclude major surgery (reimplantation), failure of multiple previous exchange arthroplasties, elderly or nonambulatory patients, and patients with polyarticular rheumatoid arthritis with limited ambulatory demands. The primary disadvantage of resection arthroplasty is the frequent occurrence of knee instability with pain during transfer or walking, with shortened limbs, poor function, and ultimately, patient dissatisfaction.[47,49]

### Arthrodesis

This procedure provides bony ankylosis of a joint. Indications for knee arthrodesis in patients with a failed TKA include high functional demand, single joint involvement, young age, failure of the reconstruc-

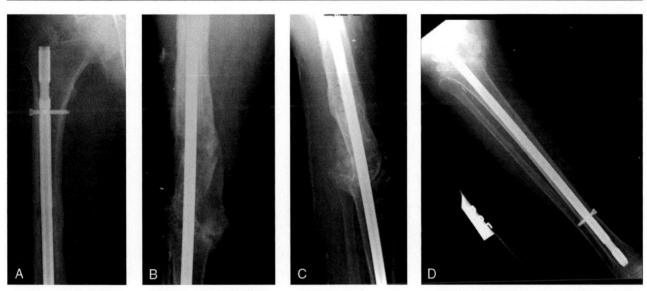

**Figure 6**  AP radiographs of the hip **(A)**, knee **(B)**, and lower extremity **(C)**, and lateral radiograph of the knee **(D)** showing a knee fusion with an intramedullary rod for fixation.

tion of the extensor mechanisms, poor soft-tissue envelope, systemic immunocompromise, and recurrent infection with virulent organisms. Inherent difficulties include inability to eradicate the infection, bone loss, and limb shortening. The hardware options include intramedullary nailing (currently favored) (Figure 6), double plating, and external fixators. Arthrodesis in patients with severe segmental bone loss can be performed with the use of Ilizarov fixation, with internal bone transport and limb lengthening. In the presence of active infection, the arthrodesis should be a staged procedure with the aim of first eradicating the infection. Overall success with eradication of infection and bony fusion can be achieved in 71% to 95% of instances.[39,47,48,50,51]

### Amputation

Above-knee amputation is indicated for recalcitrant TKA infections when all other options have been exhausted. Intractable infection associated with severe pain, soft-tissue or vascular compromise, bone loss of a severe nature that precludes using a prosthesis, and vascular compromise may be some of the indications for amputation (Figure 7). It is estimated that amputation may be the outcome in up to 5% of infected TKAs.[52,23]

### Antimicrobial Therapy

Antimicrobial therapy may be curative when the infected joint is removed and periprosthetic tissues are débrided. Antibiotics should be withheld until aspiration or intraoperative cultures are obtained, unless overwhelming sepsis is present. Ghanem and associates[54] recently reported that the initiation of intravenous antibiotics before obtaining cultures did not significantly affect the rate of positive culture results. Initial empiric therapy for most common pathogens is with the first-generation cephalosporin or vancomycin in patient populations or areas with a high incidence of methicillin-resistant *Staphylococcus aureus*. The antibiotic regimen should be tailored after identifica-

tion of the microorganism and after susceptibility testing. Antimicrobial therapy should be given for a minimum of 4 weeks systemically and locally, in some instances, by temporarily implanting antimicrobial-impregnated cement beads.

### Antibiotic-Impregnated Devices

These devices, in the form of a solid spacer, beads, or temporary arthroplasties (dynamic spacers), can be used to allow greater function.[55,56] Spacers may be commercially made or custom made in the operating room and consist entirely of cement, a cement-coated metal composite, or a sterile prosthesis, partially coated with antibiotic-impregnated cement.[57] Several types of articulating spacers can be used in the two-stage revision of a septic TKA.[5,39,58-61] One commercially available system is the antibiotic-loaded acrylic cement prosthesis, a partial load-bearing structure consisting of gentamicin-impregnated polymethylmethacrylate (PMMA) bone cement (PROSTALAC, DePuy,

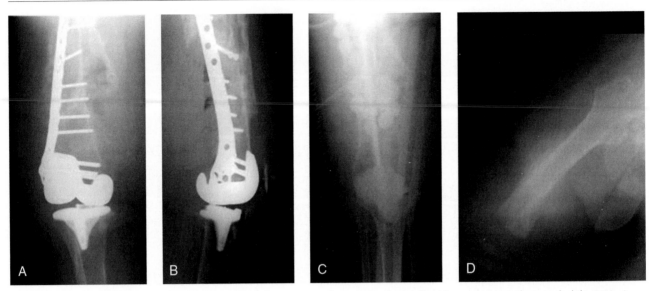

**Figure 7** Radiographs of a patient with an infected nonunion of a periprosthetic distal femur fracture that seeded the TKA. A superficial femoral arterial graft procedure was not successful, and the patient was treated with an above-knee amputation. AP **(A)** and lateral **(B)** radiographs showing the infected nonunion and arterial graft at presentation. **C,** AP radiograph of the knee with an antibiotic PMMA rod and static knee spacer after removal of the hardware. **D,** AP radiograph after an above-knee amputation.

Warsaw, IN). Such systems are costly, however, and are generally made with lower concentrations of antibiotics than normally recommended.

The cost of off-the-shelf articulating spacers can be overcome by using a composite articulating spacer. These spacers use the femoral component and polyethylene removed during the initial surgery and are sterilized and reimplanted with antibiotic-impregnated cement in a loose, nonpenetrating manner.[5,39,60,61]

The choice of antibiotics is limited to those that are thermally stable, as the polymerization of cement is an exothermic reaction that generates a substantial amount of heat. The antibiotic must be water soluble to allow diffusion into surrounding tissues, while at the same time also allowing gradual release with bactericidal effect. The most commonly used antibiotics include tobramycin, gentamicin, vancomycin, and cephalosporins, which can be combined to provide broad-spectrum coverage. Most periprosthetic infections are gram-positive (*S aureus* and *Staphylococcus epidermidis*). With a clear pathogen and antibiotic sensitivity, only one antibiotic should be used. When the pathogen is unknown, this standard becomes more difficult to apply, and complete infection eradication may require a composite set of antibiotics. The vancomycin treats methicillin-resistant *S aureus*, whereas gentamicin treats enterobacteriaceae and *Pseudomonas aeruginosa*, and cefotaxime kills the organisms that are gentamicin resistant.

It has been reported that newer antibiotics, such as daptomycin and linezolid, can be used without detriment to mechanical properties but can significantly alter the time needed for the PMMA to cure.[62,63]

Currently, PMMA that has gentamicin (SmartSet GHV, Depuy, Warsaw, IN) or tobramycin (Simplex T, Stryker Orthopaedics, Mahwah, NJ) can be used and more doses added to surgeon preference. Typically four doses of vancomycin and tobramycin per large (40-g) batch of cement can be used with most nonarticulating and articulating spacers, taking approximately three batches of cement. Concern over the total dose of antibiotics as related to the renal status of the host should be considered to safely tailor the amount of antibiotics used for each surgical spacer procedure performed.[64]

## Factors Affecting Elution of Antibiotics in PMMA Spacers

The elution of antibiotics from bone cement is dependent on several factors; the type of antibiotic, amount and number of antibiotics, type and porosity of cement, and surface area of the spacer all play a role in the release.[65] Generally, at least 3.6 g of tobramycin and 1 g of vancomycin per 40 g of bone cement have been reported. Springer and associates[64] showed the safety of combining up to 10.5 g of vancomycin with 12.5 g of gentamicin mixed in static spacers with a concurrent full 6-week course of intravenous antibiotics. In their study, there was no elevation of serum creatinine or any indication of renal dysfunction. Hand-mixing the cement also is related to a lower release of antibiotics compared with the release associated with commercially available antibiotic-loaded cements, and vacuum mixing was shown to cause only a minor change in antibiotic release. It is important when mixing to have a homogenous mixture of the antibiotic in the cement, which is the rule with commercially available formulas. With the addition of 25% dextran to cement, approximately four times as much antibiotic is released from the cement in the first 48 hours, and elution lasts for up to 10 days, compared with that of a routine preparation, which lasts for only 6 days. An advantage of the antibiotic-impregnated device is the localization of the antibiotic to the site of infection.

## Summary

Successful management of infected total knee replacement depends on several factors. Early and accurate diagnosis allows prompt treatment. Although the ideal goal is eradication of infection, alleviation of pain, and restoration of function, it is critical to individualize the treatment plan for each patient depending on the circumstances. The duration of infection, type of pathogen, patients' comorbidities, overall prognosis and function, the adequacy of local bone stock and soft tissue, and the wishes of the patient all need to be taken into consideration in the treatment plan. The treatment regimen has substantial morbidity, including multiple surgeries, prolonged intravenous antibiotic therapy, and significant cost. In more chronic and indolent infections, the treatment protocol having the highest rate of success consists of component removal, intravenous antibiotics for at least 6 weeks, and delayed reconstruction using antibiotic cement. It is hoped that with better understanding of the formation and complex interactions of the biofilm, improvements in antibiotics' penetrability and delivery, advancement in immunomodulatory agents to improve host defense, and smart self-protective implants (antibiotic coated), such periprosthetic infections someday may be treated more effectively and efficiently without the need for multiple surgeries.

## References

1. Fitzgerald RH Jr, Jones DR: Hip implant infection: Treatment with resection arthroplasty and late total hip arthroplasty. *Am J Med* 1985;78: 225-228.

2. Sartoris DJ: The role of radiology in orthopedic sepsis. *Orthop Rev* 1987; 16:271-286.

3. Morrey BF, Westholm F, Schoifet S, Rand JA, Bryan RS: Long-term results of various treatment options for infected total knee arthroplasty. *Clin Orthop Relat Res* 1989;248:120-128.

4. Schauwecker DS, Braunstein EM, Wheat LJ: Diagnostic imaging of osteomyelitis. *Infect Dis Clin North Am* 1990;4:441-463.

5. Hanssen AD, Rand JA, Osmon DR: Treatment of the infected total knee arthroplasty with insertion of another prosthesis: The effect of antibiotic-impregnated bone cement. *Clin Orthop Relat Res* 1994;309:44-55.

6. Peltola H, Vahvanen V, Aalto K: Fever, C-reactive protein and erythrocyte sedimentation rate in monitoring recovery from septic arthritis: A preliminary study. *J Pediatr Orthop* 1984; 4:170-174.

7. Spangehl MJ, Younger AS, Masri BA, Duncan CP: Diagnosis of infection following total hip arthroplasty. *Instr Course Lect* 1998;47:285-295.

8. Shih L-Y, Wu J-J, Yang D-J: Erythrocyte sedimentation rate and C-reactive protein values in patients with total hip arthroplasty. *Clin Orthop Relat Res* 1987;225:238-246.

9. Trampuz A, Hanssen AD, Osmon DR, Mandrekar J, Steckelberg JM, Patel R: Synovial fluid leukocyte count and differential for the diagnosis of prosthetic knee infection. *Am J Med* 2004;117:556-562.

10. Leone JM, Hanssen AD: Management of infection at the site of a total knee arthroplasty. *J. Bone Joint Surg Am* 2005;87:2335-2348.

11. Parvizi J, Ghanem E, Menashe S, Barrack RL, Bauer TW: Periprosthetic infection: What are the diagnostic challenges? *J Bone Joint Surg Am* 2006; 88(suppl 4):138-147.

12. Bauer TW, Parvizi J, Kobayashi N, Krebs V: Diagnosis of periprosthetic infection. *J. Bone Joint Surg Am* 2006; 88:869-882.

13. Barrack RL, Jennings RW, Wolfe MW, Bertot AJ: The value of preoperative aspiration before total knee revision. *Clin Orthop Relat Res* 1997;345:8-16.

14. Della Valle CJ, Bogner E, Desai P, et al: Analysis of frozen sections of intraoperative specimens obtained at the time of reoperation after hip or knee resection arthroplasty for the treatment of infection. *J Bone Joint Surg Am* 1999;81:684-689.

15. Lonner JH, Desai P, Dicesare PE, Steiner G, Zuckerman JD: The reliability of analysis of intraoperative frozen sections for identifying active infection during revision hip or knee arthroplasty. *J Bone Joint Surg Am* 1996;78:1553-1558.

16. Pace TB, Jeray KJ, Latham JT Jr: Synovial tissue examination by frozen section as an indicator of infection in hip and knee arthroplasty in community hospitals. *J Arthroplasty* 1997;12: 64-69.

17. Mirra JM, Marder RA, Amstutz HC: The pathology of failed total joint arthroplasty. *Clin Orthop Relat Res* 1982; 170:175-183.

18. Levitsky KA, Hozack WJ, Balderston RA, et al: Evaluation of the painful prosthetic joint: Relative value of bone scan, sedimentation rate and joint aspiration. *J Arthroplasty* 1991;6: 237-244.

19. Demopulos GA, Bleck EE, McDougall IR: Role of radionuclide imaging in the diagnosis of acute osteomyelitis. *J Pediatr Orthop* 1988;8:558-565.

20. Maurer AH, Chen DCP, Camargo EE, et al: Utility of three phase skeletal scintigraphy in suspected osteomyelitis. *J Nucl Med* 1981;22: 941-949.

21. Palestro CJ, Swyer AJ, Kim CK, Goldsmith SJ: Infected knee prosthesis: Diagnosis with In-111 leukocyte, Tc-99m sulfur colloid, and Tc-99m MDP imaging. *Radiology* 1991;179: 645-648.

22. Palestro CJ, Mehta HH, Patel M, et al: Marrow versus infection in the Charcot joint: Indium-111 leukocyte and technetium-99m sulfur colloid scintigraphy. *J Nucl Med* 1998;39: 346-350.

23. Joseph TN, Mujitaba M, Chen AL, et al: Efficacy of combined technetium-99m sulfur colloid/indium-111 leukocyte scans to detect infected total hip and knee arthroplasties. *J Arthroplasty* 2001;16:753-758.

24. Abreu SH: Skeletal uptake of In-111 labelled white blood cells. *Semin Nucl Med* 1989;19:152-155.

25. Scher DM, Pak K, Lonner JH, Fenkel JE, Zuckerman JD, Di Cesare PE: The predictive value of indium-111 leukocyte scans in the diagnosis of infected total hip, knee, or resection arthroplasties. *J Arthroplasty* 2000;15: 295-300.

26. Magnuson JE, Brown ML, Hauser MF, et al: In-111 labelled leucocyte scintigraphy in suspected orthopedic prosthetic infection: Comparison with other imaging modalities. *Radiology* 1988;168:235-239.

27. Teller RE, Christie MJ, Martin W, et al: Sequential indium labelled leucocyte and bone scans to diagnose prosthetic joint infection. *Clin Orthop*

*Relat Res* 2000;373:241-247.

28. Beltran J, Noto AM, McGhee RB, et al: Infections of the musculoskeletal systems: High field strength MR imaging. *Radiology* 1987;164: 449-454.

29. Boutin RD, Brossman J, Sartoris DJ, et al: Update on imaging of orthopedic infections. *Orthop Clin North Am* 1998;29:41-66.

30. Tarkin IS, Henry TJ, Fey PI, Iwen PC, Hinrichs SH, Garvin KL: PCR rapidly detects methicillin-resistant staphylococci periprosthetic infection. *Clin Orthop Relat Res* 2003;414:89-94.

31. Fitzgerald RH Jr, Nolan DR, Ilstrup DM, et al: Deep wound sepsis following total hip arthroplasty. *J Bone Joint Surg Am* 1977;59:847-855.

32. Tsukayama DT, Estrada R, Gustilo RB: Infection after total hip arthroplasty: A study of the treatment of one hundred and six infections. *J Bone Joint Surg Am* 1996;78:512-523.

33. Wichelhaus TA, Dingeldein E, Rauschmann M, et al: Elution characteristics of vancomycin, teicoplanin, gentamicin and clindamycin from calcium sulphate beads. *J Antimicrob Chemother* 2001;48:117-119.

34. Goldman RT, Scuderi GR, Insall JN: 2-stage reimplantation for infected total knee replacement. *Clin Orthop Relat Res* 1996;331:118-124.

35. Windsor RE, Insall JN, Urs WK, Miller DV, Brause BD: Two-stage reimplantation for the salvage of total knee arthroplasty complicated by infection: Further follow-up and refinement of indications. *J Bone Joint Surg Am* 1990;72:272-278.

36. Silva M, Tharani R, Schmalzried PT: Results of direct exchange or debridement of the infected total knee arthroplasty. *Clin Orthop Relat Res* 2002; 404:125-131.

37. Insall JN, Thompson FM, Brause BD: Two-stage reimplantation for the salvage of infected total knee arthroplasty. *J Bone Joint Surg Am* 1983;65: 1087-1098.

38. Haleem AA, Berry DJ, Hanssen AD:

Mid-term to long-term followup of two-stage reimplantation for infected total knee arthroplasty. *Clin Orthop Relat Res* 2004;428:35-39.

39. Hanssen AD, Rand JA: Evaluation and treatment of infection at the site of a total hip or knee arthroplasty. *Instr Course Lect* 1999;48:111-122.

40. Bengtson S, Knutson K: The infected knee arthroplasty: A 6-year follow-up of 357 cases. *Acta Orthop Scand* 1991; 62:301-311.

41. Bengston S, Knutson K, Lidgren L: Treatment of infected knee arthroplasty. *Clin Orthop Relat Res* 1989;245: 173-178.

42. Goulet JA, Pellicci PM, Brause BD, Salvati EM: Prolonged suppression of infection in total hip arthroplasty. *J Arthroplasty* 1988;3:109-116.

43. Tsukayama DT, Wicklund B, Gustilo RB: Suppressive antibiotic therapy in chronic prosthetic joint infections. *Orthopedics* 1991;14:841-844.

44. Segreti J, Nelson JA, Trenholme GM: Prolonged suppressive antibiotic therapy for infected orthopedic prostheses. *Clin Infect Dis* 1998;27: 711-713.

45. Schoifet SD, Morrey BF: Treatment of infection after total knee arthroplasty by débridement with retention of the components. *J Bone Joint Surg Am* 1990;72:1383-1390.

46. Perry CR, Pearson RL: Local antibiotic delivery in the treatment of bone and joint infections. *Clin Orthop Relat Res* 1991;263:215-226.

47. Rand JA: Alternatives to reimplantation for salvage of the total knee arthroplasty complicated by infection. *Instr Course Lect* 1993;42:341-347.

48. Bose WJ, Gearen PF, Randall JC, Petty W: Long-term outcome of 42 knees with chronic infection after total knee arthroplasty. *Clin Orthop Relat Res* 1995;319:285-296.

49. Falahee MH, Matthews LS, Kaufer H: Resection arthroplasty as a salvage procedure for a knee with infection after a total arthroplasty. *J Bone Joint Surg Am* 1987;69:1013-1021.

50. Knutson K, Hovelius L, Lindstrand A, Lidgren L: Arthrodesis after failed knee arthroplasty: A nation-wide multicenter investigation of 91 cases. *Clin Orthop Relat Res* 1984;191: 202-211.

51. Wiedel JD: Salvage of infected total knee fusion: The last option. *Clin Orthop Relat Res* 2002;404:139-142.

52. Isiklar ZU, Landon GC, Tullos HS: Amputation after failed total knee arthroplasty. *Clin Orthop Relat Res* 1994; 299:173-178.

53. Pring DJ, Marks L, Angel JC: Mobility after amputation for failed knee replacement. *J Bone Joint Surg Br* 1988; 70:770-771.

54. Ghanem E, Richman J, Barrack RL, Parvizi J, Purtill JJ, Sharkey, PF: Do perioperative antibiotics decrease intraoperative culture yield? *74th Annual Meeting Proceedings*. Rosemont, IL, American Academy of Orthopaedic Surgeons, 2007, p 451.

55. Hanssen AD, Spangehl MJ: Practical applications of antibiotic-loaded bone cement for treatment of infected joint replacements. *Clin Orthop Relat Res* 2004;427:79-85.

56. Haddad FS, Masri BA, Campbell D, McGraw RW, Beauchamp CP, Duncan CP: The PROSTALAC functional spacer in two-stage revision for infected knee replacements: Prosthesis of antibiotic-loaded acrylic cement. *J Bone Joint Surg Br* 2000;82: 807-812.

57. Goldstein WM, Kopplin M, Wall R, Berland K: Temporary articulating methylmethacrylate spacer (TAMMAS): A new method of intraoperative manufacturing of a custom articulating spacer. *J Bone Joint Surg Am* 2001;83:92-97.

58. Hofmann AA, Kane KR, Tkach TK, Plaster RL, Camargo MP: Treatment of infected total knee arthroplasty using an articulating spacer. *Clin Orthop Relat Res* 1995;321:45-54.

59. Calton TF, Fehring TK, Griffin WL: Bone loss associated with the use of spacer blocks in infected total knee arthroplasty. *Clin Orthop Relat Res* 1997; 345:148-154.

60. Emerson RH Jr, Muncie M, Tarbox TR, Higgins LL: Comparison of a static with a mobile spacer in total knee infection. *Clin Orthop Relat Res* 2002;404:132-138.

61. Fehring TK, Odum S, Calton TF, Mason JB: Articulating versus static spacers in revision total knee arthroplasty for sepsis. *Clin Orthop Relat Res* 2000;380:9-16.

62. Jagodzinski J, Ludwig B, Thompson J, Andes D, Squire M: Antibiotic elution of synercid, linezolid, and daptomycin from palacos bone cement. *Trans Orthop Res Soc* 2007; 32:1641.

63. Ludwig B, Jagodzinski J, Thompson J, Squire M: New antibiotic for treatment of MRSA: Inhibits PMMA polymerization. *Trans Orthop Res Soc* 2007;32:1640.

64. Springer BD, Lee GC, Osmon D, Haidukewych GJ, Hanssen AD, Jacofsky DJ: Systemic safety of high-dose antibiotic-loaded cement spacers after resection of an infected total knee arthroplasty. *Clin Orthop Relat Res* 2004;427:47-51.

65. Stevens CM, Tetsworth KD, Calhoun JH, Mader JT: An articulated antibiotic spacer used for infected total knee arthroplasty: A comparative in vitro elution study of Simplex and Palacos bone cements. *J Orthop Res* 2005;23:27-33.

# Revision Total Knee Arthroplasty: Planning, Management, and Controversies

*Thomas K. Fehring, MD
Michael J. Christie, MD
*Carlos Lavernia, MD
J. Bohannon Mason, MD
*James P. McAuley, MD, FRCSC
*Steven J. MacDonald, MD, FRCSC
Bryan D. Springer, MD

## Abstract

*The number of total knee arthroplasties (TKAs) performed annually in the United States is increasing exponentially. Even with modest annual revision rates, the number of patients requiring revision knee surgery will increase in a similar fashion. It is therefore important to have a systematic approach dealing with a patient presenting with a painful TKA. The treating physician must be able to recognize a variety of failure patterns and treat them accordingly. Surgical exploration in the absence of a definable cause is rarely successful and should be avoided. The ability to plan and execute a complex revision TKA is a challenging and rewarding aspect of adult reconstructive surgery. Commonly encountered mechanisms of failure are identified and a stepwise approach to the surgical management of these conditions is presented.*

**Instr Course Lect 2008;57:341-363.**

Common causes of a painful knee arthroplasty (TKA) include aseptic loosening, infection, instability, and particulate synovitis. Most surgeons are familiar with the clinical and radiographic findings associated with these conditions.

Radiographically, aseptic loosening of the tibial component is readily diagnosed by circumferential radiolucencies, component migration, or angulation. Femoral loosening can be much more challenging because obtaining a clear view of the complex interfaces between the components and underlying bone is difficult. Fluoroscopic radiographs can help define this interface.[1]

All painful TKAs must be presumed infected until proven otherwise. Screening blood work and aspiration should be considered in any patient presenting with a painful TKA. When cultures are positive and serology is elevated, the diagnosis is rarely in doubt. However, if cultures are negative, the cell count in the synovial fluid can be a useful diagnostic tool. Recent publications have suggested that much lower cell counts are more suggestive of infection than previously understood,[2] with greater than 2,500 white blood cells and 60% polymorphonuclear cells highly suggestive of infection.

Instability is increasingly recognized as a common factor in clinical failure. Patients with unstable TKAs are unhappy from the outset with activity-related effusions, diffuse tenderness, and variable symptoms

*Thomas K. Fehring, MD or the department with which he is affiliated has received research or institutional support from DePuy and is a consultant or employee for DePuy. Carlos Lavernia, MD or the department with which he is affiliated has received research or institutional support from Zimmer and Medtronic, holds stock or stock options in Zimmer, and is a consultant or employee for Zimmer and ORTHOsoft. James P. McAuley, MD or the department with which he is affiliated has received research or institutional support from Inova Health System and is a consultant or employee for DePuy. Steven J. MacDonald, MD or the department with which he is affiliated has received research or institutional support from DePuy and Smith & Nephew and is a consultant or employee for DePuy.

of buckling and giving way. The knee often looks good radiographically but feels uncomfortable from the patient's perspective. Instability can be categorized as varus/valgus instability, anteroposterior instability, global instability, or patellofemoral instability. These patterns can occur in isolation or in combination.

Particulate synovitis is induced by wear debris, and characterized by late-onset effusions, increasing joint stiffness, osteolysis, and even synovial pseudocysts.

When evaluating a painful TKA, the real challenge ensues when none of the common failure mechanisms previously mentioned are clearly present. A systematic approach can help sort out these difficult situations, dividing the diagnostic considerations into referred, periarticular, or intra-articular causes.

## Referred, Periarticular, or Intra-Articular Causes of Pain

Referred pain may be the most common presentation for a patient presenting with a painful TKA. Spinal stenosis or an upper lumbar disk frequently presents with anterior knee pain. A positive reverse straight-leg raise helps identify an upper lumbar radiculopathy as a source of knee pain. Referred pain can also be caused by ipsilateral hip arthritis or vascular disease. A key question to ask the patient during the examination is whether the current pain resembles the pain prior to the TKA. This question can be helpful in distinguishing knee pain from referred pain.

Heterotopic bone formation, pes anserine bursitis, and iliotibial band irritation are periarticular conditions that can produce pain after a TKA. If suspected, these can easily be confirmed either clinically or radiographically. Stress insufficiency frac-

tures can occur in osteopenic patients, even in the absence of trauma or significant changes in activity level. "End of stem" pain is surprisingly common with stemmed tibial or femoral components, either cemented or cementless.[3]

Intra-articular causes of knee pain include patellar clunk and crepitus. Patellar clunk has been recognized for some time in posterior stabilized knee designs. Patients present with a painful, palpable "clunk" that usually occurs when rising from a low chair. It results from the formation of a fibrous nodule on the undersurface of the quadriceps mechanism just proximal to the patella. This nodule catches on the anterior edge of the box of the posterior stabilized femoral component. A variation of this condition has been more recently described in which there is no clear clunk but rather an audible, palpable, painful crepitance occurring during active extension.[4] Both of these conditions are readily remedied by arthroscopic excision.

Patellofemoral arthritis can develop following a TKA with an unresurfaced patella. It clinically presents with pain during flexion activities (ascending or descending stairs, rising from chairs, etc). The pathognomonic sign is reproduction of the pain with passive knee flexion.

It is also possible for an incompletely resurfaced patella to become painful as a result of direct contact of the unresurfaced bone with the underlying femoral component. This frequently occurs when the primary surgeon places an undersized patella button far medially, in an attempt to improve tracking. Such patients tend to report well-localized lateral patellar point tenderness and pain and show a sclerotic reaction in the unresurfaced portion of the patella.

A tibial component that significantly overhangs the medial margin of the underlying tibia can occasionally result in irritation of the surrounding soft tissues. Similarly, a femoral component that is too wide can cause retinacular strain anteriorly or popliteal tendinitis if too wide posterolaterally.

Recurrent hemarthrosis is a rare entity that presents with acute, recurrent intra-articular bleeds after arthroplasty. Although an arteriovenous malformation or entrapped synovium can be a rare cause of hemarthrosis, the most common cause is prosthetic knee instability. An unstable knee will lead to repeated microtrauma to the synovium, causing recurrent bleeds.

If there is still no clear-cut cause for a painful TKA, frustration and patient pressure may result in an illadvised revision without a clear diagnosis. This is a recipe for disappointment. Arthroscopy is not a diagnostic tool in this situation and should be reserved for therapeutic indications (patellar clunk/crepitus, posterior cruciate ligament [PCL] release, and synovectomy).

## Preoperative Planning

The results of primary TKA have been excellent, with predictable and reproducible success rates well over 90% at 10-year follow-up. However, there are multiple modalities of failure leading to the necessity for revision TKA. Revision TKA can be particularly challenging to perform; complete and thorough preoperative evaluation and planning are necessary to maximize success.

It is critical to determine the mode of failure in the revision TKA scenario. The surgeon must understand why the implant failed in the first place. The most common causes for failure, listed in order of prevalence, were demonstrated by Sharkey and associates[5] to be polyethylene wear, aseptic loosening, instability, infection, arthrofibrosis, malalignment or malposition, deficient extensor mechanism, osteonecrosis of the patella, periprosthetic fracture, and isolated patellar resurfacing.

The clinical workup includes a thorough evaluation of patient history, physical examination, imaging modalities, and laboratory tests. The evaluation of the history includes a thorough knowledge and understanding of the symptoms the patient describes. These symptoms can include pain, instability, stiffness, or weakness. It is critical that throughout the clinical workup, the surgeon keeps in mind the important task of ruling out infection. A knee replacement that has always been painful, with a history of wound healing difficulty and intermittent treatment with antibiotics, is often infected.

The physical examination is equally critical to the complete clinical workup. The surgeon should rule out any other pathology, such as spine or hip conditions, that can mask as knee pain. An assessment of the patient's gait, overall limb alignment, and previous surgical incisions is required. Documenting accurately the range of motion of the knee includes any extensor mechanism issues such as quadriceps lag; assessing any evidence of mediolateral, anteroposterior, or global instability, and a thorough neurovascular examination. The patellofemoral joint should be evaluated for tracking, instability, and pain.

Routine imaging includes 3-ft standing radiographs and AP, lateral, and skyline views of the affected knee. Occasionally, the clinician will encounter a patient with a painful TKA without a definitive diagnosis.

In that scenario, it is critical to obtain, if available, the prearthroplasty radiographs. In particular, the severity of the preoperative osteoarthritic radiographic changes should be assessed to delineate the indication for the original TKA. If minimal radiographic arthritis is present, the chances for improvement are slim. Preoperative fluoroscopic evaluation, as demonstrated by Fehring and McAvoy,[1] also can help to evaluate radiolucencies that are often hidden by out-of-plane radiographs. If there is a high index of suspicion for rotational malalignment, a preoperative CT scan[6] can help determine femoral and tibial component rotation. Plain radiographs are not helpful in this regard.

Laboratory tests are used as an adjunct to rule out infection; therefore, a complete blood cell count, erythrocyte sedimentation rate (ESR), and C-reactive protein (CRP) levels are assessed in all patients. Some surgeons advocate aspiration for all knees, whereas others aspirate only those knees in which blood work is abnormal.

If available, all implant stickers, including the lot number and model number, should be obtained from previous records. It is also critical to confirm the correct operating room date if patients have undergone multiple procedures to ensure that the information is the most current. Obtaining old surgical notes also can be helpful to understand the primary surgeon's rationale and what complications occurred during the index procedure.

With the multitude of TKA devices currently on the market and that have been on the market for the past 20 years, it is imperative to be cognizant of the track record of the implant involved. If the surgeon is not familiar with the implant, then

the appropriate company representative should be contacted. If possible implant retention is planned, it is essential for all modular options to be available, including components and polyethylene inserts with varying levels of constraint. Available sterilization technique and shelf life also are important considerations. The surgeon should insist on having available all trial options and any specialized extraction devices that are required.

The surgeon should carefully plan the incision that will be required (discussed in detail later in this chapter). A standard midline incision is used in most instances; however, if multiple incisions are used, then the most laterally based incision that allows reasonable exposure to the knee should be used. The most significant blood supply to the skin and subcutaneous tissue originates medially, and therefore a lateral approach will result in less disruption. A preoperative plastic surgery consultation should be done if additional soft-tissue coverage, such as a medial gastrocnemius flap, is a possibility.

Preoperative planning also requires the surgeon to be familiar with extensile exposures. Most cases can be handled by merely subluxating the patella, using the so-called patella inversion technique.[7] If this is unsuccessful, the most commonly used extensile exposure is the quadriceps snip. Rarely a tibial tubercle osteotomy may be required to facilitate exposure in the very arthrofibrotic knee revision.

In the preoperative planning stages, the surgeon must be knowledgeable regarding the components and have available any specialized extraction devices that may be required. These include stem extractors with specific threads to engage a decoupled stem from either a tibial or a femoral component. Any specialized screwdrivers should be requested and planned for. Power equipment should be available for any metal-cutting capability required. Standard cement removal procedures and equipment, including ultrasound, osteotomes, and cement hooks, also should be available.

The reconstructive surgeon must plan ahead for any bone-grafting needs, which could include morcellized grafting, femoral heads, and, very rarely, bulk structural allografts. Along with bone grafting needs, the surgeon must plan for proper bone-grafting techniques and should have threaded wires and screws, as well as reamers for femoral head allograft preparation, available if necessary.

The surgeon must plan preoperatively for component availability and options. The radiographs should be templated for stem length and diameter and the possible need for offset stems. All constraint options, including posterior stabilized and constrained polyethylene inserts, must be available. If there is a possibility that significant collateral ligament damage may be present, a more constrained hinged implant should be available as a backup.

Controversy remains regarding the use of antibiotic cement in revision TKA. The surgeon therefore must determine if the patient is high risk and whether antibiotic cement will be used during the revision procedure. The specific cement requirements should be part of the preoperative planning process.

Many postoperative issues, such as a deep venous thrombosis prophylaxis routine, the use of prophylactic antibiotics until intraoperative cultures are negative, and a careful assessment of the potential transfusion requirements of each patient, should be planned for preoperatively.

## Exposure Options

Revision TKA is an extremely challenging procedure for the orthopaedic surgeon, especially when treating knee stiffness or ankylosis. Proper exposure and adequate visualization are key factors in the success of this procedure. Preservation of bone stock and patellar tendon integrity are paramount, while maximizing the ability to remove the implants. Exposure frequently is difficult because of scarring and lowered tissue resiliency. Quadriceps tendon thickening and contraction of the patellar tendon compound difficulties with exposure. The reconstructed knee must be properly aligned to ensure a good functional outcome. Inadequate exposure will lead to component malalignment, with subsequent early failure.

When planning the exposure, special attention should be given to previous incisions. Because the blood flow to the front of the knee is from medial to lateral, the most lateral incision should be used, if multiple incisions are present. If the most medial incision is used, regardless of the distance between the incisions, the area between the incisions is at risk for necrosis. As long as the dissection is subfascial, large flaps can be raised without risk.

Patellar tendon avulsion is a catastrophic intraoperative complication. The integrity of the patellar tendon insertion must be protected at all costs during revision knee surgery. If a patellar tendon rupture occurs, a successful functional repair can be very difficult to achieve.[8] Scar tissue formation and decreased resiliency of the soft tissue can jeopardize the patellar tendon. Various

methods have been recommended to provide adequate exposure safely.

V-Y quadricepsplasty was first described by Coonse and Adams to provide exposure to the anterior aspect of the knee.[9] This technique was modified by Insall as an extension of the standard parapatellar incision.[10] A second capsular incision is made in the extensor mechanism 45° to the proximal end of the parapatellar incision. Then the joint is exposed through a distally based flap. Scott and Siliski[11] reported on seven patients on whom this technique was used to expose joints with limited preoperative motion. Four patients exhibited a transient extensor lag, whereas three patients had permanent extensor lags of 10°, 15°, and 30°, respectively. Trousdale and associates[12] evaluated 14 patients in whom a V-Y quadricepsplasty was used for exposure. They compared V-Y quadricepsplasty with normal medial parapatellar knee patients. They found that the extensor mechanism was weaker in the V-Y group but not to a significant degree. Trousdale and associates[12] concluded that when a V-Y quadricepsplasty was used, near-normal active extension and moderate weakness in extension could be expected.

The quadriceps snip is another method of extensile exposure, which can be used in stiff revision TKAs. This technique was designed to facilitate exposure without the high risk of extensor lag noted in quadriceps turndown procedures (Figure 1). Garvin and associates reported on its use in 16 patients, 10 of whom underwent a revision TKA.[13] All 16 patients had good or excellent results. There were no significant differences in quadriceps function compared with the contralateral replaced knee in the nine patients in this category.

Tibial tubercle osteotomy was first described by Dolin in 1983.[14] He reported on the use of a 4.5-cm-long tibial tubercle osteotomy reattached with a screw anchored in bone cement. In 30 patients, there were no failures of fixation or nonunion of the tibial tubercle. Whiteside and Ohl reported similar results in 71 patients.[15] Their technique differed from Dolin's in that an 8- to 10-cm-long osteoperiosteal segment was used, leaving the lateral muscular attachments intact. This fragment was then reattached with two wires. All cases healed uneventfully, and no significant complications occurred.

Ries and Richman[16] reported on 30 patients who underwent tibial tubercle osteotomy fixed with screws. Twenty-nine patients experienced primary healing of the osteotomy. Four patients required screw removal. In one patient, postoperative displacement of the tubercle occurred, requiring revision. Another patient fractured her tibia distal to the osteotomy. Ritter and associates[17] also reported two patients with tibial shaft fractures among seven patients who underwent tibial tubercle osteotomy. They recommend sloping the distal aspect of the osteotomy to prevent this complication.

Wolff and associates[18] reported their experience with osteotomies in 26 patients; major complications related to the osteotomy occurred in 6 patients (23%). They reported three displaced osteotomized segments, all of which were only 3 cm long and fixed with a single screw. In six patients, nonmechanical complications occurred after the osteotomy. Two patients had minor wound complications, and two patients had major wound complications requiring gastrocnemius flaps for coverage. In two additional patients, a deep wound infection occurred.

The femoral peel technique described by Windsor and Insall[19] provides extensile surgical exposure, creating a soft-tissue sleeve that literally skeletonizes the distal femur. However, stability after this procedure is compromised, and therefore a constrained implant is required when this method of exposure is used.[19]

In a multicenter series, Barrack and associates[20] reported on exposure techniques in 123 patients who had revision surgery. In 60 of the 123 patients (49%), extensile exposure methods were used. The group of patients who had quadriceps snips had results equivalent to those who underwent a standard approach in every parameter measured. In contrast, those patients who had a V-Y quadricepsplasty or tibial tubercle osteotomy had significantly lower scores than the snip or standard groups. When directly comparing the V-Y group with the osteotomy group, there was no significant difference in the Knee Society scores. In a satisfaction survey, a significantly higher percentage of patients who underwent osteotomy were dissatisfied with pain relief and the ability to kneel, stoop, or perform activities of daily living.

The patellar inversion method is another alternative with which the revision surgeon should be familiar. In this technique, an early lateral retinacular release is performed, and the patella is merely subluxated laterally. The tibia is then gradually externally rotated, dissecting tissue from the posterior medial tibia. External rotation of the tibia gradually continues until the tibia is delivered from underneath the femur. Patience is required to use this method of exposure effectively. External ro-

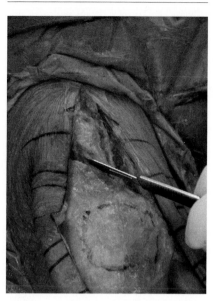

**Figure 1**  Photograph of snip quadricepsplasty used for extensile exposure.

tation of the tibia proceeds slowly, while carefully monitoring the patellar tendon and medial collateral ligament. If either structure appears in danger of injury, alternative methods of exposure should be used. This technique provided adequate exposure in 399 of 420 patients (95%) who underwent TKA performed at one institution with no episodes of patellar avulsion[7] (Figure 2). Extensile measures were used in only 5% of the patients through this technique. These results are in contrast to the study by Barrack and associates[20] in which extensile measures were used 49% of the time.

Surgical exposure should consist of a series of logical, sequential steps.[21] A stepwise progression consisting of a débridement of the suprapatellar pouch and an early lateral retinacular release, followed by gradual external rotation of the tibia without everting the patella, should be tried initially. If this course of action is not sufficient, alternative

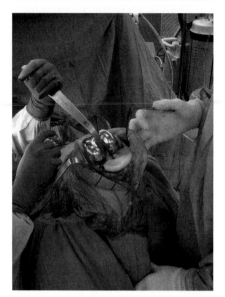

**Figure 2** Exposure without patellar eversion during revision TKA.

methods of exposure should be used.

## Component Removal

The primary goal of component removal in revision TKA is to safely and efficiently remove the component and cement without damaging underlying host bone stock. At the same time, the reconstructive surgeon must be constantly aware of other potential pitfalls during this stage of the procedure, which include damage to the extensor mechanism, collateral ligament injury, femoral condylar and tibial plateau fractures, and vascular injury. To achieve these goals, component and cement removal should be performed in a predictable and reproducible way.

Safe, reproducible component removal cannot be performed without first achieving proper exposure during the revision procedure. Various extensile exposures are described, including a quadriceps snip, quadriceps turndown, and tibial tubercle osteotomy, all of which have

been discussed in greater detail. In most revision cases, however, these exposures are not required if initial adequate exposure is performed, including clearing the femoral gutters, excision of scar tissue and adhesions, exposure of the medial tibia to at least the midcoronal point, and release of adhesions over the anterior and lateral tibia to the anterolateral corner. Patellar eversion is not required at this early stage of exposure. Simple lateral subluxation of the patella will provide adequate exposure for component removal in most patients.

The polyethylene insert is the first component to be removed, with insertion of an osteotome at the polyethylene base tray interface. Removal of the polyethylene inserts will provide the surgeon with 10 mm or more of flexion/extension laxity to enhance exposure. If a constrained polyethylene insert is being removed, anterior subluxation is usually required. In addition, there is manufacturer variability in the need for removing locking pins or posts. The surgeon should either be familiar with the system or speak to a company representative to understand the preferred method of constrained polyethylene removal.

Removal of the femoral component is performed at the implant-cement interface (in a cemented femoral component) or the implant-bone interface (in a cementless femoral component). Various techniques are described for component removal.[22] A straightforward and predictable technique uses the oscillating saw with a large blade at the anterior femoral surface, subsequently switching to the small blade to be used at the chamfer cuts and distal-cut surfaces. It is critical that the posterior condylar interface is also disrupted. Normally, a 0.25-in

curved osteotome is best used at that interface. In a cruciate-retaining femoral component or an open boxed posterior stabilized femoral component, a 0.25-in straight osteotome can be used through the notch. Once the entire interface has been freed, gentle impaction on the component is performed. If immediate movement of the component does not occur, the steps are repeated. Additionally, stacked osteotomes placed on both the medial and lateral surfaces at the distal femoral surface can be performed. Often, however, there is underlying osteolysis and osteopenia of the femur, and this osteotome technique may crush the host bone. An alternate technique involves using a Gigli saw at the anterior surface and anterior chamfer down to the level of either the distal femoral component lugs (cruciate-retaining TKA) or housing (posterior-stabilized TKA) if removing a cementless femoral component.

When removing a revision femoral component, the same steps previously outlined are used initially; however, additional steps are required to remove a stemmed femoral component. Press-fit or cementless stems do not usually pose any additional challenge for component removal. The exception to this is the scenario in which an offset stem with a coupling device has been used with cement at that interface, precluding easy disimpaction. Very rarely, a small anterior femoral cortical window may have to be performed to excise the cement that is preventing component removal.

Cemented stems create an additional challenge. In most instances, once the implant-cement bond is loosened distally around the femoral component itself, the entire component can be removed. There may, however, be occasions when, despite complete and adequate distal interface debonding, the cemented stem is still well fixed. In this situation, if there is no component movement with moderate disimpaction, an anterior femoral cortical trough may be required to facilitate cement debonding. Although techniques have been described calling this a "trap door" technique, in reality there is no significant anterior femoral soft tissue present in a revision scenario, and therefore this bone is clearly compromised with respect to its vascularity. It is critical that a femoral stem bypasses this anterior cortical window to minimize the risk of late femoral fracture. This defect can additionally be treated with bone grafting. Once the component has been removed, the surgeon should avoid the temptation to remove adherent underlying cement. This cement acts to reinforce osteopenic/osteolytic bone during tibial exposure. Furthermore, if the distal femoral bone stock is significantly osteopenic, the removed femoral component can be placed loosely back onto the distal femur to protect the bone stock during tibial component removal.

An all-polyethylene tibial component is by far the easiest to remove because an oscillating saw with a large blade is simply used at the cement-polyethylene interface, cutting through the keel-center post. The keel is then removed with a series of osteotomes or burrs.

When removing a primary modular tibial component, an oscillating saw is used at the implant-cement (cemented TKA) or implant-bone (cementless TKA) interface. Obviously any underlying keel or lugs will block access to the complete interface. A reproducible and safe technique involves passing the oscillating saw with a small blade from a posterior-medial to a posterior-lateral direction, not go-ing beyond the posterior tibial cortical margin. It is critical that a blunt posterior tibial retractor is placed to protect the neurovascular bundle. Once the entire cement implant interface has been addressed, gentle impaction of the tibial component can be performed. Once again, if there is no initial movement, the steps are repeated. Additionally, stacked osteotomes can be used as described for femoral component removal, but once again osteopenic and underlying osteolytic bone is at risk. It is critical that the tibial component is not impacted before breaking the bond at the posterior-medial and posterior-lateral corners because this can create an underlying tibial fracture.

When removing revision tibial components, the same issues that were addressed earlier with stem fixation apply. In the uncommon scenario with a solid cemented stem that is well fixed and precludes tibial component removal, a tibial tubercle osteotomy, which was described earlier in detail, may be required.

The next step involves removal of adherent cement on the femur and the tibia. Osteotomes, cement splitters, crochet hooks, and high-speed burrs all should be available. Very well-fixed cement is best removed by first using a high-speed burr to thin the cement to facilitate debonding. The cement can be harder than the underlying femoral or tibial bone, and great care must be taken in removing cement to minimize an inadvertent fracture of the underlying bone. Ultrasound devices, if available, can be very helpful in removing well-fixed cement.

Most patellar components do not require removal at the time of revision TKA. However, in the presence of infection or malposition, removal may be indicated. A cemented patellar component is removed using an oscillating saw at the polyethylene-cement interface, including sawing directly through the polyethylene pegs. The pegs and cement are then removed with a high-speed burr. Again, it is critical to avoid using osteotomes with underlying osteopenic bone.

Removing a well-fixed cementless patellar component represents a challenging scenario.[23] The surgeon must be aware that there is often underlying osteolysis of the patella, and it is critical to not pry or lever an osteotome between the implant and the bone to avoid fracture. The simplest technique is to use a high-speed metal cutting wheel to go around the periphery of the implant-bone interface. If the wheel is large enough, it will cut the metal lugs; however, it often may not be, and a metal cutting pencil-tip burr will be required to cut the lugs. Once the three lugs have each been cut with the metal cutting burr, the component is easily removed, and the lugs themselves are removed by burring around the periphery once again with a high-speed pencil-tip burr.

## Soft-Tissue Balancing

The goals of both primary and revision TKA are to eliminate pain, maximize range of motion, and provide stability throughout the gait cycle. One key to these surgical goals is proper ligament balance. Failure to obtain proper ligament balance results in asymmetric tension in the collateral ligaments in either flexion or extension and may lead to increased polyethylene wear, decreased range of motion, or anterior knee pain.[24-29] Rotational malalignment of the femur can compound ligament imbalance and lead to anterior knee pain, condylar lift-off, and increased polyethylene contact stresses.[30-32]

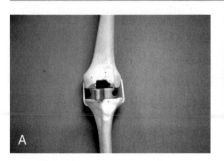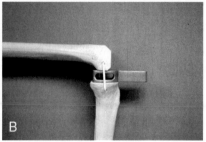

**Figure 3**  Equal extension (**A**) and flexion (**B**) gaps.

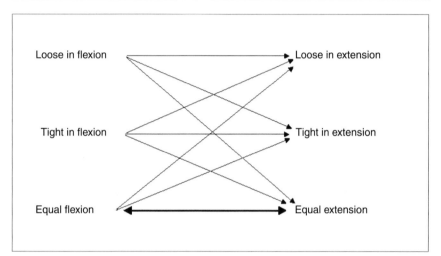

**Figure 4**  Nine gap-balancing permutations that can occur during revision TKA.

A balanced knee is attained through proper axial alignment, symmetric tension on the ligaments in flexion and extension, and equal flexion and extension gaps. An important distinction when balancing a knee is that between tension and gap size. The tension in the collateral structures is largely modulated by management of the soft-tissue envelope, including the release of contracted tissues, and the rotational position in flexion of the femoral implant. Conversely, the gap size is controlled primarily by the implant size and positioning of the implant.[33]

In a revision TKA, it is important to establish preoperatively the collateral ligament tension with an ex-

amination under anesthesia. Passive correction, with solid end point to varus or valgus stress, may indicate the level of constraint needed in revision arthroplasty. Additionally, it is important to document the extensor mechanism function before surgery. In a revision TKA, exposure and component removal can influence ligament balance. Careful removal of the implants can avoid injury to the collateral ligaments, avulsion of a condyle, or an extensor mechanism injury.

The initial bone resections customarily are minimal distal femoral resection and proximal tibial resection. It is important to obtain a 90° neutral proximal resection of the

tibia, with the slope dictated by the implant.[34] Both intramedullary and extramedullary alignment systems can easily achieve this. Once the distal femoral and proximal tibial initial resections are made, the leg is brought into full extension and the collateral ligament structures are palpated. The mechanical axis alignment is confirmed either visually or with guides. Any contracted soft tissues are released in extension to create a rectangular extension space. Spacer blocks can be helpful in assessing the collateral tension balance if the bone stock is adequate to support them.[30,35]

Once a rectangular extension space is established, the knee is brought to 90° of flexion and collateral ligament tension is reapplied medially and laterally with laminar spreaders or a tensioning device. Femoral rotation is established parallel to the cut tibial surface at 90° of flexion with the collateral structures under tension. Femoral rotation can be estimated in other ways; however, Whiteside's line is not visible in a revision setting because of the prior implant, and the transepicondylar axis may be difficult to establish because of bone loss and scarring.[35,36] A dynamic gap-balancing technique is helpful in the revision setting. Once the femoral rotational axis is determined, a cutting block is pinned to the distal femur and the AP cuts are made. The extension and flexion gaps are then measured and compared (Figure 3).

The confusion that many surgeons encounter in balancing a knee in a revision setting is summarized in Figure 4. The construct can be too loose in flexion or extension, too tight in flexion or extension, or just right. Nine permutations of this equation exist. To simplify this stability equation, the surgeon should establish the

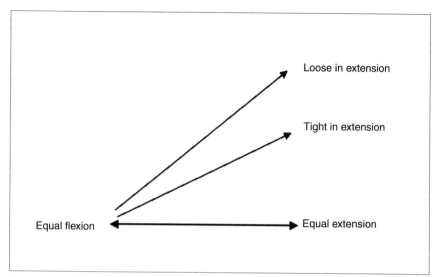

**Figure 5** By establishing the flexion gap initially, gap balancing equalization can be simplified.

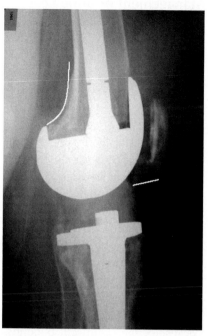

**Figure 6** Intraoperative lateral radiograph showing correct joint-line position.

flexion gap first. Femoral rotation established in the previous step yields a rectangular flexion space. The size of the flexion space is best modulated by the size of the femoral implant. The anterior to posterior dimension of femoral implants increases with the size of the implants. Therefore, the surgeon can upsize the implant by adding posterior augments and decrease the flexion space. The limit of this technique is the medial to lateral dimension of the implant. Once the flexion space is established, the stability equation is dramatically simplified (Figure 5). The knee is then brought into extension and the surgeon is yielded one of the three outcomes—either the construct is too loose in extension, too tight in extension, or just right.[37,38]

If the construct is too loose in extension relative to the flexion gap, this is typically managed with distal femoral augmentation. If the knee is too tight in extension relative to the flexion gap, options include increased distal femoral bone resection, reduction of the distal femoral augmentation, or upsizing the fe-

mur (which will tighten the flexion space).

In revision arthroplasty, compromises are often necessary to obtain appropriate reconstruction. Joint-line elevation should be avoided if possible because this can lead to mid-flexion instability, decreased range of motion, soft-tissue impingement, or anterior knee pain associated with patella infera.[39,40] Correct joint-line position is typically governed by femoral component position.[40] An intraoperative lateral radiograph is very helpful in assessing the relative joint-line position. Comparison with the contralateral extremity or the preoperative radiograph may provide guidance. The position of the inferior pole of the patella relative to the joint line and the posterior condylar sweep on the lateral film is a handy surrogate for estimating component positioning and joint-line elevation (Figure 6). To ensure accurate estimation of collateral tension and gap balance, nonvarus/valgus constrained trials are performed. In flexion, it is important to test for both AP and jump-height stability.[41]

There are situations in which balance in a revision setting is not achievable and the surgeon should consider adding prosthetic constraint. An incompetent medial collateral ligament, severe epicondylar bone loss (which may compromise the collateral ligament origin), or the inability to balance the flexion space to the extension space warrant use of higher degrees of prosthetic constraint.

Ligament balance is as important in the revision setting as it is in the primary TKA for optimal knee kinematics and pain relief. Gap-balancing techniques do not rely on bony landmarks, which are often obscured in revision arthroplasty. The surgeon should not leave the operating room without either achieving a balanced revision construct or compensating for the knee that lacks collateral stability with a constrained implant.

## Management of Bone Loss

The goals of revision TKA are the same as in primary TKA—a stable, pain-free knee with a functional range of motion sufficient to allow ambulation. Several factors contribute to achieving these goals. The patient must have sufficient motor power to support body weight. Knee stability must be achieved through proper soft-tissue tensioning or ligament substitution. Knee motion must be sufficient to support the desired function. Implants must achieve stable and durable fixation on the host skeleton. All subsequent function relies on this final tenet. Stable and durable fixation can be difficult to achieve in the failed TKA because of the significant bone loss that often accompanies knee arthroplasty failure. Periprosthetic osteolysis due to polyethylene wear debris is the most common cause of bone loss in the failed TKA, but previous component malalignment, component removal at reconstruction, and periprosthetic fracture also may decrease the amount and location of viable host bone available for the reconstruction. The degree of bone loss present will determine the reconstructive options available, as the goals of revision TKA are all subordinate to the establishment of implant stability on host bone.

Several classification systems have been described to assist with preoperative planning. The method of the Anderson Orthopaedic Research Institute (AORI) is the most frequently cited.[42] Bone defects are divided into three types: type 1 defects have intact metaphyseal bone with an intact joint line, type 2 defects have damaged metaphyseal bone, and type 3 defects compromise a major portion of either condyle or plateau. Mulhall and associates[43] compared preoperative radiographic assessment of bone loss to intraoperative assessment of bone loss and found that the AORI system predicted bone loss accurately 67% of the time for femoral defects and 82% of the time for tibial defects.

Although accurate preoperative estimation of bone loss is helpful, the key issue for the surgeon should be how the degree of bone loss determines the reconstruction. All revision arthroplasty fixation methods can be described as one of three general techniques. The underlying principles of reconstruction are the same within each category, regardless of the type of material used. "Shims" describe the use of augments, whether metal or allograft, to fill defects that are generally below the level of the epicondyles on the femoral side or are cavitary with an intact rim on the tibial side. "Sleeves," or conical metal augments or allografts that allow fixation into the metaphysis, are required if bone loss extends to the diaphysis. If bone loss extends beyond the metaphysis, then large "segments," either of metal or allograft, are required for stable fixation.

Most bone loss encountered in revision TKA can be managed with simple metal augments. A large variety of sizes and shapes are available with most implant systems, although systems vary widely as to the variety of the inventory as well as the materials, mechanical connections, and instrumentation available. Brand and associates[44] reported a series of 22 knees in 20 patients treated with modular metal tibial wedges for tibial bone stock deficiency. There were 19 primary and 3 revision arthroplasties. The primary arthroplasties included two previous unicondylar arthroplasties, two previous valgus high tibial osteotomies, and a lateral tibial plateau fracture previously treated with internal fixation. At latest follow-up (mean, 37 months; range, 24 to 59 months), there were no loose or failed arthroplasties. Pagnano and associates[45] reviewed 24 TKAs with modular tibial wedge augments at a mean of 5 years postoperatively. One TKA failed and was revised, and 13 of the remaining 23 knees had radiolucent lines at the augment interface. None of the radiolucencies were progressive and no deterioration of the wedge interfaces was seen.

Revision surgeons often encounter bone loss that extends beyond that which can be handled by simple metal augments. If the bone loss extends into the metaphyseal bone, then prostheses with modular sleeves may allow sufficient stability on host bone while restoring the joint line. Cone-shaped metallic augments, such as sleeves, fill the bony defect with metal, allowing the surgeon to bypass poor bone stock and achieve fixation in the metaphyseal flare where the implant can be wedged for stability. Several studies report the results of the S-ROM knee system (DePuy Orthopaedics, Warsaw, IN), which includes modular metaphyseal sleeves. Jones and associates reported the combined results of two retrospective reviews of the S-ROM rotating hinge system in revision TKA.[46] Thirty knees were followed for a mean of 49 months and showed no evidence of mechanical failures or radiolucent lines around the sleeves or stems at latest follow-up. Radnay and Scuderi[47] reported their early results with trabecular cones in revision TKA. Ten tibial and two femoral trabecular metal cones (nine patients) were followed for a mean of 10 months (range, 5 to 14 months).

There was no radiographic evidence of subsidence or bone resorption and no progressive radiolucent lines. One patient was resected for recurrent sepsis at 9 months, but the tibial cone appeared well incorporated with bone ingrowth at reoperation.

When bone loss is significant enough that fixation must be achieved in the diaphysis, then segments of metal or allograft must be used. The metal used for segmental replacement may be solid (titanium) or porous (tantalum; Trabecular Metal, Zimmer, Warsaw, IN). There must be sufficient diaphyseal bone to support the anticipated load, and care must be taken in assessing limb length as well as component rotation. On the tibial side, the tibial tubercle and its attachments must be protected because reattachment to standard metal implants is difficult. Allograft composites with retained tendons behave unpredictably and should be avoided. Careful assessment of rotation is important with massive tibial bone loss.

Most segmental knee replacement systems were initially designed for limb salvage after tumor resection but have been increasingly used for massive bone loss associated with failed TKA. Springer and associates[48] reported on a series of 26 knees (25 patients) treated with a Modular Segmental Kinematic Rotating Hinge prosthesis (Howmedica, Rutherford, NJ) for nonneoplastic distal femoral salvage, including 4 primary and 22 revision arthroplasties, mostly in older, low-demand patients. At mean 59 months of follow-up, 2 femoral and 2 tibial components were loose radiographically, and an additional 11 patients had isolated radiolucencies on the femoral or tibial side without evidence of progression or loosening. One patient fractured the axle component of the hinge at 101 months

postoperatively. Deep infection occurred in five patients. The authors conclude that despite a significant complication rate, this reconstructive technique expedites functional recovery, especially in the elderly, low-demand patient. There are no published results with porous metal structures in segmental knee arthroplasty.

## Fixation in Revision TKA

Revision TKA is an increasingly common procedure. It is important, therefore, to determine the best surgical techniques to manage revision complications as they are encountered. Unfortunately, no comparative information to guide the revision surgeon concerning what type of fixation option is best is currently available. The goal of stem fixation in revision TKA is to enhance the mechanical stability and fixation of the prosthesis, provide load-sharing capabilities, and protect host bone or allograft.

Options for stem fixation in revision TKA include cemented and cementless fixation. The advantages of cementless stem fixation include easy removal and preservation of bone stock if revision is required, fixation distal to the areas of metaphyseal bone loss that is often encountered in revision surgery, and the potential for favorable support and load of an allograft prosthetic composite. The main disadvantage is that a cementless stem must engage the diaphysis to provide adequate fixation. This fixation may be limited in patients with poor diaphyseal bone stock. In addition, diaphyseal-engaging stems may dictate the position of the femoral and tibial component, leading to overhang and malalignment. These conditions often may require the use of offset stems.

The advantages of cemented stem fixation are immediate fixation that is achieved at the time of the surgery, the position of the components is not dictated by the bony alignments, and better fixation is achieved in patients with poor diaphyseal bone stock. Additionally, it allows delivery of local antibiotics in the cement for patients at risk for infection or those patients with a previous infection. The main disadvantage of cement fixation is difficult removal if revision surgery is required.

Biomechanical issues with regard to stem fixation include the length of the stem, the type of fixation, concern for stress shielding, and micromotion. Several studies have focused specifically on the role of stress shielding with stem fixation. Initially, there was a concern that intramedullary stems led to stress shielding of the proximal tibia.[49] Brooks and associates, however, showed that a 70-mm stem carries 30% of the axial load and concluded that stems are load sharing, and significant stress shielding is unlikely.[50] In a biomechanical model, Jazrawi and associates[51] showed no significant decrease in the proximal tibial stresses with either cemented or cementless stems. Several studies have focused on the concern about micromotion with regard to stem fixation. Stern and associates,[52] in a cadaver study, showed that micromotion and migration were significantly less in cemented stems compared with a cementless stem construct. In a biomechanical study, Bert and McShane[53] showed that fully cemented implants have less micromotion than implants with a cemented tray and press-fit stems. Jazrawi and associates[51] showed that cemented metaphyseal-engaging stems have less micromotion than cementless stems of the same length. Additionally, longer diaphyseal-engaging stems are required to achieve the same stability as a shorter cemented stem.[51]

Murray and associates[54] published one of the first large series of cemented stems in revision TKA. Forty fully cemented revision TKAs were followed for a mean of 58.2 months. There was one loose femoral component and no loose tibial components. This initial study set the benchmark for which all other reports of cemented and cementless stems would be compared. Whaley and associates[55] looked at 38 fully cemented revision TKAs. The 11-year survivorship for aseptic loosening was 95.7%; this included one loose tibia that was of standard length and no loose femoral components. Haas and associates[56] evaluated 67 revision TKAs with cementless diaphyseal-engaging stems. The mean follow-up was only 3.5 years. Two stems were revised for aseptic loosening, and complete radiolucent lines were present in 7% of the tibias. Complete radiopaque lines were present in 38% of the cementless femoral stems and 28% of the cementless tibial stems. The authors concluded, however, that no association between radiopaque lines and clinical results were noted. Gofton and associates[57] looked at 89 revisions with cementless diaphyseal-engaging stems at an average follow-up of 5.9 years. There were seven revisions for aseptic loosening and a 93.5% survivorship at 8.6 years. Again, there were 55% femoral and 52% tibial radiopaque lines present at latest radiographic follow-up. Shannon and associates[58] reported on 60 patients with cementless diaphyseal-engaging intramedullary stems with a mean follow-up of 5.7 years. There were 12 rerevisions for aseptic loosening, and 4 radiographically loose tibial components. Their overall mechani-

cal failure rate was 16%. Radiopaque lines were present in 90% and 97% of the remaining femoral and tibial press-fit stems, respectively. In the only comparative study to date, Fehring and associates[59] compared stem fixation methods in revision TKA. All stems, whether cementless or cemented, were metaphyseal in nature and did not engage the diaphysis. There were 107 cemented stems at a mean follow-up of 53 months compared with 95 cementless stems at a mean follow-up of 61 months. In the cemented stem cohort (107 implants), 100 implants were stable, and 7 implants required close follow-up for progressive radiolucent lines. No implants were radiographically loose, and none had required revision for aseptic loosening. In the cementless stem cohort, 67 of 95 implants (71%) were stable; however, 18 required close follow-up for progression on radiographs, 10 implants were loose, and 4 implants required rerevision for aseptic loosening. This study concluded that metaphyseal-engaging stems that were implanted cementless were significantly more unstable than those implanted with cement. The authors urged caution in the use of cementless metaphyseal-engaging stems in revision TKA.

Stable fixation in revision TKA is integral to revision surgery. How to optimally achieve this fixation, however, remains controversial. Biomechanical and micromotion studies tend to favor cemented constructs. It appears evident that if cementless stems are used, they should be diaphyseal-engaging stems.

## Periprosthetic Osteolysis
Osteolysis complicating TKA was first described in modular, cementless implants in the early 1990s.[60] As in total hip arthroplasty, osteolysis is particle-induced bone resorption

that can result in severe periarticular bone stock deficiency and even periprosthetic fracture.

Plain radiographic changes of scalloped, cavitary lesions and loss of normal trabeculae frequently occur in the absence of clinical symptoms. Routine radiographic follow-up may reveal the first sign that an arthroplasty is failing. Because not all osteolysis is rapidly progressive, serial films provide invaluable insight into the progression of bone loss in a given patient.

As in other types of arthroplasty surgery, plain films significantly underestimate the extent and severity of bone loss. The situation in TKA is even more complex because reliable, reproducible wear measurements are very difficult to obtain. Furthermore, the complex geometry of knee components makes reliable plain radiographic assessment of periprosthetic osteolysis inaccurate at best.[61] The addition of oblique radiographs can be very helpful in detecting lesions not well seen on standard projections.[62]

More sophisticated three-dimensional reconstructions show promise for evaluating the true volume of an osteolytic lesion (Figure 7). Until there is a way to routinely and accurately measure wear and lysis in TKA, objective guidelines for the best timing and type of intervention will remain elusive.

It is clear that osteolysis is an increasingly common cause for revision TKA. It has been historically presumed that most wear and resultant debris generation occurs at the interface between the femoral component and the bearing surface of the tibial polyethylene. With the advent of modular components, tibial insert micromotion with the underlying tray has been documented to produce clinically significant wear and osteolysis.[63] Roughness of the tibial base-plate finish and variations in the material properties of the polyethylene (as a result of the sterilization method) can result in increased osteolysis.[64,65] Tibial post impingement in posterior-stabilized knee components can be a third source of debris contributing to failure and osteolysis[66] (Figure 8).

Once recognized, the options for treating osteolysis in knee arthroplasty surgery range from observation to full revision with or without bone grafting of defects. Because there are no validated guidelines available, basic principles must guide the surgeon in the treatment of recognized osteolytic lesions.

Observation is reasonable for small osteolytic defects ($< 1$ cm$^2$) with a compliant patient who understands the importance of routine follow-up. Osteolytic lesions are always bigger in vivo than what is seen radiographically.

Polyethylene insert exchange alone should be reserved for knees with good fixation, alignment, and soft-tissue balancing. The ideal situation is an implant that functioned well for an acceptable interval and developed expected wear with time. Osteolytic lesions should be thoroughly débrided and packed with allograft bone or augmented with cement.

If the insert has extensive delamination after a short in vivo interval, the underlying reasons for accelerated polyethylene wear (methods of manufacture, sterilization, shelf life, etc) should be examined. The surgeon should make certain that the revision components do not have the same deficiencies. The extent of osteolysis is often underestimated on radiographs, so a full revision knee system should always be available even when partial revision is contemplated.

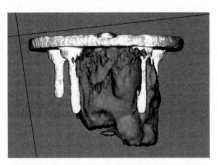

**Figure 7** Three-dimensional reconstruction of an osteolytic tibial defect.

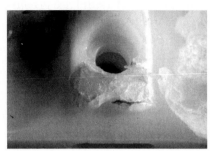

**Figure 8** Tibial post impingement-related wear in a posterior stabilized TKA.

Partial revision is acceptable if the retained implant has stable component fixation, proper alignment, and a sound clinical track record. If the tibia is retained, the reconstruction is straightforward. However, if the femur is retained, the ability to adjust the joint line to maintain proper gap balancing is compromised. Full revision should be performed if there is loss of fixation or component malalignment or if the existing implant has a poor clinical record.

Osteolysis is challenging in all aspects, from diagnosis through surgical reconstruction. One should attempt to identify all factors (technical, material, design, etc) that may have contributed to the failure and ensure these are not repeated at the time of revision. This will provide the surgeon and patient with the best potential for a long-term, successful outcome.

## Extensor Mechanism Complications

Extensor mechanism complications are quite common in TKA. Sharkey and associates reported that 12% of the revision knee procedures performed at their institution were for extensor mechanism complications.[5] The severity of the problem will vary from slight subluxation of the patella in flexion to complete

avulsion of the patellar tendon. Anatomically, these complications can occur at one of several sites—the quadriceps muscle or tendon, the patella, or the patellar tendon. The prognosis and subsequent difficulty in treating the condition depend not only on where the disruption occurs but also whether it is an acute or a chronic condition.[67-70]

The mildest form of extensor mechanism complications after TKA is patellar subluxation. It usually involves malposition of one of several components, which can ultimately lead to maltracking or frank dislocation of the patella. If either the femoral or tibial components are internally rotated, the patella will subluxate laterally or completely dislocate, depending on the magnitude of the malrotation.[67] Excessive valgus alignment can also be a cause of patellar maltracking. Error in patellar component preparation will have the same effect. An oblique patellar cut or lateral placement of the patellar component will also be problematic. The easiest way to prevent these complications is to carefully position all components during the index surgical procedure.

The presentation of a frank extensor mechanism disruption is straightforward and usually follows significant trauma.[71-76] Acute tendon ruptures are occasionally associated with exposure of a stiff knee in complicated primary or revision TKA. These ruptures may occur intraoperatively or while the patient is in rehabilitation. Late ruptures can be associated with lupus, rheumatoid disease, chronic steroid use, diabetes, or repeated steroid injections.[67]

Patients usually report the knee giving way, particularly when climbing stairs. In addition, they report difficulty rising from a chair or on occasion suffer repeated falls. Physical examination in these patients includes the inability to extend the knee completely from a flexed position, weakness to manual examination and on occasion a significant extensor lag. In addition, on physical examination there is usually a palpable defect at the site of the disruption.

The recommended approach to an acute extensor tendon rupture is direct repair and augmentation. Kollender and associates[77] recommended augmentation with synthetic strips. They reported on seven patients with a minimum of 2-year follow-up. All patients had good to excellent functional outcomes and reported no functional limitations. Other authors have used either the semitendinosus and gracilis, a medial gastrocnemius flap, or an allograft.[74,76]

Cadambi and Engh[74] reported on seven patients augmented with the semitendinosus and gracilis tendons. They augmented all reconstructions by harvesting the semitendinosus and gracilis tendons and passing these tendons through the patella. They reported excellent results with good restoration of quadriceps strength and motion of the knee. The patients' function was deemed to be good to excellent in all patients.

When dealing with chronic or late disruptions, allograft is probably the best solution because direct repair has yielded poor results.[71-73,76,78] There are five large series of extensor tendon allografts published with variable results.[71-73,76,78] The first published series of extensor tendon allografts was reported by Emerson and associates.[73] They reported on a series of 15 knees in which an extensor mechanism allograft was used to treat a ruptured extensor mechanism in a TKA. They reported excellent results in 12 of the 15 knees. Their technique involved using either a freeze-dried or a fresh-frozen specimen and tensioning the grafts in full extension. Subsequent to this report, they followed 9 knees for more than 2 years and reported extensor lag in 3 knees.[79] Leopold and associates[75] reported a high failure rate in seven patients with extensor mechanism allografts tensioned in flexion. A follow-up study compared their technique of tensioning in flexion compared with tensioning the graft in full extension.[76] The second group had good to excellent results at 2 to 4 years of follow-up. A subsequent series by Nazarian and Booth[72] reported on 36 patients with successful results in 34 patients (94%) using this technique. Crossett and associates[80] described a technique for a ruptured patellar tendon using an Achilles tendon allograft with an attached calcaneal bone graft to the tibia in nine patients. Seven of these were successful at an average follow-up of 28 months.

An infrequent but difficult complication is quadriceps tendon rupture after TKA. Dobbs and associates[70] reported an incidence of 0.1% in a cohort of 23,800 TKAs. In this series, the patients with a complete tear did not fare as well as those with a partial tear. Complications occurred in 11 of 26 patients who were surgically treated.

Revision surgery for extensor mechanism complications is not universally successful. In one reported series of revisions for this problem, the prevalence of revisions was 23%.[69] The most prudent approach to this rare but complicated condition should be prevention. Careful surgical technique and proper exposure in primary and revision surgeries are the cornerstones of prophylaxis.

## Management of the Infected TKA

Infection following TKA is uncommon, occurring in less than 2% of patients in most series. Host factors including immune deficiency or bacteremia resulting from ulcers, abscesses, or cellulitic processes often account for late infections. *Staphylococcus aureus* and *Staphylococcus epidermidis* account for nearly two thirds of the infecting organisms.[81,82] The diagnosis of infection can be quite obvious when the knee is hot and swollen. However, diagnosing infection in the painful TKA is more difficult. Clues from the patient's history include the timing and onset of pain. The lack of a pain-free interval, the presence of pain at rest, or a history of wound-healing issues following the initial arthroplasty may suggest the presence of an infection. Careful comparison of old and new radiographs often reveals the presence of progressive radiolucencies, localized osteolysis, periostitis, or subchondral resorption about the prosthesis.

Hematologic evaluation often includes a peripheral white blood cell (WBC) count with differential cell analysis. Unfortunately, a WBC count is of limited benefit in evaluating the septic knee. Morrey and associates[83] have shown that greater than 70% of infected knees have a normal WBC count. CRP is helpful in the early evaluation following TKA. Yoon and associates[84] have shown that in the uncomplicated arthroplasty, CRP levels return to normal within 3 weeks, whereas the ESR will remain elevated for up to 2 months following surgery. An elevated ESR is a helpful indicator in evaluating late sepsis.[85] Elevation of either acute phase reactant should prompt an aspiration of the suspected infected TKA.

Barrack and associates[86] reported that aspiration and culture of joint fluid in a suspected knee arthroplasty yielded a high specificity of 96%. However, sensitivity was compromised because many of the patients had received antibiotics. The authors' recommendation was to consider repeat aspiration when a patient had recently taken antibiotics. Using regression analysis, Mason and associates[2] demonstrated the utility of cell count and differential analysis of the aspiration of a suspected infected TKA. An aspirate that contained more than 2,500 white blood cells per deciliter with 60% or more polymorphonuclear cells yielded a positive predictive value of 91% with high sensitivity and specificity.

Although unnecessary in routine cases, radionuclide scanning for the diagnosis of infection can be useful in difficult cases. Technetium-99 scans, particularly with polyclonal immunoglobulin G, may be helpful in ruling out infection but may require sequential scans, limiting the use of this test.[87] Indium-111 has been shown to have an accuracy of 84%, but these scans should be carefully interpreted in the presence of massive osteolysis or rheumatoid arthritis.[88,89] Polymerase chain reaction has been advocated for the detection of infection, but the clinical utility is

limited by extreme sensitivity and a high false-positive rate.[90]

Intraoperative tests for infection include Gram stain and frozen section histopathology; however, Gram stains are associated with poor sensitivity and unreliable interpretation. The results from frozen sections are dependent on accurate sampling of the tissue submitted to the pathologist and the pathologist's experience in interpreting these sections.[91] Lonner and associates[92] and others have shown improved specificity with greater than 10 polymorphonuclear cells per high-power field in submitted specimens.[93] However, the overall histologic picture may be more important than the absolute number of polymorphonuclear cells per high-power field.

Treatment options for infected TKA include antibiotic suppression, débridement and retention of the prosthesis, resection arthroplasty, arthrodesis, amputation, and reimplantation.[94-99] The choice for each individual patient depends on a number of variables, including the length of time the infection has been present, whether the infection is deep or superficial, the status of the soft tissues (including the extensor mechanism), the infecting organism, host factors, and whether or not the implant is well fixed.

Antibiotic suppression alone should be considered only in patients unable to undergo surgery and in whom a low-virulence organism is present and a suitable oral antibiotic agent is available. Meta-analysis of the literature shows that this strategy is successful in a mere 21% of patients.[100]

Open débridement and retention of the well-fixed implant should be considered if the infection is recognized early (present for less than 3 weeks), a low-virulence organism

is present, and the implants are well positioned and well fixed. Still, meta-analysis yields only 30% success using this strategy.[100] The results of arthroscopic débridement and retention of implants are equally poor but may be improved with repeat arthroscopies for persistent fever.[101,102]

Several controversies exist regarding reimplantation of TKAs for sepsis, including the timing of reimplantation, the duration of antibiotic treatment, and the management of the joint between stages of reimplantation. Direct exchange, or the débridement of the joint with complete removal of all prosthetic material and immediate reimplantation of the new arthroplasty, has yielded encouraging results in selected patients. This strategy has been most successful when patients have few host comorbidities, the infection is detected early, and sensitive organisms are found.[103-105] However, in North America, two-stage exchange remains the gold standard.[100,106] This strategy includes removal of the infected arthroplasty and all foreign body material followed by placement of an antibiotic-impregnated polymethylmethacrylate spacer and treatment with bacteria-specific parenteral antibiotics. Hanssen and associates[107] found optimal results when patients were treated with two-stage reimplantation and antibiotic-impregnated cement was used for component fixation at the time of reimplantation.

Some authors advocate using static spacers to maintain the joint space and minimize debris generation between stages.[108,109] It is clear that the spacer must span the cortical dimensions of the distal femur and proximal tibia to prevent bone loss.[110,111] Articulating spacers may prevent interim bone loss, improve soft-tissue pliability, and facilitate reimplantation at the second surgery.[110,112-115] In both static and articulating spacers, high local concentration of antibiotic is facilitated through elution of the antibiotics placed in the cement. Several authors have shown the systemic safety of high-dose antibiotic-laden cement between stages.[112,116]

Contraindications to reimplantation include the persistence of infection that cannot be cleared despite aggressive surgical débridement, medical conditions that preclude the patient from returning to the operating room, and patients with severe immunocompromise. Relative contraindications to a reimplantation of a prosthesis include extensor mechanism disruption, very poor bone stock, and a soft-tissue envelope that challenges the healing potential of a reimplantation.

## Constraint in Revision TKA

Tibiofemoral instability is a common cause of failure in TKA. Although most revision TKAs can be made sufficiently stable with either deep-dish or posterior cruciate ligament (PCL)-substituting implant designs, greater degrees of constraint (varus-valgus constraint or hinged constraint) may be necessary. The implant that uses the least amount of constraint necessary to achieve a stable reconstruction should be used.[117,118] Constrained implants use the implant to substitute for the function of incompetent soft tissues and therefore transfer loads to the implant. This may result in load transfer that the implant is mechanically unable to withstand. Early hinged-knee designs had unacceptably high failure rates because these implants allowed movement in only one plane, therefore transferring all rotational forces about the

knee to the implant-bone interfaces. This resulted in catastrophic failures caused by implant fracture and loosening.

PCL insufficiency after cruciate-retaining TKA is a cause of patient dissatisfaction with a reconstruction that may be otherwise well aligned and well fixed to host bone. PCL insufficiency may occur early or late after TKA. These patients often present with anterior knee pain because of extensor mechanism overuse and may not describe their knees as "unstable." Stress lateral radiographs may aid in the diagnosis by revealing posterior translation of the tibia on the femur. If conservative treatment with muscle-strengthening exercises is unsuccessful, revision to a PCL-substituting implant is indicated.

Mediolateral instability must first be addressed by appropriate soft-tissue balancing before resorting to a constrained implant design. Constraint cannot substitute for soft-tissue balancing. Meticulous adherence to a stepwise approach to revision TKA requires that the surgeon achieve implant stability on adequate host bone, reestablish the joint line, and address any ligamentous imbalance issues.

Medial collateral ligament (MCL) competence will most often determine the amount of implant constraint necessary to achieve a stable reconstruction. A lax or absent MCL requires either a varus-valgus constrained or hinged implant. Varus-valgus constrained implant designs feature a taller and wider polyethylene post that is highly congruent with a deeper femoral box. This results in increased mediolateral stability as well as significant rotational constraint. This type of construct places additional stress on the polyethylene post as well as on the

bone-cement interfaces. Rodriguez and associates[119] reported a series of 44 revision TKAs with a modular constrained insert. At a mean of 5.5 years, one knee subsided and one had recurrent sepsis. Radiolucent lines were present at the interfaces of 7 femoral components and 15 tibial components. Hartford and associates[120] reported the results of 33 TKAs with constrained condylar inserts, including 16 revision TKAs. At mean 5-year follow-up, 71% of knees had either femoral or tibial radiolucencies and two components were deemed radiographically loose. Although using a mobile bearing in combination with a varus-valgus constrained insert should decrease the likelihood of complications, there are no published results to date with this type of device.

For a varus-valgus constrained implant to be a viable solution to mediolateral instability with an incompetent or absent MCL, Barrack[121,122] has delineated four minimum criteria that must be met: (1) a flexion/extension gap difference of less than 10 mm, (2) the ability to restore the joint line to within 10 mm of normal, (3) the ability to reconstruct the distal femoral anteroposterior diameter, and (4) some degree of collateral ligament stability. If these requirements are not achievable, then hinged constraint is necessary for achieving stability with the revision reconstruction. Additional indications for hinged constraint include a comminuted distal femoral periprosthetic fracture in an elderly patient, distal femoral nonunion or malunion, or a failed varus-valgus constrained implant. Jones and Barrack have both published their experiences with the S-ROM rotating hinge prosthesis (DePuy Orthopaedics).[121-125] They have reviewed 65 revision knees at a mean of 63 months. There have been no mechanical failures or radiolucent lines around the sleeves or stems.[124]

In a patient with an unstable TKA, revision to a constrained implant design can greatly improve function and satisfaction with the reconstruction. Choosing the least amount of constraint necessary to achieve a stable reconstruction will help avoid unnecessary failures.

## Management of the Stiff TKA

The goal of TKA is to relieve pain, improve function, and maximize range of motion throughout the gait cycle. Unfortunately, optimizing range of motion may be the most poorly understood element of knee replacement. Criteria for activities of daily living mandate 65° for level walking, 85° to ascend stairs, 90° to descend stairs, and 100° to rise from a chair. Those factors that maximize range of motion have been assessed in several studies, and postoperative motion correlates with preoperative motion; however, in some instances patients with limited motion improve postoperatively.[126,127] Other preoperative factors that may mitigate against physiologic range of motion include obesity and medical conditions such as fibromyalgia, depression, chronic fatigue, or anxiety disorders. In addition, those patients with minimal radiographic findings of arthritis preoperatively are particularly at risk for poor results.

Many intraoperative factors that maximize range of motion are directly under a surgeon's control. Proper ligamentous balancing may be the most important factor in maximizing range of motion. In dealing with the deformity, it is important for the surgeon to do a complete concave release to catch up with the stretched convex side or risk tightness on one side of the joint during the flexion arc. Once a rectangular extension gap has been obtained through ligamentous release, it is important for the surgeon to establish a rectangular flexion gap through proper femoral rotation. If a rectangular flexion gap is obtained, difficulties with range of motion should be minimized. However, if the femoral component is internally rotated, a trapezoidal flexion gap will ensue, and the medial structures will be much tighter during the flexion arc than the lateral structures. This leads to a "nutcracker effect" as the knee bends, which leads to painful, limited range of motion.

Once the surgeon establishes rectangular extension and flexion gaps, those gaps must be equalized. The concept of leaving the flexion gap loose to encourage range of motion leads to flexion instability and is not recommended.

Another intraoperative factor that is under a surgeon's control is the height of the patellofemoral joint. The patellofemoral joint height can be increased either by leaving the patella too thick or leaving too much bone in the anterior condyle (reverse notching). Either of these conditions leads to increased retinacular strain that contributes to limited range of motion (an overly tight extensor mechanism).

Sizing of the femoral component is also an important aspect of maximizing range of motion following TKA. Ideally, the kinematics of an individual patient could be maintained by mirroring the sagittal size of the femur with a similarly sized implant. Oversizing the femoral component in the sagittal plane will lead to an overstuffed flexion gap and subsequent loss of range of motion. Undersizing the femoral component leads to early posterior tibial impingement on the femur. The overresected posterior condyle reduces the cam effect and prevents clearance of the tibia, causing it to strike the back of the femur prematurely, limiting motion. Posterior osteophyte retention has the same effect; the posterior tibia will strike the posterior femoral osteophytes, leading to limited range of motion.

Inadequate proximal tibial resection is one technical error that can limit flexion. Most modular tibial trays range from 3 to 5 mm in thickness. Therefore, if not enough proximal tibia is resected and 10-mm-thick polyethylene is placed, the joint will be overstuffed both in flexion and extension. Additionally, if the tibia is cut in reverse slope, more bone will remain in the posterior aspect of the tibia, thus tightening the flexion gap and limiting motion.

Errors in both tibial resection and distal femoral resection can lead to a flexion contracture. Although increased tibial slope can contribute to a flexion contracture, the most common cause of a flexion contracture is inadequate distal femoral resection. In this scenario, the flexion gap is usually bigger than the extension gap. As the surgeon attempts to stabilize the flexion gap by adding polyethylene, the extension gap becomes overstuffed, leading to a flexion contracture. The simple step of resecting a few more millimeters of distal femur to equalize the flexion gap can prevent a flexion contracture.

Prosthetic design also has been implicated in range-of-motion studies. PCL-sacrificing implants have significantly greater range of motion than PCL-retaining implants.[128] PCL-substituting implants have a spine and cam mechanism that promotes rollback and subsequently improves range of motion. Kinematic studies[129] have shown that PCL-substituting implants obtain greater range of motion than PCL-retaining implants because in a PCL-retaining knee there is paradoxical rolling forward of the femur on the tibia with flexion. This causes the posterior tibia to engage the posterior femur earlier than in a substituting knee, where rollback is driven posteriorly by the spine and cam mechanism.

There appears to be no difference in the eventual range of motion regardless of surgical approach.[128] However, there is a lack of consensus in the literature as to whether closure makes any difference. In one study,[130] there was a slight increase in ultimate range of motion closing the knee in flexion, whereas another study[131] showed no significant difference.

Postoperative factors that are important in maximizing range of motion include physical therapy and continuous passive motion. Home physical therapy has the advantage of patient convenience and the disadvantage of variable quality. With office physical therapy, quality is controlled and proper equipment is accessible. The major disadvantage is patient inconvenience. One study compared physical therapy with continuous passive motion and found no difference in range of motion and lower cost with continued passive motion.[132] Multiple studies concerning continuous passive motion machines have shown no difference in ultimate motion.[133-136] However, patient expectations and comfort with this machine have led to its continuous use.

To maximize range of motion, those few patients who require manipulation following TKA must be identified early. It is therefore important to maintain a careful follow-up schedule postoperatively. All patients should be seen in the first 2 to 3 weeks following surgery to identify those patients with a predisposition to stiffness. At this point, their physical therapy efforts can be maximized and attempts made to prevent them from needing a knee manipulation by increasing the frequency of their physical therapy visits. If the patient has not regained adequate motion as determined by the surgeon, the patient's manipulation should be done in the first 6 to 8 weeks postoperatively, before maturation of fibroblasts. Manipulation has been shown to have a positive effect on those knees that were stiff during this time frame.[137] It is very important that manipulation be done carefully, with stress only on the proximal half of the tibia, to avoid putting too much force on the quadriceps tendon or distal femur. The ankle should never be used as a lever during manipulation.

Flexion contractures can also be manipulated in the early postoperative period. This is usually done in conjunction with manipulation for stiffness. If there is a small residual flexion contracture following surgery, which is not uncommon, gait training to ensure heel-toe ambulation is stressed with the patient. Also, if a 0.5-in shoe lift is placed on the nonoperated foot, this relatively lengthens the nonoperated leg. This causes the patient to stretch the posterior capsule on the surgical side when attempting to reach the floor during gait. Thus, every step becomes therapeutic. This is a simple way to hasten treatment of minor flexion contractures.

Established flexion contractures greater than 15° may require surgical treatment. Significant improvement in flexion contractures has been shown to occur through rebalancing the flexion-extension gaps.[138]

Surgical treatment of stiffness remains a controversial aspect of TKA. Arthroscopic release of the PCL to improve stiffness in PCL-retaining knees has been shown to be successful in a limited series.[139] However, arthroscopic treatment of pure arthrofibrosis has been less successful.[140,141] Open procedures such as débridement of scar tissue and polyethylene exchange have also led to mixed results. According to one study,[142] results were poor in 7 patients, whereas in another study of 18 patients,[143] there was a mean increase in range of motion of 31°. However, only two thirds of these patients had good or excellent Knee Society scores.

Three studies of revision TKA for stiffness also have shown mixed results functionally.[144-146] Most patients, however, were satisfied with the range of motion that they eventually obtained. The largest study reported on 56 knees. Significant improvement in Knee Society clinical scores was noted; 52 patients (93%) had an increase in motion. Although 37 patients (66%) had a 20° increase in range of motion, the mean increase was only from 65° to 85°. This range of motion was still well below what is required for rising from a chair.

The key to maximizing range of motion is prevention. Careful ligamentous balancing and follow-up to determine which patients require manipulation are important factors that must be understood by all knee surgeons. Late treatment is frustrating for the patient and surgeon alike.

## Summary

Revision TKA has become a commonly performed reconstructive procedure in adults. The ability to correctly identify failure mechanisms is mandatory for successful treatment. The operating surgeon must be cognizant of a variety of exposure options and methods to extract existing implants safely. It must be understood that like primary surgery, revision TKA is a soft-tissue procedure in which the importance of axial alignment, soft-tissue balancing, and gap equalization are prerequisites for success.

The modular stem and augment options currently available should help the surgeon manage most bone defects that are commonly encountered. The surgeon should be vigilant for progressive osteolysis and should intervene prior to catastrophic failure. Careful preoperative evaluation for occult infection is as important as an algorithmic approach to the management of an established prosthetic joint infection. Recognition of instability as a leading cause of failure is important when a patient presents postoperatively with symptoms of pain and normal-appearing radiographs. A systematic approach to the painful TKA should optimize outcomes for these patients.

## References

1. Fehring TK, McAvoy G: Fluoroscopic evaluation of the painful total knee arthroplasty. *Clin Orthop Relat Res* 1996;331:226-233.

2. Mason JB, Fehring TK, Odum SM, Griffin WL, Nussman DS: The value of white blood cell counts before revision total knee arthroplasty. *J Arthroplasty* 2003;18:1038-1043.

3. Barrack RL, Rorabeck C, Burt M, Sawney J: Pain at the end of the stem after revision total knee arthroplsty. *Clin Orthop Relat Res* 1999;367:216-225.

4. Pollock DC, Ammeen DJ, Engh GA: Synovial entrapment: A complication of posterior stabilized total knee arthroplasty. *J Bone Joint Surg Am* 2002;84:2174-2178.

5. Sharkey PF, Hozack WJ, Rothman RH, Shastri S, Jacoby SM: Why are total knee arthroplasties failing today? *Clin Orthop Relat Res* 2002;404:7-13.

6. Jazrawi LM, Birdzell L, Kummer FJ, DiCesare PE: The accuracy of computed tomography for determining femoral and tibial total knee arthroplasty component rotation. *J Arthroplasty* 2000;15:761-766.

7. Fehring TK, Odum S, Griffin WL, Mason JB: Patella inversion method for exposure in revision total knee arthroplasty. *J Arthroplasty* 2002;17:101-104.

8. Rand JA, Morrey BF, Bryan RS: Patellar tendon rupture after total knee arthroplasty. *Clin Orthop Relat Res* 1989;244:233-238.

9. Coonse K, Adams JD: A new operative approach to the knee joint. *Surg Gynecol Obstet* 1943;77:344-347.

10. Insall JN (ed): *Surgery of the Knee*. New York, NY, Churchill Livingstone, 1984.

11. Scott RD, Siliski JM: The use of a modified V-Y quadricepsplasty during total knee replacement to gain exposure and improve flexion in the ankylosed knee. *Orthopedics* 1985;8:45-48.

12. Trousdale RT, Hanssen AD, Rand JA, Cahalan TD: V-Y quadricepsplasty in total knee arthroplasty. *Clin Orthop Relat Res* 1993;286:48-55.

13. Garvin KL, Scuderi G, Insall JN: Evolution of the quadriceps snip. *Clin Orthop Relat Res* 1995;321:131-137.

14. Dolin MG: Osteotomy of the tibial tubercle in total knee replacement. *J Bone Joint Surg Am* 1983;65:704-706.

15. Whiteside LA, Ohl MD: Tibial tubercle osteotomy for exposure of the difficult total knee arthroplasty. *Clin Orthop Relat Res* 1990;260:6-9.

16. Ries MD, Richman JA: Extended tibial tubercle osteotomy in total knee arthroplasty. *J Arthroplasty* 1996;11:964-967.

17. Ritter MA, Carr KE, Keating M, Faris PM, Meding JB: Tibial shaft fracture following tibial tubercle osteotomy. *J Arthroplasty* 1996;11:117-119.

18. Wolff AM, Hungerford DS, Krackow KA, Jacobs MA: Osteotomy of the tibial tubercle during total knee replacement. *J Bone Joint Surg Am* 1989;71:848-852.

19. Windsor RE, Insall NJ: Exposure in revision total knee arthroplasty: The femoral peel. *Tech Orthop* 1988;3:1.

20. Barrack RL, Smith P, Munn B, Engh G, Rorabeck C: Comparison of surgical approaches in total knee arthroplasty. *Clin Orthop Relat Res* 1998;356:16-21.

21. Lotke PA, Garino JP (eds): Surgical exposures in revision total knee arthroplasty, in *Revision Total Knee Arthroplasty*. Philadelphia, PA, Lippincott-Raven, 1999.

22. Masri BA, Mitchell PA, Duncan CP: Removal of solidly fixed implants during revision hip and knee arthroplasty. *J Am Acad Orthop Surg* 2005;13:18-27.

23. Dennis DA: Removal of well-fixed cementless metal-backed patellar components. *J Arthroplasty* 1992;7:217-220.

24. Figgie HE III, Goldberg VM, Heiple KG, Moller HS III, Gordon NH: The influence of tibial-patellofemoral location on function of the knee in patients with the posterior stabilized condylar knee prosthesis. *J Bone Joint Surg Am* 1986;68:1035-1040.

25. Pagnano MW, Hanssen AD, Lewallen DG, Stuart MJ: Flexion instability after primary posterior cruciate retaining total knee arthroplasty. *Clin Orthop Relat Res* 1998;356:39-46.

26. Buechel FF: A sequential three-step lateral release for correcting fixed valgus knee deformities during total knee arthroplasty. *Clin Orthop Relat Res* 1990;260:170-175.

27. Waslewski GL, Marson BM, Benjamin JB: Early, incapacitating instability of posterior cruciate

ligament-retaining total knee arthroplasty. *J Arthroplasty* 1998;13:763-767.

28. Galinat BJ, Vernace JV, Booth RE Jr, Rothman RH: Dislocation of the posterior stabilized total knee arthroplasty: A report of two cases. *J Arthroplasty* 1988;3:363-367.

29. Gebhard JS, Kilgus DJ: Dislocation of a posterior stabilized total knee prosthesis: A report of two cases. *Clin Orthop Relat Res* 1990;254:225-229.

30. Mont MA, Delanois R, Hungerford DS: Balancing and alignment, surgical techniques on how to achieve soft-tissue balancing, in *Revision Total Knee Arthroplasty*. Baltimore, MD, Lippincott, Williams, and Wilkins, 1998, pp 173-186.

31. Ranawat CS: Technique of bone cuts with conventional instruments, in *Total Condylar Knee Arthroplasty: Techniques, Results and Complications.* New York, NY, Springer, 1985, pp 54-68.

32. Insall JN, Easley ME: Surgical techniques and instrumentation in total knee arthroplasty, in Insall JN, Scott WN (eds): *Surgery of the Knee*, ed 3. New York, NY, Churchill Livingstone, 2001, vol 2, pp 1553-1620.

33. Lotke PA, Ecker L: Influence of positioning of prosthesis in total knee replacement. *J Bone Joint Surg Am* 1977; 59:77-79.

34. Sidles JA, Matsen FA, Garlini JL, et al: Total knee arthroplasty: Functional effects of tibial resection level. *Trans Orthop Res Soc* 1986;12:263.

35. Whiteside LA: Selective ligament release in total knee arthroplasty of the knee in valgus. *Clin Orthop Relat Res* 1999;367:130-140.

36. Stiehl JB, Abbott BD: Morphology of the transepicondylar axis and its application in primary and revision total knee arthroplasty. *J Arthroplasty* 1995; 10:785-789.

37. Kelly MA: Ligament instability in total knee arthroplasty. *Instr Course Lect* 2001;50:399-401.

38. Ries MD, Haas SB, Windsor RE: Soft tissue balance in revision total knee arthroplasty. *J Bone Joint Surg Am* 2003;85:S38-S42.

39. Laskin RS: Joint line position restoration during revision total knee replacement. *Clin Orthop Relat Res* 2002; 404:169-171.

40. Martin JW, Whiteside LA: The influence of joint line position on knee stability after condylar knee arthroplasty. *Clin Orthop Relat Res* 1990;259: 146-156.

41. McDermott B: Restoration of stability, maintaining joint line, gap balancing, and constraint selection, in *Revision Total Knee Arthroplasty*. New York, NY, Springer, 2005, pp 145-151.

42. Engh GA, Ammeen DJ: Bone loss with revision total knee arthroplasty: Defect classification and alternatives for reconstruction. *Instr Course Lect* 1999;48:167-175.

43. Mulhall KJ, Ghomrawi HM, Engh GA, Clark CR, Lotke P, Saleh KJ: Radiographic prediction of intraoperative bone loss in knee arthroplasty revision. *Clin Orthop Relat Res* 2006;446:51-58.

44. Brand MG, Daley RJ, Ewald FC, Scott RD: Tibial tray augmentation with modular metal wedges for tibial bone stock deficiency. *Clin Orthop Relat Res* 1989;248:71-79.

45. Pagnano MW, Trousdale RT, Rand JA: Tibial wedge augmentation for bone deficiency in total knee arthroplasty: A followup study. *Clin Orthop Relat Res* 1995;321:151-155.

46. Jones RE, Barrack RL, Skedros J: Modular, mobile-bearing hinge total knee arthroplasty. *Clin Orthop Relat Res* 2001;392:306-314.

47. Radnay CS, Scuderi GR: Management of bone loss: Augments, cones, offset stems. *Clin Orthop Relat Res* 2006;446:83-92.

48. Springer BD, Sim FH, Hanssen AD, Lewallen DG: The modular segmental kinematic rotating hinge for nonneoplastic limb salvage. *Clin Orthop Relat Res* 2004;421:181-187.

49. Bourne RB, Finlay JB: The influence of tibial component intramedullary stems and implant-cortex contact on the strain distribution of the proximal part of the tibia: An in vitro study. *Clin Orthop Relat Res* 1986;208: 95-101.

50. Brooks PJ, Walker PJ, Scott RD: Tibial component fixation in deficient tibial bone stock. *Clin Orthop Relat Res* 1984;184:302-308.

51. Jazrawi LM, Bai B, Kummer FJ, Hiebert R, Stuchin SA: The effect of stem modularity and mode of fixation on tibial component stability in revision total knee arthroplasty. *J Arthroplasty* 2001;16:759-767.

52. Stern SH, Wills D, Gilbert JL: The effect of tibial stem design on component micromotion in knee arthroplasty. *Clin Orthop Relat Res* 1997;345: 44-51.

53. Bert JM, McShane M: Is it necessary to cement the tibial stem to improve implant stability in cemented total knee arthroplasty? *Clin Orthop Relat Res* 1998;356:73-78.

54. Murray PB, Rand JA, Hanssen AD: Cemented long-stem revision total knee arthroplasty. *Clin Orthop Relat Res* 1994;309:116-123.

55. Whaley AL, Trousdale RT, Rand JA, Hanssen AD: Cemented long-stem revision total knee arthroplasty. *J Arthroplasty* 2003;18:592-599.

56. Haas SB, Insall JN, Montgomery W, Windsor RE: Revision total knee arthroplasty with use of modular components with stems inserted without cement. *J Bone Joint Surg Am* 1995;77: 1700-1707.

57. Gofton WT, Tsigaras H, Butler RA, Patterson JJ, Barrack RL, Rorabeck CH: Revision total knee arthroplasty: Fixation with modular stems. *Clin Orthop Relat Res* 2002;404: 158-168.

58. Shannon BD, Klassen JF, Rand JA, Berry DJ, Trousdale RT: Revision total knee arthroplasty with cemented components and uncemented intramedullary stems. *J Arthroplasty* 2003;18:27-32.

59. Fehring TK, Odum S, Olekson C, Griffin WL, Mason JB, McCoy TH: Stem fixation in revision total knee

arthroplasty: A comparative analysis. *Clin Orthop Relat Res* 2003;416: 217-224.

60. Peters PC, Engh GA, Dwyer KA, Vinh TN: Osteolysis after total knee arthroplasty without cement. *J Bone Joint Surg Am* 1992;74:864-876.

61. Naudie DD, Ammeen DJ, Engh GA, Rorabeck CH: Wear and osteolysis around total knee arthroplasty. *J Am Acad Orthop Surg* 2007;15:53-64.

62. Nadaud MC, Fehring TK, Fehring K: Underestimation of osteolysis in posterior stabilized total knee arthroplasty. *J Arthroplasty* 2004;19:110-115.

63. Engh GA, Ammeen DJ: Epidemiology of osteolysis: Backside implant wear. *Instr Course Lect* 2004;53: 243-249.

64. Collier MB, Engh CA Jr, McAuley JP, Ginn SD, Engh GA: Osteolysis after total knee arthroplasty: Influence of baseplate surface finish and sterilization of polyethylene insert. *J Bone Joint Surg Am* 2005;87:2702-2708.

65. Fehring TK, Murphy JA, Hayes TD, Roberts DW, Pomeroy DL, Griffin WL: Factors influencing wear and osteolysis in press-fit condylar modular total knee replacements. *Clin Orthop Relat Res* 2004;428:40-50.

66. Puloski SK, McCalden RW, MacDonald SJ, Rorabeck CH, Bourne RB: Tibial post wear in posterior stabilized total knee arthroplasty: An unrecognized source of polyethylene debris. *J Bone Joint Surg Am* 2001;83: 390-397.

67. Rand JA: Extensor mechanism complications following total knee arthroplasty. *J Knee Surg* 2003;16:224-228.

68. Pagnano MW: Patellar tendon and quadriceps tendon tears after total knee arthroplasty. *J Knee Surg* 2003; 16:242-247.

69. Cooney WP, Sierra RJ, Trousdale RT, Pagnano MW: Revision total knees done for extensor problems frequently require reoperation. *Clin Orthop Relat Res* 2005;440:117-121.

70. Dobbs RE, Hanssen AD, Lewallen DG, Pagnano MW: Quadriceps tendon rupture after total knee arthroplasty: Prevalence, complications, and outcomes. *J Bone Joint Surg Am* 2005; 87:37-45.

71. Barrack RL, Butler RA, Valenzuela R: Extensor mechanism disruption after total knee arthroplasty: When the unthinkable happens. *Orthopedics* 2002; 25:981-982.

72. Nazarian DG, Booth RE Jr: Extensor mechanism allografts in total knee arthroplasty. *Clin Orthop Relat Res* 1999; 367:123-129.

73. Emerson RH Jr, Head WC, Malinin TI: Extensor mechanism reconstruction with an allograft after total knee arthroplasty. *Clin Orthop Relat Res* 1994;303:79-85.

74. Cadambi A, Engh GA: Use of a semitendinosus tendon autogenous graft for rupture of the patellar ligament after total knee arthroplasty: A report of seven cases. *J Bone Joint Surg Am* 1992; 74:974-979.

75. Leopold SS, Greidanus N, Paprosky WG, Berger RA, Rosenberg AG: High rate of failure of allograft reconstruction of the extensor mechanism after total knee arthroplasty. *J Bone Joint Surg Am* 1999;81:1574-1579.

76. Burnett RS, Berger RA, Paprosky WG, Della Valle CJ, Jacobs JJ, Rosenberg AG: Extensor mechanism allograft reconstruction after total knee arthroplasty: A comparison of two techniques. *J Bone Joint Surg Am* 2004; 86:2694-2699.

77. Kollender Y, Bender B, Weinbroum AA, Nirkin A, Meller I, Bickels J: Secondary reconstruction of the extensor mechanism using part of the quadriceps tendon, patellar retinaculum, and Gore-Tex strips after proximal tibial resection. *J Arthroplasty* 2004;19:354-360.

78. Barrack RL, Stanley T, Allen-Butler R: Treating extensor mechanism disruption after total knee arthroplasty. *Clin Orthop Relat Res* 2003;416: 98-104.

79. Emerson RH Jr, Head WC, Malinin TI: Reconstruction of patellar tendon rupture after total knee arthroplasty with an extensor mechanism allograft. *Clin Orthop Relat Res* 1990; 260:154-161.

80. Crossett LS, Sinha RK, Sechriest VF, Rubash HE: Reconstruction of a ruptured patellar tendon with Achilles tendon allograft following total knee arthroplasty. *J Bone Joint Surg Am* 2002;84:1354-1361.

81. Ip D, Yam SK, Chen CK: Implications of the changing pattern of bacterial infections following total joint replacements. *J Orthop Surg (Hong Kong)* 2005;13:125-130.

82. Silva M, Tharani R, Schmalzried TP: Results of direct exchange or debridement of the infected total knee arthroplasty. *Clin Orthop Relat Res* 2002; 404:125-131.

83. Morrey BF, Westholm F, Schoifet S, Rand JA, Bryan RS: Long-term results of various treatment options for infected total knee arthroplasty. *Clin Orthop Relat Res* 1989;248:120-128.

84. Yoon SI, Lim SS, Rha JD, Kim YH, Kang JS, Baek GH: The C-reactive protein (CRP) in patients with long bone fractures and after arthroplasty. *Int Orthop* 1993;17:198-201.

85. Lachiewicz PF, Rogers GD, Thomason HC: Aspiration of the hip joint before revision total hip arthroplasty. *J Bone Joint Surg Am* 1996;78:749-754.

86. Barrack RL, Jennings RW, Wolfe MW, Bertot AJ: The value of preoperative aspiration before total knee revision. *Clin Orthop Relat Res* 1997;345:8-16.

87. Demirkol MO, Adalet I, Unal SN, Tözün R, Cantez S: 99Tc(m)-polyclonal IgG scintigraphy in the detection of infected hip and knee prostheses. *Nucl Med Commun* 1997; 18:543.

88. Rand JA, Brown MD, Manuel L: The value of indium 111 leukocyte scanning in the evaluation of painful or infected total knee arthroplasties. *Clin Orthop Relat Res* 1990;259:179-182.

89. Palestro CJ, Swyer AJ, Kim CK, et al: Infected knee prosthesis: Diagnosis with In-111 leukocyte, Tc-99m sulfur colloid and Tc-99m MDP imaging. *Radiology* 1991;179:645-648.

90. Panousis K, Grigoris P, Butcher I, Rana B, Reilly JH, Hamblen DL: Poor predictive value of broad-range PCR for the detection of arthroplasty infection in 92 cases. *Acta Orthop* 2005;76:341-346.

91. Fehring TK, McAlister JA Jr: Frozen histologic section as a guide to sepsis in revision joint arthroplasty. *Clin Orthop Relat Res* 1994;304:229-237.

92. Lonner JH, Desai P, Dicesare PE, Steiner G, Zuckerman JD: The reliability of analysis of intraoperative frozen sections for identifying active infection during revision hip or knee arthroplasty. *J Bone Joint Surg Am* 1996;78:1553-1558.

93. Della Valle CJ, Bogner E, Desai P, et al: Analysis of frozen sections of intraoperative specimens obtained at the time of reoperation after hip or knee resection arthroplasty for the treatment of infection. *J Bone Joint Surg Am* 1999;81:684-689.

94. Klinger HM, Spahn G, Schultz W, Baums MH: Arthrodesis of the knee after failed infected total knee arthroplasty. *Knee Surg Sports Traumatol Arthrosc* 2006;14:447-453.

95. Crockarell JR Jr, Mihalko MJ: Knee arthrodesis using an intramedullary nail. *J Arthroplasty* 2005;20:703-708.

96. Kirpalani PA, In Y, Choi NY, Koh HS, Kim JM, Han CW: Two-stage total knee arthroplasty for non-salvageable septic arthritis in diabetes mellitus patients. *Acta Orthop Belg* 2005;71:315-320.

97. Kuo AC, Meehan JP, Lee M: Knee fusion using dual platings with the locking compression plate. *J Arthroplasty* 2005;20:772-776.

98. Cuckler JM: The infected total knee: Management options. *J Arthroplasty* 2005;20:33-36.

99. Freeman MA, Sudlow RA, Casewell MW, Radcliff SS: The management of infected total knee replacements. *J Bone Joint Surg Br* 1985;67:764-768.

100. Trousdale RT, Hanssen AD: Infection after total knee arthroplasty. *Instr Course Lect* 2001;50:409-414.

101. Waldman BJ, Mont MA, Yoon TR, Hungersford DS: Infected total knee arthroplasty treated by arthroscopic irrigation and débridement. *65th Annual Meeting Final Program*. Rosemont, IL, American Academy of Orthopaedic Surgeons, 1998, p 169.

102. Ilahi OA, Al-Habbal GA, Bocell JR, Tullos HS, Huo MH: Arthroscopic debridement of acute periprosthetic septic arthritis of the knee. *Arthroscopy* 2005;21:303-306.

103. Buechel FF, Femino FP, D'Alessio J: Primary exchange revision arthroplasty for infected total knee replacement: A long-term study. *Am J Orthop* 2004;33:190-198.

104. Goksan SB, Freeman MA: One-stage reimplantation for infected total knee arthroplasty. *J Bone Joint Surg Br* 1992;74:78-82.

105. Volin SJ, Hinrichs SH, Garvin KL: Two-stage reimplantation of total joint infections: A comparison of resistant and non-resistant organisms. *Clin Orthop Relat Res* 2004;427:94-100.

106. Hanssen AD, Trousdale RT, Osmon DR: Patient outcome with reinfection following reimplantation for the infected total knee arthroplasty. *Clin Orthop Relat Res* 1995;321:55-67.

107. Hanssen AD, Rand JA, Osmon DR: Treatment of the infected total knee arthroplasty with insertion of another prosthesis: The effect of antibiotic-impregnated bone cement. *Clin Orthop Relat Res* 1994;309:44-55.

108. Booth RE Jr, Lotke PA: The results of spacer block technique in revision of infected total knee arthroplasty. *Clin Orthop Relat Res* 1989;248:57-60.

109. Pitto RP, Spika IA: Antibiotic-loaded bone cement spacers in two-stage management of infected total knee arthroplasty. *Int Orthop* 2004;28:129-133.

110. Fehring TK, Odum SM, Calton TF, Mason JB: Articulating versus static spacers in revision total knee arthroplasty for sepsis. *Clin Orthop Relat Res* 2000;380:9-16.

111. MacAvoy MC, Ries MD: The ball

and socket articulating spacer for infected total knee arthroplasty. *J Arthroplasty* 2005;20:757-762.

112. Emerson RH Jr, Muncie M, Tarbox TR, Higgins LL: Comparison of a static with a mobile spacer in total knee infection. *Clin Orthop Relat Res* 2002;404:132-138.

113. Meek RM, Dunlop D, Garbuz DS, McGraw R, Greidanus NV, Masri BA: Patient satisfaction and functional status after aseptic versus septic revision total knee arthroplasty using the PROSTALAC articulating spacer. *J Arthroplasty* 2004;19:874-879.

114. Hendel D, Weisbort M, Garti A: "Wandering resident" surgical exposure for 1- or 2-stage revision arthroplasty in stiff aseptic and septic knee arthroplasty. *J Arthroplasty* 2004;19:757-759.

115. Hofmann AA, Goldbert TD, Tanner AM, Cook TM: Ten-year experience using an articulating antibiotic cement hip spacer for the treatment of chronically infected total hip. *J Arthroplasty* 2005;20:874-879.

116. Springer BD, Lee GC, Osmon D, Haidukewych GJ, Hanssen AD, Jacofsky DJ: Systemic safety of high-dose antiobiotic-loaded cement spacers after resection of an infected total knee arthroplasty. *Clin Orthop Relat Res* 2004;427:47-51.

117. Fehring TK, Valadie AL: Knee instability after total knee arthroplasty. *Clin Orthop Relat Res* 1994;299:157-162.

118. Naudie DD, Rorabeck CH: Managing instability in total knee arthroplasty with constrained and linked implants. *Instr Course Lect* 2004;53:207-215.

119. Rodriguez JA, Shahane S, Rasquinha VJ, Ranawat CS: Does the total condylar 3 constrained knee prosthesis predispose to failure of revision total knee replacement? *J Bone Joint Surg Am* 2003;85:153-156.

120. Hartford JM, Goodman SB, Schurman DJ, Knoblick G: Complex primary and revision total knee arthroplasty using the condylar constrained

prosthesis: An average 5-year follow-up. *J Arthroplasty* 1998;13:380-387.

121. Barrack RL: Evolution of the rotating hinge for complex total knee arthroplasty. *Clin Orthop Relat Res* 2001;392:292-299.

122. Barrack RL: Rise of the rotating hinge in revision total knee arthroplasty. *Orthopedics* 2002;25:1020-1058.

123. Jones RE: Mobile bearings in revision total knee arthroplasty. *Instr Course Lect* 2005;54:225-231.

124. Jones RE: Total knee arthroplasty with modular rotating-platform hinge. *Orthopedics* 2006;29:S80-S82.

125. Jones RE, Barrack RL, Skedros J: Modular, mobile-bearing hinge total knee arthroplasty. *Clin Orthop Relat Res* 2001;392:306-314.

126. Ritter MA, Stringer EA: Predictive range of motion after total knee replacement. *Clin Orthop Relat Res* 1979;143:115-119.

127. Parsley BS, Engh GA, Dwyer KA: Preoperative flexion: Does it influence postoperative flexion after posterior-cruciate-retaining total knee arthroplasty? *Clin Orthop Relat Res* 1992;275:204-210.

128. Hirsch HS, Lotke PA, Morrison LD: The posterior cruciate ligament in total knee surgery: Save, sacrifice, or substitute? *Clin Orthop Relat Res* 1994;309:64-68.

129. Dennis DA, Komistek RD, Colwell CE Jr, et al: In vivo anteroposterior femorotibial translation of total knee arthroplasty: A multicenter analysis. *Clin Orthop Relat Res* 1998;356:47-57.

130. Emerson RH, Ayers C, Higgins LL: Surgical closing in total knee arthroplasty: A series follow-up. *Clin Orthop Relat Res* 1999;368:176-181.

131. Masri BA, Laskin RS, Windsor RE, Haas SB: Knee closure in total knee replacement: A randomized prospective trial. *Clin Orthop Relat Res* 1996;331:81-86.

132. Worland RL, Arrendondo J, Angles F, Lopez-Jimenez F, Jessup DE: Home continuous passive motion machine versus professional physical therapy following total knee replacement. *J Arthroplasty* 1998;13:784-787.

133. Maloney WJ, Schurman DJ, Hangen D, Goodman SB, Edworthy S, Bloch A: The influence of continuous passive motion on outcome in total knee arthroplasty. *Clin Orthop Relat Res* 1990;256:162-168.

134. Lynch AF, Bourne RB, Rorabeck CH, Rankin RN, Donald A: Deep-vein thrombosis and continuous passive motion after total knee arthroplasty. *J Bone Joint Surg Am* 1988;70:11-14.

135. Ritter MA, Gandolf VS, Holston KS: Continuous passive motion versus physical therapy in total knee arthroplasty. *Clin Orthop Relat Res* 1989;244:239-243.

136. Pope RO, Corcoran S, McCaul K, Howie DW: Continuous passive motion after primary total knee arthroplasty: Does it offer any benefits? *J Bone Joint Surg Br* 1997;79:914-917.

137. Esler CNA, Lock K, Harper WM, Gregg PJ: Manipulation of total knee replacements. *J Bone Joint Surg Br* 1999;81:27-29.

138. Fehring TK, Odum S, Griffin WL, Masonis J, Springer BS: Surgical treatment of flexion contractures following total knee arthroplasty. *J Arthroplasty* 2007;22(suppl 2):62-70.

139. Williams RJ, Westrich GH, Siegel J, Windsor RE: Arthroscopic release of the posterior cruciate ligament for stiff total knee arthroplasty. *Clin Orthop Relat Res* 1996;331:185-191.

140. Bocell JR, Thorpe CD, Tullos HS: Arthroscopic treatment of symptomatic total knee arthroplasty. *Clin Orthop Relat Res* 1991;271:125-134.

141. Sprague NF III, O'Connor RL, Fox JM: Arthroscopic treatment of postoperative knee fibroarthrosis. *Clin Orthop Relat Res* 1982;166:165-172.

142. Babis GC, Trousdale RT, Pagnano MW, Morrey BF: Poor outcomes of isolated tibial insert exchange and arthrolysis for the management of stiffness following total knee arthroplasty. *J Bone Joint Surg Am* 2001;83:1534-1536.

143. Mont MA, Seyler TM, Marulanda GA, Delanois RE, Bhave A: Surgical treatment and customized rehabilitation for stiff knee arthroplasties. *Clin Orthop Relat Res* 2006;446:193-200.

144. Kim J, Nelson CL, Lotke PA: Stiffness after total knee arthroplasty. *J Bone Joint Surg Am* 2004;86:1479-1484

145. Nicholls DW, Dorr LD: Revision surgery for stiff total knee arthroplasty. *J Arthroplasty* 1990;5:S73-S77.

146. Christensen CP, Crawford JJ, Olin MD, Vail TP: Revision of the stiff total knee arthroplasty. *J Arthroplasty* 2002;17:409-415.

# Controversies and Techniques in the Surgical Management of Patellofemoral Arthritis

*William M. Mihalko, MD, PhD
Yaw Boachie-Adjei, MD
Jeffrey T. Spang, MD
*John P. Fulkerson, MD
Elizabeth A. Arendt, MD
*Khaled J. Saleh, MD

## Abstract

*Historically, the patellofemoral articulation has been a topic of less interest among orthopaedists and has been subject to fewer studies when compared with other major joints in the body. Patellofemoral arthritis is a common and debilitating condition, and greater awareness of this has led to a new interest and recent increase in the number of clinical investigations pertaining to this condition. It is hoped that an overview of patellofemoral kinematics, forces, and contact patterns will help in understanding the progression of patellofemoral arthritis. Furthermore, this understanding will ultimately allow the surgeon to apply these basic principles to more effective nonsurgical and surgical treatment options. Treatment methods for patellofemoral arthritis include both conservative as well as surgical interventions. Specifically, these treatments range from stretching and water exercises to patellar realignment procedures and the recently developed procedure of custom patellofemoral arthroplasty. In addition, many new and innovative treatments are on the horizon. This renewed interest in the patellofemoral articulation bodes well for patients who suffer from this condition.*

**Instr Course Lect 2008;57:365-380.**

The patellofemoral joint is a complex articulation that remains a relatively uncommon topic in orthopaedic literature. Most studies have been of cadavers, and there have been very few in vivo or clinical measurements.[1] The relative lack of interest in the patellofemoral joint is surprising given the fact that patellofemoral symptoms are relatively common and can be extremely debilitating.

Abnormal mechanics of the patellofemoral articulation lead to abnormal pressures on the articular surface, pain, cartilage breakdown, and severe functional limitations secondary to anterior knee pain.[2] An understanding of basic concepts regarding patellofemoral joint kinematics, forces, and contact patterns will enhance the surgeon's understanding of the progression of patellofemoral arthritis. Furthermore, this understanding should ultimately allow the surgeon to choose the appropriate option for each stage of patellofemoral disease.

## Anatomic Considerations

The patellofemoral joint comprises the patella, the femoral condyles, and the trochlear groove. The patella is a sesamoid bone that acts to redirect the forces of the quadriceps to the distal part of the femur,

*William M. Mihalko, MD, PhD or the department with which he is affiliated has received research or institutional support from Smith & Nephew and is a consultant or employee for Stryker Orthopaedics, Smith & Nephew, and Ethicon. John P. Fulkerson, MD or the department with which he is affiliated has received royalties from DJ Ortho. Khaled J. Saleh, MD, MSc(Epid), FRCSC or the department with which he is affiliated has received research or institutional support from Stryker Orthopaedics and Smith & Nephew and is a consultant or employee for Stryker Orthopaedics and Smith & Nephew.

functioning as a lever arm to increase the efficiency of the extensor mechanism. The femoral condyles have a dual articulation with the medial and lateral facets of the patella.[3] Additionally, almost 75% of people have a third articulating facet on the medial ridge of the patella that articulates with the medial femoral condyle after 120° of flexion.[4] The ridge of the lateral condyle is more prominent than the medial ridge on lateral radiographs of the knee. A deficient lateral condyle may be appreciated on lateral radiographs and may contribute to patellar instability. Between the condyles is the central sulcus, or trochlear groove. The quadriceps and the patellar tendon have a balanced, blended insertion and origin on the patella and generate most of the forces acting on the patella.

The flexion-extension pathway of the patellofemoral joint is a complex and dynamic cycle. In full extension, the patella does not come into contact with the trochlear groove. As knee flexion is initiated, the inferior pole comes into contact with the trochlea. As knee flexion continues from 0° to 90°, the area of patellofemoral contact moves proximally on the patella, from the inferior pole toward the central portion, and finally toward the superior pole. At 90° of flexion, only the superior region of the patella is in contact with the distal aspect of the trochlear groove.[5] After 120° of flexion, only the most medial and lateral aspects of the patella come into contact with the femoral condyles. The articular cartilage of the patella is the thickest of any in the body, an adaptation to the great pressures throughout the patellofemoral joint during knee flexion.[6] Most patellar motion occurs in the sagittal plane with knee flexion.

## Joint Forces

In early flexion, there is a small compressive force vector on the patellofemoral joint. As flexion increases, so do the compressive forces across the joint. The three major forces acting on the patella include (1) the pull of the quadriceps, (2) the tension in the patellar tendon, and (3) the joint reactive force of the patellofemoral joint. These forces must act through one point in the sagittal plane to be in equilibrium. Unlike a simple lever arm, the patella creates a changing fulcrum position for the quadriceps force. The patellar tendon force is therefore always less than the quadriceps force and is more pronounced in deep flexion. As detailed earlier, in early flexion this point is in the inferior pole of the patella, and in deeper flexion this point moves to the superior pole. Estimates of the forces through the patella range from 1.5 times body weight at 30° of flexion to six times body weight at 90° of flexion. Some authors[6,7] have suggested that contact between the quadriceps tendon and the distal part of the femur helps to dissipate contact forces after 90° of knee flexion.

## Patellofemoral Contact Patterns

As the contact point of the patella migrates from the inferior pole in early flexion to the superior pole in deep flexion, the contact surface area increases. There is a steady increase in contact surface area from initial contact in early flexion to about 60°. There are mixed reports regarding the area of patellofemoral contact from 60° to 90°[6]. After 90° of flexion, the reported amounts of contact area have varied, depending on individual anatomy, the amount of force applied by the quadriceps tendon, and

the thickness of the articular cartilage. It should also be noted that the quadriceps tendon plays a large role in the transfer of load. Past 90° of flexion, the tendon transfers load to the trochlear groove of the femur, providing more contact as well.[8]

## History and Physical Examination of Patients With an Arthritic Patellofemoral Joint

Examination of a patient with anterior knee pain begins, like any other medical workup, with a thorough and detailed history. Gathering information such as the duration of discomfort, the location and quality of pain, provocative or palliative factors, and functional limitation is a key portion of the patient evaluation. The summation of these facts will give the orthopaedic surgeon important clues regarding the etiology and diagnosis of the knee pain. Patients with patellofemoral arthritis often present with anterior knee pain, which may radiate medially and/or posteriorly. The pain is often worse with prolonged flexion or when the patient is descending stairs. Knee catching, locking, or giving way are less specific symptoms that may or may not represent pathologic involvement of the patellofemoral joint. The subsequent physical examination will allow the examiner to more accurately differentiate between patellofemoral disorders and other derangements of the knee.

Physical examination of the knee, particularly the patellofemoral joint, requires both static and dynamic assessment. It has been described as a three-part examination, consisting of standing, sitting, and supine assessments.[7,9]

The initial examination begins with the patient standing. Assessment of the stance position and visual gait analysis are important. The axial alignment of the lower extremities should be noted, as abnormalities of the pelvis, femur, or tibia can result in patellofemoral disorders. At the knee, genu varum and valgum alter the mechanics of the patellofemoral articulation. Measurement of the Q angle provides a key piece of information in an evaluation of a patient with knee pain, especially when the patellofemoral articulation is the suspected culprit. Briefly, the Q angle is the angle between two lines, one drawn from the middle of the tibial tubercle to the patella and the other drawn from the patella to the anterior superior iliac spine. The normal Q angle ranges from 10° to 20°, but several variations have been described.[9] Freeman[10] described a normal Q angle of 10° to 20° in females and 8° to 10° in males. Aglietti and associates[11] described a normal Q angle of 17° in females and 14° in males. Hughston[12] believed that a Q angle of greater than 10° in either gender was abnormal and should be corrected. Despite these variations, large deviations from these ranges are definitely considered relevant. An increased Q angle may lead to an increased valgus force on the patella. This may cause lateral patellar subluxation or tilt and increased compression of the lateral patellar facet. Pelvic geometry is also an important element in the examination, as a widened pelvis may increase the Q angle. The pelvic geometry in women differs slightly from that in men, as women tend to have a wider, gynecoid pelvis. Femoral anteversion may also cause increased knee valgus. This is indirectly indicated by the presence of an inward pointing, or "squinting," patella. To ensure accurate examination of the patella, it is imperative that the patient's feet be pointing forward and aligned. After observation of the axial alignment, gait is assessed. An antalgic, or painful, gait may cause a shortened stance phase of the affected lower limb. This confirms the side of the knee disorder. Limb length inequality as well as varus or valgus thrust should also be noted if present. Lastly, the patient may be asked to squat and hold that position for a few seconds. This is the half-squat test, and if it re-creates anterior knee pain, it strongly suggests a patellofemoral etiology.

The second part of the assessment is performed with the patient seated with the legs over the side of the examination table. The lower limbs should be visually inspected first. Thigh muscle girth should be evaluated for bilateral symmetry. Atrophy of the vastus medialis muscles, evidenced by flattening, contributes to patellofemoral symptoms. The anatomic position of the patella should be carefully observed because it may give clues to the cause of pain. Patella alta, or superior displacement of the patella, is common in patients with a patellofemoral disorder, particularly instability. The clinical finding of "grasshopper eyes," in which the patellae are displaced proximally and externally rotated, has been described.[10] Patella alta is radiographically confirmed with use of the Insall-Salvati ratio. Rotational malalignment is assessed by observing the relationship of the superior patellar pole to the inferior patellar pole. Most commonly, the inferior pole is lateral to the superior pole, and deviations from this are important because they may suggest patellar maltracking. Skin depressions medial and lateral to the inferior pole of the patella are normal. Their absence can signify a knee effusion, suggesting an intra-articular disorder as opposed to a patellofemoral disorder. Palpation of the knee is performed next. The important structures to evaluate include the patellar margins, the femoral epicondyles, the tibiofemoral joint line, the Gerdy tubercle, and the fibular head. Tenderness in any one or a combination of these areas may suggest a pathologic entity outside of the patellofemoral articulation.

The third portion of the examination requires the patient to lie supine. This position allows several tests to be performed to evaluate the forces acting on the patella. The patient is first asked to flex and extend the knee. Activation of the quadriceps complex permits visual recording of patellar tracking. Normally, in terminal extension, the patella lies laterally within the femoral sulcus. As the knee is flexed past 30°, the patella engages the middle of the femoral sulcus.[13] Lateral subluxation of the patella in terminal extension is known as the J sign. As the knee is subsequently flexed and extended, the patella may appear to jump in and out of the femoral sulcus. Another test is the active quadriceps pull test,[14] in which the knee is extended and the patient is asked to contract the quadriceps muscles. Normally, the patella tracks superiorly in a straight line; lateral deviation of the patella is considered abnormal. To perform the patellofemoral grind test,[13] the examiner depresses the patella in the femoral sulcus and then asks the patient to contract the quadriceps. Pain elicited from this test may represent articular injury. To elicit the patellar apprehension sign of Fairbank,[15] another indication of patellar instability, the patient is asked to flex the knee to 20° and the examiner then applies a laterally directed force on the patella. At this time, the patient may fear patellar dislocation and instinctively contract the quadriceps and extend the knee to guard against it. The passive patella glide test is performed by flexing the knee 20° to 30°. The examiner then visually divides the patella into three vertical segments, manually displaces the patella medially or laterally, and measures the degree of displacement. If the patella displaces more than three segments laterally, the medial retinaculum is probably incompetent. If the patella displaces less than one segment medially, the lateral retinaculum is tight. Both of these instances predispose the patient to lateral patellar subluxation and resultant pain. For the passive patellar tilt test, the examiner extends the patient's knee and then lifts the lateral edge of the patella away from the lateral femoral condyle. Normally, the patella will lift off slightly from the lateral femoral condyle, representing a positive tilt angle. An inability to lift the patella represents a neutral or negative tilt angle and is consistent with a tight lateral retinaculum.

The physical examination of a patient with anterior knee pain is comprehensive and, when done correctly, can give valuable clues regarding the presence or absence of a patellofemoral disorder. The clues can then be used to determine whether further evaluation is needed.

## Nonsurgical Management of Patellofemoral Arthritis

Physical therapy that includes quadriceps strengthening has been the cornerstone of nonsurgical management. The goal of any strengthening program is to improve the function of the limb while not overloading the damaged patellofemoral articu-lation. Recently improved understanding of more generalized therapy approaches has shifted focus away from just the patellofemoral joint to overall body balance and stability.

Stretching is a simple modality that may be beneficial in the management of patellofemoral arthritis. The goal of stretching is to restore passive soft-tissue balance of the patella. In most cases, the lateral tissues of the anterior aspect of the knee have become excessively tight. A directed patella mobilization program focusing on releasing the lateral tissues surrounding the patella may help to decrease excessive pressure on the lateral facet. Although attempts at relaxation of the lateral tissues may ultimately prove unsuccessful, the low morbidity associated with patellar mobilization and capsular stretching makes its inclusion in nonsurgical regimens simple.

Strengthening of the vastus medialis obliquus is a classic physical therapy modality for treatment of lateral patellar maltracking. Dysplasia of the vastus medialis obliquus has been reported in patients with problems caused by excessive lateral patellar tracking. Most physical therapy regimens involve an attempt to selectively strengthen the vastus medialis obliquus to increase medially directed forces across the patella. Despite the association between dysplasia of the vastus medialis obliquus and patellar maltracking, the utility and success of selective strengthening of the vastus medialis obliquus have not been overwhelmingly supported by the current literature.

Physical therapy ideals have shifted away from a focus on local muscle control and joint function to a focus on limb control and body positioning. In that respect, so-called core strengthening is an excellent approach to the treatment of a patient with patellofemoral arthritis. Core strengthening focuses on abdominal muscle control, trunk balance, and limb control. Exercises designed to improve limb balance focus on the hip and the knee to maximize the efficiency of the limb. In this way, alignment and balance are improved, which hopefully leads to decreased pressures on the patellofemoral articulation and improved function. One key benefit of using core-strengthening principles during rehabilitation is the avoidance of excessive repetitive strengthening exercises about the knee, which may exacerbate symptoms.

The patellar McConnell tape technique can be useful when excessive lateral patellar translation and tilt are part of the clinical presentation. This technique depends on having sufficient mobility remaining in the patellofemoral articulation to medialize the patella passively. A standard taping regimen requires understanding of the taping system, and the skin must be able to withstand multiple applications of adhesive tape.

Several braces have been designed to alleviate anterior knee pain emanating from the patellofemoral joint. Most braces are used in an attempt to drive the patella medially during the knee flexion cycle and offload the lateral facet. The success of these braces is variable and depends on the willingness of patients to reliably apply the brace each day. Some patients may also experience lessening of symptoms as a result of the heat retained by many neoprene knee braces. There are limited clinical data on patellofemoral bracing, but the easy application of such braces makes their use in a nonsurgical approach reasonable.

The rigors of land-based therapy may aggravate the problems at the patellofemoral articulation, thereby reducing any potential benefits. In such cases, water exercises may prove helpful. Obese patients may benefit the most from water therapy programs because joint forces are reduced during these exercise programs. Principles similar to those used during land-based therapy should be emphasized, including global core strengthening focusing on abdominal, hip, and knee balance.

When patellofemoral pain has elements of complex regional pain syndrome (hypersensitivity, burning pain, and pain at rest), aggressive pain management is recommended. Pertinent modalities include desensitization therapy, gabapentin or pregabapentin, local application of a lidocaine patch, and formal consultation with a pain management specialist.

## Surgical Procedures
### Role of Arthroscopy and Soft-Tissue Realignment
#### Arthroscopic Débridement
When a patient presents with mechanical symptoms and a loose body is suspected or confirmed on imaging studies, arthroscopic débridement may be warranted. A chondroplasty may also temporarily relieve discomfort and disability when patellofemoral arthritis is present and associated with swelling, crepitus, and synovitis. Removal of loose cartilage from the patella or femur may limit mechanical irritants as well. The surgeon must realize that these measures may have only temporary effects on symptoms and if underlying mechanical factors have contributed to the progression of the disease, they will continue to contribute to the clinical progression of symptoms as well.

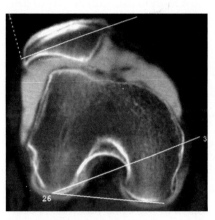

**Figure 1** Radiograph showing arthritis of the lateral facet accompanied by excessive lateral patellar tilt.

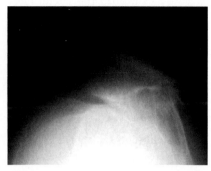

**Figure 2** A large lateral osteophyte is visible on this Merchant radiograph. This is often a finding in end-stage patellofemoral disease, and it is caused by excessive lateral tilt and/or translation of the patella.

### Arthroscopic Lateral Retinacular Release
This procedure is frequently used and is most effective for treatment of isolated lateral patellar tilt. When clinical and radiographic examinations confirm excessive lateral tilt, lateral facet arthritis may result (Figure 1). Release of the lateral retinacular structures may decrease pressure on the lateral facet and decrease pain. The tight lateral retinaculum should be confirmed on physical examination and by radiographs in a patient for whom conservative measures have failed. The procedure may be useful in patients with lateral facet arthrosis with lateral tilt but no subluxation.

When this procedure is performed, care should be taken not to release the tendinous portion of the vastus lateralis muscle from the superolateral aspect of the patella. This may cause quadriceps weakness and dynamic imbalance. Release of the lateral structures may also improve tracking, but when performed in the face of malalignment, the results are less reliable unless concurrent tightening of the medial retinacular structures is performed. Medial imbrication procedures are tradition-

ally used for treatment of patellar maltracking, but they may not be appropriate in the face of arthritis of the patellofemoral joint. In the arthritic situation, a medial imbrication may increase forces on the medial facet of the patella and the medial condyle and lead to overload of the medial aspect of the joint. Lateral release has not been shown to provide long-term benefit for patients with patellofemoral arthritis.

### Lateral Patellar Facetectomy
In patients with long-standing patellofemoral disease, excessive lateral tilt and/or translation may lead to the formation of a large lateral osteophyte visible on the Merchant radiograph (Figure 2). Some authors, including Yercan and associates,[16] support excision of the lateral facet overgrowth and retensioning of the lateral tissues. Lateral patellar facetectomy may provide pain relief and decrease the lateral overload in the patellofemoral compartment, but it may decrease bone stock necessary for future replacement.

### Proximal Soft-Tissue Realignment
Proximal soft-tissue realignment procedures have also been advocated

as a way to unload the lateral facet and improve patellar tracking. Limited success with this procedure has been reported (a 62% failure rate when signs of degenerative joint disease were present), with the belief that other alignment procedures offer more reliable results in patients with patellofemoral arthritis.[17]

These procedures are focused on arthritis affecting the lateral facet and have limited usefulness for patients with more generalized arthritis. In particular, disease of the trochlea or medial facet may lead to an increase in pain following lateral release procedures. For patients with continued symptoms emanating from the lateral aspect of the joint, more aggressive alignment procedures may be required. Soft-tissue realignment procedures alone are also indicated for skeletally immature patients with a history of recurrent dislocations. The mature patient with a high congruence angle and minimal arthrosis may benefit from proximal soft-tissue realignment if therapeutic measures have failed. A Q angle of less than 10° has also been associated with better outcomes.[18]

This technique involves a midline incision from just above the superior pole of the patella to the medial aspect of the tibial tubercle. A release of the lateral patellofemoral ligament and a retinacular release are performed, leaving the synovial tissue intact to isolate the joint. The lower fibers of the vastus lateralis are released as well, and the release is carried down to the level of the tubercle. Medially, the vastus medialis is elevated from the underlying capsule about 10 cm from its insertion. It is then advanced to the lateral free edge of the vastus lateralis, creating a sleeve around the patella. A compression dressing is applied, and

knee motion is begun at 7 to 10 days after the surgery. Insall and associates[19] reported a 91% rate of satisfactory results at 4 years after use of this procedure. Other techniques involving a lateral release with a medial imbrication have also been described.[20] They involve a similar lateral retinacular release with imbrication of the medial retinacular tissue from the medial aspect of the quadriceps tendon to the proximal aspect of the tibial tubercle. Scuderi and associates[20] reported an 81% rate of good or excellent results after 3.5 years of follow-up.

## Distal Realignment
### Osteotomy for Realignment and/or Resurfacing

Tibial tubercle transfer is recommended for treatment of patellofemoral arthritis in patients in whom unloading of discrete areas of patellar and femoral disease can lead to clinical success. Requisite for this procedure is healthy cartilage onto which patellar loading and tracking can be transferred. Tibial tubercle transfer, when combined with cartilage resurfacing, holds great promise and may reduce the need for early patellofemoral arthroplasty. Through physical and radiographic examinations, the surgeon must first determine which part of the patellofemoral joint is involved in the disease process and thus needs to be unloaded. Radiographs made with the knee in 45° of flexion combined with precise lateral radiographs, MRI scans, and arthroscopy all help the surgeon make this determination, and he or she should make sure that all of the imaging studies correlate with the findings on physical examination.

To select the correct osteotomy, one must understand that moving the tibial tubercle anteriorly decreases the flexion of the patella within the troch-

lear groove and therefore shifts contact on the patella more proximally so that this area is loaded earlier in the flexion arc. The most common areas involved in patients with malalignment are the lateral and distal articular regions.[21] Anterior and medial transfer of the tibial tubercle would thus be appropriate in these patients. It should be realized that dysplasia or atrophy of the quadriceps may also be present in patients with malalignment, and therefore a combined proximal realignment may be necessary.[22-24]

There are two main indications for tibial tubercle transfer: (1) the need to realign the patella by establishing proper alignment (this may also be accomplished with medial imbrication and lateral release, but that "pulls" the patella posteromedially and risks adding excessive load on the medial facet); and (2) when degenerative disease is limited and a realignment osteotomy can unload the affected area. The benefits provided by recent advances in allograft and autograft cartilage resurfacing procedures may also be enhanced by simultaneous tibial tubercle transfer to unload the affected areas.

Relative and absolute contraindications to tubercle transfer include inadequate patient health or obesity, poor bone quality, diffuse patellar or trochlear chondral degeneration, proximal patellar lesions (crush injuries), reflex sympathetic dystrophy or diffuse pain, poor motivation on the part of the patient, and an inadequate trial of nonsurgical measures.

### Anterior or Elevation Osteotomy of the Tibial Tubercle

This procedure, known as the Maquet osteotomy, is designed to unload the more distal areas of the patella and decrease overall forces within the joint itself. It is particularly effective in younger patients with distal patellar articular degeneration, but it does not address alignment issues in and of themselves. In general, soft-tissue release should be attempted before osteotomy. Contraindications include diffuse involvement of the proximal pole regions of the patella.

The technique is performed through a medial parapatellar incision that is extended past the tubercle. The joint, along with the fat pad, is inspected and is débrided to allow mobilization of the tendon. A 2.5- × 5-cm section of iliac crest is then harvested for the procedure. The osteotomy can be performed with use of multiple small drill holes or a thin oscillating saw blade 8 cm or greater from the superior aspect of the tubercle distally in the coronal plane. Once mobilized, the proximal segment is displaced anteriorly, allowing plastic deformation of the bone at the distal attachment. The iliac crest graft is then fashioned to allow 1.5 to 2 cm of anteriorization at the tubercle. More than 1.5 cm of anteriorization, however, is associated with a higher prevalence of skin problems postoperatively. If necessary, a cancellous screw can be used for supplemental fixation through the tubercle and the graft, into the metaphyseal aspect of the tibia. Postoperative care involves the use of crutches and partial weight bearing and passive motion. Full weight bearing is allowed at 6 weeks, when the osteotomy site is usually healed. Maquet reported a 95% rate of successful results in his series,[25] but rates as low as 31% have been reported in other series[26] (Figure 3).

### Medial Tibial Tubercle Transfer

This operation, known as the Elmslie-Trillat procedure, is a direct medial transfer procedure. It is effective for controlling instability and

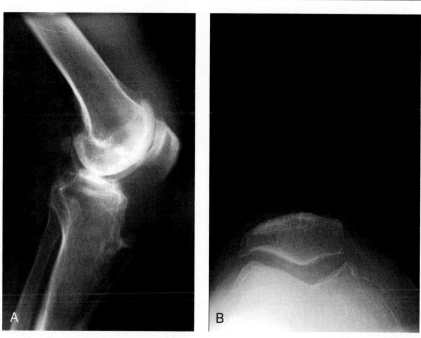

**Figure 3** **A,** Lateral and **B,** Merchant radiographs of a patient who underwent a Maquet osteotomy and had 18 years of pain relief. In the 4 months before presentation, the symptoms and pain had returned.

lateral tracking.[27-29] The operation is mainly indicated for patients with an excessive Q angle, lateral instability, and patellar and/or trochlear cartilage with grade II or less severe lesions. The procedure is contraindicated for patients with chondral lesions with a grade greater than II,[9] a normal Q angle, or an open proximal tibial physis.

The technique is performed with use of a lateral parapatellar incision extending from the proximal pole to the distal aspect of the tibial tubercle. The lateral patellofemoral ligament is then released along with the lateral retinaculum, leaving the underlying synovial layer intact and preserving the lateral geniculate blood supply to the patella.[30] The tubercle is then cut in the coronal plane with osteotomes and drill holes to aid in the osteotomy. The periosteal sleeve is left intact, and the tubercle is medialized and then fixed with a cancellous lag screw. Af-

ter the surgery, the limb is immobilized for 6 weeks and partial weight bearing is allowed. After 6 weeks, when radiographic evidence of healing has been noted, motion and strengthening exercises are begun. The rate of satisfactory results in published series[31] has been 80% or greater.

### Anteromedial Tibial Tubercle Osteotomy

This osteotomy, known as the Fulkerson procedure,[16,32] involves the transfer of the tubercle to a more anterior and medial location (Figure 4) and is more effective in diminishing or eliminating load on the distal and lateral aspects of the patella.[33] When performing a tibial tubercle transfer, the surgeon should beware of proximal lesions or medial facet or condylar lesions, as transfer procedures will increase load on the proximal part of the patella and on the medial facet and medial condyle. Thus, intact proximal and medial

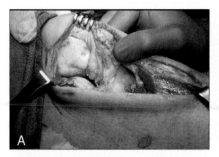
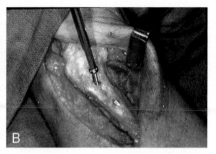
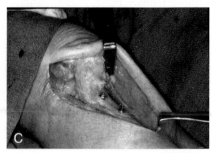

**Figure 4** Anteromedial tibial tubercle osteotomy. **A,** A distal central patellar lesion. **B,** The transfer requires exposure of the lateral aspect of the tibia by reflecting the anterior tibialis muscle. **C,** The anteromedial tibial tubercle transfer is stabilized with two cortical lag screws.

cartilage is required to obtain the maximum benefit from this procedure.

The technique is performed through an incision from the lateral inferior part of the pole of the patella to the anterior ridge of the tibia 5 cm distal to the tubercle. The lateral patellofemoral ligament and the retinaculum are released, leaving the underlying synovium intact. A small arthrotomy is used distally to inspect the joint. The tubercle is then exposed so that a set of drill holes can be made, starting from anteromedial to the tubercle and the tibial ridge and directed posterolaterally. A thin oscillating blade saw can then be used to perform the osteotomy, with angling of the proximal-lateral aspect above the tubercle and leaving the distal bone in continuity with the anterior ridge of the tibia. The tubercle is then moved medially along the osteotomy, plastically deforming the bone attached to the anterior ridge of the tibia. Once the new position of the tubercle is determined, it is fixed with a cancellous lag screw. After the surgery, the knee is immobilized, and the patient is allowed partial weight bearing. Passive motion may be permitted, depending on the strength of the fixation. At 4 to 6 weeks, when radiographic evidence of healing has occurred,

weight bearing is advanced along with strengthening therapy. Reports have described satisfactory results in more than two thirds of patients at 5 years after the surgery.[16,32-34]

### Anterolateralization of the Tibial Tubercle

This procedure may be a good therapeutic option when there is a medial lesion resulting from overimbrication during a previous medialization of the tibial tubercle. This lesion may or may not be associated with medial subluxation. Anterolateralization may also be an effective salvage procedure following failed anteriorization of the tibial tubercle. It can help to realign a medially tracking patella, unloading a medial lesion that was overloaded as a result of a previous medial tubercle transfer, and can be selectively combined with resurfacing of the patella. Anterolateralization requires an intact lateral facet.

### Autologous Cartilage Resurfacing

Autologous chondrocyte implantation may be indicated for the management of focal chondral defects in the knee of a young patient. The procedure may be considered when an intact joint space has been documented on radiographic examination and the lesion has well-shouldered margins, and when

there is no diffuse involvement of the remaining portion of the patella. It is critical that the etiology of the cartilage defect and the underlying abnormal biomechanics of the patella be accurately identified before the decision is made to move forward with this procedure. Having a proper diagnosis as well as correcting the underlying biomechanical abnormalities are paramount for a successful outcome of autologous chondrocyte implantation. The workup for these patients should include a thorough review of the history and a careful physical and radiographic examination of the axial alignment of the lower extremity as well as the patellofemoral joint. A routine series of radiographs, including anteroposterior standing, 45° posteroanterior flexion weight bearing (Rosenberg), lateral, and skyline (Merchant) radiographs, as well as a standing full-length lower extremity axial alignment radiograph, is made for all patients. When maltracking is suspected on clinical examination, a CT scan should be performed, with the leg in extension. CT scans are then obtained with and without quadriceps contraction to assess lateral patellar subluxation, the presence of dysplasia of the trochlea, and patellar height. All of these findings are extremely useful in determining the appropriateness of this procedure.

Once a patient is considered a candidate for autologous chondrocyte implantation, arthroscopic examination is performed to assess the geometry of the lesion and any pathologic motion of the joint. A cartilage biopsy specimen is also obtained from the portion of the superior aspect of the intercondylar notch that is not bearing weight. This specimen is processed and used for cell culture. Approximately 200 to 300 mg of articular cartilage is sent in a sterile transport medium to be commercially cultured and cryopreserved.[2,35]

The transplantation procedure is then performed as a second procedure. The chondrocytes are injected beneath a periosteal patch secured with resorbable sutures and fibrin glue.[35,36]

Rehabilitation after the surgery includes no weight bearing and the use of continuous passive motion for 6 to 8 hours per day for 6 weeks. The patient is allowed to progress to full weight bearing by 4 months after the surgery, but inline impact activities (running) are not permitted for 12 to 18, months and cutting sports are not allowed for at least 18 months.[35,36]

Minas and Bryant[35] performed a 7-year, prospective cohort study of 45 patients who had undergone autologous chondrocyte implantation for treatment of full-thickness chondral defects of both the patella and the trochlea, or of one surface of the joint. The average age of the patients at the time of surgery was 36.9 years, and the average duration of follow-up was 47.5 months. The patients were surveyed, and 71% were satisfied with the outcome, 16% were neutral, and 13% were dissatisfied. Eighty-seven percent

of the patients said that they would have the surgical procedure again under similar circumstances. Seventy-one percent of the patients rated the result as good to excellent, with only 7% as poor. The Short Form-36 (SF-36), the Knee Society Score, the Western Ontario and McMaster Universities Osteoarthritis Index (WOMAC), and the modified Cincinnati knee score all showed large significant improvements ($P = 0.0016$). Typically, patients started to have pain relief by 4 to 6 months after the surgery, and they were allowed to return to nonimpact sports activities at 9 months postoperatively. Full-impact activities were begun by 18 months after the surgery. The grafts failed in 8 patients (18%). Peterson and associates[36] reported similar results, up to 10 years after autologous chondrocyte implantation, regardless of whether patellar maltracking had been addressed at the time of, or corrected before, the implantation.

### Patellectomy

Patellectomy has been performed for over a century as one of the surgical treatments of severe anterior knee pain.[26,37] Its popularity has waxed and waned over time, with mixed results and opinions regarding its effectiveness. One study found that patellectomy provided adequate pain relief but with permanent loss of knee extensor power.[17] In the end, the results had deteriorated with time in most patients. The operation should be viewed as a salvage procedure, and the surgeon should warn the patient against unrealistic expectations concerning the outcome. Historically, the best results have been noted in patients with severe arthrosis of the patellofemoral joint. The technique basically involves a midline incision with a sharp dissection of the patella.

Care should be taken to repair the retinaculum to prevent an extensor lag after surgery, and tracking of the quadriceps tendon should be checked to make sure that a proximal realignment procedure is not necessary. The patient then is allowed early mobilization and weight bearing after surgery.

### Replacement
#### Patellofemoral Arthroplasty

There has been a recent resurgence of interest in patellofemoral arthroplasty. It has been indicated for endstage patellofemoral arthritis, when deterioration of the patellofemoral joint is diffuse (Figure 5). Shortterm reports have shown a high level of effectiveness, particularly when alignment issues are corrected.[38-40] Patellofemoral arthroplasty can work well in patients of normal stature with isolated patellofemoral disease and no secondary gain issues.

Isolated patellofemoral arthritis occurs in up to 10% of patients who have osteoarthritis of the knee. Over the years, several different patellofemoral implants have been designed, and previous reports of different patellofemoral implants have shown variable results.[38] The Lubinus prosthesis was reported to have a 50% failure rate at 8 years in a study of 76 cases.[39] The main reasons for failure were malalignment, wear, impingement, and disease progression. The Avon patellofemoral arthroplasty was a second-generation design with features designed to improve alignment and wear.[40]

The first Avon patellofemoral implants were placed in September 1996 and entered into a prospective review. Outcomes were assessed with use of pain scores, Bartlett's patella score, and the Oxford knee score. To date, 307 knees have been treated and 159 knees have been re-

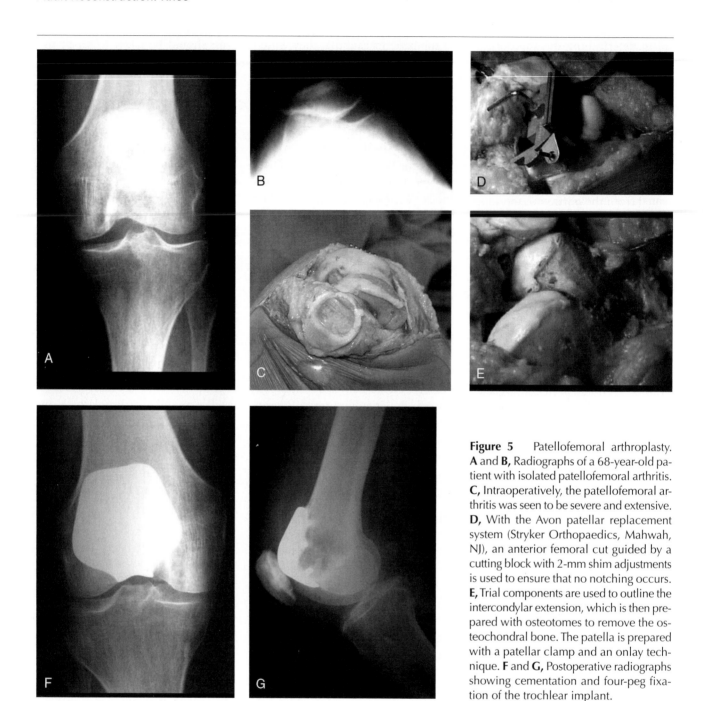

**Figure 5** Patellofemoral arthroplasty. **A** and **B,** Radiographs of a 68-year-old patient with isolated patellofemoral arthritis. **C,** Intraoperatively, the patellofemoral arthritis was seen to be severe and extensive. **D,** With the Avon patellar replacement system (Stryker Orthopaedics, Mahwah, NJ), an anterior femoral cut guided by a cutting block with 2-mm shim adjustments is used to ensure that no notching occurs. **E,** Trial components are used to outline the intercondylar extension, which is then prepared with osteotomes to remove the osteochondral bone. The patella is prepared with a patellar clamp and an onlay technique. **F** and **G,** Postoperative radiographs showing cementation and four-peg fixation of the trochlear implant.

viewed at 2 to 5 years postoperatively. The median pain score improved from 15 of 40 points preoperatively to 36 of 40 points at 5 years. The Bartlett patella score improved from 10 of 30 points to 26 of 30 points at 5 years. The Oxford knee score improved from 19 of 48 points to 39 of 48 points at 5 years. Malalignment

developed in four knees (1.3%), one of which required distal soft-tissue realignment. There have been no cases of deep infection, fracture, wear, or loosening. Evidence of disease progression developed in 18 knees (6%), 15 of which underwent revision to a total knee replacement.[40-42]

The technique involves a medial parapatellar approach to the knee and alignment of the anterior femoral resection guide (Figure 5, *C*). The alignment of this cutting block is paramount to ensure that no femoral notching or undersizing of the trochlear implant occurs. Most newer designs include an extension of the trochlear implant into the notch of the femur. This area is resected manually with either a template (Avon; Stryker Orthopaedics, Mahwah, NJ) or, in some systems, with a template and router (Journey; Smith & Nephew, Memphis, TN). Peg holes are then drilled for the template, and the patella is addressed in the usual total knee resurfacing fashion. Care should be taken not to allow excessive overstuffing of 4 mm or greater because this may affect postoperative motion. Postoperatively, patients are allowed full weight bearing and motion is initiated immediately.

Results to date suggest that the improved designs have minimized the previous problems of malalignment and early wear.[42] The functional results are comparable with those of a total knee replacement. Complication rates are low, and there is an excellent postoperative range of motion. Although disease progression remains a potential problem, these prostheses offer a reasonable alternative to total knee replacement in the small group of patients with isolated patellofemoral disease.

### Total Joint Arthroplasty

The use of total knee replacement to treat severe isolated patellofemoral arthrosis that is recalcitrant to therapeutic measures has been well established for older patients.[43-46] The procedure is not advocated for younger patients with isolated patellofemoral arthritis, but it can be used with reliable results in patients in their eighth decade of life. Total knee replacement should not be considered until nonsurgical management has failed. The exact age at which total knee arthroplasty becomes a viable option for the treatment of patellofemoral arthritis is debatable and case dependent, but certainly an age younger than 55 years should be considered a rela-

tive contraindication.[46] Careful adherence to proper techniques and component alignment is well recognized as being crucial to the success of any total knee arthroplasty, and this is no different for patients with patellofemoral arthritis. There are areas that need more emphasis in these patients to ensure a properly aligned knee replacement. Particular attention must be directed toward the correction of extensor mechanism alignment. This is evidenced by the reported rates of retinacular release in these patients, which are as high as 68%,[47-49] a threefold increase compared with the rates associated with standard total knee arthroplasty.

Complications involving the extensor mechanism and the patellofemoral joint remain the primary noninfectious indications for revision total knee arthroplasty.[50] Specifically, imbalance of the extensor mechanism and resultant poor patellar tracking are the most common causes of pain after total knee arthroplasty. Patellofemoral complications include patellar subluxation or dislocation; wear, loosening, or failure of the patellar component; and patellar fracture. Component positioning, especially rotational alignment of the femoral and tibial components, is critical to patellofemoral stability. Component malrotation is one of the most frequent causes of patellofemoral complications.[51-53]

Any surgical alteration that abnormally increases the tension in the lateral retinaculum or increases the Q angle and produces a laterally directed muscle vector will cause lateral maltracking of the patella and instability of the patellofemoral joint after total knee arthroplasty (Figure 6). Positioning of the femoral and tibial components is of supreme importance. Valgus angulation of the

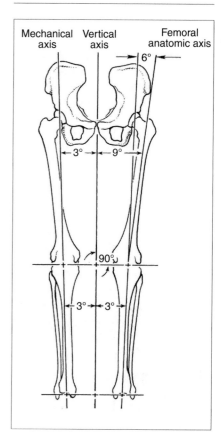

**Figure 6**  A femoral cut made perpendicular to the mechanical axis will place the femoral component in approximately 6° of valgus angulation with respect to the anatomic axis of the femur. (Medialization of the femoral component may result in lateral patellar subluxation.) (Adapted with permission from Crockarell JR, Guyton JL: Arthroplasty of ankle and knee, in Canale ST (ed): *Campbell's Surgical Orthopaedics*, ed 10. St. Louis, MO, Mosby-Year Book, 2003, p 255.)

femoral component will increase the Q angle and produce a laterally directed muscle vector. This alignment error is more common in patients with degenerative arthritis who have a preoperative valgus deformity of greater than 10° combined with loss of bone stock of the distal part of the lateral femoral condyle.[53]

Technically, the distal femoral cut should be made perpendicular to the

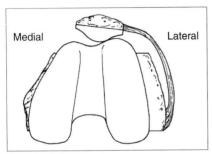

**Figure 7** Medialization of the femoral component may result in lateral patellar subluxation. (Adapted with permission from Krackow KA: The technique of total knee arthroplasty. St. Louis, MO, CV Mosby, 1990, p 139.)

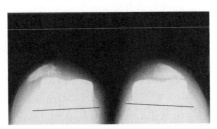

**Figure 8** Lateral patellar subluxation of the patella on the left following total knee arthroplasty. Note the lateral tilt of the patella on the right, a result of excessive resection of the lateral facet and too little resection of the medial facet.

mechanical axis of the limb (6° of valgus angulation with respect to the anatomic axis of the femur).[54] There are several pitfalls to avoid during component positioning. A medially placed prosthesis will cause increased contact stresses between the lateral flange of the femoral component and the lateral border of the patellar component, resulting in patellar subluxation (Figure 7). The femoral component should be lateralized as much as possible to reduce tension on the lateral retinaculum and reduce shearing stresses placed on the patella.

Component malrotation is the predominant cause of patellofemoral complications in patients with normal axial alignment.[51] The epicondylar axis (a line from the lateral epicondylar prominence to the medial sulcus on the medial epicondyle) is the most reliable guide to ensure correct rotational alignment of the femoral component. The anterior and posterior femoral cuts should be made parallel to the epicondylar axis. Internal rotation of the femoral component with respect to the femur will rotate the trochlear groove medially, increase tension on the lateral retinaculum, and cause

lateral patellar maltracking. Erring on the side of slight external rotation should improve patellar component tracking.

Whiteside's line (drawn from the deepest part of the patellar groove anteriorly to the center of the intercondylar notch posteriorly) is another reliable guide for rotational alignment.[55] The anterior and posterior femoral cuts should be made perpendicular to this line. The least reliable landmark for rotational alignment of the femoral component is the posterior condylar line. It is internally rotated relative to the epicondylar axis. If the posterior condylar line is used as a reference, posterior deficiency of the lateral femoral condyle (and valgus deformity) may cause the femoral component to be substantially internally rotated. This will cause lateral patellar maltracking. Studies have demonstrated that a femoral component set parallel to the posterior condylar line is more likely to be malrotated and more likely to require a lateral retinacular release to correct patellar maltracking.[56,57] Internal rotation of the tibial component will also cause patellar maltracking by forcing the tibia into external rotation and increasing the Q angle. The correct placement of the tibial component is

rotational alignment of the middle of the component's anterior border with the tibial crest or the medial third of the tibial tubercle. The combined amount of internal rotation of the femoral and tibial components is directly proportional to the severity of patellofemoral instability: 1° to 4° should be used when there is lateral tracking and patellar tilting; 3° to 8°, when there is patellar subluxation; and 7° to 17°, when there is early patellar dislocation (at less than 2 years) or late failure of the patellar prosthesis (at 2 to 6 years).

The patellar component should be placed on the medial portion of the patella, mimicking the normal anatomy of a medially oriented sagittal ridge. A laterally placed patellar button will increase the tension in the lateral retinaculum and cause lateral patellar maltracking. A centrally placed patellar component more frequently requires a lateral retinacular release to track normally than does a medially placed component.[57]

During patellar preparation, more bone must be removed from the thicker medial facet, with the patellar cut kept parallel to the plane of the medial and lateral poles of the patella. A common mistake involves resection of too much of the lateral facet and too little of the medial facet with a resultant lateral tilt of the patellar component (Figure 8).

The current literature seems to favor patellar resurfacing. Multiple studies have demonstrated success with patellar resurfacing, with good relief of pain and good overall outcomes.[58-60] However, other studies have shown success without insertion of a patellar component.[61] Ideally, a patient treated without patellar resurfacing should have no patellar arthritis, and a femoral component that was designed to accommodate the native patella should be used.

Overstuffing of the patellofemoral joint by using a femoral component that is too large (especially in the anteroposterior dimension) or resecting an inadequate amount of the patella increases tension on the lateral retinaculum.[62] The mismatch of the implant and the resected bone may also increase the circumference of the arc that the quadriceps tendon will travel in flexion, and this can affect motion as well. The patellar resection should equal the thickness of the patellar component, while maintaining at least 12 mm of bone to minimize the risk of fracture. The goal should be to maintain the overall thickness of the patellofemoral joint in the anteroposterior dimension.

Alternative surgical approaches such as the subvastus, or southern, approach potentially offer less disruption of the extensor mechanism, fewer required lateral releases, less patellar maltracking, and preservation of the medial vascular supply to the patella.[63] The technique may be difficult, however, in heavier patients or those with scarring, contractures, or large osteophytes.

Patellofemoral stability may be assessed with either the no-thumbs test or the single-suture technique. The patella should track centrally in the trochlear groove without lateral subluxation or lateral tilt through a full range of motion. Ideally, these tests should be performed with the tourniquet deflated, as binding of the extensor mechanism may lead to perceived maltracking of the patellar component. With the no-thumbs test, the knee is taken through the full flexion arc without closing the medial arthrotomy and without applying any medial force with the thumb to keep the patella located. If there is patellar tilt-

ing or slight subluxation with the no-thumbs test, the single-suture technique can be used, thus avoiding an unnecessary lateral release. With the single-suture technique, the medial tension vector of the extensor mechanism is simulated by reapproximating the medial retinaculum at the superior pole of the patella with a single number 0 suture. If the suture does not break through a full range of flexion of the knee, then a lateral release is not necessary.

Lateral retinacular release is commonly used to correct maltracking of the extensor mechanism.[47] The tight retinaculum is released approximately 2 cm lateral to the lateral patellar border, with the release extending from the vastus lateralis muscle to the proximal part of the tibia. Care should be taken to preserve the superior lateral geniculate artery. There are numerous possible complications of lateral retinacular release, including substantial vascular compromise (evident on a technetium bone scan), osteonecrosis of the patella, patellar fracture, prolonged wound healing and wound slough, an increased risk of infection, increased postoperative pain and swelling, and prolonged rehabilitation.

Patellar fracture has even been shown to be more likely after lateral release, whether or not the superior lateral geniculate artery is preserved. Mesh expansion release of the lateral retinaculum is an alternative to traditional retinacular release, with the potential benefit of less disruption to the patellar blood supply.

The results of total knee arthroplasty for the treatment of isolated patellofemoral arthritis have been very good and have included reliable pain relief. However, a high rate of residual postoperative patellar tilt, asymmetrically resurfaced patellae,

and residual subluxation has been reported in the literature.[46] These findings emphasize the need to adhere to the technical principles reviewed in this section to properly handle the inherent complexity of these cases. Studies[43-46] have demonstrated good to excellent results in terms of pain relief, and these results were superior to those achieved in comparison groups in which total knee arthroplasties had been performed for other conditions. It should be pointed out that anterior knee pain in patients with isolated patellofemoral arthritis was greater than that in patients with tricompartmental arthritis. One may view total knee replacement for arthrosis of an isolated patellofemoral articulation as excessive; however, total knee arthroplasty currently remains the most proven and predictable single procedure for this specific population of older patients with patellofemoral disease.[43-46]

## Future Directions

Increased interest and improvement in computer-assisted navigation systems for total joint arthroplasty have the potential to improve the accuracy of component alignment.[64-67] This may reduce patellofemoral complications.[66,67] It is important to note that there has not yet been any reported improvement in accuracy or variability when computer navigation, rather than conventional techniques, has been used for the critical step of rotationally aligning the femoral component in the operating room.[67]

## Summary

Patellofemoral arthritis is a common cause of anterior knee pain. When the disease is in its early stages, a careful and complete course of nonsurgical treatment may provide sufficient pain relief and functional improvement. If surgery is required, limited soft-tissue procedures such as arthroscopic lateral release and débridement may work well if the lateral portion of the joint is primarily affected. Tibial tubercle transfer, particularly anteromedialization, is a powerful way to correct malalignment and offload the lateral and distal parts of the patella. The indications for tibial tubercle transfer may expand if it proves to be a successful adjunct to cartilage resurfacing procedures.

For more severe disease, patellofemoral arthroplasty has evolved into a safe and reliable alternative. When a patient is older or when the arthritis is more diffuse, total knee arthroplasty is a reliable and reproducible way to improve function and decrease pain. Care must be taken to properly position components to avoid problems with the patellar component after surgery.

## References

1. Amis AA, Senavongse W, Darcy P: Biomechanics of patellofemoral joint prostheses. *Clin Orthop Relat Res* 2005; 436:20-29.

2. Saleh KJ, Arendt EA, Eldridge J, Fulkerson JP, Minas T, Mulhall KJ: Operative treatment of patellofemoral arthritis. *J Bone Joint Surg Am* 2005;87: 659-671.

3. Kwak SD, Colman WW, Ateshian GA, Grelsamer RP, Henry JH, Mow VC: Anatomy of the human patellofemoral joint articular cartilage: Surface curvature analysis. *J Orthop Res* 1997;15:468-472.

4. Goodfellow J, Hungerford DS, Zindel M: Patello-femoral joint mechanics and pathology: 1. Functional anatomy of the patello-femoral joint. *J Bone Joint Surg Br* 1976;58:287-290.

5. Amis AA, Farahmand F: Biomechanics of the knee extensor mechanism. *Knee* 1996;3:73-81.

6. Grelsamer RP, Weinstein CH: Applied biomechanics of the patella. *Clin Orthop Relat Res* 2001;389:9-14.

7. Scuderi GR (ed): *The Patella*. New York, NY, Springer, 1995, p 74.

8. Huberti HH, Hayes WC: Patellofemoral contact pressures: The influence of q-angle and tendofemoral contact. *J Bone Joint Surg Am* 1984;66: 715-724.

9. Insall JN, Scott WN: *Surgery of the Knee*, ed 3. Philadelphia, PA, Churchill Livingstone, 2001, p 161.

10. Freeman BL III: Recurrent dislocations, in Crenshaw AH (ed): *Campbell's Operative Orthopaedics*, ed 7. St. Louis, MO, CV Mosby, 1987, pp 2173-2218.

11. Aglietti P, Insall JN, Cerulli G: Patellar pain and incongruence: I. Measurements of incongruence. *Clin Orthop Relat Res* 1983;176:217-224.

12. Hughston JC: Subluxation of the patella. *J Bone Joint Surg Am* 1968;50: 1003-1026.

13. Scuderi GR: Surgical treatment for patellar instability. *Orthop Clin North Am* 1992;23:619-630.

14. Kolowich PA, Paulos LE, Rosenberg TD, Farnsworth S: Lateral release of the patella: Indications and contraindications. *Am J Sports Med* 1990;18:359-365.

15. Fairbank HA: Internal derangement of the knee in children. *Proc R Soc London* 1937;3:11.

16. Yercan HS, Ait Si Selmi T, Neyret P: The treatment of patellofemoral osteoarthritis with partial lateral facetectomy. *Clin Orthop Relat Res* 2005; 436:14-19.

17. Fulkerson JP: Alternatives to patellofemoral arthroplasty. *Clin Orthop Relat Res* 2005;436:76-80.

18. Hughston JC, Walsh WM: Proximal and distal reconstruction of the extensor mechanism for patellar subluxation. *Clin Orthop Relat Res* 1979;144: 36-42.

19. Insall J, Bullough PG, Burstein AH: Proximal "tube" realignment of the patella for chondromalacia patellae. *Clin Orthop Relat Res* 1979;144:63-69.

20. Scuderi G, Cuomo F, Scott WN: Lateral release and proximal realignment for patellar subluxation and dislocation: A long-term follow-up. *J Bone Joint Surg Am* 1988;70:856-861.

21. Fulkerson JP: Anteromedialization of the tibial tuberosity for patellofemoral malalignment. *Clin Orthop Relat Res* 1983;177:176-181.

22. Pidoriano AJ, Weinstein RN, Buuck DA, Fulkerson JP: Correlation of patellar articular lesions with results from anteromedial tibial tubercle transfer. *Am J Sports Med* 1997; 25:533-537.

23. Fithian DC, Meier SW: The case for advancement and repair of the medial patellofemoral ligament in patients with recurrent patellar instability. *Oper Tech Sports Med* 1999;7:81-89.

24. Kelly MA, Griffin FM: Proximal realignment of the patellofemoral joint. *Tech Orthop* 1997;12:178-184.

25. Maquet P: A biomechanical treatment of femoro-patellar arthrosis: Advancement of the patellar tendon. *Rev Rhum* 1963;30:779-783.

26. Engebretsen L, Svenningsen S, Benum P: Advancement of the tibial tuberosity for patellar pain: A 5-year follow-up. *Acta Orthop Scand* 1989; 60:20-22.

27. Post WR, Fulkerson IP: Distal realignment of the patellofemoral joint: Indications, effects, results, and recommendations. *Orthop Clin North Am* 1992;23:631-643.

28. Carney JR, Mologne TS, Muldoon M, Cox JS: Long-term evaluation of the Roux-Elmslie-Trillat procedure for patellar instability: A 26-year follow-up. *Am J Sports Med* 2005; 33:1220-1223.

29. Shelbourne KD, Porter DA, Rozzi W: Use of a modified Elmslie-Trillat procedure to improve abnormal patellar congruence angle. *Am J Sports Med* 1994;22:318-323.

30. Cox JS: An evaluation of the Elmslie-Trillat procedure for management of

patellar dislocations and subluxations: A preliminary report. *Am J Sports Med* 1976;4:72-77.

31. Brown DE, Alexander AH, Lichtman DM: The Elmslie-Trillat procedure: Evaluation in patellar dislocation and subluxation. *Am J Sports Med* 1984;12:104-109.

32. Fulkerson JP, Becker GJ: Anteromedial tibial tubercle transfer without bone graft. *Am J Sports Med* 1990;18:490-497.

33. Sakai N, Koshino T, Okamoto R: Pain reduction after anteromedial displacement of the tibial tuberosity: 5-year follow-up in 21 knees with patellofemoral arthrosis. *Acta Orthop Scand* 1996;67:13-15.

34. Morshuis WJ, Pavlov PW, de Rooy KP: Anteromedialization of the tibial tuberosity in the treatment of patellofemoral pain and malalignment. *Clin Orthop Relat Res* 1990;255:242-250.

35. Minas T, Bryant T: The role of autologous chondrocyte implantation in the patellofemoral joint. *Clin Orthop Relat Res* 2005;436:30-39.

36. Peterson L, Brittberg M, Kiviranta I, Akerlund EL, Lindahl A: Autologous chondrocyte transplantation: Biomechanics and long-term durability. *Am J Sports Med* 2002;30:2-12.

37. Ackroyd CE, Polyzoides AJ: Patellectomy for osteoarthritis: A study of eighty-one patients followed from two to twenty-two years. *J Bone Joint Surg Br* 1978;60:353-357.

38. Argenson JN, Guillaume JM, Aubaniac JM: Is there a place for patellofemoral arthroplasty? *Clin Orthop Relat Res* 1995;321:162-167.

39. Tauro B, Ackroyd CE, Newman JH, Shah NA: The Lubinus patellofemoral arthroplasty: A five- to ten-year prospective study. *J Bone Joint Surg Br* 2001;83:696-701.

40. Ackroyd CE, Newman JH: The Avon patello-femoral arthroplasty: Development and early results. *J Bone Joint Surg Br* 2001;83(suppl II):146-147.

41. Ackroyd CE, Newman JH: The Avon patellofemoral arthroplasty: Two to five year results. *J Bone Joint Surg Br* 2003;85(suppl II):162-163.

42. Ackroyd CE, Newman JH, Evans R, Eldridge JD, Joslin CC: The Avon patellofemoral arthroplasty: Five-year survivorship and functional results. *J Bone Joint Surg Br* 2007;89:310-315.

43. Thompson NW, Ruiz AL, Breslin E, Beverland DE: Total knee arthroplasty without patellar resurfacing in isolated patellofemoral osteoarthritis. *J Arthroplasty* 2001;16:607-612.

44. Laskin RS, van Steijn M: Total knee replacement for patients with patellofemoral arthritis. *Clin Orthop Relat Res* 1999;367:89-95.

45. Parvizi J, Stuart MJ, Pagnano MW, Hanssen AD: Total knee arthroplasty in patients with isolated patellofemoral arthritis. *Clin Orthop Relat Res* 2001;392:147-152.

46. Mont MA, Haas S, Mullick T, Hungerford DS: Total knee arthroplasty for patellofemoral arthritis. *J Bone Joint Surg Am* 2002;84:1977-1981.

47. Laskin RS: Lateral release rates after total knee arthroplasty. *Clin Orthop Relat Res* 2001;392:88-93.

48. Lewonowski K, Dorr LD, McPherson EJ, Huber G, Wan Z: Medialization of the patella in total knee arthroplasty. *J Arthroplasty* 1997;12:161-167.

49. Malo M, Vince KG: The unstable patella after total knee arthroplasty: Etiology, prevention, and management. *J Am Acad Orthop Surg* 2003;11:364-371.

50. Lonner JH, Lotke PA: Aseptic complications after total knee arthroplasty. *J Am Acad Orthop Surg* 1999;7:311-324.

51. Berger RA, Crossett LS, Jacobs JJ, Rubash HE: Malrotation causing patellofemoral complications after total knee arthroplasty. *Clin Orthop Relat Res* 1998;356:144-153.

52. Berger RA, Rubash HE, Seel MJ, Thompson WH, Crossett LS: Determining the rotational alignment of the femoral component in total knee arthroplasty using the epicondylar axis. *Clin Orthop Relat Res* 1993;286:40-47.

53. Merkow RL, Soudry M, Insall JN: Patellar dislocation following total knee replacement. *J Bone Joint Surg Am* 1985;67:1321-1327.

54. Krackow KA: *The Technique of Total Knee Arthroplasty.* St. Louis, MO, CV Mosby, 1990, p 139.

55. Whiteside LA, Arima J: The antero-posterior axis for femoral rotational alignment in valgus total knee arthroplasty. *Clin Orthop Relat Res* 1995;321:168-172.

56. Nagamine R, Whiteside LA, Otani T, White SE, McCarthy DS: Effect of medial displacement of the tibial tubercle on patellar position after rotational malposition of the femoral component in total knee arthroplasty. *J Arthroplasty* 1996;11:104-110.

57. Anouchi YS, Whiteside LA, Kaiser AD, Milliano MT: The effects of axial rotational alignment of the femoral component on knee stability and patellar tracking in total knee arthroplasty demonstrated on autopsy specimens. *Clin Orthop Relat Res* 1993;287:170-177.

58. Bourne RB, Burnett RS: The consequences of not resurfacing the patella. *Clin Orthop Relat Res* 2004;428:166-169.

59. Forster MC: Patellar resurfacing in total knee arthroplasty for osteoarthritis: A systematic review. *Knee* 2004;11:427-430.

60. Holt GE, Dennis DA: The role of patellar resurfacing in total knee arthroplasty. *Clin Orthop Relat Res* 2003;416:76-83.

61. Feller JA, Bartlett RJ, Lang DM: Patellar resurfacing versus retention in total knee arthroplasty. *J Bone Joint Surg Br* 1996;78:226-228.

62. Mihalko W, Fishkin Z, Krackow K: Patellofemoral overstuff and its relationship to flexion after total knee arthroplasty. *Clin Orthop Relat Res* 2006;449:283-287.

63. Matsueda M, Gustilo RB: Subvastus and medial parapatellar approaches in total knee arthroplasty. *Clin Orthop Relat Res* 2000;371:161-168.

64. Stulberg SD, Loan P, Sarin V: Computer-assisted navigation in total knee replacement: Results of an initial experience in thirty-five patients. *J Bone Joint Surg Am* 2002;84(suppl 2): 90-98.

65. Victor J, Hoste D: Image-based computer-assisted total knee arthroplasty leads to lower variability in coronal alignment. *Clin Orthop Relat Res* 2004;428:131-139.

66. Bäthis H, Perlick L, Tingart M, Lüring C, Zurakowski D, Grifka J: Alignment in total knee arthroplasty: A comparison of computer-assisted surgery with the conventional technique. *J Bone Joint Surg Br* 2004;86: 682-687.

67. Haaker RG, Stockheim M, Kamp M, Proff G, Breitenfelder J, Ottersbach A: Computer-assisted navigation increases precision of component placement in total knee arthroplasty. *Clin Orthop Relat Res* 2005;433:152-159.

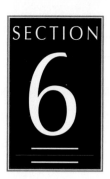

# SECTION

# 6

# Foot and Ankle

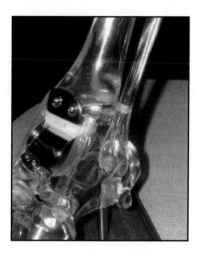

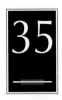

# 35

# Total Ankle Arthroplasty

*James K. DeOrio, MD
Mark E. Easley, MD

## Abstract

*Recent investigations support the belief that ankle replacement represents an attractive surgical alternative to arthrodesis for patients with advanced ankle arthritis. Although longer follow-up is necessary for total ankle arthroplasty (TAA) to displace arthrodesis as the surgical "gold standard," intermediate-term results are encouraging. Indications for TAA include primarily posttraumatic and inflammatory arthritis. Contraindications to TAA include unresectable osteonecrotic bone, peripheral vascular disease, neuropathy, active and/or recent ankle infection, nonreconstructible ankle ligaments, loss of lower leg muscular control, and severe osteopenia or osteoporosis. Young, active, high-demand patients with ankle arthritis may be better candidates for arthrodesis than for TAA. Rigorous patient selection is essential in the success of TAA, more than in other joint arthroplasty procedures.*

*Total ankle prosthetic designs (Agility, Scandinavian Total Ankle Replacement, Hintegra, Salto, and Buechel-Pappas) with a minimum of published intermediate follow-up results, and several other innovative and biomechanically supported designs (the Mobility Total Ankle System, BOX, INBONE, and Salto-Talaris) are reviewed to demonstrate the recent evolution of TAA.*

*Some TAA designs feature a nonconstrained polyethylene meniscus (mobile bearing) that articulates between the porous-coated tibial and talar components. The concern for edge loading (when the polyethylene component comes in contact with a metal edge) has been addressed in more recent designs by reducing the superior polyethylene surface area, expanding the tibial component surface, and even offering a convex tibial component. More practical, effective, and safer instrumentation for implantation has also been developed and has been essential to the success of TAA. However, complications with TAA (such as inadequate wound healing and malleolar fractures) are more frequent when compared with total hip and knee arthroplasty, irrespective of the surgeon's training method. As an individual surgeon gains more experience, the chances of a favorable outcome are increased.*

**Instr Course Lect 2008;57:383-413.**

Despite the failures of first-generation ankle prostheses implanted approximately 30 years ago, the interest in total ankle arthroplasty (TAA) has grown over the past decade. Currently, more than 20 different TAA designs are marketed worldwide, and several other designs are in development. This evolution of TAA from a procedure that was near extinction to a procedure with growing recognition can be attributed to four factors. (1) In the face of adversity, several pioneers designed ankle implants and techniques to perpetuate this procedure. Frank Alvine (Agility Ankle; DePuy, Warsaw, IN), Hakon Kofoed (Scandinavian Total Ankle Replacement [STAR]; W. Link GmbH and Co, Hamburg, Germany), and Fred Buechel (Low Contact Stress [LCS]/Buechel-Pappas Ankle; Endotec, South Orange, NJ) managed to develop and refine designs that are still currently in use; these designs have served as the foundations for current developments in TAA. Without the persistence of these individuals, the art of TAA may have ceased because of the original failures. (2) Several important studies have shown favorable outcomes with second-generation implants.[1-4]

*James K. DeOrio, MD or the department with which he is affiliated has received research or institutional support from Link Orthopaedics; miscellaneous nonincome support, commercially derived honoraria, or other nonresearch-related funding from Tornier, INBONE, and Link Orthopaedics; and is a consultant or employee for Link Orthopaedics and INBONE.*

(3) Several long-term outcome studies of ankle arthrodeses showed that although many patients do well initially with an ankle arthrodesis, some will ultimately suffer debilitating, secondary adjacent hindfoot arthritis in the subtalar and talonavicular joints.[5,6] This secondary hindfoot arthritis is so debilitating that it has prompted some surgeons to convert ankle arthrodeses to ankle replacements.[7] (4) TAA affords a nearly physiologic gait pattern in comparison with that of ankle arthrodesis using validated outcome measures.[8-10]

First-generation, cemented, constrained, two-component designs were replaced with first-generation, cementless, two-component designs, specifically the Agility Ankle[4] and the ceramic, polyethylene-lined TNK ankle (Kyocera, Kyoto, Japan).[11] Second-generation, three-component implants with minimal constraint are currently being used internationally. These implants include the STAR, Hintegra ankle replacement (New Deal SA, Lyon, France), the Salto prosthesis (Tornier SAS, Saint Ismier, France), the Buechel-Pappas ankle, Mobility (DePuy), and the Bologna Oxford (BOX) ankle (Finsbury, Leatherhead, Surrey, UK). Other three-component TAAs also have been developed, including the ESKA implant (GmbH and Co), the Ankle Evolution System (AES; Biomet, Dordrecht, Netherlands), the OSG ankle (Corin, Cirencester, England), the Albatross (Groupe Lepine, Lyon, France), and the Ramses (Fournitures Hospitaliers, Mulhouse, France). Three more designs in early trials are the CCI Evolution (van Straten Medical/Argomedical, Doets, Germany), the German Ankle System (ARGE Medizintechnik, Hannover, Germany), and the Al-

phamed ankle (Alphamed Medizintechnik Fischer GmbH, Lassnitzhöhe, Austria).

For the past decade, the Agility Ankle has been the only total ankle prosthetic design system approved by the US Food and Drug Administration (FDA). In 2006, the FDA approved three new two-component prostheses, the INBONE total ankle system (INBONE Orthopaedics, Boulder, CO), the Salto-Talaris (Tornier, Stafford, TX), and the Eclipse (Integra Life Sciences Holding Corporation, Plainsboro, NJ). To date, no three-component design has received full FDA approval; however, in April 2007 the STAR prosthesis was granted conditional FDA approval but with the need to fulfill several requirements before release to the US market.

This chapter focuses on total ankle replacement designs with FDA approval and/or available peer-reviewed outcome studies. The Agility is the only TAA system that has both FDA approval and intermediate to long-term peer-reviewed outcome data. The STAR, Buechel-Pappas, Hintegra, and Salto prostheses lack FDA approval but have more than 2 years of follow-up data in peer-reviewed outcome studies. The INBONE and Salto-Talaris prostheses also will be discussed because they are currently being used in the United States. Despite FDA approval, little information is available for the Eclipse, and it has had limited use to date. Although the Mobility and BOX implants lack both FDA approval and peer-reviewed outcomes data exceeding 2 years, these prostheses will be mentioned because these designs provide insight into recent developments in TAA.[12-14]

Whereas the hip is dislocated and the knee subluxated during arthro-

plasty procedures, TAA implants must be placed in situ.[15] The techniques to perform TAA vary with prosthetic design and the required implant-specific instrumentation. Although many complications in TAA surgery are common to all ankles, some are unique to a specific ankle replacement design. Few TAA outcome studies are available in the literature. A recent systematic meta-analysis of the three-component TAAs (1,086 patients) observed that only 18 of 1,830 citations fulfilled the eligibility criteria for a satisfactory, evidence-based study.[16] Using a standardized 100-point ankle and hindfoot score, formal data pooling was possible for only 10 trials and 497 patients. Nonetheless, many of these studies report on complications, providing knowledge about each ankle design.

## Indications/Contraindications
### Overview
Patient selection is critical in ankle arthroplasty for this relatively small but major weight-bearing joint. Good candidates for TAA have lower activity demands and are middle-aged or elderly patients with painful ankle arthritis (either traumatic or inflammatory), without osteopenia or osteoporosis. Ankle replacement is an end-stage procedure designed to relieve pain experienced with activities of daily living; it is not intended to enable patients to return to jobs requiring heavy labor or participate in impact athletics. Candidates for TAA must have satisfactory peripheral perfusion, intact sensation, and physiologic neuromuscular function. Patients with peripheral vascular disease, concomitant skin disorders, neuropathy, or Charcot joints are not suited to treatment with this procedure. Active and chronic ankle infections represent

absolute contraindications. Osteonecrosis, either of the tibial plafond or talus, is a relative contraindication (for example, patients with avascular bone segments that cannot be resected at surgery are poor candidates for TAA). However, if the avascular segment can be resected with adequate bone remaining to support an implant, TAA may be considered.

### Prior Hindfoot Arthrodesis

End-stage ankle arthritis associated with prior subtalar or triple arthrodeses may represent an ideal indication for TAA because ankle arthrodesis would add further rigidity to an already stiff ankle-hindfoot complex. However, a previous hindfoot arthrodesis that compromises the primary talar blood supply (sinus tarsi artery) may lead to subsequent talar component subsidence. Talar implants that require resection of the medial and/or lateral talar dome surfaces (such as STAR, Hintegra, and Salto) or implants that do not use the entire prepared talar surface (such as the first-generation Agility talar component) may be particularly prone to subsidence. In contrast, the INBONE, Buechel-Pappas, Mobility, and BOX talar components preserve the medial and lateral talar dome cortices and are potentially more protective against subsidence. Currently, no evidence exists to determine whether preserving medial/lateral cortical support to the talar dome or creating greater surface area for bone ingrowth with medial/lateral talar dome resection confers a greater advantage in talar component survivorship.

### Ligament Insufficiency

Similar to knee replacement, soft-tissue balancing is critical in TAA. Preoperative varus tilting in the ankle typically demands lateral ankle ligament reconstruction and potentially some deltoid ligament release. Although TAA in patients with medial (deltoid) ligament laxity is feasible, nonreconstructible ligament instability, particularly deltoid ligament absence, represents a contraindication to TAA because a satisfactory procedure for deltoid ligament reconstruction has not been perfected. Many preoperative deformities occur secondary to chronic ligament imbalance; resultant tibial plafond erosions secondary to long-standing talar tilt will create edge loading within the ankle mortise, which can result in asymmetric wear of the tibia and/or talus. Standard tibial and talar preparation with or without minor bone grafting normally addresses these bony deficiencies.

### Malalignment

Varus or valgus talar tilt in the ankle mortise in patients with end-stage ankle arthritis can be corrected with TAA. Although no absolute degree of talar tilt has been established as a limit to correction with TAA, anecdotal experience suggests that talar tilt exceeding 10° to 20° may represent a contraindication for TAA. In patients with preoperative ligament instability and/or malalignment, the surgeon should obtain preoperative informed consent to intraoperatively abandon TAA in favor of arthrodesis when satisfactory alignment and balance cannot be established. Haskell and Mann[17] suggested that patients with incongruent ankle joints (talar tilt within ankle mortise) were at greater risk for progressive edge loading of a TAA. Extra-articular deformities are generally best addressed with periarticular (supramalleolar or calcaneal) osteotomies. Although these osteotomies can be performed simultaneously with TAA, staging these procedures separately before TAA may be safer and may occasionally alleviate the patient's symptoms adequately to delay the need for TAA, similar to periarticular osteotomies for arthritis of the knee.[18-21]

### Preoperative Range of Motion

As for other joints being considered for joint arthroplasty, preoperative range of motion (ROM) of an arthritic joint typically predicts postoperative ROM. Patients with less than 10° of ankle ROM may function equally well after arthrodesis because even uncomplicated TAA in these patients may not reliably increase ROM.

## Implant Design
### Overview

The ideal ankle implant has yet to be developed. However, current expectations for TAA are (1) reproducible technique, (2) minimal bone resection, (3) rapid and adequate bone ingrowth, (4) minimal constraint, (5) replication of physiologic ankle motion (optimal soft-tissue tensioning throughout ambulation), (6) minimal complications and need for early revision, (7) long-term survivorship, and (8) predictable pain relief. In general, past experiences demonstrate that successful total hip and total knee arthroplasty designs closely mimic the anatomy of the joints they replace. Although it is logical that TAA designs and human ankle joint anatomy and function should converge, this is not necessarily the situation for all currently marketed implants. Some designs closely mimic human ankle joint morphology, whereas others differ considerably from normal anatomy. Of note, morphologic ankle joint measurements collected in 36 individuals with normal ankle anatomy show that the bones of the ankle are in direct proportion to each

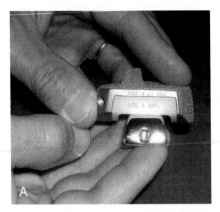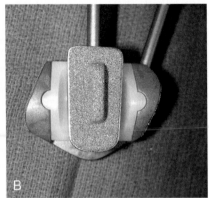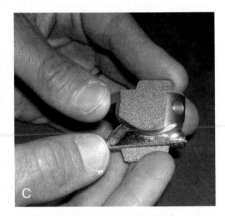

**Figure 1**   The Agility ankle prosthesis. **A,** Front view. **B,** Footprint of the talar component. **C,** View from the medial side.

other.[22] The implication with this finding is that developing an inventory of progressively larger, anatomically precise TAA component sizes is appropriate.

Currently, more than 20 different designs are either released for clinical use or are in development internationally. FDA approval for TAA implantation is currently restricted to two component designs, with the exception of the STAR, which was approved in March 2007 with some additional requirements before release. Specifically, the Agility, the INBONE, the Salto-Talaris, and the Eclipse prostheses are approved, with the Salto-Talaris being a fixed-bearing modification of the mobile-bearing Salto prosthesis. These designs are approved for use with cement only, and thus are all used "off-label." Outside the United States, the mobile-bearing, three-component prostheses have been favored over fixed-bearing, two-component designs. Implantation of three-component prostheses in the United States has been limited to select FDA-monitored clinical trials.

## Specific Implant Designs
### *Agility Prosthesis*
#### *Overview/Primary Design*
The Agility total ankle prosthesis was

designed in 1984 and is one of the few current TAA designs with FDA approval (Figure 1). Although approved for use with cement, it is routinely used off-label without cement, provided informed consent is obtained from the patient. The inventory of the Agility includes six sizes of matching tibial and talar components. Unique to this design is a titanium alloy tibial component with an ongrowth surface that rests simultaneously on the tibial plafond and inner aspects of the medial and lateral malleoli. Proper tibial component positioning requires resection of the residual tibial plafond articular surface and the articular surfaces of both malleoli. To facilitate this combined tibial/fibular support, a syndesmotic fusion is necessary for a successful outcome; a requirement unique to the Agility system.[2,4,23] This fixed-bearing implant has a size-matched, separate, high-density polyethylene insert that slides into the tibial component. This articular surface is rotated 22° externally to mimic ankle anatomy. The most recent designs afford greater tibial plafond and talar dome coverage than the original models, and a front-loading polyethylene component insert helps to facilitate polyethylene exchange. The talar component is an onlay cobalt-chromium replacement of the talar

dome, with a bone ingrowth surface facing the residual talar dome. A concern for talar component subsidence has prompted revamping of the original posteriorly tapered design to a nearly rectangular flared base (originally, the posterior taper was intended to limit posterior impingement). Currently available tibial and talar components have single fins, also with bone ingrowth surfaces, to provide greater stability. In an attempt to further limit subsidence, a broader, multifinned talar component also has been designed.

### *Revision Components*
Revision components are available for the talar and polyethylene implants. With the tibial and talar components implanted, the original polyethylene insert was difficult to exchange in revision surgery because it inserted vertically. Now, the revision polyethylene component has half columns that allow it to be inserted from the front, and it is 2 mm thicker than the standard polyethylene component. The revision talar component has a completely rectangular base and a 2-mm increase in vertical thickness relative to the primary implant. These options afford the potential to increase the total height of the revision prosthesis by 4 mm. Custom revision

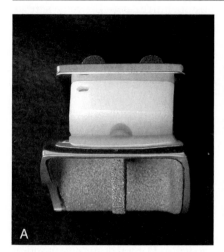
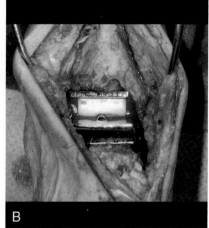
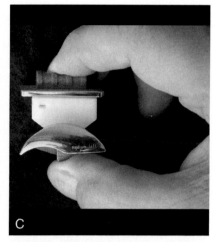

**Figure 2**    STAR prosthesis. **A,** Front view. **B,** Implanted at the time of surgery. **C,** Side view.

implants feature stemmed talar and tibial components.

### Biomechanics

Motion in the Agility ankle prosthesis is constrained by the implant's articulating surfaces and the ankle ligaments.[24-26] In a cadaver model simulating physiologic motion and loading during a walking cycle, the anterior talofibular and tibiocalcaneal ligaments proved to be reasonable guides for tibial component positioning. The anterior talofibular and tibiocalcaneal ligaments were shown to be sensitive to transverse plane and coronal plane displacements, respectively.

In another study, 10 cadaveric specimens were implanted with the Agility ankle prosthesis and axially loaded to 700 N.[27] The average contact pressure of the system was 5.6 MPa with mean peak pressures of 21.2 MPa. When physiologic ankle forces are considered for routine patient activity, peak pressures may exceed recommended contact pressures (10 MPa) and the compressive yield point (13 to 22 MPa) for polyethylene. Based on the contact pressure data, the investigators suggested that a heavy patient with a larger ankle

may be a better candidate for this procedure than a heavy patient with a small ankle.

### STAR Prosthesis
#### Overview

The STAR Prosthesis, designed in 1981, is the prototypical three-component TAA (Figure 2). The original two-piece cemented prosthesis evolved into the current three-piece, meniscal-bearing, on-growth design. The symmetrically trapezoidal tibial component is wider in the front and has two cylinders or barrels that provide an interference fit with the prepared tibial surface.

The symmetrically convex, bone ingrowth, talar component resurfaces the talar dome (including the medial and lateral aspects) so that the talar implant articulates with the polyethylene meniscus and the ankle's natural malleolar articular surfaces. To accomplish this, the medial and lateral articular surfaces of the talus are resected. Support for the talar cap is enhanced by a single bone ingrowth fin. A criticism of this talar component design is a failure to respect the relatively smaller

medial curvature and larger lateral radius of curvature of the natural talus, which may occasionally lead to relatively loose lateral ligaments and relatively tight medial ligaments after implantation. The high density polyethylene implant is concave on its inferior surface and articulates with the domed talar component. The congruent talar convexity and polyethylene concavity maintain anteroposterior polyethylene stability. The articulating dorsal talar component surface has a smooth, central, longitudinally oriented ridge that congruently articulates with a groove in the inferior polyethylene surface to maintain proper mediolateral polyethylene position. The increased constraint created by these features at the polyethylene-talar component interface is offset by the nonconstrained tibial component polyethylene interface; the flat superior polyethylene surface freely glides on the flat, polished, tibial component. The bony interfaces of the cobalt-chromium metal implants have a titanium spray coating to promote bony ingrowth; alternatively, outside the United States, a hydroxyapatite coating is available.

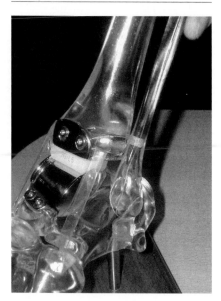

**Figure 3**    Hintegra ankle prosthesis.

Talar component inventory includes five sizes. The tibial component is available in anteroposterior dimensions of 30, 35, 40, and 45 mm, with widths only varying from 30 to 32.5 mm. The polyethylene component increases in 1-mm increments between 6 and 10 mm. Polyethylene revision components are manufactured in 1-mm increments from 11 mm to 15 mm. A revision tibial-stemmed component is available; however, to date no revision talar component is available without custom specifications.

### Biomechanics

Testing in cadavers demonstrates that optimal polyethylene thickness and sagittal plane talar component positioning maximize ankle ROM and limit polyethylene lift-off.[28] Six cadaver ankles with STAR prostheses were tested under weight-bearing conditions to determine ROM, while the strain in the ankle ligaments was monitored. Each specimen was tested with the talar component positions in neutral, 3 mm, and 6 mm of anterior and pos-

terior displacement. The sequence was repeated with an anatomic bearing thickness, as well as at 2 mm reduced and increased thicknesses. Both anterior talar component displacement and bearing thickness reduction caused a decrease in plantar flexion, associated with polyethylene lift-off. With increased bearing thickness, posterior displacement of the talar component decreased plantar flexion, whereas anterior displacement decreased dorsiflexion.

Another study evaluated the function of the ankle joint during walking before and after STAR implantation. Nine patients were evaluated both preoperatively and postoperatively in a gait analysis laboratory. Arthroplasty patients showed reduced ankle ROM compared with normal control subjects. However, postoperative arthroplasty patients had significantly improved external ankle dorsiflexion moment when compared with their preoperative status, suggesting improved function of the ankle joint.[9]

### Hintegra Prosthesis
#### Overview

The Hintegra total ankle prosthesis was designed in 2000 (Figure 3). Much like the STAR prosthesis, the Hintegra is a nonconstrained, three-component system that provides inversion/eversion stability. Axial rotation and normal flexion/extension mobility are provided by a mobile-bearing element with limits to motion imposed only by natural soft-tissue constraints. No more than 2 to 3 mm of bone removal on each side of the joint is necessary to insert the tibial and talar components.

Flat-cut tibial preparation affords apposition of the tibial component with structurally sound subchondral bone. To eliminate coronal plane micromotion in the immediate

postoperative period, two screws may be inserted through the anterior phalange of the tibial component. These screws do not lock into the oval holes of the tibial component; instead, they are inserted into the superior aspect of these holes so the benefit of axial loading is not limited in optimizing apposition between resected tibial plafond and tibial component.

The talar component caps the entire talar dome, necessitating not only superior surface resection but also medial and lateral dome subchondral bone removal for the talar implant to articulate with the natural malleolar articular surfaces. The talar component has an asymmetric dual-radius curvature, with a smaller radius of curvature on the medial rather than the lateral sides. The sides of the talar component hemiprosthetically replace medial and lateral talar facets, mimicking the morphology of the physiologic talus. An anterior extension from the talar component to the talar neck features two holes that permit screw fixation if desired. The talar component has two pegs that create greater stability, and the slightly curved medial and lateral component surfaces afford press-fit fixation, making screw fixation optional. The curved superior articular surface of the talar component is congruent with the polyethylene insert and controls sagittal plane position of the polyethylene. Medial and lateral rails on the borders of the dorsal talar surface control the coronal plane position of the polyethylene. Theoretically, the increased constraint created by these features at the polyethylene-talar component interface is offset by the nonconstrained tibial component polyethylene interface; the flat superior polyethylene surface freely glides on the flat, polished, tibial component.

## Biomechanics

In biomechanical testing, Valderrabano and associates[24-26] compared cadaver ankles that were normal, had been treated with arthrodesis, or had been implanted with either the Agility, STAR, or Hintegra prostheses, with the Hintegra most closely reproducing physiologic ankle ROM in their cadaver model. The investigation showed that the three-component ankles (Hintegra, STAR) afforded motion that approached that of the unoperated cadaver ankle.[24] In contrast, the study suggested that the fixed-bearing, two-component design (Agility) restricted talar motion within the ankle mortise, thereby increasing stress/constraint at the bone-implant interface.[24] The authors concluded that successful TAA relies on how effectively designs can mimic physiologic human ankle movement transfer, while simultaneously dissipating rotational forces and maintaining joint stability.[24-26] In particular, these investigators noted that an anatomic talar component design conferred a biomechanical advantage over nonanatomic designs.

Another study suggested that establishing physiologic hindfoot alignment is essential for optimal foot and ankle function, and preoperative malalignment should be corrected. Using the Heidelberg Foot Model, Muller and associates[29] analyzed 11 patients with the unilateral Hintegra ankle prosthesis. Although the timing of the kinematics between the physiologically normal and operated extremities appeared similar, diminished ROM was found in all operated foot segments. A limitation in hindfoot mobility, as experienced after ankle arthrodesis, was not observed. Concerning kinetics, the replaced ankle showed a decrease in power generation compensated by an increase in power in the ipsilateral knee.

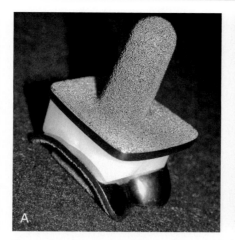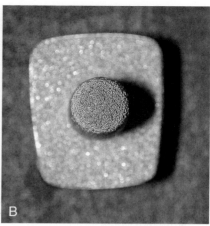

**Figure 4**    Buechal-Pappas implant. **A,** Ankle components. **B,** View from top stem.

## Buechel-Pappas Implant

### Overview

The original LCS TAA implant designed by Buechel and Pappas evolved into the current Buechel-Pappas implant[30,31] (Figure 4). The first-generation device (Mark I) was first implanted in 1978 and was modified into the second-generation device (Mark II) in 1989.[1,30-32] The Buechel-Pappas design has three components. The tibial component has a flat, polished platform that articulates with the flat superior polyethylene surface, and a central stem requires that a window be cut into the anterior tibial cortex for its implantation into the tibial metaphysis. The convex talar component has a single radius and a central sulcus that is congruent with the inferior polyethylene surface. This configuration controls coronal plane polyethylene translation and permits a mild degree of inversion/eversion while maintaining full conformity and limiting the risk of edge loading. The constraint created by the polyethylene talar implant is offset by the flat interface between the tibial component and polyethylene articulations. Modifications that have led to

the currently available design include a thicker tibial component, a second talar component backside fin for improved fixation, a titanium nitride porous coating to enhance bone ingrowth, and a deeper talar sulcus for improved polyethylene stability. A nitride ceramic film on the titanium articulating surfaces may afford improved wear characteristics with the polyethylene insert. The talar component only resurfaces the superior aspect of the talar dome; the medial and lateral cartilage is left intact to continue physiologic articulation with the malleolar articular surfaces.

### Biomechanics

A fluoroscopic evaluation of 10 patients with unilateral Buechel-Pappas implants showed an average ROM of 37.4° for normal ankles and 32.3° for implanted ankles. Implanted ankles showed rotational and translational motion but had relatively more posterior talar contact, particularly with plantar flexion, when compared with the nonoperated ankles. The authors suggested that the increased posterior contact was related to surgical technique or alterations of ligamentous tension.[33]

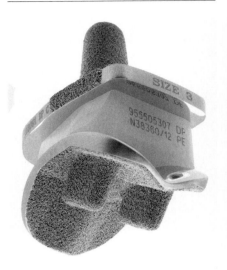

**Figure 5**    Mobility ankle prosthesis.

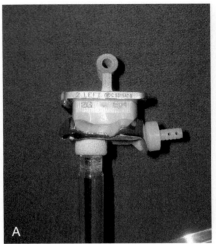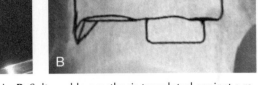

**Figure 6**    **A,** Salto ankle prosthesis. **B,** Salto ankle prosthesis templated against a radiograph.

## Mobility Total Ankle System
### Overview

The Mobility Total Ankle System was developed by a surgeon design team in collaboration with DePuy and became commercially available in October 2004 (Figure 5). The device was first implanted in September 2003 and has been released for general use in Europe, Australia, New Zealand, South Africa, and Canada. In the United States, a multicenter FDA trial comparing the Agility and Mobility prostheses has been initiated.

The Mobility unconstrained, three-component, mobile-bearing prosthesis resembles the Buechel-Pappas total ankle system. The short, conical stem, set on the central nonarticulating aspect of the tibial component, is similar to the Buechel-Pappas implant. However, the sagittal plane dimensions of the tibial component exceed those of the Buechel-Pappas implant to optimize tibial plafond coverage while being tapered posteriorly to avoid overhang and soft-tissue impingement. The talar component resurfaces only the superior dome of the talus without violating the native medial and lateral aspects of the talar dome like the Buechel-Pappas implant. The talar component also features a central, longitudinal sulcus. Talar component stability is enhanced by two fins on the non-articulating aspect of the implant. The constraint imparted by the conforming, congruent interface of the talar component and polyethylene insert is dissipated by the flat tibial component-polyethylene articulation. The porous coated, nonarticulating metal surfaces are covered with a titanium spray.

### Comparison

In simulated mechanical testing by the manufacturer, the Mobility total ankle prosthesis compares favorably with the Buechel-Pappas implant. Similar shear loads were required to dislocate the Mobility and Buechel-Pappas bearing inserts in both the sagittal and coronal planes. However, under similar circumstances, the Mobility talar component was less likely to subside when compared with the Buechel-Pappas talar component. In a comparative study of stability testing performed at Leeds University and sponsored by DePuy, researchers noted (in an internal company document) that the Mobility prosthesis demonstrated significantly higher average peak loads to failure in the coronal and sagittal planes compared with the Buechel-Pappas implant.[34] Similarly, in a simulator test, the wear rate for the Mobility ankle prosthesis was less than that of the Buechel-Pappas implant.[35]

## Salto and Salto-Talaris Prostheses
### Overview

The three-component Salto TAA prosthesis was designed in 1998 and offers a unique and optional polyethylene fibular implant to articulate with the lateral talar component (Figure 6); however, the fibular component is now rarely used. Tibial component stability is enhanced by a central pedestal-like stem that necessitates a keyhole-shaped anterior tibial cortical window for insertion. Medially, a low-profile medial rail extends vertically from the horizontal tibial surface that protects the medial malleolus and limits medial translation of the polyethylene insert.

Because of the restrictions imposed by the FDA on three-component TAA devices implanted in the United States, the two-component Salto-Talaris prosthesis (Figure 7) was recently introduced and is essentially the fixed-bearing version of the Salto prosthesis. The polyethylene component is secured to the tibial component via a locking mechanism and no fibular component is available. The Salto-Talaris prosthesis was approved for use in the United States in November 2006. The manufacturer introduced the concept of "mobile-bearing instruments." Although the tibia and talus are prepared separately, the orientation of the bony cuts are at least in part interrelated to facilitate the symmetrical articulation of the talar and fixed-bearing tibial components. With the talar component seated, an instrument unique to the Salto-Talaris system allows the surgeon to determine the ideal tibial component position relative to tracking of the talus within the ankle mortise. The tibial component is then fixed in that position. However, with larger component sizes, this "auto-alignment" feature may be limited by the ankle's coronal dimensions because the tibial component may not have sufficient space to rotate.

The concave talar component resurfaces the talar dome and mimics physiologic talar morphology, with the medial radius being shorter than the lateral radius. Although the lateral aspect of the talar component fully resurfaces the lateral talar dome, the medial side does not. Medially, the natural talar dome is not violated. The superior surface of the talar component has a central, sagittal sulcus that conforms to the

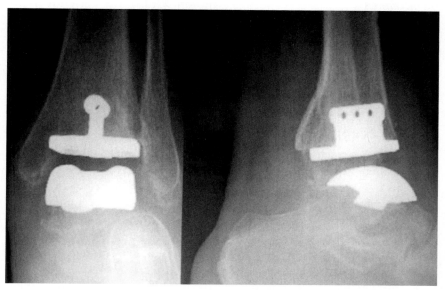

**Figure 7**   AP (left) and lateral (right) radiographic views of the Salto-Talaris ankle prosthesis.

central ridge on the inferior polyethylene surface. This configuration affords coronal plane stability and limits the risks for polyethylene dislocation while reducing edge loading. The conformity of the polyethylene to the talar component combined with the medial stop mechanism of the tibial component creates some degree of constraint. The tibial and talar components are made of cobalt-chromium and feature a titanium spray ingrowth surface; only the Salto prosthesis (not the Salto-Talaris) has a hydroxyapatite coating.

### BOX Prosthesis
#### Overview
The name BOX is derived from the joint efforts of the prostheses designers from the Istituti Ortopedici Rizzoli, Bologna, Italy, and the laboratory in Oxford, England. Like the Buechel-Pappas and Mobility prostheses, the BOX does not resurface the sides of the talus, only the superior dome. Similar to the STAR prosthesis, the BOX has ingrowth

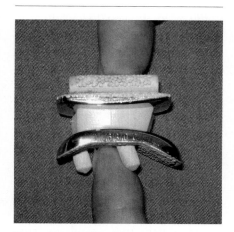

**Figure 8**   BOX ankle prosthesis.

cylinders on its tibial base plate. It has an anatomic talar component with the radius of curvature longer than that of the natural talus in the sagittal plane, and a fully conforming meniscal component. It is made of cobalt-chromium with a titanium spray coating on its surface. The BOX has a unique design with a convex tibial component that articulates with a biconcave polyethylene spacer (Figure 8).

## Biomechanics

Several researchers described how the unique BOX prosthetic design maintains optimal biomechanical behavior of coupled human ankle-hindfoot physiologic motion, while allowing complete congruence over the entire range of ankle motion. Claiming the first realistic representation of the biomechanical behavior of a prosthetic joint replacing a human ankle, researchers noted that the meniscal bearing of the BOX ankle prosthesis was observed to move 5.6 mm posteriorly during the simulated stance, and the corresponding anteroposterior displacement of the talar component was 8.3 mm.[13,14] The predicted pattern and the amount (10.6°) of internal-external rotation of the ankle complex were found to be in agreement with corresponding in vivo measurements on normal ankles. A peak contact pressure of 16.8 MPa was observed, with most of the contact pressures below 10 MPa. For most ligaments, reaction forces remain within corresponding physiologic ranges.[14] Preliminary observations in trial implantation in a few patients suggest that while reproducing physiologic ankle mobility, the new design is capable of maintaining complete congruence at the two articulating surfaces of the meniscal bearing over the entire motion arc, with the prospect of minimizing wear of this component.[12]

In another study, one of the designers of the BOX prosthesis found that rolling as well as sliding motion occurs in the natural ankle, governed by a ligamentous linkage.[36] Elongation of the tibiocalcaneal and calcaneofibular ligaments was 1.5% and 4.8%, respectively. A 13% change in lever arm length occurred for both the tibialis anterior and gastrocnemius muscles during ankle flexion. Unlike the currently available three-component designs, the newly proposed convex, tibial ligament-compatible prosthesis was found to restore the original mobility and physiologic function of the ligaments. The authors believe that the BOX prosthesis combines freedom from restraint with congruity of the components throughout the range of flexion. The designers also evaluated the kinematics of the ankle when replaced by nonconforming two-component designs and by fully conforming three-component designs with flat, concave, or convex tibial surfaces; these designs were assessed by their dynamic ankle joint simulation model. A ligament-compatible, convex-tibia, fully congruent three-component prosthesis showed the best features. The three-component prosthesis allows complete congruence over the entire ROM.[36] A convex shape for the tibial arc was preferred because of the improved degree of entrapment of the meniscal bearing. A 5-cm, convex-tibia arc radius provided 2 mm of entrapment together with 9.8 mm of tibial bone cut. Ligament elongation imposed by full congruence of the articular surfaces was less than 0.03% of the original length. The original patterns of joint kinematics and ligament tensioning were closely restored in the joint replaced by the proposed prosthesis.[37]

## INBONE Prosthesis

### Overview

The INBONE total ankle system is a fixed-bearing, two-component design with a modular stem system for both tibia and talar components (Figure 9). Multiple modular segments may be added to the tibial stem, depending on the surgeon's determination of how much stability is needed or the distance the stem should pass beyond a simultaneous supramalleolar osteotomy performed for tibial malunion. The tibia is inset into the tibial metaphysis but, unlike the Agility, does not resurface the malleoli. The talar component entirely replaces the superiormost aspect of the natural talus, after a flat dome resection. The stem of the talar component may be limited to the body of the talus or can be extended across the subtalar joint into the calcaneus if greater support for the talar component is required, or when a simultaneous subtalar arthrodesis is warranted. The longer talar component calcaneal stem is not currently FDA approved.

Unique to the INBONE total ankle system is the alignment guide placed after the ankle is exposed via an anterior approach. The device demands simultaneous alignment of the talus with the tibia in both the coronal and sagittal planes. Once that is achieved, a drill is passed from the plantar foot through the calcaneus, just anterior to the posterior facet of the subtalar joint, through the center of the talar body into the center of the tibial metaphysis; much like the guide pin for a retrograde ankle arthrodesis nail. Although many surgeons believe that it is undesirable to violate the subtalar joint when performing TAA, the designers of this alignment guide maintain that appropriate application of the device permits the 6-mm drill to safely negotiate the subtalar joint between the arterial anastomosis on the inferior talar neck and the articulation of the posterior facet with the inferior talus.

### Biomechanics

No reports are yet available documenting the kinematics of the INBONE ankle prosthesis in biomechanical testing. More information is needed to define the biome-

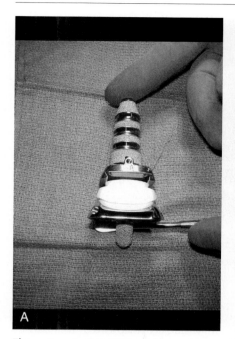

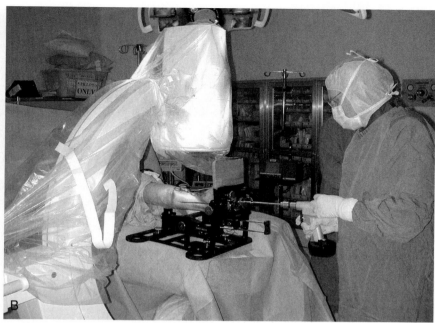

**Figure 9**   **A,** INBONE ankle prosthesis with the polyethylene component not yet inserted. **B,** Leg holder used to insert INBONE ankle prosthesis.

chanical characteristics of the INBONE total ankle system.

## Surgical Technique
### Overview
Relative to arthroplasties of other joints, the surgical technique for TAA is demanding because the soft tissue envelope is relatively vulnerable, vital neurovascular structures are in close proximity to the joint, and the ankle cannot be dislocated to improve exposure. Implant alignment determined intraoperatively under non–weight-bearing conditions is subject to tibiotalar joint distortions, the affected limb's mechanical axis, and the multiplanar function of the ankle-hindfoot complex. Similar to total knee arthroplasty in concept, bone resection alone in TAA does not determine alignment; optimal polyethylene articulation with the tibial and talar components requires proper soft-tissue balance. Soft-tissue balancing about the ankle and hindfoot for

TAA may necessitate lateral ligament reconstruction and/or a medial deltoid release and/or lengthening of the Achilles tendon either with a percutaneous triple hemisection or a gastrocnemius release. Unlike total knee arthroplasty, soft-tissue balancing techniques for TAA lack standardization but are evolving.

### Exposure and Closure
Although most TAA prostheses are implanted via an anterior approach, several implants are inserted via a transfibular approach. All prostheses mentioned in this chapter are implanted via the more conventional anterior approach except the ESKA, which is inserted laterally, and the Eclipse (Figure 10), which can be inserted medially or laterally. The other designs use a longitudinal anterior skin incision to expose the extensor retinaculum, which is divided directly medial to the extensor hallucis longus (EHL) tendon. Dis-

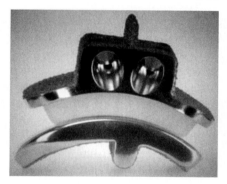

**Figure 10**   Eclipse ankle prosthesis.

tally, the superficial peroneal nerve is at risk for injury during this approach. The interval to the anterior ankle is between the tibialis anterior and EHL. By avoiding an incision directly over the tibialis anterior tendon and shifting the division of the extensor retinaculum toward the EHL tendon, less tension will be placed on the fibrous retinaculum by the tibialis anterior after closure. However, located immediately deep to the EHL is the anterior tibial

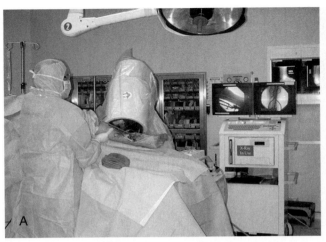
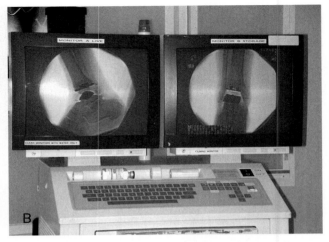

**Figure 11** **A,** Fluoroscopy is used to confirm extramedullary alignment. **B,** Fluoroscopic inspection of the STAR prosthesis at the end of the arthroplasty procedure.

artery and deep peroneal nerve. With the neurovascular structures and tendons protected, an anterior capsulotomy is performed.

A layered closure of the anterior ankle capsule, extensor retinaculum, subcutaneous tissue, and skin affords the joint more than one barrier in the event of wound dehiscence. Also, by maintaining the extensor retinaculum over the tibialis anterior, wound suction appliances and split-thickness skin grafts, in lieu of free-tissue transfer, may be feasible in situations involving wound breakdown. To minimize the risk for skin necrosis, direct skin retraction should be avoided throughout the procedure; however, deep retractors (Adson-Beckman, Langenbeck, or Gelpi) are recommended to avoid repetitive trauma or excessive tension to the skin with subsequent creation of vascular channel blockers.

### Tibial and Talar Preparation

Most surgeons familiar with TAA agree that the tibial cut must be perpendicular to the tibial shaft axis in the coronal plane, with slight dorsi-

flexion in the sagittal plane for success of the procedure. This concept is no different than that of tibial preparation in total knee arthroplasty—perpendicular in the coronal plane with a slight posterior slope in the sagittal plane. For TAA the trend is similar to findings of outcomes studies for total knee arthroplasty—a tibial cut made in varus produces a higher failure rate than neutral-symmetric tibial cuts. External tibial alignment guides align the tibial cutting block for tibial preparation. Except for a few select experts (who may even perform freehand cuts), most surgeons confirm proper tibial cutting block alignment with intraoperative fluoroscopy. The use of a large fluoroscopic C-arm to assess alignment intraoperatively facilitates instant assessment of the alignment relative to the tibia (Figure 11, *A*); a mini C-arm limits the surgeon's ability to evaluate proper alignment and is not recommended. Only a few degrees of malalignment negatively influence ligamentous tensioning and/or the compressive effect of the prosthesis on adjacent bone. Once proper

alignment is established, it is particularly important to orient the saw directly centrally and posteriorly, carefully avoiding saw blade excursion into the malleoli.

Initial talar dome preparation is typically performed by a cutting guide suspended or aligned from the same base that supported the tibial cutting block. The initial talar cut has the chance of creating a relatively serious and perhaps irreversible complication. Nowhere is the "ship in the bottle" analogy to TAA more relevant than with the initial talar preparation because the cutting guide obscures most of the joint, and visualization is further compromised by the saw that must be held directly over the joint. With minor saw blade deviation or overpenetration, the malleoli and posterior soft-tissue and/or neurovascular structures are at risk. Because the talus is not symmetrically hinged to the tibia, an assistant must maintain proper dorsiflexion and coronal plane position when applying the jigs or cutting the talus to ensure the desired talar cut. Cutting the talus in a plantar-flexed position can lead to excessive posterior talar dome resection, which is particularly true in a patient with an equinus contracture. Overresection of the posterior talus may lead to talar component subsidence. Similarly, holding the foot in excessive dorsiflexion while the talar cutting guide is secured into position or when the talus is cut can lead to anterior overresection and a plantar-flexed talar component, although this resection error is far less likely than overresection of the posterior talus. Poor coronal plane talar position during talar preparation leads to difficulties in proper varus/valgus position or tension on the collateral ligaments.

### Component Positioning

Several universal recommendations exist for TAA component positioning. After completing tibial and talar preparation, the talar component should be centered directly beneath the tibia; poorly centered components often result in polyethylene edge loading. Oversizing the prosthesis may lead to friction between the bone and components, a painful ankle, and early polyethylene wear. This is the most commonly reported complication, which is not initially recognized, following TAA. Based on anecdotal experience, the general rule is that in situations of in-between sizing, downsizing is appropriate. Although in most systems the tibial component's coronal dimensions rather than sagittal dimensions determine tibial component size, this is usually a unique feature of the chosen prosthesis. For example, the STAR prosthesis has very similar coronal dimensions and a 15-mm variance in the sagittal plane dimensions of the tibial component. The talar component, aligned with the long axis of the talus, typically parallels the second or third metatarsal.

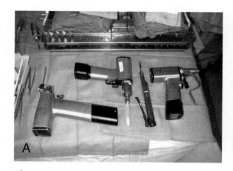 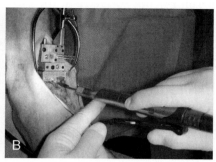

**Figure 12** **A,** A variety of saws are used to make surgery safer and easier. **B,** The small reciprocating saw can be used to cut small corners out of bone.

Ideal rotational orientation of the tibial component may be challenging, given the oblique slope of the anterior distal tibia. Placement of an osteotome in the medial gutter of the ankle joint, between the medial malleolus and the medial talar dome, will assist in determining the angle to cut the tibia. However, this technique is prosthesis dependent. For example, the Salto-Talaris instrumentation recommends "splitting" the sagittal alignment angle of the malleolar walls to find the true axis of the talus longitudinally. Because the polyethylene in mobile-bearing prostheses without stop mechanisms (STAR, Hintegra, Buechel-Pappas, and Mobility) is afforded full freedom, some minor degree of malrotation is typically tolerated, or the risk of impingement or edge loading will increase with greater malrotation. The potential for malrotation is probably greatest with the Agility prosthesis. Because the implant requires partial resections of the malleoli, errors in rotation may lead to compromise of the posterior malleolus and, in extreme circumstances, the posteromedial neurovascular bundle. If the cutting block is oriented into external rotation relative to the sagittal plane, the resultant external rotation may be dramatic because the polyethylene is designed with 22° of external rotation within the tibial component housing. Using the C-arm to confirm trial and final component positioning before leaving the operating room is currently advised (Figure 11, *B*).

### Tools

Three saws are recommended for TAA: a 1-inch nonbending 0.5-inch oscillating saw for flat tibial and talar cuts, a 0.5-inch wide × 3-cm thin reciprocating saw with circumferential and end-cutting ability, and a 0.25-inch × 1-inch reciprocating saw to remove minor bony irregularities with minimal pressure against the bone (Figure 12). A thin oscillating saw is often valuable for trimming flat areas with a ridge of bone. Osteotomes, if levered inappropriately, may lead to intraoperative malleolar fractures, some of which are not detected until postoperative radiographic evaluation. Several TAA surgeons recommend placing prophylactic malleolar guidewire; in the event an intraoperative malleolar fracture occurs, a cannulated screw may be placed over the guidewire.

### Soft-Tissue Balancing and Deformity Correction

Bone resection is critical to alignment. However, if ligamentous imbalance is not corrected at the time of surgery, varus or valgus deformity will ensue despite perfect bone cuts. Even though techniques for TAA soft-tissue balancing and corrective osteotomies about the ankle and hindfoot have not been standardized, anecdotal experience is gradually evolving into general guidelines. Simply changing the polyethylene thickness alone is not appropriate in establishing soft-tissue balance for TAA.

### Equinus Contracture

Whereas some surgeons routinely perform Achilles tendon lengthening for ankle arthritis associated with equinus, others maintain that the gastrocnemius-soleus complex will gradually stretch out if a posterior capsular release is performed at the time of surgery and proper component implantation is achieved. Typically, increased tibial resection will provide greater motion in TAA; however, there is a fine balance between appropriate and excessive resection.[38] Resecting too much bone from the tibial plafond may result in implant subsidence into the weaker proximal bone, whereas underresection may lead to inadequate dorsiflexion and increased stress on the anterior tibial cortex with weight bearing.

In patients with limited preoperative dorsiflexion, anterior osteophytes are removed and a gastrocnemius recession may be performed. Performing this procedure early in the operation avoids having to stress the "cut bone" with dorsiflexion when the prosthesis is in place and potentially damaging the newly cut surface or fracturing a malleolus. After tibial and talar resections, a posterior capsular release is performed, typically through the anterior incision. Some authors maintain a high threshold for

triple hemisection Achilles tendon lengthening, relying on the posterior capsular release and gradual Achilles tendon accommodation postoperatively. However, if at least 5° of dorsiflexion is not achieved intraoperatively during TAA, the patient will vault over their plantar-flexed forefoot when walking in shoes without heels. Bone resection performed before Achilles tendon lengthening may result in excessive resection of the posterior talus, which (based on anecdotal reports) can lead to talar component subsidence as previously described. When 5° of ankle dorsiflexion cannot be achieved despite adequate bone resection, and a posterior Achilles tendon lengthening has not already been performed, a gastrocnemius recession through a medial approach at the musculotendinous junction of the gastrocnemius-soleus complex is performed; care should be taken to avoid the sural nerve. If gastrocnemius-soleus recession fails to achieve a least 5° of ankle dorsiflexion and tibial resection is appropriate, a percutaneous triple hemisection of the Achilles tendon may be added to further lengthen the Achilles tendon.

### Varus Malalignment

Typically, a graduated deltoid ligament release and proper component positioning with appropriate sizing of the polyethylene permits satisfactory soft-tissue balance. Deltoid ligament release can be performed through the anterior approach; occasionally, a small separate incision over the posterior medial malleolus may be required to lengthen otherwise inaccessible tight deltoid fibers. Overrelease can be avoided by limiting the release to the deep deltoid fibers and preserving the superficial fibers. If it is decided that an entire deltoid ligament release is needed, taking the periosteum off the tibia in continuity with

the deltoid ligament can avoid late-term gross medial instability. Lateral ligament attenuation generally warrants lateral ligament stabilization with a modified Broström repair, Evans procedure (augmentation with the anterior third of the peroneus brevis), or a free tendon autograft or allograft reconstruction. Deltoid tightness may not always require deltoid fiber release; instead, appropriate coronal plane positioning of TAA components influences deltoid tension. Additionally, cavus or varus foot positioning may warrant osteotomies and/or arthrodeses of the foot to maintain proper ankle balance; these procedures may either be staged or performed simultaneously with TAA. Commonly performed osteotomies include a lateral closing wedge and/or lateralizing calcaneal osteotomies for valgus deformity, or dorsiflexion, first metatarsal osteotomies for forefoot-driven hindfoot varus. Tibia vara deformity proximal to the ankle may require staged or simultaneous supramalleolar medial opening or lateral closing wedge osteotomies to achieve optimal ankle alignment. Often the fibula is also cut to obtain greater correction.

### Valgus Malalignment

Unlike varus deformity, the logical approach of lateral release and medial capsular plication is not reliable or even feasible in most patients. Several techniques for deltoid ligament reconstruction have been proposed but lack objective clinical validation or even adequate anecdotal experience to recommend their use in soft-tissue balancing for TAA.[39] An intraoperative decision to convert to arthrodesis may be prudent when the deltoid ligament is incompetent. Medial displacement calcaneal osteotomies, plantar flexion osteotomies and/or arthrodeses of the medial column, or even supramalleolar medial closing wedge osteotomies may be required to appropriately treat valgus deformities that cannot be corrected with proper bone cuts for TAA and soft-tissue rebalancing alone.

## Postoperative Care

Variations in postoperative protocols are used by surgeons performing TAA. Although a surgeon confident in initial implant stability and wound resilience may recommend ROM activities and weight bearing within the first 2 weeks, a more conservative approach may involve 6 weeks of immobilization and protected weight bearing. Generally, most surgeons follow the more conservative approach of allowing patients with uncomplicated, isolated TAA to progress to regular shoe wear by 6 weeks after surgery. Routine, supervised physical therapy is not always warranted, although some patients will require such therapy to achieve maximum ROM. Usually, patients ambulate reasonably well by 3 months and return to full activities (such as golf, walking, and skiing) at 6 months. Further functional improvement is typically observed up to 24 months following successful TAA.

Bone ingrowth requires approximately 6 weeks of protected weight bearing to avoid component micromotion and associated fibrous ingrowth. Initial implant stability varies; therefore, the treating surgeon must determine when to initiate weight bearing and ROM. Enthusiasm for early ankle motion must be tempered by the potential for early manipulation of the wound resulting in delayed healing. Other factors to consider are adjunctive procedures (corrective osteotomies and ligament reconstructions), intraoperative fractures, and time to syndesmotic union (specific to the Agility prosthesis).

## Implant-Specific Aspects of Surgical Technique

### Agility Prosthesis
#### Unique Features
Intraoperative medial external fixation, syndesmotic arthrodesis, using a monoblock cutting guide for both the tibia and talus, and resurfacing the medial and lateral malleolar articular surfaces are unique features of the Agility prosthesis. Many surgeons who use other systems view the external fixator as an unnecessary and cumbersome extra step in TAA. However, for surgeons who routinely implant the Agility prosthesis, this extra step adds no more than 10 minutes to the procedure and can be applied (at least the pins) before tourniquet inflation. The advantage of the external fixator is that distraction reduces the amount of bone resection when using the recommended cutting monoblock for both tibial and talar resection. The external fixator also maintains the proper alignment for the bone cuts; if properly applied, no change in ankle position is needed between fluoroscopic confirmation and execution of the bone resections. A disadvantage is that surgeons less experienced with the Agility system may have a false sense of proper alignment with the external fixator in place. The external fixator can easily overpower or mask ankle ligamentous imbalance. Therefore, proper assessment requires release of the external fixator. Overtensioning of the external fixator may lead to an intraoperative malleolar fracture.

#### Component Positioning
For coronal plane tibial component positioning, the Agility prosthesis is subject to errors related to the resultant effects of deltoid ligament tension. The Agility is the only TAA prosthesis reviewed in this chapter that requires resection of a sizable portion of the medial malleolar articular surface. The Agility prosthesis creates a conflict for the surgeon less experienced with its recommended technique. In an attempt to avoid medial malleolar fracture (a goal in all TAA procedures) a careful surgeon may resect too little medial malleolus. The resultant tibial component lateralization forces the talus and talar component more laterally, thereby overtensioning the deltoid ligament, particularly a deltoid ligament with a preoperative contracture. The clinical effect is a varus talar tilt, edge loading, potential for talar component loosening and/or subsidence, and early polyethylene wear. Fortunately, when potential varus malalignment is observed intraoperatively, more medial malleolus can be resected, the tibial fin cut can be adjusted, and the tibial component properly positioned.

The talus must be positioned properly relative to the monoblock cutting guide of the Agility prosthesis. Direct visualization is often obscured by the instrumentation; therefore, fluoroscopic confirmation in the sagittal plane is desirable. The sagittal axis of the talar component is aligned with the second or third metatarsals. The Agility talar component has been redesigned with a wider base to avoid subsidence. Ideally, the bone interface of the talar component should be sized to cover the maximum resected talar surface without overhang, and the talar component should rest on the posterior cortex of the talar body.

### Syndesmotic Fusion
The Agility is the only prosthesis discussed in this chapter that requires syndesmotic débridement

and arthrodesis.[2,4] Although these procedures were originally performed through a separate extensile lateral incision, they may be performed via the single anterior approach. The risk of tibial component migration has been reported to increase 8.5 times if a solid syndesmotic fusion is absent.[4] Use of platelet-rich product mixed with autograft bone from the ankle, autologous concentrated growth factors, and a lateral plate has been reported to improve the syndesmotic fusion rates.[40-42]

### STAR Prosthesis

The STAR prosthesis represents the prototypical unconstrained three-component design. The surgical technique used to implant the STAR prosthesis has been described by Anderson and associates.[43]

#### Tibial Preparation

Tibial preparation is not unique to the STAR design. The cutting block must be properly aligned in the coronal, sagittal, and rotational orientations and may be confirmed using fluoroscopy. The recommended resection level is 5 mm proximal to the anterior tibia, measured after osteophyte removal. Taking into consideration the sagittal plane concavity of the tibial plafond, this generally leads to a 2-mm resection at the midtibial plafond level, similar to recommended resection levels for the most involved tibial hemiplateau in total knee arthroplasty. Proper rotation of the external tibial alignment guide cannot be assessed via fluoroscopy, but a thin osteotome inserted into the medial ankle gutter usually adequately defines rotation. The cutting block has capture guides, but divergence of the saw blade from the true sagittal plane may still result in malleolar injury.

#### Talar Preparation

Because the talar cutting guide is suspended from the tibial cutting block, it is not a monoblock as described for the Agility prosthesis. Like the surgical technique used for the Agility prosthesis, however, the talus must be positioned in the desired position for ideal resection relative to the fixed cutting guide. Osteophytes may need to be removed from the gutters to ensure that the talus can be placed in its anatomic position for dome resection (avoiding varus). Because the talar block lacks capture guides, it is advisable to place metal ribbon retractors in the gutters to protect the malleoli. Unlike the Agility prosthesis, talar preparation dictates talar component positioning because the talar component is a "talar cap," fully resurfacing the talar dome. The following observations have been made (several of which are applicable to most TAA talar components): oversizing leads to symptomatic malleolar impingement; anterior positioning increases the potential risk of untoward contact stresses, edge loading, and anterior tibial component subsidence; and inadequate posterior talar preparation leads to talar component flexion. Final talar preparation for the STAR prosthesis involves creation of a slot for the talar component fin.

A 4-mm talar resection level is desirable for the STAR prosthesis. In combination with the 5-mm tibial resection, a 9-mm space is created, which is adequate to accommodate the implants with a 6-mm or preferably 7- to 8-mm polyethylene insert. (The 6-mm polyethylene insert has been known to crack in the groove.) Next, the medial and lateral sides of the talar dome are prepared with the lateral cut 5 mm more distal than the medial cut to accommodate the longer lateral aspect of the talar component that articulates with the fibula. A tapered orientation of the medial and lateral cuts (wider anteriorly) dictates sagittal plane position of the talar component. Performed properly, the error of placing the talar component too anteriorly can be avoided.

The STAR system lacks true trial tibial and talar components, but several instruments and steps provide confirmation of appropriate joint preparation. One of these instruments serves to cap the talus to determine ideal polyethylene component thickness. In the authors' experience, the 8-mm spacer should easily fit between the trial talar cap and the tibial cut, simulating the 2-mm thickness of the tibial component, and ensuring that at least a 6-mm polyethylene component can be inserted with both the tibial and talar component implanted. If not, the tibia can be easily recut, as done in total knee arthroplasty.

#### Final Component Positioning

The tibial component must be centered under the tibial shaft axis. This necessitates proper positioning of the channels for the fixation barrels on the nonarticulating aspect of the tibial component while simultaneously ensuring appropriate tibial component balance in the coronal plane to avoid medial malleolar fracture during tibial component impaction. Because most of the stresses tend to focus on the anterior aspect of the ankle following TAA, the anterior aspect of the tibial implant should rest on the anterior tibial cortex and not be recessed beyond the cortex. Fluoroscopic confirmation of proper component position is recommended. A trial spacer is then used to determine the thickness necessary to achieve ligamentous stability. Residual coronal plane ankle instability can be corrected with lateral ligament reconstruction and/or deltoid ligament release. The trial polyethylene spacer is removed, and the true polyethylene component inserted.

### Hintegra Prosthesis

Although Hintegra cutting guides are distinct, tibial and talar preparations resemble those for the STAR prosthesis. As is common with mobile-bearing prostheses, a spacer block is available to evaluate appropriate ligamentous balance. Once proper talar preparation is confirmed, peg holes are created in the talus to accommodate pegs on the nonarticulating talar component surface. The tibial component is centered on the cut surface of the tibial plafond, and its position is clinically confirmed with an anterior phalange contacting the anterior tibial cortex. Optional screw fixation is available for both components.

### Buechel-Pappas Implant

Tibial preparation for the Buechel-Pappas implant is similar to that of the STAR and Hintegra, except that an anterior cortical window to accommodate the tibial stem must be created. Ideal tibial component positioning over the talar component (over the polyethylene bearing) avoids edge loading and contact wear. Although not ideal, the cortical window can be recut to allow adjustments in the coronal plane. Because the tibial stem is centered on the tibial component, rotation may easily be altered. Talar preparation preserves physiologic talar subchondral architecture, except that the talar trochlea is deepened to create a 5-mm, central, longitudinal sulcus and two slots to accommodate the fins on the underside of the talar component. Unlike the STAR

and Hintegra, but similar to the Mobility, the medial and lateral talar walls are left intact. Balanced talar component impaction is facilitated with the anterior tibial cortical window. Next, the tibial component is properly seated and the resected tibial window is replaced with added bone graft as needed; this prevents joint fluid from migrating to the tibial stem and backside of the tibial component, which may cause loosening. The polyethylene component of the proper thickness is then inserted.

### Mobility Total Ankle System

The instrumentation for the Mobility ankle has been refined from past experience with three-piece designs and allows for AP and lateral-medial centering of tibial and talar components. Combined with a superior tapering of the polyethylene component, optimal centering of the components is believed to result in favorable balancing with less likelihood of polyethylene component overhang. The system also allows for a visual "double check" before every important resection, thus allowing the surgeon to estimate the sufficiency of the initial tibial resection. The general technique for insertion is similar to that used for the Buechel-Pappas implant.

### Salto-Talaris Prosthesis

For the Salto-Talaris ankle prosthesis, the tibial alignment guide is stabilized to the tibia with one pin in the tibial tubercle and a second pin in the distal medial tibia. Adjustments to the tibial alignment guide are made to ensure the guide is parallel to the sagittal and coronal axis of the tibia. Optimal sagittal and coronal alignment can be confirmed fluoroscopically. Rotation of the tibial resection guide is determined vi-

sually. Rotation of the tibial component is based on the sagittal axis of the talus. Sizing of the tibial component is determined simultaneously with confirmation of talar rotation. The guide is set to allow 9-mm tibial resection from the apex of the tibial plafond. To determine this resection level, anterior tibial osteophytes must be removed beforehand. Following tibial preparation and removal of most of the cut tibial bone, the foot is held at a 90° angle to the tibia. A talar alignment pin is then placed into the talus through the guide. Next, a posterior chamfer talar dome cutting guide is placed over this pin, secured with three to four additional pins, and the posterior superior talus is cut and the bone removed. An anterior chamfer guide is then positioned, and the anterior superior portion of the talus is planed down with a milling device. Final talar preparation is performed with a third talar cutting guide that allows drilling of both a cylindrical hole to accommodate the talar stem and the cutting of lateral chamfer off the talus. The trial implants are then placed in position. The ankle is dorsiflexed and plantarflexed to allow the tibial component drill guide to rotate into the ideal position relative to the talar implant. Residual lateral tibial bone adjacent to the fibula must be removed to permit this automatic adjustment of the tibial trial implant. Trial polyethylene thicknesses allow for final adjustment of the tension. If adequate dorsiflexion is not possible, additional resection of the tibia or gastrocnemius resection is performed. Final preparation of the tibial component is achieved through pedestal drilling and pedestal strut preparation. The final implants are then inserted and the pedestal area bone grafted to avoid ingress of joint fluid.

## INBONE Prosthesis

The approach used with the INBONE prosthesis is identical to that of the other ankles between the tibialis anterior and the EHL. The leg is then placed in the leg holder, and the rotation of the ankle determined by aligning the holder parallel to a 0.25-inch osteotome in the medial mortise. The calcaneus is fixed with two pins, and the foot and lower leg secured to the leg holder with elastic bandaging. The large fluoroscopic C-arm is guided into place, and the anteroposterior rotation sites are aligned by rotating the C-arm or operating room table. This rotation confirms the center location of the guide over the talus and the tibia. Then, using a similar procedure, the lateral rotation site centering is accomplished with the C-arm in the lateral view. The AP view is then reobtained with proper centering and the cutting guide applied. Selection of the ideal cutting guide is determined using preoperative templating, intraoperative fluoroscopy, and direct visualization. The plantar calcaneal heel pad is carefully incised, a cannula is inserted through the soft tissue and locked into position, and the talus and tibia are drilled. Alignment of the monoblock cutting guide is accomplished under fluoroscopy, and the guide is pinned into position. Tibia and talus are cut through the monoblock saw guide. The saw guide is removed and the bone extracted. The tibia is reamed by applying the reamer tip into the ankle and onto the reaming rod inserted up through the calcaneus and talus. The ankle is then plantar flexed, talar component positioning is fine-tuned, and the hole for the talar stem is drilled. The tibial screw is assembled within the prepared ankle and advanced into the reamed tibia. The Morse taper

tibial component is then tamped into the modular stem's lowest cylinder and fully seated on the resected tibial surface. Next, the talar component with the 10-mm stem attached is positioned and impacted into the prepared tibia. Alternatively, a longer 14-mm stem or a not yet FDA-approved calcaneal stem is inserted first and then the talar component is inserted and locked onto this stem. Finally, the polyethylene component is inserted via a screw-pushing mechanism and then tamped into place.

## Results

### Overview

The levels of evidence and grades of recommendation remain limited to retrospective and intermediate prospective data. In the published studies, it is often difficult to determine the level of the surgeon's experience with TAA and/or the recommended surgical technique for the particular implant. The ideal study would be a prospective, randomized trial comparing TAA and ankle arthrodesis; however, expecting informed patients to accept randomized surgical options of arthrodesis versus ankle replacement is unrealistic. Currently, TAA outcomes are based on prospective, comparative studies and retrospective, case-controlled studies—some intermediate, but others have only short-term results. It is hoped that registries of TAAs will become available to provide useful data regarding particular design features, surgeon experience, institutional data, and carefully selected outcomes measures.

One concern is that currently available intermediate-term results will drive enthusiasm for TAA. Consistent long-term follow-up for current TAA implants is needed but not yet available. Most concerning is

the reported survivorship analysis. Although many implanted TAAs may maintain excellent function with long-term follow-up, there are probably an equal number that are surviving but not functioning perfectly. Reviewing the current literature with a critical eye reveals many instances of persistent malalignment, radiolucencies, osteolysis, and bone overgrowth at intermediate-term (5- to 7-year) follow-up. Nonetheless, many patients have good to excellent results in these follow-up studies. Although these patients may be functioning well at intermediate-term follow-up, it is important to remember that such positive results may not be experienced at long-term (10- to 15-year) follow-up.

Revision surgery for TAA does not necessarily mean failure of a TAA implant; if this was the situation, good to excellent results would drop to approximately 50%, rendering TAA obsolete. Many of the current studies report on successful revision surgeries. These "touch-up" surgeries include fixation of malleolar fractures not noted at the time of surgery, replacing the mobile polyethylene component with a thicker component to gain better ligamentous stability, resection of bony overgrowth causing impingement in well-fixed components, and periarticular osteotomy. The number of patients needing revision surgery may decrease as the techniques of TAA become more defined.[44,45]

### Meta-Analysis

In the meta-analysis previously mentioned, data pooling was only possible for 10 studies of three-component TAA designs ($n$ = 497).[16] These trials showed a mean improvement of 45.2 points on the American Orthopaedic Foot and

Ankle Society (AOFAS) ankle-hindfoot scoring system (95% confidence interval [CI] 39.3 to 51.1). Average ROM improved slightly (6.3°, 95% CI 2.2° to 10.5°). Weighted complication rates ranged from 1.6% (deep infections) to 14.7% (impingement). The prevalence of secondary surgery was 12.5% and secondary arthrodesis was 6.3%. The weighted 5-year prosthesis survival rate averaged 90.6%. This meta-analysis concluded that TAA improves pain and joint mobility in end-stage ankle arthritis but cautioned that its performance in comparison to ankle arthrodesis remains to be defined in a properly designed randomized trial.

## Implant-Specific Results

### Agility Prosthesis

Mean follow-up of published studies for the Agility prosthesis ranges from nearly 3 years to 9 years.[2,4,23,45] In most of these studies, patient satisfaction ranged from 90% to 97% for patients who did not have conversion to arthrodesis and were available for follow-up. One study showed an improvement in AOFAS ankle-hindfoot score from 34 to 83 points, with 49 points on the Medical Outcomes Study 36-Item Short Form physical component and 56 points on the mental component at a mean follow-up of 44 months.[23] Despite these apparently favorable results, progressive radiolucency rates (76% to 85%) have been reported.[2,23] Although it has been suggested that not all peri-implant lucency is related to failure but instead to stress shielding, high rates (24% to 45%) of component migration and subsidence have been reported.[2,4,23] One study noted a high correlation of tibial component migration with syndesmotic delayed union and particularly nonunion,

with syndesmotic nonunions occurring in 8% to 10% of Agility TAAs.[4]

One investigation suggested that not all revision surgeries represent failures.[45] In a study of 306 ankles with Agility prostheses, the authors reported a 28% revision rate, with the procedures ranging from osteophyte removal to amputation. With revision as the end point, the 5-year survival was 54%; with implant survival as the end point, the 5-year survival was 80%. If the patient cohort is limited to patients older than 54 years, the 5-year survival increased to 89%. In the study with the longest mean follow-up (9 years),[2] 11% conversion to arthrodesis was observed; in the study with the shortest mean follow-up (33 months), the amputation rate approached 3%.[45] TAA is also believed to be protective of the hindfoot articulations, particularly in comparison with ankle arthrodesis. However, despite TAA, one study noted radiographic evidence of progressive arthritis of the subtalar joint in 19% of ankles and 15% in the talonavicular joint.[2]

### STAR Prosthesis

Mean follow-up for published series for the currently available STAR prosthesis ranges from 3 to 5 years.[3,43,44,46-50] Two of the studies, with some of the same patients in their cohorts, show an AOFAS ankle-hindfoot score improvement from 25 to 84 points with 98% good to excellent results.[48] Best implant survival rates (ranging from 93% to 98%) were observed with double-coated (hydroxyapatite and titanium) cementless prostheses with optimal component fit at the implant-bone interface.[46,49] Life table survivorship analysis estimated cementless implant survival at 95% at 12 years.[3] In contrast, 5-year survival rates for

single-coating components and 12-year survivorship rates for cemented components have been reported at 70%.[3,50] Some of these less favorable outcomes may be attributable to a learning curve for surgeons and possibly by limitations in prosthetic design (a design that has remained virtually unchanged since inception of the implant more than 15 years ago).[44,46,48,50,51]

Revision rates for cementless prostheses range from 7% to 37%.[48-50] Not all revisions are indicative of prosthesis failure. In one study, no revisions involved component removal; all revision procedures were "touch-ups," again suggesting limitations of prosthetic design, characteristics common to TAA, or a learning curve for surgeons.[44] However, the rate of revision surgery for component exchange or conversion to arthrodesis is not negligible, ranging from 7% to 29% in some studies.[46,49,50]

### Hintegra Prosthesis

Only two reports of outcomes for the Hintegra prosthesis have been published, both by one of the inventors of the prosthesis.[52,53] One study of 271 Hintegra TAAs, with a mean follow-up of 3 years, reported an increase in the AOFAS ankle-hindfoot score from 40 to 85 points.[53] Revisions were performed in 14% of ankles, with 2% of TAAs being converted to arthrodesis. The revisions that did not require conversion to arthrodesis had outcomes that matched those of the residual cohort that did not undergo repeat surgery. Radiographic evaluation showed proper position without migration in 266 TAAs that were not converted to arthrodesis. Talar component positioning was deemed too posterior in 4% of the implants. The investigators, who had extensive prior clinical experience with the STAR prosthesis, reported a short, steep learning curve with the Hintegra prosthesis and noted that many revisions were not failures but instead "touch-up" procedures.

### Salto Prosthesis

The only published report on the Salto TAA is by the inventors of the prosthesis.[54] In a study of 98 consecutive Salto TAAs, with a mean follow-up of almost 3 years (minimum follow-up, 2 years), clinical and radiographic evaluation was possible for 91 patients (93 implants). Results showed an increase in the AOFAS ankle-hindfoot score from 32 to 83 points. Seventy-two patients were pain free, 54 patients could walk unlimited distances, and 25 patients had limitations but could walk more than 1 km. Sixty-seven patients had no limp but seven needed walking aids. Fifty-eight patients could walk on tiptoe, 49 patients could walk on uneven ground, 14 patients could run, 76 patients could ascend stairs normally, and 63 patients could descend stairs normally. ROM as measured on stress radiographs improved from 15.2° preoperatively to 28.3° at follow-up. Survivorship analysis (calculated at 68 months, the longest follow-up period available in the study cohort), with the end point set at implant removal, was 98% and 95% for best- and worse-case scenarios, respectively.[54]

### Buechel-Pappas Prosthesis

Mean follow-up for the currently available Buechel-Pappas prosthesis (deep sulcus design) ranges from 5 to 12 years. Two studies by the inventors of the prosthesis showed 88% good to excellent results and a 10- and 12-year survivorship rate (with revision of any component) of 93.5 and 92%, respectively.[1,32] Most patients (82% to 84%) in these stud-

ies had osteoarthritis. Results of earlier-generation Buechel-Pappas prostheses (shallow sulcus design) from these same authors showed only 70% good to excellent results and a 12-year survivorship rate of 74%.[34]

Other studies of Buechel-Pappas prostheses, either using the shallow or deep sulcus designs, report on cohorts composed solely of patients with inflammatory arthritis.[55,56] At a mean follow-up of 8 years for these studies, clinical outcome scores improved significantly, and a patient satisfaction rate of 89% was reported for those patients who underwent clinical and radiographic follow-up.[55] The outcomes did not include patients who had died or those who had undergone reoperation. In one cohort, 6% of revision surgeries were performed for aseptic loosening and another 6% for axial deformity;[55] in another study, 6% of revision surgeries were converted to ankle arthrodesis.[56] One study showed 82% acceptable radiographic alignment and ingrowth of the Buechel-Pappas prosthesis, and another study showed 18% of implants had marked component subsidence, suggestive of impending failure.[55,56] The authors reported that subsidence did not appear to correlate with radiolucent lines noted on postoperative radiographs.

### INBONE, Mobility Total Ankle, and Salto-Talaris Prostheses

At this time, published results with at least 2-year follow-up were not available for the INBONE, Mobility total ankle or Salto-Talaris prostheses.

## Complications
### Overview/Learning Curve

Despite advances in techniques, instrumentation, and implant design,

the complication rate for TAA continues to exceed that of total knee and total hip arthroplasty. Some complications require revision, with most of these revision surgeries being relatively minor procedures that are not indicative of TAA failure. In a recent investigation of complications in initial TAAs, surgeons were categorized based on their training in TAA.[57] Surgeons were classed as observers of the surgeon inventor; participants in a structured, hands-on surgical training course; and those who had completed a 1-year foot and ankle fellowship with a mentor who performed TAA. Review of surgical outcomes of these three groups was statistically indistinguishable with respect to rates of complications, revisions, or malalignment. However, experience in TAA appears to lower complication rates as shown by the experience of one surgeon who had a lower complication rate for his second 25 Agility TAAs compared with his first 25 procedures (two versus five intraoperative fractures, and zero versus five tendon/nerve lacerations, respectively). Component malalignment also decreased 9% from the first group to the second group of precedures.[15] Improved results with more experience also were found for other surgeons performing STAR TAAs.[49] However, no registry analysis has been published that shows improved outcomes and diminished complication rates based on an individual surgeon's experience and the volume of TAAs performed at an institution.

### Specific Complications and Proposed Management
#### Wound Healing

For TAAs implanted via an anterior approach, postoperative wound complications are cited along with malleolar fractures as the most common complication in TAA.[49,50,55,56]

Although wound complication rates no longer approach 40% as in early reports of TAA, some recent studies cite an incidence of postoperative wound healing complications of approximately 10%.[49,50,55,56,58] Most of these wounds involve less than 1 cm of skin necrosis and often resolve with simple immobilization and local wound care. With more extensive wound dehiscence, a negative pressure wound system may prove effective, provided the extensor retinaculum remains intact. Communication with the ankle joint typically necessitates implant removal, irrigation, débridement, and possible free-tissue transfer, with eventual conversion to arthrodesis as the prudent treatment.

Anecdotal experience has introduced four recommendations that appear to limit wound complications but do not have proven scientific support. (1) Direct skin tension should be avoided and only deep retractors (for example, Adson-Beckman or deep Gelpis) should be used. (2) Adequate exposure should be provided by making an incision long enough to avoid undue tension on the wound edges (currently precluding the use of a minimally invasive technique). (3) Four-layer closure (capsule, extensor retinaculum, subcutaneous layer, and skin) should be used. (4) A brief period of immobilization is recommended following TAA, until the wound is stable.

For the Agility prosthesis, an adequate skin bridge between the anterior and lateral incisions must be maintained. Some surgeons suggest that nasal oxygen in the immediate postoperative period may have a positive effect on wound healing. There is no current clinically proven support for perioperatively interrupting the administration of immunosuppressive medications for a patient with rheumatoid arthritis.

## Malleolar Fractures

Malleolar fractures are a relatively common complication in TAA, with the incidence significantly decreasing for surgeons with more TAA experience.[15,42,49,55,57,59] In several recent studies, the prevalence of malleolar fractures approached and sometimes exceeded 20%.[42,49,55,56,59] Such fractures can be attributed to the difficulty of performing TAA, with instrumentation that obscures already limited visualization, and a joint that narrows slightly posteriorly, making violation of the malleoli even more likely.

Malleolar fractures result from inadvertent excursion of the oscillating saw blade, levering with instrumentation, or malpositioning and improper sizing of the porous-coated tibial component.[15,42,55-57,59] Malleolar fractures may not be detected until postoperative radiographic evaluation; some are occult fractures occurring intraoperatively, and others represent postoperative stress fractures.[15,42,55-57]

Some authors suggest prophylactically pinning the malleoli before making the bone cuts.[59] This simple adjunct adds little surgical time. In the event of an intraoperative medial malleolar fracture, cannulated screw fixation and/or buttress plating is typically feasible but must be performed judiciously to avoid wound complications. A lateral malleolar fracture is generally managed with a small fragment plate, placed through a limited lateral incision with an adequate skin bridge from the anterior approach.[42]

## Malalignment

Malalignment following TAA has been reported in 4% to 45% of patients.[1,4,55,56] All prostheses with published results use extramedullary alignment instrumentation. Most techniques recommend intraoperative imaging in the coronal and sagittal planes to confirm appropriate alignment of cutting guides. Occasionally, extra-articular corrections or tendon transfers may be required to attain desired alignment, performed either simultaneously with the TAA or in a staged fashion. In select patients, residual postoperative malalignment may be effectively corrected with second-stage extra-articular osteotomies. Proper talar component alignment demands appropriate hindfoot/talar positioning when the talar cut is made.

Preexisting malalignment must be corrected with TAA. One study reported the greatest number of failures when preoperative coronal plane deformity exceeded 10°.[56] Another study reported that in patients with preoperative incongruent joints (for example, varus talar tilt within the ankle mortise in patients with end-stage arthrosis) progressive edge loading is 10 times more likely to develop than in patients with congruent joints.[17]

## Infection

Infection with TAA is a relatively uncommon complication, with an incidence similar to that of other major weight-bearing joint arthroplasties, and a reported prevalence ranging from 0% to 2%.[1,2,4,23,42,45,48-50,54-56] Management of infections associated with TAA empirically follow protocols established for infections occurring in total hip or total knee arthroplasties. Cellulitis or superficial wound infections typically respond well to irrigation, débridement, and antibiotic management, provided that an effective multilayer closure is maintained to avoid contamination of the joint. Acute joint sepsis, if detected immediately, often can be managed with irrigation and débridement, exchange of the polyethylene insert, and antibiotic therapy. Subacute or chronic infections necessitate treatment with irrigation and débridement, implant removal, a temporary antibiotic spacer, antibiotic therapy, and staged reimplantation or ankle arthrodesis. Standardized techniques for managing the infected TAA based on evidence-based outcomes have not been defined.

### Subsidence and Component Migration

Subsidence and component migration is generally a result of inadequate bone ingrowth or inadequate component support with weight bearing. A mild amount of early migration of current cementless TAA implants is anticipated, with stabilization of most components by 6 months following implantation.[60] In one study of the Buechel-Pappas tibial components, the authors suggested that the method of fixation and surgical technique (an anterior cortical window) was responsible for component settling.[60]

Progressive component migration has been associated with tibial component undersizing and preoperative deformity exceeding 10° and osteonecrosis (both specific to the Buechel-Pappas implant); and failure of syndesmotic fusion (specific to Agility prosthesis).[1,2,4,56] Occasionally, component collapse into osteopenic bone or large subchondral cysts is observed. Large subchondral cysts detected on preoperative radiographs should prompt more detailed evaluation with CT to plan bone grafting at the time of TAA.

Optimal component bone ingrowth is facilitated by congruent matching between components and prepared bony surfaces.[49] Hydroxyapatite coating, double coatings, and covering the backsides of components with platelet growth factors or mesenchymal stem cells have been studied to promote ingrowth.[3,40,46,48-50,61] With the STAR prosthesis, adding a titanium coating appears to promote more successful bony ingrowth than hydroxyapatite alone.[46,49] Initial component stability must be adequate but not excessive. Although supplemental screw fixation may limit initial micromotion at the bone-prosthesis interface, it may also restrict early component settling, which may be important for optimal bone ingrowth. If screw fixation is considered, nonlocking screws, which allow desirable minor component settling, are recommended. Even with congruent matching of component and prepared bony surfaces, stress shielding may lead to bone resorption and eventual component subsidence. For talar components that cap the prepared talar surfaces, ideal contact cannot be determined; this is another factor that may lead to inadequate bone ingrowth and/or stress shielding.

Most TAA outcome studies show a high prevalence (up to 85%) of peri-implant radiolucent lines on follow-up radiographs.[2,4,23,55] One study observed that component migration did not correlate with the presence of radiolucent lines, suggesting that progressive migration may not be solely caused by lack of bone ingrowth.[55] It is recommended that progressive peri-implant radiolucencies be followed closely for associated component migration beyond that observed with anticipated early settling. It is important to differentiate true lucency representing osteolysis from movement from gaps inherent in inserting the prosthesis (for example, asymmetric drilled holes and cylindrical barrel replacements to fill the holes in the STAR prosthesis). Many of these surgical deficiencies will be physiologically replaced with bone over time.

### Aseptic Loosening and Osteolysis

Whereas component subsidence is associated with a failure of initial component stabilization, osteolysis is caused by polyethylene particulate wear debris that stimulates an osteolytic or "bone cyst" response. Poor component alignment and incongruent polyethylene articulation with the talar and/or tibial components, including edge loading, is the primary cause leading to osteolysis (Figures 13 and 14). Two studies, one of the later-generation Buechel-Pappas implants and another of a single-coated version of the Hintegra prosthesis, show a 6% prevalence of aseptic loosening.[53,56] Conventional osteolysis should be distinguished from ballooning osteolysis that is believed to occur with component abutment against the malleoli, resulting in a loss of bone adjacent to the prosthesis (for example, the lateral malleolus in the Agility or STAR prosthesis in which one study reported a 4% prevalence of ballooning osteolysis).[48]

Newer TAA prostheses (Mobility and BOX) use a relatively small polyethylene tibial surface contact area and a larger talar articulating surface in an attempt to limit edge loading and component abutment. It may be acceptable to observe minor defects without surgical intervention; however, close follow-up is warranted to avoid missing the opportunity to salvage an ankle before gross loosening occurs. Provided component stability is maintained, larger defects (in par-

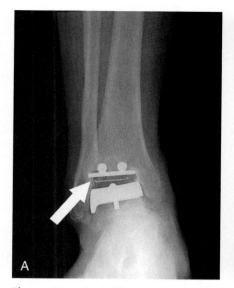 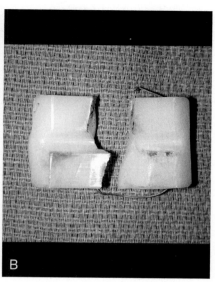

**Figure 13**    **A,** A STAR prosthesis placed in varus position in a 71-year-old man caused polyethylene wear and a cyst above the tibial component. Note the wire marker in the prosthesis is broken with small vertical piece of wire (*arrow*) in the joint of the lateral portion of ankle. **B,** Unilateral wear caused fracture of the polyethylene component.

ticular those with progression evident on serial radiographs) should be addressed with repeat surgery. Unless the cause for polyethylene wear (such as edge loading or malalignment) is rectified, recurrence of osteolysis can be expected. Although cyst débridement, bone grafting, and polyethylene exchange are appropriate, osteotomies to realign the joint may be necessary (Figure 15). Extensive osteolysis with component loosening may require revision TAA with custom implants or different designs or conversion to arthrodesis (Figure 16).

### Impingement and Bone Overgrowth and Proliferation

A high prevalence of bone overgrowth and impingement has been reported in outcome studies for TAA, with one investigation showing impingement in 63% of patients.[45,48] Based on the available literature, bone overgrowth with symptomatic impingement has prompted most revision surgeries in

TAA.[45,48,53] Exposed cancellous surfaces are believed to promote bone overgrowth. This overgrowth, combined with the anticipated early settling of components, may be responsible for impingement that was not evident at the time of the index procedure. Empirically, many surgeons recommend comprehensive débridement of the gutters. In the Agility prosthesis, exposed cancellous talar surfaces are chamfered after talar component implantation. Although some surgeons recommend bone wax on the exposed bone surfaces and/or pulsed irrigation to remove loose bone fragments, others accept bone overgrowth as a matter of course and inform their patients that repeat surgery may become necessary to address symptomatic impingement.

The risk for postoperative impingement can be minimized by proper component sizing and osteophyte removal. Occasionally, removal

of osteophytes may expose instability and the surgeon should be prepared to perform a ligament balancing/reconstruction. Downsizing the talar component in three-component designs is recommended if there is concern for impingement. Although leaving as much bone as possible is preferable, leaving metal in too close proximity to bone may create pain as the metal abuts the bone. Also, bone overgrowth can block a meniscal bearing from moving and effectively converts a mobile-bearing TAA into a fixed-bearing TAA.

### ROM and Postoperative Ankle Stiffness

Clinical assessment of ankle sagittal plane motion shows contributions from both the ankle and hindfoot. One study of the Agility TAA prosthesis used lateral ankle weight-bearing radiographs to determine ankle ROM before and after TAA.[62] Tibiotalar, midfoot, and combined ROM were measured preoperatively and 1 year postoperatively in a standardized, reproducible fashion. The preoperative tibiotalar ROM was 18.5° and combined ankle and midfoot motion was 25.1°. Isolated tibiotalar motion after an Agility TAA was 23.4°, and the combined ankle and midfoot motion was 31.3°. The average improvement in ROM in the tibiotalar joint was approximately 5°, and combined improvement in ROM was 6.1°. The authors concluded that preoperative ROM was the main determinant of eventual postoperative ROM and that TAA resulted in some, but less than expected, increase in ROM.[63] Other authors have used fluoroscopy or stress radiographs to document isolated ankle ROM after TAA with similar findings.[44,48,52-54] Although TAA rarely (if ever) restores physiologic ankle ROM, several authors

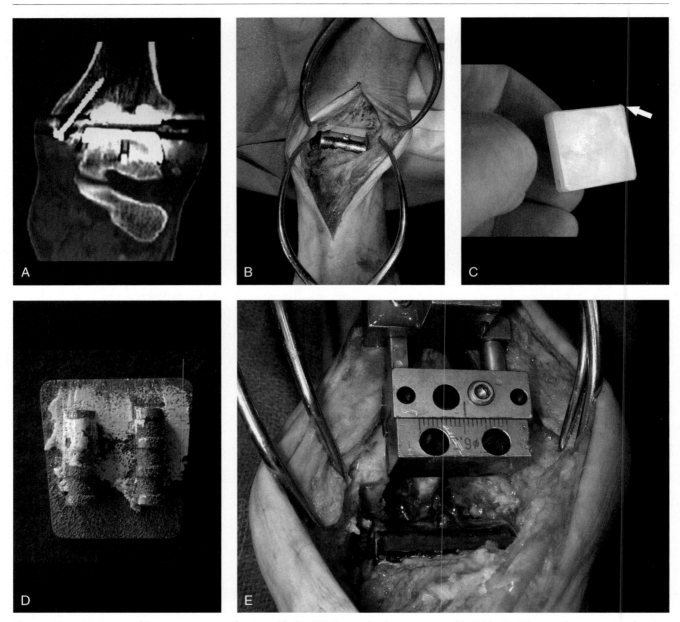

**Figure 14** A 68-year-old woman reported pain with the STAR prosthesis at 2 years after TAA. **A,** CT scan shows cystic changes from polyethylene wear particles that migrated to the medial malleolar screw inserted during previous open reduction and internal fixation. **B,** The opened ankle shows that the polyethylene component is protruding from the leading edge of the tibial component. **C,** Slight wear is seen at the anterior edge of the polyethylene component (*arrow*). **D,** The removed tibial base plate shows bony ingrowth over the anterior two thirds of component. **E,** The ankle was revised secondary to excessive dorsiflexion of the tibial component in addition to polyethylene wear. For the revision, the tibia was cut superiorly and a 12-mm revision polyethylene component was used.

have reported an improvement in ankle ROM following TAA.[44,52-54] These authors reported mean postoperative ankle ROM with TAA to be 28° to 37° (based on imaging studies of the ankle).

There is debate concerning whether to perform gastrocnemius-soleus recession or Achilles tendon lengthening for TAA in patients with an intraoperatively confirmed equinus contracture. Some surgeons believe that the gastrocnemius-soleus complex will gradually adapt after removal of anterior ankle osteophytes, comprehensive posterior capsular release, and appropriate bone resection and component sizing. If the ankle fails to achieve adequate dorsiflexion postoperatively, greater physiologic compressive forces may lead to anterior tibial cortical impaction with tibial component subsidence into extension. Therefore, at least 5° of intraoperative dorsiflexion is recommended. If this degree of dorsiflexion is not achieved, more tibial bone must be resected and/or a gastrocnemius recession and/or a percutaneous triple hemisection of the Achilles tendon should be performed.

## Instability

Ligament balancing for TAA must be achieved at the time of surgery. Although modular polyethylene inserts can enhance appropriate ligament tension, ligament repair or reconstruction may be required to establish satisfactory ankle stability with TAA. The varus ankle may require a deltoid ligament release combined with a modified Broström procedure (for mild instability), a modified Evans procedure (for mild to moderate instability), or complete or partial peroneus brevis or hamstring autograft or allograft reconstruction (for moderate instability). Because severe instability or deformity may not be reconstructible, preoperative consent should be obtained from a patient to perform arthrodesis when TAA is not appropriate based on intraoperative findings. Correction of valgus instability in conjunction with TAA remains challenging because a predictable deltoid ligament reconstruction has yet to be devised. Although several techniques of deltoid ligament reconstruction have been described, a study of their effectiveness for rebalancing valgus instability with TAA has not been published in a peer-reviewed journal. Ankle or tibiotalocalcaneal arthrodesis is currently recommended for medial ligament

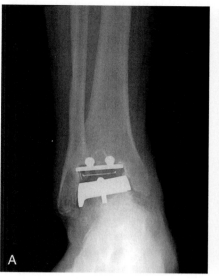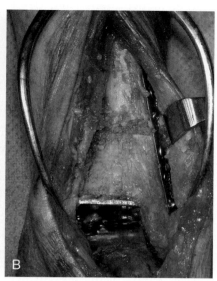

**Figure 15**   **A,** Varus malposition of STAR tibial component led to central osteolysis and fracture of the polyethylene bearing. **B,** Intraoperative view showing osteotomy used to correct malposition (polyethylene not yet implanted).

incompetence. When proper ligament balance can be achieved in conjunction with TAA, selective foot osteotomies and/or arthrodeses or supramalleolar osteotomies also ay be needed to maintain ankle balance. Fortunately, in most valgus ankles, there is lateral collapse as opposed to medial incompetence and correct alignment of the ankle, occasionally accompanied by a sliding medial calcaneal osteotomy, will effectively balance the ankle.

## Adjacent Joint Arthritis

Adjacent joint pain occurs in some patients treated with TAA. Unless the pain is symptomatic preoperatively, many of these patients will gain relief with TAA alone. However, if CT scanning or preoperative differential anesthetic blocks confirm hindfoot arthritis as a contributor to the ankle pain, arthrodeses should be performed simultaneously with TAA, or in a staged manner, particularly if associated with hindfoot malalignment. TAA does not ensure that hindfoot arthri-

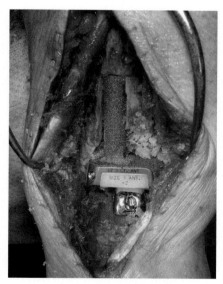

**Figure 16**   Custom tibial Agility ankle prosthesis component with stem.

tis will not develop. At an average follow-up of 9 years, hindfoot arthritis was reported in 15% of talonavicular and 19% of subtalar joints after TAA using the Agility prosthesis.[2] This finding suggests that TAA cannot completely protect hindfoot articulations from developing arthritis; however, the prevalence of hindfoot arthritis following TAA should prove to be less than that reported following ankle arthrodesis.[5,6]

### Prosthetic Breakage

As previously mentioned, malalignment may lead to eccentric, narrow, contact stresses on the components. Although component failure is uncommon, the polyethylene component is most likely to fail, and rarely, the metal or metal-backed components may fracture. Although polyethylene exchange is possible for an isolated failure of the polyethylene component, malalignment, if present, must be corrected to reduce the risk of recurrent component failure.

## Revision Surgery for Failed TAA

Few (if any) standardized techniques have been described for revision TAA. Because a full complement of revision components is not yet available, many revision surgeries require conversion to arthrodesis.[63-65] The surgeon performing revision TAA must be prepared for a full range of possible salvage options, which often requires a considerable collection of equipment, including revision and custom components, equipment for ankle arthrodesis, and structural bone graft material.

Revision TAA, even with careful removal of the primary components and judicious repeated preparation of the tibial and talar surfaces, creates a gap consistently larger than with primary TAA. Thus, the most commonly used components in revision TAA are thicker polyethylene inserts. Some systems offer augmented revision metal components to facilitate reestablishing proper joint line position and ligament

function. Full complements of revision TAA components are gradually becoming more available. Occasionally, custom prostheses must be produced, often at great expense, or consideration needs to be given to the selection of another system that can better address the larger residual gap following removal of the primary implants. One modification to available tibial and talar components is implant stem extensions. In the event only one component needs to be revised, either the tibial or talar component may be replaced, while maintaining the same articulations with a polyethylene insert of revised or increased width. The INBONE prosthesis has a patented bone-ingrowth talar-calcaneal stem extension that is placed across the subtalar joint into the calcaneus to provide talar implant support when residual talar bone stock is limited. That stem, although initially implanted as a "custom" device, is not FDA approved and is unavailable in the United States. When the residual talar bone is insufficient for a primary or an augmented talar implant, a subtalar arthrodesis may prove effective in supporting the talar prosthesis, irrespective of implant design.

Some surgeons have suggested that given the Agility prosthesis' relatively large design dimensions, it may also be used in revision situations for failed implants.[66] Recutting the tibial surface in revision TAA often rests the tibial component in weaker subchondral bone; however, adequate support can generally be achieved with syndesmotic arthrodesis. In the talus, even if the medial and lateral talar dome surfaces have been removed as part of talar preparation for other designs, the residual recut talar bone may be adequate for the Agility augmented or revision

talar components. As a custom implant, the talar component of the Agility prosthesis may be fitted with a stem extension for situations that warrant simultaneous subtalar arthrodesis. However, recognizing the difficulties of using an Agility prosthesis in ideal conditions makes surgery with the Agility as a revision prosthesis a challenging procedure. The INBONE prosthesis with its modular tibial stem design and its ingrowth calcaneal stem may be more suited for use in revision situations.

One study of revision TAA using the Hintegra prosthesis for 28 failed TAAs (STAR, 25; Buechel-Pappas, 2; Agility, 1) showed that at a mean follow-up of approximately 3 years, 23 patients (82%) were satisfied with their outcome.[67] The AOFAS hindfoot score improved from 41 points preoperatively to 86 points at follow-up. Radiographic evaluation suggested a single instance of revision tibial component loosening. However, in the absence of further symptoms, re-revision surgery was deemed unnecessary.

## Conversion of TAA to Arthrodesis

The surgical challenge of converting TAA to arthrodesis is fusing surfaces separated by a large gap that have been subjected to implants (and potentially an antibiotic spacer) while attempting to retain near-physiologic limb length, occasionally in the presence of previous infection.[49,63-65,68,69] Proponents of several three-component designs claim that in the event of implant failure, the minimal bone resection (9 mm) at the index procedure makes conversion to arthrodesis relatively straightforward. However, experience indicates that regardless of design, despite minimal initial bone resection and careful removal of bone ingrowth implants (using thin power saws to avoid damaging too much bone), a considerable gap is created. Although some patients may accept an in situ fusion with the potential need for shoe modification, many patients request that the surgeon attempt to maintain equal limb length. To do so, the surgeon is faced with the challenge of interposing a bulk allograft (often a portion of a femoral head). Occasionally, the subtalar joint can be preserved; however, this salvage procedure usually warrants a tibiotalocalcaneal arthrodesis performed with a combination plate and screws (possible through the same anterior approach), blade plate fixation (typically requiring a second lateral or posterior approach) or a retrograde intramedullary arthrodesis nail (also through a lateral or posterior approach). A midline posterior Achilles tendon-splitting approach can be used to remove the ankle components. The fibula is left in place, the ankle and subtalar surfaces are prepared, and a bulk femoral head allograft is inserted to maintain length. The structural allograft is then held with a retrograde intramedullary rod supplemented by additional bone graft in any defects (Figure 17). If infection is present, a two-stage procedure is favored, with implant removal, irrigation/débridement, antibiotic bead or spacer placement, and delayed arthrodesis. External fixation is an alternative in the presence of infection. The residual bone surfaces can be acutely opposed and compressed (after débridement), while a simultaneous proximal tibial corticotomy is performed to initiate gradual distraction to restore limb length. Regardless of the technique used, the basic principles of arthrodesis must

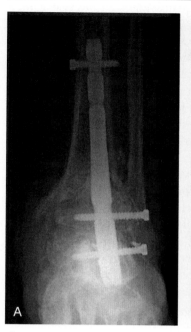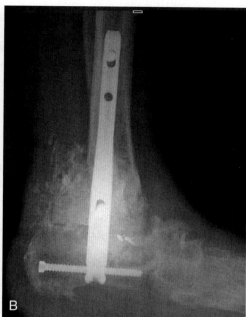

**Figure 17**    AP (**A**) and lateral (**B**) views of an intramedullary rod through femoral head used to fill the gap left by TAA prosthesis that had been removed.

be followed. All infected, nonviable tissue must be removed and bleeding surfaces established on both sides of the fusion site even if a considerable amount of bone needs to be resected.

Comprehensive studies of one institution's experience with arthrodesis and revision arthrodesis following failed TAA and failed arthrodesis after failed TAA have been published.[63-65] Using external fixation and autologous bone graft in virtually all patients, the authors reported an 89% fusion rate and little or no pain in 80% of patients at a mean follow-up of 8 years.[65] For patients undergoing revision ankle arthrodesis for nonunion following attempted conversion of failed TAA to ankle arthrodesis, outcomes were less favorable, despite successful union in most patients.[64] In another study (at a separate institution) using iliac crest bone, arthrodesis after failed TAA achieved successful fu-

sion in only two of four patients.[69] Although one of the two patients with a failed TAA had a successful union after repeat arthrodesis with an intramedullary rod, a persistent nonunion developed in the other patient. In a similar study of eight patients with failed TAA, the authors reported an 87% fusion rate and recommended an anterior plate fixation technique, reserving external fixation for patients with infection.[70]

## Future Directions
### Implant Design and Technique
The ideal TAA design has yet to be created. Despite the challenges in trying to restore physiologic, pain-free ankle function in patients with end-stage ankle arthritis, the evolution of TAA over the past decade has been extraordinary. Over the next decade several more designs currently in development will be introduced. Building on past experiences,

new designs will potentially achieve the goal of TAA results that are comparable to those achieved in total hip and total knee arthroplasty. As demonstrated with the BOX prosthesis, designs may not need to mimic human ankle anatomy to restore ankle-hindfoot function. Published results of TAA using a lateral rather than an anterior approach may confer advantages over implant designs inserted with the anterior approach. The Eclipse and ESKA are examples of such a concept, and another company is currently working on developing such a TAA. Outcomes of TAAs such as the INBONE will determine if intramedullary alignment guides confer advantages over more traditional methods using extramedullary alignment. Additionally, computer-assisted surgery with robotics and intraoperative pedobarography with TAA may improve the surgeon's ability to properly align TAA components and use a less invasive approach. Navigation systems for TAA may lag behind those for total knee and total hip arthroplasty because of industry's lack of financial incentives to develop ankle-specific software and the lower prevalence of ankle arthritis compared with that of the hip and knee.

## Cost Effectiveness

A cost-effectiveness analysis of TAA using a model that assumed a 10-year prosthetic survival suggested an incremental TAA cost-effectiveness ratio of $18,419 per quality-adjusted life year gained, and a gain of 0.52 quality-adjusted life years at a cost of $9,578 when TAA is chosen instead of fusion.[71] This ratio compares favorably when compared with other medical and surgical interventions. If the prosthesis is assumed to fail before 7 years, sensitivity analysis suggested that the cost

per quality-adjusted life year gained with TAA is more than $50,000, a figure generally associated with limited cost-effectiveness. If the theoretic functional advantages of TAA over ankle fusion are proven in future long-term clinical trials, TAA has the potential to be a cost-effective alternative to ankle fusion.

## Conversion of Ankle Fusion to TAA

In select patients with pain following ankle arthrodesis, conversion to TAA may confer advantages over correcting a malposition or adding fusions for adjacent areas of arthritis. Although no comparative studies exist, early reports of conversion of ankle arthrodesis to TAA have been published, with two studies showing similar increases in mean AOFAS ankle-hindfoot scores at short-term follow-up.[7,67] One prospective study of 19 consecutive conversions of ankle arthrodesis to Hintegra TAAs reported an improvement of the AOFAS score from 33.6 to 66.5 points.[67] The authors documented average ankle ROM (confirmed fluoroscopically) of 24°, roughly 52% of the motion of the healthy contralateral ankle. The results of the study were slightly inferior to those of studies with primary arthroplasty; however, the authors believed that ankle arthroplasty represents a valuable alternative to the current treatment for painful ankle arthrodesis. Similarly, a retrospective analysis of 16 symptomatic ankle arthrodeses converted to Agility TAAs showed an improvement of mean AOFAS hindfoot-ankle scores from a preoperative value of 42 points to 68 points at follow-up.[7] These authors observed that patients with a definitive source of pain following ankle arthrodesis, such as secondary hindfoot arthrosis,

tended to have a better outcome than patients without a distinct source of pain.[7] They also reported that patients who had the lateral malleolus resected as part of their ankle arthrodesis tended to have more complications following conversion to TAA.

## Revision TAA

As previously mentioned, the techniques for revision TAA have not been standardized and many of the available revision systems are limited, often prompting surgeons to salvage a failed primary TAA with custom implants, conversion to another TAA system, or complex arthrodesis. The challenges in revising the current generation of primary TAAs, either necessitated by complications or anticipated polyethylene wear, will bring obligatory refinements in revision TAA techniques, components, and instrumentation. Also, though less desirable, revision TAA may also include standardized recommended techniques, implants, and instrumentation to convert failed TAAs to arthrodesis.

## Summary

Adequate long-term follow-up and high levels of evidence are not available to support universal TAA over arthrodesis in the management of end-stage ankle arthritis. Although developments in TAA have been extraordinary since the procedure's inception, outcomes of TAA fall short of those reported for total hip and total ankle arthroplasty. However, the combined improvements in implants, instrumentation, patient selection, and surgical technique make 10-year implant survival of more than 90% a realistic goal. The incidence of malalignment, neurovascular injury, and material failure of

TAA implants is diminishing. Despite these improvements, impingement from bony proliferation, osteolysis/loosening, component subsidence, and failure to resolve preoperative ankle stiffness remain concerns. Further investigation will determine the cost-effectiveness of TAA and if conversion of ankle arthrodesis to arthroplasty is advisable. The future promises a full complement of revision and custom prostheses and incorporation of state-of-the-art adjuncts such as computer navigation to facilitate ideal alignment. Improved techniques, implants, and instrumentation, coupled with promising midterm results of newer prosthetic designs, make TAA a viable alternative for properly selected patients.

## References

1. Buechel FF Sr, Buechel FF Jr, Pappas MJ: Ten-year evaluation of cementless Buechel-Pappas meniscal bearing total ankle replacement. *Foot Ankle Int* 2003;24:462-472.

2. Knecht SI, Estin M, Callaghan JJ, et al: The Agility total ankle arthroplasty: Seven to sixteen-year follow-up. *J Bone Joint Surg Am* 2004;86: 1161-1171.

3. Kofoed H: Scandinavian Total Ankle Replacement (STAR). *Clin Orthop Relat Res* 2004;424:73-79.

4. Pyevich MT, Saltzman CL, Callaghan JJ, Alvine FG: Total ankle arthroplasty: A unique design: Two to twelve-year follow-up. *J Bone Joint Surg Am* 1998;80:1410-1420.

5. Coester LM, Saltzman CL, Leupold J, Pontarelli W: Long-term results following ankle arthrodesis for post-traumatic arthritis. *J Bone Joint Surg Am* 2001;83:219-228.

6. Fuchs S, Sandmann C, Skwara A, Chylarecki C: Quality of life 20 years after arthrodesis of the ankle: A study of adjacent joints. *J Bone Joint Surg Br* 2003;85:994-998.

7. Greisberg J, Assal M., Flueckiger G, Hansen ST Jr: Takedown of ankle fusion and conversion to total ankle replacement. *Clin Orthop Relat Res* 2004; 424:80-88.

8. Conti S, Lalonde KA, Martin R: Kinematic analysis of the agility total ankle during gait. *Foot Ankle Int* 2006; 27:980-984.

9. Dyrby C, Chou LB, Andriacchi TP, Mann RA: Functional evaluation of the Scandinavian Total Ankle Replacement. *Foot Ankle Int* 2004;25: 377-381.

10. Thomas R, Daniels TR, Parker K: Gait analysis and functional outcomes following ankle arthrodesis for isolated ankle arthritis. *J Bone Joint Surg Am* 2006;88:526-535.

11. Tanaka Y, Takakura Y: The TNK ankle: Short- and mid-term results. *Orthopade* 2006;35:546-551.

12. Affatato S, Leardini A, Leardini W, Giannini S, Viceconti M: Meniscal wear at a three-component total ankle prosthesis by a knee joint simulator. *J Biomech* 2007;40:1871-1876.

13. Leardini A, O'Connor JJ, Catani F, Giannini S: Mobility of the human ankle and the design of total ankle replacement. *Clin Orthop Relat Res* 2004; 424:39-46.

14. Reggiani B, Leardini A, Corazza F, Taylor M: Finite element analysis of a total ankle replacement during the stance phase of gait. *J Biomech* 2006; 39:1435-1443.

15. Myerson MS, Mroczek K: Perioperative complications of total ankle arthroplasty. *Foot Ankle Int* 2003; 24:17-21.

16. Stengel D, Bauwens K, Ekkernkamp A, Cramer J: Efficacy of total ankle replacement with meniscal-bearing devices: A systematic review and meta-analysis. *Arch Orthop Trauma Surg* 2005;125:109-119.

17. Haskell A, Mann RA: Ankle arthroplasty with preoperative coronal plane deformity: Short-term results. *Clin Orthop Relat Res* 2004;424:98-103.

18. Stamatis ED, Cooper PS, Myerson MS: Supramalleolar osteotomy for the treatment of distal tibial angular deformities and arthritis of the ankle joint. *Foot Ankle Int* 2003;24: 754-764.

19. Takakura Y, Takaoka T, Tanaka Y, Yajima H, Tamai S: Results of opening-wedge osteotomy for the treatment of a post-traumatic varus deformity of the ankle. *J Bone Joint Surg Am* 1998; 80:213-218.

20. Takakura Y, Tanaka Y, Kumai T, Tamai S: Low tibial osteotomy for osteoarthritis of the ankle: Results of a new operation in 18 patients. *J Bone Joint Surg Br* 1995;77:50-54.

21. Tanaka Y, Takakura Y, Hayashi K, Taniguchi A, Kumai T, Sugimoto K: Low tibial osteotomy for varus-type osteoarthritis of the ankle. *J Bone Joint Surg Br* 2006;88:909-913.

22. Stagni R, Leardini A, Ensini A, Cappello A: Ankle morphometry evaluated using a new semi-automated technique based on X-ray pictures. *Clin Biomech (Bristol, Avon)* 2005;20: 307-311.

23. Kopp FJ, Patel MM, Deland JT, O'Malley MJ: Total ankle arthroplasty with the Agility prosthesis: Clinical and radiographic evaluation. *Foot Ankle Int* 2006;27:97-103.

24. Valderrabano V, Hintermann B, Nigg BM, Stefanyshyn D, Stergiou P: Kinematic changes after fusion and total replacement of the ankle: Part 1. Range of motion. *Foot Ankle Int* 2003; 24:881-887.

25. Valderrabano V, Hintermann B, Nigg BM, Stefanyshyn D, Stergiou P: Kinematic changes after fusion and total replacement of the ankle: Part 2. Movement transfer. *Foot Ankle Int* 2003;24:888-896.

26. Valderrabano V, Hintermann B, Nigg BM, Stefanyshyn D, Stergiou P: Kinematic changes after fusion and total replacement of the ankle: Part 3. Talar movement. *Foot Ankle Int* 2003;24: 897-900.

27. Nicholson JJ, Parks BG, Stroud CC, Myerson MS: Joint contact character-

istics in Agility total ankle arthroplasty. *Clin Orthop Relat Res* 2004;424:125-129.

28. Tochigi Y, Rudert MJ, Brown TD, McIff TE, Saltzman CL: The effect of accuracy of implantation on range of movement of the Scandinavian Total Ankle Replacement. *J Bone Joint Surg Br* 2005;87:736-740.

29. Muller S, Wolf S, Doderlein L: Three-dimensional analysis of the foot following implantation of a HINTEGRA ankle prosthesis: Evaluation with the Heidelberg Foot Model. *Orthopade* 2006;35:506-512.

30. Buechel FF, Pappas MJ, Iorio LJ: New Jersey low contact stress total ankle replacement: Biomechanical rationale and review of 23 cementless cases. *Foot Ankle* 1988;8:279-290.

31. Pappas M, Buechel FF, DePalma AF: Cylindrical total ankle joint replacement: Surgical and biomechanical rationale. *Clin Orthop Relat Res* 1976;118:82-92.

32. Buechel FF Sr, Buechel FF Jr, Pappas MJ: Twenty-year evaluation of cementless mobile-bearing total ankle replacements. *Clin Orthop Relat Res* 2004;424:19-26.

33. Komistek RD, Stiehl JB, Buechel FF, Northcut EJ, Hajner ME: A determination of ankle kinematics using fluoroscopy. *Foot Ankle Int* 2000;21:343-350.

34. Parsons P, Leslie I, Kennard E, Barker M: *Comparative Mechanical Testing of the Mobility Total Ankle Joint Replacement Prosthesis: Talar Component Subsidence, Bearing Insert Push-Out, and Prosthesis Stability.* Leeds, UK, DePuy International, 2003.

35. Bell CJ, Fisher J: Simulation of polyethylene wear in ankle joint prostheses. *J Biomed Mater Res B Appl Biomater* 2007;81:162-167.

36. Leardini A, Moschella D: Dynamic simulation of the natural and replaced human ankle joint. *Med Biol Eng Comput* 2002;40:193-199.

37. Leardini A, Catani F, Giannini S, O'Connor JJ: Computer-assisted design of the sagittal shapes of a ligament-compatible total ankle replacement. *Med Biol Eng Comput* 2001;39:168-175.

38. Hvid I, Rasmussen O, Jensen NC, Nielsen S: Trabecular bone strength profiles at the ankle joint. *Clin Orthop Relat Res* 1985;199:306-312.

39. Deland JT, de Asla RJ, Segal A: Reconstruction of the chronically failed deltoid ligament: A new technique. *Foot Ankle Int* 2004;25:795-799.

40. Coetzee JC, Pomeroy GC, Watts JD, Barrow C: The use of autologous concentrated growth factors to promote syndesmosis fusion in the Agility total ankle replacement: A preliminary study. *Foot Ankle Int* 2005;26:840-846.

41. Jung HG, Nicholson JJ, Parks B, Myerson MS: Radiographic and biomechanical support for fibular plating of the agility total ankle. *Clin Orthop Relat Res* 2004;424:118-124.

42. Raikin SM, Myerson MS: Avoiding and managing complications of the Agility total ankle replacement system. *Orthopedics* 2006;29:930-938.

43. Anderson T, Montgomery F, Carlsson A: Uncemented STAR total ankle prostheses. *J Bone Joint Surg Am* 2004;86-A(suppl 1):103-111.

44. Hintermann B, Valderrabano V: Total ankle joint replacement. *Z Arztl Fortbild Qualitatssich* 2001;95:187-194.

45. Spirt AA, Assal M, Hansen ST Jr: Complications and failure after total ankle arthroplasty. *J Bone Joint Surg Am* 2004;86:1172-1178.

46. Carlsson A: Single- and double-coated star total ankle replacements: A clinical and radiographic follow-up study of 109 cases. *Orthopade* 2006;35:527-532.

47. Carlsson A, Markusson P, Sundberg M: Radiostereometric analysis of the double-coated STAR total ankle prosthesis: A 3-5 year follow-up of 5 cases with rheumatoid arthritis and 5 cases with osteoarthrosis. *Acta Orthop* 2005;76:573-579.

48. Valderrabano V, Hintermann B, Dick W: Scandinavian total ankle replacement: A 3.7-year average followup of 65 patients. *Clin Orthop Relat Res* 2004;424:47-56.

49. Wood PL, Deakin S: Total ankle replacement: The results in 200 ankles. *J Bone Joint Surg Br* 2003;85:334-341.

50. Anderson T, Montgomery F, Carlsson A: Uncemented STAR total ankle prostheses. Three to eight-year follow-up of fifty-one consecutive ankles. *J Bone Joint Surg Am* 2003;85-A:1321-1329.

51. Haskell A, Mann RA: Perioperative complication rate of total ankle replacement is reduced by surgeon experience. *Foot Ankle Int* 2004;25:283-289.

52. Hintermann B, Valderrabano V, Dereymaeker G, Dick W: The HINTEGRA ankle: Rationale and short-term results of 122 consecutive ankles. *Clin Orthop Relat Res* 2004;424:57-68.

53. Hintermann B, Valderrabano V, Knupp M, Horisberger M: The HINTEGRA ankle: Short- and mid-term results. *Orthopade* 2006;35:533-545.

54. Bonnin M, Judet T, Colombier JA, Buscayret F, Graveleau N, Piriou P: Midterm results of the Salto Total Ankle Prosthesis. *Clin Orthop Relat Res* 2004;424:6-18.

55. San Giovanni TP, Keblish DJ, Thomas WH, Wilson MG: Eight-year results of a minimally constrained total ankle arthroplasty. *Foot Ankle Int* 2006;27:418-426.

56. Doets HC, Brand R, Nelissen RG: Total ankle arthroplasty in inflammatory joint disease with use of two mobile-bearing designs. *J Bone Joint Surg Am* 2006;88:1272-1284.

57. Saltzman CL, Amendola A, Anderson R, et al: Surgeon training and complications in total ankle arthroplasty. *Foot Ankle Int* 2003;24:514-518.

58. Bolton-Maggs BG, Sudlow RA, Freeman MA: Total ankle arthroplasty: A long-term review of the London Hospital experience. *J Bone Joint Surg Br* 1985;67:785-790.

59. McGarvey WC, Clanton TO, Lunz

D: Malleolar fracture after total ankle arthroplasty: A comparison of two designs. *Clin Orthop Relat Res* 2004;424: 104-110.

60. Nelissen RG, Doets HC, Valstar ER: Early migration of the tibial component of the Buechel-Pappas total ankle prosthesis. *Clin Orthop Relat Res* 2006;448:146-151.

61. Ohgushi H, Kitamura S, Kotobuki N, et al: Clinical application of marrow mesenchymal stem cells for hard tissue repair. *Yonsei Med J* 2004;45: 61-67.

62. Coetzee JC, Castro MD: Accurate measurement of ankle range of motion after total ankle arthroplasty. *Clin Orthop Relat Res* 2004;424:27-31.

63. Kitaoka HB: Fusion techniques for failed total ankle arthroplasty. *Semin Arthroplasty* 1992;3:51-57.

64. Kitaoka HB: Salvage of nonunion following ankle arthrodesis for failed total ankle arthroplasty. *Clin Orthop Relat Res* 1991;268:37-43.

65. Kitaoka HB, Romness DW: Arthrodesis for failed ankle arthroplasty. *J Arthroplasty* 1992;7:277-284.

66. Assal M, Greisberg J, Hansen ST Jr: Revision total ankle arthroplasty: Conversion of New Jersey Low Contact Stress to Agility: Surgical technique and case report. *Foot Ankle Int* 2004;25:922-925.

67. Knupp M, Hintermann B: Abstract: Conversion of ankle arthrodesis into total ankle arthroplasty. *74th Annual Meeting Proceedings*, Rosemont, IL, American Academy of Orthopaedic Surgeons, 2007, p 491.

68. Gabrion A, Jarde O, Havet E, Mertl P, Olory B, de Lestang M: Ankle arthrodesis after failure of a total ankle prosthesis: Eight cases. *Rev Chir Orthop Reparatrice Appar Mot* 2004;90:353-359.

69. Zwipp H, Grass R: Ankle arthrodesis after failed joint replacement. *Oper Orthop Traumatol* 2005;17:518-533.

70. Lodhi Y, McKenna J, Herron M, Stephens MM: Total ankle replacement. *Ir Med J* 2004;97:104-105.

71. SooHoo NF, Kominski G: Cost-effectiveness analysis of total ankle arthroplasty. *J Bone Joint Surg Am* 2004; 86:2446-2455.

# Surgical Correction of Moderate and Severe Hallux Valgus: Proximal Metatarsal Osteotomy With Distal Soft-Tissue Correction and Arthrodesis of the Metatarsophalangeal Joint

*V. James Sammarco, MD

## Abstract

*Hallux valgus correction by distal soft-tissue release and proximal metatarsal osteotomy is the procedure of choice for most patients with moderate and severe hallux valgus deformity. Complications can be avoided by selecting a procedure that provides adequate correction of the intermetatarsal angle and ensuring proper balancing of the metatarsophalangeal joint though lateral soft-tissue releases and medial joint plication. Arthrodesis should be considered when revision of failed surgery is planned, degenerative joint disease is present, and where the likelihood of failure of a bunion procedure is high (such as in elderly individuals with osteoporosis, severe deformity with significant involvement of the lesser metatarsophalangeal joint, and when spasticity is present). A review of biomechanical data, clinical studies, and surgical techniques is important for successful treatment of moderate and severe hallux valgus deformity.*

**Instr Course Lect 2008;57:415-428.**

The painful bunion deformity is a common and relatively disabling condition that affects individuals of all ages. More than 150 procedures have been described for the treatment of hallux valgus, and the orthopaedic literature has focused predominantly on surgical management of this condition; however, successful treatment is often achieved with simple, off-the-shelf orthotic devices and appropriate shoe wear modifications. Given the potential for surgical complications, the substantial recovery period associated with bunion surgery, and patients' occasional dissatisfaction with the results of otherwise technically successful procedures, it is recommended that nonsurgical treatment be initiated before proceeding with surgery. It is not uncommon for a patient with an asymptomatic bunion to actively seek surgical correction because of cosmetic concerns or because of an inability to wear fashionable shoes comfortably. Although pain alone is not the only indication for surgery, it is not recommended that surgery be performed for cosmetic reasons alone. The American Orthopaedic Foot and Ankle Society (AOFAS) has issued a position statement reflecting this.[1]

Pain resulting from hallux valgus deformity is mechanical in nature and can have extrinsic and intrinsic causes. Most commonly, extrinsic pain is related to mechanical irritation of the prominent medial eminence by shoe wear or is due to impingement of the hallux on the second digit. A painful callus may develop on the medial border of the hallux as a result of pronation of the digit, and pain beneath the second metatarsal head is also common as a result of the transfer of forces as the weight-bearing function of the hallux is compromised by increasing deformity. Most extrinsic pain can

*V. James Sammarco, MD or the department with which he is affiliated has received research or institutional support from Smith & Nephew.

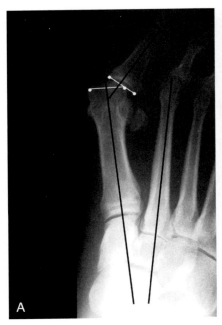 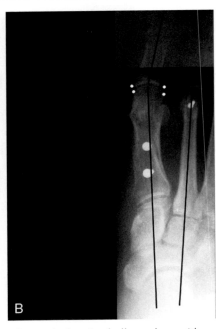

**Figure 1**   **A,** Preoperative weight-bearing radiograph showing hallux valgus with an incongruent joint. Note the lateral subluxation of the proximal phalanx and the sesamoid complex. **B,** Weight-bearing radiograph made 1 year postoperatively. The intermetatarsal angle was corrected with a proximal osteotomy of the first metatarsal, and the hallux valgus angle was corrected distally with lateral soft-tissue release and medial capsular plication.

be alleviated with nonsurgical treatment, including extra-depth shoes with a wide toe box and soft leather uppers. A silicone toe spacer between the hallux and the second toe decreases pain from impingement, and an accommodative shoe insert with a metatarsal bar can be used to diminish pain beneath the lesser metatarsal heads. Intrinsic pain is caused by abnormal joint mechanics that cause increased joint contact stresses and synovitis and can lead to cartilage degeneration. Pain intrinsic to the joint is typically reproduced with axial loading and motion of the joint and can also manifest as plantar pain with palpation of the sesamoids. Intrinsic pain is less amenable to conservative treatment but can be managed with an orthotic device that incorporates a stiff Morton extension. Corrective devices

may prevent progression of a deformity, but they will not permanently correct it. An in-depth review of conservative treatment of painful bunion deformities is beyond the scope of this chapter, and the reader is referred to a recent article in which current concepts of nonsurgical management are reviewed in greater detail.[2]

The primary indication, for surgical treatment of hallux valgus is pain that fails to respond to conservative treatment, usually within 6 to 12 months. Some conditions may not cause substantial pain but may require surgical correction because of functional problems or rapid progression. Substantial progression of a deformity by one grade or more over a 6- to 12-month period may be an indication for surgical correction, even if pain is not a major symptom.

These conditions are uncommon in patients with idiopathic hallux valgus and typically are related to neuromuscular disease or trauma.

Selection of the proper procedure for hallux valgus surgery is critical to achieving an adequate result and durable correction of the deformity. Bunion deformity has been classified, and the algorithm developed by Mann and Coughlin defines modern decision making in hallux valgus surgery.[3] The metatarsophalangeal joint should be examined radiographically for congruency (Figure 1). If the joint is congruent, surgery must be planned so that it does not alter the congruency. When the metatarsophalangeal joint is incongruent, surgery is planned to restore joint congruency. Bunion deformity is classified as mild, moderate, or severe on the basis of the radiographic findings. Other considerations are the presence of metatarsophalangeal arthritis, hypermobility of the tarsometatarsal joint complex, and the presence of hallux valgus interphalangeus. This chapter is limited to a review of two procedures: bunion correction by proximal metatarsal osteotomy with distal soft-tissue rebalancing and bunion correction by arthrodesis of the metatarsophalangeal joint. Bunion correction by proximal metatarsal osteotomy with distal soft-tissue rebalancing is indicated primarily for moderate and severe bunions when the intermetatarsal angle must be corrected by more than 5° to achieve the desired postoperative position of less than 10°. The hallux valgus angle in these cases is typically more than 30°. Mild bunion deformities with an intermetatarsal angle of 14° or less can typically be corrected with a distal osteotomy; however, in elderly individuals or those with osteoporosis, a more proximal osteotomy may be considered to im-

**Table 1**
**General Indications for Proximal Metatarsal Osteotomy
With Distal Soft-Tissue Rebalancing**

| Bunion Grade | Hallux Valgus Angle | Intermetatarsal Angle | Other Factors | Notes |
|---|---|---|---|---|
| Moderate | < 40° | ≥ 14° | Incongruent joint | Congruent joint may require double osteotomy |
| Severe | ≥ 40° | ≥ 16° | Incongruent joint | Fusion should be considered for an elderly patient, one with osteoporotic bone, and one with multiple lesser toe deformities |

**Table 2**
**Indications for Fusion in Patients
With Hallux Valgus**

Arthritis associated with hallux valgus

Neuromuscular disease/spasticity

Inflammatory arthritis

Severe deformity with osteoporosis

Salvage after failed bunion surgery or failed arthroplasty

Salvage after infection (staged reconstruction)

prove the available bone stock for fixation of the osteotomy site and to lessen the chances of osteonecrosis of the first metatarsal head. Fusion is most commonly done for the treatment of hallux valgus associated with arthritis or as a salvage procedure following failed previous bunion surgery and attempted arthroplasty. Other indications include neuromuscular conditions that cause spasticity, such as cerebral palsy and stroke, because of the high recurrence rate associated with standard procedures and the tendency for progression of the deformity with time.[4] Primary arthrodesis may also be considered for patients with severe deformity who are at high risk for failure of an osteotomy because of osteoporosis or an inability to comply with weight bearing and other activity restrictions during the postoperative period. The indications for these procedures are outlined in Tables 1 and 2.

## Proximal Osteotomy With Distal Soft-Tissue Rebalancing

Traditionally, the complication rates associated with proximal osteotomies have been higher than those associated with distal osteotomies. Many authors have noted a high prevalence of dorsal malunion following proximal metatarsal osteotomies, and this is primarily due to either loss of fixation or fracture of the metatarsal once weight bearing is initiated.[5-9] Factors that may contribute to complications include patient age, bone density, and the degree of stability of the osteotomy site. The development of newer (and more expensive) fixation devices has not necessarily improved the situation. A thorough understanding of the anatomy and biomechanics of the first ray is key to avoiding complications.

## Anatomic and Biomechanical Factors Associated With Bunion Correction Surgery

The biomechanics of the metatarsals in the human are unique in that they are the only long bones that support load perpendicular to their axis during most phases of gait and standing. The forces acting on the first metatarsal during gait were defined in the classic article by Stokes and associates,[10] who described the factors responsible for the forces in the metatarsal during gait; these include the inclination of the first metatarsal to the ground, the lengths of the first metatarsal and phalanges, the forces generated by the plantar muscles and soft tissues through the windlass mechanism, and the weight of the individual. These factors directly affect the forces that act on the first metatarsal: bending moment, shear, and axial load. For a given load, bending moment and shear forces increase with increasing metatarsal length and decreasing metatarsal inclination. Conversely, axial load increases and bending moment decreases as the metatarsal inclination increases.

Stokes and associates also calculated the effects of the tension generated by the plantar soft tissues on these forces.[10] Force at the metatarsal head is a combination of direct force through the plantar aspect of the foot and sesamoids and joint reaction forces across the metatarsophalangeal joint. This is an intrinsic mechanism whereby part of the force of weight bearing is transferred to axial load rather than shear and bending. Functionally, this is known as the "windlass mechanism" whereby dorsiflexion of the metatarsophalangeal joints causes increased tension in the longitudinal arch and raises the longitudinal arch of the foot. Increasing pull from the short and long toe flexors and increasing tension within the plantar fascia as the metatarsophalangeal joint rolls into dorsiflexion diminish bending moment and shear forces across the metatarsal while increasing axial load and the joint reaction force at the metatarsophalangeal joint. It should be noted that the calculations by Stokes and associates were based on an ideal model with a normal first metatarsophalangeal joint. Diminished motion at the metatarsophalangeal joint from arthritis or other pathologic conditions can decrease the function of the windlass mechanism and increase shear and bending forces through the metatarsal.[11]

The osseous anatomy must also be considered in the planning of a first metatarsal osteotomy. Metaphyseal osteotomies have the advantage of a larger surface area for osseous healing and screw fixation. Diaphyseal osteotomies involve less surface area and may be subject to higher strains due to disruption of the cortical architecture of the bone. A computerized finite-element analysis was performed by Kristen and associates[12] using a three-dimensional model derived from digitized cadaveric data to calculate stress and strain patterns in the first metatarsal. Simulated weight-bearing loads were applied across this model from 30° to 70° of dorsal extension, and stress and strain were visualized with use of von Mises stress analyses. Stresses were concentrated along the plantar aspect of the diaphysis and at the dorsolateral diaphyseal-metaphyseal junction, and slight dorsomedial deformation occurred. The authors suggested that, when performing an osteotomy, the surgeon should avoid violating these areas to minimize the chance for displacement.

In hallux valgus deformity, the anatomy of the first metatarsophalangeal joint becomes distorted and the subluxated joint capsule causes deforming forces that pull the hallux into further valgus and displace the first metatarsal head medially. This problem is primarily related to lateralization of the flexor hallucis longus, flexor hallucis brevis, and adductor hallucis tendons, which

occurs as the joint subluxates laterally and the hallux pronates.[13,14] Lateral and plantar migration of the abductor hallucis tendon and attenuation of the dorsomedial aspect of the joint capsule diminish the normal resistant forces to valgus deviation.[15] These changes, while flexible early in the disease process, tend to become rigid and fixed as time progresses. Contractures of the lateral aspect of the joint are accompanied by permanent shortening and fibrosis of those tissues and require meticulous surgical release for adequate correction. The combination of the lateralized moment across the metatarsophalangeal joint and loss of the normal balancing structures medially creates a medial deforming vector on the first metatarsal head. Saltzman and associates[16] performed a force vector analysis of these moments in a cadaveric model and noted an increase in medializing forces on the first metatarsophalangeal joint with increasing hallux valgus and supination. Translational and derotational osteotomies had minimal effect on these vectors. These authors concluded that normalization of these vectors through soft-tissue reconstruction was as important as realignment of the osseous structures in the prevention of recurrence of the deformity in the frontal plane. In a cadaver study, Coughlin and associates[17] demonstrated the importance of restoring the axial alignment of the osseous structures and that correction of the intermetatarsal angle with an osteotomy increased the stability of the first ray.

## Principles Governing First Metatarsal Osteotomies

Osteotomy of the first metatarsal has been studied extensively. The geometric principles used in determin-

ing correction were explored by Kummer and Jahss.[18-20] Correction of the intermetatarsal angle is increased per degree of rotation or lateral translation as the osteotomy is moved more proximally. One degree of correction is achieved on average for each millimeter of lateral translation in distal osteotomies of the metatarsal head, and only about 5° of correction can be achieved with a distal chevron-type osteotomy because further translation will result in instability of the final construct. Moving the osteotomy more proximally moves the center of rotation, and more correction is achieved per degree of rotation. Kummer and Jahss also noted that a degree of shortening and elevation of the first metatarsal head is inherent in these osteotomies. Nyska and associates[21] performed a geometric analysis of the Ludloff, Mau, Scarf, proximal chevron, proximal crescentic, and wedge osteotomies. They noted the best correction was achieved by the Ludloff osteotomy angled 16° to the shaft; however, this caused elevation and shortening. The 8° Ludloff osteotomy provided angular corrections similar to those provided by the basilar wedge and crescentic osteotomies, but with less elevation and shortening.

The stability of first metatarsal osteotomies has been studied extensively, and these osteotomies have been classified according to their geometry[11] (Figure 2). Complete osteotomies are those that divide the metatarsal into two separate fragments. These osteotomies can achieve correction through multiplanar manipulation of the distal fragment. Incomplete opening and closing wedge osteotomies leave one cortex intact to act as a hinge, which adds stability but decreases the freedom of correction. Complete osteotomies may be classified as intrinsically stable or as intrinsically unstable (Figure 3). Intrinsic stability is present when an osteotomy incorporates the direct transfer of deforming forces from the distal fragment into the proximal fragment by nature of its geometry. For displacement into dorsiflexion, which is the primary force that causes early failure, stability is related to the sagittal orientation of the osteotomy. A limb of the osteotomy that is oriented from proximal-plantar to dorsal-distal will impart intrinsic stability to the distal fragment. Osteotomies that are intrinsically unstable are those that have no osseous resistance to deforming forces and that are entirely dependent on internal fixation for maintenance of position during osseous healing. These include any osteotomy that has a single plane oriented from dorsal-proximal to plantar-distal or is perpendicular to the shaft of the metatarsal.

Consideration should be given to the method of fixation of the metatarsal osteotomy site. Fixation of all metatarsal osteotomy sites is recommended regardless of inherent stability or instability. Distal osteotomies have intrinsic stability of great enough magnitude that Kirschner wire fixation is often adequate. Because of the increased moment arm present with proximal osteotomies, simple Kirschner wire fixation is usually inadequate for definitive fixation. Screw fixation of osteotomy sites has been proven to be biomechanically superior to pin fixation in several studies and can provide rigid fixation of some otherwise unstable constructs.[22,23] The bending strength of the screw is much greater than that of a Kirschner wire because of the screw's increased diameter, and stability to rotation can be achieved

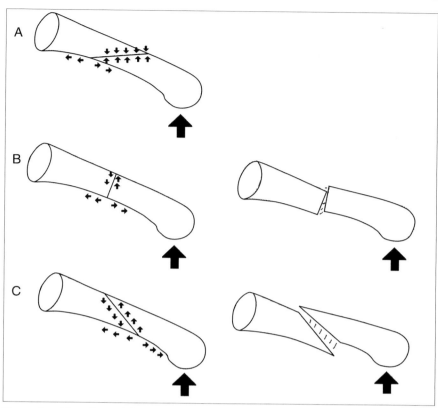

**Figure 2**    The effect of the orientation of the osteotomy on intrinsic stability. **A,** Sagittal orientation from dorsal-distal to proximal-plantar imparts inherent stability as a result of direct transfer of forces from the distal fragment into the proximal fragment. **B** and **C,** A vertical or a proximal-dorsal to distal-plantar orientation affords no intrinsic stability. (Reprinted with permission from Sammarco VJ, Acevedo J: Stability and fixation techniques in first metatarsal osteotomies. *Foot Ankle Clin* 2001;6:409-432.)

through compression of the osteotomy site itself. The predominant mechanical disadvantage of screw fixation is the stress risers created by their application. Fracture can occur through these stress risers once weight bearing is initiated. Use of a plate for primary fixation in bunion surgery is relatively uncommon despite mechanical and clinical data that show that they provide more stability than simple screw fixation.[24,25] Technically, application of small plates designed for fracture fixation can be quite time-consuming because of the need for finely adjusted contouring of the devices. Rigid fixation can be

achieved, but this technique is usually reserved for cases in which standard fixation is deemed inadequate intraoperatively because of osteoporosis or fracture. New, procedure-specific devices, including wedge plates and locking plates, have recently been marketed, but there are no published clinical data supporting their use and justifying their expense.

### Proximal Crescentic Osteotomy
To perform a proximal crescentic osteotomy, as popularized by Mann and associates,[26-28] the surgeon uses a curved oscillating saw to create an osteotomy from the proximal-dorsal

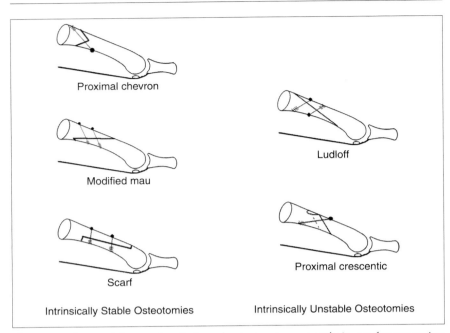

**Figure 3** Some of the proximally based osteotomies currently in use for correction of varus angulation of the first metatarsal associated with hallux valgus.

aspect of the metaphysis to the plantar aspect of the proximal part of the diaphysis. The intermetatarsal angle is corrected by rotating the distal fragment in the trough created in the base of the first metatarsal. Rather than simply rotating in a single plane, the distal fragment rolls in the inclined trough created by the saw blade, and medial or lateral angulation of the osteotomy will cause elevation or depression of the metatarsal head, respectively, as the distal fragment is rotated laterally.[29] The osteotomy site is fixed with a single compression screw from the dorsal cortex of the distal fragment to the plantar aspect of the metaphysis of the proximal fragment. Single-screw fixation provides little resistance to rotation about its axis, and some have found it necessary to augment fixation with an additional Kirschner wire or plate if fixation is questionable.[24,30] Failure tends to occur through fracture of the dorsal bone

bridge at the screw head or by loosening of the fixation screw, allowing loss of correction and elevation of the distal fragment.[21,31] Regardless of the fixation technique, the proximal crescentic osteotomy remains one of the most unstable first metatarsal osteotomies. Biomechanical studies have shown the loads to failure following a crescentic osteotomy to be lower than those following Ludloff, proximal chevron, proximal closing wedge, Scarf, and Mau osteotomies.[22,32,33] Fatigue studies have shown stability to cyclic loading after crescentic osteotomies to be relatively inferior as well.[31] Modifying this osteotomy with a proximal crescentic shelf (a dorsal dome cut and an inferior oblique cut) does not appear to improve the relative loads to failure.[34] Stability can be improved by fixing the osteotomy site with a new procedure-specific plate.[35]

Clinical data have varied widely among studies of the proximal cres-

centic osteotomy. Brodsky and associates[36] prospectively evaluated plantar pressure measurements at a mean of 29 months after proximal crescentic osteotomy in 32 patients. Twelve patients had first metatarsal elevation of more than 2 mm, and a transfer lesion developed under the second metatarsal head in five of those patients. These authors found control of the crescentic osteotomy to be unpredictable in the sagittal plane. In a prospective, randomized study, Easley and associates[6] compared proximal chevron osteotomy with proximal crescentic osteotomy for hallux valgus correction in 84 feet followed for a minimum of 1 year. Although the clinical results were good in both groups, the sites of the proximal chevron osteotomies healed faster and a higher prevalence of dorsal malunion was seen in the group treated with the proximal crescenotic osteotomy. Thordarson and Leventen[9] reported the results of 33 proximal crescentic osteotomies done to treat hallux valgus deformity. After a minimum of 2 years of follow-up, these authors reported good clinical results but noted an average dorsiflexion malunion of 6.2° through the osteotomy site. Staple fixation was noted to be more unstable and to result in more dorsiflexion. In a retrospective study of 50 patients who had undergone hallux valgus correction with either a proximal chevron or a proximal crescentic osteotomy, Markbreiter and Thompson[37] noted equivalent good results in the two groups. Okuda and associates[38] reported excellent correction of radiographic parameters and good clinical results in a study of 47 feet followed for an average of 48 months after proximal crescentic osteotomy done to treat hallux valgus. Okuda and associates[39] also reported that the

1-year results of this procedure were predictive of the 3-year results.

### Proximal Chevron Osteotomy

The distal chevron osteotomy was first described by Austin and Leventen[40] and refers to a horizontally directed V pattern that imparts inherent stability to the distal fragment. The chevron osteotomy pattern has also been used in the proximal part of the metatarsal for correction of moderate and severe metatarsus primus varus.[41,42] Biomechanically, the osteotomy site derives stability as forces are directly transferred from the distal fragment to the proximal fragment through the dorsal shelf. The osteotomy should be directed with the apex distal, as directing the apex proximally creates a stress riser in the proximal fragment adjacent to the articular surface and may result in a fracture into the first tarsometatarsal articulation.[6] Directing the apex distally moves the stress riser distally and into the distal fragmunt, thus diminishing the moment arm and eliminating the risk of intra-articular fracture should failure occur. The osteotomy site is fixed from plantar to proximal-dorsal, which provides compression on the tension side of the osteotomy. The screw should not be applied from dorsal to plantar because that concentrates stresses at the apex of the osteotomy and predisposes the bone to fracture under low loads.[32]

The chevron osteotomy has been studied biomechanically to determine its corrective potential and stability. Nyska and associates[21] found that less correction was achieved with the proximal chevron osteotomy than with the Ludloff, crescentic, and closing wedge osteotomies; however, correction was achieved by lateral translation only, without rotation. According to Kummer's analysis, the proximal chevron osteotomy can achieve high levels of correction if the distal fragment is rotated with translation, as is commonly done in clinical practice.[18] McCluskey and associates[33] compared stiffness and load to failure between cadaveric models of proximal crescentic and proximal chevron osteotomies and noted greater stability with the proximal chevron technique. In a study of the Ludloff, Scarf, biplanar closing wedge, Mau, proximal chevron, and proximal crescentic osteotomies in cadaveric preparations, Trnka and associates[32] noted less stability with the proximal chevron osteotomy than with the others tested except for the proximal crescentic osteotomy; however, the fixation screw was placed dorsally rather than plantarly, which allows distraction of the plantar cortex during loading. It is possible that this study demonstrated the importance of using a plantar-based screw rather than identifying an inherent problem with the osteotomy. Acevedo and associates[31] studied five osteotomies in a cyclic loading model and found the site of the proximal chevron osteotomy to be stronger than all others tested in both Sawbones and cadaveric models with a screw placed from plantar to dorsal.

Correction of hallux valgus with the proximal chevron osteotomy has reportedly yielded good clinical results with few complications. Sammarco and associates[41] reported on 43 patients who had undergone surgical correction of hallux valgus with a proximal chevron osteotomy for correction of the intermetatarsal angle.[41] No malunions were found, and the AOFAS score improved significantly. Sammarco and Russo-Alesi[43] reported the results of 72 consecutive procedures after an average duration of follow-up of 41 months. Again, dorsal malunion was not observed, and improvement in the AOFAS scores was noted. Easley and associates[6] reported good clinical results after both the proximal chevron and the proximal crescentic osteotomy but noted a lower complication rate and faster healing of the osteotomy site after the proximal chevron osteotomy. Those authors thought that improved stability of the osteotomy site was responsible for these outcomes. Markbreiter and Thompson[37] reported the results in 50 feet in which either a proximal crescentic or a chevron osteotomy had been done for the correction of hallux valgus. Excellent results were reported in both groups, but the proximal chevron osteotomy was thought to be technically easier to perform because of its inherent stability.

### Scarf Osteotomy

The Scarf osteotomy was introduced to the surgical community by Zygmunt and associates,[44] and its use for the correction of moderate and severe metatarsus primus varus has steadily increased in Europe and elsewhere. As originally described, the osteotomy is horizontal in the distal part of the diaphysis, with a limb exiting superiorly at the distal end of the metatarsal and a limb exiting proximally at the midpart of the diaphysis. The osteotomy provides tremendous inherent stability to displacement as a result of the long dorsal shelf afforded with the horizontal saw cut. The originally described osteotomy achieved correction by lateral translation of the distal fragment. Barouk[45] and Weil[46] proposed numerous modifications, including lengthening or shortening of the metatarsal, rotation of the distal fragment, raising or lowering of the metatarsal head, and correction of the distal metatarsal articular angle by rotation of the distal fragment. Nyska and associates[21] noted less correction of the intermetatarsal angle with the Scarf osteotomy than with the Ludloff, closing wedge, and crescentic osteotomies.

Barouk's modifications extend the osteotomy proximally, which allows greater correction of the intermetatarsal angle but also increases the moment arm on the dorsal shelf, and fracture of the metatarsal has been reported as a complication.[47,48] Trnka and associates[32] performed static load-to-failure testing in cadavers in which the Scarf osteotomy had been performed and compared the results with those after five other osteotomies of the first metatarsal. They found that the osteotomy site was stable and concluded that it should be acceptable for patients with normal bone density to immediately bear weight in a postoperative shoe. In their study, however, the osteotomy did not include the proximal extension that is currently used to achieve greater corrections of the intermetatarsal angle. Acevedo and associates[31] performed cyclic loading of the sites of Scarf osteotomies in Sawbones models and found substantial problems with fracture of the metatarsal at the proximal part of the dorsal limb. There may also be problems with positioning of the final construct as a result of the diaphyseal nature of the osteotomy. Because the osteotomy divides the metatarsal horizontally along its length, the distal fragment may rotate axially as the medial cortex of the distal fragment slides into the medullary canal of the proximal fragment, causing undesired elevation and supination of the distal articular surface (so-called troughing).[11,47]

Clinical studies of the Scarf osteotomy have demonstrated mixed results. Aminian and associates[49] evaluated the results of 27 consecutive Scarf osteotomies at an average of 16 months. The complication rate was low, and the AOFAS scores improved. Fracture of the metatarsal was not noted. Jones and associates[50] reviewed the results at a mean of 20 months after 35 Scarf osteotomies were done for hallux valgus correction. Excellent correction was achieved, as demonstrated radiographically and clinically, and pedobarographic measurements made after more than 1 year were noted to be normalized. One intraoperative fracture was noted, but no postoperative stress fractures occurred. The authors concluded that the procedure is effective, with reproducible results, for correction of moderate and severe deformity. Coetzee[47] reported less promising clinical results after 20 Scarf osteotomies. Malunion from troughing, malrotation, and fracture were responsible for major complications despite postoperative immobilization in a short leg cast for 6 weeks. Forty-five percent of the patients were dissatisfied with the result of the surgery after 1 year. At an average of 22 months following 84 Scarf osteotomies, Crevoisier and associates[51] noted improvement in radiographic parameters and AOFAS scores, although 11% of the patients were not satisfied and required additional procedures. Problems with the fixation of the osteotomy site and stiffness of the first metatarsophalangeal joint occurred. Fracture was not reported.

### Ludloff Osteotomy

The metatarsal osteotomy described by Ludloff extends from the dorsal aspect of the metaphysis proximally to the plantar aspect of the diaphysis distally. Despite the inherent instability of its geometry, the Ludloff osteotomy affords a broad surface for screw fixation, which substantially increases the relative strength of the construct. Some biomechanical studies have shown the load-to-failure values after the Ludloff osteotomy to be superior to those after the proximal chevron or crescentic osteotomies. Lian and associates[22] noted that a Ludloff osteotomy site fixed with two screws was 82% stronger than the site of a crescentic osteotomy fixed with a single screw. Using a cadaver model, Trnka and associates[32] noted that, compared with five other constructs, the Ludloff osteotomy provided excellent stability and stiffness. Acevedo and associates[31] noted that the Ludloff osteotomy resulted in excellent fatigue endurance under cyclic loading in both a cadaver and a Sawbones model. The osteotomy site is fixed with two screws, which compress the proximal and distal fragments in diaphyseal bone. When loaded to failure, the osteotomy site fails either by fracture of the metatarsal at the proximal screw head or from pullout of the screw threads. In a Sawbones model, Nyska and associates[21] noted that the sagittal inclination of the Ludloff osteotomy plays a large role in the amount that the intermetatarsal angle can be corrected.[52] A 16° angulation allowed the most correction but also caused shortening and elevation of the first metatarsal head, whereas an 8° angulation afforded correction comparable with that provided by other proximal osteotomies without substantial shortening or elevation. Beischer and associates[53] noted that 10° is the ideal orientation for correction without shortening or elevation.

The Ludloff osteotomy with screw fixation for correction of hallux valgus has had excellent clinical results to date. Chiodo and associates[54] reviewed the results of 70 procedures for correction of moderate and severe hallux valgus. After an average duration of follow-up of 30 months, the satisfaction rate was 94% and few complications had developed. The authors noted that fixation was inadequate in two patients who had required a steeper osteotomy in the sagittal plane. These two osteotomy sites healed with callus formation and slight shortening, and elevation of the first metatarsal was noted on the final follow-up radiographs. Improved fixation methods may negate these issues.[30,55-57] Petroutsas and Trnka[58] reported the results in 70 patients at a minimum of 2 years after they had undergone a Ludloff osteotomy for hallux valgus repair. Radiographic measurements had improved. Evaluation with a four-point clinical scale showed that 81% of the patients were satisfied or very satisfied, but 5% had continued pain.

### Mau Osteotomy

The osteotomy described by Mau and Lauber[59] is an oblique diaphyseal osteotomy that is directed from proximal-plantar to distal-dorsal. With this procedure, as originally described, the angular correction that can be achieved by rotation of the distal fragment is less than that possible with the more proximal osteotomies. Nyska and associates[21] showed that both the 8° and the 16° Mau osteotomies provide angular correction without substantial elevation but the correction is greater with the Ludloff osteotomy, probably because of the more proximal center of rotation. Although clinical comparison studies of the Mau osteotomy are lacking, mechanical testing has shown that it provides superior stability. Both static and dy-

namic fatigue studies have shown Mau osteotomy sites to be more stable than the sites of other proximal and shaft osteotomies, including the Scarf and the Ludloff procedures.[31,32] In one clinical study with a short follow-up (18 weeks), Neese and associates[60] noted a low prevalence of shortening and malunion. More long-term prospective trials are needed to determine the clinical efficacy of the procedure. This osteotomy was modified with a second cut through the plantar metaphyseal cortex, which allows it to be extended more proximally to gain more substantial correction while taking advantage of its superior biomechanical properties (Figure 4). A detailed description of the author's preferred surgical technique for the modified Mau osteotomy was recently published.[61] **(DVD 36.1)**

### Arthrodesis of the Hallux Metatarsophalangeal Joint for Treatment of Hallux Valgus

Arthrodesis of the first metatarsophalangeal joint for the treatment of hallux valgus is a salvage procedure that is primarily used when more standard bunion correction procedures will not provide durable results or pain relief or have a high risk of early failure. Coughlin and associates[62] reported the results of arthrodesis for the treatment of 21 moderate or severe cases of idiopathic hallux valgus. Arthrodesis was considered for moderate bunions if degenerative changes of the first metatarsophalangeal joint were seen radiographically or if there was advanced deformity of the lesser metatarsophalangeal joints. Primary arthrodesis was considered for severe deformity in which the hallux valgus angle was more than 40°, regardless of the presence of degenerative changes or involvement of the

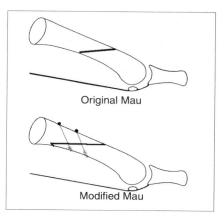

**Figure 4** Modification of the Mau osteotomy moves the osteotomy proximally into the metaphysis and the proximal part of the diaphysis of the bone. This allows greater correction of the intermetatarsal angle and provides more predictable healing. (Reprinted with permission from Sammarco VJ: Surgical strategies: Mau osteotomy for correction of moderate and severe hallux valgus deformity. *Foot Ankle Int* 2007;28:857-864.)

lesser metatarsophalangeal joints. Three nonunions occurred; two were asymptomatic and one was revised to a fusion, which was successful. All patients were considered to have a good or excellent result at the time of final follow-up, at an average of 8.2 years (range, 24 to 272 months). Similarly, Riggs and Johnson[63] noted that in most cases arthrodesis for the treatment of hallux valgus was successful at the time of short- or long-term follow-up (range, 1 to 15 years), with resolution of pain in 92% of patients. Overall satisfaction was rated at 86%, although hardware frequently had to be removed (in 30% of the cases) and the rate of complications, including infection and failure, was 8%. Tourné and associates[64] suggested that arthrodesis of the metatarsophalangeal joint was a predictable method for managing hallux valgus deformity in elderly individuals. Ar-

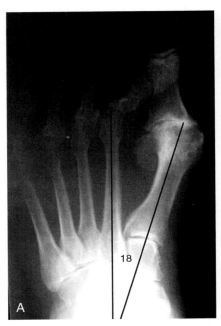 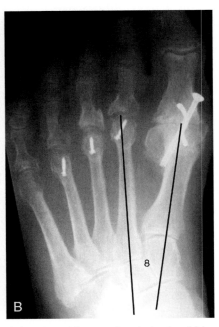

**Figure 5**  **A,** Correction of hallux valgus deformity with an arthrodesis should be considered if there is substantial arthritis of the metatarsophalangeal joint. **B,** Note the correction of the intermetatarsal angle without osteotomy of the first metatarsal.

throdesis should also be considered the primary treatment of hallux valgus in patients with clinically relevant osteoarthritis or inflammatory arthritis of the metatarsophalangeal joint, as reconstructive procedures designed to restore axial alignment do not address the underlying loss of cartilage or destruction of the normal supporting structures.[65,66] Hallux valgus associated with spasticity, as is commonly seen in patients with cerebral palsy, has a high recurrence rate when treated with standard techniques. Davids and associates[4] reviewed 26 cases of hallux valgus managed with arthrodesis of the first metatarsophalangeal joint in children with cerebral palsy. They noted high satisfaction among both patients and caregivers, with excellent radiographic and clinical correction. They recommended fusion for primary treatment in children with a spastic foot deformity.

Salvage following failed bunion surgery is technically demanding, and attempts at revision are associated with increased failure rates. If a specific cause for the failure can be identified, it may be possible to revise the previous bunion surgery successfully, but arthrodesis can usually be used for salvage in difficult cases in which nonunion, osteonecrosis, or extensive arthritis is present. Grimes and Coughlin[67] reported 33 cases in which a failure of hallux valgus surgery was treated with arthrodesis of the metatarsophalangeal joint. Four nonunions resulted, three of which were asymptomatic. Radiographic correction was excellent in all cases. Although the patients with failed bunion surgery had improvement following the arthrodesis, the final results were worse than the final results of successful primary bunion surgery. Kitaoka and Patzer[68] noted that, compared with successful primary procedures, arthrodeses done

to revise failed bunion surgery resulted in similar improvements in scores but less patient satisfaction. These authors also observed that the results of the arthrodeses were slightly better than those of resection arthroplasties for salvage following failed bunion surgery. Myerson and associates[69] described staged arthrodesis for the management of failed bunion surgery associated with osteomyelitis. Several studies have shown that arthrodesis of the first metatarsophalangeal joint will correct an even substantially increased intermetatarsal angle, and metatarsal osteotomy is typically not necessary[70] (Figure 5).

Biomechanical studies may help surgeons to select the appropriate technique for arthrodesis of the metatarsophalangeal joint. A more stable construct theoretically allows a higher fusion rate and permits earlier weight bearing. Joint preparation is usually done through a dorsal or medial incision. Preparation with matched cuts made with a straight or crescentic saw or a "cup-in-cone" arthrodesis bed prepared with a high-speed burr or with matched conical reamers has been reported. In cadaveric models of arthrodeses of the first metatarsophalangeal joint, Curtis and associates[71] noted that machined conical reaming followed by fixation with interfragmentary screws provided more strength than preparation with matched planar cuts regardless of the fixation technique, including the use of a dorsal plate. In a study involving mechanical testing of five fusion models in cadavers, Politi and associates[72] similarly noted that conical reaming provided improved strength compared with that provided by planar excision. The strongest construct in this study was created by matched conical reaming and use

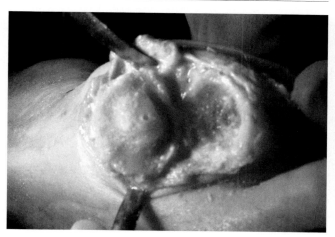

**Figure 6** The cup-in-cone arthrodesis bed is created by denuding cartilage and subchondral bone with a 5-mm burr to create matching fusion surfaces.

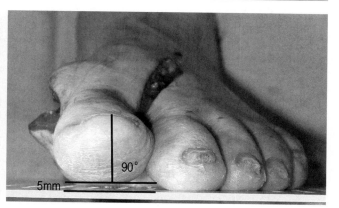

**Figure 7** A lid from an instrument set can be used to gauge dorsiflexion intraoperatively. Approximately 5 mm of clearance of the pulp of the digit from the floor is desired to allow roll-off of the hallux. Care should be taken to fix the toe rotation so that it is neutral to the axis of the foot.

of a dorsal compression plate and a single oblique lag screw. A review of the available mechanical data shows plate-and-screw fixation to be the most stable, followed by interfragmentary or intramedullary screw fixation, both of which are superior to fixation with Kirschner wires or compression staples.[73-75]

## Author's Preferred Technique: Cup-in-Cone Arthrodesis With Crossed Screws

The preferred technique is based on an attempt to balance the available biomechanical data with current constraints imposed by implant cost and the surgical time required for the procedure. The costs of specialized plates, compression staples, and cannulated screws must be balanced against the surgeon's ability to achieve successful results with less expensive, generic solid screws and fracture plates. It has been my experience that even the use of precontoured plates substantially increases operating room time and can be associated with incorrect alignment of the arthrodesis. At least three commercially manufactured conical reaming systems are currently available for this procedure, but they must usually be rented or purchased or are paired with an implant system. Surgeons must take care when learning to use these systems because fractures of both the metatarsal head and the proximal phalanx have been seen with use of these reamers. The cup-in-cone preparation described by Myerson is done through a dorsal incision and with use of a standard, inexpensive 5-mm burr[76] (Figure 6). The first metatarsal head is denuded of any remaining cartilage and subchondral bone until the underlying cancellous bone is exposed. The proximal phalanx is similarly prepared to create the recipient "cup," following removal of cartilage and subchondral bone. Final adjustments are made with the burr for positioning, and the metatarsophalangeal joint is stabilized with a Kirschner wire and checked for alignment. The arthrodesis site can be secured with two 4.0-mm cannulated or noncannulated cancellous screws. If stability is poor secondary to osteoporosis or bone loss, a contoured one-third tubular plate will substantially improve fixation.

Final positioning should consist of 10° to 20° of hallux valgus, but care must be taken to allow clearance of the second toe by 1 to 2 mm. Dorsiflexion should be 15° to 30° from the first metatarsal, or 5° to 10° from the floor. A good way to assess the final position intraoperatively is to press the foot flat on a sterile plate (an instrument case lid) (Figure 7). The hallux should not impinge on the second toe, rotation should be neutral with the axis of the floor, and there should be approximately 5 mm of space between the plate and the pulp of the hallux. Malpositioning is the most common complication associated with this surgery. Plantar flexion and malrotation are associated with secondary arthritis of the interphalangeal joint. Excessive dorsiflexion may cause difficulty with shoe wear and transfer lesions at the lesser metatarsophalangeal joints. After the surgery, the patient wears a postoperative shoe with weight bearing on the heel for 4 to 6 weeks or until fusion is evident radiographically.

## Summary

Hallux valgus correction with distal soft-tissue release and proximal metatarsal osteotomy is the procedure of choice for most patients with a symptomatic moderate or severe hallux valgus deformity. Complications can be avoided by selecting a procedure that provides adequate correction of the intermetatarsal angle and ensuring proper balancing of the first metatarsophalangeal joint through lateral soft-tissue releases and medial joint plication. Arthrodesis of the first metatarsophalangeal joint should be considered when revision of failed bunion surgery is planned or when degenerative joint disease is present. Arthrodesis should also be considered if the likelihood of failure of a standard bunion procedure is high, such as in elderly individuals with osteoporosis, patients with severe deformity and substantial involvement of the lesser metatarsophalangeal joints, and those with neuromuscular spasticity.

## References

1. Position statement on cosmetic foot surgery. American Orthopaedic Foot and Ankle Society; Rosemont, Illinois. 2003. Available at: http://www.aofas.org/i4a/pages/index.cfm?pageid=367 2. Accessed August 8, 2007.

2. Sammarco VJ, Nichols R: Orthotic management for disorders of the hallux. *Foot Ankle Clin* 2005;10:191-209.

3. Mann RA, Coughlin MJ (eds): *Surgery of the Foot and Ankle.* St. Louis, MO, Mosby, 1993, pp 167-296.

4. Davids JR, Mason TA, Danko A, Banks D, Blackhurst D: Surgical management of hallux valgus deformity in children with cerebral palsy. *J Pediatr Orthop* 2001;21:89-94.

5. Acevedo JI: Fixation of metatarsal osteotomies in the treatment of hallux valgus. *Foot Ankle Clin* 2000;5: 451-468.

6. Easley ME, Kiebzak GM, Davis WH, Anderson RB: Prospective, randomized comparison of proximal crescentic and proximal chevron osteotomies for correction of hallux valgus deformity. *Foot Ankle Int* 1996;17:307-316.

7. Gill LH: Distal osteotomy for bunionectomy and hallux valgus correction. *Foot Ankle Clin* 2001;6:433-453.

8. Pearson SW, Kitaoka HB, Cracchiolo A, Leventen EO: Results and complications following a proximal curved osteotomy of the hallux metatarsal. *Contemp Orthop* 1991;23:127-132.

9. Thordarson DB, Leventen EO: Hallux valgus correction with proximal metatarsal osteotomy: Two-year follow-up. *Foot Ankle* 1992;13: 321-326.

10. Stokes IA, Hutton WC, Stott JR: Forces acting on the metatarsals during normal walking. *J Anat* 1979;129: 579-590.

11. Sammarco VJ, Acevedo J: Stability and fixation techniques in first metatarsal osteotomies. *Foot Ankle Clin* 2001;6:409-432.

12. Kristen KH, Berger K, Berger C, Kampla W, Anzbšck W, Weitzel SH: The first metatarsal bone under loading conditions: A finite element analysis. *Foot Ankle Clin* 2005;10:1-14.

13. Alvarez R, Haddad RJ, Gould N, Trevino S: The simple bunion: Anatomy at the metatarsophalangeal joint of the great toe. *Foot Ankle* 1984;4:229-240.

14. Jahss MH: Hallux valgus: Further considerations: The first metatarsal head. *Foot Ankle* 1981;2:1-4.

15. Scranton PE Jr, Rutkowski R: Anatomic variations in the first ray: Part II. Disorders of the sesamoids. *Clin Orthop Relat Res* 1980;151:256-264.

16. Saltzman CL, Aper RL, Brown TD: Anatomic determinants of first metatarsophalangeal flexion moments in hallux valgus. *Clin Orthop Relat Res* 1997;339:261-269.

17. Coughlin MJ, Jones CP, Viladot R, et al: Hallux valgus and first ray mobility: A cadaveric study. *Foot Ankle Int* 2004;25:537-544.

18. Kummer FJ: Mathematical analysis of first metatarsal osteotomies. *Foot Ankle* 1989;9:281-289.

19. Jahss MH, Troy AI, Kummer F: Roentgenographic and mathematical analysis of first metatarsal osteotomies for metatarsus primus varus: A comparative study. *Foot Ankle* 1985;5: 280-321.

20. Kummer F, Jahss M: Mathematical analysis of foot and ankle osteotomies, in Jahss M (ed): *Disorders of the Foot and Ankle: Medical and Surgical Management.* Philadelphia, PA, WB Saunders, 1991, pp 541-563.

21. Nyska M, Trnka HJ, Parks BG, Myerson MS: Proximal metatarsal osteotomies: A comparative geometric analysis conducted on sawbone models. *Foot Ankle Int* 2002;23:938-945.

22. Lian GJ, Markolf K, Cracchiolo A III: Strength of fixation constructs for basilar osteotomies of the first metatarsal. *Foot Ankle* 1992;13:509-514.

23. Shereff MJ, Sobel MA, Kummer FJ: The stability of fixation of first metatarsal osteotomies. *Foot Ankle* 1991;11: 208-211.

24. Rosenberg GA, Donley BG: Plate augmentation of screw fixation of proximal crescentic osteotomy of the first metatarsal. *Foot Ankle Int* 2003;24: 570-571.

25. Campbell JT, Schon LC, Parks BG, Wang Y, Berger BI: Mechanical comparison of biplanar proximal closing wedge osteotomy with plantar plate fixation versus crescentic osteotomy with screw fixation for the correction of metatarsus primus varus. *Foot Ankle Int* 1998;19:293-299.

26. Mann RA, Rudicel S, Graves SC: Repair of hallux valgus with a distal soft-tissue procedure and proximal metatarsal osteotomy: A long-term follow-up. *J Bone Joint Surg Am* 1992;74: 124-129.

27. Mann RA: Distal soft tissue procedure and proximal metatarsal osteotomy for correction of hallux valgus deformity. *Orthopedics* 1990;13: 1013-1018.

28. Mann RA: Hallux valgus. *Instr Course Lect* 1986;35:339-353.

29. Jones C, Coughlin M, Villadot R, Golanó P: Proximal crescentic metatarsal osteotomy: The effect of saw blade orientation on first ray elevation. *Foot Ankle Int* 2005;26:152-157.

30. Jung HG, Guyton GP, Parks BG, et al: Supplementary axial kirschner wire fixation for crescentic and Ludloff proximal metatarsal osteotomies: A biomechanical study. *Foot Ankle Int* 2005;26:620-626.

31. Acevedo JI, Sammarco VJ, Boucher HR, Parks BG, Schon LC, Myerson MS: Mechanical comparison of cyclic loading in five different first metatarsal shaft osteotomies. *Foot Ankle Int* 2002;23:711-716.

32. Trnka HJ, Parks BG, Ivanic G, et al: Six first metatarsal shaft osteotomies: Mechanical and immobilization comparisons. *Clin Orthop Relat Res* 2000; 381:256-265.

33. McCluskey LC, Johnson JE, Wynarsky GT, Harris GF: Comparison of stability of proximal crescentic metatarsal osteotomy and proximal horizontal "V" osteotomy. *Foot Ankle Int* 1994;15:263-270.

34. Earll M, Wayne J, Caldwell P, Adelaar R: Comparison of two proximal osteotomies for the treatment of hallux valgus. *Foot Ankle Int* 1998;19: 425-429.

35. Jones C, Coughlin M, Petersen W, Herbot M, Paletta J: Mechanical comparison of two types of fixation for proximal first metatarsal crescentic osteotomy. *Foot Ankle Int* 2005;26: 371-374.

36. Brodsky JW, Beischer AD, Robinson AH, Westra S, Negrine JP, Shabat S: Surgery for hallux valgus with proximal crescentic osteotomy causes variable postoperative pressure patterns. *Clin Orthop Relat Res* 2006;443: 280-286.

37. Markbreiter LA, Thompson FM: Proximal metatarsal osteotomy in hallux valgus correction: A comparison of Crescentic and Chevron procedures. *Foot Ankle Int* 1997;18:71-76.

38. Okuda R, Kinoshita M, Morikawa J, Jotoku T, Abe M: Distal soft tissue procedure and proximal metatarsal osteotomy in hallux valgus. *Clin Orthop Relat Res* 2000;379:209-217.

39. Okuda R, Kinoshita M, Morikawa J, Yasuda T, Abe M: Proximal metatarsal osteotomy: Relation between 1- to greater than 3-years results. *Clin Orthop Relat Res* 2005;435:191-196.

40. Austin DW, Leventen EO: A new osteotomy for hallux valgus: A horizontally directed "V" displacement osteotomy of the metatarsal head for hallux valgus and primus varus. *Clin Orthop Relat Res* 1981;157:25-30.

41. Sammarco GJ, Brainard BJ, Sammarco VJ: Bunion correction using proximal Chevron osteotomy. *Foot Ankle* 1993;14:8-14.

42. Sammarco GJ, Conti SF: Proximal Chevron metatarsal osteotomy: Single incision technique. *Foot Ankle* 1993;14:44-47.

43. Sammarco GJ, Russo-Alesi FG: Bunion correction using proximal chevron osteotomy: A single-incision technique. *Foot Ankle Int* 1998;19: 430-437.

44. Zygmunt KH, Gudas CJ, Laros GS: Z-bunionectomy with internal screw fixation. *J Am Podiatr Med Assoc* 1989; 79:322-329.

45. Barouk LS: Scarf osteotomy for hallux valgus correction: Local anatomy, surgical technique, and combination with other forefoot procedures. *Foot Ankle Clin* 2000;5:525-558.

46. Weil LS: Scarf osteotomy for correction of hallux valgus: Historical perspective, surgical technique, and results. *Foot Ankle Clin* 2000;5:559-580.

47. Coetzee JC: Scarf osteotomy for hallux valgus repair: The dark side. *Foot Ankle Int* 2003;24:29-33.

48. Miller JM, Stuck R, Sartori M, Patwardhan A, Cane R, Vrbos L: The inverted Z bunionectomy: Quantitative analysis of the scarf and inverted scarf bunionectomy osteotomies in fresh cadaveric matched pair specimens. *J Foot Ankle Surg* 1994;33:455-462.

49. Aminian A, Kelikian A, Moen T: Scarf osteotomy for hallux valgus deformity: An intermediate followup of clinical and radiographic outcomes. *Foot Ankle Int* 2006;27:883-886.

50. Jones S, Al Hussainy HA, Ali F, Betts RP, Flowers MJ: Scarf osteotomy for hallux valgus: A prospective clinical and pedobarographic study. *J Bone Joint Surg Br* 2004;86:830-836.

51. Crevoisier X, Mouhsine E, Ortolano V, Udin B, Dutoit M: The scarf osteotomy for the treatment of hallux valgus deformity: A review of 84 cases. *Foot Ankle Int* 2001;22:970-976.

52. Nyska M, Trnka HJ, Parks BG, Myerson MS: The Ludloff metatarsal osteotomy: Guidelines for optimal correction based on a geometric analysis conducted on a sawbone model. *Foot Ankle Int* 2003;24:34-39.

53. Beischer AD, Ammon P, Corniou A, Myerson M: Three-dimensional computer analysis of the modified Ludloff osteotomy. *Foot Ankle Int* 2005;26:627-632.

54. Chiodo CP, Schon LC, Myerson MS: Clinical results with the Ludloff osteotomy for correction of adult hallux valgus. *Foot Ankle Int* 2004;25: 532-536.

55. Schon LC, Dom KJ, Jung HG: Clinical tip: Stabilization of the proximal Ludloff osteotomy. *Foot Ankle Int* 2005;26:579-581.

56. Bae SY, Schon LC: Surgical strategies: Ludloff first metatarsal osteotomy. *Foot Ankle Int* 2007;28:137-144.

57. Stamatis ED, Navid DO, Parks BG, Myerson MS: Strength of fixation of Ludloff metatarsal osteotomy utilizing three different types of Kirschner wires: A biomechanical study. *Foot Ankle Int* 2003;24:805-811.

58. Petroutsas J, Trnka HJ: The Ludloff osteotomy for correction of hallux valgus. *Oper Orthop Traumatol* 2005; 17:102-117.

59. Mau C, Lauber HJ: Die operative behandlung des hallux valgus. *Deutsche Zeit Orthop* 1926;197:361-377.

60. Neese DJ, Zelichowski JE, Patton GW: Mau osteotomy: An alternative procedure to the closing abductory base wedge osteotomy. *J Foot Surg* 1989;28:352-362.

61. Sammarco VJ: Surgical strategies: Mau osteotomy for correction of moderate and severe hallux valgus deformity. *Foot Ankle Int* 2007;28: 857-864.

62. Coughlin MJ, Grebing BR, Jones CP: Arthrodesis of the first metatarsophalangeal joint for idiopathic hallux valgus: Intermediate results. *Foot Ankle Int* 2005;26:783-792.

63. Riggs SA Jr, Johnson EW Jr: McKeever arthrodesis for the painful hallux. *Foot Ankle* 1983;3:248-253.

64. Tourné Y, Saragaglia D, Zattara A, et al: Hallux valgus in the elderly: Metatarsophalangeal arthrodesis of the first ray. *Foot Ankle Int* 1997;18: 195-198.

65. Mann RA, Thompson FM: Arthrodesis of the first metatarsophalangeal joint for hallux valgus in rheumatoid arthritis: 1984. *Foot Ankle Int* 1997;18: 65-67.

66. Lipscomb PR: Arthrodesis of the first metatarsophalangeal joint for severe bunions and hallux rigidus. *Clin Orthop Relat Res* 1979;142:48-54.

67. Grimes JS, Coughlin MJ: First metatarsophalangeal joint arthrodesis as a treatment for failed hallux valgus surgery. *Foot Ankle Int* 2006;27:887-893.

68. Kitaoka HB, Patzer GL: Salvage treatment of failed hallux valgus operations with proximal first metatarsal osteotomy and distal soft-tissue reconstruction. *Foot Ankle Int* 1998;19: 127-131.

69. Myerson MS, Miller SD, Henderson MR, Saxby T: Staged arthrodesis for salvage of the septic hallux metatarsophalangeal joint. *Clin Orthop Relat Res* 1994;307:174-181.

70. Cronin JJ, Limbers JP, Kutty S, Stephens MM: Intermetatarsal angle after first metatarsophalangeal joint arthrodesis for hallux valgus. *Foot Ankle Int* 2006;27:104-109.

71. Curtis MJ, Myerson M, Jinnah RH, Cox QG, Alexander I: Arthrodesis of the first metatarsophalangeal joint: A biomechanical study of internal fixation techniques. *Foot Ankle* 1993;14: 395-399.

72. Politi J, John H, Njus G, Bennett GL, Kay DB: First metatarsal-phalangeal joint arthrodesis: A biomechanical assessment of stability. *Foot Ankle Int* 2003;24:332-337.

73. Neufeld SK, Parks BG, Naseef GS, Melamed EA, Schon LC: Arthrodesis of the first metatarsophalangeal joint: A biomechanical study comparing memory compression staples, cannulated screws, and a dorsal plate. *Foot Ankle Int* 2002;23:97-101.

74. Molloy S, Burkhart BG, Jasper LE, Solan MC, Campbell JT, Belkoff SM: Biomechanical comparison of two fixation methods for first metatarsophalangeal joint arthrodesis. *Foot Ankle Int* 2003;24:169-171.

75. Rongstad KM, Miller GJ, Vander Griend RA, Cowin D: A biomechanical comparison of four fixation methods of first metatarsophalangeal joint arthrodesis. *Foot Ankle Int* 1994;15: 415-419.

76. Myerson MS (ed): Foot and ankle disorders, in *Arthrodesis of the Midfoot and Forefoot Joints*. Philadelphia, PA, WB Saunders, 2000, pp 972-998.

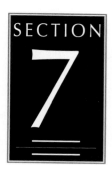

# SECTION
# 7

# Spine

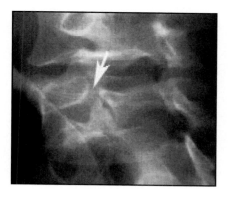

# Spondylolisthesis and Spondylolysis

*Serena S. Hu, MD
*Clifford B. Tribus, MD
Mohammad Diab, MD
*Alexander J. Ghanayem, MD

## Abstract

*Spondylolisthesis is a common condition that can be managed both nonsurgically and surgically. More than 80% of children treated nonsurgically have resolution of symptoms. For those patients requiring surgical treatment, fusion in situ may provide adequate treatment for young patients. Patients with neural compression may require decompression to relieve symptoms, and fusion is also usually indicated. High-grade and degenerative spondylolisthesis require care that is unique to those conditions.*

*Spondylolysis is a defect in the pars interarticularis that occurs in approximately 5% of the general population. Approximately 15% of individuals with a pars interarticularis lesion have progression to spondylolisthesis.*

**Instr Course Lect 2008;57:431-445.**

The term spondylolisthesis refers to slipping, or olisthesis, of a vertebra (spondylos in Greek) relative to an adjacent vertebra. The term spondylolysis refers to dissolution of, or a defect in, the pars interarticularis of a vertebra. To these original terms has been added spondyloptosis, from the Greek "ptosis" (falling off or down) to indicate a vertebra that is completely or essentially completely dislocated.

There are five types of spondylolisthesis: dysplastic, isthmic, degenerative, traumatic, and pathologic.[1] In the dysplastic type, facet joints allow anterior translation of one vertebra on another. Because the neural arch of the olisthetic vertebra is intact, it can compress the cauda equina as it translates. This type accounts for the only reported case of spondylolisthesis at birth.[2] "Isthmic" is from the Greek, meaning "narrow." The isthmic type involves a lesion of the pars interarticularis (the narrow part of bone between the superior and inferior articular processes) (Figure 1). There are three subclasses: type A, which is caused by a stress fracture of the pars interarticularis; type B, an elongation of the pars interarticularis; and type C, which is caused by an acute fracture of the pars interarticularis. Dysplastic and isthmic are the two subtypes found in children, with the latter accounting for approximately 85% of cases.

Degenerative spondylolisthesis is secondary to osteoarthritis leading to facet incompetence and disk degeneration. This condition allows anterior translation of one vertebra on another. Traumatic spondylolisthesis is caused by a fracture of the posterior elements, other than the pars interarticularis, leading to instability and olisthesis. A pathologic spondylolisthesis is caused by a tumor or another primary disease of bone affecting the pars interarticularis or the facet joints and leads to instability and olisthesis.

The dysplastic and isthmic patterns can be classified as congenital, whereas the degenerative, traumatic, and pathologic patterns are considered acquired.[3] The dysplastic type is considered to be high if L5 is abnormal and low if L5 is normal. The low types are higher-grade deformities, with domed-shaped S1 end plates and a trapezoidal L5 vertebral body. The severity of spondylolisthesis is graded on the basis of the percentage of translation of one vertebra relative to the caudal vertebra.[4] Grade I is translation of up to 25%; grade II, 26% to 50%; grade III, 51% to 75%; grade IV, 76% to 100%; and grade V, more than 100% (spondyloptosis). Most cases of spondylolis-

*Serena S. Hu, MD or the department with which she is affiliated has received research or institutional support from Medtronic and DePuy. Clifford B. Tribus, MD or the department with which he is affiliated has received research or institutional support from Medtronic and St. Francis; miscellaneous nonincome support, commercially-derived honoraria, or other nonresearch-related funding from Medtronic, Stryker, St. Francis, and Kyphon; royalties from Stryker; holds stock or stock options in St. Francis; and is a consultant or employee for Kyphon and Stryker. Alexander J. Ghanayem, MD or the department with which he is affiliated has received research or institutional support from DePuy, Synthes, and Medtronic.

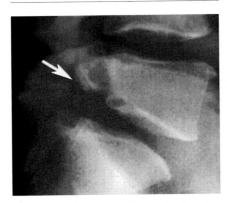

**Figure 1** Lateral radiograph showing isthmic spondylolisthesis. The arrow points to the pars interarticularis defect.

thesis (75%) are grade I, and 20% are grade II. A simpler classification system divides spondylolisthesis into cases with translation of 50% or less (stable) and those with translation of more than 50% (unstable).[5]

## Pathophysiology

When the lumbar spine extends, the inferior articular process of the cranial vertebra impacts the pars interarticularis of the caudal vertebra.[6,7] Repeated impacts can produce a stress or fatigue fracture of the pars interarticularis. Lumbar hyperextension activities, such as gymnastics and American football, and lumbar hyperextension secondary to spinal deformity, such as Scheuermann disease, are associated with spondylolysis, findings that support the traumatic mechanism.[8-10] This mechanism is consistent with the observation that spondylolysis never has been reported in individuals who cannot walk and the fact that up to 40% of athletes with spondylolysis recall a specific back injury.[11,12] This direct compression by means of a "nutcracker" mechanism is one explanation, but another is that the pars interarticularis fails in tension through a traction mechanism.[13,14]

Which of the two mechanisms is more likely to be present in a given individual is believed to be determined by the lordosis of the spine and the lumbosacral relationship. More recently, reviews of surgical and radiographic findings in patients with high-grade spondylolisthesis as well as biomechanical studies have suggested that abnormalities of the sacral growth plate may be an etiology of high-grade slippage. Yue and associates[15] found that the only constant abnormal anatomic feature in 27 patients treated for spondyloptosis was rounding of the proximal sacral end plate. Biomechanical studies of immature calf spines placed under shear loads showed the growth plate to be the site of failure in all patients.[16] These studies have raised the question of which of these abnormalities, the pars interarticularis defect or the sacral growth plate, is the primary cause of spondylolysis and spondylolisthesis.

## Genetics

Family history, gender, and race all are implicated. Spondylolysis occurs in 15% to 70% of first-degree relatives of individuals with the disorder.[17-19] Lysis is two to three times more frequent in boys than girls, but slippage affects girls two to three times more often than boys.[20] The prevalence of spondylolysis is approximately 6% in the white population, a rate that is two to three times higher than that in the black population.[21,22] In the Inuit population, the rate is as high as 25%.[23]

## Natural History

The prevalence of a defect in the pars interarticularis is approximately 5% in the general population. Fredrickson and associates[22] started a prospective study of 500 first-grade

children in 1955. The prevalence of spondylolysis was 4.4% at 6 years of age and 6% in adulthood. It was twice as common in males. Pain was not associated with the development of the pars interarticularis defect. Approximately 15% of individuals with a pars interarticularis lesion had progression to a spondylolisthesis. The slip was seen predominantly during the growth spurt, with minimal change after age 16 years. Progression to a slip did not cause pain. After these individuals had been followed for 45 years, 30 had a pars interarticularis defect (22 of the 30 individuals had final lumbar radiographs).[24] No slip was greater than 40%. Slip progression also appeared to slow with each decade and, of particular note, the results from a back pain questionnaire and a Medical Outcomes Study 36-Item Short Form survey were no different from those for an age-matched general population control group.

Patients with low dysplastic spondylolisthesis have a lower prevalence of progression than those with high dysplastic spondylolisthesis. Patients with higher grades of spondylolisthesis and higher slip angles, a measure of lumbosacral kyphosis, have a higher risk of progression.[25-27] Low-grade isthmic spondylolisthesis can progress in an adult, but the progression is believed to be secondary to progressive degeneration of the L5-S1 intervertebral disk.[28]

## Clinical Presentation

In most children with back pain (75%), the cause is idiopathic or so-called overuse.[29,30] The most common identifiable cause of back pain in a child is spondylolysis. The child typically describes a history of activity-related pain, and 40% recall a specific traumatic event.[12]

The child may have lumbar hyperlordosis, which may be the cause of the spondylolysis, or lumbar flattening if he or she has severe pain or a high-grade spondylolisthesis. A high-grade spondylolysis in a child is characterized by a palpable lumbosacral step-off as well as lumbosacral kyphosis with a retroverted sacrum that results in a heart-shaped buttocks. Hyperextension of the lumbar spine may cause pain, particularly during single-limb stance. Hamstring contracture is common, although its mechanism is unknown, but it resolves with spinal fusion. In severe cases, the child has a gait disturbance characterized by crouching, a short stride length, and an incomplete swing phase, as described by Phalen and Dickson.[31]

The child may have a radiculopathy that manifests as changes in sensation, a motor deficit, or tension signs distinct from the hamstring contracture. When a child has high-grade olisthesis (translation of > 50%), a rectal examination should be performed. An abnormal finding suggests compromise of the sacral roots. The importance of this finding is highlighted by reports of cauda equina syndrome after surgery, presumably caused by the loss of reflex protection under anesthesia, which makes the patient more vulnerable to nerve root injury.[32-34]

Scoliosis may be associated with spondylolysis.[35] When the scoliosis is caused by pain, the scoliosis usually resolves spontaneously following successful treatment of the spondylolysis.

When an adult with low-grade isthmic spondylolisthesis seeks medical attention, pain, usually lower limb pain, is invariably the chief symptom.[36] It is important to correlate the pain pattern with the findings of the diagnostic work up, because adults may have other spinal disease that is causing the pain.

## Imaging
### Radiography
Collimated lateral and angled (according to the inclination of the L5-S1 intervertebral disk) AP radiographs of the lumbosacral spine reduce parallax and provide the best detail.[27,28,31] Oblique lumbar views highlight the "Scotty dog," the ear of which is the superior articular process, the eye is the pedicle, the nose is the transverse process, the neck is the pars interarticularis, and the front limb is the inferior articular process. Spondylolysis is seen as a broken neck or a collar (Figure 2). Full-length radiographs of the spine are essential to determine spinal balance, especially in the sagittal plane, and to evaluate for associated deformity. Flexion and extension lateral radiographs help to determine how much postural reduction of the lumbosacral angulation and translation can be obtained.

The degree of slip, slip angle, sacral inclination, chronicity of the slip, and pelvic incidence are all seen on the lateral radiograph.[13,14,37-39] The degree of slip is the percentage of displacement, with a slip of more than 50% considered unstable and associated with progression and lumbosacral kyphosis. The slip angle is the angle between a perpendicular drawn along the posterior aspect of the sacrum and a line drawn along the inferior end plate of L5, and a positive value is defined as lumbosacral lordosis. The sacral inclination is the angle between the posterior aspect of the sacrum and the vertical, and a value of more than 60° is associated with progression. The chronicity of the slip is reflected by blunting of the osseous

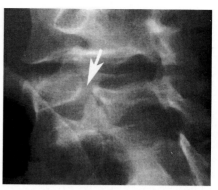

**Figure 2** An oblique radiograph showing a "collar" (*arrow*), or "broken neck," of the "Scotty dog." The nose of the Scotty dog is the transverse process, the eye is the pedicle, the neck is the pars interarticularis, the ear is the superior articular facet, the front leg is the inferior articular facet, and the body is the lamina.

margins; a trapezoidal L5 and a domed shape or rounding of the superior end plate of S1 indicates long-standing alterations. The pelvic incidence is the angle between a line drawn between the center of the femoral head to the midpoint of the sacral end plate and a line perpendicular to the center of the sacral end plate; it is increased in patients with spondylolisthesis, and it correlates with the slip angle.[13,14] There is controversy about the relevance of this measurement.[40-42]

### Single-Photon Emission CT
Tomography of a scintigram enables localization of the signal to the posterior vertebral elements, specifically the pars interarticularis.[43] In addition to facilitating a diagnosis, the study may aid in the treatment of spondylolysis. Increased signal intensity suggests osseous activity and healing potential, whereas absence of an increased signal suggests a nonunion and diminished healing potential.[44]

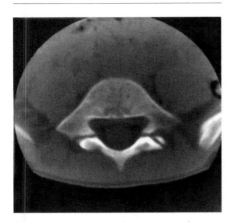

**Figure 3** CT scan showing a right pars interarticularis defect.

### Computed Tomography

CT scans may play several roles.[45-47] When the pars interarticularis appears normal on the CT scan but there is increased activity on the single-photon emission CT scan, a stress response, or "prelysis" defect, is the diagnosis. This is akin to the "preslip" condition in slipped capital femoral epiphysis. Prelysis may be evaluated further with MRI. On the other hand, when the pars interarticularis is seen to have a defect on the CT scan and there is no increased activity on the single-photon emission CT scan, the patient probably has a nonunion with little healing potential. CT scans are also excellent for the follow-up evaluation of healing, to rule out another lesion (such as osteoid osteoma) when there is an atypical presentation, and for surgical planning in patients with dysplastic vertebrae or associated anomalies (Figure 3).

### Magnetic Resonance Imaging

MRI is useful to evaluate an atypical presentation, including prelysis, when the CT scan shows normal findings.[48] MRI is indicated for patients with high-grade spondylolisthesis and for those with a radiculopathy.[49,50]

### Medical Treatment

Activity modification, including cessation of inciting sports activities, and nonsteroidal anti-inflammatory agents are combined with an exercise regimen aimed principally at the reduction of lumbar lordosis as well as the treatment of hip flexion and hamstring contracture.[51] This is sufficient for a child in whom it alleviates symptoms or reduces them to an acceptable level. The child should be evaluated annually through maturity because of the risk of progression during adolescent growth acceleration.[52]

Physical therapy should be the first line of treatment for adults with symptoms from spondylolisthesis. Hamstring stretching, trunk strengthening, and avoidance of inciting activities are beneficial for adults. Steroid injections, at the nerve root and/or the pars interarticularis, can be both diagnostic and therapeutic in adults.

The key role of spinal orthotics in the treatment of spondylolysis is reduction of the lumbar lordosis. The orthotic device is typically molded at 15° of flexion of the lumbar spine.[53,54] It is indicated for a child with unacceptable symptoms and for one with positive findings on a single-photon emission CT scan, which suggests healing potential. The typical recommendation is 3 months of full-time wear (more than 20 hours per day) with no sports activities followed by 3 months of full-time wear with sports activities allowed.[55] The patient is evaluated at the conclusion of each phase, principally to confirm that the pain has been alleviated. If the pain persists, surgical intervention should be considered.

### Nonsurgical Management

More than 80% of children treated nonsurgically have resolution of symptoms. There is no consensus in the literature on the healing rate of spondylolysis, but it has been estimated that 75% to 100% of acute lesions heal, all unilateral acute lesions heal, 50% of bilateral acute lesions heal, but no chronic defects heal. There is an intermediate defect, with MRI findings only, that has a variable healing rate.[48] Cephalad lumbar defects heal more often than do L5 lesions. Even with these numbers, most children (≥ 90%) return to their previous levels of activity.[56] This suggests that the stability of a fibrous union can be acceptable.

### Surgical Options

An L5-S1 in situ fusion with an autogenous posterior iliac crest bone graft is the standard of care for patients with a symptomatic L5 spondylolysis.[57-60] Instrumentation is not necessary because the spine is inherently stable. The procedure may be performed through a midline approach or a paraspinous muscle-splitting approach.[61] The former approach has the advantages of familiarity to surgeons and a greater surface area for fusion, whereas the latter approach is associated with less blood loss and preserves the soft-tissue stabilizers. Postoperative protocols vary widely, from no immobilization to the use of a lumbosacral orthotic with unilateral hip immobilization. We are not aware of any data supporting the efficacy of one bracing protocol over another, but we prefer to use at least a lightweight rigid brace for most patients, with a greater degree of immobilization for younger patients who have a greater slip and a lesser degree of immobilization for older adolescents or young adults with a lesser degree of slip.

A repair of the pars interarticularis is recommended for adolescents and young adults with L4 or

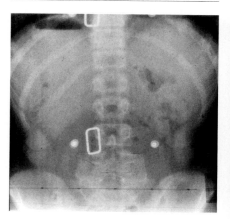

**Figure 4** AP plain radiograph made after a bilateral lateral fusion to treat a spondylolysis between L5 and L6.

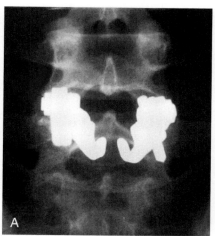
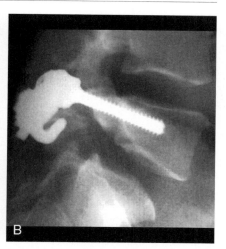

**Figure 5** AP (**A**) and lateral (**B**) radiographs made following internal fixation of a pars interarticularis defect.

more cephalad spondylolysis and a normal intervertebral disk. The transverse process, which may serve as an anchor site or a site for fusion, is sufficiently large compared with a relatively small L5 transverse process (Figure 4). In addition, loss of motion from a fusion cephalad to L4 is more relevant clinically than a loss between L5 and S1. Instrumentation techniques include placement of a screw across the lytic defect in the pars interarticularis, placement of a wire between the transverse process and the spinous process, or attachment of a pedicle screw to the spinous process with a rod and hook or a wire[62-68] (Figure 5).

Kakiuchi[66] reported on 16 patients treated with bilateral L5 transpedicular fixation with rod and sublaminar hook fixation. Preoperatively, the patients had persistent pain and a positive response to lidocaine infiltrated into the pars interarticularis defect. Thirteen patients reported having no back pain after healing, and the other three had only occasional back pain without limitations in their activity.

In adults with a potentially reparable pars interarticularis defect, it is important to establish that the defect

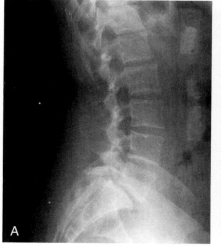
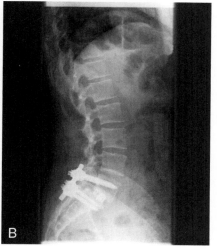

**Figure 6** An adult with severe lower limb pain secondary to spondylolisthesis and a herniated disk at L5-S1. **A,** Preoperative lateral radiograph. **B,** Postoperative lateral radiograph made after posterior spinal fusion with transforaminal interbody fusion performed because removal of the herniated disk had increased the instability of the spine.

is the source of pain.[69] Pain relief after a lidocaine injection at the pars interarticularis supports the concept that the defect is the cause of the pain. When the L5-S1 intervertebral disk appears normal on an MRI scan and there is minimal dynamic instability, a pars interarticularis repair can be considered. The most common technique is excision of the nonunion site, placement of a pedicle screw, bone grafting, placement of a sublaminar hook with connection of each hook by means of a rod to the ipsilateral pedicle screw (Figure 6).

Surgical decompression is indicated when the patient has neural

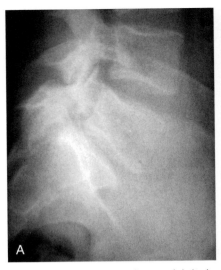
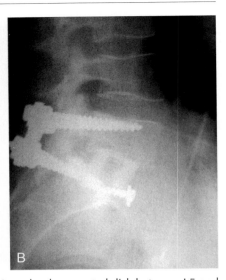

**Figure 7**    A patient with spondylolisthesis and a degenerated disk between L5 and S1. **A,** Preoperative lateral radiograph. **B,** Postoperative radiograph. Stability has been obtained with posterior instrumentation, and the disk height has been restored with a bone graft placed from an anterior approach.

compromise, with a radiculopathy or bowel or bladder dysfunction.[34,70,71] Decompression must be wide and bilateral with removal of the loose lamina (a Gill procedure) and a foraminotomy, possibly including a facetectomy. Decompression increases the rate of pseudarthrosis and increases instability, which can result in progression of deformity if instrumentation is not used.[72] In the literature, there is both support for and advice against concomitant decompression and fusion for patients with spondylolisthesis.[70-76] Decompression with instrumentation at the time of fusion if there is any lower-limb pain or neural compression.

Carragee[72] enrolled 46 adults with symptomatic low-grade isthmic spondylolisthesis into a randomized prospective study to evaluate the effect of decompression. All smokers were treated with transpedicular instrumentation, whereas the nonsmokers had no instrumentation. Patients were randomized with regard to whether or not they underwent a formal decompression. Only one of the 24 patients without decompression had an unsatisfactory result. Obtaining fusion was more important than the decompression, and use of instrumentation was found to improve the fusion rate.

### Instrumentation

The use of instrumentation in the treatment of low-grade isthmic spondylolisthesis in adults increased with the widespread use of pedicle screws and the belief that a fusion is necessary to obtain a good result. Transpedicular fixation increases the rate of fusion, and there is a positive correlation between successful fusion and clinical outcome.[77-83] On the other hand, it was found that instrumentation offered no advantage when a comparison was made between patients treated with in situ fusion with transpedicular fixation and those treated with in situ fusion without transpedicular fixation.[84,85] Furthermore, the patients who were treated with instrumentation had greater blood loss and a longer surgical time.[84,85] Therefore, an in situ arthrodesis without instrumentation remains a reasonable option, particularly in patients with osteoporotic bone. Despite this, and because of better fusion rates and at least a suggestion of better outcomes with a solid fusion, we recommend instrumentation with transpedicular fixation, especially when a decompression is done.

### Interbody Fusion

There are several theoretic advantages to adding anterior column support to the standard posterolateral fusion. These include providing a larger surface area for bone graft incorporation, placing the bone graft under compression, obtaining an indirect reduction of foraminal stenosis by using the graft to restore the height of the intervertebral disk, improving lumbar lordosis, and ablating the degenerated disk (a potential source of pain) (Figure 7). The interbody device or bone graft may be placed through a transforaminal lumbar interbody fusion approach or a posterolateral approach. The disadvantages of performing the interbody fusion through a posterolateral approach are the additional surgical time compared with that needed for posterior-only surgery and the risk of injury to the neural elements with the retraction required for disk excision and placement of the interbody device.[86-90]

The interbody fusion can be done through an anterior approach without a posterior fusion. This is called an anterior lumbar interbody fusion. Proponents of this approach prefer it because it provides the same treatment advantages of the interbody fusion while avoiding disruption of the posterior paraspinal muscles and the exposure of the neural elements.[91-93] An anterior-only interbody fusion in a patient with spondylolisthesis must achieve inherent stability or it will displace. One of the authors (CBT) had encouraging results in a small group of patients after using an anterior plate and an interbody component to fuse the site of an isthmic spondylolisthesis with an anterior-only approach. The anterior approach adds the risk of retrograde ejaculation in males and vascular complications. Aunoble and associates[92] reported successful outcomes of anterior lumbar interbody fusion in a series of 20 patients.

Combining both posterior and anterior approaches in the treatment of low-grade isthmic spondylolisthesis in an adult has both advantages and disadvantages compared with the single approaches. The anterior approach allows better reduction of the deformity than is possible with the posterior approach, whereas the posterior approach allows a direct decompression of compressed nerve roots, and transpedicular fixation increases the rigidity of the construct. The combined approach addresses the pars interarticularis defect, foraminal stenosis, degenerative disk disease, a "loose lamina," and dynamic instability. The disadvantage is that this technique requires two separate procedures, with increased surgical time and morbidity. In a prospective study, patients who had undergone the combined approach had better outcome measures in all categories at 6 and 12 months postoperatively compared with patients treated with posterior fusion only.[94] The differences were less pronounced at 2 years.

The treatment approach for a high-grade spondylolisthesis should differ from that for a low-grade spondylolisthesis (Figure 8). The management of patients with more than 50% slippage (grade III or higher) or lumbosacral kyphosis is more complex. High-grade spondylolisthesis can be associated with dysplastic L5-S1 facets without a pars interarticularis defect and therefore is more likely to cause severe stenosis. With the displacement of the vertebral body, the posterior lamina is pulled forward rather than remaining posteriorly (separated from the vertebral body), as occurs if there is a pars interarticularis defect. Although the preferred surgical treatment is fusion in situ, that procedure is associated with a higher rate of slip progression, pseudarthrosis, neurologic injury, and, if instrumentation is used, failure of the hardware even in young patients.[95-98]

Even without reduction, management of a high-grade spondylolisthesis presents risks.[32,34] The management of an adult with a high-grade spondylolisthesis should start with nonsurgical methods that include physical therapy and epidural steroids. A child with a high-grade spondylolisthesis or an adult who does not respond to nonsurgical care should have surgical stabilization. An in situ fusion can be successful in many young patients. Because these patients often have a dysplastic L5 transverse process and an L5-S1 fusion would place the fusion bed under tension, inclusion of L4 is generally required to achieve a successful fusion. A paramedian Wiltse approach is preferred to maintain the integrity of the midline structures. An external brace is usually applied until the fusion site heals. Patients followed over the long term after an in situ fusion generally have good function and pain relief, although the surgery does not affect their appearance.[99,100] Although the hamstring tightness that many of these patients exhibit is suspected to be related to neurologic compression, it usually resolves without decompression when a successful fusion has been achieved. This may take up to 18 months, however, and some authors believe that a subtle gait abnormality persists.[59]

Reduction of high-grade spondylolisthesis has become more common, probably because of the availability of smaller implants, which are needed in these patients, as well as the higher prevalence of unsuccessful fusion in patients with high-grade spondylolisthesis.[100] A patient who is considered for a reduction of a spondylolisthesis should have substantial angulation of L5 over S1 (a slip angle of > 45°, lumbosacral kyphosis, or an inability to stand upright with the head balanced over the pelvis), require a decompression, have demonstrated progression of the slip angle, have demonstrated progression after an attempted fusion, or have an unacceptable clinical appearance. It is important that the patient and his or her family understand and accept the risks associated with a reduction.

Reduction can be done with external cast techniques, particularly in very young patients in whom pedicle screw fixation may not be possible.[101] The reduction is performed after the bone graft is placed and the wound is closed. The patient is placed on a spica table or Stryker frame and should be awake so that he or she can report any neurologic changes. A padded support is placed over the sacrum, and the spine is allowed to extend to reduce the lumbosacral kyphosis. The trunk and at least one thigh are then incorporated into a spica cast. A brace with a thigh extension can be used when early healing is apparent on radiographs, usually at 6 to 12 weeks.

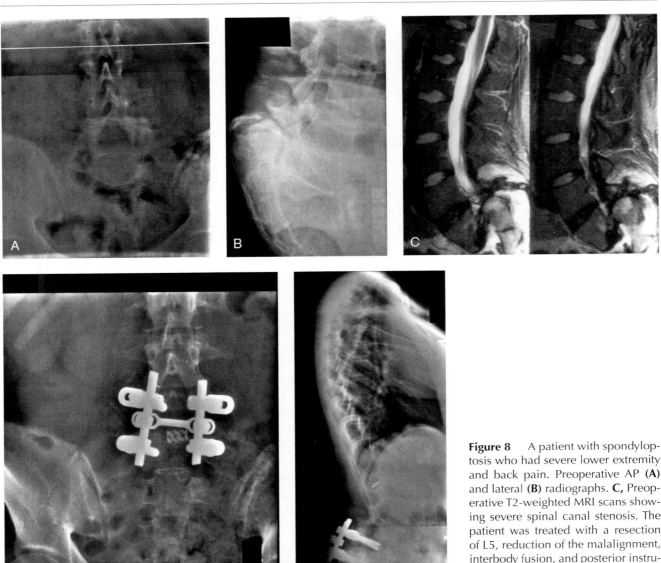

**Figure 8** A patient with spondyloptosis who had severe lower extremity and back pain. Preoperative AP (**A**) and lateral (**B**) radiographs. **C,** Preoperative T2-weighted MRI scans showing severe spinal canal stenosis. The patient was treated with a resection of L5, reduction of the malalignment, interbody fusion, and posterior instrumentation. Postoperative AP (**D**) and lateral (**E**) radiographs.

Open reduction with instrumentation is used for patients who require a decompression or for whom a fusion attempt without instrumentation has failed, with progression of the slip. A wide surgical decompression is performed, with care taken to adequately decompress the nerve roots (usually L5). A temporary distraction rod is applied from L3 to the sacrum, usually with temporary hooks. Pedicle screws are then placed in L4 and L5, and sacral screws are directed to the sacral promontory, where maximal purchase in the sacrum is achieved, or the sacral screws can be drilled through the sacrum into L5. Neurophysiologic monitoring is advised. We have found that it helps to monitor several muscle groups, both motor and sensory, as well as electromyographic activity and sphincter activity. Removal of the L5-S1 disk and/or osteotomy of the sacral dome can be done to improve the reduction. The reduction maneuvers of distraction and translation should be performed slowly. The final millimeters of translation and the final degrees of angular reduction are the most risky, and partial reduction is an option.[102] Care should be taken during the reduction, not only because of the neurologic risk but also because of the risk of pedicle screw pullout. This is particularly true for the caudal fixation. Transsacral screws, iliac screws, and Jackson intrasacral buttress rods have all been used to improve the strength of the caudal fixation with varying degrees of success. Once correction has been achieved, a decision regarding whether to perform an interbody fusion is made. A standard interbody cage filled with bone or a transsacral fibular graft provides additional stability during the posterior approach.[103-105] An alternative surgical option is combined anterior and posterior fusion, with the anterior fusion done first to release the anterior structures and thus make the reduction and placement of the interbody spacer easier.[106,107]

The long-term results of the different treatment options for high-grade spondylolisthesis are relatively good. In one study of 67 children and adolescents, the results of posterolateral, anterior, and circumferential fusion were compared at an average of 17 years postoperatively, and the best clinical outcome, as measured with the Oswestry Disability Index, was found after circumferential fusion.[108] A review of the results of posterolateral decompression and fusion with transsacral placement of a fibular graft in 14 patients demonstrated complete neurologic recovery in patients in whom neurologic deficits had developed after surgery, and incorporation of the fibular graft and achievement of a solid fusion in all but one of the patients.[105] In a similar series, one patient was not satisfied with the cosmetic result and one patient had a nonunion and continued back pain.[109] The results after reduction of high-grade spondylolisthesis are generally good.[103,110-113]

When a patient has complete spondyloptosis, particularly with L5 below the level of the sacral end plate, resection of L5 and reduction of L4 onto the sacrum, through a combined anterior and posterior approach (the Gaines procedure), can be considered.[114] Although this is a spine-shortening procedure and thus intended to be associated with decreased neurologic injury in this particularly high-risk patient group, the rate of neurologic injury was 76% in Gaines' original series;[114] however, only 2 of the 30 patients in that series required lower-extremity bracing at the time of long-term follow-up.[115]

## Degenerative Spondylolisthesis

Unlike isthmic spondylolisthesis, degenerative spondylolisthesis occurs most often (in 85% of patients) at L4-L5. The L3-L4 level is the next most common level (Figure 9), with L5-S1 rarely being involved. Degenerative spondylolisthesis is most common in the sixth decade of life and is more common in females than in males (a ratio of 6:1).

The pathophysiology of this type of spondylolisthesis has been postulated to be a combination of disk and facet joint degeneration. Patients with degenerative spondylolisthesis have more sagittally oriented facet joints than do patients without degenerative spondylolisthesis; however, it is unclear whether the facet orientation is a primary cause or a secondary effect.[116,117] The slip rarely progresses beyond grade I.

Patients usually present with neurogenic claudication or radicular symptoms from the spinal stenosis, and some patients recount a long history of back pain prior to the development of lower extremity symptoms. Evaluation of a patient with degenerative spondylolisthesis is similar to that of any patient with a back condition, with a careful neu-

rologic examination and evaluation of the spine, including the patient's stance and sagittal balance. Vascular insufficiency and peripheral neuropathy need to be considered as alternative causes of the symptoms. Patients whose symptoms do not correspond to the level of the stenosis should have a complete neurologic work-up or electromyographic studies. Patients who do not have palpable peripheral pulses, do not have relief of pain with sitting, or do not need to sit to relieve the claudication are more likely to have vascular insufficiency. Spinal tumors, infection, and nonspinal etiologies also need to be considered. As is the case with isthmic spondylolisthesis, upright radiographs are necessary to determine the degree of degenerative spondylolisthesis.[118] MRI scans are ideal for assessing the severity of spinal canal and foraminal narrowing.

Conservative management may help many patients with symptoms of degenerative spondylolisthesis. Nonsteroidal anti-inflammatory medications, physical therapy, and cardiovascular conditioning, as well as alternative treatments such as acupuncture, may relieve symptoms to the point where surgery is not necessary. Patients with substantial radicular or claudication symptoms often benefit from epidural steroid injections or selective nerve root blocks.

Surgical management is offered when nonsurgical options have not adequately relieved symptoms. Although both nonsurgical and surgical treatment can substantially decrease symptoms, surgery seems to provide faster and greater improvement for patients with severe symptoms and associated severe stenosis.[119] The most common surgical treatment options are a limited decompression (laminoforaminotomy

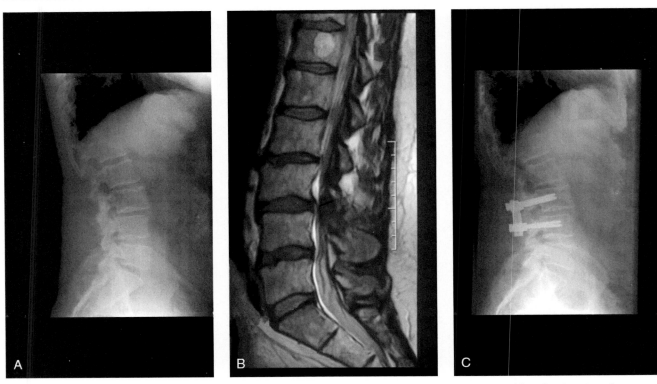

**Figure 9** A patient with degenerative spondylolisthesis at L3-L4 and severe lower extremity and low back pain refractory to conservative treatment. **A,** Preoperative lateral radiograph. **B,** Preoperative T2-weighted sagittal MRI scan showing moderately severe stenosis at L3-L4. **C,** Postoperative lateral radiograph.

or interlaminar decompression), laminectomy, or laminotomy with fusion (with or without instrumentation). The severity of the stenosis and where it is located (foraminal, lateral recess, central, or, most commonly, a combination of these sites) determine the extent of decompression required and, therefore, the likelihood of slip progression without fusion. A limited decompression may be considered for patients who have unilateral disease without evidence of motion on flexion-extension radiographs.[120] At least 50% of the facet joints and the interspinous ligaments need to be preserved during the decompression to maintain inherent stability.

Most patients who undergo surgery should have a laminectomy and fusion. Studies have shown that patients who have a laminectomy and fusion do significantly better than patients who have a laminectomy alone.[121-125] Short-term follow-up did not show an advantage to using instruments with the fusion, which increased the prevalence of complications. However, longer follow-up showed that patients did better if a fusion had been achieved, and fusion was achieved more reliably with internal fixation. Patients with substantial comorbidities or with osteoporosis and/or substantial disk space narrowing may be better treated by fusion without internal fixation. Most symptomatic patients with degenerative spondylolisthesis who are in reasonable health and for whom nonsurgical treatment has failed should have a laminectomy and fusion with instrumentation.

Such an approach has resulted in a high fusion rate and excellent clinical success.[124,126]

To improve the fusion rate and patient outcomes, some surgeons are including interbody fusion in their surgical approach. Posterior-based transforaminal interbody fusion or posterolateral interbody fusion may improve restoration of disk and foraminal height.[127,128] However, to our knowledge there are no published studies that demonstrate improved outcomes with the addition of posterior-based transforaminal interbody fusion or posterolateral interbody fusion to the surgical procedure in patients with degenerative spondylolisthesis.

Currently, motion-preservation and nonfusion devices are receiving tremendous attention in the lay press. While early, preclinical investigational device exemption studies have shown favorable results,[129,130] the use of these devices in patients with degenerative spondylolisthesis has yet to be validated in independent, randomized prospective studies. Because of the selection criteria used in the preclinical studies, only a small number of cases of degenerative spondylolisthesis were included.

## Summary

Spondylolisthesis is a common condition and most patients are successfully treated without surgery. Patients for whom surgery is indicated usually have good outcomes. Young patients may require only a fusion in situ; however, patients who have evidence of neural compression may need a decompression to relieve symptoms, and fusion is usually also indicated in these patients. Additional adjuncts have been proposed to improve outcomes, but there are few randomized, prospective trials to demonstrate superiority of one technique over another.

## References

1. Wiltse LL, Newman PH, MacNab I: Classification of spondylolysis and spondylolisthesis. *Clin Orthop Relat Res* 1976;117:23-29.

2. Borkow SE, Kleiger B: Spondylolisthesis in the newborn. A case report. *Clin Orthop Relat Res* 1971;81:73-76.

3. Marchetti PG, Bartolozzi P: Classification of spondylolisthesis as a guideline for treatment, in Bridwell KH, DeWald RL (eds): *The Textbook of Spinal Surgery*, ed 2. Philadelphia, PA, Lippincott-Raven, 1997, p 1212.

4. Meyerding H: Spondylolisthesis. *Surg Gynecol Obstet* 1932;54:371-377.

5. Taillard WF: Les spondylolisthesis chez l'enfant et l'adolescent. (Etude de 50 cas). *Acta Orthop Scand* 1955;24:115-144.

6. Farfan HF, Osteria V, Lamy C: The mechanical etiology of spondylolysis and spondylolisthesis. *Clin Orthop Relat Res* 1976;117:40-55.

7. Wiltse LL, Widell EH Jr, Jackson DW: Fatigue fracture: The basic lesion in isthmic spondylolisthesis. *J Bone Joint Surg Am* 1975;57:17-22.

8. Ferguson RJ, McMaster JH, Stanitski CL: Low back pain in college football linemen. *J Sports Med* 1974;2:63-69.

9. Jackson DW, Wiltse LL, Cirincoine RJ: Spondylolysis in the female gymnast. *Clin Orthop Relat Res* 1976;117:68-73.

10. Ogilvie JW, Sherman J: Spondylolysis in Scheuermann's disease. *Spine* 1987;12:251-253.

11. Rosenberg NJ, Bargar WL, Friedman B: The incidence of spondylolysis and spondylolisthesis in nonambulatory patients. *Spine* 1981;6:35-38.

12. el Rassi G, Takemitsu M, Woratanarat P, Shah SA: Lumbar spondylolysis in pediatric and adolescent soccer players. *Am J Sports Med* 2005;33:1688-1693.

13. Labelle H, Roussouly P, Berthonnaud E, Dimnet J, O'Brien M: The importance of spino-pelvic balance in L5-S1 developmental spondylolisthesis: A review of pertinent radiologic measurements. *Spine* 2005;30(suppl 6):S27-S34.

14. Labelle H, Roussouly P, Berthonnaud E, et al: Spondylolisthesis, pelvic incidence, and spinopelvic balance: A correlation study. *Spine* 2004;29:2049-2054.

15. Yue WM, Brodner W, Gaines RW: Abnormal spinal anatomy in 27 cases of surgically corrected spondyloptosis: Proximal sacral endplate damage as a possible cause of spondyloptosis. *Spine* 2005;30(6 suppl):S22-S26.

16. Kajiura K, Katoh S, Sairyo K, Ikata T, Goel VK, Murakami RI: Slippage mechanism of pediatric spondylolysis: Biomechanical study using immature calf spines. *Spine* 2001;26:2208-2213.

17. Albanese M, Pizzutillo PD: Family study of spondylolysis and spondylolisthesis. *J Pediatr Orthop* 1982;2:496-499.

18. Friberg S: Studies on spondylolisthesis. *Acta Chir Scand* 1939;(suppl):55.

19. Wynne-Davies R, Scott JH: Inheritance and spondylolisthesis: A radiographic family survey. *J Bone Joint Surg Br* 1979;61:301-305.

20. Roche MB, Rowe GG: The incidence of separate neural arch and coincident bone variations: A summary. *J Bone Joint Surg Am* 1952;34:491-494.

21. Baker DR, McHolick W: Spondyloschisis and spondylolisthesis in children. *J Bone Joint Surg Am* 1956;38:933-934.

22. Fredrickson BE, Baker D, McHollick WJ, Yuan HA, Lubicky JP: The natural history of spondylolysis and spondylolisthesis. *J Bone Joint Surg Am* 1984;66:699-707.

23. Stewart TD: The incidence of neural-arch defects in Alaskan natives, considered from the standpoint of etiology. *J Bone Joint Surg Am* 1953;35:937-950.

24. Beutler WJ, Fredrickson BE, Murtland A, Sweeney CA, Grant WD, Baker D: The natural history of spondylolysis and spondylolisthesis: 45-year follow-up evaluation. *Spine* 2003;28:1027-1035.

25. Frennered AK, Danielson BI, Nachemson AL: Natural history of symptomatic isthmic low-grade spondylolisthesis in children and adolescents: A seven-year follow-up study. *J Pediatr Orthop* 1991;11:209-213.

26. Saraste H: Long-term clinical and radiological follow-up of spondylolysis and spondylolisthesis. *J Pediatr Orthop* 1987;7:631-638.

27. Seitsalo S, Osterman K, Hyvarinen H, Tallroth K, Schlenzka D, Poussa M: Progression of spondylolisthesis in children and adoles-

cents: A long term follow-up of 272 patients. *Spine* 1991;16:417-421.

28. Floman Y: Progression of lumbosacral isthmic spondylolisthesis in adults. *Spine* 2000;25:342-347.

29. Feldman DS, Hedden DM, Wright JG: The use of bone scan to investigate back pain in children and adolescents. *J Pediatr Orthop* 2000;20:790-795.

30. Feldman DS, Straight JJ, Badra MI, Mohaideen A, Madan SS: Evaluation of an algorithmic approach to pediatric back pain. *J Pediatr Orthop* 2006;26:353-357.

31. Phalen GS, Dickson JA: Spondylolisthesis and tight hamstrings. *J Bone Joint Surg Am* 1961;43:505-512.

32. Maurice HD, Morley TR: Cauda equina lesions following fusion in situ and decompressive laminectomy for severe spondylolisthesis: Four case reports. *Spine* 1989;14:214-216.

33. Newman PH: A clinical syndrome associated with severe lumbo-sacral subluxation. *J Bone Joint Surg Br* 1965;47:472-481.

34. Schoenecker PL, Cole HO, Herring JA, Capelli AM, Bradford DS: Cauda equina syndrome after in situ arthrodesis for severe spondylolisthesis at the lumbosacral junction. *J Bone Joint Surg Am* 1990;72:369-377.

35. Seitsalo S, Osterman K, Poussa M: Scoliosis associated with lumbar spondylolisthesis: A clinical survey of 190 young patients. *Spine* 1988;13:899-904.

36. Möller H, Sundin A, Hedlund R: Symptoms, signs, and functional disability in adult spondylolisthesis. *Spine* 2000;25:683-690.

37. Lowe RW, Hayes TD, Kaye J, Bagg RJ, Leukens CA: Standing roentgenograms in spondylolisthesis. *Clin Orthop Relat Res* 1976;117:80-84.

38. Wiltse LL, Guyer RD, Spencer CW, Glenn WV, Porter IS: Alar transverse process impingement of the L5 spinal nerve: The far-out syndrome. *Spine* 1984;9:31-41.

39. Wiltse LL, Winter RB: Terminology and measurement of spondylolisthesis. *J Bone Joint Surg Am* 1983;65:768-772.

40. Legaye J, Duval-Beaupere G, Hecquet J, Marty C: Pelvic incidence: A fundamental pelvic parameter for three-dimensional regulation of spinal sagittal curves. *Eur Spine J* 1998;7:99-103.

41. Mac-Thiong JM, Labelle H: A proposal for a surgical classification of pediatric lumbosacral spondylolisthesis based on current literature. *Eur Spine J* 2006;15:1425-1435.

42. Huang RP, Bohlmann HH, Thompson GH, Poe-Kochert C: Predictive value of pelvic incidence in progression of spondylolisthesis. *Spine* 2003;28:2381-2385.

43. Read MT: Single photon emission computed tomography (SPECT) scanning for adolescent low back pain: A sine qua non? *Br J Sports Med* 1994;28:56-57.

44. van den Oever M, Merrick MV, Scott JHS: Bone scintigraphy in symptomatic spondylolysis. *J Bone Joint Surg Br* 1987;69:453-456.

45. Gregory PL, Batt ME, Kerslake RW, Scammell BE, Webb JF: The value of combining single photon emission computerised tomography and computerised tomography in the investigation of spondylolysis. *Eur Spine J* 2004;13:503-509.

46. Grogan JP, Hemminghytt S, Williams AL, Carrera GF, Haughton VM: Spondylolysis studied with computed tomography. *Radiology* 1982;145:737-742.

47. McAfee PC, Yuan HA: Computed tomography in spondylolisthesis. *Clin Orthop Relat Res* 1982;166:62-71.

48. Sairyo K, Katoh S, Takata Y, et al: MRI signal changes of the pedicle as an indicator for early diagnosis of spondylolysis in children and adolescents: A clinical and biomechanical study. *Spine* 2006;31:206-211.

49. Birch JG, Herring JA, Maravilla KR: Splitting of the intervertebral disc in spondylolisthesis: A magnetic resonance imaging finding in two cases. *J Pediatr Orthop* 1986;6:609-611.

50. Szypryt EP, Twining P, Mulholland RC, Worthington BS: The prevalence of disc degeneration associated with neural arch defects of the lumbar spine assessed by magnetic resonance imaging. *Spine* 1989;14:977-981.

51. Pizzutillo PD, Hummer CD III: Nonoperative treatment for painful adolescent spondylolysis or spondylolisthesis. *J Pediatr Orthop* 1989;9:538-540.

52. Sairyo K, Katoh S, Ikata T, Fujii K, Kajiura K, Goel VK: Development of spondylytic olisthesis in adolescents. *Spine J* 2001;1:171-175.

53. Bell DF, Ehrlich MG, Zaleske DJ: Brace treatment for symptomatic spondylolisthesis. *Clin Orthop Relat Res* 1988;236:192-198.

54. Blanda J, Bethem D, Moats W, Lew M: Defect of pars interarticularis in athletes: A protocol for nonoperative treatment. *J Spinal Disord* 1993;6:406-411.

55. Steiner ME, Micheli LJ: Treatment of symptomatic spondylolysis and spondylolisthesis with the modified Boston brace. *Spine* 1985;10:937-943.

56. Sys J, Michielsen J, Bracke P, Martens M, Verstreken J: Nonoperative treatment of active spondylolysis in elite athletes with normal X-ray findings: Literature review and results of conservative treatment. *Eur Spine J* 2001;10:498-504.

57. Hensinger RN, Lang JR, MacEwen GD: Surgical management of spondylolisthesis in children. *Spine* 1976;1:207-217.

58. Lenke LG, Bridwell KH, Bullis D, Betz RR, Baldus C, Schoenecker PL: Results of in situ fusion for isthmic spondylolisthesis. *J Spinal Disord* 1992;5:433-442.

59. Pizzutillo PD, Mirenda W, MacEwan GD: Posterolateral fusion for spondylolisthesis in adolescence. *J Pediatr Orthop* 1986;6:311-316.

60. Sherman FC, Rosenthal RK, Hall JE: Spine fusion for spondylolysis and

spondylolisthesis in children. *Spine* 1979;4:59-66.

61. Wiltse LL, Jackson DW: Treatment of spondylolisthesis and spondylolysis in children. *Clin Orthop Relat Res* 1976; 117:92-100.

62. Buck JE: Direct repair of the defect in spondylolisthesis: Preliminary report. *J Bone Joint Surg Br* 1970;52:432-437.

63. Buck JE: Further thoughts on direct repair of the defect in spondylolysis. *J Bone Joint Surg Br* 1979;61:123.

64. Bradford DS, Iza J: Repair of the defect in spondylolysis or minimal degrees of spondylolisthesis by segmental wire fixation and bone grafting. *Spine* 1985;10:673-679.

65. Scott JHS: The Edinburgh repair of isthmic (Group II) spondylolysis. *J Bone Joint Surg Br* 1987;69:491.

66. Kakiuchi M: Repair of the defect in spondylolysis: Durable fixation with pedicle screws and laminar hooks. *J Bone Joint Surg Am* 1997;79:818-825.

67. Morscher E, Gerber B, Fasel J: Surgical treatment of spondylolisthesis by bone grafting and direct stabilization of spondylolysis by means of a hook screw. *Arch Orthop Trauma Surg* 1984; 103:175-178.

68. Songer MN, Rovin R: Repair of the pars interarticularis defect with a cable-screw construct: A preliminary report. *Spine* 1998;23:263-269.

69. Suh PB, Esses SI, Kostuik JP: Repair of pars interarticularis defect: The prognostic value of pars infiltration. *Spine* 1991;16(suppl 8):S445-S448.

70. Gill GG: Long-term follow-up evaluation of a few patients with spondylolisthesis treated by excision of the loose lamina with decompression of the nerve roots without spinal fusion. *Clin Orthop Relat Res* 1984;182: 215-219.

71. Gill GG, Manning JG, White HL: Surgical treatment of spondylolisthesis without spine fusion: Excision of the loose lamina with decompression of the nerve roots. *J Bone Joint Surg Am* 1955;37:493-520.

72. Carragee EJ: Single-level posterolateral arthrodesis, with or without posterior decompression, for the treatment of isthmic spondylolisthesis in adults: A prospective, randomized study. *J Bone Joint Surg Am* 1997;79: 1175-1180.

73. Davis IS, Bailey RW: Spondylolisthesis: Long-term follow-up study of treatment with total laminectomy. *Clin Orthop Relat Res* 1972;88:46-49.

74. McGuire RA, Amundson GM: The use of primary internal fixation in spondylolisthesis. *Spine* 1993;18: 1662-1672.

75. Peek RD, Wiltse LL, Reynolds JB, Thomas JC, Guyer DW, Widell EH: In situ arthrodesis without decompression for grade III or IV isthmic spondylolisthesis in adults who have severe sciatica. *J Bone Joint Surg Am* 1989;71:62-68.

76. de Loubresse CG, Bon T, Deburge A, Lassale B, Benoit M: Posterolateral fusion for radicular pain in isthmic spondylolisthesis. *Clin Orthop Relat Res* 1996;323:194-201.

77. Zdeblick TA: A prospective, randomized study of lumbar fusion: Preliminary results. *Spine* 1993;18:983-991.

78. Yuan HA, Garfin SR, Dickman CA, Mardjetko SM: A historical cohort study of pedicle screw fixation in thoracic, lumbar, and sacral spinal fusions. *Spine* 1994;19(20 suppl): 2279S-2296S.

79. Bjarke Christensen F, Stender Hansen E, Laursen M, Thomsen K, Bünger CE: Long-term functional outcome of pedicle screw instrumentation as a support for posterolateral spinal fusion: Randomized clinical study with a 5-year follow-up. *Spine* 2002;27:1269-1277.

80. Deguchi M, Rapoff AJ, Zdeblick TA: Posterolateral fusion for isthmic spondylolisthesis in adults: Analysis of fusion rate and clinical results. *J Spinal Disord* 1998;11:459-464.

81. Ricciardi JE, Pflueger PC, Isaza JE, Whitecloud TS III: Transpedicular fixation for the treatment of isthmic

spondylolisthesis in adults. *Spine* 1995;20:1917-1922.

82. Chang P, Seow KH, Tan SK: Comparison of the results of spinal fusion for spondylolisthesis in patients who are instrumented with patients who are not. *Singapore Med J* 1993;34: 511-514.

83. Bono CM, Lee CK: Critical analysis of trends in fusion for degenerative disc disease over the past 20 years: Influence of technique on fusion rate and clinical outcome. *Spine* 2004;29: 455-463.

84. Möller H, Hedlund R: Surgery versus conservative management in adult isthmic spondylolisthesis: A prospective randomized study. Part 1. *Spine* 2000;25:1711-1715.

85. Möller H, Hedlund R: Instrumented and noninstrumented posterolateral fusion in adult spondylolisthesis: A prospective randomized study. Part 2. *Spine* 2000;25:1716-1721.

86. Dehoux E, Fourati E, Madi K, Reddy B, Segal P: Posterolateral versus interbody fusion in isthmic spondylolisthesis: Functional results in 52 cases with a minimum follow-up of 6 years. *Acta Orthop Belg* 2004;70: 578-582.

87. Harris BM, Hilibrand AS, Savas PE, et al: Transforaminal lumbar interbody fusion: The effect of various instrumentation techniques on the flexibility of the lumbar spine. *Spine* 2004;29:E65-E70.

88. Kwon B, Zaremski J, Kim D, Tromanhauser S, Banco R, Jenis L: Surgical outcomes after treatment of spondylolytic spondylolisthesis: Analysis of three techniques. The Spine Journal Website. Available at: http://www.thespinejournalonline.com/article/PIIS1529943006004396/abstract. Accessed January 2008.

89. Suk SI, Lee CK, Kim WJ, Lee JH, Cho KJ, Kim HG: Adding posterior lumbar interbody fusion to pedicle screw fixation and posterolateral fusion after decompression in spondylolytic spondylolisthesis. *Spine* 1997; 22:210-220.

90. Holly LT, Schwender JD, Rouben DP, Foley KT: Minimally invasive transforaminal lumbar interbody fusion: Indications, technique, and complications. *Neurosurg Focus* 2006;20:E6.

91. Cheng CL, Fang D, Lee PC, Leong JC: Anterior spinal fusion for spondylolysis and isthmic spondylolisthesis: Long term results in adults. *J Bone Joint Surg Br* 1989;71:264-267.

92. Aunoble S, Hoste D, Donkersloot P, Liquois F, Basso Y, Le Huec JC: Video-assisted ALIF with cage and anterior plate fixation for L5-S1 spondylolisthesis. *J Spinal Disord Tech* 2006;19:471-476.

93. Pavlov PW, Spruit M, Havinga M, Anderson PG, van Limbeek J, Jacobs WC: Anterior lumbar interbody fusion with threaded fusion cages and autologous bone grafts. *Eur Spine J* 2000;9:224-229.

94. Swan J, Hurwitz E, Malek F, et al: Surgical treatment for unstable low-grade isthmic spondylolisthesis in adults: A prospective controlled study of posterior instrumented fusion compared with combined anterior-posterior fusion. *Spine J* 2006;6: 606-614.

95. Boxall D, Bradford DS, Winter RB, Moe JH: Management of severe spondylolisthesis in children and adolescents. *J Bone Joint Surg Am* 1979;61: 479-495.

96. Matthiass HH, Heine J: The surgical reduction of spondylolisthesis. *Clin Orthop Relat Res* 1986;203:34-44.

97. Molinari RW, Bridwell KH, Lenke LG, Ungacta FF, Riew KD: Complications in the surgical treatment of pediatric high-grade isthmic dysplastic spondylolisthesis: A comparison of three surgical techniques. *Spine* 1999; 24:1701-1711.

98. Newton PO, Johnston CE II: Analysis and treatment of poor outcomes following in situ arthrodesis in adolescent spondylolisthesis. *J Pediatr Orthop* 1997;17:754-761.

99. Johnson JR, Kirwan EO: The long-term results of fusion in situ for se-vere spondylolisthesis. *J Bone Joint Surg Br* 1983;65:43-46.

100. Seitsalo S, Osterman K, Hyvarinen J, Schlenzka D, Poussa M: Severe spondylolisthesis in children and adolescents: A long-term review of fusion in situ. *J Bone Joint Surg Br* 1990; 72:259-265.

101. Burkus JK, Lonstein JE, Winter RB, Denis F: Long-term evaluation of adolescents treated operatively for spondylolisthesis: A comparison of in situ arthrodesis only with in situ arthrodesis and reduction followed by immobilization in a cast. *J Bone Joint Surg Am* 1992;74:693-704.

102. Petraco DM, Spivak JM, Cappadona JG, Kummer FJ, Neuwirth MG: An anatomic evaluation of L5 nerve stretch in spondylolisthesis reduction. *Spine* 1996;21:1133-1139.

103. Shufflebarger HL, Geck MJ: High-grade isthmic dysplastic spondylolisthesis: Monosegmental surgical treatment. *Spine* 2005;30(6 suppl): S42-S48.

104. Bohlman HH, Cook SS: One-stage decompression and posterolateral and interbody fusion for lumbosacral spondyloptosis through a posterior approach: Report of two cases. *J Bone Joint Surg Am* 1982;64:415-418.

105. Hanson DS, Bridwell KH, Rhee JM, Lenke LG: Dowel fibular strut grafts for high-grade dysplastic isthmic spondylolisthesis. *Spine* 2002;27: 1982-1988.

106. Bradford DS, Boachie-Adjei O: Treatment of severe spondylolisthesis by anterior and posterior reduction and stabilization: A long-term follow-up study. *J Bone Joint Surg Am* 1990;72:1060-1066.

107. Muschik M, Zippel H, Perka C: Surgical management of severe spondylolisthesis in children and adolescents: Anterior fusion in situ versus anterior spondylodesis with posterior transpedicular instrumentation and reduction. *Spine* 1997;22: 2036-2043.

108. Remes V, Lamberg T, Tervahartiala P, et al: Long-term outcome after pos-terolateral, anterior, and circumferential fusion for high-grade isthmic spondylolisthesis in children and adolescents: Magnetic resonance imaging findings after average of 17-year follow-up. *Spine* 2006;31:2491-2499.

109. Roca J, Ubierna MT, Cáceres E, Iborra M: One-stage decompression and posterolateral and interbody fusion for severe spondylolisthesis: An analysis of 14 patients. *Spine* 1999;24: 709-714.

110. Ruf M, Koch H, Melcher RP, Harms J: Anatomic reduction and monosegmental fusion in high-grade developmental spondylolisthesis. *Spine* 2006; 31:269-274.

111. Bartolozzi P, Sandri A, Cassini M, Ricci M: One-stage posterior decompression-stabilization and trans-sacral interbody fusion after partial reduction for severe L5-S1 spondylolisthesis. *Spine* 2003;28: 1135-1141.

112. Fabris DA, Costantini S, Nena U: Surgical treatment of severe L5-S1 spondylolisthesis in children and adolescents: Results of intraoperative reduction, posterior interbody fusion, and segmental pedicle fixation. *Spine* 1996;21:728-733.

113. Smith JA, Deviren V, Berven S, Kleinstueck F, Bradford DS: Clinical outcome of trans-sacral interbody fusion after partial reduction for high-grade L5-S1 spondylolisthesis. *Spine* 2001;26:2227-2234.

114. Gaines RW, Nichols WK: Treatment of spondyloptosis by two stage L5 vertebrectomy and reduction of L4 onto S1. *Spine* 1985;10:680-686.

115. Gaines RW: L5 vertebrectomy for the surgical treatment of spondyloptosis: Thirty cases in 25 years. *Spine* 2005;30 (6 suppl):S66-S70.

116. Boden SD, Riew KD, Yamaguchi K, Branch TP, Schellinger D, Wiesel SW: Orientation of the lumbar facet joints: Association with degenerative disc disease. *J Bone Joint Surg Am* 1996;78:403-411.

117. Love TW, Fagan AB, Fraser RD: Degenerative spondylolisthesis: Devel-

opmental or acquired? *J Bone Joint Surg Br* 1999;81:670-674.

118. Bendo JA, Ong B: Importance of correlating static and dynamic imaging studies in diagnosing degenerative lumbar spondylolisthesis. *Am J Orthop* 2001;30:247-250.

119. Weinstein JN, Lurie JD, Tosteson TD, et al: Surgical versus nonsurgical treatment for lumbar degenerative spondylolisthesis. *N Engl J Med* 2007; 356:2257-2270.

120. Epstein NE: Decompression in the surgical management of degenerative spondylolisthesis: Advantages of a conservative approach in 290 patients. *J Spinal Disord* 1998;11:116-123.

121. Fischgrund JS, Mackay M, Herkowitz HN, Brower R, Montgomery DM, Kurz LT: Degenerative lumbar spondylolisthesis with spinal stenosis: A prospective, randomized study comparing decompressive laminectomy and arthrodesis with and without spinal instrumentation. *Spine* 1997;22:2807-2812.

122. Herkowitz HN, Kurz LT: Degenerative lumbar spondylolisthesis with spinal stenosis: A prospective study comparing decompression with decompression and intertransverse process arthrodesis. *J Bone Joint Surg Am* 1991;73:802-808.

123. Kornblum MB, Fischgrund JS, Herkowitz HN, Abraham DA, Berkower DL, Ditkoff JS: Degenerative lumbar spondylolisthesis with spinal stenosis: A prospective long-term study comparing fusion and pseudarthrosis. *Spine* 2004;29: 726-734.

124. France JC, Yaszemski MJ, Lauerman WC, et al: A randomized prospective study of posterolateral lumbar fusion: Outcomes with and without pedicle screw instrumentation. *Spine* 1999; 24:553-560.

125. Mardjetko SM, Connolly PJ, Shott S: Degenerative lumbar spondylolisthesis: A meta-analysis of literature 1970-1993. *Spine* 1994;19(20 suppl): 2256S-2265S.

126. Nork SE, Hu SS, Workman KL, Glazer PA, Bradford DS: Patient outcomes after decompression and instrumented posterior spinal fusion for degenerative spondylolisthesis. *Spine* 1999;24:561-569.

127. Lauber S, Schulte TL, Liljenqvist U, Halm H, Hackenberg L: Clinical and radiologic 2-4-year results of transforaminal lumbar interbody fusion in degenerative and isthmic spondylolisthesis grades 1 and 2. *Spine* 2006;31: 1693-1698.

128. Potter BK, Freedman BA, Verwiebe EG, Hall JM, Polly DW Jr, Kuklo TR: Transforaminal lumbar interbody fusion: Clinical and radiographic results and complications in 100 consecutive patients. *J Spinal Disord Tech* 2005;18:337-346.

129. Zigler J, Delamarter R, Spivak JM, et al: Results of the prospective, randomized, multicenter Food and Drug Administration investigation device exemption study of the ProDisc-L total disc replacement versus circumferential fusion for the treatment of 1-level desenerative disc disease. *Spine* 2007;32:1155-1163.

130. Kondrashov DG, Hannibal M, Hsu KY, Zucherman JF: Interspinous process decompression with X-STOP device for lumbar spinal stenosis: A 4-year follow-up study. *J Spinal Disord Tech* 2006;19:323-327.

# Degenerative Cervical Spondylosis: Clinical Syndromes, Pathogenesis, and Management

Raj D. Rao, MD
*Bradford L. Currier, MD
*Todd J. Albert, MD
Christopher M. Bono, MD
Satyajit V. Marawar, MD
Kornelis A. Poelstra, MD, PhD
Jason C. Eck, DO, MS

## Abstract

*Degenerative changes in the cervical spinal column are ubiquitous in the adult population, but infrequently symptomatic. The evaluation of patients with symptoms is facilitated by classifying the resulting clinical syndromes into axial neck pain, cervical radiculopathy, cervical myelopathy, or a combination of these conditions. Although most patients with axial neck pain, cervical radiculopathy, or mild cervical myelopathy respond well to initial nonsurgical treatment, those who continue to have symptoms or patients with clinically evident myelopathy are candidates for surgical intervention.*

**Instr Course Lect 2008;57:447-469.**

Spondylosis refers to age-related degenerative changes within the spinal column. Radiographic evidence of cervical spondylosis is frequent in asymptomatic adults.[1,2] Approximately 25% of individuals younger than 40 years of age, 50% of individuals older than 40 years of age, and 85% of individuals older than 60 years of age have some degree of disk degeneration.[2,3] Occupations that place increased loads on the head predispose individuals to the development of cervical spondylosis. Activities such as rugby, soccer, and horseback riding and occupations such as flying fighter jets may also predispose individuals to the development of cervical spondylosis.[4-8]

Symptoms caused by cervical spondylosis can be categorized broadly into three clinical syndromes: axial neck pain, cervical radiculopathy, and cervical myelopathy. Patients can have a combination of these syndromes. Axial posterior neck pain occasionally radiates to the shoulder or periscapular region in a nondermatomal distribution. Axial neck pain is more common in women, has a lifetime prevalence of 66% in North American adults, and 5% of the population has disabling pain at any given time.[9-11] Cervical radiculopathy refers to pain, sensory findings, or a neurologic deficit in a dermatomal distribution in the upper extremity, with or without neck pain. The annual incidence of cervical radiculopathy was reported to be 83 per 100,000 population, whereas the prevalence was found to be 3.5 per 1,000 population with a peak incidence in the sixth decade of life.[12,13] Cervical myelopathy refers to the syndrome of long-tract clinical findings in the upper and lower extremities arising from involvement of the spinal cord by the spondylotic changes in the cervical

*Bradford L. Currier, MD or the department with which he is affiliated has received research or institutional support from Synthes Spine and royalties from DePuy Spine and Stryker Spine. Todd J. Albert, MD is a consultant or employee for DePuy Spine.

spinal column. The true incidence is difficult to ascertain because of the subtle findings in its early stages.

## Pathogenesis of Symptoms
### Neck Pain

Subaxial neck pain is most often caused by muscular and ligamentous factors related to improper posture, poor ergonomics, and muscle fatigue. Numerous potential causes have been reported, but their contribution is unclear. Low levels of high-energy phosphates such as adenosine triphosphate (ATP), adenosine diphosphate, and phosphoryl creatine have been found in the trapezius muscles of patients with fibromyalgic neck pain.[14] Patients with chronic trapezius myalgia have shown lower muscle blood flow and higher intramuscular tension on the symptomatic side when compared with the contralateral, asymptomatic side of the same patient and with healthy controls.[15] Prior neck injury has been found to be an independent risk factor.[16] Degenerative changes at the cervical disk and facet joints can be a source of symptoms. Nerve fibers and nociceptive nerve endings are present in the peripheral portions of the disk and in the capsule and synovium of the facet joints.[17-20] Findings of diskography and provocative injections of the facet joint have supported the role of these structures in the causation of neck pain.[21,22]

### Cervical Radiculopathy

Biochemical and biomechanical changes that occur with age result in a degenerative cascade. The intervertebral disk gradually loses height, posterior portions of the disk bulge into the spinal canal and the neuroforamina, the ligamentum flavum and facet joint capsule infold, and osteophytes form. All of this leads to decreases in canal and foraminal size. Subluxation and hypermobility between vertebral bodies may occur.

It is not clear why compression of a nerve causes pain. It is generally believed that only an inflamed or irritated nerve root can result in radicular pain on compression. Neurogenic chemical mediators of pain released from the cell bodies of the sensory neurons and non-neurogenic mediators released from disk tissue may play a role in initiating and perpetuating an inflammatory response.[23,24] Chronic edema and fibrosis within the nerve root caused by compression can also potentially alter the response threshold and increase the sensitivity of the nerve root to pain.[25] It may be that the dorsal root ganglion is the source of pain, as it is exquisitely sensitive to deformation.[26] In addition to mechanical compression of the dorsal root ganglion, the prolapsed nucleus pulposus elutes inflammatory mediators, initiating a local inflammatory response that leads to increased permeability at the dorsal root ganglion and pain.[27]

### Cervical Myelopathy

Mechanical compression of the spinal cord is widely held to be the primary pathophysiologic mechanism of cervical myelopathy. Animal studies have shown that at least 40% cord compression was necessary to produce reversible neurologic deficits.[28] Patients with less than 40% compression and myelopathy are likely to have additional factors such as a developmentally reduced anteroposterior diameter of the spinal canal, dynamic cord compression, dynamic changes in the intrinsic morphology of the spinal cord, or an impaired vascular supply of the spinal cord. The anteroposterior diameter of the subaxial spine in normal adults measures 17 to 18 mm. Individuals with an anteroposterior diameter of the canal of less than 13 mm are considered to have developmental stenosis and may be predisposed to the development of cervical myelopathy.[29] The shape and cross-sectional area of the spinal canal are important predictors of the development of cervical myelopathy. A cross-sectional area of the spinal cord of less than 60 mm$^2$ and a banana-shaped cord both have been found to be associated with the development of clinical signs or symptoms of myelopathy.[30,31] An anteroposterior cord compression ratio (the ratio of the anteroposterior to the transverse cord diameter) of less than 40% suggested substantial flattening of the cord and also was found to be associated with worse neurologic dysfunction.[32] Changes in the dimensions of the spinal canal during normal neck movement or as a result of abnormal segmental mobility may play a role in the development of cervical myelopathy by causing dynamic cord compression. The segmental anteroposterior diameter as well as the volume of the cervical spinal canal have been found to be reduced in extension.[33,34] Retrolisthesis of C3 on C4 could accentuate cord compression in elderly individuals with myelopathy.[35] Instability at a segment cephalad to a motion segment with severe disk degeneration may lead to dynamic cord compression.[36]

Morphologic changes also occur within the spinal cord with flexion and extension. Breig and associates[37] previously showed that the spinal cord stretches with flexion of the cervical spine and shortens and thickens with extension of the cervical spine. Thickening of the cord in extension makes it more susceptible to pressure from the infolded ligamentum flavum or the lamina. In flexion, the stretched cord may be prone to higher intrinsic pressure if it abuts against a disk or a vertebral body anteriorly.

Experimental studies have shown that ischemia of the cord has an additive effect on the clinical manifestations of myelopathy resulting from compression.[38,39] Tenting of the anterior spinal arteries as well as reduced flow in the anterior radicular arteries and especially the transverse intramedullary arterioles arising from the anterior sulcal artery can lead to ischemia of the anterior horn and the adjacent lateral columns.[37,40] Abnormal movement of a motion segment can trigger a vasospastic response that can also compromise the cord's intrinsic blood supply.[41]

## Clinical Evaluation
### Neck Pain
Localized pain and tenderness in the posterior muscles of the neck suggest a muscle sprain or a soft-tissue injury. Deep palpation of "trigger points" produces referred patterns of pain along the course of the myofascial structures. Determining a position of maximal discomfort may also provide a clue to the underlying pathologic entity. Pain in the posterior neck muscles that is worsened by flexion of the head suggests a myofascial etiology. Pain in the posterior aspect of the neck that is aggravated by extension, and especially by rotation of the head to one side, suggests a discogenic component. Predominant suboccipital pain radiating to the back of the ear, occiput, or neck raises the possibility of pathologic involvement of the upper cervical spine. Restricted rotation of the head to one side suggests involvement of the ipsilateral atlantoaxial articulation.

Pain in the neck and shoulder girdle can be referred from the heart, lungs, and abdominal viscera. Morning stiffness, polyarticular involvement, rigidity, or cutaneous manifestations accompanying the neck pain suggest a systemic inflammatory arthritic process. Fever, weight loss, or nonmechanical neck pain may point to an infectious or neoplastic lesion in the cervical spine, causing neck pain.

### Cervical Radiculopathy
Henderson and associates[42] reviewed the clinical presentations in 736 patients with cervical radiculopathy and reported that 99% had arm pain, 85% had sensory deficits, 80% had neck pain, 71% had reflex deficits, 68% had motor deficits, 52% had scapular pain, 18% had anterior chest pain, 10% had headaches, and 1% presented with left-sided chest and arm pain ("cervical angina"). The symptoms are usually aggravated by extension or lateral rotation of the head to the side of the pain (the Spurling maneuver). Patients with radicular pain may obtain some relief by elevating the arm overhead (the shoulder abduction sign) and sometimes by flexing and tilting the neck to the contralateral side.[43]

Upper cervical radiculopathies occasionally present as suboccipital pain with referral to the back of the ear. C4 radiculopathy can present as neck and shoulder pain with accompanying ipsilateral diaphragmatic palsy.[44] Paresthesias along the superior border of the trapezius are a clue to a radicular etiology. Nonspondylotic pathologic conditions can occasionally simulate cervical radiculopathy (Figure 1, Table 1).

### Cervical Myelopathy
Patients with cervical myelopathy generally present with clumsiness or a loss of fine motor skills in the hands. An increasingly awkward gait or difficulty with maintaining balance may have been noted by the patient or family members. Patients may report urinary urgency, hesitation, or frequency but rarely incontinence or retention of urine. Concomitant axial neck pain and/or radiculopathy are frequent. Motor weakness and wasting may be present in the upper or lower extremities. Pain, temperature, proprioception and vibratory sensations, and touch all may be diminished in the extremities and the trunk, depending on the location of the spinal cord compromise. Abnormal reflex findings include hyperreflexia or clonus of normal deep tendon reflexes, absence of superficial reflexes, or the presence of pathologic reflexes (the inverted radial reflex, the Hoffmann reflex, and the extensor plantar response) (Figure 1). Myelopathy hand is a term used to refer to a constellation of findings, including loss of dexterity, diffuse numbness, wasting of the intrinsic hand muscles, inability to rapidly grasp and release the fist, and ulnar and flexor drift of the ulnar two digits while attempting to keep the fingers adducted and extended (finger escape sign).[32,45] Myelopathy resulting from a cord level cephalad to C3 may result in a hyperactive scapulohumeral reflex—that is, tapping of the spine of the scapula or acromion results in scapular elevation and/or abduction of the humerus.

## Investigations
Patients with warning signs and symptoms of serious pathologic involvement of the cervical spine, such as tumor, infection, fracture, or neurologic injury, should undergo appropriate imaging studies without delay (Table 2). For all other

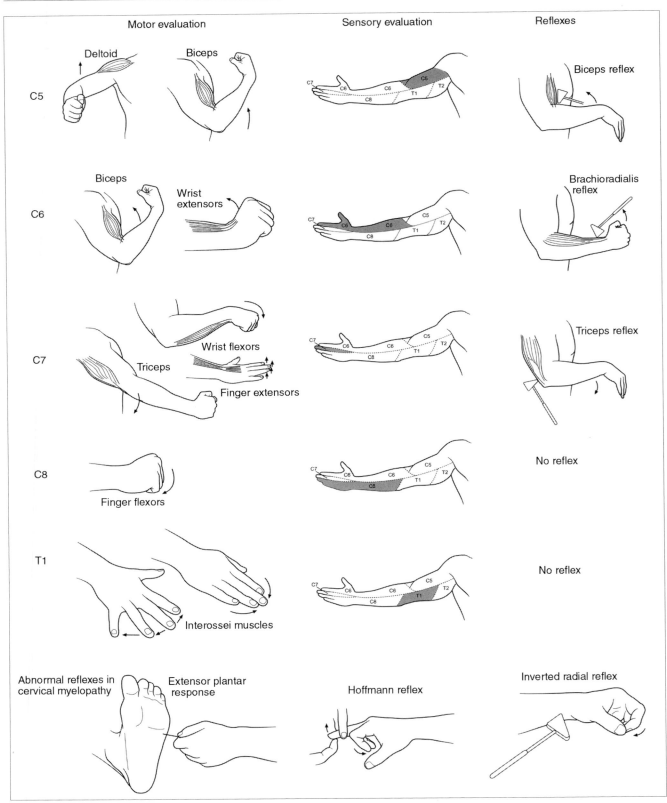

**Figure 1**   Neurologic evaluation of a patient with cervical radiculopathy and myelopathy.

**Table 1**
**Differential Diagnosis of Cervical Radiculopathy**

Peripheral entrapment syndromes

Rotator cuff/shoulder abnormalities

Brachial plexitis

Herpes zoster

Thoracic outlet syndrome

Sympathetic mediated pain syndrome

Intraspinal or extraspinal tumor

Epidural abscess

Cardiac ischemia

**Table 2**
**Warning Signs of Serious Cervical Spine Disorders Necessitating Immediate Imaging Studies**

| Potential Cause | Clinical Characteristics |
| --- | --- |
| Fracture | Clinically relevant trauma in adolescent or adult; minor trauma in elderly patient; ankylosing spondylitis |
| Neoplasm | Pain worse at night; unexplained weight loss; history of neoplasm; age older than 50 years or younger than 20 years |
| Infection | Fever, chills, night sweats; unexplained weight loss; history of recent systemic infection; recent invasive procedure; immunosuppression; intravenous drug use |
| Neurologic injury | Progressive neurologic deficit; upper and lower extremity symptoms; bowel or bladder dysfunction |

patients, imaging studies are delayed for 4 to 6 weeks to allow time for spontaneous recovery.

### Plain Radiographs

Plain radiographs should be made with the patient in an upright position when possible. Degenerative changes such as intervertebral disk space narrowing, osteoarthrosis of the facet and uncovertebral joints, osteophytes, and end plate sclerosis are ubiquitous in the adult population and are not diagnostic.[46] The Pavlov ratio is calculated by dividing the anteroposterior diameter of the spinal canal by the anteroposterior diameter of the vertebral body. A normal value is 1.0. A value of less than 0.8 suggests developmental canal stenosis but does not correlate with the space available for the spinal cord.[47,48] Lateral flexion-extension radiographs are used to measure the cervical range of motion and to identify ankylosed segments and cervical instability (translation of > 3.5 mm and relative sagittal plane angulation of > 11°).[49]

### Computed Tomography With Myelography

Compressive osteophytes, foraminal stenosis, and ossification of the posterior longitudinal ligament are best identified with use of CT scans. CT myelography, an invasive procedure,

is reportedly better than MRI in distinguishing osseous from soft-tissue impingement of neural structures and in detecting foraminal stenosis.[50,51] Shafaie and associates[52] found that concordance between CT and MRI findings was only moderately good in the interpretation of degenerative cervical spine changes that led to radiculopathy or myelopathy. CT myelography tended to upgrade the degree of spinal canal compromise, neural foraminal encroachment, and cord diameter reduction. They concluded that, while CT myelography and MRI should be considered complementary studies, CT myelography may be preferable to MRI because of its superior differentiation of bone and soft tissues.[52] CT myelography also provides better imaging detail in patients with postoperative metal artifacts or scoliotic deformity.

### Magnetic Resonance Imaging

MRI is the diagnostic standard for evaluation of the soft tissues of the cervical spine, including the neural elements, disk, joint capsule, and ligaments. Abnormalities are frequently seen on the MRIs of adults, and it is important to correlate imaging and clinical findings. Teresi and associates[53] found disk degeneration on the MRIs of 5 of 25 asymptomatic individuals between 45 and

54 years of age and those of 24 of 42 asymptomatic individuals who were older than 64 years. Spinal cord compression was found on the images of 9 of 58 individuals who were younger than 64 years and on those of 11 of 42 individuals who were older than 64 years.[53] Boden and associates[1] detected foraminal stenosis on the images of 1 of 40 asymptomatic patients who were younger than 40 years and on those of 5 of 23 patients who were older than 40 years.

MRI also allows direct visualization of intramedullary cord changes. Ohshio and associates[54] reported a direct correlation between histopathologic features and intramedullary signal changes on MRI. Isolated areas of high signal intensity on T2-weighted images indicate edema, which may resolve. A combination of low signal intensity on T1-weighted images and high signal intensity on T2-weighted images indicates severe lesions in gray matter with necrosis, myelomalacia, or spongiform changes.

Intramedullary signal changes in the cord have been detected in more than 60% of patients with symptomatic cervical myelopathy.[55-57] It is, however, not clear if the presence and the type of intramedullary signal changes in patients with symptomatic cervical myelopathy can be

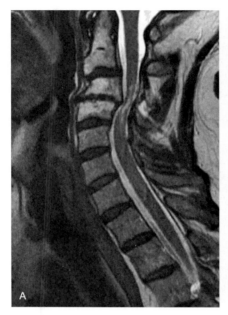

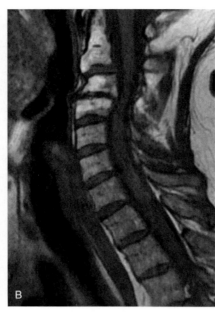

**Figure 2** Sagittal MRIs of the cervical spine of a patient with cervical myelopathy. **A,** T2-weighted image showing a well-circumscribed and extensive high signal intensity lesion at the site of compression in the cephalad part of the cervical spinal cord. **B,** T1-weighted image showing low signal intensity change at the site of compression.

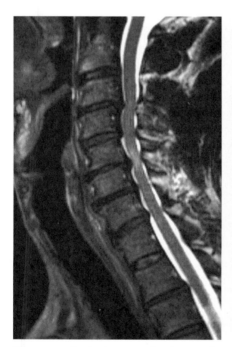

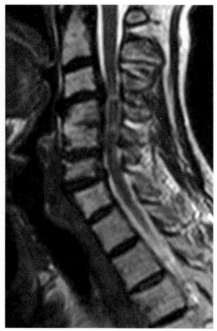

**Figure 3** Sagittal T2-weighted MRI of a patient with cervical myelopathy. A high signal intensity lesion with a faint and ill-defined border is seen at the site of spinal cord compression at the level of the C5-C6 disk space.

**Figure 4** Sagittal T2-weighted MRI of the cervical spine showing compression over several levels and multisegmental areas of high signal intensity.

used to predict either the prognosis or the outcome of treatment with any accuracy. High-intensity signal changes on T2-weighted images are found frequently and can be diffuse or well demarcated, focal or multisegmental; however, their clinical relevance is unclear (Figures 2 through 4). Well-demarcated high-intensity signal changes on T2-weighted images combined with low-intensity signal changes on T1-weighted images are rare; they usually are found in late stages of cervical myelopathy and indicate a more severe, irreversible pathologic condition such as late-stage myelomalacia and cystic necrosis.[58,59] Bednarik and associates[58] found high-intensity intramedullary signal changes on T2-weighted images of 23 of 66 asymptomatic patients with cervical stenosis, but they identified no patients with a combination of high-intensity intramedullary signal changes on T2-weighted images and low-intensity intramedullary signal changes on T1-weighted images. The presence of intramedullary signal changes does not predict a poor outcome after nonsurgical treatment in patients with mild myelopathy.[56]

Morio and associates[55] identified intramedullary signal changes in 71 of 73 patients who underwent surgery for clinically evident myelopathy. They concluded that, while low-intensity signal changes on T1-weighted images may indicate a poor prognosis, high-intensity signal changes on T2-weighted images can be caused by a broad spectrum of compressive myelomalacic pathologic conditions and reflect a broad spectrum of spinal cord recuperative potentials. In another surgical series, Suri and associates[57] identified intramedullary signal changes in 121 of 146 symptomatic patients. Of these 121 patients, 33% had changes only on the T2-weighted images and 67% had changes on both the T1- and the T2-weighted images. Patients without intramedullary signal changes or with changes only on T2-weighted images had significantly better postoperative motor strength than did patients with changes on both T1- and T2-weighted images ($P < 0.05$). There have also been reports that patients with focal high-intensity intramedullary signal changes on T2-weighted images have better clinical outcomes following surgery than do patients with multisegmental high-intensity intramedullary signal changes on T2-weighted images.[60,61]

The transverse area and shape of the spinal cord at the compressed segment may predict outcomes, with a preoperative transverse spinal cord area of less than 0.45 cm² correlating with poor surgical results.[62] With progressive compression, the cross section of the spinal cord changes from a boomerang shape to a teardrop shape to a triangular shape.[63] The boomerang and teardrop shapes have a better potential for recovery than do the triangular shape.

Metabolic neuroimaging technology recently has been applied to the spinal cord. Uchida and associates[64] compared findings on preoperative high-resolution[18] F-fluorodeoxy-glucose-positron emission tomography (FDG-PET) with Japanese Orthopaedic Association (JOA) scores and findings on MRI in 23 patients undergoing surgery for myelopathy. FDG-PET findings correlated with preoperative JOA scores, postoperative JOA scores, and the rate of postoperative improvement, but they had no correlation with high-intensity intramedullary signal changes on T2-weighted images. Currently, the major limitation of this technology is the

poor resolution of PET scans. (Accurate measurements of glucose utilization are difficult to obtain.) Future technologic advancements in PET scanning may facilitate evaluation of early spinal cord damage and provide indications for surgical intervention.

### Electrodiagnostic Studies

Electrodiagnostic studies may help to differentiate between various causes of symptoms, including myelopathy, radiculopathy, peripheral entrapment syndromes, peripheral neuropathy, shoulder dysfunction, and brachial plexopathy. Recommended investigations for neurophysiologic examination of patients with cervical myelopathy include testing of somatosensory-evoked potentials by stimulation of the tibial nerve and motor evoked potentials from the upper and lower extremities.[65] Both motor-evoked potentials and somatosensory-evoked potentials can be abnormal in patients with spinal cord compression who have no clinical features of myelopathy.[66,67] Bednarik and associates[67] prospectively followed 30 patients with evidence of spinal cord compression on MRI, but no clinical evidence of cervical myelopathy, by testing motor- and somatosensory-evoked potentials for a period of 2 years. The authors detected electrophysiologic abnormalities in 15 of the 30 patients at the beginning of the study. Clinical signs of cervical myelopathy were detected in 5 of these 15 patients over the next 2 years, with at least one test of evoked potentials showing deterioration at the time of the appearance of the signs of cervical myelopathy. Myelopathy did not develop in any of the patients with normal motor- and somatosensory-evoked potentials at the beginning of the study. Bednarik and associates

concluded that there was a significant association between abnormal findings on evoked-potential studies and the development of cervical myelopathy in patients with spinal cord compression ($p = 0.02$).

Studies of motor- and somatosensory-evoked potentials might be useful in detecting subclinical myelopathy. In patients with evidence of spinal cord compression on MRI and symptoms but no definitive signs of myelopathy, motor-evoked potentials are more commonly abnormal than are somatosensory-evoked potentials.[66] Clinical features of cervical myelopathy can be masked in patients with peripheral neuropathy, and studies of evoked potentials can detect clinically silent myelopathy in these patients.[68] In patients with diagnosed cervical spondylotic myelopathy, upper extremity motor-evoked potentials are most commonly abnormal. Patients who have normal preoperative median somatosensory-evoked potentials may have better recovery rates after surgery for myelopathy than patients who have abnormal somatosensory evoked potentials.[69] A decrease in motor-evoked potentials of 50% or more correlates well with a postoperative motor deficit.[70]

Electromyography can show increased insertional activity, fibrillations, and fasciculations and diminished motor unit recruitment, which are signs of denervation caused by pathologic changes at the nerve root or anterior horn cells. Electromyography in combination with nerve conduction velocity studies can help to distinguish cervical radiculopathy from peripheral neuropathy or peripheral root entrapment syndromes in some patients. The value of electromyography as a primary diagnostic modality for patients with clinical signs of radiculopathy is offset by its low sensitivity.[71,72] Its concordance with MRI findings in patients is low. Nardin and associates[73] reported that, in 19 of 47 patients with cervical radiculopathy, electromyographic results did not correlate with findings on MRI. Additionally, electromyography is less likely to show abnormal findings in patients with predominantly sensory radiculopathy.[73,74] It may be possible to improve the sensitivity of electromyography for detecting cervical radiculopathy by the addition of paraspinal muscles to the electromyography screen.[75]

## Nonsurgical Management

Narcotic analgesics, nonsteroidal anti-inflammatory agents, corticosteroids, muscle relaxants, and antidepressants are commonly used to relieve neck pain and radiculopathy. A short period of rest or cessation of pain-provoking activities and the use of a soft collar with the neck in mild flexion may sometimes alleviate acute pain and spasm. In a metaanalysis of the literature, physical modalities such as heat, cold, therapeutic ultrasound, massage, use of transcutaneous electrical nerve stimulation (TENS), and cervical traction were not found to have any reproducible benefit in the treatment of acute or chronic neck pain.[76] A 4- to 6-week program of physical therapy, including isometric exercises, active range-of-motion exercises, aerobic conditioning, and resistive exercises has been found to be helpful for patients with chronic neck pain.[77,78] There have been a few reports of substantial relief of radicular pain and improved functional outcome after the use of cervical traction for the treatment of cervical radiculopathy.[79,80] Long-term success has been reported in 40% to

70% of patients who received translaminar or transforaminal epidural corticosteroid injections for treatment of cervical radiculopathy.[81-83] Rare but potentially catastrophic complications can be associated with these injection techniques.[84] In a cohort of patients with neck pain or radicular symptoms in the upper extremities followed for 10 to 25 years, Gore and associates[85] found that nonsurgical management resulted in complete resolution of symptoms in 43% of the patients and partial resolution in 25%, whereas 32% had continued moderate or severe pain.

Patients with mild myelopathy are occasionally offered a trial of observation or nonsurgical management, but nonsurgical management is generally not successful in reversing or permanently halting the progress of myelopathy. Conservative treatment includes intermittent cervical immobilization in a soft collar; anti-inflammatory medications and bed rest; and active discouragement of high-risk activities, manipulation therapies, and vigorous or prolonged flexion of the head.[86] A greater anteroposterior diameter of the spinal canal, a transverse area of the spinal cord greater than 70 mm$^2$, and age older than 56 years are factors that seem to be associated with a better response to conservative treatment by patients with mild myelopathy.[87]

## Indications for Surgical Intervention

Success rates for nonsurgical management of neck pain and cervical radiculopathy may vary depending on the patient population studied. Even in a referral practice, 70% to 80% of patients with neck pain respond favorably to nonsurgical treatment.[88,89] Surgical intervention

is considered for the following patients with predominantly axial neck pain.

1. Those with severely limiting pain caused by cervical degenerative disease that is not relieved by nonsurgical treatment of more than 12 months. It is difficult to identify the symptomatic level in these patients with MRI alone,[90,91] and objective confirmation of the disk as the "pain generator" with use of both MRI and provocative diskography should be considered to improve the clinical success rates. A nonorganic component to the pain should be absent. Anterior discectomy and fusion is the surgical intervention of choice for these patients with discogenic neck pain.

2. Patients with C3 or C4 nerve root impingement can present with features simulating axial neck pain. Patients with such "pseudoaxial" neck pain who do not respond to nonsurgical measures for 6 to 12 weeks may be candidates for surgical intervention.

3. Patients with pseudarthrosis of the cervical spine with graft collapse or hardware migration and disabling axial neck pain are candidates for revision anterior surgery. Patients without implant failure may have higher fusion rates and superior clinical outcomes after posterior cervical fusion with instrumentation than after anterior revision.[92,93]

Surgery is an option for patients with persistent cervical radiculopathy following failure of a 3-month trial of nonsurgical measures to relieve disabling radicular pain. These patients must have neuroimaging studies that show a pathologic condition that corresponds to the clinical features. Surgery is also an option for patients with a progressive motor deficit or a disabling motor deficit from the radiculopathy.[94]

Studies of the natural history of cervical myelopathy suggest that most patients with clinically established disease will have progression of symptoms, possibly in a stepwise fashion with time.[95-98] Bednarik and associates[58] found that clinical signs or symptoms of myelopathy developed in 13 of 66 patients with asymptomatic spinal cord compression seen on MRI in a study with a minimum 2-year follow-up. Patients with mild myelopathy probably do not benefit from surgery. In a prospective randomized study with a duration of follow-up of 3 years, patients with mild to moderate nonprogressive or slowly progressive myelopathy were found to have similar outcomes after either nonsurgical or surgical treatment.[86] A trial of nonsurgical treatment did not decrease the potential for ultimate recovery of patients with mild myelopathy.[99] Patients with severe or progressive myelopathy are candidates for surgical intervention. Several factors are considered in the decision regarding when to proceed with surgery in patients with myelopathy; these include the degree of neurologic dysfunction, patient disability, findings on radiographs and MRI, duration of symptoms, and presence of comorbidity.

## Surgical Options and Techniques

The two options typically considered for the surgical management of cervical radiculopathy are (1) anterior cervical diskectomy and fusion and (2) posterior laminotomy-foraminotomy. An anterior approach is preferred for patients with a central or bilateral disk lesion, whereas a lateral cervical disk herniation can be approached either anteriorly or posteriorly. The long-term results of the two procedures are comparable, but anterior cervical diskectomy and fusion is preferred for patients who have substantial neck pain associated with radicular symptoms.[100-102] Patients with myelopathy should be treated with anterior cervical diskectomy or corpectomy when there is pathologic compression at up to three levels or when cervical lordosis is reversed.[103] A laminectomy or laminoplasty is used in patients requiring decompression at four or more segments, those with a developmentally narrow canal, and those in whom the anterior column is already fused. Cervical lordosis is critical for a posterior approach because it allows the cord to migrate dorsally after the decompression.

### Anterior Cervical Diskectomy and Corpectomy

A subtotal diskectomy with removal of cartilaginous end plates and anterior osteophytes is done through a Smith-Robinson approach[104] (Figure 5). We prefer to use a left-sided approach because the course of the recurrent laryngeal nerve is more sheltered within the tracheoesophageal groove on this side.

After removal of disk material within the interspace, posterior osteophytes may need to be removed to adequately decompress the spinal cord and nerve root. Removal of posterior osteophytes increases the risk of injury to the spinal cord, and large osteophytes may be removed more safely with a partial corpectomy.[105] Osteophytes may resorb after a successful anterior fusion, but this theory is controversial.[106,107] Removal of the posterior longitudinal ligament similarly increases the risk of cord contusion and postoperative epidural hematoma,[108] but it should be done if a rent in the posterior longitudinal ligament is detected or if there is clinical or imaging-based suspicion of an extruded fragment posterior to the ligament.

During the corpectomy, a 15- to 19-mm central trough is removed from the anterior aspect of the vertebral body with a rongeur or a high-speed burr. A thin residue of posterior wall and the posterior longitudinal ligament are resected with use of a diamond-tipped burr, small curets, and a 1-mm Kerrison rongeur as required. The adequacy of the decompression is assessed by visual inspection of the decompressed posterior longitudinal ligament or dura.

Anterior cervical diskectomy without fusion results in a higher prevalence of postoperative neck pain, can lead to a reduction in the neuroforaminal area, and is rarely advised.[109,110]

### Anterior Fusion

All cartilaginous material is removed, but the integrity of the osseous end plate is preserved to provide mechanical stability to the inserted graft. Four or five tiny perforations are created within the cephalad and caudad osseous end plates with use of a small curet or burr to facilitate fusion across the interspace. Some surgeons remove the osseous end plates and seat the inserted graft within the exposed cancellous bone, with the aim of improving fusion rates.[111] The graft should be 2 mm taller than the measured height of the disk space to maintain sagittal alignment. The graft is recessed 2 mm posterior to the anterior cortical margin of the adjacent vertebral bodies.

Following anterior diskectomy, the placement of a tricortical horseshoe-shaped autograft harvested from the anterior iliac crest has led to excellent fusion rates.[112-114]

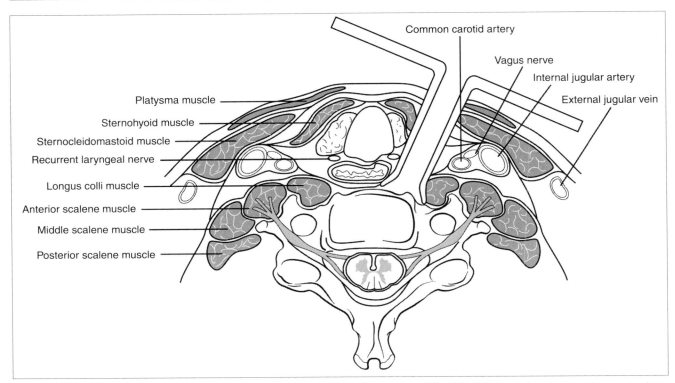

**Figure 5**  Cross-sectional anatomy through the midcervical spine, illustrating the fascial planes used in the anterior cervical approach. The strap muscles, the trachea, and the esophagus are retracted medially while the carotid sheath is retracted laterally. (Reproduced from Rao RD, Bagario V: Anterior approaches to the cervical and cervicothoracic spine, in *Orthopaedic Knowledge Online*. Rosemont, IL, American Academy of Orthopaedic Surgeons, 2005.)

Equivalent fusion rates have been reported after allografting and autografting, combined with use of anterior plates and segmental screw fixation, for intervertebral fusions of up to three levels.[115,116] Longer-term results are required before definite recommendations can be made regarding the use of titanium cages, carbon-fiber cages, and polyetheretherketone (PEEK) cages.[117-119]

Tricortical iliac crest autograft struts are the best option for anterior column reconstruction after a one- or two-level anterior cervical corpectomy, but they are associated with donor site morbidity. A fibular strut is preferred when the iliac crest is mechanically insufficient or for corpectomy defects that are longer than two levels. The use of longer strut grafts after multilevel corpectomies is associated with complications. Settling of the graft with kyphotic change in the angulation and fracture of the fibular strut graft has been reported after the use of long fibular grafts.[120,121] Wang and associates[122] found the risk of graft displacement and migration to be higher as the number of removed vertebral bodies increased and when the fusion extended down to C7. Use of metallic cages and synthetic spacers in conjunction with local autograft or allograft after single- or multiple-level corpectomies (Figure 6) has resulted in comparable fusion rates, but the long-term results are still unclear.[123,124] High rates of early failure of the reconstruction, cage subsidence, and plate loosening have been reported following the use of titanium mesh cages in multilevel corpectomies.[125,126]

### Anterior Cervical Plates

After either diskectomy or corpectomy, anterior osteophytes are removed from the margins of the adjacent vertebrae to prepare a flat bed for the plate. The length of the plate is selected so that a minimum distance of 5 mm is maintained between the ends of the plate and the adjacent disks (Figure 7). This helps to decrease adjacent-level disk ossification.[127] The use of screws locked to the plate obviates the need for bicortical purchase in the vertebral body. When multisegmental fixation is performed, an attempt should be made to fix the plate to all vertebral levels.

The use of an anterior cervical plate in an anterior cervical diskectomy and fusion involving two or more levels improves fusion rates, reduces the need for postoperative stabilization, reduces graft-related complications, and is associated with less postoperative kyphosis.[128,129] Use of an anterior cervical plate after a single-level anterior cervical diskectomy and fusion with autograft bone does not improve clinical results or fusion rates but reduces graft collapse.[130,131] An anterior plate may be beneficial when allograft bone is used for a single-level anterior cervical diskectomy and fusion.[132] Fusion occurs in approximately 90% of patients who have a single-level anterior cervical diskectomy.[133,134] The prevalence of pseudarthrosis increases with the number of levels that are operated on.[112]

The use of an anterior plate has been found to reduce pseudarthrosis rates following single-level corpectomy.[135] Failure rates ranging from 6 of 12 to 5 of 7 have been reported following corpectomy involving three or more levels, even with use of an anterior plate, and supplemental posterior instrumentation should be considered for such patients.[136,137]

### Cervical Disk Replacement

Artificial disk replacement has not yet been approved by the US Food and Drug Administration for clinical use. Cervical disk replacement has been proposed as an alternative to anterior cervical diskectomy and fusion in patients with pathologic involvement of a cervical disk. Although the causes of deterioration of motion segments adjacent to a "stiff" fusion are unclear, a theoretic benefit of disk replacement is a reduction in this risk of adjacent segment

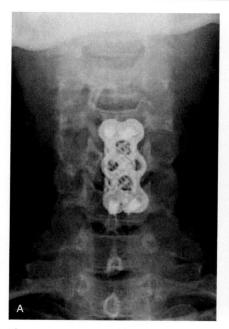 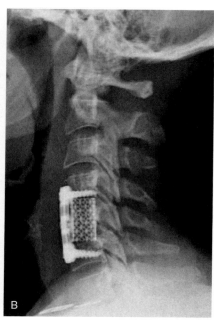

**Figure 6**   AP **(A)** and lateral **(B)** radiographs of the cervical spin of a patient with cervical spondylotic myelopathy treated with C5 corpectomy, insertion of a titanium mesh cage packed with local autogenous bone in the trough, and application of an anterior cervical plate from C4 to C6.

deterioration.[138-140] Cadaver and clinical studies with a 2-year follow-up have demonstrated maintenance of motion at a surgical segment following disk replacement.[141,142] Selection of patients for cervical disk replacement currently is not standardized. Common exclusion criteria mentioned in the current literature are substantial cervical deformity, radiographic findings of segmental instability, isolated axial neck pain, a lack of motion at the segment preoperatively, and severe facet arthrosis.[143-145] In a series of 49 patients with a one-level disk replacement, 32 had an excellent result; 2, a good result; 10, a fair result; and 5, a poor result.[142] Comparable clinical outcomes were reported 2 years following Bryan artificial disk replacement and 2 years following anterior cervical diskectomy and fusion. Other early results have been similar.[146,147] In one study, the prevalence of symptomatic

adjacent-level degenerative disk disease in patients treated with fusion was reported to be significantly higher than that in patients treated with disk replacement ($p = 0.009$).[148] Heterotopic ossification, persistent pain, prosthetic migration, segmental kyphosis, and device failure have been reported following cervical disk replacement.[142,145,149,150]

### Posterior Laminotomy-Foraminotomy

The keyhole foraminotomy technique was originally described by Scoville[151] and is used for patients with unilateral radicular findings caused by a lateral or foraminal soft cervical disk herniation or foraminal stenosis. The procedure involves removal of the lateral one third of the superior and inferior hemilaminae with removal of the medial one third of the facet joint. In the case of a soft cervical disk, the foraminot-

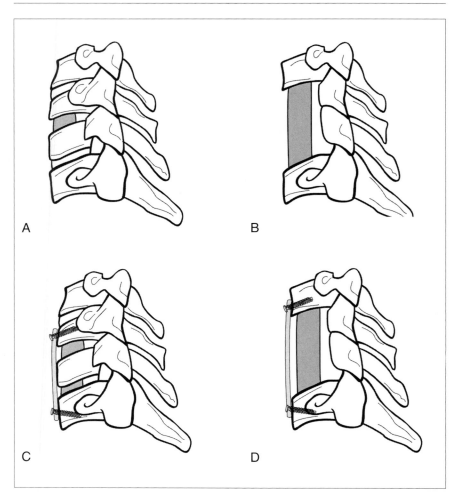

**Figure 7** Common anterior surgical interventions used for cervical spondylosis. **A,** Anterior cervical diskectomy and insertion of a spacer for fusion. **B,** Anterior cervical corpectomy and insertion of a strut bone graft. **C,** Anterior cervical diskectomy followed by insertion of a bone spacer for fusion and application of an anterior plate. **D,** Anterior cervical corpectomy, insertion of a strut graft, and application of an anterior plate. (Reproduced with permission from Rao RD, Gourab K, David KS: Surgical treatment of cervical spondylotic myelopathy. *J Bone Joint Surg Am* 2006;88:1624.)

the risk of kyphosis, limits constriction of the dura from extradural scar formation, and obviates the need for fusion.[154,155]

Intraoperatively, visible expansion of the dural sac and pulsation of the dura after opening of the laminoplasty doors or following laminectomy suggest good canal expansion.[156] A laminoplasty opening gap of 8 to 10 mm and an average increase in the canal diameter of approximately 5 mm usually result in adequate decompression.[157,158] Foraminotomy is considered following a laminoplasty or laminectomy in patients who show foraminal stenosis from a disk protrusion or foraminal osteophytes and concordant radicular symptoms. A prophylactic C5 foraminotomy can be performed to reduce the prevalence of C5 palsy from posterior translation of the cord, although there is no clear evidence that it reduces the prevalence of C5 palsy.

The laminoplasty door is held open by anchoring the spinous process to the facet joint on the hinge side with use of suture or wire, or by insertion of autograft, allograft, or ceramic spacers on the open side. Stabilization of the open door with use of mini-plates fixed to the lamina and the lateral mass without major complications has been reported by multiple authors[159,160] (Figure 8).

omy is followed by excision of the extruded disk fragment with use of a small, blunt-tipped nerve hook. Foraminotomy alone is adequate in patients with foraminal stenosis because of an osteophytic ridge.[152] Microendoscopic posterior cervical foraminotomy techniques may further reduce the postoperative pain and disability associated with muscle stripping during an open foraminotomy.[153]

## Laminoplasty

Laminoplasty increases the effective diameter of the spinal canal from C3 to C7 by shifting the laminae dorsally with use of either a so-called single door with a single lateral hinge or a double door with lateral hinges on both sides. In contrast to laminectomy, laminoplasty retains a covering of posterior laminar bone and ligamentum flavum over the spinal cord, minimizes the instability and

## Laminectomy

Laminectomy can be considered when decompression is required at more than three levels, particularly in elderly patients, in whom comorbidities increase surgical risk. All levels with radiographic evidence of stenosis should be included in the decompression. Limiting the number of segments that are decompressed does not influence the development of postlaminectomy

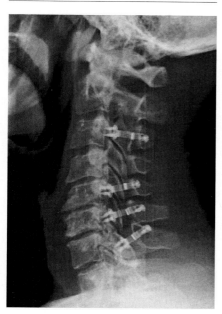

**Figure 8** Lateral radiograph of the cervical spine of a patient with cervical spondylotic myelopathy managed with C3-C7 laminoplasty and mini plate fixation.

kyphosis or instability, but inclusion of C2 and T1 in the laminectomy increases the likelihood of kyphosis and instability developing.[161,162] Concern about postlaminectomy kyphosis and instability has led to the development of the laminectomy with fusion and posterior instrumentation.

Laminectomy without instrumentation should be restricted to patients with preserved cervical lordosis. In patients with a flexible cervical kyphosis, laminectomy may be combined with application of posterior instrumentation with the neck extended to restore cervical lordosis and maximize posterior shift of the spinal cord.

### Posterior Cervical Instrumentation

Instrumentation options for posterior cervical fixation after laminectomy include sublaminar and facet wires connected to a longitudinal rod or a rectangular construct, and interspinous wires.[163,164] Lateral mass and cervical pedicle-based screw fixation systems are alternative options for patients with deficient posterior elements, but they have not yet been approved by the Food and Drug Administration for clinical use in the United States.[165-167] To reduce the risk of spinal cord injury during the use of lateral mass or pedicle screws, the screw holes should be drilled before the laminectomy. Pedicle screws may be preferable at C2 and C7 because the lateral masses are poorly developed at these levels. The reported prevalence of fusion in patients treated with instrumentation is better than that in patients treated with bone grafting alone.[166,168,169]

### Outcomes Following Cervical Surgery

#### Neck Pain

Most patients with axial neck pain respond favorably to nonsurgical management.[85,88,89,96] Clinical outcomes in patients with predominantly axial neck pain may be influenced by psychological factors.[114,170] The benign natural history of neck pain, difficulty in identifying an accurate pain generator, and the lack of randomized controlled studies comparing surgical and nonsurgical management have led many surgeons to recommend nonsurgical management for patients with axial neck pain, but some studies have demonstrated a substantial decrease in pain and improved function following anterior cervical diskectomy and fusion for axial neck pain.[91,171] Use of both MRI and provocative diskography to determine whether fusion should be performed in patients with axial neck pain has been found to reduce the number of levels that need to be fused, and sometimes painful levels are revealed to be morphologically normal on the MRI.[91]

#### Cervical Radiculopathy

Anterior cervical diskectomy and fusion is an excellent surgical option for the treatment of cervical radiculopathy, with good to excellent clinical results in 70% to 90% of patients.[112,172,173] The age of the patient, the duration of symptoms, and the type of disk (soft or hard) have not been found to affect the clinical outcome.[174,175] Nonsmokers tend to have significantly more relief of arm pain and a better clinical outcome than smokers ($p < 0.01$).[133] Additionally, male gender, greater segmental kyphosis, a greater preoperative range of motion of the neck, greater right and left hand grip strength, an organic type of pain drawing, and a low disability score on the Neck Disability Index (NDI) have been significantly correlated with better postoperative pain relief in patients with radiculopathy ($p < 0.1$).[176]

Wirth and associates[101] found no significant difference between the clinical outcomes following anterior cervical diskectomy and fusion and those following posterior foraminotomy for the treatment of cervical radiculopathy. Recurrence of radiculopathy at the same level was more common after foraminotomy, whereas recurrence at other levels was more common after anterior cervical diskectomy and fusion. Patients treated with posterior foraminotomy more frequently have persistent neck pain postoperatively.[100] Herkowitz and associates[102] concluded that there was not a significant difference between the results of anterior cervical diskectomy and fusion and those of posterior foraminotomy, although there was a trend for better clinical outcomes after anterior cervical diskectomy and fusion.

### Cervical Myelopathy

Good restoration of spinal canal dimensions, earlier decompression, lack of comorbidity, and either a complete lack of intramedullary cord changes or only isolated changes on T2-weighted MRIs predict better outcomes following anterior decompression for the treatment of cervical myelopathy.[57,177,178] Emery and associates[179] reported on 106 patients with cervical myelopathy who had undergone either anterior diskectomy or corpectomy and fusion without instrumentation. Eighty-two of these patients had preoperative gait abnormalities; 38 of them recovered normal gait, and an additional 33 had an improvement in gait. Substantial improvements in hand function and sensory deficits also have been reported after anterior decompression for the treatment of myelopathy.[177,179,180]

A meta-analysis revealed that 55% of more than 2,000 patients showed some neurologic recovery following laminoplasty.[181] The neurologic outcome was not influenced by the laminoplasty technique and was similar after laminoplasty and laminectomy.

In a study comparing 23 patients treated with cervical corpectomy and 24 patients treated with cervical laminoplasty for multilevel spondylotic myelopathy, no significant difference in neurologic recovery was found between the groups at 1 year, at 5 years, or at the time of final follow-up, which ranged from 10 to 14 years.[182] Longer surgical times and more blood loss were reported with the anterior cervical surgery, whereas frequent axial neck pain and more postoperative stiffness were reported after the laminoplasties.

## Common Complications of Surgical Intervention
### Neurologic Complications

Flynn[183] reported 311 neurologic complications following more than 36,000 anterior cervical diskectomy and fusion procedures done by 704 neurosurgeons. Radiculopathy accounted for 40% of the complications; substantial permanent myelopathy, 25%; and recurrent laryngeal nerve palsy, 17%. Recurrent laryngeal nerve palsy has been reported in 2% to 11% of patients following an anterior cervical approach.[184,185] A prospective study in which preoperative and postoperative laryngoscopy was performed in 123 patients who underwent single- or multiple-level anterior cervical diskectomy or corpectomy with fusion demonstrated a 24% initial prevalence of recurrent laryngeal nerve palsy with persistence of the palsy at 3 months in 13%.[186] Comparative studies have not shown any significant correlation between the side of the approach and the prevalence of recurrent laryngeal nerve palsy.[187] Avoidance of prolonged retraction, knowledge of the anatomy, careful dissection, and deflation of the endotracheal tube cuff after placement of the retractor may all help to diminish the prevalence of this complication.

Postoperative C5 radiculopathy can occur after laminoplasty or laminectomy, presumably as a result of traction on the short C5 nerve root due to posterior migration of the cord after posterior decompression or as a result of closure of the laminoplasty door causing nerve impingement. The complication is equally frequent following anterior surgery, possibly because of impingement of the ventral aspect of the spinal cord against the edges of a corpectomy trough. C5 radiculopa-

thy occurred in approximately 4% of patients after anterior surgery or laminoplasty and in 1% of patients after laminectomy.[188] Patients with a postoperative C5 palsy were found to have more severe cord compression at the C3-C4 and C4-C5 levels than did patients without palsy.[189] Spontaneous recovery is expected in most patients, but it may be delayed for up to 12 months.[105,189] Concurrent foraminotomy and intraoperative electromyographic monitoring of the C5 nerve root may help to diminish the prevalence of this condition.[190,191] Injury to the superior laryngeal nerve leading to easy voice fatigue and difficulty with high-pitched tones, and Horner syndrome from injury to the sympathetic nerves, occur infrequently after anterior surgery.

### Neck Pain

More than half of patients experience posterior neck and shoulder girdle pain after laminoplasty, and the pain may be severe.[192] The prevalence of axial pain and stiffness following multilevel posterior decompression has been reportedly lowered by preservation of the extensor muscle and ligament attachments by performing partial or complete laminectomies or interlaminar decompression at a few levels or by reattaching osteotomized spinous processes after laminoplasty, and by early postoperative mobilization.[182,193-196] In addition, restricting the laminoplasty to the C3-C6 level and avoiding the inclusion of C7 in the procedure reduce the prevalence of early postoperative axial neck pain.[197]

### Neck Stiffness

Neck stiffness is common after laminoplasty or laminectomy with fusion and instrumentation. In a meta-analysis of laminoplasty, approximately half of the range of motion of the neck was found to be lost postoperatively.[181] Postoperative interlaminar osseous fusion, which occurs most frequently at C2-C3, may be one of the major causes of restriction of the range of motion following laminoplasty.[198] Substantial postoperative stiffness is not common following anterior cervical diskectomy and fusion. Stiffness following corpectomy and fusion is more pronounced in patients who have undergone a three- or four-level procedure.[199]

### Instability and Kyphosis

Laminectomy alone, especially in children and young adults or in patients with preexisting kyphosis or segmental mobility, can result in postoperative instability, kyphosis, and worsening of the neurologic deficit.[200] Laminectomy with fusion and instrumentation maintains lordosis that is close to its preoperative value.[165] Kyphosis can also result following laminoplasty, especially when C2 is included, when preoperative lordosis is less than 10°, and when the range of preoperative flexion is greater than the range of preoperative extension.[181,201,202]

### Dysphagia

Hematoma, local edema, denervation of the pharyngeal plexus, adhesions between the esophagus, trachea, and prevertebral fascia, and a displaced graft or instrumentation are potential causes of dysphagia after anterior surgery. A prevalence of dysphagia of as high as 50% at 1 month, but with gradual improvement over time, has been reported.[203,204] The risk of dysphagia is higher after multilevel procedures and in patients with long-standing neck pain, but the type of procedure (diskectomy or corpectomy) and the

use of an anterior plate do not influence the prevalence of postoperative dysphagia.[203,204]

### Adjacent Segment Deterioration

The prevalence of adjacent segment degeneration increases each year following anterior cervical fusion, with about 25% of patients having symptomatic adjacent segment disease at 10 years.[205] The facts that segments most prone to adjacent-segment deterioration are C5-C6 and C6-C7, which are also most likely to naturally show degenerative changes, and that this prevalence is similar to that found following foraminotomy without fusion, suggest that adjacent segment disease may be a consequence of the natural evolution of spondylotic disease and not necessarily related to the adjacent fusion.

### Complications With Instrumentation

Breakage or loosening of a plate or screws has been reported in 35% of patients after anterior surgery.[206] Hardware failure was more common when the screws were not locked to the plate.[206] Migration of the loosened screws into the esophagus is a potential complication.[207,208]

Nerve root injury is the most common complication after posterior instrumentation, but it occurs in fewer than 1% of patients. In one study, cortical penetration was reported in association with 10 of 190 pedicle screws inserted (5%), with no resulting neurovascular complications in these patients.[167]

### Summary

Degenerative cervical spondylosis can present clinically as axial neck pain, cervical radiculopathy, or cervical myelopathy. Pathoanatomic changes are generally well visualized

on imaging studies and must be correlated with the clinical findings. Most patients with axial neck pain, cervical radiculopathy, or mild cervical myelopathy respond well to an initial trial of nonsurgical management.

Anterior cervical diskectomy and fusion and laminotomy-foraminotomy are options for the surgical management of cervical radiculopathy. The clinical outcome after the performance of either of these procedures to treat cervical radiculopathy is excellent. Surgical considerations in patients with cervical myelopathy include the number of levels involved, the alignment of the cervical spine, and the dimensions of the spinal canal. The clinical outcome following surgery for cervical myelopathy depends primarily on the duration since the onset of symptoms, the presence and pattern of intramedullary signal changes on MRI, and the adequacy of decompression. Both anterior and posterior decompressions of the cervical spinal cord result in satisfactory outcomes. Approach-related complications such as dysphagia and injury to the laryngeal nerves are concerns with the anterior neck approach, whereas persistent neck pain, stiffness, and the development of instability are concerns with the posterior approach.

Instrumentation is frequently used in conjunction with anterior or posterior fusion to increase the rigidity of the construct and to enhance the success of the fusion. The use of a plate following anterior fusion improves fusion rates after multilevel anterior cervical diskectomy or single-level corpectomy and can reduce the prevalence of postoperative dislodgment of the graft and the development of kyphosis even following single-level diskectomy. The prevalence of complications remains high after multilevel anterior cervical corpectomies, despite the addition of an anterior cervical plate, and supplemental posterior stabilization ought to be considered for these patients. Artificial disk replacement in the cervical spine is still in its infancy, and long-term outcomes are required before it can be recommended.

## References

1. Boden SD, McCowin PR, Davis DO, Dina TS, Mark AS, Wiesel S: Abnormal magnetic-resonance scans of the cervical spine in asymptomatic subjects: A prospective investigation. *J Bone Joint Surg Am* 1990;72:1178-1184.

2. Lehto IJ, Tertti MO, Komu ME, Paajanen HE, Tuominen J, Kormano MJ: Age-related MRI changes at 0.1 T in cervical discs in asymptomatic subjects. *Neuroradiology* 1994;36:49-53.

3. Matsumoto M, Fujimura Y, Suzuki N, et al: MRI of cervical intervertebral discs in asymptomatic subjects. *J Bone Joint Surg Br* 1998;80:19-24.

4. Mahbub MH, Laskar MS, Seikh FA, et al: Prevalence of cervical spondylosis and musculoskeletal symptoms among coolies in a city of Bangladesh. *J Occup Health* 2006;48:69-73.

5. Berge J, Marque B, Vital JM, Senegas J, Caille JM: Age-related changes in the cervical spines of front-line rugby players. *Am J Sports Med* 1999;27:422-429.

6. Kartal A, Yildiran I, Senkoylu A, Korkusuz F: Soccer causes degenerative changes in the cervical spine. *Eur Spine J* 2004;13:76-82.

7. Tsirikos A, Papagelopoulos PJ, Giannakopoulos PN, et al: Degenerative spondyloarthropathy of the cervical and lumbar spine in jockeys. *Orthopedics* 2001;24:561-564.

8. Hendriksen IJ, Holewijn M: Degenerative changes of the spine of fighter pilots of the Royal Netherlands Air Force (RNLAF). *Aviat Space Environ Med* 1999;70:1057-1063.

9. Cote P, Cassidy JD, Carroll LJ, Kristman V: The annual incidence and course of neck pain in the general population: A population-based cohort study. *Pain* 2004;112:267-273.

10. Cote P, Cassidy JD, Carroll L: The Saskatchewan Health and Back Pain Survey: The prevalence of neck pain and related disability in Saskatchewan adults. *Spine* 1998;23:1689-1698.

11. Cote P, Cassidy JD, Carroll L: The factors associated with neck pain and its related disability in the Saskatchewan population. *Spine* 2000;25:1109-1117.

12. Radhakrishnan K, Litchy WJ, O'Fallon WM, Kurland LT: Epidemiology of cervical radiculopathy: A population-based study from Rochester, Minnesota, 1976 through 1990. *Brain* 1994;117:325-335.

13. Salemi G, Savettieri G, Meneghini F, et al: Prevalence of cervical spondylotic radiculopathy: A door-to-door survey in a Sicilian municipality. *Acta Neurol Scand* 1996;93:184-188.

14. Bengtsson A, Henriksson KG, Larsson J: Reduced high-energy phosphate levels in the painful muscles of patients with primary fibromyalgia. *Arthritis Rheum* 1986;29:817-821.

15. Larsson R, Oberg PA, Larsson SE: Changes of trapezius muscle blood flow and electromyography in chronic neck pain due to trapezius myalgia. *Pain* 1999;79:45-50.

16. Croft PR, Lewis M, Papageorgiou AC, et al: Risk factors for neck pain: A longitudinal study in the general population. *Pain* 2001;93:317-325.

17. Ferlic DC: The nerve supply of the cervical intervertebral disc in man. *Bull Johns Hopkins Hosp* 1963;113:347-351.

18. McLain RF: Mechanoreceptor endings in human cervical facet joints. *Spine* 1994;19:495-501.

19. Chen C, Lu Y, Kallakuri S, Patwardhan A, Cavanaugh JM: Distribution of A-delta and C-fiber receptors in the cervical facet joint capsule and their response to stretch. *J Bone Joint Surg Am* 2006;88:1807-1816.

20. Inami S, Shiga T, Tsujino A, Yabuki T, Okado N, Ochiai N: Immunohistochemical demonstration of nerve fibers in the synovial fold of the human cervical facet joint. *J Orthop Res* 2001;19:593-596.

21. Grubb SA, Kelly CK: Cervical discography: Clinical implications from 12 years of experience. *Spine* 2000;25:1382-1389.

22. Dwyer A, Aprill C, Bogduk N: Cervical zygapophyseal joint pain patterns: I. A study in normal volunteers. *Spine* 1990;15:453-457.

23. Chabot MC, Montgomery DM: The pathophysiology of axial and radicular neck pain. *Semin Spine Surg* 1995;7:2-8.

24. Cornefjord M, Olmarker K, Farley DB, Weinstein JN, Rydevik B: Neuropeptide changes in compressed spinal nerve roots. *Spine* 1995;20:670-673.

25. Cooper RG, Freemont AJ, Hoyland JA, et al: Herniated intervertebral disc-associated periradicular fibrosis and vascular abnormalities occur without inflammatory cell infiltration. *Spine* 1995;20:591-598.

26. Rydevik BL, Myers RR, Powell HC: Pressure increase in the dorsal root ganglion following mechanical compression. Closed compartment syndrome in nerve roots. *Spine* 1989;14:574-576.

27. Murata Y, Onda A, Rydevik B, Takahashi I, Takahashi K, Olmarker K: Changes in pain behavior and histologic changes caused by application of tumor necrosis factor-alpha to the dorsal root ganglion in rats. *Spine* 2006;31:530-535.

28. Hukuda S, Mochizuki T, Ogata M, Shichikawa K, Shimomura Y: Operations for cervical spondylotic myelopathy: A comparison of the results of anterior and posterior procedures. *J Bone Joint Surg Br* 1985;67:609-615.

29. Bohlman HH: Cervical spondylosis and myelopathy. *Instr Course Lect* 1995;44:81-97.

30. Penning L, Wilmink JT, van Woerden HH, Knol E: CT myelographic findings in degenerative disorders of the cervical spine: Clinical significance. *AJR Am J Roentgenol* 1986;146: 793-801.

31. Houser OW, Onofrio BM, Miller GM, Folger WN, Smith PL: Cervical spondylotic stenosis and myelopathy: Evaluation with computed tomographic myelography. *Mayo Clin Proc* 1994;69:557-563.

32. Ono K, Ebara S, Fuji T, Yonenobu K, Fujiwara K, Yamashita K: Myelopathy hand: New clinical signs of cervical cord damage. *J Bone Joint Surg Br* 1987;69:215-219.

33. Gu R, Zhu Q, Lin Y, Yang X, Gao Z, Tanaka Y: Dynamic canal encroachment of ligamentum flavum: An in vitro study of cadaveric specimens. *J Spinal Disord Tech* 2006;19:187-190.

34. Holmes A, Han ZH, Dang GT, Chen ZQ, Wang ZG, Fang J: Changes in cervical canal spinal volume during in vitro flexion-extension. *Spine* 1996; 21:1313-1319.

35. Mihara H, Ohnari K, Hachiya M, Kondo S, Yamada K: Cervical myelopathy caused by C3-C4 spondylosis in elderly patients: A radiographic analysis of pathogenesis. *Spine* 2000; 25:796-800.

36. Wang B, Liu H, Wang H, Zhou D: Segmental instability in cervical spondylotic myelopathy with severe disc degeneration. *Spine* 2006;31: 1327-1331.

37. Breig A, Turnbull I, Hassler O: Effects of mechanical stresses on the spinal cord in cervical spondylosis: A study on fresh cadaver material. *J Neurosurg* 1966;25:45-56.

38. Gooding MR, Wilson CB, Hoff JT: Experimental cervical myelopathy: Effects of ischemia and compression of the canine cervical spinal cord. *J Neurosurg* 1975;43:9-17.

39. Hukuda S, Wilson CB: Experimental cervical myelopathy: Effects of compression and ischemia on the canine cervical cord. *J Neurosurg* 1972;37: 631-652.

40. Doppman JL: The mechanism of ischemia in anteroposterior compression of the spinal cord 1975. *Invest Radiol* 1990;25:444-452.

41. Gooding MR: Pathogenesis of myelopathy in cervical spondylosis. *Lancet* 1974;2:1180-1181.

42. Henderson CM, Hennessy RG, Shuey HM Jr, Shackelford EG: Posterior-lateral foraminotomy as an exclusive operative technique for cervical radiculopathy: A review of 846 consecutively operated cases. *Neurosurgery* 1983;13:504-512.

43. Davidson RI, Dunn EJ, Metzmaker JN: The shoulder abduction test in the diagnosis of radicular pain in cervical extradural compressive monoradiculopathies. *Spine* 1981;6:441-446.

44. Cloward RB: Diaphragm paralysis from cervical disc lesions. *Br J Neurosurg* 1988;2:395-399.

45. Ebara S, Yonenobu K, Fujiwara K, Yamashita K, Ono K: Myelopathy hand characterized by muscle wasting: A different type of myelopathy hand in patients with cervical spondylosis. *Spine* 1988;13:785-791.

46. Gore DR, Sepic SB, Gardner GM: Roentgenographic findings of the cervical spine in asymptomatic people. *Spine* 1986;11:521-524.

47. Pavlov H, Torg JS, Robie B, Jahre C: Cervical spinal stenosis: Determination with vertebral body ratio method. *Radiology* 1987;164:771-775.

48. Prasad SS, O'Malley M, Caplan M, Shackleford IM, Pydisetty RK: MRI measurements of the cervical spine and their correlation to Pavlov's ratio. *Spine* 2003;28:1263-1268.

49. White AA III, Panjabi MM: Update on the evaluation of instability of the lower cervical spine. *Instr Course Lect* 1987;36:513-520.

50. Modic MT, Masaryk TJ, Mulopulos GP, Bundschuh C, Han JS, Bohlman H: Cervical radiculopathy: Prospective evaluation with surface coil MR imaging, CT with metrizamide, and metrizamide myelography. *Radiology* 1986;161:753-759.

51. Jahnke RW, Hart BL: Cervical stenosis, spondylosis, and herniated disc disease. *Radiol Clin North Am* 1991;29: 777-791.

52. Shafaie FF, Wippold FJ II, Gado M, Pilgram TK, Riew KD: Comparison of computed tomography myelography and magnetic resonance imaging in the evaluation of cervical spondylotic myelopathy and radiculopathy. *Spine* 1999;24:1781-1785.

53. Teresi LM, Lufkin RB, Reicher MA, et al: Asymptomatic degenerative disk disease and spondylosis of the cervical spine: MR imaging. *Radiology* 1987; 164:83-88.

54. Ohshio I, Hatayama A, Kaneda K, Takahara M, Nagashima K: Correlation between histopathologic features and magnetic resonance images of spinal cord lesions. *Spine* 1993;18:1140-1149.

55. Morio Y, Teshima R, Nagashima H, Nawata K, Yamasaki D, Nanjo Y: Correlation between operative outcomes of cervical compression myelopathy and MRI of the spinal cord. *Spine* 2001;26:1238-1245.

56. Matsumoto M, Toyama Y, Ishikawa M, Chiba K, Suzuki N, Fujimura Y: Increased signal intensity of the spinal cord on magnetic resonance images in cervical compressive myelopathy: Does it predict the outcome of conservative treatment? *Spine* 2000;25: 677-682.

57. Suri A, Chabbra RP, Mehta VS, Gaikwad S, Pandey RM: Effect of intramedullary signal changes on the surgical outcome of patients with cervical spondylotic myelopathy. *Spine J* 2003;3:33-45.

58. Bednarik J, Kadanka Z, Dusek L, et al: Presymptomatic spondylotic cervical cord compression. *Spine* 2004;29: 2260-2269.

59. Wada E, Ohmura M, Yonenobu K: Intramedullary changes of the spinal cord in cervical spondylotic myelopathy. *Spine* 1995;20:2226-2232.

60. Wada E, Yonenobu K, Suzuki S, Kanazawa A, Ochi T: Can intramedullary signal change on magnetic

resonance imaging predict surgical outcome in cervical spondylotic myelopathy? *Spine* 1999;24:455-462.

61. Papadopoulos CA, Katonis P, Papagelopoulos PJ, Karampekios S, Hadjipavlou AG: Surgical decompression for cervical spondylotic myelopathy: Correlation between operative outcomes and MRI of the spinal cord. *Orthopedics* 2004;27: 1087-1091.

62. Fukushima T, Ikata T, Taoka Y, Takata S: Magnetic resonance imaging study on spinal cord plasticity in patients with cervical compression myelopathy. *Spine* 1991;16 (10 suppl): S534-S538.

63. Matsuyama Y, Kawakami N, Yanase M, et al: Cervical myelopathy due to OPLL: Clinical evaluation by MRI and intraoperative spinal sonography. *J Spinal Disord Tech* 2004;17:401-404.

64. Uchida K, Kobayashi S, Yayama T, et al: Metabolic neuroimaging of the cervical spinal cord in patients with compressive myelopathy: A high-resolution positron emission tomography study. *J Neurosurg Spine* 2004;1: 72-79.

65. Dvorak J, Sutter M, Herdmann J: Cervical myelopathy: Clinical and neurophysiological evaluation. *Eur Spine J* 2003;12(suppl 2):S181-S187.

66. Simo M, Szirmai I, Aranyi Z: Superior sensitivity of motor over somatosensory evoked potentials in the diagnosis of cervical spondylotic myelopathy. *Eur J Neurol* 2004;11: 621-626.

67. Bednarik J, Kadanka Z, Vohanka S, et al: The value of somatosensory and motor evoked potentials in preclinical spondylotic cervical cord compression. *Eur Spine J* 1998;7: 493-500.

68. Chistyakov AV, Soustiel JF, Hafner H, Kaplan B, Feinsod M: The value of motor and somatosensory evoked potentials in evaluation of cervical myelopathy in the presence of peripheral neuropathy. *Spine* 2004;29: E239-E247.

69. Lyu RK, Tang LM, Chen CJ, Chen CM, Chang HS, Wu YR: The use of evoked potentials for clinical correlation and surgical outcome in cervical spondylotic myelopathy with intramedullary high signal intensity on MRI. *J Neurol Neurosurg Psychiatry* 2004;75:256-261.

70. Nakagawa Y, Tamaki T, Yamada H, Nishiura H: Discrepancy between decreases in the amplitude of compound muscle action potential and loss of motor function caused by ischemic and compressive insults to the spinal cord. *J Orthop Sci* 2002;7: 102-110.

71. Ashkan K, Johnston P, Moore AJ: A comparison of magnetic resonance imaging and neurophysiological studies in the assessment of cervical radiculopathy. *Br J Neurosurg* 2002;16: 146-148.

72. Berger AR, Busis NA, Logigian EL, Wierzbicka M, Shahani BT: Cervical root stimulation in the diagnosis of radiculopathy. *Neurology* 1987;37: 329-332.

73. Nardin RA, Patel MR, Gudas TF, Rutkove SB, Raynor EM: Electromyography and magnetic resonance imaging in the evaluation of radiculopathy. *Muscle Nerve* 1999;22: 151-155.

74. Wilbourn AJ, Aminoff MJ: AAEE minimonograph #32: The electrophysiologic examination in patients with radiculopathies. *Muscle Nerve* 1988;11:1099-1114.

75. Dillingham TR, Lauder TD, Andary M, et al: Identification of cervical radiculopathies: Optimizing the electromyographic screen. *Am J Phys Med Rehabil* 2001;80:84-91.

76. Philadelphia Panel: Philadelphia Panel evidence-based clinical practice guidelines on selected rehabilitation interventions for neck pain. *Phys Ther* 2001;81:1701-1717.

77. Wang WT, Olson SL, Campbell AH, Hanten WP, Gleeson PB: Effectiveness of physical therapy for patients with neck pain: An individualized approach using a clinical decision-

making algorithm. *Am J Phys Med Rehabil* 2003;82:203-221.

78. Chiu TT, Lam TH, Hedley AJ: A randomized controlled trial on the efficacy of exercise for patients with chronic neck pain. *Spine* 2005;30: E1-E7.

79. Olivero WC, Dulebohn SC: Results of halter cervical traction for the treatment of cervical radiculopathy: Retrospective review of 81 patients. *Neurosurg Focus* 2002;12:ECP1.

80. Joghataei MT, Arab AM, Khaksar H: The effect of cervical traction combined with conventional therapy on grip strength on patients with cervical radiculopathy. *Clin Rehabil* 2004;18: 879-887.

81. Bush K, Hillier S: Outcome of cervical radiculopathy treated with periradicular/epidural corticosteroid injections: A prospective study with independent clinical review. *Eur Spine J* 1996;5:319-325.

82. Cicala RS, Thoni K, Angel JJ: Long-term results of cervical epidural steroid injections. *Clin J Pain* 1989;5: 143-145.

83. Vallee JN, Feydy A, Carlier RY, Mutschler C, Mompoint D, Vallee CA: Chronic cervical radiculopathy: Lateral-approach periradicular corticosteroid injection. *Radiology* 2001; 218:886-892.

84. Rathmell JP, Aprill C, Bogduk N: Cervical transforaminal injection of steroids. *Anesthesiology* 2004;100: 1595-1600.

85. Gore DR, Sepic SB, Gardner GM, Murray MP: Neck pain: A long-term follow-up of 205 patients. *Spine* 1987; 12:1-5.

86. Kadanka Z, Mares M, Bednanik J, et al: Approaches to spondylotic cervical myelopathy: Conservative versus surgical results in a 3-year follow-up study. *Spine* 2002;27:2205-2211.

87. Kadanka Z, Mares M, Bednarik J, et al: Predictive factors for spondylotic cervical myelopathy treated conservatively or surgically. *Eur J Neurol* 2005;12:55-63.

88. DePalma AF, Subin DK: Study of the cervical syndrome. *Clin Orthop Relat Res* 1965;38:135-142.

89. Rothman RH, Rashbaum RF: Pathogenesis of signs and symptoms of cervical disc degeneration. *Instr Course Lect* 1978;27:203-215.

90. Schellhas KP, Smith MD, Gundry CR, Pollei SR: Cervical discogenic pain: Prospective correlation of magnetic resonance imaging and discography in asymptomatic subjects and pain sufferers. *Spine* 1996;21:300-312.

91. Zheng Y, Liew SM, Simmons ED: Value of magnetic resonance imaging and discography in determining the level of cervical discectomy and fusion. *Spine* 2004;29:2140-2146.

92. Carreon L, Glassman SD, Campbell MJ: Treatment of anterior cervical pseudoarthrosis: Posterior fusion versus anterior revision. *Spine J* 2006;6:154-156.

93. Kuhns CA, Geck MJ, Wang JC, Delamarter RB: An outcomes analysis of the treatment of cervical pseudarthrosis with posterior fusion. *Spine* 2005;30:2424-2429.

94. Albert TJ, Murrell SE: Surgical management of cervical radiculopathy. *J Am Acad Orthop Surg* 1999;7:368-376.

95. Clarke E, Robinson PK: Cervical myelopathy: A complication of cervical spondylosis. *Brain* 1956;79:483-510.

96. Lees F, Turner JW: Natural history and prognosis of cervical spondylosis. *BMJ* 1963;2:1607-1610.

97. Nurick S: The natural history and the results of surgical treatment of the spinal cord disorder associated with cervical spondylosis. *Brain* 1972;95:101-108.

98. Symon L, Lavender P: The surgical treatment of cervical spondylotic myelopathy. *Neurology* 1967;17:117-127.

99. Matsumoto M, Chiba K, Ishikawa M, Maruiwa H, Fujimura Y, Toyama Y: Relationships between outcomes of conservative treatment and magnetic resonance imaging findings in patients with mild cervical myelopathy caused by soft disc herniations. *Spine* 2001;26:1592-1598.

100. Onimus M, Destrumelle N, Gangloff S: Surgical treatment of cervical disk displacement: Anterior or posterior approach?. *Rev Chir Orthop Reparatrice Appar Mot* 1995;81:296-301.

101. Wirth FP, Dowd GC, Sanders HF, Wirth C: Cervical discectomy: A prospective analysis of three operative techniques. *Surg Neurol* 2000;53:340-348.

102. Herkowitz HN, Kurz LT, Overholt DP: Surgical management of cervical soft disc herniation: A comparison between the anterior and posterior approach. *Spine* 1990;15:1026-1030.

103. Rao RD, Gourab K, David KS: Operative treatment of cervical spondylotic myelopathy. *J Bone Joint Surg Am* 2006;88:1619-1640.

104. Robinson RA, Smith GW: Anterolateral cervical disc removal and interbody fusion for cervical disc syndrome. *Bull Johns Hopkins Hosp* 1955;96:223-224.

105. Yonenobu K, Okada K, Fuji T, Fujiwara K, Yamashita K, Ono K: Causes of neurologic deterioration following surgical treatment of cervical myelopathy. *Spine* 1986;11:818-823.

106. Connolly ES, Seymour RJ, Adams JE: Clinical evaluation of anterior cervical fusion for degenerative cervical disc disease. *J Neurosurg* 1965;23:431-437.

107. Stevens JM, Clifton AG, Whitear P: Appearances of posterior osteophytes after sound anterior interbody fusion in the cervical spine: A high-definition computed myelographic study. *Neuroradiology* 1993;35:227-228.

108. Bertalanffy H, Eggert HR: Complications of anterior cervical discectomy without fusion in 450 consecutive patients. *Acta Neurochir (Wien)* 1989;99:41-50.

109. Yamamoto I, Ikeda A, Shibuya N, Tsugane R, Sato O: Clinical long-term results of anterior discectomy without interbody fusion for cervical disc disease. *Spine* 1991;16:272-279.

110. Lieu AS, Howng SL: Clinical results of anterior cervical discectomy without interbody fusion. *Kaohsiung J Med Sci* 1998;14:212-216.

111. Emery SE, Bolesta MJ, Banks MA, Jones PK: Robinson anterior cervical fusion comparison of the standard and modified techniques. *Spine* 1994;19:660-663.

112. Bohlman HH, Emery SE, Goodfellow DB, Jones PK: Robinson anterior cervical discectomy and arthrodesis for cervical radiculopathy: Long-term follow-up of one hundred and twenty-two patients. *J Bone Joint Surg Am* 1993;75:1298-1307.

113. Clements DH, O'Leary PF: Anterior cervical discectomy and fusion. *Spine* 1990;15:1023-1025.

114. Riley LH Jr, Robinson RA, Johnson KA, Walker AE: The results of anterior interbody fusion of the cervical spine: Review of ninety-three consecutive cases. *J Neurosurg* 1969;30:127-133.

115. Papadopoulos EC, Huang RC, Girardi FP, Synnott K, Cammisa FP Jr: Three-level anterior cervical discectomy and fusion with plate fixation: Radiographic and clinical results. *Spine* 2006;31:897-902.

116. Samartzis D, Shen FH, Matthews DK, Yoon ST, Goldberg EJ, An HS: Comparison of allograft to autograft in multilevel anterior cervical discectomy and fusion with rigid plate fixation. *Spine J* 2003;3:451-459.

117. Moreland DB, Asch HL, Clabeaux DE, et al: Anterior cervical discectomy and fusion with implantable titanium cage: Initial impressions, patient outcomes and comparison to fusion with allograft. *Spine J* 2004;4:184-191.

118. Frederic S, Benedict R, Payer M: Implantation of an empty carbon fiber cage or a tricortical iliac crest autograft after cervical discectomy for single-level disc herniation: A prospective comparative study. *J Neurosurg Spine* 2006;4:292-299.

119. Sekerci Z, Ugur A, Ergun R, Sanli M: Early changes in the cervical forami-

nal area after anterior interbody fusion with polyetheretherketone (PEEK) cage containing synthetic bone particulate: A prospective study of 20 cases. *Neurol Res* 2006;28:568-571.

120. Hughes SS, Pringle T, Phillips F, Emery S: Settling of fibula strut grafts following multilevel anterior cervical corpectomy: A radiographic evaluation. *Spine* 2006;31:1911-1915.

121. Jones J, Yoo J, Hart R: Delayed fracture of fibular strut allograft following multilevel anterior cervical spine corpectomy and fusion. *Spine* 2006;31: E595-E599.

122. Wang JC, Hart RA, Emery SE, Bohlman HH: Graft migration or displacement after multilevel cervical corpectomy and strut grafting. *Spine* 2003;28:1016-1022.

123. Woiciechowsky C: Distractable vertebral cages for reconstruction after cervical corpectomy. *Spine* 2005;30: 1736-1741.

124. Sevki K, Mehmet T, Ufuk T, Azmi H, Mercan S, Erkal B: Results of surgical treatment for degenerative cervical myelopathy: Anterior cervical corpectomy and stabilization. *Spine* 2004; 29:2493-2500.

125. Daubs MD: Early failures following cervical corpectomy reconstruction with titanium mesh cages and anterior plating. *Spine* 2005;30:1402-1406.

126. Hee HT, Majd ME, Holt RT, Whitecloud TS III, Pienkowski D: Complications of multilevel cervical corpectomies and reconstruction with titanium cages and anterior plating. *J Spinal Disord Tech* 2003;16:1-8.

127. Park JB, Cho YS, Riew KD: Development of adjacent-level ossification in patients with an anterior cervical plate. *J Bone Joint Surg Am* 2005;87: 558-563.

128. Wang JC, McDonough PW, Endow KK, Delamarter RB: Increased fusion rates with cervical plating for two-level anterior cervical discectomy and fusion. *Spine* 2000;25:41-45.

129. Connolly PJ, Esses SI, Kostuik JP: Anterior cervical fusion: Outcome

analysis of patients fused with and without anterior cervical plates. *J Spinal Disord* 1996;9:202-206.

130. Wang JC, McDonough PW, Endow K, Kanim LE, Delamarter RB: The effect of cervical plating on single-level anterior cervical discectomy and fusion. *J Spinal Disord* 1999;12: 467-471.

131. Samartzis D, Shen FH, Lyon C, Phillips M, Goldberg EJ, An HS: Does rigid instrumentation increase the fusion rate in one-level anterior cervical discectomy and fusion? *Spine J* 2004; 4:636-643.

132. Kaiser MG, Haid RW Jr, Subach BR, Barnes B, Rodts GE Jr: Anterior cervical plating enhances arthrodesis after discectomy and fusion with cortical allograft. *Neurosurgery* 2002;50: 229-238.

133. Cauthen JC, Kinard RE, Vogler JB, et al: Outcome analysis of noninstrumented anterior cervical discectomy and interbody fusion in 348 patients. *Spine* 1998;23:188-192.

134. Martin GJ Jr, Haid RW Jr, MacMillan M, Rodts GE Jr, Berkman R: Anterior cervical discectomy with freeze-dried fibula allograft: Overview of 317 cases and literature review. *Spine* 1999;24:852-859.

135. Epstein NE: The management of one-level anterior cervical corpectomy with fusion using Atlantis hybrid plates: Preliminary experience. *J Spinal Disord* 2000;13:324-328.

136. Vaccaro AR, Falatyn SP, Scuderi GJ, et al: Early failure of long segment anterior cervical plate fixation. *J Spinal Disord* 1998;11:410-415.

137. Sasso RC, Ruggiero RA Jr, Reilly TM, Hall PV: Early reconstruction failures after multilevel cervical corpectomy. *Spine* 2003;28:140-142.

138. Hilibrand A, Berta S, Daffner S: The impact of anterior cervical fusion upon overall range of motion and neck flexibility. *Proceedings of the Annual Meeting of the North American Spine Society*. Burr Ridge, IL, North American Spine Society, 2005.

139. Rao RD, Wang M, McGrady LM, Perlewitz TJ, David KS: Does anterior plating of the cervical spine predispose to adjacent segment changes? *Spine* 2005;30:2788-2793.

140. Dmitriev AE, Cunningham BW, Hu N, Sell G, Vigna F, McAfee PC: Adjacent level intradiscal pressure and segmental kinematics following a cervical total disc arthroplasty: An in vitro human cadaveric model. *Spine* 2005;30:1165-1172.

141. Puttlitz CM, Rousseau MA, Xu Z, Hu S, Tay BK, Lotz JC: Intervertebral disc replacement maintains cervical spine kinetics. *Spine* 2004;29:2809-2814.

142. Goffin J, Van Calenbergh F, van Loon J, et al: Intermediate follow-up after treatment of degenerative disc disease with the Bryan Cervical Disc Prosthesis: Single-level and bi-level. *Spine* 2003;28:2673-2678.

143. Pracyk JB, Traynelis VC: Treatment of the painful motion segment: Cervical arthroplasty. *Spine* 2005;30 (16 suppl):S23-S32.

144. Anderson PA, Sasso RC, Rouleau JP, Carlson CS, Goffin J: The Bryan Cervical Disc: Wear properties and early clinical results. *Spine J* 2004;4 (6 suppl):303S-309S.

145. Pickett GE, Sekhon LH, Sears WR, Duggal N: Complications with cervical arthroplasty. *J Neurosurg Spine* 2006;4:98-105.

146. Coric D, Finger F, Boltes P: Prospective randomized controlled study of the Bryan Cervical Disc: Early clinical results from a single investigational site. *J Neurosurg Spine* 2006;4:31-35.

147. Sasso RC, Hacker R, Heller JG: Artificial disc versus fusion: Abstract: A prospective, randomized study with 2-year follow-up on 99 patients. *Final Program: The 34th Annual Meeting of the Cervical Spine Research Society*. Rosemont, IL, Cervical Spine Research Society, 2006, p 66.

148. Robertson JT, Papadopoulos SM, Traynelis VC: Assessment of adjacent-segment disease in patients treated with cervical fusion or arthro-

plasty: A prospective 2-year study. *J Neurosurg Spine* 2005;3:417-423.

149. Leung C, Casey AT, Goffin J, et al: Clinical significance of heterotopic ossification in cervical disc replacement: A prospective multicenter clinical trial. *Neurosurgery* 2005;57:759-763.

150. Shim CS, Lee SH, Park HJ, Kang HS, Hwang JH: Early clinical and radiologic outcomes of cervical arthroplasty with Bryan Cervical Disc prosthesis. *J Spinal Disord Tech* 2006;19:465-470.

151. Scoville WB: Types of cervical disk lesions and their surgical approaches. *JAMA* 1966;196:479-481.

152. Russell SM, Benjamin V: Posterior surgical approach to the cervical neural foramen for intervertebral disc disease. *Neurosurgery* 2004;54:662-666.

153. Adamson TE: Microendoscopic posterior cervical laminoforaminotomy for unilateral radiculopathy: Results of a new technique in 100 cases. *J Neurosurg* 2001;95(1 suppl): 51-57.

154. Mikawa Y, Shikata J, Yamamuro T: Spinal deformity and instability after multilevel cervical laminectomy. *Spine* 1987;12:6-11.

155. Ishida Y, Suzuki K, Ohmori K, Kikata Y, Hattori Y: Critical analysis of extensive cervical laminectomy. *Neurosurgery* 1989;24:215-222.

156. Naito M, Ogata K, Kurose S, Oyama M: Canal-expansive laminoplasty in 83 patients with cervical myelopathy: A comparative study of three different procedures. *Int Orthop* 1994;18:347-351.

157. Itoh T, Tsuji H: Technical improvements and results of laminoplasty for compressive myelopathy in the cervical spine. *Spine* 1985;10:729-736.

158. Hirabayashi K, Toyama Y, Chiba K: Expansive laminoplasty for myelopathy in ossification of the longitudinal ligament. *Clin Orthop Relat Res* 1999;359:35-48.

159. Deutsch H, Mummaneni PV, Rodts GE, Haid RW: Posterior cervical laminoplasty using a new plating system: Technical note. *J Spinal Disord Tech* 2004;17:317-320.

160. O'Brien MF, Peterson D, Casey AT, Crockard HA: A novel technique for laminoplasty augmentation of spinal canal area using titanium miniplate stabilization: A computerized morphometric analysis. *Spine* 1996;21:474-484.

161. Guigui P, Benoist M, Deburge A: Spinal deformity and instability after multilevel cervical laminectomy for spondylotic myelopathy. *Spine* 1998;23:440-447.

162. Kaptain GJ, Simmons NE, Replogle RE, Pobereskin L: Incidence and outcome of kyphotic deformity following laminectomy for cervical spondylotic myelopathy. *J Neurosurg* 2000;93(2 suppl):199-204.

163. Kumar VG, Rea GL, Mervis LJ, McGregor JM: Cervical spondylotic myelopathy: Functional and radiographic long-term outcome after laminectomy and posterior fusion. *Neurosurgery* 1999;44:771-778.

164. Epstein NE: Laminectomy with posterior wiring and fusion for cervical ossification of the posterior longitudinal ligament, spondylosis, ossification of the yellow ligament, stenosis, and instability: A study of 5 patients. *J Spinal Disord* 1999;12:461-466.

165. Houten JK, Cooper PR: Laminectomy and posterior cervical plating for multilevel cervical spondylotic myelopathy and ossification of the posterior longitudinal ligament: Effects on cervical alignment, spinal cord compression, and neurological outcome. *Neurosurgery* 2003;52:1081-1088.

166. Heller JG, Edwards CC II, Murakami H, Rodts GE: Laminoplasty versus laminectomy and fusion for multilevel cervical myelopathy: An independent matched cohort analysis. *Spine* 2001;26:1330-1336.

167. Abumi K, Kaneda K, Shono Y, Fujiya M: One-stage posterior decompression and reconstruction of the cervical spine by using pedicle screw fixation systems. *J Neurosurg* 1999;90(1 suppl):19-26.

168. Callahan RA, Johnson RM, Margolis RN, Keggi KJ, Albright JA, Southwick WO: Cervical facet fusion for control of instability following laminectomy. *J Bone Joint Surg Am* 1977;59:991-1002.

169. Hamanishi C, Tanaka S: Bilateral multilevel laminectomy with or without posterolateral fusion for cervical spondylotic myelopathy: Relationship to type of onset and time until operation. *J Neurosurg* 1996;85:447-451.

170. Peolsson A, Vavruch L, Oberg B: Predictive factors for arm pain, neck pain, neck specific disability and health after anterior cervical decompression and fusion. *Acta Neurochir (Wien)* 2006;148:167-173.

171. Palit M, Schofferman J, Goldthwaite N, et al: Anterior discectomy and fusion for the management of neck pain. *Spine* 1999;24:2224-2228.

172. Gore DR, Sepic SB: Anterior cervical fusion for degenerated or protruded discs. A review of one hundred forty-six patients. *Spine* 1984;9:667-671.

173. Goldberg EJ, Singh K, Van U, Garretson R, An HS: Comparing outcomes of anterior cervical discectomy and fusion in workman's versus non-workman's compensation population. *Spine J* 2002;2:408-414.

174. Arnasson O, Carlsson CA, Pelletieri L: Surgical and conservative treatment of cervical spondylotic radiculopathy and myelopathy. *Acta Neurochir (Wien)* 1987;84:48-53.

175. Lunsford LD, Bissonette DJ, Jannetta PJ, Sheptak PE, Zorub DS: Anterior surgery for cervical disc disease: Part 1. Treatment of lateral cervical disc herniation in 253 cases. *J Neurosurg* 1980;53:1-11.

176. Peolsson A, Hedlund R, Vavruch L, Oberg B: Predictive factors for the outcome of anterior cervical decompression and fusion. *Eur Spine J* 2003;12:274-280.

177. Fujiwara K, Yonenobu K, Ebara S, Yamashita K, Ono K: The prognosis of surgery for cervical compression my-

elopathy: An analysis of the factors involved. *J Bone Joint Surg Br* 1989;71: 393-398.

178. Kawaguchi Y, Kanamori M, Ishihara H, Ohmori K, Abe Y, Kimura T: Pathomechanism of myelopathy and surgical results of laminoplasty in elderly patients with cervical spondylosis. *Spine* 2003;28:2209-2214.

179. Emery SE, Bohlman HH, Bolesta MJ, Jones PK: Anterior cervical decompression and arthrodesis for the treatment of cervical spondylotic myelopathy: Two to seventeen-year follow-up. *J Bone Joint Surg Am* 1998; 80:941-951.

180. Prabhu K, Babu KS, Samuel S, Chacko AG: Rapid opening and closing of the hand as a measure of early neurologic recovery in the upper extremity after surgery for cervical spondylotic myelopathy. *Arch Phys Med Rehabil* 2005;86:105-108.

181. Ratliff JK, Cooper PR: Cervical laminoplasty: A critical review. *J Neurosurg* 2003;98(3 suppl):230-238.

182. Wada E, Suzuki S, Kanazawa A, Matsuoka T, Miyamoto S, Yonenobu K: Subtotal corpectomy versus laminoplasty for multilevel cervical spondylotic myelopathy: A long-term follow-up study over 10 years. *Spine* 2001;26:1443-1448.

183. Flynn TB: Neurologic complications of anterior cervical interbody fusion. *Spine* 1982;7:536-539.

184. Apfelbaum RI, Kriskovich MD, Haller JR: On the incidence, cause, and prevention of recurrent laryngeal nerve palsies during anterior cervical spine surgery. *Spine* 2000;25:2906-2912.

185. Heeneman H: Vocal cord paralysis following approaches to the anterior cervical spine. *Laryngoscope* 1973;83: 17-21.

186. Jung A, Schramm J, Lehnerdt K, Herberhold C: Recurrent laryngeal nerve palsy during anterior cervical spine surgery: A prospective study. *J Neurosurg Spine* 2005;2:123-127.

187. Kilburg C, Sullivan HG, Mathiason MA: Effect of approach side during anterior cervical discectomy and fusion on the incidence of recurrent laryngeal nerve injury. *J Neurosurg Spine* 2006;4:273-277.

188. Yonenobu K, Hosono N, Iwasaki M, Asano M, Ono K: Neurologic complications of surgery for cervical compression myelopathy. *Spine* 1991;16: 1277-1282.

189. Ikenaga M, Shikata J, Tanaka C: Radiculopathy of C-5 after anterior decompression for cervical myelopathy. *J Neurosurg Spine* 2005;3:210-217.

190. Komagata M, Nishiyama M, Endo K, Ikegami H, Tanaka S, Imakiire A: Prophylaxis of C5 palsy after cervical expansive laminoplasty by bilateral partial foraminotomy. *Spine J* 2004;4: 650-655.

191. Jimenez JC, Sani S, Braverman B, Deutsch H, Ratliff JK: Palsies of the fifth cervical nerve root after cervical decompression: Prevention using continuous intraoperative electromyography monitoring. *J Neurosurg Spine* 2005;3:92-97.

192. Hosono N, Yonenobu K, Ono K: Neck and shoulder pain after laminoplasty: A noticeable complication. *Spine* 1996;21:1969-1973.

193. Yoshida M, Otani K, Shibasaki K, Ueda S: Expansive laminoplasty with reattachment of spinous process and extensor musculature for cervical myelopathy. *Spine* 1992;17:491-497.

194. Shiraishi T, Fukuda K, Yato Y, Nakamura M, Ikegami T: Results of skip laminectomy-minimum 2-year follow-up study compared with open-door laminoplasty. *Spine* 2003; 28:2667-2672.

195. Kawaguchi Y, Kanamori M, Ishiara H, Nobukiyo M, Seki S, Kimura T: Preventive measures for axial symptoms following cervical laminoplasty. *J Spinal Disord Tech* 2003;16:497-501.

196. Takeuchi K, Yokoyama T, Aburakawa S, et al: Axial symptoms after cervical laminoplasty with C3 laminectomy compared with conventional C3-C7

laminoplasty: A modified laminoplasty preserving the semispinalis cervicis inserted into axis. *Spine* 2005;30: 2544-2549.

197. Hosono N, Sakaura H, Mukai Y, Yoshikawa H: Abstract: The source of axial pain after cervical laminoplasty-C7 is more crucial than deep extensor muscles. *Final Program: The 34th Annual Meeting of the Cervical Spine Research Society*. Rosemont, IL, Cervical Spine Research Society, 2006, p 112.

198. Iizuka H, Iizuka Y, Nakagawa Y, et al: Interlaminar bony fusion after cervical laminoplasty: Its characteristics and relationship with clinical results. *Spine* 2006;31:644-647.

199. Hanai K, Fujiyoshi F, Kamei K: Subtotal vertebrectomy and spinal fusion for cervical spondylotic myelopathy. *Spine* 1986;11:310-315.

200. Kaptain GJ, Simmons NE, Replogle RE, Pobereskin L: Incidence and outcome of kyphotic deformity following laminectomy for cervical spondylotic myelopathy. *J Neurosurg* 2000;93(2 suppl):199-204.

201. Takeshita K, Seichi A, Akune T, Kawamura N, Kawaguchi H, Nakamura K: Can laminoplasty maintain the cervical alignment even when the C2 lamina is contained? *Spine* 2005; 30:1294-1298.

202. Suk K-S, Kim K-T, Lee J-H, Lee S-H: Sagittal alignment of the cervical spine after laminoplasty. *Proceedings of the North American Spine Society 21st Annual Meeting*. Burr Ridge, IL, North American Spine Society, 2006.

203. Bazaz R, Lee MJ, Yoo JU: Incidence of dysphagia after anterior cervical spine surgery: A prospective study. *Spine* 2002;27:2453-2458.

204. Riley LH III, Skolasky RL, Albert TJ, Vaccaro AR, Heller JG: Dysphagia after anterior cervical decompression and fusion: Prevalence and risk factors from a longitudinal cohort study. *Spine* 2005;30:2564-2569.

205. Hilibrand AS, Carlson GD, Palumbo MA, Jones PK, Bohlman HH: Radiculopathy and myelopathy at seg-

ments adjacent to the site of a previous anterior cervical arthrodesis. *J Bone Joint Surg Am* 1999;81:519-528.

206. Lowery GL, McDonough RF: The significance of hardware failure in anterior cervical plate fixation: Patients with 2- to 7-year follow-up. *Spine* 1998;23:181-186.

207. Geyer TE, Foy MA: Oral extrusion of a screw after anterior cervical spine plating. *Spine* 2001;26:1814-1816.

208. Pompili A, Canitano S, Caroli F, et al: Asymptomatic esophageal perforation caused by late screw migration after anterior cervical plating: Report of a case and review of relevant literature. *Spine* 2002;27:E499-E502.

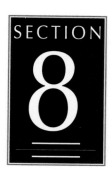

# SECTION 8

# Pediatrics

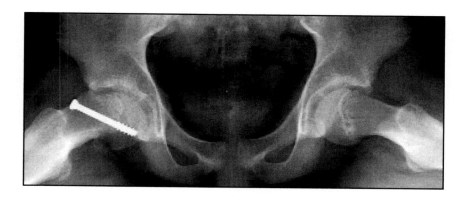

# Slipped Capital Femoral Epiphysis

Randall T. Loder, MD
David D. Aronsson, MD
Stuart L. Weinstein, MD
Gert J. Breur, DVM, PhD
Reinhold Ganz, MD
Michael Leunig, MD

## Abstract

*Slipped capital femoral epiphysis (SCFE) is a common adolescent hip disorder. The etiology of SCFE includes biomechanical and biochemical factors. SCFEs are classified as stable and unstable and are more common in boys than girls and in certain racial groups; most children with SCFEs are obese. Bilateral SCFEs may have a simultaneous or sequential presentation.*

*Imaging studies show a posterior slip of the epiphysis relative to the metaphysis, seen early on lateral radiographs. The most common and effective initial treatment for stable SCFEs is in situ central single-screw fixation; other options include epiphysiodesis, and osteotomy with or without surgical dislocation of the hip. Later reconstruction options, typically reserved for the child with functional abnormalities, include proximal femoral osteotomy, or surgical dislocation of the hip with removal of metaphyseal prominent bone to remove the source of femoroacetabular impingement. Unstable SCFEs have an increased risk of osteonecrosis; the role of reduction, methods of fixation, and decompression are controversial. The natural history of untreated SCFEs is associated with the risk of progression and later degenerative joint disease.*

*Based on treatment methods of 30 to 40 years ago, in situ fixation provided the best long-term function with the lowest risk of complications and the most effective delay of degenerative arthritis regardless of the severity of the SCFE. Newer technologies and techniques are allowing the reevaluation of the role of either acute or later reconstructive osteotomy. It has not yet been determined if these improved techniques will result in better outcomes than in the past. Surgical dislocation of the hip with epiphyseal orientation is a considered treatment option for those technically adept at the procedure; however, the long-term outcome compared with in situ fixation is still unknown.*

**Instr Course Lect 2008;57:473-498.**

Slipped capital femoral epiphysis (SCFE) is an adolescent hip disorder in which there is a displacement of the capital femoral epiphysis from the metaphysis through the physis. The term SCFE is a misnomer because it is actually the metaphysis that moves superiorly and anteriorly, with the epiphysis held in the acetabulum by the ligamentum teres (Figure 1). An apparent varus relationship between the epiphysis and metaphysis exists in most patients, but occasionally the epiphysis displaces laterally and superiorly in relation to the metaphysis (valgus SCFE).[1-4] Most SCFEs have an idiopathic etiology, although they also can occur from a known endocrine disorder, renal failure osteodystrophy, or previous radiation therapy.[5-10] This chapter is limited to a discussion of idiopathic SCFE.

## Epidemiology and Demographics

The incidence of SCFE is not completely known. The reported incidence ranges from 0.2 per 100,000 people in eastern Japan, 2.13 per 100,000 in the southwestern United States, and 10.08 per 100,000 people in the northeastern United States.[11,12] Recent studies indicate that the overall incidence of SCFE in the United States is 10.8 per 100,000 people, but in Japan has increased to 2.22 per 100,000 for boys and 0.76 per 100,000 for girls.[13,14] Although most studies show a male predominance, as seen early in this century when 90% of all SCFE incidents occurred in males, recent studies show that males account for only 60% of patients with SCFE.[15] The average duration of symptoms for children with chronic SCFEs, with no difference noted by gender, is 5 months; however, two recent

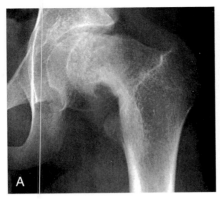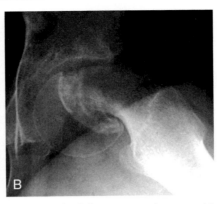

**Figure 1** AP (**A**) and frog-lateral (**B**) radiographs of a left SCFE in a boy age 13 years, 7 months. Note the superior and anterior displacement of the metaphysis relative to the epiphysis and the remodeling with a bony callus/buttress inferiorly and posteriorly.

studies noted a decrease to between 2 and 3 months.[16,17] The average age at diagnosis is 13.5 years for boys and 12.0 years for girls, with a typical range for both genders from 9 to 16 years.[18] Newer data indicate a younger age at diagnosis for children with SCFE, likely a result of the earlier maturation of children.[13] Most children with SCFE are obese; at least 50% of the children with SCFE are above the 95th percentile for weight based on age.[18,19] Using body mass index to evaluate body habitus, more recent studies have shown an average body mass index of between 25 and 30 kg/m$^2$ (above the 85th percentile).[17,20-24] Children with bilateral SCFE have an even greater average body mass index (31.1 kg/m$^2$) than children with unilateral SCFE (26.8 kg/m$^2$).[22] The age of onset decreases with increasing obesity; onset occurs at 12.4 years for those above the 95th percentile for weight based on age, and at 14.3 years for those under the 10th percentile for weight based on age.[18] Although variability in chronologic age exists, SCFE occurs in a more narrow physiologic age range—the "narrow window" of bone age.[25,26] In latitudes north of 40°, SCFE presents more frequently in the late summer and fall months[27-33] (Figure 2, A).

The reported incidence of bilateral SCFE is variable and depends on the study, method of radiographic measurement, the child's race, and treatment method. Most studies report an incidence of between 18% and 50%; however, recent studies with follow-up into adulthood describe the incidence of bilaterality as high as 63%.[18,30,34,35] The percentage of bilaterality is higher in blacks (34%) than in Hispanics (17%), whites (17%), or Asians (18%).[18] Treatment may affect the incidence of bilaterality; the prevalence of bilaterality in those treated with in situ fixation in one study was 36%, and 7% in those treated with a spica cast.[36] Therefore, close attention to the opposite normal hip is mandatory in those children with a unilateral SCFE treated with in situ fixation. Children who are physiologically younger at the initial presentation of unilateral SCFE are at higher risk for development of a contralateral SCFE. In a study of 50 children with unilateral SCFE, Stasikelis and associates[37] used a modified Oxford hip score to correlate bone age with the subsequent development of a contralateral SCFE and found an occurrence of 85% in hips with a score of 16, 11% in hips with a score of 21, and no occurrence of contralateral SCFE with a score of 22 or more.

Of those with bilateral SCFE, 50% to 60% of patients present with bilateral involvement. In the 40% with sequential bilateral progression, 80% to 90% of the second SCFEs occur within the first 18 months after the first SCFE.[18,30,38-41] The age at presentation is younger in children who present with a unilateral SCFE and have later development of bilateral SCFEs compared with those with a unilateral SCFE who do not have later development of bilateral SCFEs.[27,37,40-42] This age difference is seen in both the chronologic age (12 versus 13 years of age) as well as in the pelvic bone age. Of those with unilateral SCFEs, 60% occur in the left hip.

There is racial variability in the incidence of SCFE. The relative racial frequency of SCFE is 1.0 for whites, 4.5 for Pacific Islanders, 2.2 for blacks, 1.05 for Amerindian peoples (Native Americans and Hispanics), 0.5 for Indonesian-Malay (such as Chinese, Japanese, Thai, Vietnamese), and 0.1 for Indo-Mediterranean people (Near East, North African, or Indian subcontinent ancestry).[18] More recent data indicate that these numbers, relative to occurrence in whites (1.0) is 5.6 for Polynesians, 3.9 for blacks, and 2.5 for Hispanics[13,43] (Figure 2, B). These racial differences most likely reflect the average body weights for each racial group and further support the major role that obesity and mechanical stress play in the etiology of SCFE.[18] A less likely explanation for the differences is racial variability in acetabular depth and femoral head coverage. One study showed that the acetabular depth in black children was greater than in white children; however, another study did not support this finding.[44,45]

## Classification

SCFE is classified both by its clinical nature and by its magnitude. The traditional clinical classification is preslip, acute, chronic, and acute-on-chronic and is based on the patient's history, physical examination, and radiographs.[46-50]

In the preslip stage, patients usually report weakness in the leg, limping, or exertional pain in the groin or the knee, which are further provoked by prolonged standing or walking. On physical examination, the most consistent positive finding is lack of internal rotation. On radiographs, generalized bone atrophy of the hemipelvis and upper femur is noted in patients with limited activity or limp, as well as potential for widening and irregularity of the physis.[51]

An acute SCFE is defined as that occurring in patients with symptoms for fewer than 3 weeks with an abrupt displacement through the proximal physis in which there was a preexisting epiphyseolysis.[46] In 67% of patients with acute SCFEs, a 1- to 3-month history of mild prodromal symptoms occurs before an acute episode, indicating that a preslip or a mild SCFE existed before the acute episode.[1,46,49,50,52] The acute episode may consist of an activity as trivial as turning over in bed. Physical examination shows an external rotation deformity, shortening, and marked limitation of motion secondary to pain that is usually severe enough to prevent weight bearing. Acute SCFEs represent

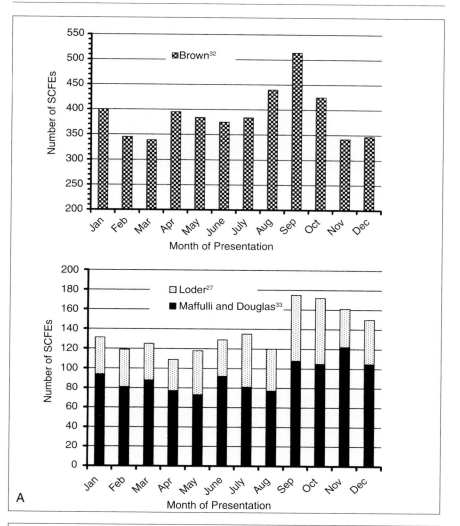

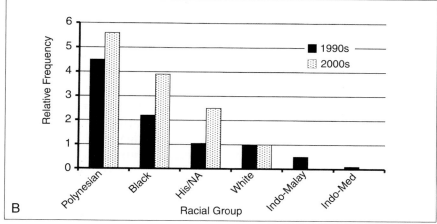

**Figure 2**  **A,** Seasonal variation in the month of presentation of children with SCFE north of the 40 N° latitude; data combined from three recent studies. **B,** The relative racial frequency of children with SCFE using the white population as a norm of 1.0. The studies were either published in the 1990s or 2000s; note the increase in frequency in the Polynesian, black, and Hispanic/Native American groups between the 1990s and the first decade of the 21st century.

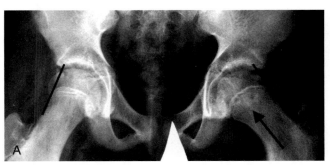
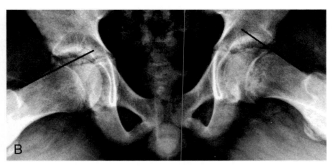

**Figure 3** Radiographs of a 15-year-old boy with a mild left SCFE. **A,** The metaphyseal blanch sign is a radiographic double density seen on the AP view at the level of the metaphysis (*arrow*); this double density reflects the posterior cortical lip of the epiphysis as it is beginning to slip posteriorly and is radiographically superimposed on the metaphyseal density. Klein's line is a line along the anterior or superior aspect of the femoral neck; the epiphysis should normally intersect this line (right hip). In an early SCFE the epiphysis will be flush with or even below this line (left hip). **B,** The frog-lateral radiograph shows early slipping and step-off at the physeal level and also an abnormal Klein's line on the left compared with the right.

10% to 15% of SCFEs in most large studies.[41,50]

Chronic SCFEs account for 85% of all slips; patients usually present with more than 3 weeks of groin, thigh, and knee pain and often have a history of exacerbations and remissions of the pain and limp.[41] The initial symptom is frequently knee or lower thigh pain, emphasizing the importance of a hip examination in a child reporting knee pain.[16,53,54] Physical examination shows an antalgic gait, with loss of internal rotation, abduction, and flexion of the hip.[55] In severe instances, there is a limb-length discrepancy with the lower extremity in external rotation. As the hip is flexed, the lower extremity spontaneously assumes an increased external rotation position. Acute-on-chronic SCFEs are those with initial chronic symptoms and the subsequent development of acute symptoms.

The traditional classification is based on the memory of the child and parent and may be inaccurate. Newer, more clinically useful classifications are based on physeal stability, which provide a prognosis regarding subsequent hip osteonecrosis. There are two such classifications:

clinical and radiographic. The clinical classification is based on the degree to which the child is able to ambulate.[56] A stable SCFE is defined as one in which the child is able to ambulate with or without crutches, whereas an unstable SCFE is defined as one in which the child cannot ambulate with or without crutches. By contrast, the radiographic classification system is based on the presence or absence of a hip effusion on ultrasonography.[57,58] The absence of metaphyseal remodeling and the presence of an effusion define an unstable SCFE; the presence of metaphyseal remodeling and the absence of an effusion define a stable SCFE.

Unstable SCFEs have a much higher incidence of osteonecrosis (up to 50% in some studies) compared with stable SCFEs (nearly 0%).[56] The high complication rates associated with unstable slip are most likely secondary to vascular injury caused at the time of the initial displacement.[56,59] Osteonecrosis correlates with results of pretreatment bone scans. A "cold" bone scan (showing the absence of vascularity) essentially is seen with unstable SCFEs. When a cold bone scan is present, the subsequent develop-

ment of osteonecrosis is 80% to 100%.[60] A child with unstable SCFE has symptoms similar to those of a child with a hip fracture, and the SCFE may be considered as a type of Salter-Harris I fracture. The child is in severe pain and resists any passive or active attempts to move the lower extremity, which is held in a flexed and externally rotated position.

## Imaging

Radiographs of SCFEs show an inferior and posterior slip of the proximal femoral epiphysis relative to the metaphysis. In a gradual slip, radiographic signs of remodeling on the superior and anterior femoral metaphysis are present along with periosteal new bone formation at the epiphyseal-metaphyseal junction posteriorly and inferiorly. In the early SCFE, the changes can be subtle with only posterior displacement.[55] As such, it is often only seen early on the lateral view, and both AP and lateral radiographs must be obtained. Other radiographic signs of an early SCFE are the metaphyseal blanch sign of Steel and Klein's line[61,62] (Figure 3). The metaphyseal blanch sign of Steel is a radiographic double density seen on the AP view

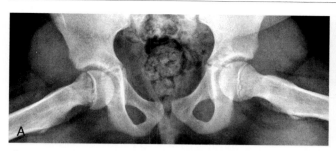
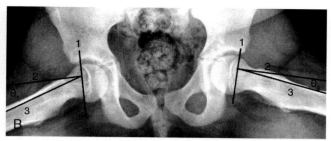

**Figure 4**    The lateral epiphyseal-shaft angle of the Southwick angle is measured on a frog-lateral radiograph. **A,** Frog-lateral radiograph of a 9-year-old girl with a mild right SCFE. **B,** Line 1 is drawn between the anterior and posterior physis; line 2 is perpendicular to line 1; line 3 is an axial line along the shaft of the femur. The angle defined by the intersection of line 2 and 3 is the lateral epiphyseal shaft angle (θ). The slip angle is calculated by subtracting the lateral epiphyseal shaft angle of the normal hip from the slip side. In this example, the angle on the right hip ($\theta_1$) created by lines 2 and 3 is 20°, and on the angle ($\theta_2$) on the left hip is 7°. The magnitude of the SCFE is 20° − 7° = 13° (a mild SCFE).

at the level of the metaphysis; this double density reflects the posterior cortical lip of the epiphysis as it is beginning to slip posteriorly and is radiographically superimposed on the metaphyseal density. Klein's line is drawn along the anterior or superior aspect of the femoral neck; the epiphysis should normally intersect this line, whereas in an early SCFE, the epiphysis will be level with or even below the level of this line.

Other imaging methods are occasionally used in children with SCFE. Bone scans and MRI scans allow earlier diagnosis of osteonecrosis and chondrolysis, whereas ultrasonography allows early visualization of an effusion in the hip.[60] The CT scan has improved the three-dimensional understanding of a SCFE and can be used in preoperative planning of an osteotomy and when determining whether there is joint penetration by internal fixation.[63]

SCFE magnitude is described by two different methods. The first describes magnitude by the amount of displacement of the epiphysis on the metaphysis. A mild SCFE is defined as epiphyseal-metaphyseal displacement less than one third the width of the metaphysis, a moderate SCFE

is defined as displacement one third to one half the width of the metaphysis, and a severe SCFE is defined as greater than one half the width of the metaphysis.[54] This first method to describe SCFE magnitude by degree of displacement is less accurate because distinct landmarks are difficult to determine as a result of metaphyseal remodeling in the gradually stable SCFE.[64] Angular measurement, the second method, is more accurate. The epiphyseal-shaft angle on the frog-lateral radiograph is measured and categorized into three groups: mild, less than 30°; moderate, 30° to 50°; and severe, greater than 50°[50,65] (Figure 4). This classification is important for long-term prognosis because mild and moderate slips have a much better long-term prognosis than severe slips, in which degenerative hip disease more rapidly develops.[53,66]

## Etiology

The etiology of idiopathic SCFE is a combination of both biomechanical and biochemical factors, the combined effect of which results in a weakened physis with subsequent failure[67] (Figure 5). Mechanical factors associated with SCFE are obesity, femoral retroversion, and in-

creased physeal obliquity.[18,19,68-71] Obesity and femoral retroversion increase shear stress across the physis.[70] The average anteversion in adolescents of normal weight is 10.6° and 0.4° in obese adolescents.[68] Children with SCFE also have a more vertical proximal femoral physis, even in the contralateral normal hip (8° to 11° increase compared with children without SCFE). The increase in physeal shear force resulting from femoral retroversion and increased physeal slope is enough to cause a SCFE.[70] The average shear load to failure of the proximal femoral physis in adolescents of normal weight is 4.0 times body weight; the average shear load to failure in obese adolescents with neutral version and who are running is 5.1 times body weight, higher than the 4.0 body weight threshold. Similarly, finite element analysis studies have shown that a varus load on the proximal femoral physis in an overweight child with femoral retroversion creates physeal shear strains above the yield point and can result in a slip.[72] In one study, children with SCFE were found to have greater acetabula depth than a group of children without SCFE (center-edge angle of Wiberg 37° versus 33°,

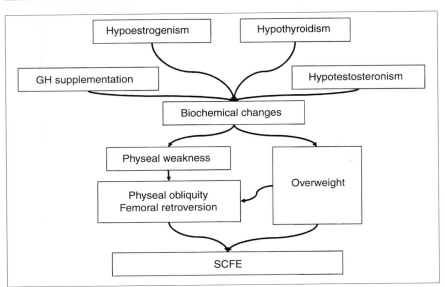

**Figure 5**  Proposed pathophysiology of SCFE across all species, including humans. GH = growth hormone.

respectively), demonstrating greater coverage of the femoral head yields more shearing stress across the physis.[44] However, this concept recently has been questioned.[45]

Biochemical and endocrine factors also are components of the disorder. SCFE is a disease of puberty, with rapid longitudinal growth occurring in response to growth hormone.[73] This growth is a result of increased physiologic activity of the physis and is associated with widening of the physis. Decreased physeal strength also occurs at puberty; the cause is not clear but may result from increased cartilage width of the zones of hypertrophy and provisional calcification.[29,74]

Many other hormonal changes occur during this time.[29] The increased incidence of SCFE in children with hypothyroidism, during growth hormone supplementation, and hypogonadal states also suggests an association between SCFE and endocrine dysfunction. The effects of the gonadotropins on the physis may explain the male predominance in SCFE, given that testosterone reduces physeal strength, whereas estrogen reduces physeal width and increases physeal strength.[29,75] This effect explains why the incidence of SCFE is extremely rare in girls after the onset of menarche.[39] Although most children with SCFE do not have demonstrable endocrine disorders, a subtle but as-yet undiagnosable endocrinopathy may be present.[76-81] In some children there is a delay in bone age compared with chronologic age, further supporting this concept.[29,39]

The role of genetics and heredity is variable. Rennie[82] discovered that the risk of SCFE to a second family member was 7.1% and that 14.5% of patients with SCFE were related to a close relative who also had SCFE. In a few families with members who have SCFE, there may be an autosomal dominant inheritance with incomplete penetrance.[82] Tightly knit communities (such as the Amish community) with little change in gene pools may have more familial tendencies in SCFE.[83] Human leukocyte antigen typing in children with SCFE is variable.[84-87]

Routine histology and electron microscopy show both cellular and matrical abnormalities in the proliferative and hypertrophic zones. Cellular abnormalities consist of a decreased number of chondrocytes and chondrocyte clustering and disarray; this decrease in chondrocyte number is the result of an abnormal frequency and distribution of chondrocytes undergoing apoptosis.[88-90] Reported histologic changes in the matrix include deficiency and abnormality in the supporting collagenous and proteoglycan framework of the physis. Changes in proteoglycan and glycoprotein concentrations with an increased glycoprotein staining in the territorial matrix and increased proteoglycan staining in the interterritorial matrix were seen in the proliferative zone. Ultrastructural studies have shown defective collagen fibrils and defects in collagen banding in the matrix of the hypertrophic zone.[91] Whether these abnormalities represent the cause or effect of the SCFE is not known.

## SCFE in Animals and Insights Into Etiology

Naturally occurring SCFE has been reported in cats, pigs, dogs, coypus, and cattle. These occurrences of SCFE in animal models suggest that biochemical changes precede both physeal changes and subsequent SCFE; animal models may further elucidate the pathophysiology of SCFE.

### Cats

SCFE has been reported in cats.[92-94] In the most detailed study, 26 cases with spontaneous, often insidious, femoral capital physeal fractures were examined, 9 of which were bilateral (35%).[92] The mean age of the cats was 22.5 months; 25 of 26 were neutered males with an average weight of 5.6 kg compared with a weight of 4.5 kg in an age- and sex-matched control group. Of the 16 cats with a recorded age at the time of neutering, 14 had been neutered before 6 months of age (prepubescent). Radiographically, more severe metaphyseal osteolysis and sclerosis scores were seen in chronic separations; 72% had radiographically open femoral capital physes. Histopathologically, the capital epiphysis contained cartilage and bone. Physeal tissue attached to the capital epiphysis lacked the normal chondrocyte columnar arrangement, and chondrocytes were clustered within the extracellular matrix. It was concluded that this feline condition mimics SCFE in children. Collectively, these studies identified obesity, gender (male), castration (particularly prepubescent castration), and delayed physeal closure as risk factors for feline SCFE.[92,93] Prepubertal or postpubertal castration in cats results in delayed physeal closure in a set of steps that are hypothesized to begin with hypotestosteronism resulting from castration with subsequent delayed physeal closure, followed by increased shear forces to the capital physis, resulting in a spontaneous, nontraumatic slippage of the capital femoral epiphysis[95,96] (Figure 6).

### Pigs

Separation of the femoral head also occurs in sows and boars (epiphysiolysis capitis femoris), and morphologic changes of the femoral head and neck have been described.[97,98] Although epiphysiolysis in pigs does not mimic SCFE in children, the condition may provide insight into the mechanisms of growth plate weakening, metaphyseal slippage

and separation, and the effect of obesity on hip development. The associated lameness varies from moderate to severe in unilateral lesions, to an inability to rise or walk in bilaterally affected animals. It has been suggested that osteochondritis weakens the growth plate, which ultimately results in slippage and separation. Causative factors of osteochondrosis (genetics, rapid growth) and trauma (such as fighting, copulation,) are considered risk factors for epiphysiolysis.

### Coypus

SCFE in the coypu *(Myocastor coypus)*, a large rodent (approximately 8 to 10 kg) commercially raised for fur, has been reported as a cause of lameness. In two reports, the onset of SCFE occurred during puberty (8 of 10 cases), and gross pathologic and histologic changes were consistent with SCFE in children.[99,100] These studies suggest that gender (female), pregnancy, and being overweight are risk factors for SCFE in coypus but do not explain whether the risk associated with pregnancy is a result of endocrine-related or mechanical factors. Because the incidence of SCFE in the coypu is low, and basic endocrine and skeletal physiology information is lacking, the coypu is not a good animal model for the study of SCFE.

### Dogs and Cattle

Recently, bilateral SCFE was reported in five dogs.[101,102] SCFE may also have caused other reported canine cases of capital femoral physeal fractures with insidious onset.[103] SCFE also has been reported in calves.[104] However, in 21 of 29 of the affected calves, the separation was attributed to difficult parturition and forced traction delivery. More recently, bovine SCFE was reported in older

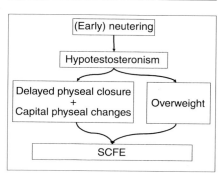

**Figure 6**  Proposed pathophysiology of SCFE in the cat.

calves and young adult cattle without a history of trauma.[105] The limited number of reported cases and limited information about canine and bovine SCFE currently make either animal model unsuitable for future investigations.

Although the pathologic changes of SCFE across species are the same, it appears that the etiology and pathophysiology are different. Common findings are trauma and physeal changes. In children these physeal changes include physeal obliquity and femoral retroversion, both the result of asymmetric physeal growth during development, which is the result of physeal trauma secondary to obesity. Slippage appears to occur during a limited bone age window when the perichondrial ring of the proximal capital femoral epiphysis is weakened.[25,26] Biochemical changes include endocrine alterations. Whereas in children no direct relationship has been established between SCFE and biochemical and mechanical changes, a very clear relationship between endocrine (hypotestosteronism) and physeal (delayed closure) changes exists in the cat model. It is not known why delayed physeal closure in cats can result in increased vulnerability and whether this vulnerability is a result of increased physeal obliquity, femoral retroversion, and perichondrial weakness. It is possible that physeal changes in children are also the result of both biochemical changes and obesity, which result in asymmetric physeal growth (Figure 5). Because biochemical changes are often minimal, and the time of onset of physeal closure is difficult to determine, weight control may be the most important measure to prevent SCFE. Further studies regarding the genesis of the physeal changes are needed.

## Treatment

Once a diagnosis of SCFE is made, treatment is indicated to prevent slip progression and to avoid complications, especially osteonecrosis and chondrolysis.[16,17,106] Several treatment methods exist, each characterized by particular advantages and disadvantages.

The treatment of SCFE has changed with improvements in imaging techniques. The development of intraoperative fluoroscopy to assist in the placement of internal fixation has markedly lowered the complication rate of internal fixation. Previously, patients were often treated by in situ multiple pin fixation using intraoperative spot radiographs to control pin placement. Using this technique, pin placement was not always ideal, and malpositioned pins were associated with complications including further slippage, chondrolysis, and osteonecrosis in 20% to 40% of patients. This high complication rate led to increased use of the hip spica cast, open epiphysiodesis, or femoral osteotomy as treatment. The hip spica cast, multiple pins, and, to a large extent, epiphysiodesis currently are treatments of historic interest only.[47,48,107-109]

### Stable SCFE

Treatment methods for a patient with a stable (chronic) SCFE include (1) in situ stabilization with a single screw,[47,48,110,111] (2) epiphysiodesis,[108,112,113] (3) open reduction with corrective osteotomy through the physis and internal fixation,[114-117] (4) treatment with a bilateral hip spica cast, (5) in situ fixation with multiple pins, (6) basilar neck osteotomy,[118,119] (7) intertrochanteric osteotomy,[63,65,120-122] and (8) surgical dislocation of the hip with transphyseal callus removal, reduction, and fixation.[123-127]

### In Situ Fixation Using a Single Central Screw

Since O'Brien and Fahey[128] reported on the remodeling potential of the proximal femur in patients with SCFE, internal fixation in situ has been the most popular treatment method. Long-term follow-up studies have shown that postoperative remodeling occurs, and the loss of internal rotation of the hip after in situ fixation in many patients is not clinically relevant.[129,130]

Because of femoral head vascularity and the blind spot, the ideal position for a screw is in the center of the epiphysis (Figure 7). The major contribution of the blood supply to the femoral head is derived from the lateral epiphyseal vessels, which enter the femoral head in the posterosuperior quadrant and anastomose with vessels from the round ligament at the junction of the medial and central thirds of the femoral head.[131,132] If fixation is placed in the posterosuperior quadrant, there is an increased risk of damage to the epiphyseal blood supply. This risk is minimized by a single screw in the center of the epiphysis and perpendicular to the physis.[47]

The blind spot is the area in which fixation devices radiographically appear to be within the femoral head but in reality are penetrating into the joint.[133] Often unrecognized pin protrusion results in subsequent development of chondrolysis and degenerative changes. The use of multiple pins increases the possibility that one or more pins will protrude into the joint; this risk is lowered by using a single screw.[48,134,135] Because single-screw fixation is 77% as stable as double-screw fixation in a calf model, single-screw fixation is recommended because the small gains in stiffness with a second screw do not offset the increased risk of joint penetration.[136]

The technique for the percutaneous insertion of a single screw has been described.[47,135] The patient is positioned supine on a fracture or radiolucent table to allow simultaneous biplane AP and lateral fluoroscopic imaging. The authors prefer a fracture table for single screw fixation, although others report good results and reduced surgical time on a radiolucent table.[137,138] It is important to emphasize that the technique is image dependent; therefore, excellent visualization of the femoral head and neck is required before beginning the procedure. Because the procedure is performed percutaneously through a small skin incision using a cannulated screw, it is critical to locate the proper starting position for the guide pin. To determine the starting point, a guide pin is placed on the skin overlying the proximal femur and, under anteroposterior fluoroscopic guidance, the pin is positioned such that it projects over the center of the femoral epiphysis, crossing the physis in a perpendicular fashion. Once this pin position has been obtained, a marking pen is used to draw a line on the skin that reflects the pin position on the AP image. The same procedure is used for the lateral fluoroscopic image, and a 1-cm skin incision is made at the intersection of the two lines. The guide pin is advanced in a free-hand manner through the soft tissues to the anterolateral femoral cortex. Using fluoroscopic guidance, the position and angulation of the guide pin are adjusted to obtain the proper alignment before the guide pin is drilled into the bone. It is ideal to advance the guide pin into the center of the epiphysis, perpendicular to the physis, on both the AP and lateral fluoroscopic images on the first attempt because multiple drill holes can weaken the bone, causing a fracture through an unused hole.[139] After the appropriate screw length has been determined, a 6.5-mm to 7.3-mm stainless steel cannulated screw is placed in a routine manner and advanced until approximately five threads engage the epiphysis (Figure 7). Carney and associates[140] reported progression of the SCFE greater than 10° in 9 of 22 hips (41%) when fewer than five threads engaged the epiphysis. When five or more threads engaged the epiphysis, no progression was reported. The screw should not be left protruding beyond the lateral aspect of the femoral shaft where it can be toggled by the soft tissues, leading to screw loosening.[141]

At this point in the procedure, it must be confirmed that the screw tip is not in the joint space by using either variations on the "approach-withdraw" maneuver or arthrography.[142-146] The approach-withdraw maneuver indicates the position of the screw tip and helps avoid unrecognized screw penetration, which is associated with the blind spot that exists with individual views on the image intensifier. As the screw ap-

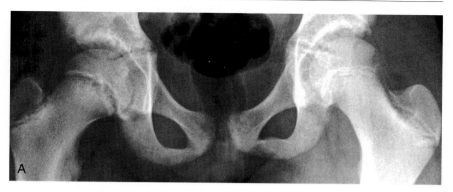

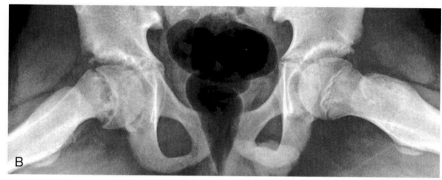

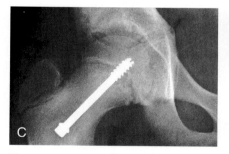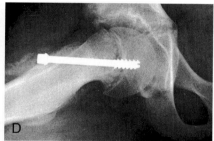

**Figure 7**   **A,** Initial AP radiograph of the pelvis of a boy age 11 years, 11 months with a stable right SCFE. **B,** Frog-lateral pelvic radiograph showing the right SCFE. **C,** Postoperative AP view of the pelvis shows screw placement perpendicular to the physis. **D,** Postoperative frog-lateral radiograph of the pelvis shows screw placement perpendicular to the physis.

proaches the subchondral bone of the femoral head, and with the surgeon observing the image intensifier screen, the lower extremity is rotated from maximum internal rotation to maximum external rotation. During the first part of the rotation, the screw tip appears to move closer to the subchondral bone (approach), then moves away (withdraw). The instant of change from approach to withdrawal identifies the view in

which the screw tip is shown in its true position. After surgery, the patient begins partial weight-bearing ambulation using crutches and gradually advances to full weight bearing after 4 to 6 weeks.

The results of single-screw fixation for patients with SCFE are good. Aronson and Carlson[47] reported excellent or good results in 36 of 38 mild slips (95%), in 10 of 11 moderate slips (91%), and in 8 of 9 severe slips (89%).[91] Osteonecrosis developed in only one patient (2%) with an unstable SCFE, and chondrolysis developed in none. Ward and associates[48] reported on 42 patients (53 hips) with a SCFE treated by single screw fixation. After an average follow-up of 32 months, 92% demonstrated physeal fusion and participated in full activities. No patient developed chondrolysis or osteonecrosis. The advantages of single-screw fixation for a patient with a stable SCFE include a high success rate, a low incidence of further slippage, and a low incidence of complications.[47,147,148] It is currently the most common treatment of SCFE in North America.

### Bone Graft Epiphysiodesis With Iliac Crest or Allograft Bone Graft

In 1931, Ferguson and Howorth[28] first reported open epiphysiodesis with iliac crest bone graft to stabilize a SCFE. The surgical technique is characterized by an anterior iliofemoral exposure of the hip joint and removal of a rectangular window of bone from the anterior aspect of the femoral neck. A hollow mill is used to create a tunnel across the physis, and multiple corticocancellous strips of iliac crest bone graft are driven into the tunnel as bone pegs across the proximal femoral physis.

Epiphysiodesis avoids the complications associated with internal fixation including unrecognized pin protrusion, damage to the lateral epiphyseal vessels, and hardware failure. The graft is not inserted as deep as recommended for internal fixation; therefore, there is less risk of graft protrusion into the hip joint. However, the fixation provided by the iliac crest bone graft is not as secure as that achieved by internal fixation. Rao and associates[108] evaluated 43 patients (64 hips) treated by open

bone peg epiphysiodesis. At the time of healing, further slippage developed in 27 hips (42%). Osteonecrosis developed in 4 hips (6%), chondrolysis in 3 (5%), and additional complications in 14 (22%). Adamczyk and associates[109] reported their 50-year experience with bone graft epiphysiodesis in 43 patients with 45 incidences of unstable SCFE, and 225 patients with 278 incidences of stable SCFE. Slip progression occurred in 6 of the patients (13%) with unstable SCFE and in 17 of the patients (6%) with stable SCFE. Other disadvantages of bone graft epiphysiodesis include increased blood loss, a longer duration of anesthesia, and a larger scar. As a result of these complications, open bone peg epiphysiodesis is no longer recommended as the initial treatment of SCFE.[108,109]

Adamczyk and associates[109] believe that the rate of reslippage with iliac crest bone graft is unacceptable and that the use of a fibular allograft should be considered for increased stability. Schmidt and associates[113] have recently developed a technique to percutaneously place a freeze-dried irradiated cortical strut allograft across the physis. The technique is similar to that used for the percutaneous insertion of a single screw, but instead of inserting a screw, a 10-mm cannulated reamer is placed over the guide pin to ream a channel to within 2 mm of the subchondral bone. A cortical strut allograft is then passed into the channel and advanced until at least 1 cm lay across the physis. Schmidt and associates[113] evaluated 33 patients (40 hips) after a mean follow-up of 3 years, 6 months and reported excellent Harris hip scores in 35 hips, good scores in 1, and fair in 2. Major complications developed in 6 hips (15%), including one each

of osteonecrosis, chondrolysis, femoral neck fracture, subtrochanteric hip fracture, bilateral coxa vara deformity, and unilateral coxa vara deformity. Despite these complications, the authors recommend this technique, particularly for patients with severe SCFE.

### Open Reduction With Corrective Osteotomy Through the Physis and Internal Fixation Using Multiple Pins

A cuneiform osteotomy through the physis is the ideal method to correct the retroversion deformity of the femoral neck, but the question of safety is relevant. The surgical technique is characterized by an anterior Smith-Peterson or anterolateral exposure of the hip.[114,115] A cuneiform-shaped wedge of bone is removed from the metaphysis of the femoral neck, which allows the epiphysis to be anatomically repositioned on the metaphysis without creating tension on the epiphyseal vasculature. After the femoral neck is sufficiently shortened, reduction and fixation of the epiphysis is accomplished internally using three pins. In one study, a cuneiform osteotomy was performed on 61 patients (66 hips) with 55 excellent results (83%), 6 good (9%), 2 fair (3%), and 3 poor (5%).[117] DeRosa and associates[114] evaluated 23 patients (27 hips) with a severe SCFE treated by cuneiform osteotomy. At an average follow-up of 8 years, 5 months, there were no excellent results, 19 good (70%), 4 fair (15%), and 4 poor (15%). Osteonecrosis developed in four hips (15%) and chondrolysis in eight (30%). Two patients (7%) lost fixation and required further surgery, a skin erosion over one of the pins developed in one patient and required pin removal, and a pressure sore developed in the buttock of another patient. Despite a 15% rate of osteonecrosis, DeRosa and associates[114] recommended cuneiform osteotomy for patients with severe SCFE.

Velasco and associates[115] evaluated 65 patients (66 hips) treated with open reduction of the SCFE. In 60 hips, the open reduction of the slip was combined with a cuneiform subcapital wedge resection of the femoral neck according to the technique described by Dunn and Angel.[149] At an average follow-up of 16 years, chondrolysis developed in 8 hips (12%), and osteonecrosis developed in 7 (11%). The results in 48 hips with a minimum follow-up of 10 years (average follow-up, 20.6 years) were good in 46%, moderate in 33%, and poor in 21%. Degenerative arthritis occurred in 19 of the 48 hips (40%). Because of the high risk of osteonecrosis and subsequent poor results in most studies, a physeal cuneiform osteotomy is not recommended as the initial treatment of SCFE.

### Bilateral Hip Spica Cast

Hip spica cast immobilization provides prophylactic treatment of the opposite hip and avoids surgical complications. Hurley and associates[36] compared 169 patients treated with in situ fixation with 30 patients treated with a spica cast. In the in situ fixation group, a contralateral SCFE developed in 61 patients (36%) at a mean follow-up of 2.8 years. In the spica cast group, a contralateral SCFE developed in two patients (7%) at a mean follow-up of 3.6 years. Betz and associates[150] evaluated 32 patients (37 hips) treated with a hip spica cast without reduction. The cast was used until the metaphyseal lucency adjacent to the physis was no longer radiographically visible on the radiographs at an average follow-up of 12 weeks. Osteonecrosis did not develop in any of the patients, but progression of the slip occurred in two hips (5%), and chondrolysis in seven (19%). Meier and associates[107] evaluated 13 patients (17 hips) treated with a spica cast for an average of 12 weeks. Progression of the slip occurred in three hips (18%), chondrolysis in nine (53%), and full-thickness cast pressure sores in two (12%). There were a total of 14 complications in the 17 hips (82%). In addition to the high complication and slip progression rate, a hip spica cast is awkward and cumbersome for the wearer and family, particularly when the patient is obese. Spica cast treatment of SCFE is not recommended.

### In Situ Fixation With Multiple Pins

Complications associated with multiple pins stemmed from a lack of understanding of the three-dimensional anatomy of SCFE and from poor intraoperative imaging techniques. As a result, fixation was often started on the lateral aspect of the femoral shaft, similar to the technique of treating a hip fracture in an adult. Because the proximal femur is retroverted in a patient with a SCFE, the fixation was often placed in the anterosuperior aspect of the epiphysis, achieving suboptimal fixation. To improve fixation, clinicians would angle the pin more posteriorly, often exiting the posterior aspect of the femoral neck and entering the epiphysis in the posterosuperior quadrant. This technique jeopardized the blood supply to the femoral head and also led to unrecognized pin protrusion with subsequent chondrolysis or osteonecrosis. Given the superior results of single central screw fixation, multiple pin fixation is now used infrequently in the treatment of a stable SCFE.

After the initial treatment of SCFE, the external rotational deformity of the lower extremity gradually improves as the inflammation resolves and the proximal femoral retroversion deformity remodels. The retroversion deformity may occasionally cause pain and loss of motion for the patient and may cause anterior femoroacetabular impingement, which can contribute to the early development of osteoarthritis.[123-127] When the retroversion deformity causes pain or loss of motion, the clinician may choose intertrochanteric osteotomy, basilar neck osteotomy, or open surgical dislocation with femoral neck osteoplasty as treatment.

### Compensating Base-of-Neck Osteotomy With Stabilization In Situ of the SCFE Using Multiple Pin Fixation

Kramer and associates[119] described an anterosuperior-based wedge osteotomy at the base of the femoral neck with both the osteotomy and the SCFE stabilized with multiple pins. Barmada and associates[118] described an extracapsular basilar neck osteotomy implemented in an attempt to avoid osteonecrosis. The incidence of osteonecrosis is lower with basilar neck osteotomies compared with the cuneiform osteotomy; however, only 35° to 55° of correction is possible.[151] One benefit of the basilar neck osteotomy is improvement in hip motion; a disadvantage is that the procedure shortens the femoral neck, which may result in the greater trochanter impinging against the lateral aspect of the acetabulum during hip abduction. This femoral neck shortening may aggravate a limb-length discrepancy when there is premature closure of the proximal femoral physis, as is often seen in patients with SCFE.

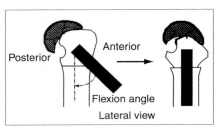

**Figure 8** The Imhäuser flexion closing wedge intertrochanteric osteotomy for a SCFE. (Reproduced with permission from Kamegaya M, Saisu T, Ochiai N, Moriya H: Preoperative assessment for intertrochanteric femoral osteotomies in severe chronic slipped capital femoral epiphysis using computed tomography. *J Pediatr Orthop* 2005;14:71-78.)

### Intertrochanteric Osteotomy With Internal Fixation

Southwick[65] described an intertrochanteric osteotomy through the lesser trochanter with flexion, abduction, and internal rotation of the distal fragment. This osteotomy improves hip motion and is not associated with osteonecrosis. The osteotomy is fixed with a compression hip screw and, if unstable, the SCFE is fixed with a cannulated screw. The intertrochanteric osteotomy is also a compensating osteotomy with correction limited to 45° on the AP radiograph and 60° on the lateral radiograph.[152] Because an anterolateral wedge of bone is removed, this osteotomy is also a shortening procedure. A risk of limb-length discrepancy exists when considerable correction is desired. Schai and associates[120] evaluated 51 patients with 30° to 60° slips treated with an intertrochanteric osteotomy at an average follow-up of 24 years. Moderate osteoarthritis developed in 14 patients (28%) and severe osteoarthritis in 9 patients (17%). In 35 patients (69%), the affected limb was shorter than the opposite side, and 2 patients (4%) underwent a limb-

length equalization procedure. There was only one instance of osteonecrosis. The authors believed their results were superior to those treated with in situ fixation.[153] However, their results are at odds with the results of the long-term study of Carney and associates[53] in which those with realignment showed poorer results than those without realignment. In most studies, the results of intertrochanteric osteotomy using the Southwick technique are relatively poor compared with results using the current technique of in situ single-screw fixation; therefore, intertrochanteric osteotomy is not ideal for the initial treatment of SCFE.[65,120,152]

The Southwick osteotomy has now been replaced by the simpler Imhäuser flexion intertrochanteric osteotomy[63,121,122] (Figure 8). This osteotomy relies on the concept that the slip is essentially posterior, with secondary rotational deformity and minimal valgus or varus displacement.[55,69,154] The results of such an osteotomy are disparate. Kartenbender and associates[122] reviewed 39 severe SCFEs treated with an Imhäuser osteotomy at an average follow-up of 23.4 years. Three patients had severe degenerative disease and osteonecrosis developed in two patients. The number of excellent or good clinical results was 77%, whereas the excellent or good radiographic results using the Southwick classification were only 67%. Parsch and associates[121] noted one patient with osteonecrosis in stable SCFEs greater than 50°, yet concluded that they were unable to prove the advantage of osteotomy in late adult life.

Jerre and associates[155] evaluated the results of different realignment procedures in 36 patients (37 hips) at an average follow-up of 33.8 years (range, 26 to 42 years). Serious

short-term complications developed in 7 of 22 hips (32%) treated with subcapital osteotomy, 3 of 11 hips (27%) with intertrochanteric osteotomy, and 3 of 4 hips (75%) treated with manipulative reduction. Long-term excellent or good results were reported in 9 of 22 hips (41%) treated with subcapital osteotomy, 4 of 11 (36%) treated with intertrochanteric osteotomy, and in none of the 4 hips (0%) treated with manipulative reduction.

### Unstable SCFE

The treatment of an unstable SCFE is considerably more controversial than that of the stable SCFE. There is debate concerning an emergent or urgent reduction versus an elective reduction, an incidental reduction (improvement in the SCFE that occurs with positioning the patient on the operating table) versus a complete reduction, the magnitude of reduction, the role of joint decompression, and fixation with one or two screws. There is an increased risk of complications, particularly osteonecrosis, in patients with unstable SCFE.

This controversy regarding reduction was well documented by Mooney and associates[156] who surveyed the Pediatric Orthopaedic Society of North America membership about the treatment of unstable SCFE. Of the respondents; 57% favored urgent reduction (< 8 hours), 31% favored emergent reduction, and 12% favored elective treatment. An incidental reduction was favored by 84% of respondents, whereas 12% favored a formal (complete) manipulative reduction. Capsular decompression of the hematoma was not recommended by 65% of respondents, whereas 35% recommended decompression; 26% of those recommending decompression performed open decompression and 73% used a closed aspiration technique. Single-screw fixation was used by 57% of respondents, whereas 40% used double-screw fixation.

In the initial study that describes unstable SCFE and its increased risk for osteonecrosis, 25 acute stable SCFEs (24 patients) with 30 acute unstable SCFEs (30 patients) were compared.[56] There were 96% satisfactory results with no osteonecrosis in the 25 stable SCFEs, and 47% satisfactory results in the 30 unstable SCFEs. Osteonecrosis developed in 14 of 30 (47%) of the unstable SCFEs. Those with an acute slip were separated into two groups based on the time interval between the onset of symptoms and surgical stabilization. In the group that had surgical stabilization less than 48 hours after the onset of symptoms, the incidence of osteonecrosis was 88%. In the group that had surgical stabilization more than 48 hours after the onset of symptoms, the incidence of osteonecrosis was 32%. However, the data were inadequate to develop guidelines regarding the exact timing of surgical stabilization because the cause-effect relationship between the timing of surgical stabilization and the development of osteonecrosis could not be determined. It was possible that the more severe unstable SCFEs, which would likely have a higher risk of osteonecrosis, were stabilized sooner in an effort to reduce the child's discomfort as quickly as possible; the less severe unstable SCFEs, which theoretically had a lower risk of osteonecrosis, were stabilized later because the child was more comfortable.

Several authors have attempted to answer the questions regarding timing and surgical stabilization. The authors of one study evaluated 70 patients (81 hips) who had an un-stable SCFE treated with gentle closed reduction and fixation using one or two screws or pins.[157] They reported complications in eight hips: three with chondrolysis (4%), three wound infections (4%), and two with osteonecrosis (2%). The authors concluded that a gentle reduction with percutaneous single-screw fixation is a stable, safe, and reliable method for treating patients with an unstable SCFE. Herman and associates[158] evaluated 15 unstable SCFEs (> 50% displacement) at an average follow-up of 2.8 years. Nine were treated by a gentle closed reduction and internal fixation, using either one or two screws. Five hips had a complete reduction of the SCFE, and osteonecrosis developed in three, whereas four hips had an incomplete reduction, and none developed osteonecrosis. The authors hypothesized that injury to the epiphyseal vasculature occurs at the time of the acute SCFE.

Peterson and associates[159] evaluated 91 patients with unstable SCFEs at an average follow-up of 44 months and especially evaluated the timing of the reduction and outcome regarding osteonecrosis. In 42 hips, a closed reduction was performed in less than 24 hours after presentation; osteonecrosis developed in 3 hips (7%). In 49 hips, a closed reduction was performed more than 24 hours after presentation, and osteonecrosis developed in 10 hips (20%). The authors hypothesized that the acute displacement of the femoral head may kink the posterior blood vessels, compromising the blood flow to the epiphysis. In this situation, a timely reduction of the SCFE may restore blood flow to the epiphysis. Gordon and associates[160] confirmed this concept with no occurrences of osteonecrosis in 10 unstable SCFEs treated within 24 hours with reduction, ar-throtomy, and two-screw fixation.

Animal studies support the concept of early reduction and joint decompression. Beck and associates[161] evaluated the effects of increased intra-articular pressure on the blood flow to the femoral head. In 11 patients treated with open surgical dislocation for the femoroacetabular impingement, saline was injected into the intact intracapsular space while monitoring the blood flow to the femoral head with laser Doppler flowmetry. After an average intracapsular saline injection of 20 mL, loss of the pulsatile signal occurred with an average intra-articular pressure of 58 mm Hg. Aspiration of the joint caused a return of the pulsatile flow. These results support the recommendation to perform an urgent decompression of the intracapsular hematoma to optimize blood flow to the femoral head. Similarly, in the juvenile goat, Svalastoga and associates[162] showed that a joint pressure of 75 mm Hg resulted in a decrease in oxygen tension from 48 mm Hg to 29 mm Hg; traction in extension further decreased the oxygen tension. This study highlights the risks of treating a hip joint with an effusion by traction and indicates that aspiration should be strongly considered.

Several studies evaluated the question of how many screws should be used in the unstable SCFE; however, nearly all of the studies used in vitro animal models and were relatively far removed from the clinical situation. Karol and associates[136] compared one- and two-screw fixation in a calf model (testing a single load to failure) and found that single-screw fixation was 77% as stable as double-screw fixation. Kibiloski and associates[163] used the same model but studied the effects of physiologic shear loading, simulating slow walking and fast walking. The rates of creep were larger for the single-screw fixation group, particularly with fast walking, but the results were not statistically significant. The authors concluded that regardless of whether one or two screws are used, protected weight bearing is advisable in the postoperative period in the unstable SCFE. In an immature porcine model, Snyder and associates[164] studied torsional strength after removal of the perichondrium at the physeal level (analogous to the situation of the unstable SCFE in which the perichondrium at the physeal level has been compromised). This study differed from the studies done by both Karol and associates[136] and by Kibiloski and associates[163] who studied shear to failure, not torsion. Snyder and associates[164] found that two-screw fixation after removal of the perichondrium provided 43% of the stiffness and 74% of the strength of the intact physis in torsion. In an immature bovine model, Kishan and associates[165] evaluated one- and two-screw fixations in varying configurations at physiologically relevant loads and found no significant differences among three different screw configurations but did find that two-screw constructs were 66% stiffer and 66% stronger than single screw constructs.

Based on the literature to date, the authors recommend closed reduction, urgent hip joint aspiration/decompression, and single- or double-screw fixation for patients with unstable SCFE. One screw may not provide adequate fixation, but two screws may increase the risk of osteonecrosis and chondrolysis. In either situation, not bearing weight on the affected limb and the use of crutches for 6 to 8 weeks is recommended to prevent progression.

## Prophylactic Fixation of the Contralateral Hip

The risk of a contralateral SCFE in a patient with unilateral SCFE is reported to be 2,335 times higher than the risk of an initial SCFE.[166] Schultz and associates[166] developed a decision analysis model with probabilities for the occurrence of a contralateral SCFE and concluded that prophylactic fixation of the contralateral hip was beneficial to the long-term outcome of that hip. The authors cautioned that the clinician must use sound judgment with respect to the age, gender, and endocrine status of the patient, including the preferences of the patient and family, before recommending prophylactic fixation of the contralateral hip. By contrast, Kocher and associates[167] also used a decision analysis model with probabilities for the occurrence of a contralateral SCFE but described a more limited group for whom the procedure would be beneficial. In their model, prophylactic fixation of the contralateral hip is favored for those in whom the probability of a contralateral SCFE is greater than 27% or in patients for whom reliable follow-up is not feasible. The difference in these studies is that Schultz and associates[166] used values from the literature for various incidences and probabilities of events (such as osteonecrosis, chondrolysis, severity of SCFE,), whereas Kocher and associates[167] used a questionnaire to determine patient preferences in a group of children without SCFE; the questionnaire posed scenarios for different outcomes and asked the children to rate preferences regarding prophylactic fixation from the context of the scenario.

Epidemiologic data also provide conflicting opinions regarding prophylactic fixation, with. prophylactic fixation recommended by some

physicians and close observation recommended by others.[34,168-171] A Pediatric Orthopaedic Society of North America membership survey recommended prophylactic fixation of the contralateral hip only 12.2% of the time.[156]

## Complications
### Osteonecrosis

Osteonecrosis is a devastating complication, occurring infrequently in a stable SCFE but more frequently in an unstable SCFE[56] (Figure 9). Factors associated with osteonecrosis are an unstable SCFE, anterior physeal separation, overreduction of an unstable SCFE, attempted reduction of a stable SCFE, the placement of pins in the posterosuperior quadrant of the epiphysis, and cuneiform osteotomy.[53,56,131,132,172-175]

The patient with osteonecrosis typically reports pain in the groin or knee. On physical examination, a loss of range of motion of the hip (particularly internal rotation) exists, and the hip is irritable to passive internal and external rotation. The plain radiographs are unremarkable early in the course of the disorder, but changes diagnostic of osteonecrosis (collapse of the femoral head with cyst formation and sclerosis) develop after a few months. Osteonecrosis after SCFE will be radiographically apparent in all patients within 1 year. An early bone scan or an MRI scan will often show asymmetry between the femoral heads, predicting the eventual development of osteonecrosis.[176] Krahn and associates[173] evaluated 22 patients with osteonecrosis after a mean follow-up of 31 years. Nine patients (41%) had reconstructive surgery, four during adolescence and five during adulthood. The remaining 13 patients had not yet had reconstructive surgery, but all had

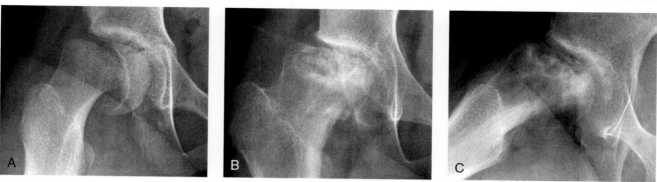

**Figure 9** **A,** The AP radiograph of an unstable right SCFE in a girl age 11 years, 2 months. Emergent reduction and fixation was performed, but by the age of 12 years, 8 months, osteonecrosis was apparent on the AP (**B**) and lateral (**C**) radiographs.

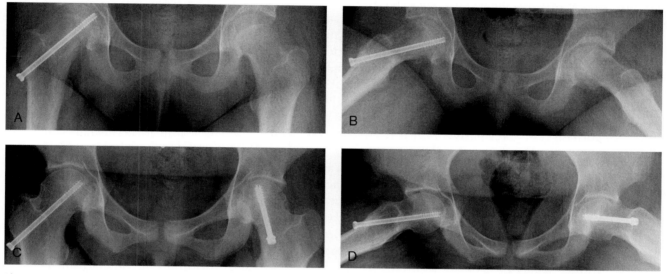

**Figure 10** AP (**A**) and frog pelvis lateral (**B**) radiographs of a girl age 13 years, 6 months, who had previously undergone in situ fixation for a right SCFE. Note the protrusion of the screw into the joint space and the joint space narrowing, indicative of chondrolysis. Also note the opposite left SCFE. The right screw was slightly withdrawn along with in situ fixation of the left SCFE. At age 15 years, 5 months, the AP (**C**) and frog-lateral (**D**) radiographs show physeal closure of both hips and improvement in the joint space narrowing of the right hip.

radiographic degenerative changes.

The treatment of osteonecrosis includes not bearing weight by using crutches, range-of-motion exercises, and anti-inflammatory medication. Internal fixation that protrudes into the joint should be repositioned in the epiphysis if the physis is open or removed if the physis is closed. Ten-year survivorship of the hip may approach 75% when an arthrogram and examination under anesthesia indicate that

an osteotomy would result in a more congruous joint in a noninvolved portion of the femoral head.[177]

### Chondrolysis

Chondrolysis is defined as a narrowing of the joint space by at least 50% compared with the opposite hip with unilateral chondrolysis, and less than 3 mm joint space with bilateral chondrolysis.[178-180] Chondrolysis may already be present when the patient first presents with

SCFE. However, in most patients with SCFE, the etiology of chondrolysis is secondary to unrecognized pin penetration of the femoral head at the time of surgery (Figure 10). In patients without pin penetration, an autoimmune phenomenon or some factor that interferes with cartilage nutrition may contribute to the chondrolysis. Factors associated with chondrolysis include unrecognized pin penetration, treatment in a hip spica cast, intertrochanteric osteotomy, severe SCFE, and prolonged symptoms before treatment.

The incidence of chondrolysis in patients with a SCFE was historically 5% to 7%, but many recent studies now support a far lower 1% to 2% incidence.[47,48] The patient usually reports pain in the groin or knee, and loss of hip motion, particularly internal rotation, is shown on physical examination. The diagnosis is confirmed by radiographs that show decreased joint width. An early bone scan that shows increased uptake in the hip with premature closure of the greater trochanter has been associated with an increased risk for the development of chondrolysis.[181] The incidence of chondrolysis increases with increasing severity of the SCFE. It is not increased in the black population as previously reported.[180,182-187] The frequency of chondrolysis is less with single-screw fixation than with fixation using multiple screws or pins.[188]

The treatment of chondrolysis, as with the treatment of osteonecrosis, is not particularly rewarding for the patient or the clinician. Non–weight-bearing ambulation with crutches, range-of-motion exercises, and anti-inflammatory medication may help alleviate symptoms. When there is screw protrusion, backing the screw out of the joint, or removing it if the physis is closed, will help minimize hip damage (Figure 10). Lengthening of the contracted muscle is recommended by some physicians for a hip with contracture, with arthrodesis required in severe situations.

Patients with chondrolysis have a better long-term prognosis than those with osteonecrosis. Tudisco and associates[189] evaluated nine patients with chondrolysis at a mean follow-up of 14 years and noted

gradual regression of hip pain with restoration of the joint space after a mean of 10 months. At follow-up, five patients had mild pain after prolonged activity; all had some limitation of abduction and internal rotation.

### Internal Fixation

The frequency of problems related to internal fixation (slip progression, implant breakage, and joint penetration) is decreasing with the use of fluoroscopically guided, cannulated single-screw fixation. The risk of fracture through an unused pinhole can be avoided by using fluoroscopy to position the guide pin correctly on the first attempt and by entering the bone proximal to the lesser trochanter.

## Natural History Without Treatment

Two major issues arise with the untreated SCFE: the risk of further progression and the risk of degenerative joint disease in adult life. Unfortunately, there are few long-term studies of patients with SCFE and even fewer studies that also include untreated patients with SCFEs.[50,51,53,66,190-192]

### Risk of Progression

The natural history of SCFE is unpredictable, and the risk of further progression is difficult to ascertain. Ordeberg and associates[193] reviewed studies of SCFEs without primary treatment 20 to 40 years after diagnosis. Although few patients had restrictions in their working capacity or social life, there was a risk of slip progression if the physis remained open.[194] Carney and associates[53] reported on 35 SCFEs that were initially observed; additional displacement occurred in 6 SCFEs (17%) after initial diagnosis, and 5 SCFEs

became severe. Eleven of the 35 patients (31%) had an acute episode of SCFE superimposed on the chronic SCFE; these 11 slips all progressed to severe displacement and required surgical stabilization.

### Risk of Degenerative Joint Disease

Howorth[195] stated that SCFE is likely the most frequent cause of degenerative joint disease of the hip in middle life and a common source of pain and disability. This conclusion is not necessarily supported by other studies. In reviewing a large study of patients with degenerative joint disease, the number of patients with known SCFE is low, averaging approximately 5%.[196-198] Murray[197] reported an association with SCFE in 80 of 200 patients (40%) believed to have primary degenerative joint disease. He described a tilt deformity caused by bone resorption laterally with new bone formation medially and believed this disorder to be compatible with an old SCFE. Stulberg and associates[199] also described a similar deformity, the pistol grip deformity, in 40% of patients without known prior hip disease undergoing total hip arthroplasty. This deformity was also believed to be compatible with an old SCFE. Resnick[200] refuted this theory in a pathologic study of 48 femoral heads of patients with a tilt deformity on radiographs that suggested the deformity was solely related to the remodeling changes of osteoarthritis. Whether subclinical forms of SCFE led to early osteoarthritis remains uncertain.

It is known that the severity of deformity in the untreated SCFE correlates with the long-term prognosis regarding degenerative joint disease.[53,66,153,191,192,201] Oram[191] reported on 22 untreated SCFEs, 11 of which were observed for more than 15 years. Those with moderate SCFEs retained good function for years, whereas degenerative joint disease with resultant poor function developed within 15 years in patients with severe SCFEs. Jerre[153,201] and Ross and associates[192] reported increasingly poor results with longer follow-up. Both groups reported many patients doing well early in the disease process; however, increasing symptoms and decreasing function developed with increasing age.

Carney and Weinstein[66] studied the natural history of the untreated, chronic SCFE in an evaluation of 31 hips in 28 patients at an average age of 55 years and at an average follow-up of 41 years. The average Iowa Hip Rating for the entire group was 89 points; the scores were: 92 in the 17 mild SCFEs, 87 in the 11 moderate SCFEs, and 75 in the 3 severe SCFEs. Although patients with mild SCFE appear to have a favorable prognosis, patients with moderate and severe SCFE have a high incidence of degenerative joint disease. At 41-year follow-up, an Iowa Hip Rating greater than 80 points was present in 100% of mild SCFEs and 64% of moderate and severe SCFEs. Degenerative changes were noted in 36% of the mild SCFEs and 100% of the moderate and severe SCFEs. However, poor results can occasionally occur even with minimal SCFEs.[50,53,66,192] The natural history of chronic (stable) SCFE is favorable, provided that displacement is mild and remains so.

There are few data on the natural history of untreated acute SCFEs. Progression begins with an acute episode, which is followed by a 2- to 3-week period of intolerance to weight bearing. As the pain and spasm subside, a degree of motion returns, although the hip remains moderately painful in a position of external rotation. Degenerative changes (joint space narrowing, subchondral bone cysts, epiphyseal collapse) develop within a few months, and the patient is left with residual flexion, adduction, and external rotation contractures.[51]

## Long-Term Results of Treatment

Wilson and associates[38] reviewed 300 hips in 240 patients treated between 1936 and 1960; 187 were treated by fixation in situ with 81% good clinical results and 77% good radiographic results. Poorer results occurred in the 76 hips in which correction of the deformity had been attempted (60% good clinical results and 55% good radiographic results). Hall[190] reported on 138 patients, with the best results obtained with the use of multiple pins; 16 of 20 patients (80%) had excellent results. The worst results were seen after realignment had been attempted with manipulation or osteotomy; osteotomy of the femoral neck, in particular, led to poor results in 36% of the hips and osteonecrosis in 38%.

Patients with SCFE in southern Sweden were followed for more than 30 years.[193] Symptomatic treatment or fixation in situ resulted in high clinical ratings and few radiographic changes, with only 2% of the hips needing a secondary reconstructive procedure. When closed reduction and a spica cast were used, the combined rate of osteonecrosis and chondrolysis was 13%, and reconstructive procedures were needed in 35% of the hips. Femoral neck osteotomy was followed by a combined rate of osteonecrosis and chondrolysis of 30%, and reconstructive procedures were necessary in 15% of the hips.

Carney and associates[53] reported

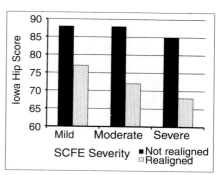

**Figure 11** The graph shows worsening scores on the Iowa Hip Rating Scale for children with SCFE at 41-year average follow-up. Deterioration over time becomes more pronounced as slip severity increases.

on 155 hips in 124 patients at a mean follow-up of 41 years using the Iowa Hip Rating and radiographic classification of degenerative joint disease (0 = no degenerative disease, 3 = severe degenerative disease). The SCFEs were mild in 42% of patients, moderate in 32%, and severe in 26%. Management of the chronic SCFEs involved symptomatic treatment in 25% of patients, a spica cast in 30%, fixation in situ in 24%, and osteotomy in 20%. Poorer results were associated with more severe slips and realignment (Figure 11). Osteonecrosis (12%) and chondrolysis (16%) were more common with increasing slip severity. Reduction was performed in 39 hips and realignment in 65 hips. For the 116 hips that had not been reduced, the mean Iowa Hip Rating was 85 points and the mean radiographic grade was 1.7. Osteonecrosis developed in 7 hips (6%) and chondrolysis in 14 (12%). For the 39 SCFEs that had been reduced, the mean Iowa Hip Rating was 72 points and the mean radiographic degenerative score was 2.4. Osteonecrosis developed in 12 hips (31%) and chondrolysis in 11 (28%). Twenty-seven hips with a chronic SCFE pinned in situ showed

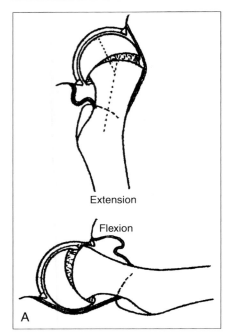 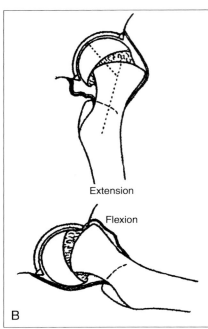

**Figure 12** Schematic lateral drawings of varying types of degrees of SCFE in extension and flexion. **A,** Mild to moderate SCFE causes jamming of the femoral metaphysis against the acetabular cartilage in flexion. **B,** Severe SCFE with an impingement of the femoral neck against the acetabular rim in flexion. (Reproduced with permission from Leunig M. Casillas MM, Hamlet M, Hersche O, Nötzli H, Slongo T, Ganz R: Slipped capital femoral epiphysis: Early mechanical damage to the acetabular cartilage by a prominent femoral metaphysis. *Acta Orthop Scand* 2000;71:370-375.)

a mean hip rating of 90 points and a mean radiographic grade of 1.5. Osteonecrosis developed in one hip and chondrolysis in none.[53] These long-term study results support the use of in situ fixation as the treatment of choice for SCFE. Realignment was associated with appreciable complications and adversely affected the outcome. Regardless of slip severity, fixation in situ provided the best long-term function and delay of degenerative arthritis with the lowest risk of complications (Figure 11). Although limb-length discrepancy and motion in abduction and internal rotation were affected by the severity of the slip, function was not significantly impaired.

The conclusion from these studies is that regardless of the slip severity, fixation in situ provides the best

long-term function, lowest complication risk, and most effective delay of degenerative arthritis. Many patients with SCFE do well with this treatment at long-term follow-up when the SCFE is of mild or moderate severity, good congruity between the femoral head and the acetabulum is maintained, and osteonecrosis and chondrolysis do not occur. In severe SCFEs or those with osteonecrosis or chondrolysis, a more rapid deterioration with degenerative changes occurs. SCFE differs from other pediatric hip disorders such as Legg-Calvé-Perthes disease and developmental hip dysplasia in that SCFE occurs at an age when most of the acetabular development is completed. Because of this acetabular maturity, adaptation to head deformity cannot occur.

## Possible Future Directions

With newer technology that includes improved implants and intraoperative imaging, some surgeons are revisiting the role of transphyseal osteotomy, reduction, and fixation. This advancement has been brought about by the advent of surgical dislocation of the hip. As noted earlier, children treated with in situ fixation had better results than those treated with realignment. However, the realignment procedures used in those patients were either closed reductions in stable SCFEs, which should not be performed, or osteotomies done at a time when present-day improvements in intraoperative radiography and internal fixation did not exist. Therefore, will a realignment osteotomy performed today have a better outcome than those described in the long-term study of Carney and associates,[53] and, if so, will an osteotomy using current methods in a severe SCFE improve the natural history? This question is now being vigorously debated because of increasing evidence of potential mechanical damage that can occur from the prominent femoral metaphysis in a severe SCFE on the acetabular cartilage or femoracetabular impingement.[55,123,154,202]

In 14 adolescent hips with SCFE, Leunig and associates[123] noted labral and acetabular cartilage damage had occurred when the anterior femoral metaphysis was level with or extended past the epiphysis (Figures 12 and 13). This damage consisted of scars, tears, and erosions in the acetabular cartilage and ranged from partial to full-thickness loss. The femoral head cartilage was intact. These findings suggest that degenerative hip disease in children with SCFE can be triggered by early mechanical damage of the acetabular cartilage and that femoroacetabular impingement, which increases with SCFE severity, will result in significant long-term deterioration of the hip.

The technique of surgical dislocation of the hip with epiphyseal reorientation has been developed.[123,124] This technique involves a trochanteric osteotomy, gentle dislocation after a wide Z-capsulotomy, subperiosteal exposure of the posterior femoral neck, separation of the epiphysis through the physis, resection of the medial and posterior callus off the femoral neck, removal of the epiphyseal physis, reduction of the epiphysis without retinacular tension, and fixation of the epiphysis to the femoral neck.[124] The concept is that, with a properly and gently performed surgical dislocation of the hip, epiphyseal perfusion can be maintained during epiphyseal reorientation and avoid the high incidence of osteonecrosis that occurs when physeal resection with epiphyseal reduction is performed without surgical dislocation. Since 1996, Ganz has performed this procedure in 32 hips with a minimum follow-up of 18 months. Complications have included two fixation failures, the need for one varus/extension intertrochanteric osteotomy, and, most remarkably, no occurrence of osteonecrosis. (R. Ganz, MD, Chicago, IL, unpublished data, 2006.) This technique is demanding and should be performed by those appropriately trained. It still remains to be seen whether this new approach will result in improvement in long-term prognosis compared with results in a 41-year retrospective review by Carney and associates.[53]

## Summary

The etiology of the idiopathic SCFE is a combination of both biomechanical and biochemical factors,

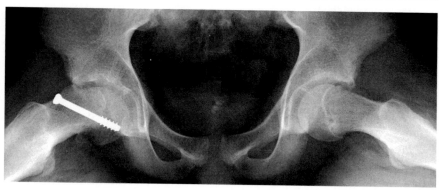

**Figure 13**  An example of impaction of the metaphysis on the acetabular rim when the hip is in the flexed position in a severe right SCFE in boy age 15 years, 5 months, after in situ single-screw central fixation. Note the early mild SCFE in the left hip.

whereas the role of genetics and heredity is variable. Naturally occurring SCFEs in animal models suggest that biochemical changes precede both physeal changes and subsequent SCFEs. Although pathologic changes of SCFE across species are the same, it appears that the etiology and pathophysiology are different. Several treatment modes, improved because of advances in imaging, exist for the stable SCFE, with single-screw fixation the most common treatment of SCFE currently used in North America. In the unstable SCFE, treatment is more controversial because of the increased risk of complications, especially osteonecrosis. Complications include osteonecrosis and chondrolysis, with better long-term prognosis for those with chondrolysis. Natural history without treatment entails the risk of progression and later degenerative joint disease of the hip. The conclusion drawn for long-term results of treatment is that regardless of severity, fixation in situ provides the best long-term function, lowest complication risk, and most effective delay of degenerative arthritis. Newer technologies include improved implants and in-

traoperative imaging, allowing surgeons to revisit the role of transphyseal osteotomy, reduction, and fixation. A current question is whether a realignment osteotomy performed today has a better outcome than that performed in the past. Finally, the technique of surgical dislocation of the hip with epiphyseal reorientation is considered; however, the long-term outcome is unknown.

## References

1. Schein AJ: Acute severe slipped capital femoral epiphysis. *Clin Orthop Relat Res* 1967;51:151-166.

2. Segal LS, Weitzel PP, Davidson RS: Valgus slipped capital femoral epiphysis: Fact or fiction? *Clin Orthop Relat Res* 1996;322:91-98.

3. Loder RT, O'Donnell PW, Didelot WP, Kayes KJ: Valgus slipped capital femoral epiphysis. *J Pediatr Orthop* 2006;26:594-600.

4. Yngve DA, Moulton DL, Evans EB: Valgus slipped capital femoral epiphysis. *J Pediatr Orthop B* 2005;14:172-176.

5. Loder RT, Wittenberg B, DeSilva G: Slipped capital femoral epiphysis associated with endocrine disorders. *J Pediatr Orthop* 1995;15:349-356.

6. Wells D, King JD, Roe TF, Kaufman FR: Review of slipped capital femoral epiphysis associated with endocrine disease. *J Pediatr Orthop* 1993;13: 610-614.

7. McAfee PC, Cady RB: Endocrinologic and metabolic factors in atypical presentations of slipped capital femoral epiphysis: Report of four cases and review of the literature. *Clin Orthop Relat Res* 1983;180:188-196.

8. Loder RT, Hensinger RN: Slipped capital femoral epiphysis associated with renal failure osteodystrophy. *J Pediatr Orthop* 1997;17:205-211.

9. Loder RT, Hensinger RN, Alburger PD, et al: Slipped capital femoral epiphysis associated with radiation therapy. *J Pediatr Orthop* 1998;18: 630-636.

10. Liu S-C, Tsai C-C, Huang C-H: Atypical slipped capital femoral epiphysis after radiotherapy and chemotherapy. *Clin Orthop Relat Res* 2004;426:212-218.

11. Ninomiya S, Nagasaka Y, Tagawa H: Slipped capital femoral epiphysis: A study of 68 cases in the eastern half area of Japan. *Clin Orthop Relat Res* 1976;119:172-176.

12. Kelsey JL, Keggi KJ, Southwick WO: The incidence and distribution of slipped capital femoral epiphysis in Connecticut and southwestern United States. *J Bone Joint Surg Am* 1970;52:1203-1216.

13. Lehmann CL, Arons RP, Loder RT, Vitale MG: The epidemiology of slipped capital femoral epiphysis: An update. *J Pediatr Orthop* 2006;26: 286-290.

14. Noguchi Y, Sakamaki T: Epidemiology and demographics of slipped capital femoral epiphysis in Japan: A multicenter study by the Japanese Paediatric Orthopaedic Association. *J Orthop Sci* 2002;7:610-617.

15. Hansson LI, Hägglund G, Ordeberg G: Slipped capital femoral epiphysis in southern Sweden 1910-1982. *Acta Orthop Scand Suppl* 1987;226:1-67.

16. Kocher MS, Bishop JA, Weed B, et al: Delay in diagnosis of slipped capital femoral epiphysis. *Pediatrics* 2004;113: e322-e325.

17. Loder RT, Starnes T, Dikos G, Aronsson DD: Demographic predictors of severity of stable slipped capital femoral epiphyses. *J Bone Joint Surg Am* 2006;88:97-105.

18. Loder RT: The demographics of slipped capital femoral epiphysis: An international multicenter study. *Clin Orthop Relat Res* 1996;322:8-27.

19. Kelsey JL, Acheson RM, Keggi KJ: The body build of patients with slipped capital femoral epiphysis. *Am J Dis Child* 1972;124:276-281.

20. KeepKidsHealty Website. Calculator BMI. Available at: http://www. keepkidshealthy.com/welcome/ bmicalculator.html. Accessed September 10, 2007.

21. Centers for Disease Control and Prevention Website. Body Mass Index. www.cdc.gov/nccdphp/dnpa/bmi/ bmi-for-age.html. Accessed September 10, 2007.

22. Bhatia NN, Pirpiris M, Otsuka NY: Body mass index in patients with slipped capital femoral epiphysis. *J Pediatr Orthop* 2006;26:197-199.

23. Manoff EM, Banffy MB, Winell JJ: Relationship between body mass index and slipped capital femoral epiphysis. *J Pediatr Orthop* 2005;25: 744-746.

24. Poussa M, Schlenzka D, Yrjönen T: Body mass index and slipped capital femoral epiphysis. *J Pediatr Orthop B* 2003;12:369-371.

25. Loder RT, Farley FA, Herzenberg JE, Hensinger RN, Kuhn JL: Narrow window of bone age in children with slipped capital femoral epiphyses. *J Pediatr Orthop* 1993;13:290-293.

26. Loder RT, Starnes T, Dikos G: The narrow window of bone age in children with slipped capital femoral epiphysis: A reassessment one decade later. *J Pediatr Orthop* 2006;26: 300-306.

27. Loder RT: A worldwide study on the seasonal variation of slipped capital femoral epiphysis. *Clin Orthop Relat Res* 1996;322:28-36.

28. Ferguson AB, Howorth MB: Slipping of the upper femoral epiphysis. *JAMA* 1931;97:1867-1872.

29. Morscher E: Strength and morphology of growth cartilage under hormonal influence of puberty: Animal experiments and clinical study on the etiology of local growth disorders during puberty. *Reconstr Surg Traumatol* 1968;10:3-104.

30. Hägglund G, Hansson LI, Ordeberg G: Epidemiology of slipped capital femoral epiphysis in southern Sweden. *Clin Orthop Relat Res* 1984;191: 82-94.

31. Andrén L, Borgström KE: Seasonal variation of epiphysiolysis of the hip and possibility of causal factor. *Acta Orthop Scand* 1958;28:22-26.

32. Brown D: Seasonal variation of slipped capital femoral epiphysis in the United States. *J Pediatr Orthop* 2004;24:139-143.

33. Maffulli N, Douglas AS: Seasonal variation of slipped capital femoral epiphysis. *J Pediatr Orthop B* 2002;11: 29-33.

34. Jerre R, Billing L, Hansson G, Wallin J: The contralateral hip in patients primarily treated for unilateral slipped upper femoral epiphysis. *J Bone Joint Surg Br* 1994;76:563-567.

35. Jerre R, Billing L, Hansson G, Karlsson J, Wallin J: Bilaterality in slipped capital femoral epiphysis: Importance of a reliable radiographic method. *J Pediatr Orthop B* 1996;5: 80-84.

36. Hurley JM, Betz RR, Loder RT, Davidson RS, Alburger PD, Steel HH: Slipped capital femoral epiphysis: The prevalence of late contralateral slip. *J Bone Joint Surg Am* 1996;78: 226-230.

37. Stasikelis PJ, Sullivan CM, Phillips WA, Polard JA: Slipped capital femoral epiphysis: Prediction of contralateral involvement. *J Bone Joint Surg Am* 1996;78:1149-1155.

38. Wilson PD, Jacobs B, Schecter L: Slipped capital femoral epiphysis: An

end-result study. *J Bone Joint Surg Am* 1965;47:1128-1145.

39. Sørensen KH: Slipped upper femoral epiphysis: Clinical study on aetiology. *Acta Orthop Scand* 1968;39:499-517.

40. Dreghorn CR, Knight D, Mainds CC, Blockey NJ: Slipped upper femoral epiphysis: A review of 12 years of experience in Glasgow (1972-1983). *J Pediatr Orthop* 1987;7: 283-287.

41. Loder RT, Aronson DD, Greenfield ML: The epidemiology of bilateral slipped capital femoral epiphysis: A study of children in Michigan. *J Bone Joint Surg Am* 1993;75:1141-1147.

42. Segal LS, Davidson RS, Robertson WWJ, Drummond DS: Growth disturbance after pinning of juvenile slipped capital femoral epiphysis. *J Pediatr Orthop* 1991;11:631-637.

43. Stott S, Bidwell T: Epidemiology of slipped capital femoral epiphysis in a population with a high proportion of New Zealand Maori and Pacific children. *N Z Med J* 2003;116:U647.

44. Kitadai HK, Milani C, Nery CAS, Filho JL: Wiberg's center-edge angle in patients with slipped capital femoral epiphysis. *J Pediatr Orthop* 1999;19: 97-105.

45. Loder RT, Mehbod AA, Meyer CA, Meisterling M: Acetabular depth and race in young adults: A potential explanation of the differences in the prevalence of slipped capital femoral epiphysis (SCFE) between different racial groups? *J Pediatr Orthop* 2003; 23:699-702.

46. Fahey JJ, O'Brien ET: Acute slipped capital femoral epiphysis. *J Bone Joint Surg Am* 1965;47:1105-1127.

47. Aronson DD, Carlson WE: Slipped capital femoral epiphysis: A prospective study of fixation with a single screw. *J Bone Joint Surg Am* 1992;74: 810-819.

48. Ward WT, Stefko J, Wood KB, Stanitski CL: Fixation with a single screw for slipped capital femoral epiphysis. *J Bone Joint Surg Am* 1992;74:799-809.

49. Aadalen RJ, Weiner DS, Hoyt W, Herndon CH: Acute slipped capital femoral epiphysis. *J Bone Joint Surg Am* 1974;56:1473-1487.

50. Boyer DW, Mickelson MR, Ponseti IV: Slipped capital femoral epiphysis: Long-term follow-up of one hundred and twenty-one patients. *J Bone Joint Surg Am* 1981;63:85-95.

51. Ponseti I, Barta CK: Evaluation of treatment of slipping of the capital femoral epiphysis. *Surg Gynecol Obstet* 1948;86:87-97.

52. Casey BH, Hamilton HW, Bobechko WP: Reduction of acutely slipped capital femoral epiphysis. *J Bone Joint Surg Br* 1972;54:607-614.

53. Carney BT, Weinstein SW, Noble J: Long-term follow-up of slipped capital femoral epiphysis. *J Bone Joint Surg Am* 1991;73:667-674.

54. Jacobs B: Diagnosis and natural history of slipped capital femoral epiphysis. *Instr Course Lect* 1972;21:167-173.

55. Rab GT: The geometry of slipped capital femoral epiphysis: Implications for movement, impingement, and corrective osteotomy. *J Pediatr Orthop* 1999;19:419-424.

56. Loder RT, Richards BS, Shapiro PS, Reznick LR, Aronson DD: Acute slipped capital femoral epiphysis: The importance of physeal stability. *J Bone Joint Surg Am* 1993;75:1134-1140.

57. Kallio PE, Paterson DC, Foster BK, Lequesne GW: Classification in slipped capital femoral epiphysis: Sonographic assessment of stability and remodeling. *Clin Orthop Relat Res* 1993;294:196-203.

58. Kallio PE, Mah ET, Foster BK, Paterson DC, LeQuesne GW: Slipped capital femoral epiphysis: Incidence and assessment of physeal instability. *J Bone Joint Surg Br* 1995;77:752-755.

59. Aronsson DD, Loder RT: Treatment of the unstable (acute) slipped capital femoral epiphysis. *Clin Orthop Relat Res* 1996;322:99-110.

60. Rhoad RC, Davidson RS, Heyman S, Dormans JP, Drummond DS: Pretreatment bone scan in SCFE: A predictor of ischemia and avascular necrosis. *J Pediatr Orthop* 1999;19: 164-168.

61. Steel HH: The metaphyseal blanch sign of slipped capital femoral epiphysis. *J Bone Joint Surg Am* 1986;68: 920-922.

62. Klein A, Joplin RJ, Reidy JA, Hanelin J: Slipped capital femoral epiphysis: Early diagnosis and treatment facilitated by "normal" roentgenograms. *J Bone Joint Surg Am* 1952;34:233-239.

63. Kamegaya M, Saisu T, Ochiai N, Moriya H: Preoperative assessment for intertrochanteric femoral osteotomies in severe chronic slipped capital femoral epiphysis using computed tomography. *J Pediatr Orthop B* 2005;14: 71-78.

64. Loder RT, Blakemore LC, Farley FA, Laidlaw AT: Measurement variability of slipped capital femoral epiphysis. *J Orthop Surg (Hong Kong)* 2000;7: 33-42.

65. Southwick WO: Osteotomy through the lesser trochanter for slipped capital femoral epiphysis. *J Bone Joint Surg Am* 1967;49:807-835.

66. Carney BT, Weinstein SL: Natural history of untreated chronic slipped capital femoral epiphysis. *Clin Orthop Relat Res* 1996;322:43-47.

67. Weiner D: Pathogenesis of slipped capital femoral epiphysis: Current concepts. *J Pediatr Orthop B* 1996;5: 67-73.

68. Galbraith RT, Gelberman RH, Hajek PC, et al: Obesity and decreased femoral anteversion in adolescence. *J Orthop Res* 1987;5:523-528.

69. Gelberman RH, Cohen MS, Shaw BA, Kasser JR, Griffin PP, Wilkinson RH: The association of femoral retroversion with slipped capital femoral epiphysis. *J Bone Joint Surg Am* 1986; 68:1000-1007.

70. Pritchett JW, Perdue KD: Mechanical factors in slipped capital femoral epiphysis. *J Pediatr Orthop* 1988;8: 385-388.

71. Mirkopulos N, Weiner DS, Askew M: The evolving slope of the proximal femoral growth plate relationship

to slipped capital femoral epiphysis. *J Pediatr Orthop* 1988;8:268-273.

72. Fishkin Z, Armstrong D, Shah H, Patra A, Mihaldo WM: Proximal femoral physis shear in slipped capital femoral epiphysis: A finite element study. *J Pediatr Orthop* 2006;26:291-294.

73. Exner GU: Growth and pubertal development in slipped capital femoral epiphysis: A longitudinal study. *J Pediatr Orthop* 1986;6:403-409.

74. Speer DP: Experimental epiphysiolysis: Etiologic models of slipped capital femoral epiphysis, in Nelson JP (ed): *The Hip: Proceedings of the 12th Open Scientific Meeting of the Hip Society.* St. Louis, MO, CV Mosby, 1982, pp 68-88.

75. Harris WR: The endocrine basis for slipping of the upper femoral epiphysis. *J Bone Joint Surg Br* 1950;32:5-11.

76. Brenkel IJ, Dias JJ, Iqbal SJ, Gregg PJ: Thyroid hormone levels in patients with slipped capital femoral epiphysis. *J Pediatr Orthop* 1988;8:22-25.

77. Eisenstein A, Rothschild S: Biochemical abnormalities in patients with slipped capital femoral epiphysis and chondrolysis. *J Bone Joint Surg Am* 1976;58:459-467.

78. Mann DC, Weddington J, Richton S: Hormonal studies in patients with slipped capital femoral epiphysis without evidence of endocrinopathy. *J Pediatr Orthop* 1988;8:543-545.

79. Razzano CD, Nelson C, Eversman J: Growth hormone levels in slipped capital femoral epiphysis. *J Bone Joint Surg Am* 1972;54:1224-1226.

80. Wilcox PG, Weiner DS, Leighlye B: Maturation factors in slipped capital femoral epiphysis. *J Pediatr Orthop* 1988;8:196-200.

81. Nicolai RD, Grasemann H, Oberste-Berghaus C, Hövel M, Hauffa BP: Serum insulin-like growth factors IGF-1 and IGFBP-3 in children with slipped capital femoral epiphysis. *J Pediatr Orthop B* 1999;8:103-106.

82. Rennie AM: The inheritance of slipped upper femoral epiphysis.

*J Bone Joint Surg Br* 1982;64:180-184.

83. Loder RT, Nechleba J, Sanders JO, Doyle P: Idiopathic slipped capital femoral epiphysis in Amish children. *J Bone Joint Surg Am* 2005;87:543-549.

84. Günal I, Ates E: The HLA phenotype in slipped capital femoral epiphysis. *J Pediatr Orthop* 1997;17:655-656.

85. Bednarz PA, Stanitski CL: Slipped capital femoral epiphysis in identical twins: HLA predisposition. *Orthopedics* 1998;21:1291-1293. Medline

86. Wong-Chung J, Al-Aali Y, Farid I, Al-Aradi A: A common HLA phenotype in slipped capital femoral epiphysis? *Int Orthop* 2000;24:158-159.

87. Flores M, Satish SG, Key T: Slipped capital femoral epiphysis in identical twins: Is there an HLA predisposition? *Bull Hosp Jt Dis* 2006;63:158-160. Medline

88. Agamanolis DP, Weiner DS, Lloyd JK: Slipped capital femoral epiphysis: A pathological study: I. A light microscopic and histochemical study of 21 cases. *J Pediatr Orthop* 1985;5:40-46.

89. Ponseti IV, McClintock R: Pathology of slipping of the upper femoral epiphysis. *J Bone Joint Surg Am* 1956;38:71-83.

90. Adamczyk MJ, Weiner DS, Nugent A, McBurney D, Horton WE Jr: Increased chondrocyte apoptosis in growth plates from children with slipped capital femoral epiphysis. *J Pediatr Orthop* 2005;25:440-444.

91. Agamanolis DP, Weiner DS, Lloyd JK: Slipped capital femoral epiphysis: A pathological study: II. An ultrastructural study of 23 cases. *J Pediatr Orthop* 1985;5:47-58.

92. McNicholas WT Jr, Wilkens BE, Blevins WE, et al: Spontaneous femoral capital physeal fractures in adult cats: 26 cases (1996-2001). *J Am Vet Med Assoc* 2002;221:1731-1736.

93. Craig LE: Physeal dysplasia with slipped capital femoral epiphysis in 13 cats. *Vet Pathol* 2001;38:92-97.

94. Queen J, Bennett D, Carmichael S: Femoral neck metaphyseal osteopa-

thy in the cat. *Vet Rec* 1998;142:159-162.

95. Root MV, Johnston SD, Olson PN: The effect of prepuberal and postpuberal gonadectomy on radial physeal closure in male and female domestic cats. *Vet Radiol Ultrasound* 1997;38:42-47.

96. Stubbs WP, Bloomberg MS, Scruggs SL, Shille VM, Lane TJ: Effects of prepubertal gonadectomy on physical and behavioral development in cats. *J Am Vet Med Assoc* 1996;209:1864-1871.

97. Hill MA: Skeletal system and feet, in Leman AD, Straw BE, Mengeling WL, D'Allaire S, Taylor DJ, (eds): *Diseases of Swine,* ed 7. Ames, Iowa, Iowa State University Press, 1992, pp163-195.

98. Reiland S: Morphology of osteochondrosis and sequelae in pigs. *Acta Radiol Suppl* 1978;358:45-90.

99. Holmes RG: Separation of the upper femoral epiphysis in the coypu (*Myocastor coypus*). *Vet Rec* 1967;80:405-407.

100. Blenkinsopp WK, Blenkinsopp EC, Flack MB: Slipped femoral epiphysis in the coypu. *J Pathol Bacteriol* 1967;93:690-693.

101. Dupuis J, Breton L, Drolet R: Bilateral epiphysiolysis of the femoral heads in two dogs. *J Am Vet Med Assoc* 1997;210:1162-1165.

102. Moores AP, Owen MR, Coe RJ, Brown PJ, Butterworth SJ: Slipped capital femoral epiphysis in dogs. *J Small Anim Pract* 2004;45:602-608.

103. Lee R: Proximal femoral epiphyseal separation in the dog. *J Small Anim Pract* 1976;17:669-679.

104. Hamilton GF, Turner AS, Ferguson JG, Pharr JW: Slipped capital femoral epiphysis in calves. *J Am Vet Med Assoc* 1978;172:1318-1322.

105. Hull BL, Koenig GJ, Monke DR: Treatment of slipped capital femoral epiphysis in cattle: 11 cases (1974-1988). *J Am Vet Med Assoc* 1990;197:1509-1512.

106. Rahme D, Comley A, Foster B, Cundy P: Consequences of diagnos-

tic delays in slipped capital femoral epiphysis. *J Pediatr Orthop B* 2006;15: 93-97.

107. Meier MC, Meyer LC, Ferguson RL: Treatment of slipped capital femoral epiphysis with a spica cast. *J Bone Joint Surg Am* 1992;74:1522-1529.

108. Rao SB, Crawford AH, Burger RR, Roy DR: Open bone peg epiphyseodesis for slipped capital femoral epiphysis. *J Pediatr Orthop* 1996;16:37-48.

109. Adamczyk MJ, Weiner DS, Hawk D: A 50-year experience with bone graft epiphyseodesis in the treatment of slipped capital femoral epiphysis. *J Pediatr Orthop* 2003;23:578-583.

110. Aronson DD, Peterson DA, Miller DV: Slipped capital femoral epiphysis: The case for internal fixation in situ. *Clin Orthop Relat Res* 1992;281: 115-122.

111. Strong M, Lejman T, Michno P, Sulko J: Fixation of slipped capital femoral epiphyses with unthreaded 2-mm wires. *J Pediatr Orthop* 1996;16: 53-55.

112. Weiner DS, Weiner S, Melby A, Hoyt WH Jr: A 30-year experience with bone graft epiphysiodesis in the treatment of slipped capital femoral epiphysis. *J Pediatr Orthop* 1984;4:145-152.

113. Schmidt TL, Cimino WG, Seidel FG: Allograft epiphysiodesis for slipped capital femoral epiphysis. *Clin Orthop Relat Res* 1996;322:61-76.

114. DeRosa GP, Mullins RC, Kling TF Jr : Cuneiform osteotomy of the femoral neck in severe slipped capital femoral epiphysis. *Clin Orthop Relat Res* 1996;322:48-60.

115. Velasco R, Schai PA, Exner GU: Slipped capital femoral epiphysis: A long-term follow-up study after open reduction of the femoral head combined with subcapital wedge resection. *J Pediatr Orthop B* 1998;7:43-52.

116. Fish JB: Cuneiform osteotomy of the femoral neck in the treatment of slipped capital femoral epiphysis. *J Bone Joint Surg Am* 1984;66:1153-1168.

117. Fish JB: Cuneiform osteotomy of the femoral neck in the treatment of slipped capital femoral epiphysis. *J Bone Joint Surg Am* 1994;76:46-59.

118. Barmada R, Bruch RF, Gimbel JS, Ray RD: Base of the neck extracapsular osteotomy for correction of deformity in slipped capital femoral epiphysis. *Clin Orthop Relat Res* 1978;132: 98-101.

119. Kramer WG, Craig WA, Noel S: Compensating osteotomy at the base of the femoral neck for slipped capital femoral epiphysis. *J Bone Joint Surg Am* 1976;58:796-800.

120. Schai PA, Exner GU, Hansch O: Prevention of secondary coxarthrosis in slipped capital femoral epiphysis: A long-term follow-up study after corrective intertrochanteric osteotomy. *J Pediatr Orthop B* 1996;5:135-143.

121. Parsch K, Bühl T, Weller S: Intertrochanteric corrective osteotomy for moderate and severe chronic slipped capital femoral epiphysis. *J Pediatr Orthop B* 1999;8:223-230.

122. Kartenbender K, Cordier W, Katthagen B-D: Long-term follow-up study after corrective Imhäuser osteotomy for severe slipped capital femoral epiphysis. *J Pediatr Orthop* 2000;20:749-756.

123. Leunig M, Casillas MM, Hamlet M, et al: Slipped capital femoral epiphysis: Early mechanical damage to the acetabular cartilage by a prominent femoral metaphysis. *Acta Orthop Scand* 2000;71:370-375.

124. Ganz R, Gill TJ, Gautier E, Ganz K, Krügel N, Berlemann U: Surgical dislocation of the adult hip: A technique with full access to the femoral head and acetabulum without the risk of avascular necrosis. *J Bone Joint Surg Br* 2001;83:1119-1124.

125. Spencer S, Millis MB, Kim Y-J: Early results of treatment for hip impingement syndrome in slipped capital femoral epiphysis and pistol grip deformity of the femoral head-neck junction using the surgical dislocation technique. *J Pediatr Orthop* 2006;26: 281-285.

126. Beck M, Leunig M, Parvizi J, Boutier V, Wyss D, Ganz R: Anterior femoroacetabular impingement: Part II. Midterm results of surgical treatment. *Clin Orthop Relat Res* 2004;418: 67-73.

127. Lavigne M, Parvizi J, Beck M, Siebenrock KA, Ganz R, Leunig M: Anterior femoroacetabular impingement: Part 1. Techniques of joint preserving surgery. *Clin Orthop Relat Res* 2004;418: 61-66.

128. O'Brien ET, Fahey JJ: Remodeling of the femoral neck after in-situ pinning for slipped capital femoral epiphysis. *J Bone Joint Surg Am* 1977;59:62-68.

129. Bellemans J, Fabry G, Molenaers G, Lammens J, Moens P: Slipped capital femoral epiphysis: A long-term follow-up, with special emphasis on the capacities for remodeling. *J Pediatr Orthop B* 1996;5:151-157.

130. Jerre R, Billing L, Karlsson J: Loss of hip motion in slipped capital femoral epiphysis: A calculation from the slipping angle. *J Pediatr Orthop B* 1996;5: 144-150.

131. Claffey TJ: Avascular necrosis of the femoral head: An anatomical study. *J Bone Joint Surg Br* 1960;42:802-809.

132. Brodetti A: The blood supply of the femoral neck and head in relation to the damaging effects of nails and screws. *J Bone Joint Surg Br* 1960;42: 794-801.

133. Walters R, Simon SR: Joint destruction: A sequel of unrecognized pin penetration in patients with slipped capital femoral epiphyses, in *The Hip: Proceedings of the Eighth Open Scientific Meeting of the Hip Society*. St. Louis, MO, CV Mosby, 1980, pp 145-164.

134. Blanco JS, Taylor B, Johnston CE II: Comparison of single pin vs multiple pin fixation in treatment of slipped capital femoral epiphysis. *J Pediatr Orthop* 1992;12:384-389.

135. Morrissy RT: Slipped capital femoral epiphysis: Technique of percutaneous in situ fixation. *J Pediatr Orthop* 1990;10:347-350.

136. Karol LA, Doane RM, Cornicelli SF, Zak PA, Haut RC, Manoli A II:

Single versus double screw fixation for treatment of slipped capital femoral epiphysis: A biomechanical analysis. *J Pediatr Orthop* 1992;12:741-745.

137. Lee FY, Chapman CB: In situ pinning of hip for stable slipped capital femoral epiphysis on a radiolucent operating table. *J Pediatr Orthop* 2003; 23:27-29.

138. Blasier RD, Ramsey JR, White RR: Comparison of radiolucent and fracture tables in the treatment of slipped capital femoral epiphysis. *J Pediatr Orthop* 2004;24:642-644.

139. Canale ST, Azar F, Young J, Beaty JH, Warner WC, Whitmer G: Subtrochanteric fracture fixation of slipped capital femoral epiphysis: A complication of unused drill holes. *J Pediatr Orthop* 1994;14:623-626.

140. Carney BT, Birnbaum P, Minter C: Slip progression after in situ single screw fixation for stable slipped capital femoral epiphysis. *J Pediatr Orthop* 2003;23:584-589.

141. Maletis GB, Bassett GS: Windshield-wiper loosening: A complication of in situ screw fixation of slipped capital femoral epiphysis. *J Pediatr Orthop* 1993;13:607-609.

142. Mosely C: The "approach-withdraw phenomenon" in the pinning of slipped capital femoral epiphysis. *Orthop Trans* 1985;9:947.

143. Burke JG, Sher JL: Intra-operative arthrography facilitates accurate screw fixation of a slipped capital femoral epiphysis. *J Bone Joint Surg Br* 2004;86: 1197-1198.

144. Koval KJ, Lehman WB, Rose D, Koval RP, Grant A, Strongwater A: Treatment of slipped capital femoral epiphysis with a cannulated-screw technique. *J Bone Joint Surg Am* 1989; 71:1370-1377.

145. Lehman WB, Grant A, Rose D, Pugh J, Norman A: A method of evaluating possible pin penetration in slipped capital femoral epiphysis using a cannulated internal fixation device. *Clin Orthop Relat Res* 1984;186:65-70.

146. Lehman WB, Menche D, Grant A, Norman A, Pugh J: The problem of

evaluating in situ pinning of slipped capital femoral epiphysis: An experimental model and review of 63 consecutive cases. *J Pediatr Orthop* 1984;4: 297-303.

147. Goodman WW, Johnson JT, Robertson WW Jr: Single screw fixation for acute and acute-on-chronic slipped capital femoral epiphysis. *Clin Orthop Relat Res* 1996;322:86-90.

148. Stevens DB, Short BA, Burch JM: In situ fixation of the slipped capital femoral epiphysis with a single screw. *J Pediatr Orthop B* 1996;5:85-89.

149. Dunn DM, Angel JC: Replacement of the femoral head by open operation in severe adolescent slipping of the upper femoral epiphysis. *J Bone Joint Surg Br* 1978;60-B:394-403.

150. Betz RR, Steel HH, Emper WD, Huss GK, Clancy M: Treatment of slipped capital femoral epiphysis: Spica cast immobilization. *J Bone Joint Surg Am* 1990;72:587-600.

151. Crawford AH: Role of osteotomy in the treatment of slipped capital femoral epiphysis. *J Pediatr Orthop B* 1996; 5:102-109.

152. Southwick WO: Compression fixation after biplane intertrochanteric osteotomy for slipped capital femoral epiphysis. *J Bone Joint Surg Am* 1973; 55:1218-1224.

153. Jerre T: A study in slipped upper femoral epiphysis with special reference to late functional and roentgenological results and the value of closed reduction. *Acta Orthop Scand* 1950;(suppl 6).

154. Cooperman DR, Charles LM, Pathria M, Latimer B, Thompson GH: Postmortem description of slipped capital femoral epiphysis. *J Bone Joint Surg Br* 1992;74:595-599.

155. Jerne R, Hansson G, Wallin J, Karlsson J: Long-term results after realignment operations for slipped upper femoral epiphysis. *J Bone Joint Surg Br* 1996;78:745-750.

156. Mooney JF III, Sanders JO, Browne RH, et al: Management of unstable/ acute slipped capital femoral epiphysis: Results of a survey of the POSNA

membership. *J Pediatr Orthop* 2005;25: 162-166.

157. de Sanctis N, Di Gennaro G, Pempinello C, Della Corte S, Carannante G: Is gentle manipulative reduction and percutaneous fixation with a single screw the best management of acute and acute-on-chronic slipped capital femoral epiphysis? *J Pediatr Orthop B* 1996;5:90-95.

158. Herman MJ, Dormans JP, Davidson RS, Drummond DS, Gregg JR: Screw fixation of grade III slipped capital femoral epiphysis. *Clin Orthop Relat Res* 1996;322:77-85.

159. Peterson MD, Weiner DS, Green NE, Terry CL: Acute slipped capital femoral epiphysis: The value and safety of urgent manipulative reduction. *J Pediatr Orthop* 1997;17:648-654.

160. Gordon JE, Abrahams MS, Dobbs MB, Luhmann SJ, Schoenecker PL: Early reduction, arthrotomy, and cannulated screw fixation in unstable slipped capital femoral epiphysis treatment. *J Pediatr Orthop* 2002;22: 352-358.

161. Beck M, Siebenrock KA, Affolter B, Nützli H, Parvizi J, Ganz R: Increased intraarticular pressure reduces blood flow to the femoral head. *Clin Orthop Relat Res* 2004;424:149-152.

162. Svalastoga E, Kiær T, Jensen PE: The effect of intracapsular pressure and extension of the hip on oxygenation of the juvenile femoral epiphysis. *J Bone Joint Surg Br* 1989;71:222-226.

163. Kibiloski LJ, Doane RM, Karol LA, Haut RC, Loder RT: Biomechanical analysis of single- versus double-screw fixation in slipped capital femoral epiphysis at physiological load levels. *J Pediatr Orthop* 1994;14:627-630.

164. Snyder RR, Williams JL, Schmidt TL, Salsbury TL: Torsional strength of double- versus single-screw fixation in a pig model of unstable slipped capital femoral epiphysis. *J Pediatr Orthop* 2006;26:295-299.

165. Kishan S, Upasani V, Mahar A, et al: Biomechanical stability of single-screw versus two-screw fixation of an

unstable slipped capital femoral epiphysis model: Effect of screw position in the femoral neck. *J Pediatr Orthop* 2006;26:601-605.

166. Schultz WR, Weinstein JN, Weinstein SL, Smith BG: Prophylactic pinning of the contralateral hip in slipped capital femoral epiphysis: Evaluation of long-term outcome for the contralateral hip with use of decision analysis. *J Bone Joint Surg Am* 2002;84-A:1305-1314.

167. Kocher MS, Bishop JA, Hresko MT, Millis MB, Kim Y-J, Kasser JR: Prophylactic pinning of the contralateral hip after unilateral slipped capital femoral epiphysis. *J Bone Joint Surg Am* 2004;86-A:2658-2665.

168. Hägglund G: The contralateral hip in slipped capital femoral epiphysis. *J Pediatr Orthop B* 1996;5:158-161.

169. MacLean JGB, Reddy SK: The contralateral slip. *J Bone Joint Surg Br* 2006;88:1497-1501.

170. Seller K, Raab P, Wild A, Krauspe R: Risk-benefit analysis of prophylactic pinning in slipped capital femoral epiphysis. *J Pediatr Orthop B* 2001;10:192-196.

171. Castro FP Jr, Bennett JT, Doulens K: Epidemiological perspective on prophylactic pinning in patients with unilateral slipped capital femoral epiphysis. *J Pediatr Orthop* 2000;20:745-748.

172. Dietz FR: Traction reduction of acute and acute-on-chronic slipped capital femoral epiphysis. *Clin Orthop Relat Res* 1994;302:101-110.

173. Krahn TH, Canale ST, Beaty JH, Warner WC, Lourenco P: Long-term follow-up of patients with avascular necrosis after treatment of slipped capital femoral epiphysis. *J Pediatr Orthop* 1993;13:154-158.

174. Tokmakova KP, Stanton RP, Mason DE: Factors influencing the development of osteonecrosis in patients treated for slipped capital femoral epiphysis. *J Bone Joint Surg Am* 2003;85-A:798-801.

175. Ballard J, Cosgrove AP: Anterior physeal separation: A sign indicating a high risk for avascular necrosis after slipped capital femoral epiphysis. *J Bone Joint Surg Br* 2002;84:1176-1179.

176. Strange-Vognsen H, Wagner A, Dirksen K, et al: The value of scintigraphy in hips with slipped capital femoral epiphysis and the value of radiography and MRI after 10 years. *Acta Orthop Belg* 1999;65:33-38.

177. Mullins MM, Sood M, Hashemi-Nejad A, Catterall A: The management of avascular necrosis after slipped capital femoral epiphysis. *J Bone Joint Surg Br* 2005;87:1669-1674.

178. Maurer RC, Larsen IJ: Acute necrosis of cartilage in slipped capital femoral epiphysis. *J Bone Joint Surg Am* 1970;52:39-50.

179. Vrettos BC, Hoffman EB: Chondrolysis in slipped upper femoral epiphysis. *J Bone Joint Surg Br* 1993;75:956-961.

180. Ingram AJ, Clarke MS, Clark CS Jr, Marshall WR: Chondrolysis complicating slipped capital femoral epiphysis. *Clin Orthop Relat Res* 1982;165:99-109.

181. Mandell GA, Keret D, Harcke HT, Bowen JR: Chondrolysis: Detection by bone scintigraphy. *J Pediatr Orthop* 1992;12:80-85.

182. Aronson DD, Loder RT: Slipped capital femoral epiphysis in Black children. *J Pediatr Orthop* 1992;12:74-79.

183. Bishop JO, Oley TJ, Stephenson CT, Hullos HS: Slipped capital femoral epiphysis: A study of 50 cases in Black children. *Clin Orthop Relat Res* 1978;135:93-96.

184. Spero CR, Masciale JP, Tornetta P III, Star MJ, Tucci JJ: Slipped capital femoral epiphysis in Black children: Incidence of chondrolysis. *J Pediatr Orthop* 1992;12:444-448.

185. Kennedy JP, Weiner DS: Results of slipped capital femoral epiphysis in the Black population. *J Pediatr Orthop* 1990;10:224-227.

186. Orofino C, Innis JJ, Lowrey CW: Slipped capital femoral epiphysis in Negroes: A study of ninety-five cases. *J Bone Joint Surg Am* 1960;42:1079-1083.

187. Tillema DA, Golding JSR: Chondrolysis following slipped capital femoral epiphysis. *J Bone Joint Surg Am* 1971;53:1528-1540.

188. Gonzalez-Moran G, Carsi B, Abril JC, Albinana J: Results after preoperative traction and pinning in slipped capital femoral epiphysis: K wires versus cannulated screws. *J Pediatr Orthop B* 1998;7:53-58.

189. Tudisco C, Caterini R, Farsetti P, Potenza V: Chondrolysis of the hip complicating slipped capital femoral epiphysis: Long-term follow-up of nine patients. *J Pediatr Orthop B* 1999;8:107-111.

190. Hall JE: The results of treatment of slipped upper femoral epiphysis. *J Bone Joint Surg Br* 1957;39-B:659-673.

191. Oram V: Epiphysiolysis of the head of the femur: A follow-up examination with special reference to end results and the social prognosis. *Acta Orthop Scand* 1953;23:100-120.

192. Ross PM, Lyne ED, Morawa LG: Slipped capital femoral epiphysis: Long term results after 10-38 years. *Clin Orthop Relat Res* 1979;141:176-180.

193. Ordeberg G, Hansson LI, Sandström S: Slipped capital femoral epiphysis in southern Sweden. *Clin Orthop Relat Res* 1987;220:148-154.

194. Jerre R, Hansson G, Wallin J, Karlsson J: Does a single device prevent further slipping of the epiphysis in children with slipped capital femoral epiphysis? *Arch Orthop Trauma Surg* 1997;116:348-351.

195. Howorth B: Slipping of the capital femoral epiphysis: History. *Clin Orthop Relat Res* 1966;48:11-32.

196. Johnston RC, Larson CB: Results of treatment of hip disorders with cup arthroplasty. *J Bone Joint Surg Am* 1969;51:1461.

197. Murray RO: The etiology of primary osteoarthritis of the hip. *Br J Radiol* 1965;38:810-824.

198. Solomon L: Patterns of osteoarthritis of the hip. *J Bone Joint Surg Br* 1976;58:176-183.

199. Stulberg SD, Cordell LD, Harris WH: Unrecognized childhood hip disease: A major cause of idiopathic osteonecrosis of the hip, in *The Hip: Proceedings of the Third Open Scientific Meeting of The Hip Society*. St. Louis, MO, CV Mosby, 1975, pp 212-230.

200. Resnick D: The "tilt" deformity of the femoral head in osteoarthritis of the hip: A poor indicator of previous epiphysiolysis. *Clin Radiol* 1976;27:355-363.

201. Jerre T: Early complications of osteosynthesis with a three flanged nail in situ for slipped epiphysis. *Acta Orthop Scand* 1958;27:126.

202. Richolt JA, Teschner M, Everett PC, Millis MB, Kikinis R: Impingement simulation of the hip in SCFE using 3D models. *Comput Aided Surg* 1999;4:144-151.

# Subcapital Realignment in Slipped Capital Femoral Epiphysis: Surgical Hip Dislocation and Trimming of the Stable Trochanter to Protect the Perfusion of the Epiphysis

Michael Leunig, MD
Theddy Slongo, MD
Reinhold Ganz, MD

## Abstract

*Based on the recognition that even minor slip displacement in patients with slipped capital femoral epiphysis can regularly produce acetabular cartilage damage and early clinical symptoms, subcapital realignment of the epiphysis should be considered, although a substantial risk of osteonecrosis has been reported.*

*A modified surgical technique can be used in which the perfusion of the epiphysis via the medial femoral circumflex artery is actively protected during surgery by executing surgical dislocation of the joint and by developing a soft-tissue flap consisting of the retinaculum and the external rotator muscles. This flap allows mobilization of the epiphysis within the growth plate as well as complete callus resection of the neck without stretching the retinaculum. The dislocation of the head allows manual fixation of the epiphysis while curettage of the residual growth plate is performed, as well as manual reduction of the epiphysis onto the metaphysis under visual control of the retinaculum. With the head dislocated, any uncontrolled manipulation of the leg will result in less risk to the integrity of the retinaculum than would be the case if the head was reduced in the socket.*

**Instr Course Lect 2008;57:499-507.**

Although the best long-term outcomes for patients with slipped capital femoral epiphysis (SCFE) can be achieved with surgical treatment leading to normal perfusion and proper anatomic position of the epiphysis on the metaphysis, such surgery is rarely performed because of the risk of osteonecrosis and the presumed technical difficulties involved. Such concerns have favored the use of pinning in situ, which is a much less demanding technique. Several studies have reported good midterm results using this technique; however, some controversy exists because hips treated with pinning in situ may not become symptomatic until the patient reaches adulthood.[1-3]

Based on long-term experience with the use of osteotomies to treat SCFE, including the technique of subcapital wedge osteotomy, a clinical study was initiated because of the development of immediate postoperative joint narrowing in one patient.[4,5] This study showed that even minor slips of less than 30° can often lead to early and substantial acetabular cartilage damage.[6] Such damage is the result of a femoral or cam-type impingement between the prominent metaphysis and the acetabulum.[7] Intraoperative evidence has shown that the prominent metaphyseal bone with multiple callus spicas are squeezed into the acetabulum in flexion and in flexion-internal rotation. As a consequence, the undersurface of the labrum and the adjacent cartilage in the anterosuperior acetabulum show marks of abrasion, which may extend down to the subchondral bone (Figure 1). The extent of the acetabular damage is high in the early stages of the slippage and again when remodeling of the metaphyseal bump has been completed. These morphologic changes allow the metaphysis to penetrate into the acetabulum, while a clear posterior translation from epiphysis to metaphysis will lead to a stop at the acetabular rim rather than allowing the metaphysis to enter the joint. A three-dimensional simulation by Rab[3] indicated that in patients with SCFE, the metaphysis must come in contact with the

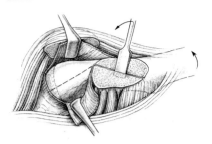

**Figure 1** Development of the retinaculum provides vascularity to the femoral head. The posterior portion of the greater trochanter is reduced through the apophysis down to the femoral neck. Distally, the short external rotators are subperiosteally released from the bone. At the cranial end of the osteotomy, the retinaculum is incised in line with the femoral neck axis to avoid uncontrolled tearing (*dashed line*).

acetabular cartilage; however, the deleterious consequence of motion was not considered. In a study of cadaver hips by Goodman and associates,[2] the most severe osteoarthritis in a group of younger adults was found in patients with silent slip morphology.

Osteotomies distant to the slip, which are described for angular correction of major deformities, may normalize the spatial orientation between the acetabulum and epiphysis, but they cannot sufficiently eliminate the impinging subcapital bump.[8] Screws inserted from the anterior neck into the head to eliminate further slippage have an even more deleterious effect.[9] The heads of these screws may increase the risk for impingement, even when they are only slightly above the level of the bone. Since 1998, the authors used a technique that allowed surgical dislocation of the hip without the risk of osteonecrosis in combination with the technique for open replacement of the displaced femoral head according to Dunn.[10-12] This combined technique allowed precise

mapping of the patient's cartilage damage. The safety of the combined procedure with respect to osteonecrosis was further improved with the addition of two steps. First, subperiosteal trimming of the stable trochanter down to the level of the neck allows safe exposure of the posterior aspect of the neck. This creates a soft-tissue flap of all external rotators and the retinaculum containing the deep branch of the medial femoral circumflex artery and its retinacular end branches, allowing perfusion of the epiphysis.[11,13] This rather large flap substantially reduces the danger of stretching or rupturing the retinaculum during removal of the callus formation around the neck.[14] The second step that improves the procedure is the dislocation of the femoral head, which allows visually controlled disconnection of the epiphysis and precise curettage of residuals of the former growth plate and debris using manual fixation of the epiphysis and a manual, anatomic repositioning of the epiphysis under visual control of the retinaculum. Real-time, dynamic recording of the perfusion of the epiphysis using laser Doppler flowmetry is possible.[15] The procedure normally does not lead to a shortening of the neck because only the femoral neck callus is removed.

## Goals of Treatment

The goals of subcapital realignment in patients with SCFE are to correct the position of the epiphysis at the level of the tilt, obtain mechanically undisturbed hip motion, and prevent further mechanical damage to the joint cartilage. The execution of the procedure is demanding, and detailed knowledge of the vascular anatomy of the hip is needed. This procedure may be indicated for all

chronic slips in which isolated trimming of the metaphyseal bump for impingement-free motion would exceed one third of the neck diameter.[16] The technique is also useful for all acute slips. Symptomatic slips after closure of the growth plate are better treated with a femoral neck osteotomy; however, most aspects of the procedures are identical. Because healing of a femoral neck osteotomy may take more time, stronger fixation is needed. Only partial weight bearing is allowed for the first 10 weeks after surgery. The prognosis for the hip undergoing surgery depends on the precision of the surgery and the amount of cartilage damage present at the time of surgery.

## Imaging Studies

Surgery for a chronic slip is a planned procedure, whereas treatment of an acute slip should be considered emergency surgery that should be performed within 6 to 8 hours after the event. An AP radiograph of the pelvis and axial views of both hips to define angulation and translation of the epiphysis in the frontal and sagittal plane should be obtained. A radial MRI of the hip allows the evaluation of the preexisting cartilage damage. Standard MRI and CT have little preoperative value for this procedure.

## Approach and Surgical Technique

A lateral decubitus position is used and the patient's leg is draped free. A sterile bag in which the leg is temporarily placed is fixed on the front of the operating table. A Gibson approach is used with posterior retraction of the gluteus maximus; this approach allows an exposure similar to the Kocher-Langenbeck approach but produces results that are cosmetically more acceptable.[17] Retracting the fascial layer between the maximus and medius muscles together with the gluteus maximus preserves optimal innervation and blood supply of this muscle.[18] The leg is then internally rotated and the posterior border of the gluteus medius is identified by dissecting the overlying adipose tissue. The level and direction of the trochanteric osteotomy are marked with a knife, creating a line from the posterosuperior edge to the posterior border of the vastus lateralis. The line is placed anterior to the trochanteric crest to avoid injury to the insertion of the external rotators. After the osteotomy, the gluteus medius, the vastus lateralis, and the long tendon of the gluteus minimus will remain attached to the trochanteric fragment. In patients with SCFE, the contracture of the joint in external rotation, by producing a closed vicinity of the tip of the greater trochanter to the posterior acetabular wall, may lead to a palpatory impression different from normal trochanteric anatomy, and may cause difficulties in executing the osteotomy. The maximum thickness of the trochanteric fragment should not exceed 1.5 cm. At its proximal end, the osteotomy should exit just anterior to the most posterior inserting fibers of the gluteus medius. This will keep most of the piriformis insertion on the femur and not on the fragment. Further dissection to expose the capsule takes place between the piriformis tendon and the gluteus minimus, an interval that offers the best protection for the blood supply to the femoral head and allows preservation of the constant anastomosis between the inferior gluteal artery and deep branch of the medial femoral circumflex artery. This anastomosis courses along the

distal border of the piriformis muscle and can provide sufficient perfusion of the femoral head when the deep branch of the medial femoral circumflex artery is violated.[11] The greater trochanteric fragment is then flipped anteriorly by elevating the vastus lateralis along its posterior border to the middle of the gluteus maximus tendon insertion onto the femoral shaft. Proximally, the few gluteus medius fibers remaining on the stable trochanter are cut, allowing further anterior mobilization of the trochanteric fragment. Flexion and external rotation of the leg facilitates the exposure of the capsule within the gap between the piriformis and the gluteus minimus. The anterosuperior capsular insertion of the gluteus minimus muscle is released while preserving the long tendon of the gluteus minimus that inserts anteriorly on the trochanteric fragment. Up to this point in the surgery, all external rotators remain attached to the stable trochanter and protect the medial femoral circumflex artery. The capsule is first incised close to the anterosuperior edge of the stable trochanter in a direction axial to the neck. With a perpendicular extension along the anterior neck insertion, a flap can be lifted up, allowing further insideout capsulotomy that provides protection from cutting into cartilage and labrum. The Z-shaped capsulotomy (for the right side) is extended along the posterosuperior border of the acetabulum. The anteroinferior extension of the capsulotomy is directed toward the anteroinferior border of the acetabulum. This extension must remain anterior to the lesser trochanter to avoid damage to the main branch of the medial femoral circumflex artery, which is located in the vicinity of the femur just superior and posterior to the

lesser trochanter. The anteromedial capsular flap is retracted using a small, spiked Hohmann retractor that is driven into the supraacetabular bone just lateral to the anteroinferior iliac spine. With the use of two additional Langenbeck retractors, the joint can be inspected for synovitis, color and quantity of synovial fluid, degree of femoral head tilt, and stability of the epiphysis on the metaphysis. If the epiphysis is mobile or stability is questionable, prophylactic pinning is recommended; however, any attempt at reducing a mobile epiphysis anatomically should be avoided at this time because there is a high risk of pathologic stretching of the retinaculum before removal of the posterior callus. Before surgical dislocation, a 2-mm drill hole is placed in the femoral head to document its blood perfusion.[19] Using laser Doppler flowmetry, dynamic control of the perfusion is possible and can be used throughout the operation.[15] The hip is then flexed and externally rotated; the leg is placed into a sterile bag over the anterior side of the table. During this maneuver, the femoral head subluxates; the view into the joint can be further improved using a bone hook around the calcar femoris.

The damage pattern to the labrum and cartilage of the acetabulum can now be documented, and the creation of the damage by the anterior metaphysis above the level of the epiphyseal contour can be reproduced by again reducing the head and driving it through flexion and flexion internal rotation. If the epiphyseal tilt is small (< 30°) in a stable situation, and if trimming of the anterior metaphysis would be sufficient without creating a too thin neck, full dislocation is not necessary.[16] Surgery then proceeds with

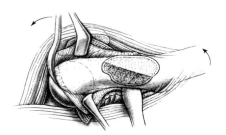

**Figure 2** The retinaculum is mobilized further proximally and dorsally while carefully respecting the vascular foramina at the head/neck junction. After transepiphyseal separation of the epiphysis from the metaphysis, the posterior callus can be resected down the original bone of the neck. The retinaculum should not be under any tension.

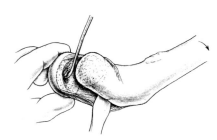

**Figure 3** Using manual control, the remaining cartilage from the physis is débrided.

the creation of a normal offset by trimming the metaphyseal contour and pinning the epiphysis in situ.

If the amount of slippage does not permit the use of this technique, the next step is dislocation of the femoral head. With the head in a subluxated position, the round ligament can be sectioned using curved scissors. By manipulations of the leg, and with the help of special retractors on the acetabular rim and around the teardrop area, 360° of the acetabulum can be viewed. When the retractors are removed, lowering of the knee exposes the femoral head for inspection. Different surfaces of the head can be visualized by rotating the leg, and the actual amount of epiphyseal slip can be recorded. The retinaculum protecting the terminal branches of the medial femoral circumflex artery to the femoral epiphysis is clearly visible on the posterosuperior contour of the neck as a somewhat mobile layer of connective tissue. The femoral head cartilage should be constantly moistened during exposure. The femoral head is again reduced in the socket for the creation of the soft-

tissue flap consisting of retinaculum and external rotators and containing the blood supply for the epiphysis. The area of the stable trochanter proximal to the visible growth plate is carefully mobilized using an osteotome (Figure 1). This fragment is then subperiosteally excised in an inside-out fashion. The periosteum of the neck is incised anterior to the visible retinaculum from the anterosuperior edge of the trochanteric growth plate toward the head. The periosteum is now elevated from the posterior neck using a knife and sharp periosteal elevators. Care must be taken to avoid rupture of the anterior insertion of the retinaculum near the femoral epiphysis. The periosteal release is extended distally to the base of the lesser trochanter. Any remaining osseous ledge of the trochanteric base is leveled. In a similar manner, the anteromedial periosteum is freed, a step that is easier to perform with the femoral head dislocated. Care must be taken to prevent disruption of the periosteal tube from the epiphysis (Figure 2). At this point in the procedure, the perfusion of the epiphysis may again be checked with the previously described techniques. With the head still dislocated, two blunt retractors are used to expose the femoral neck medially and later-

ally, avoiding any stretching of the retinaculum. The epiphysis will be mobilized in a stepwise fashion using a curved 10-mm osteotome that is anteriorly placed into the epiphyseal growth plate.

It should be noted that the growth plate is located proximal to the distal border of the epiphyseal joint cartilage. Normally, no wedge resection is necessary. By simultaneous levering with the osteotome and with controlled external rotation of the leg, the metaphyseal stump will emerge from the periosteal tube while the epiphysis remains in a posteromedial position. Removal of a posteromedial callus bridge in flexion-external rotation may facilitate this step in the process. Spontaneous reduction of the isolated epiphysis into the socket may occur at this time. Redislocation is difficult even when using Kirschner wires introduced into the epiphysis; however, a small swab placed in the socket can help to avoid this complication. Next, the visible or palpable callus formation on the posterior and posteromedial aspect of the neck is removed. Such callus formation is present even in acute slips with brief symptomatology. To provide a large contact area with the epiphysis, the front surface of the metaphyseal stump is rounded; actual neck shortening is rarely indicated. Controlled rotational maneuvers of the shaped femoral neck allow manual fixation of the epiphysis while curettage of the remainder of the growth plate is performed (Figure 3). Normally, the exposed epiphyseal bone shows clear bleeding as a sign of intact perfusion. After removal of all callus particles, the epiphysis is reduced onto the neck under visual control of the retinacular tension. The reduction is facilitated by internal rotation of the leg. If any tension in the retinaculum occurs during this maneuver, the maneuver is immediately stopped. Occasionally, parts of the posterior soft-tissue flap are inverted and must be unfolded. The height of the metaphysis rarely requires reduction. It is very important to determine the correct spatial orientation of the epiphysis. The border of the epiphysis should have an equal distance to the neck in all planes, which can be controlled using a palpating instrument or with intraoperative fluoroscopy. Correct rotation may be checked visually with the relative localization of the retinaculum and the fovea capitis. The most difficult realignment involves obtaining the correct varus-valgus position; this must be controlled with fluoroscopy. The accepted position is temporarily fixed using a fully threaded Kirschner wire that is inserted in a retrograde direction via the fovea capitis and which perforates the lateral cortex of the femur just distal to the vastus lateralis ridge (Figure 4). After this wire is pulled back so far that its tip levels the femoral head cartilage, the head is carefully reduced into the socket to allow final control of alignment with fluoroscopy. If perfect alignment of the epiphysis is achieved, one or two additional fully threaded Kirschner wires are introduced from the lateral cortex of the subtrochanteric bone. The correct wire length can be visually controlled with another dislocation of the joint or with the use of fluoroscopy. The threaded pins should be optimally distributed within the epiphysis (Figure 4).

Bone grafting at the epimetaphyseal step is not necessary because existing gaps will be filled spontaneously. At the end of the procedure, the perfusion of the epiphysis again can be controlled. The periosteal tube is closed with a few stitches, avoiding any tension. The capsular closure also should avoid tension. If the tendon of the piriformis muscle

is producing tension on the capsule, it should be released. Refixation of the trochanteric fragment is performed with two 3.5-mm screws (Figure 4). With careful closure of the subcutaneous adipose tissue in several layers, suction drainage is not necessary. Continuous passive motion is used during the postoperative hospital stay. The patient is instructed on the use of crutches for toe-touch walking. Deep venous thrombosis prophylaxis using low-dose heparin is administered only to obese patients.

Radiographic follow-up is done after 8 weeks; at this time, the trochanteric osteotomy should be healed. Full weight bearing is allowed after 8 to 10 weeks, when AP and lateral radiographs show sufficient consolidation. Training of the gluteus medius starts at 6 to 8 weeks, and full muscle strength should be achieved at 10 to 12 weeks. If hardware removal is required, it should not be done until at least 1 year after surgery. **(DVD 40.1)**

## Results of the Authors' Experience

In 1992, the authors first used the original Dunn and Angel[12] surgical procedure for open realignment of the displaced femoral head to treat 19 hips. From 1996 to 1998, a surgical subluxation or dislocation technique was added to the procedure to allow inspection of the acetabular rim area (used on 18 hips). No osteonecrosis occurred in either group. The modification of the Dunn and Angel procedure, including dislocation of the hip and the creation of a soft-tissue flap for more active protection of the femoral head perfusion, was first performed by the authors in 1998. From 1998 until August 2004, 33 hips were surgically treated with the technique. Three hips were ex-

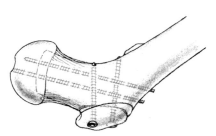

**Figure 4**      With the joint dislocated, the epiphysis is reduced without tension on the retinaculum. The reduction is stabilized with fully threaded wires.

cluded from the results—two hips in a patient with chronic renal insufficiency who had bilateral slip realignment and one hip in a patient with established necrosis of the hip. The 30 remaining patients (30 hips) in the series were surgically treated for classic SCFE (Figure 5).

A summary of the patients treated in this consecutive series is shown in Table 1. Outcomes include one hip in which the epiphysis slipped again 1 year after pins from an earlier fixation had been removed before closure of the growth plate was completed. Twenty-three procedures were performed on the left hip and seven on the right hip. Patients ranged in age from 10 to 17 years (mean age of girls, 12 years; mean age of boys, 14 years). The posterior tilt of the epiphysis ranged from 30° to 70°. An additional linear shift of the epiphysis was especially prevalent with minor angulations but was a more crucial factor in the impingement process. In six hips, an "acute-on-chronic" slip made quantification of the slip impossible. In one hip (No. 8), radiography was performed shortly before the acute slip. Another hip (No. 18) was asymptomatic before a high-energy traumatic injury and was therefore diagnosed as traumatic growth plate separation. However, the intraoperative findings of callus formation on

**Table 1**
**Summary of a Consecutive Series of 30 Patients With SCFE Who Were Treated With the Described Surgical Technique to Protect Perfusion of the Epiphysis**

| Patient No. | Age at Surgery (years) | Sex | Side Right (R) Left (L) | Duration of Symptoms | Slip | Linear Translation |
|---|---|---|---|---|---|---|
| 1 | 11 | F | R | 3 weeks | 30° | +++ |
| 2 | 14 | M | L | 6 weeks | -- | -- |
| 3 | 13 | M | L | Unknown | 30° | + |
| 4 | 15 | M | L | Unknown | 20° | +++ |
| 5 | 13 | F | L | 3 to 4 months | 50° | +++ |
| 6 | 11 | F | L | 2 weeks | -- | -- |
| 7 | 14 | M | L | 6 months | -- | -- |
| 8 | 12 | M | L | 3 months | 15°* | ++* |
| 9 | 11 | F | L | 3 months | 70° | +++ |
| 10 | 11 | F | L | 2 months | 35° | +++ |
| 11 | 13 | F | L | 4 weeks | 70° | +++ |
| 12 | 12 | F | L | 6 months | 50° | ++ |
| 13 | 13 | M | L | 2 months | 70° | +++ |
| 14 | 17 | M | R | 2 months | 50° | + |
| 15 | 11 | F | R | 5 months | 50° | +++ |
| 16 | 13 | M | L | 2 months | -- | -- |
| 17 | 15 | M | R | 9 months | 40° | +++ |
| 18 | 16 | M | R | Unknown | -- | -- |
| 19 | 13 | M | L | 2 months | 35° | ++ |
| 20 | 15 | F | L | 3 months | 60° | +++ |
| 21 | 15 | M | L | 6 weeks | 30° | +++ |
| 22 | 14 | M | L | 4 months | 35° | ++ |
| 23 | 15 | M | L | 3 years | 45° | + |
| 24 | 14 | M | R | 3 months | 50° | ++ |
| 25 | 10 | F | L | 2 weeks | -- | -- |
| 26 | 11 | F | L | 5 weeks | 40° | +++ |
| 27 | 12 | F | L | 5 months | 30° | +++ |
| 28 | 13 | M | L | Unknown | 40° | ++ |
| 29 | 10 | F | R | 12 months | 30° | +++ |
| 30 | 15 | F | R | 18 months | 50° | +++ |

**Table 1 (cont)**
**Summary of a Consecutive Series of 30 Patients With SCFE Who Were Treated With the Described Surgical Technique to Protect Perfusion of the Epiphysis**

| Chronicity | Labral Damage | Acetabular Cartilage Damage | Miscellaneous | LDF | Complications | Follow-up (months) |
|---|---|---|---|---|---|---|
| Chronic | ++ | +++ | 0 | | 0 | 24 |
| Acute-on-chronic | + | ++ | 0 | | 0 | 24 |
| Chronic | + | ++ | 0 | Yes | 0 | 26 |
| Chronic | ++ | ++ | 0 | | 0 | 29 |
| Chronic | 0 | +++ | 0 | Yes | 0 | 32 |
| Acute-on-chronic | + | ++ | 0 | Yes | 0 | 32 |
| Acute | ++ | + | 0 | | 0 | 44 |
| Acute-on-chronic | + | + | 0 | | 0 | 4 |
| Chronic | 0 | + | 0 | | 0 | 44 |
| Chronic | +++ | +++ | 0 | Yes | 0 | 45 |
| Chronic | + | ++ | 1 year after pin removal | | 0 | 46 |
| Chronic | ++ | ++ | 0 | Yes | 0 | 50 |
| Chronic | +++ | + | 0 | Yes | 0 | 52 |
| Chronic | ++ | + | 0 | Yes | 0 | 55 |
| Chronic | + | ++ | 0 | Yes | 0 | 58 |
| Acute-on-chronic | ++ | + | Intraoperative no femoral head perfusion | Yes | Revision caused by second dislocation after 6 weeks; perfusion of femoral head | 60 |
| Chronic | + | ++ | 0 | | 0 | 60 |
| Acute-on-chronic | +++ | + | -- | Yes | -- | 64 |
| Chronic | ++ | ++ | -- | | -- | 67 |
| Chronic | +++ | +++ | Bell-shaped epiphysis | | Revision after 2 years caused by residual FAI | 67 |
| Chronic | ++ | ++ | 0 | | 0 | 68 |
| Chronic | ++ | ++ | -- | | 0 | 68 |
| Chronic | ++ | +++ | Curved femoral neck | | 0 | 68 |
| Chronic | -- | +++ | -- | | 0 | 70 |
| Acute-on-chronic | -- | -- | -- | | 0 | 79 |
| Chronic | + | ++ | -- | | 0 | 87 |
| Chronic | ++ | +++ | -- | | 0 | 90 |
| Chronic | -- | -- | -- | | 0 | 95 |
| Chronic | +++ | +++ | Bell-shaped epiphysis | | Revision after 8 weeks caused by hardware breakage | 96 |
| Chronic | ++ | +++ | -- | | Revision after 6 weeks caused by hardware breakage | 96 |

*Radiograph of prior acute slip
FAI = femoroacetabular impingement, LDF = laser Doppler flowmetry;
-- = no information, + = mild, ++ = moderate, +++ = severe, 0 = none

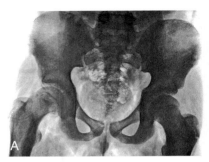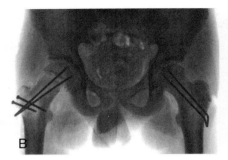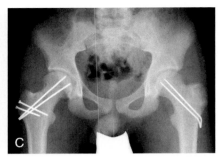

**Figure 5**     **A,** Radiograph of the pelvis of a 14-year-old boy with acute-on-chronic SCFE of the right hip. **B,** The postoperative radiograph shows an anatomic reduction and fixation with two threaded wires. The greater trochanter is fixed by two screws. **C,** A radiograph taken 1 year postoperatively shows that the step at the head-neck junction has remodelled into a smooth waist.

the posteromedial neck indicated a preexisting chronic slip. One hip (No. 16) with "acute-on-chronic" slip was surgically treated only 2 days after the acute slip. Intraoperatively, the epiphysis was not bleeding. Laser Doppler flowmetry measurements showed pulsatile signals over the retinaculum but not within the epiphysis. Six weeks after surgery, the patient was readmitted with loss of correction after a fall. During surgery, brisk bleeding from the epiphysis was seen along with clear pulsatile signals with laser Doppler flowmetry. On 5-year follow-up of this hip, no signs of osteonecrosis were present. Another hip (No. 23) showed marked bending of the neck indicating chronic slipping, which corresponded with the long duration of the patient's symptoms.

Intraoperatively, labral damage in the hips ranged from roughening of the undersurface to complete destruction when the labrum was squeezed by the impacting step of the femoral metaphysis. Abrasions of the acetabular cartilage had a tendency to appear larger with smaller slips. This finding may be explained by the fact that large slips do not allow the metaphysis to enter into the acetabular socket. Follow-up on patients in the study ranged from 24 months to 96 months (average follow-up, 58 months). No

hips showed osteonecrosis within the period of observation. Three hips underwent successful resurgical treatment for loss of correction caused by either bending of the fully threaded 3.0-mm wires or failure of the 3.5-mm screws. The authors prefer the use of wires because of their material properties and design, which may allow bending, but fatigue fracture has never been observed. One hip with a chronic slip that occurred over a 2-year period showed a bell-shaped epiphysis at the time of surgery that continued to impinge even with anatomic realignment. The critical relationship of the deformity near the retinaculum did not allow trimming of the nonspherical extension. The acetabular cartilage destruction was rather extensive. Because the patient had ongoing symptoms accompanied by limited internal rotation, the hip was reopened more than 1 year after the index surgery, when the nonspherical extension of the epiphysis could be sufficiently trimmed. The hip showed clinical improvement, but symptoms did not completely resolve.

## Summary

Subcapital realignment in SCFE is believed to achieve a higher level of standardization with the use of surgical steps involving surgical dislo-

cation of the hip and trimming of the stable trochanter to protect the perfusion of the epiphysis. A comparison of the modified procedure and the Dunn procedure[4,12,20] showed a lower risk of osteonecrosis with the modified procedure; however, the value of the procedure and its precise indications need further evaluation involving larger case studies and longer follow-up periods. The execution of the modified procedure is demanding and requires careful training based on a detailed knowledge of anatomy, especially the vascular anatomy of the hip. Knowledge beyond that needed to achieve classic surgical exposures is required. Nevertheless, the development of new and improved reconstructive techniques for SCFE in young patients is a worthwhile investment.

## References

1. Carney BT, Weinstein SL, Noble J: Long-term follow-up of slipped capital femoral epiphysis. *J Bone Joint Surg Am* 1991;73:667-674.

2. Goodman DA, Feighan JE, Smith AD, Latimer B, Buly RL, Cooperman DR: Subclinical slipped capital femoral epiphysis: Relationship to osteoarthrosis of the hip.

*J Bone Joint Surg Am* 1997;79:1489-1497.

3. Rab GT: The geometry of slipped capital femoral epiphysis: Implications for movement, impingement, and corrective osteotomy. *J Pediatr Orthop* 1999;19:419-424.

4. Ballmer PM, Gilg M, Aebi B, Ganz R: Results following sub-capital and Imhauser-Weber osteotomy in femur head epiphyseolysis. *Z Orthop Ihre Grenzgeb* 1990;128:63-66.

5. Muller ME: Diagnosis and therapy of mechanic hip dysfunctions in children as prevention of secondary arthrosis. *Minerva Ortop* 1968;19:267-273.

6. Leunig M, Fraitzl CR, Ganz R: Early damage to the acetabular cartilage in slipped capital femoral epiphysis: Therapeutic consequences. *Orthopade* 2002;31:894-899.

7. Ganz R, Parvizi J, Beck M, Leunig M, Notzli H, Siebenrock KA: Femoroacetabular impingement: A cause for osteoarthritis of the hip. *Clin Orthop Relat Res* 2003;417:112-120.

8. Imhauser G: Imhauser's osteotomy in the florid gliding process: Observations on the corresponding work of B.G. Weber. *Z Orthop Ihre Grenzgeb* 1966;102:327-329.

9. Weber BG: Imhauser osteotomy for epiphysiolysis. *Z Orthop Ihre Grenzgeb* 1965;100:312-320.

10. Ganz R, Gill TJ, Gautier E, Ganz K, Krugel N, Berlemann U: Surgical dislocation of the adult hip: A technique with full access to the femoral head and acetabulum without the risk of avascular necrosis. *J Bone Joint Surg Br* 2001;83:1119-1124.

11. Gautier E, Ganz K, Krugel N, Gill T, Ganz R: Anatomy of the medial femoral circumflex artery and its surgical implications. *J Bone Joint Surg Br* 2000;82:679-683.

12. Dunn DM, Angel JC: Replacement of the femoral head by open operation in severe adolescent slipping of the upper femoral epiphysis. *J Bone Joint Surg Br* 1978;60-B:394-403.

13. Sevitt S, Thompson RG: The distribution and anastomoses of arteries supplying the head and neck of the femur. *J Bone Joint Surg Br* 1965;47:560-573.

14. Leunig M, Südkamp N, Trentz O, Ganz R. Severely displaced mal- and nonunion of the femoral neck in the younger age group: An approach to facilitate the preservation of the vital femoral head during reconstructive surgery, in Marti RK, Van Hertward R (eds): *Osteonecrosis for Posttraumatic Deformities.* Stuttgart, Germany, Thieme, 2008.

15. Notzli HP, Siebenrock KA, Hempfing A, Ramseier LE, Ganz R: Perfusion of the femoral head during surgical dislocation of the hip: Monitoring by laser Doppler flowmetry. *J Bone Joint Surg Br* 2002;84:300-304.

16. Mardones RM, Gonzalez C, Chen Q, Zobitz M, Kaufman KR, Trousdale RT: Surgical treatment of femoroacetabular impingement: Evaluation of the effect of the size of the resection. *J Bone Joint Surg Am* 2005;87:273-279.

17. Gibson A: A posterior exposure of the hip. *J Bone Joint Surg Br* 1950;32:183-186.

18. Nork SE, Schar M, Pfander G, et al: Anatomic considerations for the choice of surgical approach for hip resurfacing arthroplasty. *Orthop Clin North Am* 2005;36:163-170.

19. Gill TJ, Sledge JB, Ekkernkamp A, Ganz R: Intraoperative assessment of femoral head vascularity after femoral neck fracture. *J Orthop Trauma* 1998;12:474-478.

20. Fish JB: Cuneiform osteotomy of the femoral neck in the treatment of slipped capital femoral epiphysis: A follow-up note. *J Bone Joint Surg Am* 1994;76:46-59.

# Surgical Management of Forearm and Distal Radius Fractures in Children and Adolescents

Charles T. Price, MD

## Abstract

*Closed reduction with cast immobilization is the preferred method of treatment for most fractures of the forearm and distal radius in children and adolescents. Nonunion of these fractures is exceptionally rare, and remodeling restores alignment for minor incomplete reductions. Most closed reductions can be performed in the emergency department with the patient sedated or with regional anesthesia. However, reduction in an operating room with the patient under general anesthesia lowers the threshold for surgical stabilization to avoid the need for repeat reductions under general anesthesia. Surgical management with fixation is often indicated for unstable fractures, open fractures, refractures, and in circumstances involving multiple trauma and other complex injuries.*

**Instr Course Lect 2008;57:509-514.**

Closed management is more likely to produce satisfactory outcomes for children younger than 8 years (regardless of the location of fracture) and in patients of all ages with distal to midshaft fractures.[1,2] Immobilization incorporating the thumb with the elbow in extension may facilitate closed treatment in younger children because of the propensity toward volar bow when the elbow is flexed and swelling subsides.[3] Acceptable alignment for patients younger than 8 years is complete displacement, 15° of angulation, and 45° of malrotation. In children age 8 years to 13 years, acceptable alignment is complete displacement, 10° of angulation, and 30° of malrotation.[4]

## Forearm Shaft Fractures

Closed management may be difficult for severely displaced fractures because of loss of soft-tissue re-straints. Patients treated with closed reduction and cast immobilization require frequent follow-up visits with cast changes, or molding of the forearm cast to maintain alignment within acceptable guidelines. This process may be difficult, painful, or time consuming, and parents may be wary of the potential for remodeling. For these and other reasons, reduction in the operating room with intramedullary fixation may be preferred as the initial form of treatment, especially in older children. However, surgical treatment may lead to complications, and surgical skill is required to achieve satisfactory results.[5]

Open reduction with fixation is recommended as the initial treatment for displaced forearm fractures proximal to the midshaft in patients older than 8 years (Figure 1). Patients with proximal forearm fractures who are managed with closed reduction have a greater risk for loss of forearm rotation because smaller degrees of angulation are more likely to limit the arc of forearm rotation (Figure 2).[2,6]

When surgical treatment is appropriate, intramedullary nailing is recommended for fixation of forearm fractures in skeletally immature patients.[7] This method is minimally invasive, provides excellent callus formation, and allows removal of implants without extensive surgical exposure or the risk of refracture. The principles of elastic, stable, intramedullary pinning were outlined in 1985.[8] In the forearm, small intramedullary wires provide adequate stability to maintain alignment during healing.[9] A 1.5- to 2.5-mm diameter stainless steel Steinmann pin or titanium nail may be used. The tip of the pin should be dull and the distal 2 to 3 mm should be bent approximately 30° to facilitate passage into the medullary canal and across the fracture site. A Rush rod (Berivon Inc, Meridian, MS) also may be substituted for fixation of the ulna.

With the patient under general anesthesia, an initial reduction is performed to achieve the best alignment before fixation. The first bone to be fixed is the bone with the best reduction, or the bone that will be easiest to stabilize with intramedullary fixation (often the ulna). For

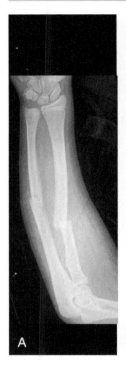
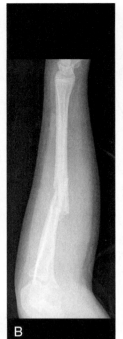
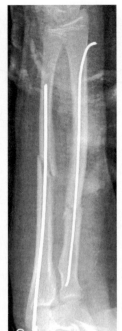
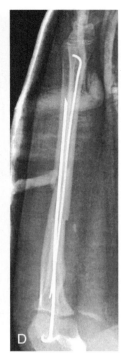

**Figure 1** Radiographs of the forearm of a 13-year-old girl. AP **(A)** and lateral **(B)** radiographs show displaced diaphyseal fractures of the radius and ulna. The ulna fracture is midshaft, but the fracture of the radius is at the junction of the proximal and middle third of the forearm. Proximal fractures of the forearm that are treated by closed reduction are more likely to lose motion than distal fractures unless anatomic reduction is obtained and maintained. AP **(C)** and lateral **(D)** postoperative radiographs show intramedullary nailing with a 2.0-mm diameter titanium nail in the radius and a 3-mm Rush rod in the ulna. Open reduction of the radius and ulna were performed through small incisions to facilitate fixation. The fracture united without complications and the patient regained full range of motion.

fixation of the ulna, a 1-cm incision is made lateral to the tip of the olecranon. A 2.5- to 3.5-mm drill hole is made through the apophysis. This rod insertion does not interfere with growth potential of the olecranon. The nail is introduced into the hole and advanced to the fracture site. Attempts are made to pass the pin or nail across the fracture site; open reduction is recommended if difficulty is encountered. Only a small incision is required to assist with the reduction and this incision facilitates passage of the nail. For fixation of the radius, a 1-cm incision is made on the lateral side of the distal forearm proximal to the styloid process of the radius. Blunt dissection is used to protect the dorsal branch of the radial nerve. The extensor tendons are retracted dorsally, exposing the flat lateral surface of the distal radial metaphysis. An oblique drill

hole is made at a 45° angle through the lateral cortex proximal to the growth plate. This hole is slightly larger than the pin that will be inserted. Care should be taken to avoid touching the opposite cortex with the drill bit so that the elastic wire will slide easily along the opposite cortex. The nail is introduced into the drill hole and advanced to the fracture site. The fracture is reduced. The angulated tip of the nail is used by rotating the nail to engage the proximal fragment so that the nail can be advanced into the proximal fragment. Only one or two passes are recommended; care should be taken to avoid excessive penetration of the soft tissues of the proximal forearm. Multiple attempts at passage of the nail combined with tourniquet use for more than 1 hour have been associated with compartment syndrome.[10] If

passage of the nail is difficult, a 3- to 4-cm forearm incision is made and the fracture is reduced through a volar approach along the ulnar border of the brachioradialis muscle. The radial artery is retracted medially and the superficial branch of the radial nerve is protected on the deep surface of the brachioradialis muscle. The forearm is fully supinated and the shaft can be palpated for incision of the periosteum in the area of the fracture. Reduction is then performed under direct vision and the nail is advanced into the proximal fragment.

The nails are cut off so that they can be buried under the skin without causing irritation. Because early nail removal has been associated with refracture, the nails are left in place until the union is mature.[9] Immobilization in a loosely applied splint or bivalved cast is recommended during the initial postoperative period. After swelling has subsided, an above-elbow cast is used for approximately 6 weeks postoperatively for added stability and comfort.

## Distal Radius Metaphyseal Fractures

Metaphyseal fractures of the distal radius are common injuries in children and adolescents. The location of the fractures will usually advance distally with advancing age.[11] Younger children have a more elastic radius, with a gradual transition from diaphysis to metaphysis. Adolescents and adults have a stiffer shaft and a more abrupt metaphyseal transition. Distal radius fractures in skeletally immature patients are remarkably benign because of the excellent remodeling capacity in this anatomic location. Most of these injuries can be treated by closed reduction with local or regional anesthetic block or conscious sedation. Acceptable alignment for children younger than 8 years is complete displacement, 25° of dorsal or volar tilt, and 15° of radial tilt. In patients who are older than 8 years, attempts should be made to reduce the fracture displacement to less than 50%, with no more than 20° dorsal tilt and 15° of radial tilt. This degree of deformity will remodel if the patient has at least 2 years of remaining bone growth.[12-15]

Completely displaced fractures of the distal radius and ulna are the most challenging to treat. These injuries in older children are most likely to benefit from reduction under general anesthesia followed by pin fixation. Completely displaced distal radius fractures are difficult to reduce and may be unstable following reduction. Loss of acceptable reduction occurs in 20% to 60% of pa-

tients depending on the guidelines for acceptable alignment and the quality of cast application.[15-20] In randomized trials evaluating above-elbow versus below-elbow casts, no difference was found in maintenance of alignment; however, a poorly molded cast or excessive swelling may lead to redisplacement regardless of the elbow's inclusion in or exclusion from the cast.[21,22] Although above-elbow casts do not reduce the risk of redisplacement, they may provide more comfort for the patient in the early stages of healing.

The risk of redisplacement is greater for completely displaced distal radius fractures when the initial reduction is incomplete.[16,17] Proctor and associates[17] reported that redisplacement occurred in 20% of patients following anatomic reduction and in 73% of patients with incomplete reduction. McLauchlan and associates[18] used a randomized controlled trial to evaluate cast immobilization compared with pin fixation following reduction of completely displaced fractures of the distal radius. These authors found that no remanipulations were required in the group treated with pin fixation, but that 20% of the patients in the cast group required remanipulation. The final clinical results were equal in both groups regardless of method of treatment.

For patients with completely displaced fractures of the distal radius, closed reduction should be attempted in the clinic or emergency department with regional, local, or intravenous analgesia. If the fracture redisplaces, or reangulates, or the initial reduction is inadequate, closed reduction and pinning should be performed with the patient under general anesthesia. Pinning is used primarily to maintain

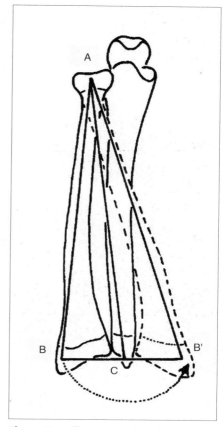

**Figure 2**     Illustration showing rotation of the radius on the ulna. The mechanical triangle of rotation (ABC) has an axis from the center of the radial head (A) to the ulnar styloid (C). The radial styloid (B) rotates around to a pronated position (B'), subtending a semicircular cone. (Reproduced with permission from Ogden JA: *Skeletal Injury in the Child,* ed 3. New York, NY, Springer-Verlag, 2000.)

alignment for fractures with incomplete but acceptable alignment (Figure 3). When the fracture reduces anatomically, pinning is rarely needed. The Kapandji or pin leverage technique may facilitate reduction and fixation in difficult situations (Figure 4); however, simple pinning across the fracture site is most commonly used. The safety of transphyseal pinning has not been proved; therefore, care should be taken to avoid multiple penetrations of the

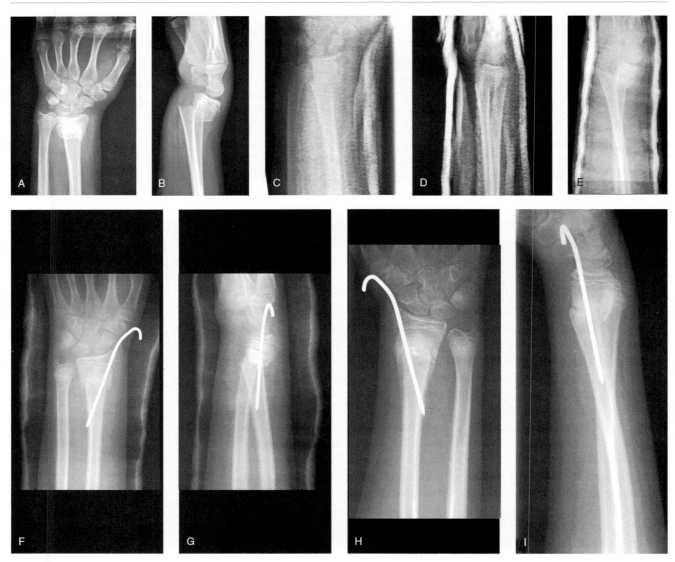

**Figure 3** Radiographs of a completely displaced metaphyseal fracture of the distal radius and ulna in a 14-year-old boy. Initial AP **(A)** and lateral **(B)** radiographs show complete displacement. AP **(C)** and lateral **(D)** radiographs following reduction in the emergency department show incomplete reduction with acceptable alignment. Early follow-up was recommended because redisplacement is more common after incomplete reduction than after anatomic reduction. Lateral **(E)** radiograph taken 7 days later shows complete redisplacement and malalignment. Secondary reduction was then performed with the patient under general anesthesia. AP **(F)** and lateral **(G)** radiographs following re-reduction show pinning performed with a single percutaneous transphyseal pin to reduce the risk of further displacement caused by incomplete reduction. AP **(H)** and lateral **(I)** radiographs at the time of pin removal 6 weeks later show excellent callus formation and maintenance of satisfactory alignment.

growth plate if this technique is used.[5,23] Pinning from the intact proximal ulna to the distal radius is another alternative for fixation.

Fractures through the growth plate of the distal radius and ulna are treated similarly to metaphyseal fractures. Parents should be warned of the potential for growth disturbances, and patients should be reevaluated for potential growth arrest.[24] Injuries involving the growth plate of the distal ulna are especially prone to growth disturbance.[25]

## Summary

Closed reduction with cast immobilization is the preferred method for the initial management of most fractures of the forearm and distal radius in children and adolescents. The remodeling potential of the distal ra-

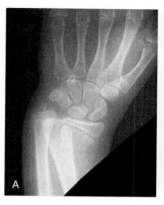
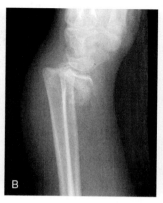
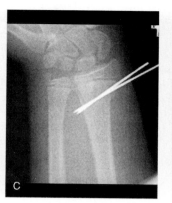
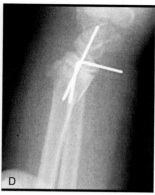

**Figure 4**    Radiographs of a displaced distal radius fracture in a 14-year-old boy. AP (**A**) and lateral (**B**) radiographs show volar and radial displacement of the distal radius. This is an unstable fracture pattern. The percutaneous pin leverage technique was used to obtain reduction and stabilization. AP (**C**) and lateral (**D**) radiographs after reduction and pinning show satisfactory alignment and fixation.

dius is excellent. Surgical stabilization with pins or intramedullary nails is recommended for unstable fractures, when loss of reduction occurs, or in patients with polytrauma or complex fractures.

## References

1. Zionts LE, Zalavras C, Gerhardt MB: Closed treatment of displaced diaphyseal both-bone forearm fractures in older children and adolescents. *J Pediatr Orthop* 2005;25:507-512.

2. Price CT, Scott DS, Kurzner ME, Flynn JC: Malunited forearm fractures in children. *J Pediatr Orthop* 1990;10:705-712.

3. Walker JL, Rang M: Forearm fractures in children: Cast treatment with the elbow extended. *J Bone Joint Surg Br* 1991;73:299-301.

4. Noonan KJ, Price CT: Forearm and distal radius fractures in children. *J Am Acad Orthop Surg* 1998;6: 146-156.

5. Shoemaker SD, Comstock CP, Mubarak SJ, Wenger DR, Chambers HG: Intramedullary Kirschner wire fixation of open or unstable forearm fractures in children. *J Pediatr Orthop* 1999;19:329-337.

6. McHenry TP, Pierce WA, Lais RL, Schacherer TG: Effect of displacement of ulna-shaft fractures on forearm rotation: A cadaveric model. *Am J Orthop* 2002;31:420-424.

7. Fernandez FF, Egenolf M, Carsten C, Holz F, Schneider S, Wentzensen A: Unstable diaphyseal fractures of both bones of the forearm in children: Plate fixation versus intramedullary nailing. *Injury* 2005;36:1210-1216.

8. Ligier JN, Metaizeau J, Prevot J, Lascombes P: Elastic stable intramedullary pinning of long bone shaft fractures in children. *Z Kinderchir* 1985; 40:209-212.

9. Lascombes P, Prevot J, Ligier JN, Metaizeau JP, Poncelet T: Elastic stable intramedullary nailing in forearm shaft fractures in children: 85 cases. *J Pediatr Orthop* 1990;10: 167-171.

10. Yuan PS, Pring ME, Gaynor TP, Mubarak SJ, Newton PO: Compartment syndrome following intramedullary fixation of pediatric forearm fractures. *J Pediatr Orthop* 2004;24: 370-375.

11. Tredwell SJ, Van Peteghem K, Clough M: Pattern of forearm fractures in children. *J Pediatr Orthop* 1984;4:604-608.

12. Fuller DJ, McCullough CJ: Malunited fractures of the forearm in children. *J Bone Joint Surg Br* 1982;64:364-367.

13. Johari AN, Sinha M: Remodeling of forearm fractures in children. *J Pediatr Orthop B* 1999;8:84-87.

14. Larsen E, Vittas D, Torp-Pedersen S: Remodeling of angulated distal forearm fractures in children. *Clin Orthop Relat Res* 1988;237:190-195.

15. Roy DR: Completely displaced distal radius fractures with intact ulnas in children. *Orthopedics* 1989;12:1089-1092.

16. Zamzam MM, Khoshhal K: Displaced fracture of the distal radius in children. *J Bone Joint Surg Br* 2005;87:841-843.

17. Proctor MT, Moore DJ, Paterson JM: Redisplacement after manipulation of distal radial fractures in children. *J Bone Joint Surg Br* 1993;75:453-454.

18. McLauchlan GJ, Cowan B, Annan IH, Robb JE: Management of completely displaced metaphyseal fractures of the distal radius in children: A prospective randomised control trial. *J Bone Joint Surg Br* 2002; 84:413-417.

19. Bhatia M, Housden P: Redisplacement of paediatric forearm fractures: Role of plaster moulding and padding. *Injury* 2006;37:259-268.

20. Chan C, Meads B, Nicol R: Remanipulation of forearm fractures in children. *N Z Med J* 1997;110: 249-250.

21. Webb GR, Galpin R, Armstrong DG: Comparison of short and long arm plaster casts for displaced fractures in the distal third of the forearm in children. *J Bone Joint Surg Am* 2006; 88:9-17.

22. Bohm ER, Bubber V, Hing KY, Dzus A: Above and below-the-elbow plaster casts for distal forearm fractures in children: A randomized controlled trial. *J Bone Joint Surg Am* 2006;88:1-8.

23. Yung PS, Lam CY, Ng BK, Lam TP, Cheng JC: Percutaneous transphyseal intramedullary Kirschner wire pinning: A safe and effective procedure for treatment of displaced diaphyseal forearm fracture in children. *J Pediatr Orthop* 2004;24:7-12.

24. Cannata G, DeMaio F, Mancini F, Ippolito E: Physeal fractures of the distal radius and ulna: Long-term prognosis. *J Orthop Trauma* 2003;17: 172-180.

25. Golz RJ, Grogan DP, Greene TL, Belsole RJ, Ogden JA: Distal ulnar physeal injury. *J Pediatr Orthop* 1991;11:318-326.

# Surgical Treatment of Carpal and Hand Injuries in Children

Peter M. Waters, MD

## Abstract

*Most carpal and hand injuries in children are treated nonsurgically. However, surgical treatment is often required for certain clinical situations. Complications resulting from pediatric hand fractures, dislocations, and soft-tissue injuries are most commonly caused by a failure to identify and treat an injury requiring surgery.*

**Instr Course Lect 2008;57:515-524.**

This chapter will review surgical techniques for specific injuries of the carpus and hand in children. With regard to the wrist, this discussion will include the indications for open reduction of scaphoid fractures, treatment of scaphoid nonunions, and arthroscopic examination and treatment of chondral and ligamentous injuries. Distal injuries that are treated surgically include Seymour fractures, phalangeal neck injuries, and intra-articular fractures.

## Scaphoid Fractures

A scaphoid fracture is the most common carpal injury in children, and it has become more common over the past two decades.[1-3] The increased participation in competitive youth sports may account for the increased incidence of these fractures. As in adults, scaphoid fractures are classified by the location, degree, and direction of fracture displacement. Distal pole, waist, and proximal fractures all occur in children, with waist fractures being the most common.[4,5] As in adults, displacement beyond 1 to 2 mm is associated with malunion or nonunion in children.[6] Determining the amount of displacement can be difficult, and CT or MRI scans are important evaluation tools for this purpose and can be of help as a guide in the treatment of these fractures.[7-10] Osteonecrosis also occurs in children, especially in those with a displaced proximal waist or proximal pole fracture.[11]

Nondisplaced distal pole fractures usually heal without complications.[12-19] Plain radiographs or, if appropriate, CT scans are closely inspected to detect distal intra-articular extension or displacement. Immobilization in a long or short arm-thumb spica cast for up to 6 weeks is recommended to protect healing of the distal pole fracture. Nondisplaced waist fractures in a child or adolescent are also generally treated with cast immobilization, and there is some evidence that initial use of a long arm cast is more efficacious.[15] CT scans are indicated to confirm three-dimensional anatomic alignment. Cast immobilization is continued until complete healing has occurred. At times, a CT scan is required to confirm healing. Because there is a risk of both nonunion and osteonecrosis even with nondisplaced waist fractures, and as a result of concerns about prolonged immobilization, percutaneous intraosseous screw fixation has been used more commonly in adults with nondisplaced scaphoid fractures.[20,21] This technique has been carried over to the treatment of adolescents who desire earlier mobilization. Under fluoroscopic guidance, a cannulated screw can be placed from distal-volar to proximal-dorsal or vice versa. The technique is demanding, and its use depends on the fracture's location and the surgeon's skills. The pin and cannulated screw must be placed centrally in both the anteroposterior and the lateral plane. Misplacement of the screw increases the risk of nonunion, with osteolysis about the screw.

Displaced waist fractures require anatomic reduction and stable fixation. This is usually performed by open reduction and internal fixation.[6,17,22-26] A volar approach to the scaphoid is the most common because the dorsal blood supply is protected, and the flexion displacement can be reduced. On rare occasions, bone graft is required in the acute setting to correct a humpback

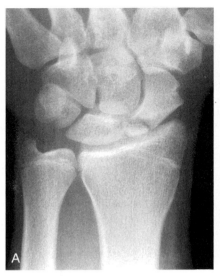 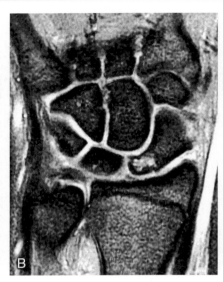 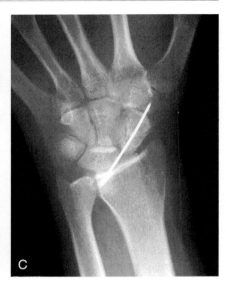

**Figure 1**   **A,** Radiograph of a nonunion of the proximal pole of the scaphoid. This injury, which is rare in children and adolescents, is associated with a high risk of necrosis of the proximal pole and persistence of the nonunion. The increased density of the proximal pole is virtually diagnostic of necrotic bone. **B,** MRI scan revealing osteonecrosis of the proximal pole. The signal characteristics of the proximal pole confirm the necrosis. **C,** Pedicle vascularized bone grafting and pin fixation led to union. (Reproduced with permission from Children's Orthopaedic Surgery Foundation, Boston, MA.)

deformity caused by volar fracture comminution. Smooth wire or intraosseous screw fixation has been used after anatomic reduction. More recently, arthroscopic-assisted reduction and fixation has been performed for acutely displaced scaphoid fractures. This is more technically demanding. Arthroscopic inspection and manipulation of the fracture site to obtain anatomic alignment for cannulated pin and screw placement is performed under both fluoroscopic guidance and arthroscopic visualization.

A splint or cast is used after surgery as deemed necessary by the surgeon to prevent excessive stress on the healing fracture. Generally, postfracture stiffness from prolonged immobilization is not as much of a risk in an adolescent as it is in an adult.

The proximal fragment of a proximal pole scaphoid fracture is at high risk of being necrotic and of not healing to the body of the scaphoid. Percutaneous screw fixation before fracture displacement or fragmentation may be useful in the treatment of this rare fracture in an adolescent. Perfect placement of the screw, centrally in both planes, is necessary in this situation to lessen the risk of complications. An established proximal pole nonunion with displacement may require reduction, vascularized bone grafting, and internal fixation to achieve healing (Figure 1).[11] Nonvascularized grafting and internal fixation is not recommended because it has a high rate of failure.

Treatment of scaphoid nonunions in adolescents is similar to treatment in adults.[2,27-34] If the fracture is truly nondisplaced, prolonged cast treatment or percutaneous screw fixation can be considered. Adjunctive electrical stimulation has been used. Most scaphoid fracture nonunions, however, are displaced and may have a necrotic proximal pole fragment. This situation requires internal fixation and bone grafting (Figure 2).

Smooth wire fixation was used in the past, but screw fixation currently is preferred. Autologous bone grafting techniques are most often used to restore structural integrity and expedite healing.[30,31,33,34] Most nonunions treated with reduction, internal fixation, and bone graft heal in children and adolescents. The reason to treat a nonunion surgically is to prevent long-term complications such as pain, stiffness, and arthrosis.[35,36]

## Hand Fractures

The hand is the most commonly injured body part of a child. In the toddler, the fracture is usually a crush injury, such as occurs when a hand gets caught in a door.[37-45] In the older child, the fracture is usually secondary to recreational sports. Most of these injuries heal without complications.[46] However, there is a subset of fractures, dislocations, and soft-tissue injuries that have dire consequences if not treated appropriately initially.

## Distal Phalangeal Injuries

A crush injury to the distal aspect of the finger is the most common hand injury in a toddler. The distal tip can be partially or completely amputated by the injury. Nail bed and nail plate injuries are usually associated with distal phalangeal fractures, which range from minor avulsions to comminuted open fractures. The growth plate is usually not involved except in the case of a Seymour fracture, which will be discussed below. Most of these injuries can be cared for in the emergency department with local anesthesia and/or conscious sedation, but more complicated injuries should be repaired in an operating room with the patient under general anesthesia. With partial amputations, the dorsal skin, nail bed, and eponychial regions are usually lacerated but there is an intact, viable volar skin bridge. With adequate facilities in the emergency department and with the aid of loupe magnification, the nail bed can be anatomically and delicately repaired with absorbable suture after removal of the nail plate.[47-50] Most of these injuries heal without permanent nail deformity. Parents and primary care physicians are advised to obtain a reevaluation if there is a nail deformity at 6 months after the injury.

Complete amputations of the distal tip are treated with various techniques, depending on the surgeon's experience and preference as well as the size and orientation of the defect.[51-56] If the skin loss is minimal, irrigation and débridement as well as coverage with a sterile nonadherent dressing is appropriate. Healing by secondary intention will be relatively rapid and uncomplicated in a young patient. At times, acute treatment requires minimal débridement of exposed bone with a rongeur. Because the proximal phy-

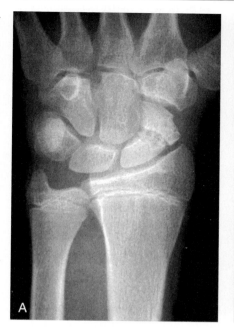
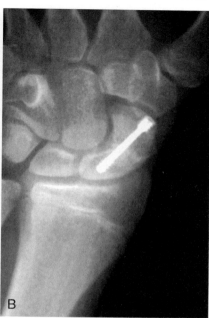

**Figure 2**   **A,** Radiograph of a nonunion in the waist region of the scaphoid in an adolescent athlete. **B,** Surgical treatment with bone graft and internal fixation with an intraosseous screw. (Reproduced with permission from Children's Orthopaedic Surgery Foundation, Boston, MA.)

sis has not been violated, longitudinal growth will be unimpaired and the length of the digit eventually will be nearly normal. More extensive loss can be treated with composite grafting with use of the amputated part, pedicle grafting such as with an advancement or a thenar flap, or skin or composite grafting from distant donor sites. Attachment of the amputated part as a composite graft can be performed acutely in the emergency department after débridement of both the part and the amputation site. Healing following use of this technique is more prolonged than that following use of local dressings alone, but it may result in greater bulk and less risk of nail deformity from an extensive injury. Injuries through the proximal quarter to third of the nail area are candidates for surgical correction. Flap or donor grafting is usually performed semiacutely.

A mallet finger deformity in a child is similar to one in an adult, with disruption of the extensor tendon as it inserts onto the dorsum of the distal phalanx. The extensor tendon inserts on the epiphysis in a child, whereas the flexor digitorum profundus inserts on the metaphysis. A true mallet injury occurs either through an osseous avulsion or through an intrasubstance tendon injury, whereas a Seymour fracture, which occurs through the physis, is not a true mallet injury. A true mallet injury, regardless of type, can be treated with immobilization of the distal interphalangeal joint in an extension splint while allowing motion of the proximal interphalangeal joint. Successful healing can be expected if the patient complies with instructions for splint wear. This is true even for treatment of a chronic mallet finger deformity, although there are rare instances of chronic

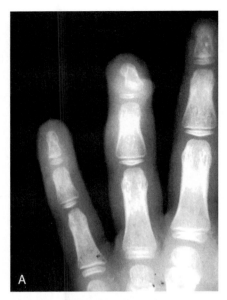

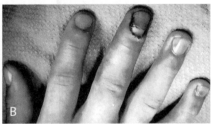

**Figure 3** **A,** AP radiograph of a displaced physeal fracture (Seymour fracture) of the distal phalanx of the ring finger. The extensor tendon is intact, inserting onto the nondisplaced epiphysis. The germinal matrix of the nail can become entrapped in the physeal fracture site. **B,** Clinical appearance of a Seymour fracture with physeal displacement and entrapment of the germinal matrix. The nail plate and eponychium are displaced, requiring repair of the nail bed and reduction of the physis. (Reproduced with permission from Children's Orthopaedic Surgery Foundation, Boston, MA.)

mallet injuries requiring reconstruction to achieve improved active extension. Tenodermodesis involves advancement and repair of the disrupted tendon with advancement and suture repair of the skin and subcutaneous tissues to the tendon.[57] The risk of this procedure is

loss of flexion or the creation of a nail plate deformity, but active extension can be improved.

A flexion injury in a child that results in a physeal separation between the extensor tendon dorsally and the flexor digitorum profundus insertion volarly is called a Seymour fracture.[58] The germinal matrix of the nail bed may be interposed in the physeal fracture site and prevent reduction (Figure 3). Often, the flexed digit is misinterpreted as a mallet finger and incorrectly treated with dorsal splinting. These open wounds can become infected if left without appropriate treatment. Optimum treatment requires early recognition and management. Treatment includes removal of the nail plate, delicate removal of the entrapped germinal matrix from the physis, reduction of the fracture, and repair of the nail bed. Usually, the phalangeal fracture is stable after the soft-tissue repair. At times, pin fixation of the distal phalanx and interphalangeal joint for 3 to 4 weeks protects the nail bed repair and maintains fracture alignment.

### Phalangeal Neck Fractures

Injuries to the subchondral region of the proximal or middle phalanx are common with more proximal crush injuries, such as closure of a door on a child's finger. As the child attempts to extract the digit from the door, the greatest force occurs across the subchondral region and it fractures. The resultant phalangeal neck fracture can displace dorsally and into extension (Figure 4).[59] Radiographically, the distal fragment appears small because much of the articular surface is cartilaginous in young patients; therefore, the severity of displacement and its effect on adjacent interphalangeal joint motion can be underappreciated. Fail-

ure to treat this injury with anatomic reduction and pin stabilization can result in a malunion that limits digital flexion. At the proximal interphalangeal joint, obliteration of the subcondylar fossa can result in marked loss of digital motion. There also can be an element of malrotation to the fracture. It is imperative that these injuries be recognized and treated early. They are usually unstable injuries that redisplace after closed reduction and cast immobilization. This is difficult to appreciate on radiographs made with the hand in a cast. Closed reduction and stabilization with one or more distal to proximal oblique pins for 3 to 4 weeks is the recommended treatment. Children who present with an incipient malunion can frequently be treated either with percutaneous pin reduction and stabilization[60] or with a careful open reduction that protects the blood supply to the distal fragment through the collateral ligaments. Treatment of an established malunion is more complex. In a very young patient, it may remodel with growth, especially at the middle phalanx.[60,61] However, as the physis is proximal, this process will be slow (1 to 2 years) and may not be sufficient. Subchondral fossa reconstruction through a volar approach will improve but not normalize motion.[62] Clearly, the best option is accurate recognition and treatment of this injury in the acute setting.

### Malrotation Fractures

Any phalangeal or metacarpal fracture can result in digital malrotation regardless of its radiographic appearance (Figure 5). It is imperative to perform a clinical examination to inspect digital alignment. Through a tenodesis effect, passive wrist extension results in passive digital flexion and allows assessment of digital

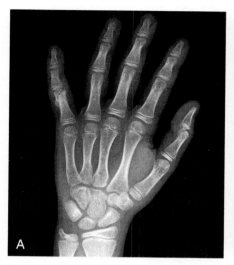
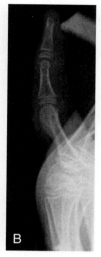
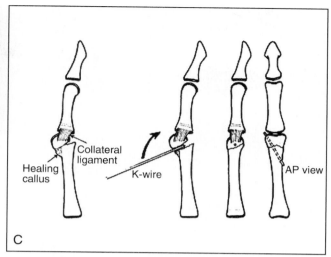

**Figure 4**    AP **(A)** and lateral **(B)** radiographs of a displaced fracture of the neck of the proximal phalanx with incipient malunion. The subchondral fossa is blocked by the extension displacement of the condylar fragment. If left untreated, this will lead to a flexion block at the interphalangeal joint. (Reproduced with permission from Children's Orthopaedic Surgery Foundation, Boston, MA.) **C,** These drawings illustrate osteoclasis with percutaneous pin reduction and fixation. (Reproduced with permission from Waters PM, Taylor BA, Kuo AY: Percutaneous reduction of incipient malunion of phalangeal neck fractures in children. *J Hand Surg Am* 2004;29:710.)

alignment. Asymmetric convergence or divergence of the fractured digit will be apparent even in the acute setting with this examination. All malrotated digits require anatomic reduction and surgical stabilization. Most commonly, malrotation is caused by oblique phalangeal and metacarpal fractures involving the border digits. However, physeal, transverse, and intra-articular fractures all can lead to malrotation. Treatment consists of smooth pin stabilization or internal fixation. A high index of suspicion and careful clinical examination are critical to identify a potential malunion.

### Intra-Articular Fractures

Any intra-articular fracture requires anatomic alignment and stability during healing. Some injuries are nondisplaced and stable and can be treated with closed means. However, careful follow-up clinically and radiographically during the healing phase is necessary to be certain that there is no loss of alignment. This may require out-of-cast radiographs to accurately assess joint alignment. Displaced fractures require reduction and pin or screw stabilization.[40,63,64] At the middle phalanx, these injuries can involve central osteochondral fragmentation. Careful surgical dissection and anatomic reduction is necessary to lessen the already real risk of osteonecrosis in these fractures. At times, acute bone grafting is necessary to achieve stability. The olecranon distal to the apophysis is a reasonable source of cortical bone graft in a child.

These injuries can be unicondylar, bicondylar, or comminuted. The interphalangeal joint is always at risk for permanent loss of motion with any juxta-articular or intra-articular injury. Permanent articular incongruity clearly increases that risk, and anatomic reduction is the treatment of choice for these injuries. Most often, this can be achieved in children with percutaneous pin reduction and fixation. If reduction or stabilization cannot be achieved with

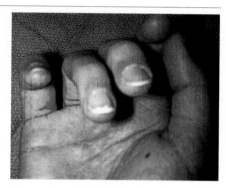

**Figure 5**    Clinical malrotation of the ring finger noted on the passive tenodesis examination. (Reproduced with permission from Children's Orthopaedic Surgery Foundation, Boston, MA.)

closed means, an open procedure involving pin or screw stabilization should be done. Extreme comminution requiring distraction treatment is rare in children and adolescents.[65,66] Postoperative rehabilitation to regain interphalangeal joint motion is necessary to lessen the risk of a flexion contracture. Intra-articular malunion is a difficult problem to manage, with loss of

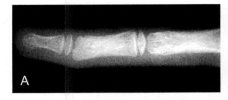

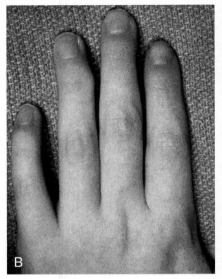

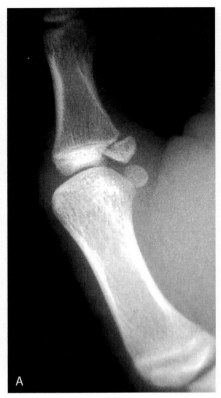

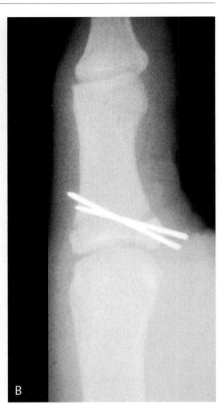

**Figure 6** **A,** Radiograph showing intra-articular malunion of a middle phalangeal unicondylar fracture. This fracture requires reduction and fixation in the acute setting. **B,** Clinical appearance of the malunion with ulnar deviation of the ring finger through the distal interphalangeal joint. (Reproduced with permission from Children's Orthopaedic Surgery Foundation, Boston, MA.)

**Figure 7** **A,** AP radiograph of a displaced Salter-Harris type III intra-articular fracture of the proximal phalanx of the thumb. This is the equivalent of a gamekeeper's thumb in an adult. **B,** Open reduction and internal fixation is indicated to restore articular and physeal congruity and joint stability. The AP radiograph demonstrates smooth pin fixation. (Reproduced with permission from Children's Orthopaedic Surgery Foundation, Boston, MA.)

motion and pain being common and a substantial risk of arthrosis (Figure 6). Unfortunately, intra-articular osteotomies performed late result in less-than-desired results in terms of motion, even when the radiographic appearance is improved.

Displaced Salter-Harris type III intra-articular fractures of the thumb are the pediatric equivalent of the gamekeeper's injury in the adult.[67,68] Rather than the ulnar collateral ligament of the metacarpophalangeal joint being injured in a fall, such as in downhill skiing, the epiphysis fractures. A displaced epi-

physeal fracture of the proximal phalanx results in articular and physeal incongruity. Open reduction and pin fixation is required (Figure 7). Surgical dissection into the joint should be through the fracture site and distal to the intact ulnar collateral ligament insertion. When anatomically realigned, these injuries heal in 4 to 6 weeks without complications. When unrecognized or left malreduced, they can result in a nonunion or malunion that is painful and limits motion and function. Similarly, displaced intra-articular fractures of the base of the first metacarpal require anatomic articular reduction and pin stabiliza-

tion. The oblique ligament between the first and second metacarpals holds the ulnar basilar fragment in place while the abductor pollicis longus dynamically displaces the larger radial fragment. Reduction involves restoration of length and correction of the angulation and malrotation. Two or three percutaneous pins placed into the adjacent metacarpal base and the carpus provide stability until the fracture heals. The rare comminuted intra-articular fracture requires careful open reduction. Severely comminuted injuries that are best treated with distraction techniques in adults almost never occur in children.

## Dislocations

Most interphalangeal joint injuries are "jammed fingers" at the proximal interphalangeal joint secondary to a hyperextension force such as from a thrown basketball. This results in a volar plate injury and, at times, a minor avulsion fracture of the volar aspect of the middle phalangeal epiphysis. These injuries can be overtreated with immobilization, which can result in stiffness of the interphalangeal joint. Complete dislocations can usually be reduced with distraction without complications. If the joint is reduced and stable with motion, treatment involves brief splint protection and mobilization within 5 to 10 days.[69] Buddy taping is frequently used for protection, while active and passive mobility is stressed. The rare avulsion fracture of the base of the middle phalanx that results in a displaced, unstable joint is drastically different (Figure 8). This injury requires joint reduction and mobilization only within the stable flexion-extension arc.[70] Fluoroscopic examination is necessary to determine the safe arc of motion. Dorsal splint or pin extension blocking is used to prevent joint subluxation. Progressive extension as stability is restored with healing is performed carefully to maintain joint reduction while achieving maximum interphalangeal motion. These injuries heal over 6 weeks, and therapy to regain maximal motion can be prolonged. Periarticular swelling often lasts 3 to 6 months.

Most interphalangeal joint dislocations are uncomplicated. Dorsal dislocations are most common and often are treated at the site of the injury with reduction with gentle distraction by the patient, trainer, parent, or coach. These injuries are usually stable after reduction as long as another hyperextension force is

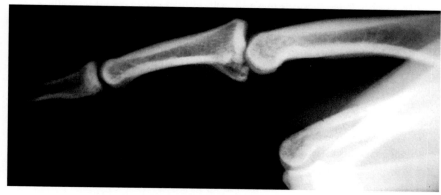

**Figure 8** Lateral radiograph of an incomplete reduction of a volar intra-articular fracture-dislocation. Congruent reduction of this injury needs to be achieved, and the arc of stable motion must be determined. (Reproduced with permission from Children's Orthopaedic Surgery Foundation, Boston, MA.)

avoided during volar plate and collateral ligament healing. Again, early protected mobilization is advocated to lessen the risk of long-term stiffness. A metacarpophalangeal joint dislocation is more likely to be irreducible (a so-called complex dislocation).[71-76] An irreducible dorsal dislocation of either the interphalangeal or the metacarpophalangeal joint is usually secondary to volar plate entrapment. In the metacarpophalangeal joint, this may be evident radiographically by sesamoid interposition or bayonet apposition alignment. Closed reduction is not feasible. Open reduction through either a volar or a dorsal approach is necessary.[72,73,77-82] If a volar approach to an irreducible metacarpophalangeal joint dislocation is used, extreme care is necessary to protect the displaced radial digital neurovascular bundle. Early protected mobilization is important to lessen the risk of stiffness.[80,81]

## Soft-Tissue Injuries

The most common mechanism of a flexor tendon injury in a child is a laceration from broken glass. In these injuries, the skin wound often appears minor relative to the severity of the underlying soft-tissue injury. Failure to perform isolated tendon and nerve testing can result in a delayed or missed diagnosis. Wrist lacerations often involve multiple tendon and, at times, major nerve or blood vessel lacerations. Obviously, an ischemic digit is a surgical emergency. Acute surgical exploration and repair of these soft-tissue lacerations in a young child are recommended because of the limited ability to thoroughly examine the child. Palmar or digital lacerations require careful examination to detect partial or complete nerve, tendon, or arterial lacerations. Too often, digital nerve or isolated flexor tendon injuries are missed acutely. A repair delayed for up to 2 to 3 weeks can be uncomplicated, but beyond that the prognosis for recovery is worse. Microscopic digital nerve repairs in children and adolescents generally enable the full recovery of discriminatory sensibility. Postoperative protection is necessary for only 2 weeks or so. Flexor tendon repairs are more complicated, but the results are generally better than they are in adults. There is debate about cast immobilization compared with protected mobilization after a flexor tendon repair. Cast immobilization for 4 weeks has been found to have more favorable results than protected flexor tendon mobilization protocols with regard to the return of a total active arc of motion and a lower incidence of tendon rupture in children.[83]

So-called jersey finger avulsions of the flexor digitorum profundus insertion occur in children and adolescents. The fusiform swelling in the flexor tendon sheath can be mistaken for a jammed or sprained finger. Because the flexor digitorum superficialis is intact, the patient can move or flex the digit at the proximal interphalangeal joint when asked. Unless isolated profundus tendon function is tested, the tendon rupture will be missed in the acute or semiacute setting. A true lateral radiograph may show the distal phalangeal avulsion fracture and the location of the proximally displaced tendon. Acute repair involves reinsertion of the tendon or the attached osseous fragment into the volar aspect of the distal phalanx. This may require repair over a dorsal button. Because the injury is in zone I, acute repair usually has an excellent result. Late reconstruction, however, is much more complicated. There is insufficient information in the literature to determine whether it is better to leave the patient with a superficialis-only finger or to perform a complicated free tendon-graft reconstruction. Therefore, the surgeon's and patient's preferences still play a large role in the decision making.

A complete amputation proximal to the level of the trifurcation of the digital arteries in a child is considered an indication for replantation. A crush injury that results in an amputation is associated with a higher rate of failure of replantation than is an amputation caused by a sharp laceration.[84] Microscopic repair that results in prompt capillary refill and instantaneous restoration of arterial flow intraoperatively is a positive sign of viability of the replanted digit. The techniques of replantation in a child are the same as those in an adult. Digital survival after replantation is most probable with sharp amputations, a body weight in excess of 11 kg, repair of more than one vein, bone shortening and interosseous wire fixation, and vein grafting of arteries and veins as needed.[84]

## Summary

Although most carpal and hand injuries in children can be treated nonsurgically, it is imperative that the treating physician identify those clinical situations that require surgical intervention. The injuries that require surgery include intra-articular fractures, phalangeal neck fractures, malrotated fractures, scaphoid fractures, and tendon injuries. Prompt and appropriate surgical treatment of these selected injuries usually leads to an excellent outcome.

## References

1. Beatty E, Light TR, Belsole RJ, Ogden JA: Wrist and hand skeletal injuries in children. *Hand Clin* 1990;6: 723-738.

2. Christodoulou AG, Colton CL: Scaphoid fractures in children. *J Pediatr Orthop* 1986;6:37-39.

3. Greene MH, Hadied AM, LaMont RL: Scaphoid fractures in children. *J Hand Surg Am* 1984;9:536-541.

4. London PS: Sprains and fractures involving the interphalangeal joints. *Hand* 1971;3:155-158.

5. Weber ER, Chao EY: An experimental approach to the mechanism of scaphoid waist fractures. *J Hand Surg Am* 1978;3:142-148.

6. Mintzer CM, Waters PM: Surgical treatment of pediatric scaphoid fracture nonunions. *J Pediatr Orthop* 1999;19:236-239.

7. Brydie A, Raby N: Early MRI in the management of clinical scaphoid fracture. *Br J Radiol* 2003;76:296-300.

8. Dorsay TA, Major NM, Helms CA: Cost-effectiveness of immediate MR imaging versus traditional follow-up for revealing radiographically occult scaphoid fractures. *AJR Am J Roentgenol* 2001;177:1257-1263.

9. Mack MG, Keim S, Balzer JO, et al: Clinical impact of MRI in acute wrist fractures. *Eur Radiol* 2003;13:612-617.

10. Sanders WE: Evaluation of the humpback scaphoid by computed tomography in the longitudinal axial plane of the scaphoid. *J Hand Surg Am* 1988;13:182-187.

11. Waters PM, Stewart SL: Surgical treatment of nonunion and avascular necrosis of the proximal part of the scaphoid in adolescents. *J Bone Joint Surg Am* 2002;84:915-920.

12. Amadio PC, Berquist TH, Smith DK, Ilstrup DM, Cooney WP III, Linscheid RL: Scaphoid malunion. *J Hand Surg Am* 1989;14:679-687.

13. Bora FW Jr, Culp RW, Osterman AL, Skirven T: A flexible wrist splint. *J Hand Surg Am* 1989;14:574-575.

14. Burge P: Closed cast treatment of scaphoid fractures. *Hand Clin* 2001; 17:541-552.

15. Gellman H, Caputo RJ, Carter V, Aboulafia A, McKay M: Comparison of short and long thumb-spica casts for non-displaced fractures of the carpal scaphoid. *J Bone Joint Surg Am* 1989;71:354-357.

16. Hambidge JE, Desai VV, Schranz PJ, Compson JP, Davis TR, Barton NJ: Acute fractures of the scaphoid: Treatment by cast immobilisation with the wrist in flexion or extension? *J Bone Joint Surg Br* 1999;81:91-92.

17. McLaughlin HL: Fracture of the carpal navicular (scaphoid) bone: Some observations based on treatment by

open reduction and internal fixation. *J Bone Joint Surg Am* 1954;36:765-774.

18. Thomaidis VT: Elbow-wrist-thumb immobilisation in the treatment of fractures of the carpal scaphoid. *Acta Orthop Scand* 1973;44:679-689.

19. Yanni D, Lieppins P, Laurence M: Fractures of the carpal scaphoid: A critical study of the standard splint. *J Bone Joint Surg Br* 1991;73:600-602.

20. Adolfsson L, Lindau T, Arner M: Acutrak screw fixation versus cast immobilisation for undisplaced scaphoid waist fractures. *J Hand Surg Br* 2001;26:192-195.

21. Yip HS, Wu WC, Chang RY, So TY: Percutaneous cannulated screw fixation of acute scaphoid waist fracture. *J Hand Surg Br* 2002;27:42-46.

22. Herbert TJ: Use of the Herbert bone screw in surgery of the wrist. *Clin Orthop Relat Res* 1986;202:79-92.

23. Herbert TJ, Fisher WE: Management of the fractured scaphoid using a new bone screw. *J Bone Joint Surg Br* 1984;66:114-123.

24. Mintzer C, Waters PM: Acute open reduction of a displaced scaphoid fracture in a child. *J Hand Surg Am* 1994;19:760-761.

25. Muramatsu K, Doi K, Kuwata N, Kawakami F, Ihara K, Kawai S: Scaphoid fracture in the young athlete: Therapeutic outcome of internal fixation using the Herbert screw. *Arch Orthop Trauma Surg* 2002;122:510-513.

26. Rettig ME, Raskin KB: Retrograde compression screw fixation of acute proximal pole scaphoid fractures. *J Hand Surg Am* 1999;24:1206-1210.

27. De Boeck H, Van Wellen P, Haentjens P: Nonunion of a carpal scaphoid fracture in a child. *J Orthop Trauma* 1991;5:370-372.

28. Larson B, Light TR, Ogden JA: Fracture and ischemic necrosis of the immature scaphoid. *J Hand Surg Am* 1987;12:122-127.

29. Light TR: Injury to the immature carpus. *Hand Clin* 1988;4:415-424.

30. Littlefield WG, Friedman RL, Urbaniak JR: Bilateral non-union of the carpal scaphoid in a child: A case report. *J Bone Joint Surg Am* 1995;77:124-126.

31. Maxted MJ, Owen R: Two cases of non-union of carpal scaphoid fractures in children. *Injury* 1982;13:441-443.

32. Onuba O, Ireland J: Two cases of non-union of fractures of the scaphoid in children. *Injury* 1983;15:109-112.

33. Pick RY, Segal D: Carpal scaphoid fracture and non-union in an eight-year-old child: Report of a case. *J Bone Joint Surg Am* 1983;65:1188-1189.

34. Southcott R, Rosman MA: Nonunion of carpal scaphoid fractures in children. *J Bone Joint Surg Br* 1977;59:20-23.

35. Mack GR, Bosse MJ, Gelberman RH, Yu E: The natural history of scaphoid non-union. *J Bone Joint Surg Am* 1984;66:504-509.

36. Watson HK, Ballet FL: The SLAC wrist: Scapholunate advanced collapse pattern of degenerative arthritis. *J Hand Surg Am* 1984;9:358-365.

37. Barton NJ: Fractures of the phalanges of the hand in children. *Hand* 1979;11:134-143.

38. Fischer MD, McElfresh EC: Physeal and periphyseal injuries of the hand: Patterns of injury and results of treatment. *Hand Clin* 1994;10:287-301.

39. Grad JB: Children's skeletal injuries. *Orthop Clin North Am* 1986;17:437-449.

40. Hastings H II, Simmons BP: Hand fractures in children: A statistical analysis. *Clin Orthop Relat Res* 1984;188:120-130.

41. Leonard MH, Dubravcik P: Management of fractured fingers in the child. *Clin Orthop Relat Res* 1970;73:160-168.

42. Mahabir RC, Kazemi AR, Cannon WG, Courtemanche DJ: Pediatric hand fractures: A review. *Pediatr Emerg Care* 2001;17:153-156.

43. Rajesh A, Basu AK, Vaidhyanath R, Finlay D: Hand fractures: A study of their site and type in childhood. *Clin Radiol* 2001;56:667-669.

44. Worlock P, Stower M: Fracture patterns in Nottingham children. *J Pediatr Orthop* 1986;6:656-660.

45. Worlock PH, Stower MJ: The incidence and pattern of hand fractures in children. *J Hand Surg Br* 1986;11:198-200.

46. Kozin SH, Waters PM: Fractures and dislocations of the hand and carpus in children, in Beaty JH, Kasser JR, (eds): *Rockwood and Wilkins' Fractures in Children*, ed 6. Philadelphia, PA, Lippincott Williams and Wilkins, 2006, pp 257-336.

47. Ersek RA, Gadaria U, Denton DR: Nail bed avulsions treated with porcine xenografts. *J Hand Surg Am* 1985;10:152-153.

48. Ruggles DL, Peterson HA, Scott SG: Radial growth plate injury in a female gymnast. *Med Sci Sports Exerc* 1991;23:393-396.

49. Sandzen SC, Oakey RS: Crushing injury of the fingertip. *Hand* 1972;4:253-256.

50. Zook EG, Guy RJ, Russell RC: A study of nail bed injuries: Causes, treatment, and prognosis. *J Hand Surg Am* 1984;9:247-252.

51. Atasoy E, Ioakimidis E, Kasdan ML, Kutz JE, Kleinert HE: Reconstruction of the amputated finger tip with a triangular volar flap: A new surgical procedure. *J Bone Joint Surg Am* 1970;52:921-926.

52. Clayburgh RH, Wood MB, Cooney WP: Nail bed repair and reconstruction by reverse dermal grafts. *J Hand Surg Am* 1983;8:594-598.

53. Gatewood J: A plastic repair of finger defects without hospitalization. *JAMA* 1926;87:1479.

54. Kappel DA, Burech JG: The cross-finger flap: An established reconstructive procedure. *Hand Clin* 1985;1:677-683.

55. Shepard GH: Nail grafts for reconstruction. *Hand Clin* 1990;6:79-103.

56. Zook EG, Russell RC: Reconstruction of a functional and esthetic nail.

*Hand Clin* 1990;6:59-68.

57. De Boeck H, Jaeken R: Treatment of chronic mallet finger deformity in children by tenodermodesis. *J Pediatr Orthop* 1992;12:351-354.

58. Seymour N: Juxta-epiphysial fracture of the terminal phalanx of the finger. *J Bone Joint Surg Br* 1966;48:347-349.

59. Dixon GL, Moon NF: Rotational supracondylar fractures of the proximal phalanx in children. *Clin Orthop Relat Res* 1972;83:151-156.

60. Cornwall R, Waters PM: Remodeling of phalangeal neck fracture malunions in children: Case report. *J Hand Surg Am* 2004;29:458-461.

61. Hennrikus WL, Cohen MR: Complete remodelling of displaced fractures of the neck of the phalanx. *J Bone Joint Surg Br* 2003;85:273-274.

62. Simmons BP, Peters TT: Subcondylar fossa reconstruction for malunion of fractures of the proximal phalanx in children. *J Hand Surg Am* 1987;12:1079-1082.

63. Blair WF, Marcus NA: Extrusion of the proximal interphalangeal joint: Case report. *J Hand Surg Am* 1981;6:146-147.

64. Segmuller G, Schonenberger F: Fracture of the hand, in Weber BG, Brunner C, Freuler F (eds): *Treatment of Fractures in Children and Adolescents,* New York, NY, Springer-Verlag, 1980, pp 218-225.

65. Agee JM: Unstable fracture dislocations of the proximal interphalangeal joint of the fingers: A preliminary report of a new treatment technique. *J Hand Surg Am* 1978;3:386-389.

66. Schenck RR: Dynamic traction and early passive movement for fractures of the proximal interphalangeal joint. *J Hand Surg Am* 1986;11:850-858.

67. Mintzer CM, Waters PM: Late presentation of a ligamentous ulnar collateral ligament injury in a child. *J Hand Surg Am* 1994;19:1048-1049.

68. White GM: Ligamentous avulsion of the ulnar collateral ligament of the thumb of a child. *J Hand Surg Am* 1986;11:669-672.

69. Eaton RG, Dobranski AI, Littler JW: Marginal osteophyte excision in treatment of mucous cysts. *J Bone Joint Surg Am* 1973;55:570-574.

70. McElfresh EC, Dobyns JH: Intra-articular metacarpal head fractures. *J Hand Surg Am* 1983;8:383-393.

71. Campbell RM Jr : Operative treatment of fractures and dislocations of the hand and wrist region in children. *Orthop Clin North Am* 1990;21:217-243.

72. Gilbert A: Dislocation of the MCP joints in children, in Tubiana R (ed): *The Hand.* Philadelphia, PA, WB Saunders, 1985.

73. Light TR, Ogden JA: Complex dislocation of the index metacarpophalangeal joint in children. *J Pediatr Orthop* 1988;8:300-305.

74. Robins RH: Injuries of the metacarpophalangeal joints. *Hand* 1971;3:159-163.

75. Smith RJ: Post-traumatic instability of the metacarpophalangeal joint of the thumb. *J Bone Joint Surg Am* 1977;59:14-21.

76. Stuart HC, Pyle SI, Cornoni J, Reed RB: Onsets, completions and spans of ossification in the 29 bone-growth centers of the hand and wrist. *Pediatrics* 1962;29:237-249.

77. Barenfeld PA, Weseley MS: Dorsal dislocation of the metacarpophalangeal joint of the index finger treated by late open reduction: A case report. *J Bone Joint Surg Am* 1972;54:1311-1313.

78. Blount WP: Fractures in children. *Schweiz Med Wochenschr* 1954;84:986-988.

79. Green DP, Terry GC: Complex dislocation of the metacarpophalangeal joint: Correlative pathological anatomy. *J Bone Joint Surg Am* 1973;55:1480-1486.

80. Kaplan EB: Dorsal dislocation of the metacarpophalangeal joint of the index finger. *J Bone Joint Surg Am* 1957;39:1081-1086.

81. McLaughlin HL: Complex "locked" dislocation of the metacarpophalangeal joints. *J Trauma* 1965;5: 683-688.

82. Becton JL, Christian JD Jr, Goodwin HN, Jackson JG III: A simplified technique for treating the complex dislocation of the index metacarpophalangeal joint. *J Bone Joint Surg Am* 1975;57:698-700.

83. O'Connell SJ, Moore MM, Strickland JW, Frazier GT, Dell PC: Results of zone I and zone II flexor tendon repairs in children. *J Hand Surg Am* 1994;19:48-52.

84. Baker GL, Kleinert JM: Digit replantation in infants and young children: Determinants of survival. *Plast Reconstr Surg* 1994;94:139-145.

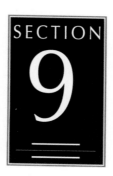

# SECTION 9

# Sports Medicine

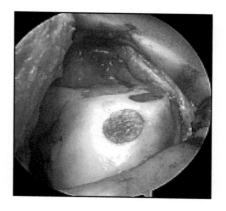

# Biceps Tendon and Superior Labrum Injuries: Decision Making

F. Alan Barber, MD, FACS
*Larry D. Field, MD
*Richard K.N. Ryu, MD

## Abstract

*Although the anatomy of the biceps tendon and the restraining structures within the rotator interval are well defined, biceps function is not clearly understood. Biceps pathology is often associated with rotator cuff disease. Although careful clinical examinations along with diagnostic testing can accurately identify patients with biceps pathology, arthroscopy is extremely valuable in the diagnosis and treatment of biceps pathology. Surgical treatment options for biceps pathology include decompression, débridement, tenotomy, and tenodesis. Several factors must be considered in this decision. The most important factors when deciding between tenodesis or tenotomy are the activity expectations of the patient, cosmesis, patient compliance, associated pathology, and patient age. Those older than 60 years tolerate a tenotomy with the fewest adverse effects. Various arthroscopic tenodesis techniques exist, including an interference screw in bone, suture anchor fixation, and suture to adjacent tissue fixation. An open subpectoral tenodesis is another option and appropriate for a retracted biceps rupture or when the biceps disease extends distal to the bicipital groove. A superior labrum anterior and posterior (SLAP) lesion at the attachment site of the biceps tendon to the superior glenoid labrum is uncommon. Clinically significant SLAP lesions are found in about 5% of all shoulder arthroscopies and may be mistaken for normal superior labral variations. Clinical examinations and diagnostic imaging tests for SLAP lesions are often unreliable, and the ultimate diagnostic confirmation is made by arthroscopy. Surgical treatment is focused on the reattachment of the unstable biceps-labral complex.*

**Instr Course Lect 2008;57:527-538.**

The biceps tendon originates from the labrum and the supraglenoid tubercle of the scapula. The structure is intra-articular yet extrasynovial. It is widest at its origin and progressively narrows as it exits the bicipital groove. The proximal third of the biceps tendon has a high degree of innervation, with substance P and calcitonin gene-related peptides present, suggesting a rich sympathetic network.[1]

## Biceps Anatomy and Function

There is a spectrum of pathologic conditions of the proximal part of the biceps, including tendinitis, superior labrum anterior and posterior (SLAP) lesions, biceps instability, and partial or complete ruptures. The origin of the long head of the biceps is variable and is approximately 9 cm long.[2] The proximal portion of the long head receives its blood supply primarily from the anterior circumflex humeral artery.[3] The biceps tendon passes posterior to the coracohumeral ligament and beneath the transverse humeral ligament as it courses distally. The capsuloligamentous structures of the rotator interval are responsible for restraining the biceps tendon within its proper anatomic location as it passes into the bicipital groove.[4,5] The coracohumeral ligament and the superior glenohumeral ligament are the two most important structures within the rotator interval for

*Larry D. Field, MD or the department with which he is affiliated has received royalties from Smith & Nephew and is a consultant or employee for Smith & Nephew. Richard K.N. Ryu, MD is a consultant or employee for KFx Medical Corporation.*

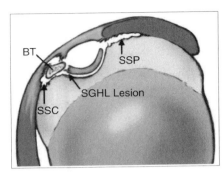

**Figure 1** Medial subluxation or dislocation of the biceps tendon (BT) can occur with repetitive wear or trauma to the superior glenohumeral ligament (SGHL) and is commonly associated with rotator cuff disease, especially subscapularis tears (SSC) as well as supraspinatus (SSP) tears. (Reproduced with permission from Habermeyer P, Magosch P, Pritsch M, Scheibel MT, Lichtenberg S: Anterosuperior impingement of the shoulder as a result of pulley lesion: A prospective arthroscopic study. *J Shoulder Elbow Surg* 2004;13:5-12.)

securing the biceps tendon.[2] The superior glenohumeral ligament forms an anterior sling about the biceps. The more distal transverse humeral ligament is not believed to play a primary role in securing the biceps tendon.[5]

The exact function of the long head of the biceps tendon in the shoulder is controversial. The angular orientation of the biceps relative to the humeral head appears to be adaptive in nature, and it diminishes the capacity for arm elevation, perhaps placing the biceps at risk for instability. The proximal part of the biceps tendon probably has at least a passive shoulder stabilizing function. Although several authors have observed that the proximal part of the biceps tendon has an active stabilizing effect, others have not.[6-9] Cadaveric biomechanical evidence indicates that the contribution of the biceps to glenohumeral stability may depend on the

position of the elbow.[10]

Problems related to the biceps tendon can be classified as inflammatory, instability, or traumatic.[11] Bicipital tenosynovitis is closely associated with impingement. Neer[12] demonstrated that the biceps tendon is subject to the same mechanical wear beneath the coracoacromial arch as is the rotator cuff. Because the biceps tendon sheath is continuous with the glenohumeral joint, any inflammatory process affecting the intra-articular environment can also affect the biceps. Biceps instability may occur more commonly than would be expected on the basis of clinical and arthroscopic examinations. The biceps tendon passes through an angle of approximately 30° as it exits the shoulder.[13] Medial subluxation or dislocation of the tendon can occur with repetitive wear or trauma to the restraining structures and is commonly associated with rotator cuff lesions, especially subscapularis tears[2,14] (Figure 1). Finally, although traumatic biceps tendon lesions including rupture are uncommon, other traumatic disruptions such as SLAP lesions do occur.

## Biceps Tendinitis and Instability

Biceps tendinitis is a relatively common cause of anterior shoulder pain. The tendinitis can be primary or secondary. Primary bicipital tendinitis is the isolated inflammation of the long head of the biceps tendon in the intertubercular groove, with no associated pathologic changes in the shoulder. It has been estimated to represent only 5% of the cases of biceps tendinitis.[4] Secondary biceps tendinitis occurs in conjunction with pathologic changes in the adjacent osseous, ligamentous, and muscular structures. This type of tendinitis often results in tendon fraying and even failure as the biceps tendon undergoes wear. As a result of repetitive wear or trauma, the soft-tissue restraints surrounding the biceps tendon can lose their stabilizing function, and medial subluxation or dislocation of the tendon can occur.

Patients with biceps tendinitis or instability present with pain primarily in the bicipital groove. The history and the results of the physical examination are usually compatible with an impingement syndrome, although the pain may be more anterior and may radiate down the biceps itself. Usually, there is no history of trauma. Patients with biceps instability occasionally report popping and an audible or palpable snap during the arc of shoulder motion. Biceps tendon instability is almost always associated with pathologic changes in the subscapularis tendon and rarely occurs in the absence of at least some subscapularis tearing.

On physical examination, the most common finding in patients with biceps tendinitis or instability is point tenderness in the bicipital groove. Several provocative tests have been described for isolating a pathologic condition of the biceps, including the Yergason test, the Speed test, the biceps instability test, the lift-off test, and the O'Brien active compression test.[15-18] As an adjunct to these provocative tests, selective injections can be very helpful in differentiating the source of shoulder pain. Unfortunately, there is no single physical finding that is conclusive evidence of a symptomatic pathologic condition of the biceps. Coexisting impingement and rotator cuff-related symptoms may make the diagnosis difficult.

Radiographic evaluation is usually not helpful and almost always reveals normal findings in patients with primary biceps tendinitis. Secondary causes, such as an avulsion fragment from the tuberosity, suggest a biceps dislocation, and a large anterior acromial spur may suggest an impingement syndrome. Additional radiographic views can be used to evaluate the bicipital groove. Ultrasonography has become a useful tool in some centers for evaluation of the biceps and the rotator cuff.[19] However, ultrasonography is heavily operator dependent and can be limited by osseous anatomy.

MRI is an excellent tool for evaluating the biceps tendon and the superior labral complex. An MRI arthrogram continues to be the most appropriate noninvasive diagnostic study available for confirming a pathologic condition of the biceps. Oblique and sagittal images can demonstrate subluxation and dislocation of the long head of the biceps tendon. Edema associated with bicipital tendinitis produces an increased signal intensity on T2-weighted images. Biceps tendon ruptures also are relatively easy to detect on MRI.

Boileau and associates[20] described an hourglass-shaped biceps tendon that causes typical tendinitis symptoms. It can be seen on arthrography. It results from an inflamed, thickened intra-articular segment, which can block tendon excursion during shoulder motion because the thickened part cannot traverse the bicipital groove. This so-called shoulder trigger finger can cause anterior shoulder pain and a loss of 10° to 20° of passive elevation as a result of mechanical locking, but it is difficult to recognize clinically. A thickened tendon can disrupt the pulley and destabilize the biceps over time. The treatment is excision of the thickened part of the biceps and tenodesis if necessary.

When a pathologic condition of the biceps is suspected but confirmation proves elusive, arthroscopic evaluation is the most accurate means of verifying the diagnosis. During the arthroscopy, it is imperative that the tendon be inspected thoroughly, and this requires pulling the biceps into the joint to completely visualize the portion within the bicipital groove. Testing for instability of the biceps tendon should be done.

### Instability of the Biceps Tendon

The biceps tendon makes a 30° to 40° turn into the bicipital groove as it exits the shoulder and is stabilized by a pulley system[2] (Figure 2). This pulley system is made up of the coracohumeral ligament and the superior glenohumeral ligament along with both supraspinatus and subscapularis tendon fibers (Figure 1). Progressive disruption of the pulley leads to biceps instability with medial subluxation, which in turn leads to progressive damage of the pulley itself. The biceps can dislocate immediately on top of the subscapularis, under the subscapularis if the subscapularis tendon is torn, or even laterally.[21] A clear understanding of the anatomy of the rotator interval is necessary to appreciate the variations of biceps instability in association with rotator cuff lesions.

The coracohumeral ligament arises from the coracoid process and separates into two bands. It invests the biceps at this critical angle as it exits the joint.[7] The superior glenohumeral ligament travels from the labrum to the humeral head. It becomes a U-shaped sling that supports the biceps tendon at this critical exit angle.[5] Also, rotator cuff fibers reinforce the pulley system. The transverse humeral ligament appears to be much less important to biceps stability. In fact, its more dis-

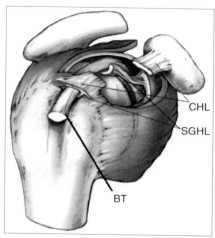

**Figure 2** The biceps tendon (BT) makes a 30° to 40° turn into the bicipital groove as it exits the shoulder and is stabilized by a pulley system. CHL = coracohumeral ligament, SGHL = superior glenohumeral ligament. (Reproduced with permission from Habermeyer P, Magosch P, Pritsch M, Scheibel MT, Lichtenberg S: Anterosuperior impingement of the shoulder as a result of pulley lesions: A prospective arthroscopic study. *J Shoulder Elbow Surg* 2004;13: 5-12.)

tal location means that the critical angle of biceps passage occurs more proximally, and any subluxation would likely occur more proximally. The description of progressive damage to the pulley system by Habermeyer and associates[2] has been labeled "pulley lesions." These lesions can be traumatic or degenerative, and the pulley is susceptible to rotator cuff degeneration as is the biceps tendon itself.

Damage to the pulley system often occurs in a series of steps and is usually initiated by an articular-sided supraspinatus tear, which then leads to a tear of the superior glenohumeral ligament.[13,14] The tear of the superior glenohumeral ligament in turn allows subtle subluxation of the long head of the biceps, which can, in turn, cause a partial articular subscapularis tear.

Progressive subluxation of the long head of the biceps causes more damage to the subscapularis tendon (Figure 1). This cycle of progressive subluxation leading to subscapularis damage can ultimately lead to medial dislocation of the biceps and even anterosuperior instability with the occurrence of labral lesions. The possibility of a subscapularis tear occurring in conjunction with biceps instability cannot be overemphasized. Recognition of these tears is important as they often cause substantial anterior shoulder pain along with the biceps instability.

## Nonsurgical Treatment of Bicipital Tendinitis and Biceps Instability

The initial treatment of primary and secondary bicipital tendinitis is nonsurgical. Initially, rest and nonsteroidal anti-inflammatory drugs are recommended. Subacromial steroid injections can help to treat both primary and secondary tendinitis.[3] Injections into the glenohumeral joint can reduce intra-articular biceps irritation. Finally, injections into the bicipital sheath anteriorly, with care taken to avoid the biceps tendon itself, can be of benefit.[3] Once the symptoms begin to decrease, gentle range-of-motion exercises are begun. When a patient has secondary bicipital tendinitis caused by impingement syndrome, treatment should be directed toward the rotator cuff lesion. Exercises can be advanced as dictated by the status of the rotator cuff.

Nonsurgical treatment of biceps instability is limited and should be directed toward the management of the rotator cuff lesions. Intra-articular injections are sometimes beneficial for older, sedentary patients. Younger, more active individuals almost always require surgery to address the rotator cuff lesions and the biceps instability.

## Surgical Treatment of Biceps Tendinitis and Instability

The most important aspect of treating a pathologic condition of the biceps tendon is to determine its cause, define the degree of structural compromise, and detect associated pathologic conditions, such as rotator cuff disease and impingement, that need to be addressed concomitantly. Surgical intervention for biceps tendinitis is generally indicated if the patient continues to have symptoms after 3 months of conservative management or if there is biceps instability.

The surgical options available include tendon débridement, a release of a constricted synovial sheath, a tenodesis, or a tenotomy.

## Biceps Débridement

A simple débridement of the tendon in association with an arthroscopic subacromial decompression is appropriate for the treatment of mild tendon fraying. If the patient has a partial tear, involving less than 50% of the tendon, and an inactive lifestyle, a simple débridement and decompression may be sufficient. In younger active patients, partial tears should be treated more aggressively, with any tear involving more than 25% of the tendon being managed with tenodesis. Tenotomy should be avoided in younger active patients, whereas it is a reasonable option for more sedentary patients. A so-called Popeye deformity may develop after a tenotomy, but it will not develop after a tenodesis.

## Biceps Decompression

Biceps tendon decompression can relieve the symptoms of primary biceps tendinitis through a tenosynovial release. A release of the transverse humeral ligament, sparing the coracohumeral ligament, and an arthroscopic or open release of the bicipital tendon sheath in the absence of other pathologic entities will decrease symptoms. This surgical option is applicable only for inflammation of an otherwise intact tendon in the absence of other substantial pathologic entities. If the tenosynovitis is severe and unrelenting, and occurs above as well as below the bicipital groove, a tenotomy in a less active patient or a subpectoral tenodesis in a more active individual is recommended.

## Tenotomy

There is controversy about the choice of tenotomy or tenodesis.[22] Tenotomy is currently a more popular option for the treatment of a diseased biceps tendon,[23,24] but the decision regarding treatment of an inflamed but otherwise intact biceps tendon is not an easy one. Associated pathologic entities and surgery may render the decision regarding whether to perform a tenotomy and a tenodesis moot because the prolonged immobilization necessary after an arthroscopic rotator cuff repair, into which a tenotomy can be easily incorporated, reduces the benefits of a tenodesis.

Tenotomy has obvious advantages. It is technically very easy to perform, rehabilitation is simple, and there is no need for immobilization. The disadvantage of a tenotomy is the potential for a residual Popeye deformity caused by retraction of the biceps muscle distally. In addition to this deformity, cramping and weakness with vigorous use of the biceps may be encountered. In many instances, one can predict the possibility of deformity by carefully inspecting the proximal end of the biceps. In cases of chronic inflammation in which the biceps origin is substantially thickened, simple tenotomies rarely lead to deformity because the proximal end of the biceps is too large to pass through the bicipital groove.

Clinical studies of simple tenotomies have revealed that pain relief is achieved and the satisfaction rate usually exceeds 90%, but the Popeye deformity occurs in up to 70% of patients, and as many as 40% of patients experience fatigue or soreness with resisted elbow flexion. In several studies, patients older than 60 years did not experience this fatigue.[25,26] Osbahr and associates[27] noted no significant difference in terms of the cosmetic result, pain relief, or muscle spasms between tenodesis and tenotomy, but the patients who were treated with a tenodesis were younger than those who were treated with a tenotomy. Walch and associates[23] reviewed the outcomes of 307 patients who had had a biceps tenotomy because of an irreparable rotator cuff tear or because they were unwilling to undergo the lengthy rehabilitation associated with an arthroscopic rotator cuff repair. Eighty-seven percent were satisfied, although a subacromial decompression was often performed as well. Preoperative fatty infiltration of the rotator cuff muscles and a high-riding humeral head were prognostic of a poor outcome.

### Tenodesis

Tenodesis can be performed either open or arthroscopically, with use of soft-tissue or osseous fixation, and above or below the bicipital groove. The advantages of a biceps tenodesis are a better cosmetic result and restoration of strength, whereas the disadvantages include a more difficult operation, the possible need for

costly implants, a longer rehabilitation, a period of immobilization, and the possibility of the tenodesis failing. Several alternatives for arthroscopic fixation are available. The tendon can be secured with use of an interference screw in a bone tunnel or with suture anchors in the bicipital groove, or by suturing it to the rotator interval.[28,29] Suturing the biceps remnant to the conjoint tendon has also been described.[30] An open subpectoral approach in which a keyhole type of fixation is achieved can be used. Investigators comparing the mechanical strength values following tenodesis fixation techniques concluded that the interference screw and bone tunnel technique provides the greatest initial fixation strength.[31]

Tenodesis for treatment of disease of the long head of the biceps is usually performed in conjunction with the treatment of concomitant rotator cuff disease. Isolated biceps tenodesis has historically been uncommon, and the results have been modest at best, perhaps reflecting neglected underlying pathologic conditions such as an impingement phenomenon. Studies in which a biceps tenodesis was done in conjunction with a decompression have uniformly revealed satisfactory results,[32] although Walch and associates[23] reported no difference in the success rates of tenodeses done with and without an accompanying decompression.

In the case of a complete biceps rupture, tenodesis is appropriate for a younger active patient and can be accomplished through an open subpectoral approach. Technically, reestablishing the proper resting length to the tenodesed biceps tendon is critical if strength and a good cosmetic appearance are to be restored. The subpectoral approach helps the

surgeon to find the ruptured proximal stump and permits direct visualization so that the musculotendinous portion of the biceps can be lined up with the pectoralis insertion site to reproduce the optimal resting length. Furthermore, with any open approach, a keyhole-type fixation technique, in which the stump of the tendon is fixed and delivered into the humeral shaft, helps to avoid the need for costly implants. Older patients with lower functional demands have tolerated benign neglect well.[33] Isolated pathologic involvement of the biceps is uncommon, and if a rupture occurs the presence of associated rotator cuff disease should be considered.

### Biceps Instability

Subluxation or dislocation of the biceps tendon is almost invariably associated with rotator cuff tearing, particularly of the subscapularis, and pathologic involvement of the rotator interval.[2] It is important to determine the direction of the instability, which is most commonly medial, and the instability is usually fixed rather than dynamic. The superior portion of the subscapularis tendon is usually torn and must be addressed in addition to the biceps disease. The treatment options for biceps instability include tenotomy, tenodesis, or reconstruction of the stabilizing structures that support the biceps tendon. The indications for tenotomy and tenodesis parallel those for patients with moderate to severe tendinitis and are the more common choices.

Tenodesis of the biceps, in conjunction with a subscapularis repair, is appropriate if a patient is young and active, whereas a tenotomy is an appropriate intervention for a less active patient even when the subscapu-

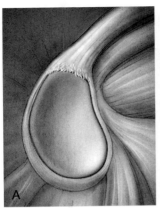 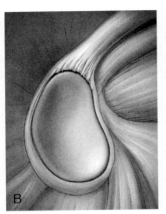 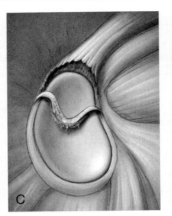 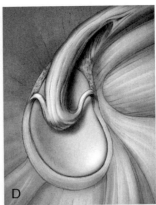

**Figure 3**    The classification system for SLAP lesions. **A,** A type 1 SLAP lesion consists of degenerative fraying on the inner margin of the superior aspect of the labrum. **B,** With a type 2 SLAP lesion, the biceps attachment and the adjacent superior aspect of the labrum have pulled off the superior glenoid tubercle. **C,** A type 3 SLAP lesion is a superior labral bucket-handle tear. **D,** A type 4 SLAP lesion is a superior labral bucket-handle tear that extends into the biceps tendon. (Reproduced with permission from Powell SE, Nord KD, Ryu RK: The diagnosis, classification, and treatment of SLAP lesions. *Oper Tech Sports Med* 2004;12:99-110.)

laris is being repaired. Not treating the unstable biceps definitely leads to rupture of the subscapularis repair. These anterior-superior tears that include the biceps and subscapularis often also involve the supraspinatus. Furthermore, careful evaluation of the subcoracoid space is recommended because subcoracoid impingement may have led to the cumulative injury to the rotator interval structures.[34,35] Reconstruction of the stabilizing structures in the rotator interval, with attention paid to the superior glenohumeral ligament and the coracohumeral ligament, and the creation of a sling around the tendon can be performed. However, recurrent instability can be a problem, and a stenosed, painful tendon may result.

### Overview of Surgical Treatments of the Biceps Tendon

Both tenodesis and tenotomy can yield good results.[22] Interestingly, several authors have found that acromioplasty alone relieved anterior shoulder pain despite a preoper-

ative diagnosis of biceps tenosynovitis.[36] Although there is much controversy regarding surgical management of a symptomatic biceps tendon, we typically sacrifice the biceps tendon only when there is a substantial partial tear, extensive tenosynovitis, or tendon instability. The decision to perform a tenodesis or tenotomy is usually based on several factors. Tenotomy is routinely performed in sedentary patients and in those for whom the cosmetic result is not a concern. However, tenodesis is almost always performed in younger, more active patients or any patient for whom the cosmetic result is an issue, particularly those with thin arms.

### The SLAP Injury

Superior glenoid labrum injuries were apparently first defined as SLAP tears by Snyder and associates[37] in 1990. Although the recognized varieties of SLAP injuries have expanded over time, the challenge is to differentiate between the labral variations that are clinically relevant lesions and those that are normal

variations or simply the effects of aging.

SLAP lesions can be created by various mechanisms of injury, including a biceps traction overload caused by the long head of the biceps acting as a decelerator of the arm during the follow-through phase of throwing; arm acceleration during the late cocking phase; a tight posterior aspect of the capsule; falling on the outstretched arm, creating shearing forces on the superior biceps labral complex;[38] sudden forced abduction and external rotation of the shoulder; and passive disruption during a motor vehicle crash when the shoulder-lap belt restrains the ipsilateral chest wall, causing the shoulder to roll around the seat belt.

Any classification system should provide a logical method for evaluating the injury that can positively affect the treatment algorithm. The classification system now includes many more types than had been initially described.[37] A type 1 SLAP lesion has fraying on the inner margin of the superior aspect of the labrum

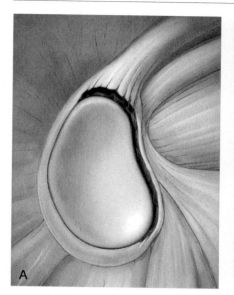
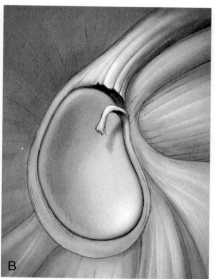
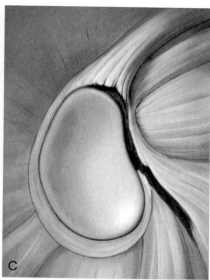

**Figure 4** The SLAP classification system was expanded to include injuries associated with dislocation. **A,** A type 5 SLAP lesion is a Bankart lesion that extends superiorly to the biceps attachment. **B,** A type 6 SLAP lesion has an anterior or posterior labral flap with a type 2 biceps elevation. **C,** A type 7 SLAP lesion is a separation of the biceps attachment that extends into the middle glenohumeral ligament. (Reproduced with permission from Powell SE, Nord KD, Ryu RK: The diagnosis, classification, and treatment of SLAP lesions. *Oper Tech Sports Med* 2004;12:99-110.)

(Figure 3, *A*) and probably represents normal degenerative changes associated with increased age and the retreat of blood supply from the superior aspect of the labrum. This may be confused with a meniscoid superior part of the labrum, which is a normal variant.

A type 2 SLAP lesion is the most common clinically relevant abnormality. It occurs when the superior labral attachment of the biceps tendon pulls off the superior glenoid tubercle (Figure 3, *B*). Burkhart and Morgan[39] further defined the type 2 SLAP lesion according to three subtypes based on the anatomic location of this elevation: anterior, posterior, and combined anterior and posterior. The most common of these subtypes is the anterior lesion, which involves a labral avulsion from the anterosuperior quadrant of the glenoid. The posterior subtype involves the posterosuperior quadrant of the glenoid and is most com-

monly seen in throwing athletes. The combined (anterior and superior) subtype is the least common. When traction is applied to the biceps tendon of a patient with a labral separation from the posterosuperior quadrant of the glenoid, the force on the tendon shifts from an anterior-horizontal to a posterior-vertical position. This force is transmitted to the labrum at the base of the biceps tendon and results in the detached labrum sliding medially or peeling off the posterior-superior aspect of the glenoid; this has been called the "peel-back" phenomenon.[39]

A type 3 SLAP lesion is a superior labral bucket-handle tear often extending from anterior to posterior at the biceps insertion (Figure 3, *C*). In contrast to the type 2 lesion, the biceps-labral attachment is not elevated from the glenoid. In a type 4 SLAP lesion, the bucket-handle tear extends into the biceps tendon, splitting the tendon attachment

(Figure 3, *D*). Additional SLAP lesions (types 5 through 10) have also been described[40-42] (Figures 4 and 5).

Maffet and associates[40] expanded this classification system to include shoulder instability injuries. Their type 5 SLAP lesion is a Bankart lesion extending superiorly to the biceps attachment (Figure 4, *A*). A type 6 SLAP lesion has a labral flap with a type 2 biceps elevation (Figure 4, *B*), and a type 7 SLAP lesion is a lesion of the middle glenohumeral ligament extending to the biceps attachment (Figure 4, *C*). Powell and associates[41] further expanded this classification system to include a type 8 lesion, which is a type 2 SLAP lesion with posterior labral extension (Figure 5, *A*); a type 9 lesion, which is a type 2 SLAP lesion with circumferential labral tearing (Figure 5, *B*); and a type 10 lesion, which is a type 2 SLAP lesion with a posterior-inferior labral separation (Figure 5, *C*). An additional variation of labral disease in-

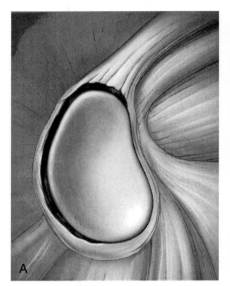
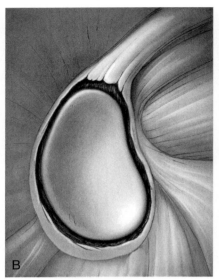
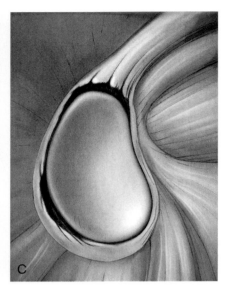

**Figure 5**    Additional types of SLAP lesions have been identified. **A,** A type 8 SLAP lesion is a type 2 lesion with posterior labral extension. **B,** A type 9 SLAP lesion is a type 2 lesion with circumferential separate labral tearing. **C,** A type 10 SLAP lesion is a type 2 lesion with a posterior-inferior labral separation. (Reproduced with permission from Powell SE, Nord KD, Ryu RK: The diagnosis, classification, and treatment of SLAP lesions. *Oper Tech Sports Med* 2004;12:99-110.)

cludes a type 2 SLAP injury with articular cartilage avulsions and loose bodies as described by Choi and Kim.[42]

Approximately half of clinically relevant SLAP lesions are type 2. Also, except in series dealing principally with shoulder instability, the overall prevalence of SLAP tears is very low.[37,43-45] In the original study in which SLAP lesions were defined,[38] they accounted for only 4% of 700 cases in a consecutive series of shoulder arthroscopic procedures, and a review of 2,375 patients in another series of consecutive shoulder arthroscopic procedures demonstrated a 5.9% prevalence of SLAP lesions.[43-45]

### Clinical Presentation
Clinically relevant SLAP lesions are most often found after trauma, in swimmers, or in long-time overhead throwing athletes.[37,39,40] The patients describe clicking and popping often associated with anterior shoulder pain and reduced function, including decreased throwing or serving velocity or slower swimming speed. The symptoms may appear suddenly or gradually. The dead arm syndrome is characterized by the inability to throw at the preinjury velocity.[46]

The key elements to be considered in differentiating a clinically relevant superior labral injury from normal variations or changes due to aging include the patient, the mechanism of injury, the findings of the clinical examination, and the findings of appropriate imaging studies. Demonstrated improvement after surgical treatment confirms the diagnosis.

Proper patient selection is critical. A SLAP lesion should be anticipated before surgery so that it is not an unexpected finding at arthroscopy. True type 2 SLAP injuries are seldom associated with substantial glenohumeral arthritis or rotator cuff tears. When degenerative changes are found, the labral abnormality is likely to be part of a degenerative process.

Clinically relevant SLAP injuries are most often found in the dominant arm of a man younger than age 40 years who has participated in high-performance overhead activities for many years, a patient with a specific history of shoulder trauma, or a patient with shoulder instability. A fall on an outstretched hand or a prior motor vehicle crash during which the patient was wearing a shoulder-lap belt is also suggestive of a SLAP injury.[12,47]

### Physical Examination
Several tests have been proposed for the diagnosis of a clinically relevant SLAP injury. However, these tests often provide inconsistent results and are not consistently diagnostic.[18,48-54] The modified O'Brien test, the crank test, the anterior slide test, the Jobe relocation test, the biceps load test, and the pain provocation test are advocated by some and

dismissed by others.[54] A positive Speed test and a loss of internal rotation that has not resolved following a short course of physical therapy have been said to indicate a SLAP lesion.[39] Despite the concerns about the reliability of these tests, they do play a role in the physical examination of the shoulder. However, no single test should be completely relied upon.

Diagnostic imaging also provides inconsistent results. Plain radiographs reveal osseous problems. The superior aspect of the glenoid labrum can be seen on a gadolinium-enhanced MRI scan, but correct interpretation requires special expertise. The variability of the normal superior aspect of the labrum reduces the diagnostic value of this test. However, the presence of a sublabral ganglion cyst is very suggestive of a SLAP lesion.[55]

### Nonsurgical Treatment

The initial treatment of a SLAP lesion should include rest, anti-inflammatory medication, stretching, and strengthening to address muscular imbalances. Decreased internal rotation is often found in athletes who throw overhead. A reduction in shoulder rotation to less than 180° or a loss of internal rotation suggests a tight posterior aspect of the capsule. Scapular dyskinesis or weakness of the scapular stabilizers may result in scapular winging and asymmetric arm motion. Stretching to attain full motion (internal rotation) should be performed before surgical intervention. If symptoms persist after 3 months of nonsurgical treatment, surgery may be indicated.

### Surgical Treatment

The arthroscopic treatment of a SLAP lesion depends on the type of lesion. A type 1 SLAP lesion is treat-ed with débridement of the area of labral fraying. A type 2 lesion should be treated with reattachment of the superior aspect of the labrum to achieve a stable biceps-superior labral anchor. A type 3 SLAP lesion requires removal of the bucket-handle tear. A type 4 lesion requires débridement of any flap or bucket-handle tear and repair of the associated biceps tear or a biceps tenodesis. Types 5, 6, and 7 SLAP lesions are associated with shoulder instability, which should be corrected at the same time as the SLAP lesion is repaired, and any flap should be débrided. For types 8, 9, and 10, the labrum should be reattached, and any flap should be débrided. The goal of surgical repair is to securely reattach the biceps-labral complex and to eliminate the peel-back and drive-through signs.

Half of all SLAP lesions that require surgery are type 2. Although various techniques have been used in the past, suture anchors are currently the preferred method of biceps-labral fixation. An anterior type 2 SLAP lesion requires one suture anchor placed either beneath or slightly anterior to the biceps tendon origin. In this location, a mattress suture (or two simple sutures) can fix both sides of the biceps origin. A posterior or combined type 2 SLAP lesion requires a suture anchor posterior to the biceps origin to fully stabilize the posterior-superior aspect of the labrum.

The initial step in a repair of a SLAP lesion is to carefully probe and assess the biceps and the superior labral injury and to débride any degenerative tissue. After the superior aspect of the labrum has been elevated to expose the glenoid neck, this area is débrided to prepare it for biceps-labral reattachment. Roughening the bone surface to create a bleeding bed, rather than decorticating the superior glenoid tubercle, is sufficient. The appropriate suture anchor or anchors are inserted into the superior glenoid articular cartilage margin at an angle (usually 45°) that places the anchor into the bone without it cutting out either medially or laterally. Once the anchor is in place, the sutures are passed through the labral tissue, and either a simple or a mattress stitch is used.

### Postoperative Treatment

SLAP repairs are often followed by stiffness in the postoperative period, as the repair can substantially decrease motion, including internal and external rotation and translation.[56] Thus, a sling is used for only 3 weeks, and the patient is encouraged to remove the sling and perform rotation movements to stretch the capsule during this period. After use of the sling is discontinued, pendulum exercises with elbow flexion and extension are recommended and should be performed. At 6 weeks, strengthening of the rotator cuff, scapular stabilizers, biceps, and deltoid muscle is initiated. Throwing athletes begin an interval-throwing program at 4 months on a level surface. Stretching (of the posterior aspect of the capsule) and strengthening are continued, and throwing from the mound begins at 6 months. A return to full activity is permitted at 7 months. Nonthrowing athletes may return to their sports at 4 months.

### Summary

Although the anatomy of the biceps tendon and the restraining structures within the rotator interval have been well defined, biceps function and the importance of the long head of the biceps are not clearly understood at this time. Pathologic involvement of the biceps, when encountered, is usually associated with rotator cuff disease and possibly an impingement process. Functionally, some humeral head stability may be imparted through the biceps tendon. Although careful clinical examination along with diagnostic testing can accurately identify a pathologic condition of the biceps, arthroscopy is an extremely valuable tool with which to establish the accurate diagnosis and treatment of biceps disease.

Options for the surgical treatment of pathologic biceps conditions include decompression, débridement, tenotomy, and tenodesis. Several factors must be considered in this decision. The most important factors to be taken into account when choosing between tenodesis and tenotomy are the activity expectations of the patient, the importance of the cosmetic result, patient compliance, associated pathologic entities requiring a surgical procedure that may allow easy incorporation of a tenodesis, and the patient's age. Those older than 60 years appear to tolerate a tenotomy with the fewest adverse effects.

There are various techniques for arthroscopic tenodesis, including interference screw fixation to bone, suture anchor fixation, and suture fixation to adjacent tissue. The interference screw technique yields the best initial fixation, although soft-tissue fixation can also lead to a satisfactory result and is easier to perform. An open subpectoral tenodesis is the appropriate choice for patients with a retracted ruptured tendon or for those with biceps disease extending distal to the bicipital groove.

The SLAP lesion at the attachment of the biceps tendon to the superior aspect of the glenoid labrum is uncommon. A clinically relevant SLAP lesion is found during about 5% of all shoulder arthroscopies and may be confused with a normal anterior labral variation. Clinical examinations and imaging tests for the diagnosis of SLAP lesions are often unreliable, and the ultimate diagnostic confirmation is made with arthroscopy. Surgical treatment is focused on the reattachment of the unstable biceps-labral complex.

## References

1. Curtis AS, Snyder SJ: Evaluation and treatment of biceps tendon pathology. *Orthop Clin North Am* 1993;24:33-43.

2. Habermeyer P, Magosch P, Pritsch M, Scheibel MT, Lichtenberg S: Anterosuperior impingement of the shoulder as a result of pulley lesions: A prospective arthroscopic study. *J Shoulder Elbow Surg* 2004; 13:5-12.

3. Burkhead WZ Jr, Arcand MA, Zeman C, Habermeyer P, Walch G: The biceps tendon, in Rockwood CA Jr, Matsen FA III, Wirth MA, Lippitt SB (eds): *The Shoulder*, ed 3. Philadelphia, PA, Saunders, 2004, vol 2, pp 1059-1119.

4. Favorito PJ, Harding WG III, Heidt RS Jr: Complete arthroscopic examination of the long head of the biceps tendon. *Arthroscopy* 2001;17: 430-432.

5. Pfahler M, Branner S, Refior HJ: The role of the bicipital groove in tendopathy of the long biceps tendon. *J Shoulder Elbow Surg* 1999;8:419-424.

6. Pagnani MJ, Deng XH, Warren RF, Torzilli PA, O'Brien SJ: Role of the long head of the biceps brachii in glenohumeral stability: A biomechanical study in cadavera. *J Shoulder Elbow Surg* 1996;5:255-262.

7. Itoi E, Kuechle DK, Newman SR, Morrey BF, An KN: Stabilising function of the biceps in stable and unstable shoulders. *J Bone Joint Surg Br* 1993;75:546-550.

8. Warner JJ, McMahon PJ: The role of the long head of the biceps brachii in superior stability of the glenohumeral joint. *J Bone Joint Surg Am* 1995;77: 366-372.

9. Yamaguchi K, Riew KD, Galatz LM, Syme JA, Neviaser RJ: Biceps activity during shoulder motion: An electromyographic analysis. *Clin Orthop Relat Res* 1997;336:122-129.

10. Gowan ID, Jobe FW, Tibone JE, Perry J, Moynes DR: A comparative electromyographic analysis of the shoulder during pitching: Professional versus amateur pitchers. *Am J Sports Med* 1987;15:586-590.

11. Yamaguchi K, Bindra R: Disorders of the biceps tendon, in Iannotti JP, Williams GR Jr (eds): *Disorders of the Shoulder: Diagnosis and Management.* Philadelphia, PA, Lippincott Williams and Wilkins, 1999, pp 159-190.

12. Neer CS II: Anterior acromioplasty for the chronic impingement syndrome in the shoulder: A preliminary report. *J Bone Joint Surg Am* 1972;54: 41-50.

13. Bennett WF: Visualization of the anatomy of the rotator interval and bicipital sheath. *Arthroscopy* 2001;17: 107-111.

14. Bennett WF: Arthroscopic repair of isolated subscapularis tears: A prospective cohort with 2- to 4-year follow-up. *Arthroscopy* 2003;19:131-143.

15. Yergason RM: Supination sign. *J Bone Joint Surg Am* 1931;13:160.

16. Bennett WF: Arthroscopic repair of anterosuperior (supraspinatus/subscapularis) rotator cuff tears: A prospective cohort with 2- to 4-year follow-up: Classification of biceps subluxation/instability. *Arthroscopy* 2003;19:21-33.

17. Gerber C, Krushell RJ: Isolated rupture of the tendon of the subscapularis muscle: Clinical features in 16 cases. *J Bone Joint Surg Br* 1991;73:389-394.

18. O'Brien SJ, Pagnani MJ, Fealy S, McGlynn SR, Wilson JB: The active compression test: A new and effective test for diagnosing labral tears and acromioclavicular joint abnormality. *Am J Sports Med* 1998;26:610-613.

19. Iannotti JP, Ciccone J, Buss DD, et al: Accuracy of office-based ultrasonography of the shoulder for the diagnosis of rotator cuff tears. *J Bone Joint Surg Am* 2005;87:1305-1311.

20. Boileau P, Ahrens PM, Hatzidakis AM: Entrapment of the long head of the biceps tendon: The hourglass biceps. A cause of pain and locking of the shoulder. *J Shoulder Elbow Surg* 2004;13:249-257.

21. Bennett WF: Subscapularis, medial, and lateral head coracohumeral ligament insertion anatomy: Arthroscopic appearance and incidence of "hidden" rotator interval lesions. *Arthroscopy* 2001;17:173-180.

22. Berlemann U, Bayley I: Tenodesis of the long head of biceps brachii in the painful shoulder: Improving results in the long term. *J Shoulder Elbow Surg* 1995;4:429-435.

23. Walch G, Edwards TB, Boulahia A, Nové-Josserand L, Neyton L, Szabo I: Arthroscopic tenotomy of the long head of the biceps in the treatment of rotator cuff tears: Clinical and radiographic results of 307 cases. *J Shoulder Elbow Surg* 2005;14:238-246.

24. Wolf RS, Zheng N, Weichel D: Long head biceps tenotomy versus tenodesis: A cadaveric biomechanical analysis. *Arthroscopy* 2005;21:182-185.

25. Kelly AM, Drakos MC, Fealy S, Taylor SA, O'Brien SJ: Arthroscopic release of the long head of the biceps tendon: Functional outcome and clinical results. *Am J Sports Med* 2005;33:208-213.

26. Gill TJ, McIrvin E, Mair SD, Hawkins RJ: Results of biceps tenotomy for treatment of pathology of the long head of the biceps brachii. *J Shoulder Elbow Surg* 2001;10:247-249.

27. Osbahr DC, Diamond AB, Speer KP: The cosmetic appearance of the biceps muscle after long-head tenotomy versus tenodesis. *Arthroscopy* 2002;18:483-487.

28. Boileau P, Krishnan SG, Coste JS, Walch G: Arthroscopic biceps tenodesis: A new technique using bioabsorbable interference screw fixation.

*Arthroscopy* 2002;18:1002-1012.

29. Romeo AA, Mazzocca AD, Tauro JC: Arthroscopic biceps tenodesis. *Arthroscopy* 2004;20:206-213.

30. Verma NN, Drakos M, O'Brien SJ: Arthroscopic transfer of the long head biceps to the conjoint tendon. *Arthroscopy* 2005;21:764.

31. Ozalay M, Akpinar S, Karaeminogullari O, et al: Mechanical strength of four different biceps tenodesis techniques. *Arthroscopy* 2005;21:992-998.

32. Klepps S, Hazrati Y, Flatow E: Arthroscopic biceps tenodesis. *Arthroscopy* 2002;18:1040-1045.

33. Mariani EM, Cofield RH, Askew LJ, Li GP, Chao EY: Rupture of the tendon of the long head of the biceps brachii: Surgical versus nonsurgical treatment. *Clin Orthop Relat Res* 1988; 228:233-239.

34. Richards DP, Burkhart SS, Campbell SE: Relation between narrowed coracohumeral distance and subscapularis tears. *Arthroscopy* 2005;21:1223-1228.

35. Burkhart SS, Brady PC: Arthroscopic subscapularis repair: Surgical tips and pearls A to Z. *Arthroscopy* 2006;22:1014-1027.

36. Neviaser RJ: Lesions of the biceps and tendinitis of the shoulder. *Orthop Clin North Am* 1980;11:343-348.

37. Snyder SJ, Karzel RP, Del Pizzo W, Ferkel RD, Friedman MJ: SLAP lesions of the shoulder. *Arthroscopy* 1990;6:274-279.

38. Clavert P, Bonnomet F, Kempf JF, Boutemy P, Braun M, Kahn JL: Contribution to the study of the pathogenesis of type II superior labrum anterior-posterior lesions: A cadaveric model of a fall on the outstretched hand. *J Shoulder Elbow Surg* 2004;13: 45-50.

39. Burkhart SS, Morgan CD: The peel-back mechanism: Its role in producing and extending posterior type II SLAP lesions and its effect on SLAP repair rehabilitation. *Arthroscopy* 1998; 14:637-640.

40. Maffet MW, Gartsman GM, Moseley B: Superior labrum-biceps tendon complex lesions of the shoulder. *Am J Sports Med* 1995;23:93-98.

41. Powell SE, Nord KD, Ryu RK: The diagnosis, classification, and treatment of SLAP lesions. *Oper Tech Sports Med* 2004;12:99-110.

42. Choi NH, Kim SJ: Avulsion of the superior labrum. *Arthroscopy* 2004;20: 872-874.

43. Snyder SJ, Banas MP, Karzel RP: An analysis of 140 injuries to the superior glenoid labrum. *J Shoulder Elbow Surg* 1995;4:243-248.

44. Handelberg F, Willems S, Shahabpour M, Huskin JP, Kuta J: SLAP lesions: A retrospective multicenter study. *Arthroscopy* 1998;14:856-862.

45. Kim TK, Queale WS, Cosgarea AJ, McFarland EG: Clinical features of the different types of SLAP lesions: An analysis of one hundred and thirty-nine cases. Superior labrum anterior posterior. *J Bone Joint Surg Am* 2003;85:66-71.

46. Burkhart SS, Morgan CD, Kibler WB: Shoulder injuries in overhead athletes: The "dead arm" revisited. *Clin Sports Med* 2000;19:125-158.

47. Ruotolo C, Nottage WM, Flatow EL, Gross RM, Fanton GS: Controversial topics in shoulder arthroscopy. *Arthroscopy* 2002;18(2, Suppl 1):65-75.

48. Liu SH, Henry MH, Nuccion SL: A prospective evaluation of a new physical examination in predicting glenoid labral tears. *Am J Sports Med* 1996;24:721-725.

49. Kibler WB: Specificity and sensitivity of the anterior slide test in throwing athletes with superior glenoid labral tears. *Arthroscopy* 1995;11:296-300.

50. Stetson WB, Templin K: The crank test, the O'Brien test, and routine magnetic resonance imaging scans in the diagnosis of labral tears. *Am J Sports Med* 2002;30:806-809.

51. McFarland EG, Kim TK, Savino RM: Clinical assessment of three common tests for superior labral anterior-posterior lesions. *Am J Sports Med*

2002;30:810-815.

52. Jobe CM: Superior glenoid impingement: Current concepts. *Clin Orthop Relat Res* 1996;330:98-107.

53. Kim SH, Ha KI, Ahn JH, Kim SH, Choi HJ: Biceps load test II: A clinical test for SLAP lesions of the shoulder. *Arthroscopy* 2001;17:160-164.

54. Mimori K, Muneta T, Nakagawa T, Shinomiya K: A new pain provocation test for superior labral tears of the shoulder. *Am J Sports Med* 1999;27: 137-142.

55. Westerheide KJ, Karzel RP: Ganglion cysts of the shoulder: Technique of arthroscopic decompression and fixation of associated type II superior labral anterior to posterior lesions. *Orthop Clin North Am* 2003;34:521-528.

56. Panossian VR, Mihata T, Tibone JE, Fitzpatrick MJ, McGarry MH, Lee TQ: Biomechanical analysis of isolated type II SLAP lesions and repair. *J Shoulder Elbow Surg* 2005; 14:529-534.

# Sports Injuries in Women: Sex- and Gender-Based Differences in Etiology and Prevention

Kimberly J. Templeton, MD
Sharon L. Hame, MD
*Jo A. Hannafin, MD, PhD
Letha Y. Griffin, MD, PhD
Laura L. Tosi, MD
Naomi N. Shields, MD

## Abstract

*There has been a significant increase in the participation of women in sports at all levels, especially after the enactment of the Title IX Education Amendment in 1972. This increased participation at all levels has resulted in more women sustaining sports injuries. Data on sex- and gender-based differences in all organ systems, including the musculoskeletal system, are being gathered. It is important to review some of the areas of sex- and gender-based differences in sports injuries for which there is significant research, such as osteoporosis, the female athlete triad, and anterior cruciate ligament injuries. It is also necessary to examine those areas in which more information is needed, such as injuries to the shoulder, foot, and ankle.*

**Instr Course Lect 2008;57:539-552.**

There has been a significant increase in the participation of women in sports from recreational to Olympic levels.[1] Title IX of the Education Amendment to the Civil Rights Act of 1964 was signed into law in 1972, paving the way for increased female participation in organized athletics. The number of women participating in college sports has increased from approximately 294,000 in the 1970-1971 school year to 2,520,000 in the 1998-1999 academic year. Women of all ages are participating in athletic activities in large numbers. Younger female athletes often are competing at high levels before skeletal maturity, often in multiple sports or on multiple teams (such as club, traveling, and school teams). Choosing one sport and participating throughout the year leads to overuse of specific anatomic areas and provides little cross training. This is a different situation from that of the athlete 10 to 15 years ago who often participated in multiple sports requiring different biomechanical and physical efforts. At the other end of the spectrum are geriatric athletes who compete in athletic events at the local, national, and international levels. With growth in the popularity of sports participation, the incidence of female athletic injuries has increased considerably.

There is growing evidence that female athletes are at a higher risk for certain types of injuries than male athletes.[2-7] Musculoskeletal health has been recognized as one area of medicine in which an individual's sex has a significant influence on the prevalence of disease and/or disability. Osteoporosis, osteoarthritis, spinal disorders, and fractures are known to occur more commonly in women than men. It has been argued that recognition that anterior cruciate ligament (ACL) injuries occur two to eight times more frequently in young female athletes than in male athletes

*Jo A. Hannafin, MD, PhD or the department with which she is affiliated has received research or institutional support from Lifecell.*

was the catalyst for the orthopaedic community to explore why these differences occur.

To date, there is no explanation for the numerous examples of sexual dimorphism seen in orthopaedic practice. However, the successful completion of the Human Genome Project has allowed researchers to elucidate some aspects of the genetic basis of disease and identify innate differences between men and women. Scientists now recognize that every cell in the body, not just the reproductive system, responds differently on the basis of sex. These responses result from chromosomes, not just hormones. A male cell is not the same as a female cell, and sex chromosome-linked genes can be expressed in germ lines and somatic cells.

This chapter examines how the recognition of sexual dimorphism in athletes impacts quality of care. It is essential to clarify the language of sexual dimorphism, namely sex and gender. According to the Institute of Medicine, sex is "the classification of living things, generally male or female, according to their reproductive organs and functions assigned by the chromosomal complement."[8] Gender is defined as "a person's self-perception as male or female, or how that person is responded to by social institutions on the basis of the individual's gender presentation."[8] Thus, sex determines the inner workings of an individual's growth and development, whereas gender takes into consideration the environment in which an individual grows and lives.

Sex is certainly relevant in sports medicine, but so is gender. Sex influences the individual's athletic ability as well as his or her risk of injury. Gender influences how an athlete is perceived and frequently influences

access to training, equipment, or coaching. As science and care in sports medicine advance, it is essential to differentiate between the terms sex and gender.

## The Female Athlete Triad and Stress Fractures

Yeager and associates[9] first defined the female athlete triad in 1993. The three components of the triad are eating disorders, amenorrhea, and osteoporosis.[9,10] It is important to understand that the development of the syndrome is a continuum, and each of the three components of the syndrome occur on a spectrum. In addition, the three components do not have to occur at the same time; bone changes may occur at a later date. The incidence of this disorder varies among different groups of female athletes, with the highest rates (up to 62%) occurring in those athletes who participate in sports in which appearance is judged, such as figure skating, gymnastics, and ballet, and in which a low body fat percentage is beneficial.[11,12]

### Pathogenesis

A negative energy balance in which calories expended outweigh calories consumed is an important component of the female athlete triad. Inadequate calorie intake appears to be the primary mechanism that predisposes female athletes to menstrual dysfunction and results in detrimental effects on bone.[13] The role of inadequate calorie intake in men is not as well understood. Bachrach and associates[14] reported that nearly 75% of adolescent girls with anorexia nervosa have a bone mineral density (BMD) more than two standard deviations below the normal value. Another study showed that women with anorexia nervosa are at an increased risk for stress fractures.[15] In

men with anorexia nervosa, the association with stress fractures has not been as thoroughly studied.

### Disordered Eating

Disordered eating occurs along a spectrum ranging from apparently normal eating in combination with excessive caloric expenditure to anorexia nervosa and bulimia nervosa. It can occur in both male and female athletes, and it spans all ethnic groups and socioeconomic classes. Disordered eating behaviors include binging, purging, caloric restriction, excessive exercise, and using diuretics/laxatives and diet pills. Distorted body image, unrealistic fears of weight gain, and preoccupation with food may occur. Disordered eating occurs more commonly in female athletes, particularly those who participate in aesthetic or weight-dependent sports. Males also are at risk in these types of sports, especially weight-dependent sports such as wrestling and horse racing.[16] Sundgot-Borgen and Torstveit[17] reported the prevalence of eating disorders in males in antigravitation sports (such as long jumping and pole vaulting) to be 22% compared with 42% in female athletes involved in aesthetic sports. The common factor in all of these manifestations is the presence of a negative energy balance.

### Amenorrhea

Primary amenorrhea is defined as the absence of menses (menarche has not begun) by age 16 years along with the delayed development of secondary sexual characteristics, whereas secondary amenorrhea is defined as an absence of menses for more than 3 consecutive months after menarche has begun. Amenorrhea is more prevalent in the athletic population (3% to 66%) than in the general female population (2% to 5%).[18] Any factor that may influence the hypothalamus-pituitary-ovarian axis can affect menses. Such factors include energy deficit, low leptin (a protein hormone involved in metabolism and reproductive function) during caloric restriction, and the physical and psychological stress of training and competing. In men, a decrease in bone mass has been reported in those with a history of constitutional delay of puberty.[19] The mechanism for delayed puberty is not fully understood, and data in this area are conflicting.[20]

### Osteoporosis

Osteoporosis or low BMD is the third component of the female athlete triad. Lower BMD in affected female athletes is related to the presence of eating disorders or a negative energy balance, as well as estrogen deficiency and menstrual dysfunction. Lower BMD also has been reported in male athletes and may be a risk factor for stress fractures. The mechanism of decreased BMD in male athletes is not well understood. Research concerning BMD in men is focusing on the roles of testosterone and energy deficit.

### Diagnosis

All athletes should be screened for components of the female athlete triad in their preparticipation examinations. A thorough history including nutritional status, weight changes, gynecologic disorders, exercise routine, psychiatric issues, and a record of stress fractures should be obtained. Careful attention during the physical examination for signs of the triad is imperative. These signs include low weight, bradycardia, dry hair and skin, lanugo hair, hirsutism, parotid

gland enlargement, Russell's sign, and erosion of dental enamel. Laboratory and radiologic testing also is important.

### Treatment

The treatment of patients with the female athlete triad generally should include encouraging a positive energy balance, setting weight goals, frequently consultating with health care workers, and developing a written contract with the athlete. Levels of serum osteocalcin, a measure of osteoblast activity, frequently normalize once the patient's energy balance has been reversed, even before the resumption of menses. Nutritional supplements including calcium (1,200 to 1,500 mg/day) and vitamin D (400 to 800 IU/day) also can help improve bone mass. A multidisciplinary approach including physicians, trainers, psychiatrists or psychologists, coaches, and parents can provide effective treatment. However, despite these multidisciplinary efforts, the prognosis for patients with female athlete triad is still unknown. Even with correction of energy balance, young athletes with a history of female athlete triad may never attain peak bone mass.

## Stress Fractures

Stress fractures are defined as skeletal defects that result from repeated application of stress lower than that required to fracture a bone in a single loading but greater than the bone's ability to fully recover. Microdamage occurs when bone fails to remodel adequately with the application of repetitive, subthreshold stress. More than 95% of all stress fractures occur in the lower extremity, which reflects the high repetitive loads typically experienced by a weight-bearing bone. The most common sites are the tibia, metatar-

sals, and fibula.[21,22] In female collegiate athletes, the incidence of stress fractures is highest for participants in track-and-field sports.[23] Male participants in track-and-field sports also have a high incidence of stress fractures.[23] In a recent study of 5,900 Division 1 collegiate athletes, there was no significant difference between men and women in the incidence of all fractures (0.0438 and 0.0461, respectively), but the incidence of stress fractures was nearly double in women athletes compared with men.[23]

Factors influencing the risks of stress fractures include biomechanical factors, bone geometry and morphology, muscle mass, strength, changes in training, and BMD. Particularly in the tibia, polar moments of inertia, section modulus, and anteroposterior and mediolateral widths may have some effect on the development of stress fractures. Female runners with a history of tibial stress fractures show more rapid lower extremity muscle fatigue compared with runners without previous stress fractures. Significant increases in activity often are a triggering event for many stress injuries and explain the high rate of stress fractures among military recruits during boot camp.

The patient history may include activity-related pain, worsening pain over time, and a previous stress fracture. Physical examination typically demonstrates pain with palpation, edema, and pain with percussion. Imaging studies should include radiographs of the affected area. Plain radiographs may not show callus formation and early fracture healing until 2 to 3 weeks after the onset of symptoms. Nuclear medicine scintigraphy (bone scanning) is sensitive for diagnosing early stress remodeling and fractures. Acute stress frac-

**Table 1**
**Recommended Testing for Athletes With Multiple Stress Fractures**

Thyroid-stimulating hormone

Complete blood count

Chemistry panel

Dual energy x-ray absorptiometry

**Additional Testing If the Female Athlete Triad Is Suspected**

Follicle-stimulating hormone

Luteinizing hormone

Estradiol

Urine pregnancy

Testosterone

Dexamethasone suppression testing

tures show increased uptake in all three phases of a technetium Tc 99m diphosphonate bone scan.[24] When initial radiographs are negative, MRI often is the next imaging step. MRI is sensitive at detecting endosteal marrow edema, one of the earliest signs of stress remodeling.[25] Arendt and associates[26] proposed a grading system that helps predict time to return to play. They reported athletes with grade I fractures take 3.3 weeks to return to play, whereas those with grades II, III, or IV fractures take 5.5, 11.4, and 14.3 weeks, respectively, to return to play.

All athletes with multiple stress fractures should undergo some routine laboratory testing, including assessment of thyroid-stimulating hormone level, complete blood count, and routine chemistry panel. A dual-energy x-ray absorptiometry scan to evaluate BMD is also recommended. Athletes suspected of having female athlete triad should undergo additional laboratory testing for levels of follicle-stimulating hormone, luteinizing hormone, estradiol, urine pregnancy testing (if amenorrheic), and dexamethasone suppression testing (Table 1).

The management of athletes with stress fractures requires an individu-

alized postinjury course of treatment that may include bracing, surgical or nonsurgical care, bone stimulation, nutritional changes, and medication. Careful evaluation of the athlete for other components of the female athlete triad is important.

## The Role of Sex in Shoulder Injury

Shoulder injuries in female athletes are common and frequently are attributed to a combination of increased joint laxity, relatively weaker upper body strength, and shorter bone length compared with male athletes.[27] However, published data that evaluate the role of sex in the incidence, etiology, prevention, and treatment of female shoulder injuries are limited.

Shoulder instability and impingement syndrome are common conditions seen in the athlete's shoulder; however, the frequency of shoulder instability (both traumatic and atraumatic) and impingement syndrome (primary and secondary) in female athletes is unknown. Numerous studies report the prevalence of male and female injuries, but few evaluate sex-specific variables affecting the type or incidence of injury.

The National Collegiate Athletic Association (NCAA) injury surveillance system reports sport-specific data categorized by the injured body part and the injury mechanism.[28] Shoulder injuries are common injuries in women's softball, totaling 10% to 20% of softball injuries. The NCAA injury surveillance system currently includes data on 8 of 16 women's collegiate sports (soccer, volleyball, field hockey, basketball, gymnastics, ice hockey, lacrosse, and softball), with new datasets being collected for swimming, tennis, golf, and rowing.

Military studies have evaluated sex as a variable affecting injury rates. A study of Army parachutists from 1985 to 1994 found that rates of injury did not differ significantly by sex; however, the sites of injury differed, with upper extremity injuries reported in 43% of injured men compared with 27% of the injured women.[29] Frequent shoulder dislocations in men were also reported in an Israeli military study.[30] There was a male predominance of shoulder injuries (30% of total injuries) compared with 5% of total injuries in women. The authors postulated that the 6:1 ratio may reflect the role of trauma in recurrent shoulder dislocation.

Evidence to correlate sex with athletic shoulder injury is inconclusive. Kocher and associates[31] reported that 11% of total injuries in Alpine skiers were shoulder injuries (accounting for 39% of all upper extremity injuries), with a male-to-female ratio of 3:1. Aargard and Jorgensen,[32] in a study of elite Danish volleyball players, found overuse shoulder injuries in females more common than in males, whereas the incidences of overall shoulder injuries were similar. In a study of an NCAA Division III college sports program from 1980 to 1995, Sallis and associates[33] reported more frequent shoulder injuries (52.5 per 100 participant-years) in women than in men (47.7 per 1,000 participant-years). A significant increase in injury rates was seen in female swimmers and water polo players. Studies have shown that shoulder injuries are common in both male and female elite swimmers;[33] however, the published data do not explore the role of sex as an independent variable in the etiology of the injury or response to treatment. These studies concern the occurrence of injuries in competitive athletes; there is even less information available concerning the incidence of shoulder injury in the larger population of women who are recreational athletes.

### Multidirectional Instability

Multidirectional instability (MDI) is believed to be more common in women than in men and it may be related to increased ligamentous laxity in women. Women demonstrate more anterior glenohumeral joint laxity, less anterior joint stiffness, and more joint hypermobility than do men.[34] McFarland and associates[35] reported that asymptomatic high school and collegiate female athletes showed an increase in posterior and inferior laxity compared with male athletes: more female shoulders (65%) could be subluxated posteriorly than could male shoulders (51%). However, insufficient data are available to confirm that the shoulders of female athletes exhibit more laxity than the shoulders of male athletes. Female athletes also may be more prone to overuse and repetitive microtrauma of the shoulder, with an increased risk of converting global laxity to symptomatic instability.

Overhead throwing athletes tend to have greater joint laxity on average than do nonthrowing athletes.[36,37] These data suggest that female athletes participating in sports such as swimming, water polo, softball, volleyball, and tennis may have greater joint laxity when compared with their male counterparts. There also is evidence that proprioception is reduced in overhead throwing athletes or those with recurrent anterior dislocation. Dover and associates[38] reported a significant decrease in external joint position sense in female softball players when compared with nonthrowing female athletes (soccer and track), suggesting that joint position sense is reduced in female overhead athletes.

### Nonsurgical and Surgical Treatment of Shoulder Instability

Nonsurgical management of shoulder instability has been evaluated in multiple studies, but the role of sex in treatment outcomes has not been addressed. Buss and associates[39] evaluated the effectiveness of nonsurgical treatment for in-season athletes with symptomatic instability. Twenty-four men and six women (age 14 to 20 years) were treated with physical therapy in which range of motion and rotator cuff strengthening exercises were emphasized. Eighty-seven percent of the athletes successfully returned to competition within the season, without any period of immobilization. In this study, sex was not evaluated as an independent variable.

Literature on the outcome of surgical management of shoulder instability also does not consistently stratify results by sex. Neer and Foster[40] reported the results of treating patients with MDI with an anterior capsular shift with 1 of 36 patients experiencing recurrent subluxation. The study included equal numbers of male and female patients. Although sex was not evaluated as a factor in treatment response, the study suggests that it was not a significant variable. Cooper and Brems[41] evaluated 38 patients (22 females and 16 males) treated with an anteroinferior capsular shift. Improvement occurred in 86% of the patients, despite the fact that generalized ligamentous laxity was found in 76% of the patients. Steinbeck and Jerosch[42] evaluated the outcomes of a modified capsular shift as a treatment of MDI in 19 patients

(17 females and 2 males). The authors reported no recurrent dislocations in 17 of the 19 patients. Recent results of thermal capsular shrinkage have been reported; however, sex has not been examined as a variable related to outcome. Hayashida and associates[43] reported the results of arthroscopic transglenoid suture repair for traumatic anterior shoulder instability in 82 patients (63 males and 19 females). The authors reported 67% excellent, 17% good, and 16% poor results. Sex was not a statistically significant parameter related to outcome.

In most of the literature discussing surgical treatment of MDI, including results for open capsular shifts, arthroscopic stabilization, and thermal capsulorrhaphy, the number of female patients is significantly lower than the number of male patients. Hiemstra and Kirkley[44] reviewed the available literature examining the surgical treatment of anterior instability and MDI. Of the 43 studies reporting results for surgical treatment of anterior instability, women accounted for 22.3% of all patients. Hiemstra and Kirkley[44] noted that males may be more likely to participate in overhead throwing sports or high-risk activities, thus predisposing them to shoulder injury and subsequent treatment.

In 14 studies reporting surgical treatment of MDI, 35.7% of patients were female. With the increasing number of women participating in sports, including overhead throwing activities, it is unclear why there is not an equal percentage of female patients in these studies. Is there a selection bias in surgical treatment? Do females respond better to non-surgical treatment than males? Are women undertreated for MDI and thus underreported? These questions remain to be answered.

## Impingement Syndrome

There are few data available regarding the impact of sex on impingement syndrome among athletes. Gill and associates[45] reviewed the results of 523 patients who had arthroscopic or open shoulder surgery and reported that a larger proportion of male patients (76.4%, $P = 0.019$) had full-thickness rotator cuff tears than did female patients. There was an independent association between rotator cuff pathology and sex in this study, but this does not necessarily imply causation.

Morrison and associates[46] examined the outcomes of nonsurgical treatment of impingement syndrome in 616 patients. The patients were of mixed age, activity level, and sex and were treated with a uniform rehabilitation protocol. Sex did not affect outcome, with 262 of 386 men (68%) and 152 of 230 women (66%) achieving satisfactory results. This appears to be the only published study that evaluates the role of sex in response to nonsurgical treatment of impingement syndrome. Mechanism of injury or response to nonsurgical treatment may vary by sex, but data are inconclusive at this time. In both of these studies, patients were included from the general population and were not athletes. Sperling and associates[47] examined the long-term success of full-thickness rotator cuff repair in young patients (50 years of age or younger). Sex did not appear to be a significant variable affecting outcome in this small study.

## Noncontact ACL Injuries

Noncontact ACL injuries also exhibit sex differences in musculoskeletal injury expression. The ACL is a small ligament, but it has been the focus of much scientific investigation and is a premier topic at most sports medical meetings and in the sports medicine literature. It was reported that ACL reconstruction ranked sixth among the most common surgical procedures performed by all sports medicine fellows sitting for part II of the Orthopaedic Boards examination and was the third most common procedure among those surgeons who sat for the Boards and stated they were generalists (W Garret, MD, unpublished data, 2004).

## Epidemiology

The incidence of noncontact ACL injury in sports involving pivoting or cutting appears to be two to eight times greater in women than in men.[7,48] Epidemiologic studies estimate that 1 of every 100 high school female athletes will sustain an ACL injury during her 4-year playing career; in college athletes the number is approximately 1 in 10 during their playing careers.[49] The incidence of injury in the general population is reported to be 1 in 3,000, with the preponderance of these injuries occurring in young people 15 to 25 years of age.[50] This group of young athletes sustains approximately one half of the ACL injuries that occur yearly in the United States.[50]

## Impact of ACL Injury

With an estimated 100,000 to 150,000 ACL reconstructions performed annually in the United States, at an estimated cost of $10,000 to $17,000 per reconstruction, the minimal total yearly cost for surgical treatment of this injury is approximately $1 billion.[51-53] Moreover, this number does not include the cost of diagnosis, rehabilitation for those who elect no surgical intervention, or the significant estimated cost for treating the degenerative arthritis that appears to be a natural consequence of this injury, even in those successfully treated with reconstruction.

In the 1990s there was a concern that women would have poorer outcomes than men following reconstruction procedures; however, this concern has proven to be unfounded. The functional outcome and laxity measures in men and women following reconstruction with patellar tendon or hamstring autografts or patellar tendon or Achilles tendon allografts appear to be equivalent.[54-58] Posttraumatic, degenerative arthritis following ACL injury may develop in both men and women. It is unclear whether this arthritis is a consequence of injury to the articular cartilage at the time of the initial incident or results from the inadequacies of current reconstructive techniques to effectively restore normal joint kinematics. Because noncontact ACL injuries are common in young people, and surgical stabilization of the knee does not appear to effectively reduce the incidence of posttraumatic arthritis, decreasing the incidence of injury through effective prevention strategies appears prudent.

## Injury Mechanism and Risk Factors for Injury

Understanding the mechanism of the injury or at least the risk factors leading to injury is a logical initial step in developing an injury prevention program. Although risk factors and the mechanism of injury have not been well defined for noncontact ACL injuries, research initiatives over the previous 10 years have brought investigators closer to the answers. Risk factors associated with injury can be divided into intrinsic factors, those coming from within the body, and extrinsic factors, those coming from outside the body. Risk factors also can be categorized as environmental, anatomic, hormonal, neuromuscular, and familial.

### Environmental Risk Factors

Environmental risk factors include weather conditions, type of playing surface, type of footwear, the interaction of footwear with the type of playing surface, and the use of protective equipment or braces. Because braces effectively decreased the injury risk for ankle injuries, it was hoped that prophylactic bracing either with off-the-shelf or custom-fit braces would decrease the risk of ACL injury. Early research did not support this hypothesis. Functional knee braces can reduce anteroposterior laxity of the ACL-deficient knee to within the limits of the normal knee during non–weight-bearing or weight-bearing activities. However, in the ACL-deficient knee, braces cannot reduce the abnormal anterior displacement of the tibia relative to the femur that is produced as the knee transitions from non–weight-bearing to weight-bearing conditions.[59,60] In a recent prospective randomized study of 100 military cadets who sustained an ACL tear and underwent reconstruction, functional bracing had no marked effect on the incidence of reinjury of the ACL graft.[61] However, there were only five reinjuries (two in the braced and three in the nonbraced knees of athletes).

In contrast to these findings, a prospective 2003 study of 180 ACL-deficient knees in skiers identified from a screening of 9,410 professional skiers reported that a significantly higher proportion of injuries occurred in skiers without knee braces compared with those with braces ($P = 0.005$).[62] One group of investigators reported that a new brace hinge design featuring increasing resistance over a range of

motion before the final stop in motion resulted in a decrease in the flexion angle of the knee on landing.[63] Whether this decreased flexion angle will translate into a positive effect by decreasing noncontact ACL injuries has not been evaluated in clinical trials.

With regard to shoe-surface interaction, a retrospective analysis of 53 ACL injuries in Norwegian team handball players found that women had an increased risk of ACL injury in games played on artificial floors relative to natural wood floors, whereas men did not.[64] A higher coefficient of friction was found on the artificial floors compared with natural wood floors, suggesting that shoe-surface traction on these floors is increased.[65] Why women are more affected than men by this factor is not understood.

In another study of Australian football players, an increased risk for noncontact ACL injury during periods of high evaporation and low rainfall was reported.[66] Presumably, the hard ground condition increased shoe-surface traction and the risk of injury. Injury rates in this study were not reported by sex. Decreasing shoe-surface traction by watering the ground, playing on natural grass, and wearing shoes with shorter cleats appeared to decrease injuries. Because shoe-surface conditions may be an easily modifiable risk factor, future research on this subject should be encouraged.

### Anatomic Risk Factors

Because women are at a greater risk for developing ACL injury than men and because the musculoskeletal anatomy of males and females is different, researchers have examined these differences as possible risk factors for noncontact ACL injury. The Q angle of the knee, dynamic and

static knee valgus, foot pronation, body mass index, and geometry of the ACL and the notch in which it is housed have been studied for their potential as risk factors for noncontact injury. Most studies comparing Q angles in adult women with those of adult men have reported that women have greater Q angle than men.[68] A study of 45 basketball athletes found that the average Q angle of the athletes sustaining an ACL injury was significantly larger than Q angles of players who were not injured (14° versus 10°).[67]

Studies on the association of foot pronation with knee injury have not consistently demonstrated a correlation, even though research suggests that marked pronation could increase the risks for injury by increasing internal tibial rotation.[68]

A prospective study of cadets at a US military academy found that women with a higher than average body mass index had an increased injury risk, a finding consistent with a prior study by Brown and associates.[69] However, other studies have not verified this finding.

One study involving notch sizes as related to noncontact ACL injury found that notch width in bilateral and unilateral ACL-injured knees was smaller than the notch width of normal control subjects, implying an association between notch width and injury.[70] However, there is variability in the literature concerning this association, with several studies showing no correlation of notch size and injury risk. A study by Anderson and associates[71] that used MRI to measure the size of the ACL found that the ACL in young women is smaller than that in young men even when normalized for body weight. Shelbourne and associates[72] demonstrated a positive correlation between small ACLs and injury risk.

However, other studies do not consistently demonstrate an association between ACL size and injury risk.[73] Multiple measurements and comparisons of notch sizes and the size of the ACL within the notch adds to the confusion when trying to interpret studies on these anatomic factors. A study reported at the 29th Annual Meeting of the American Society of Biomechanics found that compared with male ACLs, the female ACL has a lower mechanical quality (8.3% lower strain at failure and a 22.49% lower module of elasticity).[74] This finding is interesting, but further investigation for verification and potential clinical impact is warranted.

Anatomic risk factors are an intriguing area of study and reflect sex differences. To date, conflicting data exist regarding the role of Q angle, dynamic and static knee valgus, foot pronation, body mass index, the width of the femoral notch, and the geometry and strength of the ACL as injury risk factors in noncontact ACL injuries. Further research is justified.

### Hormonal Risk Factors

Sex hormones play a role in collagen synthesis and degradation. However, whether certain variations in sex hormones are related to the risk of noncontact ACL injury is not clear. A connection between sex hormones and injury was theorized because the distribution of ACL injuries in females is not random throughout the month as would be suspected if monthly hormonal variations did not influence injury occurrences. Instead these injuries are clustered typically in the perimenstrual and preovulatory stage.

Estrogen receptors have been found on the ACL in animal studies. However, the results of in vitro and in vivo animal studies on the impact of estrogen on the mechanical properties of the ACL have not been consistent. Two separate studies in animals have shown no material or mechanical differences in ACLs from animals that underwent ovariectomy and those that underwent sham surgical procedures, implying that the presence of estrogen in these animals did not alter the material properties of the ACL.[75,76] In sheep no difference in collagen fibroblast synthesis relative to a physiologic range of estradiol levels was found.[77]

The relevance of these studies to humans is uncertain because only humans and the great apes have menstrual cycles; all other animals have estrous cycles. Studies on human ACL tissue are suggestive but not confirmatory of an association of sex hormones and noncontact ACL injury. Some studies have shown an association between the phase of the menstrual cycle or sex hormone levels and knee laxity, but the association between knee laxity and ACL injury is not well established.

### Neuromuscular Risk Factors

Research on neuromuscular factors as risk factors for ACL injury is intertwined with research into the mechanisms of injury and centers around investigations into altered movement patterns, altered neuromuscular activation patterns, and inadequate muscle stiffness as related to injury occurrences.

Eighty percent to 85% of all noncontact ACL injuries sustained in sports that involve pivoting and jumping have been reported to occur during landing a jump, decelerating, or pivoting or cutting to change directions. ACL injuries are believed to be associated with abnormal loading of the knee and occur when unsuccessful postural adjustments result in abnormal dynamic loading across the knee. Hewett and associates[52] theorized that females lack a neuromuscular spurt to match their growth spurt and suggested that the rapid increase in size and weight at puberty is not accompanied by a proportional increase in neuromuscular power and control; this may be a predisposing factor in ACL noncontact injuries. Analyses of videotapes taken at the time of ACL injury show a relatively extended hip and knee, hip internal rotation, tibial external rotation, apparent knee valgus, and foot pronation. In landings associated with injury, the athlete typically lands flat-footed rather than on the toes.

Research on altered movement patterns in jump landings and cutting and pivoting in females and males has shown that females have less knee and hip flexion, increased knee valgus, increased internal rotation of the hip, increased external rotation of the tibia, and less knee stiffness during these activities.[68] Females also display high quadriceps activity relative to hamstring activity (a quadriceps dominant contraction). Aggressive quadriceps loading of the knee, more a characteristic of women than men, can result in significant anterior translation of the tibia on the femur.[78] Fatigue appears to decrease neuromuscular control in both males and females and also may be a risk factor.

### Familial Risk Factors

Two studies have investigated the occurrence of noncontact ACL injuries in families. In a retrospective review of 31 patients who sustained bilateral ACL injuries, Harner and associates[79] found a significant difference ($P < 0.01$) in the incidence of ACL injuries in immediate family members when compared with control patients matched by age, height, weight, sex, and activity level. In a study of 191 patients with verified ACL tears, Flynn and associates[80] found that patients with an ACL tear are twice as likely to have a relative with an ACL tear than control subjects who had not sustained an ACL injury.

### Prevention Programs

To decrease the incidence of ACL injury, which occurs all too frequently in young people and results in significant sequelae, multiple prevention programs have been developed. However, few programs have been organized as randomized controlled trials. Most studies have evaluated injury prevention in women only, and many have had small cohorts. Although most studies to date have been based on altering neuromuscular risk factors, few of these studies have actually tested patients who have participated in a prevention program to ascertain whether the program alters the neuromuscular risk factors and, if so, whether these alterations are temporary or long lasting.[81]

Questions still remain regarding the appropriate time to initiate a prevention program relative to the playing season and on the duration needed to obtain positive benefits. In most studies, compliance and contamination are issues that must be considered when assessing results.

Several prevention programs involve small group instruction sessions before the season begins, whereas others are intended to be done on the field or court before games and practices. Effective prevention programs include one or several of the following components: strengthening and stretching exercises; aerobic conditioning; bal-ance, agility, or proprioception drills; plyometric activities with attention to proper landing techniques; and awareness of injury mechanisms.[82]

### Foot and Ankle Injuries

Foot and ankle injuries, disease, and dysfunction are common in women. However, there is limited literature on these conditions in the female athlete. Women have some unique anatomic characteristics that affect the biomechanics of the lower extremity. Women have wider hips, increased genu valgum leading to increased foot pronation, increased ligamentous laxity (which is accentuated with the hormonal and weight changes associated with child bearing), and a different center of gravity than men. However, muscle strength at the foot and ankle in weight-bearing conditions does not differ significantly between the sexes, when normalized by body size (product of weight and height).[83] Women tend to have tighter Achilles tendons, which may lead to forefoot and midfoot overload. Women have been shown to land differently from jumps, especially with their hips and knees extended and their feet flat. The foot and ankle function both as a shock absorber and as a lever to propel the athlete forward or upward. Many athletes who present with more proximal lower extremity (such as hip and/or knee) injuries may have an underlying biomechanical foot and ankle disorder that needs correction.

One of the biggest challenges for the female athlete is finding appropriately sized and supportive shoes. Appropriate shoe fit not only affects comfort but also may play a role in injury prevention.[84] However, most studies in this area do not address the role of shoe wear in athletic injuries.[85] In the past, shoe manufacturers have simply downsized a male lathe to make shoes for women. However, women's feet have different proportions than those of men. Wunderlich and Cavanagh[84] found that when foot length and width were normalized to stature, men had longer and wider feet than women. Another premise has been that as feet get larger, the heel gets wider; this is not true in women. Women also have a higher arch, shallower hallux, shorter ankle length, and a smaller instep circumference.[85] The decline in availability of combination lathed shoes (narrow heel, wider forefoot) has contributed to shoe fitting issues. Recently, some manufacturers have begun to produce women's shoes using a woman's lathe. There also has been a trend to remove midfoot support from many athletic shoes, which has manifested itself in increased heel and midfoot disorders. Some sports-specific shoes such as cleats for soccer, softball, or track do not provide adequate (if any) support and often lack space for an orthosis.

Common foot and ankle disorders in female athletes include fractures, dislocations, tendon pathology (posterior tibial, anterior tibial, and flexor hallux longus, with Achilles and peroneal being the most common), ligamentous instability (primarily ankle, metatarsotarsal, and metatarsophalangeal), heel pain (plantar fasciitis, heel pad atrophy, tarsal tunnel syndrome), nail pathology, forefoot disorders (metatarsalgia, metatarsophalangeal instability, hallux rigidus, hallux valgus, bunions, and hammer toes), and disorders related to underlying foot shape (planovalgus, cavovarus).

Fractures can be caused by a single traumatic event. Stress fractures occur as a result of multiple factors including training errors, inappropriate shoe wear, training surface changes, osteoporosis, foot type, and Achilles tendon contracture. All women with stress fractures should be evaluated for underlying conditions, such as the female athlete triad or other metabolic or endocrine abnormalities. An increased incidence of stress fractures occurs in impact athletes and athletes participating at an increased level of competition or training. Stress fractures commonly occur within 2 to 6 weeks of the onset of training or the competitive season. Coaches contribute to the risk of stress fractures with early double-training impact sessions or punitive training sessions in which athletes must participate in two workouts for each workout missed. This policy makes it difficult for athletes with injuries such as a stress fracture to return to play. Shoes provided by the school may not be appropriate for an individual's foot shape or type and may contribute to stress fractures if adequate support is not provided.

Common foot and ankle stress fractures seen in female athletes include distal fibular and tibial stress fractures; calcaneal stress fractures, which must be differentiated from plantar fasciitis; navicular stress fractures; second and third metatarsal fractures; base of the fifth metatarsal fractures; and sesamoid fractures. Elite female runners land primarily striking the midfoot, which may increase the risk of stress fractures in this area.[86] A careful patient history documenting changes in training intensity or duration within the previous weeks, shoe wear changes, training surface changes (for example, from treadmill to street running), nutritional status, menstrual cycle irregularities, and previous injuries should be obtained. Second and third metatarsal fractures often occur in patients with a tight Achilles or gastrocnemius complex, first metatarsotarsal hypermobility, hallux valgus or bunion deformity, and longer second or third metatarsals relative to the first. Wearing shoes with flexible soles can contribute to second and third metatarsal overload. A retrospective review of foot and ankle injuries in elite female gymnasts showed that these injuries can end an athlete's career.[87]

The shape of feet can be categorized as neutral, cavovarus, and planovalgus. The athlete with a neutral foot has many shoe choices and experiences less foot pathology. The cavovarus foot is more rigid with decreased shock absorption and often is associated with increased ankle pathology (ankle sprains, ankle instability, peroneal tendinitis, and peroneal tendon tears) and increased forefoot overload pathology (sesamoiditis, sesamoid fractures, metatarsal injuries, and toe deformities). The subtle cavovarus foot with a varus heel without the claw toes and typical high arch may be mistaken for a pronating or flatfoot as the forefoot compensates for the varus heel. These athletes have many of the same conditions as those with a typical cavovarus foot. A unilateral cavovarus foot, especially if progressive, must be evaluated for an underlying neurologic disorder. The planovalgus or pes planus foot is much more hypermobile and often is associated with more overuse-type injuries such as posterior tibial tendinitis, "shin splints," medial knee pain, flexor hallux longus tendinitis, Achilles tendinitis, hallux valgus, and bunion deformities. Shoe wear may be problematic for both groups. Orthotics to return the foot to a neutral position by controlling heel varus or valgus and accommodating the forefoot supination or pronation may be helpful in decreasing chronic injuries.

Posterior ankle pain is common in equinus athletes such as dancers, gymnasts, swimmers, and soccer players. Posteromedial ankle pain may represent flexor hallucis longus tendon pathology. Posterolateral pain often occurs with a symptomatic os trigonum. Posterior heel pain is associated with Achilles tendinosus or tendinitis and may be nodular or insertional. Retrocalcaneal bursitis or a symptomatic Haglund deformity also may be present and can create additional difficulties with shoe wear.

The differential diagnosis for plantar heel pain includes plantar fasciitis, calcaneal pad atrophy, tarsal tunnel, lateral calcaneal (Baxter) nerve entrapment, and stress fracture. A good history and physical examination will help to differentiate these disorders.

Lateral ankle pain may be secondary to lateral ankle or subtalar instability, peroneal tendon pathology, lateral impingement, or talar coalition. Fractures at the base of the fifth metatarsal also may occur with inversion injuries or in chronic stress fracture situations. Proprioceptive deficits often occur in patients with recurrent ankle sprains, many of whom have an underlying cavus foot.

Forefoot disorders include hallux valgus or bunion deformities, hammer toes, claw toes, hallux rigidus, sesamoiditis or stress fractures, second or third metatarsophalangeal joint instability and synovitis, neuromas, corns, calluses, and toenail pathologies. Many of these disorders can be treated with appropriately fitting shoes and the use of orthotics. A good Achilles tendon stretching program also will help offload the forefoot, reducing forefoot pressures.

Most foot and ankle disorders are not specific to athletes but occur more commonly in active women than inactive women. To return athletes to participation in their sport, it is important to obtain a good history, including training regimen, training changes, shoe wear used, surface trained on, previous injury, and previous treatment and response. It is also necessary to perform a careful physical examination that looks at the lower extremity biomechanics and the athlete's foot type; evaluate the athlete's training and competition shoe wear and their daily shoe wear and orthotics; learn as much as possible about their sport and the stresses placed on the lower extremity; and work with each athlete to maximize cross training during healing of the injury.

## Summary

Most research evaluating sports-related injuries has focused on differences among sports rather than between the sexes. Although some conditions, such as stress fractures and noncontact ACL injuries, are more prevalent in female athletes, sex as a contributing factor to other conditions, such as shoulder or foot and ankle injuries, is not as well understood. Sex has routinely been ignored in the research of incidence and response to treatment of these injuries.

Even for those conditions that occur more often in females, the etiology of sex-based differences has not been clearly defined. Sex-based differences in shoe-surface interactions, various anatomic parameters, hormonal levels, and movement and muscle activation patterns may influence the noted differences in injury

rates for noncontact ACL injuries. Foot and ankle injuries are more common in women, but those seen in female athletes are not isolated to that population. Enhanced knowledge of the impact of sex on these sports-related injuries can improve injury prevention and treatment for all patients. As the gap in participation rates between male and female athletes narrows, sex is an increasingly important variable that warrants careful investigation and remains a wide-open field of research. These injuries may serve as an appropriate showcase for studying sex-based differences in musculoskeletal health, improving the health and function of all patients.

## References

1. Olympic Movement Website. International Olympic Committee: Promotion of Women in Sport: New Record Participation of Women at the Olympic Games. August 19, 2004. Available at: http://www.olympic.org/uk/organisation/missions/women/full_story_uk.asp?id=1017. Accessed January 26, 2006.

2. Arendt E, Dick R: Knee injury patterns among men and women in collegiate basketball and soccer: NCAA data and review of literature. *Am J Sports Med* 1995;23:694-701.

3. Zelisko JA, Noble HB, Porter M: A comparison of men's and women's professional basketball injuries. *Am J Sports Med* 1982;10:297-299.

4. Hutchinson MR, Ireland ML: Knee injuries in female athletes. *Sports Med* 1995;19:288-302.

5. Hewett TE, Myer GD, Ford KR: Anterior cruciate ligament injuries in female athletes: Part 1. Mechanisms and risk factors. *Am J Sports Med* 2006;34:299-311.

6. Engström B, Johansson C, Törnkvist H: Soccer injuries among elite female

players. *Am J Sports Med* 1991;19:372-375.

7. Agel J, Arendt EA, Bershadsky B: Anterior cruciate ligament injury in National Collegiate Athletic Association basketball and soccer: A 13-year review. *Am J Sports Med* 2005;33:524-531.

8. Wizemann TM, Pardue ML (eds): *Institute of Medicine (US) Committee on Understanding the Biology of Sex and Gender Differences: Exploring the Biological Contributions to Human Health: Does Sex Matter?* Washington, DC, National Academy Press, 2001.

9. Yeager KK, Agostini R, Nattiv A, Drinkwater B: The female athlete triad: Disordered eating, amenorrhea, osteoporosis. *Med Sci Sports Exerc* 1993;25:775-777.

10. Otis CL, Drinkwater B, Johnson M, Loucks A, Wilmore J: American College of Sports Medicine position stand: The female athlete triad. *Med Sci Sports Exerc* 1997;29:1669-1671.

11. Rosen LW, Hough DO: Pathogenic weight-control behaviors of female college gymnasts. *Phys Sportsmed* 1988;19:141.

12. Nattiv A, Agostini R, Drinkwater B, et al: The female athlete triad: The inter-relatedness of disordered eating, amenorrhea, and osteoporosis. *Clin Sports Med* 1994;13:405-418.

13. Pepper M, Akuthota V, McCarty EC: The pathophysiology of stress fractures. *Clin Sports Med* 2006;25:1-16.

14. Bachrach LK, Guido D, Katzman K, et al: Decreased bone density in adolescent girls with anorexia nervosa. *Pediatrics* 1990;86:440-447.

15. Nattiv A, Puffer JC, Green GA: Lifestyles and health risks of collegiate athletes: A multicenter study. *Clin J Sport Med* 1997;7:262-272.

16. Baum A: Eating disorders in the male athlete. *Sports Med* 2006;36:1-6.

17. Sundgot-Borgen J, Torstveit MK: Prevalence of eating disorders in elite athletes is higher than the general population. *Clin J Sport Med* 2004;14:25-32.

18. Otis CL: Exercise-associated amenorrhea. *Clin Sports Med* 1992;11: 351-362.

19. Finkelstein JS, Neer RM, Biller BMK, et al: Osteopenia in men with a history of delayed puberty. *N Engl J Med* 1992;326:600-604.

20. Bertelloni S, Baroncelli GI, Ferdeghini M, Perri G, Saggese G: Normal volumetric bone mineral density and bone turnover in young men with histories of constitutional delay of puberty. *J Clin Endocrinol Metab* 1998;83: 4280-4283.

21. Bennell KL, Malcolm SA, Thomas SA, et al: The incidence and distribution of stress fractures in competitive track and field athletes. *Am J Sports Med* 1996;24:211-217.

22. Bruckner PD, Bradshaw C, Khan KM, et al: Stress fractures: A review of 180 cases. *Clin Sports Med* 1996;6: 85-89.

23. Hame SL, LaFemina JM, McAllister DR, Schaadt GW, Dorey FJ: Fractures in the collegiate athlete. *Am J Sports Med* 2004;32:446-451.

24. Prather JL, Nusynowitz ML, Snowdy HA, Hughes AD, McCartney WH, Bagg RJ: Scintigraphic findings in stress fractures. *J Bone Joint Surg Am* 1977;59:869-874.

25. Kiuru MJ, Niva M, Reponen A, et al: Bone stress injuries in asymptomatic elite recruits: A clinical and magnetic resonance imaging study. *Am J Sports Med* 2005;33:272-276.

26. Arendt E, Agel J, Heikes C, Griffiths H: Stress injuries to bone in college athletes: A retrospective review of experience at a single institution. *Am J Sports Med* 2003;31:959-968.

27. Holschen JC: The female athlete. *South Med J* 2004;97:852-858.

28. National Collegiate Athletic Association Website. Injury Surveillance System: Sport-specific injury data 2003-2004, Women's softball, Injury summary 1986-2003. Available at: http://www1.ncaa.org/membership/ed_outreach/health-safety/iss/Injury_Reports_2004/Softball_Summary_2004.pdf. Accessed January 26, 2006.

29. Amoroso PJ, Bell NS, Jones BH: Injury among female and male army parachutists. *Aviat Space Environ Med* 1997;68:1006-1011.

30. Milgrom C, Mann G, Finestone A: A prevalence study of recurrent shoulder dislocations in young adults. *J Shoulder Elbow Surg* 1998;7:621-624.

31. Kocher MS, Dupre MM, Feagin JA Jr: Shoulder injuries from alpine skiing and snowboarding: Aetiology, treatment and prevention. *Sports Med* 1998;25:201-211.

32. Aagaard H, Jorgensen U: Injuries in elite volleyball. *Scand J Med Sci Sports* 1996;6:228-232.

33. Sallis RE, Jones K, Sunshine S, Smith G, Simon L: Comparing sports injuries in men and women. *Int J Sports Med* 2001;22:420-423.

34. Borsa PA, Sauers EL, Herling DE: Patterns of glenohumeral joint laxity and stiffness in healthy men and women. *Med Sci Sports Exerc* 2000;32: 1685-1690.

35. McFarland EG, Campbell G, McDowell J: Posterior shoulder laxity in asymptomatic athletes. *Am J Sports Med* 1996;24:468-471.

36. Bigliani LU, Codd TP, Connor PM, Levine WN, Littlefield MA, Hershon SJ: Shoulder motion and laxity in the professional baseball player. *Am J Sports Med* 1997;25:609-613.

37. Kvitne RS, Jobe FW, Jobe CM: Shoulder instability in the overhand or throwing athlete. *Clin Sports Med* 1995;14:917-935.

38. Dover GC, Kaminski TW, Meister K, Powers ME, Horodyski M: Assessment of shoulder proprioception in the female softball athlete. *Am J Sports Med* 2003;31:431-437.

39. Buss DD, Lynch GP, Meyer CP, Huber SM, Freehill MQ: Nonoperative management for in-season athletes with anterior shoulder instability. *Am J Sports Med* 2004;32:1430-1433.

40. Neer CS, Foster CR: Inferior capsular shift for involuntary inferior and multidirectional instability of the shoulder. *J Bone Joint Surg Am* 1980; 62:897-908.

41. Cooper RA, Brems JJ: The inferior capsular-shift procedure for multidirectional instability of the shoulder. *J Bone Joint Surg Am* 1992;74: 1516-1521.

42. Steinbeck J, Jerosch J: Surgery for atraumatic anterior-inferior shoulder instability: A modified capsular shift evaluated in 20 patients followed for 3 years. *Acta Orthop Scand* 1997;68: 447-450.

43. Hayashida K, Yoneda M, Nakagawa S, Okamura K, Fukushima S: Arthroscopic Bankart suture repair for traumatic anterior shoulder instability: Analysis of the causes of a recurrence. *Arthroscopy* 1998;14:295-301.

44. Hiemstra LA, Kirkley A: Shoulder instability in female athletes. *Sports Med Arthrosc Rev* 2002;10:50-57.

45. Gill TJ, McIrvin E, Kocher MS, Homa K, Mair SD, Hawkins RJ: The relative importance of acromial morphology and age with respect to rotator cuff pathology. *J Shoulder Elbow Surg* 2002;11:327-330.

46. Morrison DS, Frogameni AD, Woolworth P: Non-operative treatment of subacromial impingement syndrome. *J Bone Joint Surg Am* 1997;79:732-737.

47. Sperling JW, Cofield RH, Schleck C: Rotator cuff repair in patients fifty years of age and younger. *J Bone Joint Surg Am* 2004;86:2212-2215.

48. Arendt E, Dick R: Knee injury patterns among men and women in collegiate basketball and soccer. *Am J Sports Med* 1995;23:694-701.

49. Huston LJ, Vibert B, Ashton-Miller JA, et al: Gender differences in knee angle when landing from a drop-jump. *Am J Knee Surg* 2001;14: 215-219.

50. Garrick J, Requa R: Anterior cruciate ligament injuries in men and women: How common are they?, in Griffin LY (ed): *Prevention of Noncontact ACL Injuries*. Rosemont, IL, American Academy of Orthopaedic Surgeons, 2001, pp 1-10.

51. De Carlo MS, Sell KE: The effects of the number and frequency of physical therapy treatments on selected outcomes of treatment in patients with anterior cruciate ligament reconstructions. *J Orthop Sports Phys Ther* 1997; 26:332-339.

52. Hewett TE, Stroupe AL, Nance TA, et al: Plyometric training in female athletes: Decreased impact forces and increased hamstring torques. *Am J Sports Med* 1996;24:765-773.

53. Kao JT, Giangarra CE, Singer G, Martin S: A comparison of outpatient and inpatient anterior cruciate ligament reconstruction surgery. *Arthroscopy* 1995;11:151-156.

54. Barber-Westin SD, Noyes FR, Andrews M: A rigorous comparison between the sexes of results and complications after anterior cruciate ligament reconstruction. *Am J Sports Med* 1997;25:514-526.

55. Colombet P, Allard M, Bousquet V, deLavigne C, Flurin RH, Lachaud C: Anterior cruciate ligament reconstruction using four-strand semitendinosus and gracilis tendon grafts and metal interference screw fixation. *Arthroscopy* 2002;18:232-237.

56. Corry IS, Web JM, Clingeleffer AJ, Pinczewski LA: Arthroscopic reconstruction of the anterior cruciate ligament: A comparison of patella tendon autograft and four-strand hamstring tendon autograft. *Am J Sports Med* 1999;27:444-454.

57. Ferrari JD, Bach BR, Bush-Joseph CA, Wang T, Bojchuk J: Anterior cruciate ligament reconstruction in men and women: An outcome analysis comparing gender. *Arthroscopy* 2001;17:588-596.

58. Siegel MG, Barber-Westin SD: Arthroscopic-assisted outpatient anterior cruciate ligament reconstruction using the semitendinosus and gracilis tendons. *Arthroscopy* 1998;14: 268-277.

59. Beynnon BD, Fleming BC, Churchill DL, et al: The effect of anterior cruciate ligament deficiency and functional bracing on translation of the tibia relative to the femur during nonweightbearing and weightbearing. *Am J Sports Med* 2003;31: 99-105.

60. Beynnon BD, Fleming BC, Labovitch R, et al: Chronic anterior cruciate ligament deficiency is associated with increased anterior translation of the tibia during the transition from non-weightbearing to weightbearing. *J Orthop Res* 2002;20:332-337.

61. McDevitt ER, Taylor DC, Miller MD, et al: Functional bracing after anterior cruciate ligament reconstruction: A prospective, randomized, multicenter study. *Am J Sports Med* 2004;32:1887-1892.

62. Kocher MS, Sterett WI, Briggs KK, Zurakowski D, Stedman JR: Effective functional bracing on subsequent knee injury in ACL-deficient professional skiers. *J Knee Surg* 2003;16:87-92.

63. Yu B, Herman D, Preston J, et al: Immediate effects of a knee brace with a constraint to knee extension on knee kinematics and ground reaction forces in a stop-jump task. *Am J Sports Med* 2004;32:1136-1143.

64. Meyers MC, Barnhill BS: Incidences, causes, and severity of high school football injuries on field turf versus natural grass: A 5-year prospective study. *Am J Sports Med* 2004;32: 1626-1638.

65. Olsen OE, Myklebust G, Engebretsen L, et al: Relationship between floor type and risk of ACL injury in team handball. *Scand J Med Sci Sports* 2003;13:299-304.

66. Orchard J: Is there a relationship between ground and climatic conditions and injuries in football? *Sports Med* 2002;32:419-432.

67. Shambaugh JP, Klein A, Herbert JH: Structural measures as predictors of injury in basketball players. *Med Sci Sports Exerc* 1991;23:522-527.

68. Woodford-Rogers B, Cyphert L, Denegar CR: Risk factors for anterior cruciate ligament injury in high school and college athletes. *J Athl Train* 1994;29:343-346.

69. Brown CN, Yu B, Kirkendall D, et al: Effects of increased body mass index on lower extremity motion patterns in a stop-jump task. *J Athl Train* 2005; 404(suppl):5.

70. Arendt E: Relationship between notch width index and risk of noncontact ACL injury, in Griffin LY (ed): *Prevention of Noncontact ACL Injuries.* Rosemont, IL, American Academy of Orthopaedic Surgeons, 2001, pp 33-44.

71. Anderson AF, Dome PC, Gautam S, et al: Correlation of anthropometric measurements, strength, anterior cruciate ligament size, and intercondylar notch characteristic to sex differences in anterior cruciate ligament tear rates. *Am J Sports Med* 2001; 29:58-66.

72. Shelbourne KD, Davis TJ, Klootwyk TE: The relationship between intercondylar notch width of the femur and incidence of anterior cruciate ligament tears: A prospective study. *Am J Sports Med* 1998;26:402-408.

73. Yu B, Kirkendall D, Garrett W: ACL injuries in female athletes: Anatomy, physiology, and motor control. *Sports Med Arthros Rev* 2002;10:58-68.

74. Chandrashekar N, Mansouri H, Slauterbeck J, Hashemi J: Sex-based differences in tensile properties of human anterior cruciate ligament. *J Biomech* 2006;39:2943-2950.

75. Wentorf FA, Sudoh K, Moses C, Arendt EA, Carlson CS: The effects of estrogen on material and mechanical properties of the intra- and extra-articular knee structure. *Am J Sports Med* 2006;34:1948-1952.

76. Strickland S, Belknap T, Turner S, Wright T, Hannafin J: Lack of hormonal influences on mechanical properties of sheep knee ligaments. *Am J Sports Med* 2003;31:210-215.

77. Seneviratne A, Attia E, Williams RJ, Rodeo SA, Hannafin JA: The effect of estrogen on ovine anterior cruciate ligament fibroblasts: Cell proliferation and collagen synthesis. *Am J Sports Med* 2004;32:1613-1618.

78. White KK, Lee SS, Cutuk A, Hargens AR, Pedowitz RA: EMG power spectra of intercollegiate athletes and anterior cruciate ligament injury risk in females. *Med Sci Sports Exerc* 2003;35: 371-376.

79. Harner CD, Paulos LE, Greenwald AE, Rosenberg TD, Cooley VC: Detailed analysis of patients with bilateral anterior cruciate ligament injuries. *Am J Sports Med* 1994;22:37-43.

80. Flynn RK, Pedersen CL, Birmingham TB, Kirkley A, Jackowski D, Fowler PJ: The familial predisposition toward tearing the anterior cruciate ligament: A case control study. *Am J Sports Med* 2005;33:23-28.

81. Hewett TE, Ford KR, Myer GD: Anterior cruciate ligament injury in female athletes: Part 2. A meta-analysis of neuromuscular interventions aimed at injury prevention. *Am J Sports Med* 2006;34:490-498.

82. Griffin LY, Albohm MJ, Arendt EA, et al: Understanding and preventing non-contact ACL injuries: A review of the Hunt Valley II Meeting, January 2005. *Am J Sports Med* 2006;34: 1512-1532.

83. Ottaviani RA, Ashton-Miller JA, Wojtys EM: Inversion and eversion strengths in the weightbearing ankle of young women: Effects of plantar flexion and basketball shoe height. *Am J Sports Med* 2001;29:219-225.

84. Wunderlich RE, Cavanagh PR: Gender differences in adult shoe shape: Implications for shoe design. *Med Sci Sports Exerc* 2001;33:605-611.

85. O'Connor K, Bragdon G, Baumhauer JF: Sexial dimorphism of the foot and ankle. *Orthop Clin North Am* 2006;37:569-574.

86. Frey C: Foot health and shoewear for women. *Clin Orthop Relat Res* 2000; 372:32-44.

87. Chilvers M, Donahue M, Nassar L, Manoli A: Foot and ankle injuries in elite female gymnasts. *Foot Ankle Int* 2007;28:214-218.

# Cartilage Repair Procedures: Clinical Approach and Decision Making

*Riley J. Williams III, MD
Robert H. Brophy, MD

## Abstract

*Articular cartilage lesions present a clinical challenge, but treatment options for these lesions are changing and expanding. The size of the lesion, the physical demands of the patient, and treatment history all are important factors to consider when selecting a surgical approach. It is important for the surgeon to understand the physiology of the selected cartilage repair method and to be aware of its effects on the postoperative rehabilitation program. Attention to surgical technique and selection of the most appropriate rehabilitation protocol will provide patients with the best chance of optimal results.*

**Instr Course Lect 2008;57:553-561.**

Articular cartilage injuries often are encountered during knee arthroscopy, particularly in younger patients.[1,2] Articular cartilage has a poor intrinsic capacity for healing following injury because of its avascular nature and the extracellular matrix structure of collagen and proteoglycan.[3-7] The lack of blood flow within the cartilage matrix limits the intrinsic healing process by inhibiting transport of inflammatory mediators to the defect, and the extracellular matrix does not allow cellular migration to the sites of cartilage injury.[8,9] As a result, even though chondrocytes initially respond to tissue injury, they are not capable of repopulating the defect; ultimately these cells cease their attempts at healing the area of injured cartilage, resulting in poor defect fill.[10] These lesions can become symptomatic; continued cartilage erosion and osteoarthritis may occur over time.[9-12]

Although isolated articular cartilage lesions often cause debilitating knee pain, there is no validated treatment algorithm for the management of these lesions. This emerging subspecialty is evolving rapidly, making the development of a treatment standard even more difficult. The overall treatment goal of cartilage reconstruction is to fill the defect to provide a durable return of joint function. Currently, there are several surgical options for the treatment of articular cartilage lesions. Although there is some discrepancy as to which procedures work best in certain patients, an extensive body of evidence exists showing that procedures such as microfracture, autologous osteochondral transplantation, autologous chondrocyte implantation (ACI), and osteochondral allograft transplantation are effective in restoring knee functions.[13-25]

A validated approach to the treatment of such lesions remains elusive, and decision making in these circumstances is highly variable among practitioners. Although no treatment algorithm yet has been validated for cartilage repair surgery, this chapter describes a systematic method of approaching symptomatic cartilage lesions of the knee.

## Cartilage Repair Strategies

The repair strategies currently available for treating an articular cartilage lesion can be classified into one of the following categories: palliative, enhancement of intrinsic repair, whole tissue transplantation,

*Riley J. Williams III, MD or the department with which he is affiliated has received research or institutional support from Smith & Nephew.*

## Table 1
**Current Cartilage Repair Strategies**

| Approach | Treatment | Repair Tissue | Fill | Known Durability |
|---|---|---|---|---|
| Palliative | Arthroscopic débridement | None | None | < 2 years |
| Enhancement of intrinsic repair | Mesenchymal stem cell-based repair Microfracture Abrasion arthroplasty Drilling | Fibrocartilage | Partial | 2 to 6 years |
| Whole tissue | Autologous osteochondral transplantation Mosaicplasty | Hyaline cartilage | Near total | 2 to 10 years |
| | Osteochondral allograft Fresh allograft | Hyaline cartilage | Near total | 5 to 20 years |
| Cell-based | Autologous chondrocyte implantation (ACI) | Hyaline-like | Partial | 2 to 11 years |
| Cell-based plus scaffold | Matrix-induced autologous chondrocyte implantation (MACI) | Hyaline-like | Near total | 2 years |
| | Hyalograft C | Hyaline-like | Near total | 3 years |
| Scaffold alone | Synthetic osteoarticular reconstruction TruFit | Hyaline-like | Near total | Unknown |

cell-based repair, scaffold-based repair, and combined cell-based and scaffold-based repair. Each of these strategies has specific treatment objectives, advantages, and disadvantages that should be considered in the development of a surgical plan. Palliative options focus on the relief of mechanical symptoms and include débridement, lavage, and chondroplasty.[26-28] These strategies attempt to remove the mechanical sources of pain but do not result in lesion fill. The enhancement of intrinsic cartilage repair strategy relies on recruiting marrow-based, pluripotent stem cells to the site of an articular cartilage lesion for the purpose of forming repair tissue. Specific treatment options in this group include abrasion arthroplasty, microfracture, and drilling.[16-19,29-35] Cell-based cartilage repair methods involve the local implantation of chondrogenic cells at the defect site for the purpose of forming hyaline-

like cartilage tissue. ACI (also known as autologous chondrocyte transplantation) falls into this category. To date, periosteal patches (ACI) and type I/III collagen patches (collagen associated chondrocyte implantation) have been used in cell-based methods.[13,14,36] Recently, the cell-based repair strategy has expanded to include the use of chondrocyte-matrix composites such as Matrix-Induced Autologous Chondrocyte Implantation (MACI, Verigen AG, Leverkusen, Germany) and Hyalograft C (Fidia, Abane Terme, Italy).[37-39] Scaffolds alone also can be used as an effective method of treating both chondral and osteochondral defects. A biphasic resorbable synthetic implant (TruFit, Smith & Nephew, San Antonio, TX) is currently available for primary cartilage repair in Europe; this implant also is available in the United States, with an indication for filling bony defects, including the

backfill of donor sites during mosaicplasty procedures.[40,41] The whole-tissue transplantation strategy relies on the implantation of mature osteoarticular tissue into a chondral or osteochondral defect. This tissue can be delivered as a single plug or multiple plugs, which typically are derived from an autologous source or from an allograft donor.[15,24,42-44]

These strategies can be further described according to the type of repair tissue that each approach aims to create, the resulting fill of the lesion, and the durability of the repair tissue (Table 1).

### Palliative Approach

In the authors' algorithm (Figure 1), the palliative approach is indicated for older patients with low functional demands with grade III or IV lesions covering 0.5 to 2 cm². The goals of this technique are to improve the congruency of the articular lesion with the opposing articular surface and to minimize further delamination of the joint surface cartilage. Although this is an expedient and cost-efficient technique, it does not result in tissue fill and is a temporizing treatment at best. This approach should be considered as a first-line treatment option only in patients age 45 years or older with low physical demands and more generalized cartilage pathology.

In a study by Dozin and associates,[45] more than 30% of patients had good to excellent results after simple débridement and 6 months of rehabilitation. Despite the study's limitations, this finding suggests there is a role for simple débridement in treating these lesions, particularly in low-demand patients or patients who may not be ready to face the demands of more extensive reconstructive surgery. At the same time, it is important to emphasize

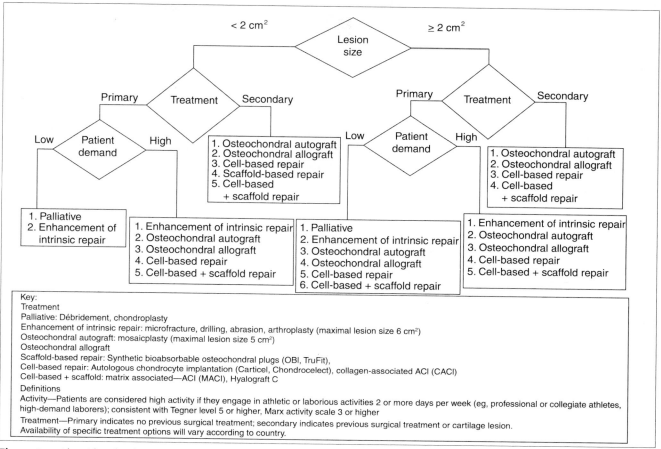

**Figure 1**    Algorithm for the surgical treatment of symptomatic articular cartilage lesions of the knee.

that the probability of success is low with débridement alone.

### Enhancement of Intrinsic Repair

Enhancement of intrinsic repair is an appropriate first-stage strategy for grade III or IV lesions of the femur covering 0.5 to 5 cm²; lesions considered for this method should possess a normal cartilage rim around the lesion for blood clot stabilization within the defect. High-demand patients with small lesions (smaller than 2 cm²), and low-demand patients with larger lesions (2 cm² or larger) are appropriate candidates for this treatment approach. Patients with a body mass index greater than 30 should not be considered for this approach.[21]

Both microfracture and drilling of the subchondral bone stimulate the intrinsic repair process by facilitating the formation of a fibrin clot rich with stem cells within the lesion, ultimately resulting in the creation of reparative fibrocartilage.[46] Use of the microfracture technique with this repair strategy is recommended because of concerns about the thermal effect of drilling on the subchondral bone and local marrow cells. This approach is a single-stage, arthroscopic technique that is technically easy, cost-effective, and results in tissue fill. However, tissue fill can be unpredictable, and bony overgrowth can occur. The durability of the fill created by this repair

technique is estimated to be 2 to 5 years in high-demand patients.[47] Overall, this is a safe, effective, first-line treatment with little morbidity. Increasingly effective results have been reported in the literature.[17,20,21,29,30,48,49]

The results from prospective, comparative studies of microfracture have been mixed. Although the comparison of microfracture to ACI by Knutsen and associates[50] essentially demonstrated no difference between the two techniques, the results of this study suggest that better results are obtained with the microfracture method. The Medical Outcomes Study 36-Item Short Form (SF-36) physical component score was higher in the microfracture group than in the ACI group. The histology findings, although not statistically significant, suggested a trend toward better results with microfracture. This study reported a correlation between lesion size and outcome among patients treated with microfracture, with worse outcomes in patients with a lesion size larger than 4 cm². Younger patients (age younger than 30 years) and more active patients (Tegner score greater than 4 points) also did better with microfracture compared with older or less active patients.

Microfracture did not perform as well as mosaicplasty in the treatment of cartilage lesions in a young, athletic cohort. In the study by Gudas and associates,[51] young athletes treated with microfracture demonstrated significantly worse clinical outcomes, poor-looking reparative cartilage, and lower rates of return to play compared with young athletes treated with mosaicplasty. This study also found significantly worse results among athletes treated with microfracture who had lesions larger than 2 cm². Patients younger than 30 years did better with microfracture than patients older than 30 years.

### Whole Tissue Transplantation
#### Autologous Osteochondral Transplantation

Cartilage resurfacing using autologous osteochondral transplantation can be accomplished using multiple, small osteochondral cylinders (mosaicplasty) or a single large plug.[15,44] Autologous osteochondral transplantation is indicated for focal, traumatic lesions 1 to 5 cm² in size; such lesions need not be contained. One advantage of this technique is that it can be used for lesions on the patella as well as the femur. This approach uses autogenous tissue to recreate the hyaline cartilage surface; this is a cost-effective approach with a recovery period that is similar to that of microfracture. Because autogenous osteochondral donor plugs typically are harvested from non–weight-bearing portions of the ipsilateral femur, such as the trochlea and notch, the supply of donor tissue is limited. Autologous osteochondral transplantation is a technically demanding procedure that usually requires an arthrotomy for a reliable three-dimensional reconstruction of the cartilage surface.[52] Despite the technical demands, it is a good option for first-line treatment of focal defects or for the treatment of smaller cartilage lesions in high-demand patients.[43]

Autologous osteochondral transplantation, specifically mosaicplasty, has generally performed well in comparative studies.[45,51,53,54] The one exception is the study by Bentley and associates,[53] which demonstrated worse clinical outcomes and International Cartilage Repair Society scores in a mosaicplasty cohort compared with an ACI cohort. An important technical aspect of this study was that the plugs were left slightly proud relative to the surrounding native articular surface. This method of plug placement is not typically recommended, and most studies describe leaving the plugs flush with the surrounding articular surface.[43,44]

Horas and associates,[54] using a technique that places the osteochondral plugs flush with the surrounding cartilage, reported quicker and more significant recovery of Lysholm scores in a mosaicplasty cohort compared with an ACI cohort. They also found a predominance of hyaline cartilage in patients treated with mosaicplasty compared with a predominance of fibrocartilage in patients treated with ACI. Dozin and associates[45] also reported a trend toward better clinical outcomes among patients treated with mosaicplasty compared with ACI ($P = 0.09$).

As mentioned previously, Gudas and associates[51] found mosaicplasty superior to microfracture for a young, athletic cohort. Mosaicplasty led to better clinical outcomes, better histology, and a higher rate of return to play. Patients younger than age 30 years had better clinical results compared with older patients treated with mosaicplasty. Unlike microfracture, there was no difference in outcome based on lesion size among patients treated with mosaicplasty.

### Osteochondral Allograft Transplantation

Fresh osteochondral allograft transplantation typically is used for large osteochondral lesions (2 to 12 cm² or larger). Large uncontained chondral lesions, osteochondral lesions, osteochondritis dissecans lesions, osteonecrotic lesions, and posttraumatic lesions can all be treated with this approach.[24,42] Osteochondral allograft transplantation also can be used as a salvage procedure for failed first-line treatments. This technique offers the advantages of bony fixation of the graft and the presence of intact functional hyaline cartilage that contains viable, matrix-maintaining chondrocytes. There is no donor site morbidity with this approach. However, allograft specimens are limited in supply and are costly. Fresh osteochondral allografts can elicit a local host immune response that may compromise bony healing, and disease transmission remains a remote but real possibility. This method of cartilage resurfacing has the longest history of any method; good long-term results have been reported.[22,42,55] Osteochondral allograft transplantation should be considered a primary option for large osteochondral lesions (osteochondritis dissecans, osteonecrosis), and secondary treatment for other failed cartilage repair treatments.

Because osteochondral allograft transplantation typically is considered an option of last resort, studies rarely compare this technique to other cartilage restoration techniques. A recent study reported clinical outcomes after osteochondral allograft transplantation using commercially available, fresh, cold-stored allograft tissue. The authors reported good results based on prospective outcome scores and MRI findings.[56] In the cohort of 19 patients with a mean lesion size of 5.9 cm², at a mean follow-up of 48 months (minimum 24 months), mean SF-36 scores increased from 51 to 66, and the mean activities of daily living score increased from 56 to 70. MRIs were obtained for 18 patients at a mean follow-up of 25 months. In all 18 patients, the allograft showed normal articular cartilage thickness; in 8 patients, the allograft cartilage signal properties were isointense relative to normal articular cartilage. The mean preimplantation storage time of the grafts used in this study was 30 days (range, 17 to 42 days). In this cohort, no correlation was found between clinical outcome scores and graft storage time, patient age, body mass index, and lesion size or location.

### Cell-Based Repair

ACI is indicated for large lesions (2 to 10 cm²) as a first- or second-stage treatment in patients with high physical demands. Chondral lesions of the femur, trochlea, patella, and tibia can be treated with this technique.[25,57] Treatable lesions can be uncontained, and multiple lesions can be treated at one setting. Osteochondral lesions can be treated if there is less than 6 mm of bone loss; lesions with more than 6 mm of bone loss should be treated with staged bone grafting before the ACI procedure. Patients should be between 15 and 55 years of age, have normal or correctable knee alignment, and a body mass index of less than 30. The ACI method is a two-stage technique that uses autologous chondrocytes that are expanded in culture following harvest. At implantation, these cells are secured within the cartilage defect using either a periosteal or collagen patch. Good clinical results have been reported, even in athletes.[58,59] However, these cell-based repair procedures are technically challenging, have a high revision rate (9% to 20%), and are expensive. ACI is a reasonable first-line therapy for patients with large cartilage lesions or for patients in whom other treatment modalities have failed.

Like microfracture, ACI has mixed results when compared with other treatment alternatives. Whereas Bentley and associates[53] demonstrated better results with ACI than with mosaicplasty, the described technique used for mosaicplasty in this study (plugs left proud) may have compromised their clinical results. Horas and associates[54] showed better clinical results and cartilage repair tissue with a hyaline cartilage appearance in mosaicplasty patients compared with ACI patients. Dozin and associates[45] reported a trend toward better clinical outcomes in patients treated with mosaicplasty compared with ACI. Knutsen and associates[50] demonstrated better clinical outcomes with microfracture compared with ACI. In this study, patients treated with microfracture did worse if they had lesions that were larger than 4 cm²; however, there was no correlation between lesion size and outcome among the patients treated with ACI. Similar to patients treated with microfracture, patients treated with ACI did better if they were younger than 30 years and more active (Tegner activity score greater than 4).

### Cell-Based Repair With a Scaffold

The emerging technology in the field of cartilage repair has further expanded the options available to clinicians. Cartilage repair techniques are beginning to include the use of genetically selected chondrocytes, matrix scaffolds, and growth factors.[3,4,60-63] In Europe and Australia, there has been extensive clinical experience with cell-based repair strategies that combine expanded autologous chondrocytes with matrix scaffolds. These so-called third-generation ACI techniques include the Hyalograft C chondrocyte-seeded implant and the MACI method, among others.[37,38,64,65] The Hyalograft C implant uses a hyaluronic acid-based scaffold for the delivery of autologous chondrocytes to the site of a cartilage lesion.[66-68] This cartilage repair method has created great interest because the implant requires no suture stabilization and can be placed arthroscopically. Studies on this cell-based technique have reported good clinical results with hyaline-like cartilage lesion fill.[37,69]

MACI is another third-generation method that is gaining popularity in both Europe and Australia. In this technique, cultured chondrocytes are seeded onto a type I/III porcine collagen membrane. After the membrane is fashioned to the appropriate lesion size, it is implanted into the articular cartilage defect.[39,70] The MACI membrane is easily handled and requires only fibrin glue and a few stabilizing sutures for fixation; it can be implanted on the femur, patella, or potentially the tibia using a limited arthrotomy. The MACI method results in nearly total lesion fill; good clinical results have been reported at short-term follow-up.[39,71] These third-generation ACI techniques have advanced the applications for the use of autologous cells in cartilage repair.

Both the MACI and Hyalograft C implants are technically easier to place than the original "first-generation" ACI implants. Although long-term follow-up is still needed to validate the use of the Hyalograft C and MACI matrices for the treatment of symptomatic articular cartilage lesions, these repair methods are promising.

One study comparing ACI with MACI found that clinical outcomes, International Cartilage Repair Society scores, complications, and reoperation rates were all comparable at 1-year follow-up.[38] The mean modified Cincinnati knee score increased 17.6 points from 41.4 to 59.0 in the ACI group and by 19.6 from 44.5 to 64.1 in the MACI group ($P = 0.32$). Among the patients who had second-look arthroscopy, excellent or good results were reported in 79.2% of ACIs and 66.6% of MACI grafts ($P = 0.3$). There were four instances of graft hypertrophy in the ACI group compared with three in the MACI group. In each group, three patients required manipulation of the knee under anesthesia. Two grafts failed in the MACI group, and one superficial infection was noted in the MACI group com-

pared with no graft failures or infections in the ACI group.

## Treatment Selection

The authors' treatment algorithm shown in Figure 1 is a modification of an algorithm by Alford and Cole.[72] The lesion size should be considered when developing a treatment plan. Lesion size is estimated from preoperative MRI, prior surgical reports, or at the time of surgery. Prior treatments and patient demand also are important considerations. High-demand patients are those who wish to return to athletic activities or high-demand labor. In the described approach, a lesion area of 2 cm² is critical. Once lesion size has been established, patient demand is determined (high versus low), typically using the Tegner[73] and Marx[74] knee activity rating scales. For the purposes of the algorithm, high activity is defined as 2 or more days of athletic participation or heavy labor per week and is consistent with level 5 or higher on the Tegner scale or a score of 3 or more on the Marx scale. The surgeon should determine whether the proposed treatment is a primary or secondary (revision) treatment.

## Summary

The treatment of isolated articular cartilage lesions remains a difficult clinical challenge. Treatment options for these lesions continue to evolve and expand. Lesion size, patient demand, and the treatment history are considered when selecting a surgical approach. Surgeons should understand the physiology of the cartilage repair method used and how this relates to the postoperative rehabilitation program. The clarification of other relevant conditions (such as obesity or limb malalignment) before treating articular carti-

lage defects will greatly increase the likelihood of a successful outcome. Appropriate attention should be paid to surgical technique and rehabilitation protocol to give patients the best chance for an optimal outcome.

## References

1. Curl WW, Krome J, Gordon ES, Rushing J, Smith BP, Poehling GG: Cartilage injuries: A review of 31,516 knee arthroscopies. *Arthroscopy* 1997;13:456-460.

2. Hjelle K, Solheim E, Strand T, Muri R, Brittberg M: Articular cartilage defects in 1,000 knee arthroscopies. *Arthroscopy* 2002;18:730-734.

3. Hunziker EB: Articular cartilage repair: Basic science and clinical progress. A review of the current status and prospects. *Osteoarthritis Cartilage* 2002;10:432-463.

4. Martinek V, Ueblacker P, Imhoff A: Current concepts of gene therapy and cartilage repair. *J Bone Joint Surg Br* 2003;85:782-788.

5. Vangsness CT, Kurzweil PR, Lieberman JR: Restoring articular cartilage in the knee. *Am J Orthop* 2004;33 (suppl 2):29-34.

6. Mankin HJ: The response of articular cartilage to mechanical injury. *J Bone Joint Surg Am* 1982;64:460-466.

7. Newman AP: Articular cartilage repair. *Am J Sports Med* 1998;26:309-324.

8. Buckwalter JA: Articular cartilage injuries. *Clin Orthop Relat Res* 2002;402:21-37.

9. Buckwalter JA, Mankin HJ: Articular cartilage: Degeneration and osteoarthritis, repair, regeneration, and transplantation. *Instr Course Lect* 1998;47:487-504.

10. Buckwalter JA, Mankin HJ: Articular cartilage: Tissue design and chondrocyte-matrix interactions. *Instr Course Lect* 1998;47:477-486.

11. Caplan AI, Elyaderani M, Mochi-

zuki Y, Wakitani S, Goldberg VM: Principles of cartilage repair and regeneration. *Clin Orthop Relat Res* 1997; 342:254-269.

12. Lefkoe TP, Trafton PG, Ehrlich MG, et al: An experimental model of femoral condylar defect leading to osteoarthrosis. *J Orthop Trauma* 1993; 7:458-467.

13. Brittberg M, Lindhal A, Nilsson A, Ohlsson C, Isaksson O, Peterson L: Treatment of deep cartilage defects in the knee with autologous chondrocyte transplantation of the knee. *N Engl J Med* 1994;331:889-895.

14. Peterson L, Minas T, Brittberg M, Nilsson A, Sjogren-Jansson E, Lindhal A: Two- to 9-year outcome after autologous chondrocyte transplantation of the knee. *Clin Orthop Relat Res* 2000;374:212-234.

15. Hangody L, Kish G, Karpati Z, Udvarhelyi I, Szigeti I, Bely M: Mosaicplasty for the treatment of articular cartilage defects: Application in clinical practice. *Orthopedics* 1998;21: 751-756.

16. Johnson LL: Arthroscopic abrasion arthroplasty: A review. *Clin Orthop Relat Res* 2001;(suppl 391):S306-S317.

17. Marder R, Hopkins G, Timmerman L: Arthroscopic microfracture of chondral defects of the knee: A comparison of two postoperative treatments. *Arthroscopy* 2005;21:152-158.

18. Rae PJ, Noble J: Arthroscopic drilling of osteochondral lesions of the knee. *J Bone Joint Surg Br* 1989;71:534.

19. Bert JM: Role of abrasion arthroplasty and debridement in the management of osteoarthritis of the knee. *Rheum Dis Clin North Am* 1993;19:725-739.

20. Steadman JR, Rodkey WG, Rodrigo JJ: Microfracture: Surgical technique and rehabilitation to treat chondral defects. *Clin Orthop Relat Res* 2001;391:S362-S369.

21. Mithoefer K, Williams R, Warren R, et al: The microfracture technique for the treatment of articular cartilage lesions in the knee: A prospective cohort study. *J Bone Joint Surg Am* 2005;87:1911-1920.

22. Meyers MH, Akeson W, Convery FR: Resurfacing of the knee with fresh osteochondral allograft. *J Bone Joint Surg Am* 1989;71:704-713.

23. Minas T, Chiu R: Autologous chondrocyte implantation. *Am J Knee Surg* 2000;13:41-50.

24. Bugbee WD, Convery FR: Osteochondral allograft transplantation. *Clin Sports Med* 1999;18:67-75.

25. Brittberg M, Tallheden T, Sjogren-Jansson B, Lindhal A, Peterson L: Autologous chondrocytes used for articular cartilage repair: An update. *Clin Orthop Relat Res* 2001;391:S337-S348.

26. Ogilvie-Harris DJ, Bauer M, Corey P: Prostaglandin inhibition and the rate of recovery after arthroscopic meniscectomy. *J Bone Joint Surg Br* 1985;67:567-571.

27. Evans CH, Mazzocchi RA, Nelson DD, Rubash HE: Experimental arthritis induced by intra-articular injection of allogeneic cartilaginous particles into rabbit knees. *Arthritis Rheum* 1984;27:200-207.

28. O'Connor RL: The arthroscope in the management of crystal-induced synovitis of the knee. *J Bone Joint Surg Am* 1973;55:1443-1449.

29. Steadman JR, Briggs KK, Rodrigo JJ, Kocher MS, Gill TJ, Rodkey WG: Outcomes of microfracture for traumatic chondral defects of the knee: Average 11-year follow-up. *Arthroscopy* 2003;19:477-484.

30. Blevins FT, Steadman JR, Rodrigo JJ, Silliman J: Treatment of articular cartilage defects in athletes: An analysis of functional outcome and lesion appearance. *Orthopedics* 1998;21: 761-767.

31. Bert JM, Maschka K: The arthroscopic treatment of unicompartmental gonarthrosis: A five-year follow-up study of abrasion arthroplasty plus arthroscopic debridement and arthroscopic debridement alone. *Arthroscopy* 1989;5:25-32.

32. Friedman MJ, Berasi CC, Fox JM, Del Pizzo W, Snyder SJ, Ferkel RD: Preliminary results with abrasion ar-

throplasty in the osteoarthritic knee. *Clin Orthop Relat Res* 1984;182: 200-205.

33. Insall J: The Pridie debridement operation for osteoarthritis of the knee. *Clin Orthop Relat Res* 1974;101:61-67.

34. Pridie K: A method of resurfacing osteoarthritic knee joints. *J Bone Joint Surg Br* 1959;41:618-619.

35. Childers JC, Ellwood SC: Partial chondrectomy and subchondral bone drilling for chondromalacia. *Clin Orthop Relat Res* 1979;144:114-120.

36. Gooding CR, Bartlett W, Bentley G, Skinner JA, Carrington R, Flanagan A: A prospective, randomised study comparing two techniques of autologous chondrocyte implantation for osteochondral defects in the knee: Periosteum covered versus type I/III collagen covered. *Knee* 2006;13: 203-210.

37. Marcacci M, Berruto M, Brocchetta D, et al: Articular cartilage engineering with Hyalograft C: 3-year clinical results. *Clin Orthop Relat Res* 2005;435:96-105.

38. Bartlett W, Skinner J, Gooding C, et al: Autologous chondrocyte implantation versus matrix-induced autologous chondrocyte implantation for osteochondral defects of the knee: A prospective, randomized study. *J Bone Joint Surg Br* 2005;87: 640-645.

39. Marlovits S, Singer P, Zeller P, Mandl I, Haller J, Trattnig S: Magnetic resonance observation of cartilage repair tissue (MOCART) for the evaluation of autologous chondrocyte transplantation: Determination of interobserver variability and correlation to clinical outcome after 2 years. *Eur J Radiol* 2005;57:16-23.

40. Slivka MA, Leatherbury NC, Kieswetter K, Niederauer GG: Porous, resorbable, fiber-reinforced scaffolds tailored for articular cartilage repair. *Tissue Eng* 2001;7:767-780.

41. Niederauer GG, Slivka MA, Leatherbury NC, et al: Evaluation of multiphase implants for repair of focal osteochondral defects in goats.

*Biomaterials* 2000;21:2561-2574.

42. Gross AE, Shasha N, Aubin P: Long-term followup of the use of fresh osteochondral allografts for posttraumatic knee defects. *Clin Orthop Relat Res* 2005;435:79-87.

43. Marcacci M, Kon E, Zaffagnini S, et al: Multiple osteochondral arthroscopic grafting (mosaicplasty) for cartilage defects of the knee: Prospective study results at 2-year follow-up. *Arthroscopy* 2005;21:462-470.

44. Hangody L, Rathonyi GK, Duska Z, Vasarhelyi G, Fules P, Modis L: Autologous osteochondral mosaicplasty: Surgical technique. *J Bone Joint Surg Am* 2004;86:65-72.

45. Dozin B, Malpeli M, Cancedda R, et al: Comparative evaluation of autologous chondrocyte implantation and mosaicplasty: A multicentered randomized clinical trial. *Clin J Sport Med* 2005;15:220-226.

46. Minas T, Nehrer S: Current concepts in the treatment of articular cartilage defects. *Orthopedics* 1997;20:525-538.

47. Mithoefer K, Williams RJ III, Warren RF, Wickiewicz TL, Marx RG: High-impact athletics after knee articular cartilage repair: A prospective evaluation of the microfracture technique. *Am J Sports Med* 2006;34:1413-1418.

48. Steadman JR, Rodkey WG, Briggs KK: Microfracture to treat full-thickness chondral defects: Surgical technique, rehabilitation, and outcomes. *J Knee Surg* 2002;15:170-176.

49. Steadman JR, Miller BS, Karas SG, Schlegel TF, Briggs KK, Hawkins RJ: The microfracture technique in the treatment of full-thickness chondral lesions of the knee in National Football League players. *J Knee Surg* 2003;16:83-86.

50. Knutsen G, Engebretsen L, Ludvigsen TC, et al: Autologous chondrocyte implantation compared with microfracture in the knee: A randomized trial. *J Bone Joint Surg Am* 2004;86:455-464.

51. Gudas R, Kalesinskas RJ, Kimtys V, et al: A prospective randomized clinical study of mosaic osteochondral autologous transplantation versus microfracture for the treatment of osteochondral defects in the knee joint in young athletes. *Arthroscopy* 2005;21:1066-1075.

52. Morelli M, Nagamori J, Miniaci A: Management of chondral injuries of the knee by osteochondral autogenous transfer (mosaicplasty). *J Knee Surg* 2002;15:185-190.

53. Bentley G, Biant LC, Carrington RW, et al: A prospective, randomised comparison of autologous chondrocyte implantation versus mosaicplasty for osteochondral defects in the knee. *J Bone Joint Surg Br* 2003;85:223-230.

54. Horas U, Pelinkovic D, Herr G, Aigner T, Schnettler R: Autologous chondrocyte implantation and osteochondral cylinder transplantation in cartilage repair of the knee joint: A prospective, comparative trial. *J Bone Joint Surg Am* 2003;85:185-192.

55. Chu CR, Convery FR, Akeson WH, Meyers M, Amiel D: Articular cartilage transplantation: Clinical results in the knee. *Clin Orthop Relat Res* 1999;360:159-168.

56. Williams RJ III, Ranawat AS, Potter HG, Carter T, Warren RF: Fresh stored allografts for the treatment of osteochondral lesions of the knee. *J Bone Joint Surg Am* 2007;89:718-726.

57. Minas T: Autologous chondrocyte implantation for focal chondral defects of the knee. *Clin Orthop Relat Res* 2001;391:S349-S361.

58. Mithofer K, Peterson L, Mandelbaum BR, Minas T: Articular cartilage repair in soccer players with autologous chondrocyte transplantation: Functional outcome and return to competition. *Am J Sports Med* 2005;33:1639-1646.

59. Mithofer K, Minas T, Peterson L, Yeon H, Micheli LJ: Functional outcome of knee articular cartilage repair in adolescent athletes. *Am J Sports Med* 2005;33:1147-1153.

60. Chen Y: Orthopedic applications of gene therapy. *J Orthop Sci* 2001;6:199-207.

61. Blunk T, Sieminski A, Gooch K, et al: Differential effects of growth factors on tissue-engineered cartilage. *Tissue Eng* 2002;8:73-84.

62. Frenkel SR, Saadeh PB, Mehrara BJ, et al: Transforming growth factor beta superfamily members: Role in cartilage modeling. *Plast Reconstr Surg* 2000;105:980-990.

63. Trippel SB: Growth factors as therapeutic agents. *Instr Course Lect* 1997;46:473-476.

64. Solchaga LA, Dennis JE, Goldberg VM, Caplan AI: Hyaluronic acid-based polymers as cell carriers for tissue-engineered repair of bone and cartilage. *J Orthop Res* 1999;17:205-213.

65. Solchaga LA, Yoo JU, Lundberg M, et al: Hyaluronan-based polymers in the treatment of osteochondral defects. *J Orthop Res* 2000;18:773-780.

66. Campoccia D, Doherty P, Radice M, Brun P, Abatangelo G, Williams D: Semisynthetic resorbable materials from hyaluronan esterification. *Biomaterials* 1998;19:2101-2127.

67. Grigolo B, Roseti L, Fiorini M, et al: Transplantation of chondrocytes seeded on a hyaluronan derivative (hyaff 11) into cartilage defects in rabbits. *Biomaterials* 2001;22:2417-2424.

68. Brun P, Abatangelo G, Radice M, et al: Chondrocyte aggregation and reorganization into three-dimensional scaffolds. *J Biomed Mater Res* 1999;46:337-346.

69. Pavesio A, Abatangelo G, Borrione A, et al: Hyaluronan-based scaffolds (Hyalograft C) in the treatment of knee cartilage defects: Preliminary clinical findings, in *Novartis Foundation Symposia: Tissue Engineering of Cartilage and Bone*. London, England, Novartis Foundation, 2003, pp 203-217.

70. Behrens P, Ehlers E, Kochermann K, Rohwedel J, Russlies M, Plotz W: New therapy procedure for localized cartilage defects: Encouraging results with autologous chondrocyte implan-

tation. *MMW Fortschr Med* 1999;141: 49-51.

71. Bachmann G, Basad E, Lommel D, Steinmeyer J: MRI in the follow-up of matrix-supported autologous chondrocyte transplantation (MACI) and microfracture. *Radiologe* 2004;44: 773-782.

72. Alford JW, Cole BJ: Cartilage restoration, part 2: Techniques, outcomes, and future directions. *Am J Sports Med* 2005;33:443-460.

73. Tegner Y, Lysholm J: Rating systems in the evaluation of knee ligament injuries. *Clin Orthop Relat Res* 1985;198: 43-49.

74. Marx RG, Stump TJ, Jones EC, Wickiewicz TL, Warren RF: Development and evaluation of an activity rating scale for disorders of the knee. *Am J Sports Med* 2001;29:213-218.

# Articular Cartilage Repair Using a Resorbable Matrix Scaffold

*Riley J. Williams III, MD
Seth C. Gamradt, MD

## Abstract

*The creation of cartilage repair tissue relies on the implantation or neosynthesis of cartilage matrix elements. One cartilage repair strategy involves the implantation of bioabsorbable matrices that immediately fill a chondral or osteochondral defect. Such matrices support the local migration of chondrogenic or osteogenic cells that ultimately synthesize new ground substance. One such matrix scaffold, a synthetic resorbable biphasic implant (TruFit Plug; Smith & Nephew, San Antonio, TX), is a promising device for the treatment of osteochondral voids. The implant is intended to serve as a scaffold for native marrow elements and matrix ingrowth in chondral defect repair. The device is a resorbable tissue regeneration scaffold made predominantly from polylactide-coglycolide copolymer, calcium sulfate, and polyglycolide. It is approved in Europe for the treatment of acute focal articular cartilage or osteochondral defects but is approved by the US Food and Drug Administration only for backfill of osteochondral autograft sites. Preclinical studies demonstrated restoration of hyaline-like cartilage in a goat model with subchondral bony incorporation at 12 months. Early clinical results of patients enrolled in the Hospital for Special Surgery Cartilage Registry have been favorable, with a good safety profile.*

**Instr Course Lect 2008;57:563-571.**

Adult articular cartilage has a limited capacity for healing,[1] and cartilage injury in the knee can result in the development of painful osteoarthritis and joint degeneration,[2-5] making restoration of articular cartilage an important focus in both orthopaedics and tissue engineering.[6,7] Multiple techniques have been described for surgical cartilage repair or reconstruction,[3] but the ideal method for restoring cartilage has not been identified, despite significant advances in applying tissue engineering strategies to clinical practice.[8] Each surgical technique aims to improve the cartilage quality at the site of the defect to limit pain, improve function, and prevent degenerative joint disease. No consensus exists among surgeons as to the indications for each procedure. The basic science and clinical data supporting each treatment are incomplete and occasionally conflicting, and the quality of the repair tissue (hyaline-like cartilage, fibrocartilage) formed by each repair strategy varies among techniques and studies.[9-13] The durability of repair cartilage formed by current techniques also is believed to deteriorate over time.[3]

## Current Surgical Strategies for Cartilage Restoration

Currently, six strategies are used to treat cartilage lesions: palliative (for example, débridement); enhancement of intrinsic healing response (for example, microfracture); whole tissue transplantation (for example, osteochondral autograft or allograft); cell-based repair (for example, autologous chondrocyte implantation); cell-based plus scaffold repair (for example, matrix-based autologous chondrocyte implantation); and scaffolds alone. The indications and results of these six strategies are discussed in chapter 45.

Osteochondral autograft trans-

*Riley J. Williams III, MD or the department with which he is affiliated has received research or institutional support from Smith & Nephew.*

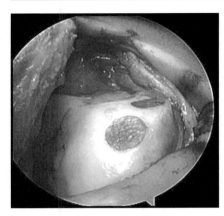

**Figure 1** Intraoperative photograph of the lateral femoral condyle of a knee undergoing mosaicplasty for a symptomatic full-thickness cartilage defect. A biphasic, resorbable TruFit osteochondral plug has been used to fill the autograft donor sites.

plantation, also known as mosaicplasty, involves the transfer of normal, mature osteochondral plugs into a site of cartilage injury.[14] Such plugs typically are taken from the superolateral trochlear region or from the femoral notch.[3,14] Although it is believed that these areas have low joint reactive forces during normal knee kinematics, contact pressures exist at all locations of donor graft harvest.[15] As such, the morbidity of removing these osteochondral grafts is unknown. In the largest series of osteochondral autografts,[16] few long-term symptoms were attributable to the donor site following mosaicplasty; only 18 of 597 patients (3%) had symptoms attributable to the donor graft sites. However, Jakob and associates[17] reported that 3 of 7 patients with larger femoral defects treated with autogenous grafts from the contralateral knee had pain and functional limitations after harvest of osteochondral grafts from the contralateral knee. Backfilling of donor sites is commonly done during mosaicplasty, usually with bone taken from the lesion site. This graft source

is not optimal because the bony volume usually is not sufficient to fill the donor defect. More recently, resorbable biphasic osteoconductive matrices have been developed for this purpose, such as the TruFit plug (Smith & Nephew, San Antonio, TX) (Figure 1). These synthetic plugs are designed to fill the donor defect during autologous osteochondral transplantation procedures and support the creation of bone and cartilage repair tissue at the site of implantation. Feczko and associates[18] investigated several biodegradable materials in a dog model of osteochondral autograft transplantation and harvest and concluded that the quality of fibrocartilaginous repair tissue was best when donor sites were backfilled with a matrix implant consisting of compressed collagen.

The primary indication for mosaicplasty is the treatment of symptomatic focal chondral and osteochondral lesions.[14,19] Patients typically are younger than age 50 years and have normal meniscal volume and tibial cartilage with no ligamentous instability or malalignment.[20] In a study of 831 mosaicplasty patients, 92% good to excellent results were reported for femoral condylar lesions, and 79% good to excellent results were reported for patellofemoral lesions.[16]

Mosaicplasty usually is done with commercially available chisels to harvest the autogenous grafts as dowels. The recipient site is prepared with a matching chisel or drill, and the grafts are delivered to the recipient site within the defect. These autogenous grafts are then manually pressed into position or gently tapped flush with the surrounding cartilage.[14] Because of the limited amount of osteochondral autograft available from the ipsilateral knee, traditional mosaicplasty usually is limited to smaller cartilage lesions no larger than 2.0 to 5.0 cm².[3,14] Un-

contained lesions larger than 5.0 cm² should be treated with autologous chondrocyte implantation or osteochondral allograft.[21] In theory, a synthetic osteochondral graft that could be implanted into a cartilage defect would have obvious advantages. Such a synthetic implant could be used to fill symptomatic lesions, much as autogenous plugs currently are used for mosaicplasty. A synthetic osteochondral plug would expand the indications for the mosaicplasty procedure because there would be no limit on the amount of material available to fill a cartilage defect, and there would be no donor site morbidity. In addition, the local cartilage architecture would be more easily re-created with synthetic implants. Harvesting and implanting autograft plugs at the defect site to successfully re-create the contour of the femoral condyle or patellar surface is technically demanding.[22] The surface of an osteochondral autograft plug cannot be contoured without damaging the cartilage surface.[23] Synthetic matrix implants, however, can be contoured (via tamping) to match the shape of the native articular surface without compromising the structural integrity of the plug.

## Tissue Engineering of Cartilage With Bioabsorbable Scaffolds

In an attempt to improve the quality of cartilage repair tissue after surgery, extensive laboratory investigations and preclinical animal studies have focused on the use of biodegradable matrix scaffolds alone and in combination with chondrogenic cells.[6] Three-dimensional porous scaffolds are most commonly used in cartilage repair models because they encourage cellular attachment and local tissue ingrowth at the site of repair.[24,25] Muschler and associates[26] extensively reviewed the engineering principles behind scaffold selection in tissue engineering and identified the variables important in scaffold structure and function: material, architecture, surface chemistry, mechanical strength, and degradation characteristics.

Variations of these types of materials are most commonly used as scaffolds in cartilage tissue engineering. Polylactides and polyglycolides, bioabsorbable materials commonly used in orthopaedic surgery for suture material (for example, Vicryl; Ethicon, Somerville, NJ), interference screws, and suture anchors[27] have been used in cartilage repair models in laboratory and animal studies.[25,28-36] Hydrogels, polymer networks that have the ability to absorb significant quantities of water,[37] and collagen also have been used as scaffolds for cartilage tissue engineering.[38-40] The optimal scaffold for articular cartilage repair is not yet known, but an ideal scaffold material would allow the attachment of cells, facilitate the ingrowth of reparative tissue, provide substantial initial mechanical strength, and ultimately incorporate into the host tissue.[26]

## Poly(α-hydroxy esters) as Scaffolds for Cartilage Repair

The physical and mechanical properties of a given matrix scaffold profoundly affect the healing response and the type of cartilage repair tissue formed in a treated defect; this effect is even more pronounced in a weight-bearing environment.[41] Mechanical strength of the scaffold implant is essential for stable initial fixation and resistance to deformation during weight bearing.[26] Designing a synthetic implant for cartilage repair (in this circumstance the mosaicplasty procedure) involves an attempt to re-create two types of tissue: articular cartilage and sub-

chondral bone. In designing a multiphase implant, the stability of the underlying subchondral area of the defect site is critical to support the overlying neocartilage regenerate.

Poly(α-hydroxy esters), including polylactic acid (PLA), polyglycolic acid, and polylactic-coglycolic acid (PLGA), have been used extensively in cartilage tissue engineering studies.[6] Basic science studies using such scaffolds have documented the preservation of chondrocyte phenotypes and the production of a cartilage extracellular matrix.[29,30,42,43] The degradation characteristics of these scaffolds can be modified by altering the composition of the scaffold materials.[26] The TruFit CB (Cartilage/Bone) (Smith & Nephew) is a resorbable implant composed of semiporous 75:25 poly(D,L-lactide-coglycolide) (PLG) copolymer, calcium sulfate, polyglycolide (PGA) fibers, and surfactant.[44] Designed to fill osteochondral defects, the functions of this scaffold are to re-create the mechanical properties of subchondral bone in one phase (deep) and facilitate cartilage regeneration on the surface of the implant in a second phase (superficial). The two phases are designed to initially approximate the mechanical properties of the adjacent cartilage (superficial) and bone (deep).[44] The superficial cartilage phase is softer and malleable enough to be contoured to the joint curvature. The bone phase incorporates calcium sulfate in the scaffold design to improve initial strength. Slivka and associates[45] showed that incorporating chopped polyglycolic acid fibers improved the early structural integrity of the scaffold after implantation.[45] In Europe, the TruFit CB plug is approved for primary bone and cartilage repair, but in the United States, it is approved only for the backfill of

autogenous osteochondral harvest site defects and bony voids.

Although no clinical studies have examined the efficacy of the TruFit CB scaffold in restoring articular cartilage or treating symptomatic cartilage defects, the implant has been examined in the femoral condyles and trochleas of goats. Goat knees have a cartilage thickness of approximately 0.9 to 1.2 mm and are an effective large animal model for testing cartilage repair methods.[46-48] Jackson and associates[48] created 6 × 6 mm defects in the medial femoral condyles of goats and found that at 26 weeks untreated defects became cavitary lesions with an overlying thin layer of fibrocartilage on the sclerotic walls of the defects (Figure 2). To test the efficacy of the TruFit CB scaffolds in this preclinical in vivo model, osteochondral defects (5 × 5 mm) were created through bilateral arthrotomies in 12 Spanish goats. Two defects were created in the joint: one in the medial femoral condyle and one in the trochlea (Figure 3). The TruFit CB cylindrical implants were press-fit into the osteochondral defects flush with the articular surface. After scaffold implantation, immediate, full weight bearing was allowed. Animals were sacrificed at 6 weeks, 6 months, and 12 months, and retrieved scaffolds were subjected to mechanical testing and histology. There were no surgical complications, and all animals returned to normal activity. Evaluations at necropsy indicated no gross joint abnormalities. Gross observation of treated defects at 12 months showed that the repair tissue had integrated well with the native cartilage, the surface of the repair sites was smooth, and the defects were almost entirely filled in all instances (Figure 4). Mechanical testing revealed

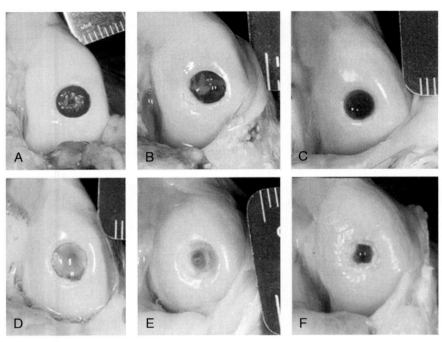

**Figure 2**  Gross appearance of 6 × 6 mm articular cartilage defect in the medial femoral condyle of a goat at selected time intervals after creation of the defect. **A,** Time zero (immediately after creation of the lesion). **B,** One week. **C,** Two weeks. **D,** Six weeks. **E,** Twenty-six weeks. **F,** Fifty-two weeks. (Reprinted with permission from Jackson DW, Lalor PA, Aberman HM, Simon TM: Spontaneous repair of full-thickness defects of articular cartilage in a goat model: A preliminary study. *J Bone Joint Surg Am* 2001;83A:53-64.)

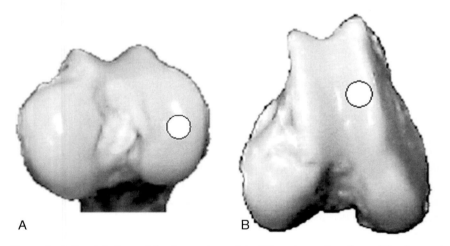

**Figure 3**  Cranial view of the femoral condyle (**A**) and anterior view of the femoral trochlear surface of the right knee joint of an adult goat (**B**); 5 × 5-mm defect sites were created on the medial femoral condyle and medial aspect of the trochlea.

that the stiffness of the repair tissue ranged from 93% to 101% of the value for healthy cartilage.

Histologic evaluation of retrieved specimens demonstrated that all groups had a high percentage of

hyaline-like cartilage and good bony restoration (Figure 5). Healing of the osteochondral defect continued to improve from the 6-week to the 12-month end point. Integration of healed tissue showed a smooth transition to the native cartilage, and the repair cartilage thickness was very close to that of adjacent cartilage, with no observable differences between condylar and trochlea lesions. The 12-month specimens showed nearly complete incorporation into cancellous bone in the subchondral bone region and hyaline-like cartilage in the overlying region. In comparison to historical, untreated control specimens, the scaffold provided mechanical support for the tissue to heal and prevented the collapse of the adjacent defect walls.[48] This preclinical study demonstrated that hyaline-like cartilage can be restored in osteochondral defects in the knee joints of goats using a synthetic biphasic matrix (Industry Study, Smith & Nephew, London).

At the Hospital for Special Surgery, these implants were initially used for backfill of osteochondral donor sites during traditional osteochondral autograft transplantation (mosaicplasty). No adverse events and only minimal donor site morbidity occurred in treated patients. On follow-up cartilage-sensitive MRI studies of these patients (by the Hospital for Special Surgery Cartilage Registry protocol), the appearance of the donor sites filled with synthetic biphasic matrices demonstrated good surface contour and cartilage phase signal intensity.[49,50] Because of the excellent fill and contour noted on the follow-up MRIs of the donor sites, surgeons at the Hospital for Special Surgery decided to prospectively evaluate the effectiveness of the TruFit CB implant for the direct treatment of patients with symptomatic, full-thickness chondral injuries of the knee. These patients continue to be prospectively evaluated as part of the Hospital for Special Surgery Cartilage Registry maintained by the senior author (RJW). Since 2005, the device has been implanted in more than 100 patients for the treatment of femoral condylar and patellar lesions. These patients are being followed with clinical examinations; outcomes questionnaires (Medical Outcomes Study Short Form-36, International Knee Documentation Committee, and activities of daily living scores) at baseline and 3, 6, 12, and 24 months following surgery; and serial MRI examinations at 3 months, 1 year, and 2 years following implantation. These data continue to be collected. The safety profile of these implants has been good; there have been no overt implant

failures in the direct treatment group or in patients who had mosaicplasty with TruFit CB backfill. No

persistent effusions or loose implants have been documented. To date, subjective clinical results have

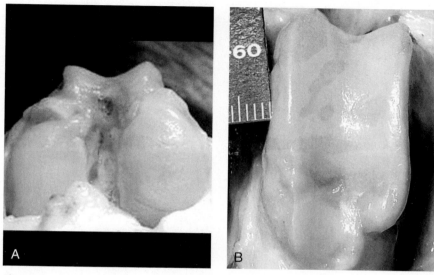

**Figure 4**  Gross images of goat joint surface at 12 months after treatment of osteochondral defects with synthetic biphasic matrices: **A,** Femoral condyle. **B,** Trochlear groove.

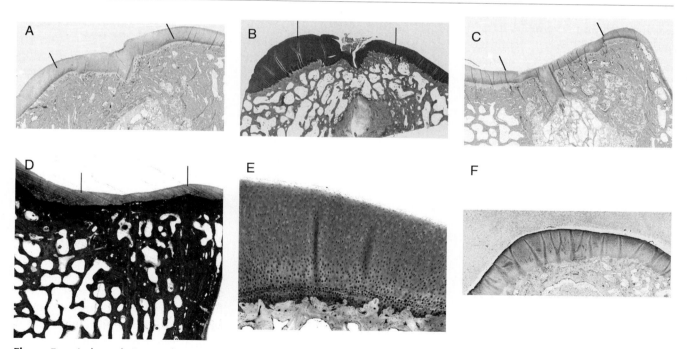

**Figure 5**  A through **F,** Histologic appearance of 5 × 5 mm osteochondral defect in goat femur. Sections of femoral (**A**) and trochlear (**C**) lesions treated with the TruFit CB matrix stained with Goldner's TriChrome at 6 months of healing. Hatch marks show original lesion size. Toluidine blue stained sections of femoral (**B**) and trochlear (**D**) lesions treated with the TruFit CB matrix at 12 months of healing. (A through **D,** magnification ×4). **E,** Safranin O/Fast Green staining at 12 months of healing (magnification ×20). **F,** Uniform appearance of type II collagen immunohistochemical staining at 12 months.

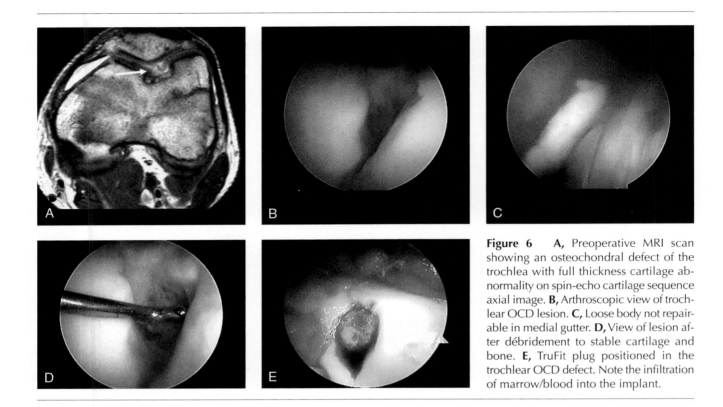

**Figure 6** **A,** Preoperative MRI scan showing an osteochondral defect of the trochlea with full thickness cartilage abnormality on spin-echo cartilage sequence axial image. **B,** Arthroscopic view of trochlear OCD lesion. **C,** Loose body not repairable in medial gutter. **D,** View of lesion after débridement to stable cartilage and bone. **E,** TruFit plug positioned in the trochlear OCD defect. Note the infiltration of marrow/blood into the implant.

been good, with most patients reporting early improvements in pain and function. Serial cartilage-sequence MRI and T2 cartilage mapping have documented good fill of the cartilage defects and gradual but incomplete bony incorporation at approximately 1 year.

## Clinical Case No. 1

A 17-year-old player on a National Collegiate Athletic Association Division I lacrosse team injured his left knee during practice and presented with a painful effusion. Radiographs of the knee showed no abnormality. On examination, there was a large effusion, and the patient's active range of motion was 0 to 110°. No instability or joint line tenderness was observed. Tenderness on the medial and lateral facets of the patella was noted. Cartilage-sensitive MRI demonstrated an osteochondral defect in the medial trochlea, resulting from a displaced osteochondritis dissecans (OCD) lesion, with full thickness cartilage loss. The lesion size was approximately 1 cm². Diagnostic arthroscopy revealed a 9 × 9 mm Outerbridge grade 4 chondral injury to the trochlea with a small amount of bone loss. A loose body (OCD fragment) was removed from the medial gutter; after examination of the fragment, it was determined that the piece could not be fixed back in the defect. The osteochondral defect was treated with a single 9-mm TruFit CB plug (Figure 6). Cryotherapy and toe-touch weight bearing were prescribed for 1 week. Continuous passive motion was initiated immediately for 6 hours per day and continued for 6 weeks; the patient was allowed to bear weight to tolerance with a brace locked in extension through week 6. The patient participated in outpatient physical therapy from weeks 2 through 8 postoperatively. Normal ambulation was allowed after 6 weeks. Return to sport was allowed 6 months following surgery. The patient was evaluated with cartilage-sensitive MRI at 3 months and 12 months postoperatively (Figure 7). He regained full range of motion without effusion and returned to play Division I lacrosse at his previous level with no limitations.

## Clinical Case No. 2

A 46-year-old man who had undergone previous anterior cruciate ligament (ACL) reconstruction, partial medial meniscectomy, and microfracture for a medial femoral condylar cartilage lesion presented with a gradual onset of medial knee pain, mechanical symptoms, and effusion. He reported pain with walking and activities of daily living. Microfracture surgery done 8 months earlier had failed to relieve his symptoms. MRI revealed an intact ACL graft and full-thickness cartilage loss on the weight-bearing surface of the medial femoral condyle (Figure 8). Diagnostic arthroscopy revealed a degenerative Outerbridge grade 4 lesion measuring approximately 20 × 10 mm over the medial femoral condyle with minimal fibrocartilage formation in the area of previous microfracture. This lesion was treated with two 11-mm TruFit CB implants through a medial parapatellar arthrotomy (no patellar eversion).

The MRI at 3 months showed the implant flush with the native articular surface with incomplete "fill" of the repaired articular surface. Cartilage-sequence MRI at 14 months showed maturation of the repair tissue at the site of the implant, with nearly full restoration of the contour of the medial femoral condyle. Incomplete cancellous osseous integration also was seen. Slight hyperintensity was noted in the superficial phase of the treated site when compared to the native articular cartilage, but no discernable

fissures were noted at the interface with the native cartilage.

At 24-month follow-up, the patient had full range of motion without pain, could perform activities of daily living pain free, and was able to bike and swim.

## Summary

The TruFit implant is a synthetic biphasic matrix implant that is commercially available for filling osteochondral defects in the United States. Industry-based, preclinical studies in a goat model demonstrated excellent tissue fill, the formation of hyaline-like repair tissue,

and incorporation into host bone. To date, no safety issues or loose implants have been noted. A review of the Hospital for Special Surgery Cartilage Registry database identified no adverse events or implant loosening in patients treated with a backfill or direct lesion indication. It must be emphasized that using this implant for the direct treatment of chondral defects is an off-label indication for the product in the United States; it is approved only for the filling of bony voids, such as those created at the donor site during traditional osteochondral autograft transplantation. Although optimistic

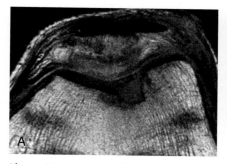
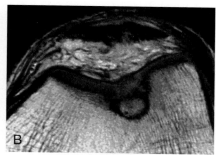

**Figure 7**  **A,** Spin-echo cartilage-sensitive postoperative MRI scan at 3 months. **B,** Cartilage-sensitive MRI scan 12 months after implantation.

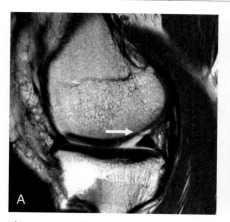
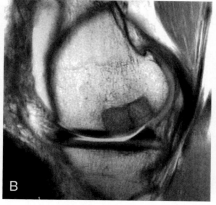
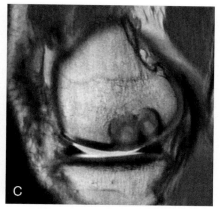

**Figure 8**  **A,** Preoperative MRI demonstrating poor fill 6 months after microfracture of the medial femoral condyle with full-thickness cartilage loss on spin-echo cartilage sequence MRI scan (*arrow*). The defect was treated with two 11-mm TruFit CB plugs. **B,** Three-month postoperative spin-echo cartilage-sequence MRI scan. This MRI scan shows incomplete fill of the cartilage defect and minimal incorporation of the plug into subchondral bone. **C,** Twelve-month postoperative spin-echo cartilage-sequence MRI scan. Note the increased fill of the defect compared with image **(B)**.

about the clinical results of patients treated for symptomatic articular cartilage lesions with this implant, the senior author continues to prospectively collect clinical and MRI data. To date, no patient has required a second-look arthroscopy during which probing and biopsy of the repair tissue could be done. Serial MRI has been used to assess the repair tissue; these MRI studies, although sensitive, do not provide direct evidence of the quality of the tissue filling the site of cartilage injury. Therefore, with only short-term follow-up and no human biopsy studies, the quality and durability of repair tissue formed with the TruFit implant are unknown. Although complications of bioabsorbable implants made from poly($\alpha$-hydroxy esters)[27] have been reported, including inflammatory reaction,[51,52] persistent effusion, early resorption, and breakage,[53] to date no device-related complications have been observed; however, the complication rate with widespread use and long-term follow-up cannot be predicted.

## References

1. Shapiro F, Koide S, Glimcher MJ: Cell origin and differentiation in the repair of full-thickness defects of articular cartilage. *J Bone Joint Surg Am* 1993;75:532-553.

2. Alford JW, Cole BJ: Cartilage restoration: Part 1. Basic science, historical perspective, patient evaluation, and treatment options. *Am J Sports Med* 2005;33:295-306.

3. Alford JW, Cole BJ: Cartilage restoration: Part 2. Techniques, outcomes, and future directions. *Am J Sports Med* 2005;33:443-460.

4. Buckwalter JA, Mankin HJ, Grodzinsky AJ: Articular cartilage and osteoarthritis. *Instr Course Lect* 2005;54:465-480.

5. Mankin HJ: The response of articular cartilage to mechanical injury. *J Bone Joint Surg Am* 1982;64:460-466.

6. Kuo CK, Li WJ, Mauck RL, Tuan RS: Cartilage tissue engineering: Its potential and uses. *Curr Opin Rheumatol* 2006;18:64-73.

7. Tuli R, Li WJ, Tuan RS: Current state of cartilage tissue engineering. *Arthritis Res Ther* 2003;5:235-238.

8. Brittberg M, Peterson L, Sjogren-Jansson E, Tallheden T, Lindahl A: Articular cartilage engineering with autologous chondrocyte transplantation: A review of recent developments. *J Bone Joint Surg Am* 2003;85-A (suppl 3):109-115.

9. Bentley G, Biant LC, Carrington RW, et al: A prospective, randomised comparison of autologous chondrocyte implantation versus mosaicplasty for osteochondral defects in the knee. *J Bone Joint Surg Br* 2003;85:223-230.

10. Knutsen G, Engebretsen L, Ludvigsen TC, et al: Autologous chondrocyte implantation compared with microfracture in the knee: A randomized trial. *J Bone Joint Surg Am* 2004;86-A:455-464.

11. Breinan HA, Martin SD, Hsu HP, Spector M: Healing of canine articular cartilage defects treated with microfracture, a type-II collagen matrix, or cultured autologous chondrocytes. *J Orthop Res* 2000;18:781-789.

12. Horas U, Pelinkovic D, Herr G, Aigner T, Schnettler R: Autologous chondrocyte implantation and osteochondral cylinder transplantation in cartilage repair of the knee joint: A prospective, comparative trial. *J Bone Joint Surg Am* 2003;85-A:185-192.

13. Steadman JR, Rodkey WG, Briggs KK: Microfracture to treat full-thickness chondral defects: Surgical technique, rehabilitation, and outcomes. *J Knee Surg* 2002;15:170-176.

14. Hangody L, Rathonyi GK, Duska Z, Vasarhelyi G, Fules P, Modis L: Autologous osteochondral mosaicplasty: Surgical technique. *J Bone Joint Surg Am* 2004;86-A(suppl 1):65-72.

15. Simonian PT, Sussmann PS, Wickiewicz TL, Paletta GA, Warren RF: Contact pressures at osteochondral donor sites in the knee. *Am J Sports Med* 1998;26:491-494.

16. Hangody L, Fules P: Autologous osteochondral mosaicplasty for the treatment of full-thickness defects of weight-bearing joints: Ten years of experimental and clinical experience. *J Bone Joint Surg Am* 2003;85-A (suppl 2):25-32.

17. Jakob RP, Franz T, Gautier E, Mainil-Varlet P: Autologous osteochondral grafting in the knee: Indication, results, and reflections. *Clin Orthop Relat Res* 2002;401:170-184.

18. Feczko P, Hangody L, Varga J, et al: Experimental results of donor site filling for autologous osteochondral mosaicplasty. *Arthroscopy* 2003;19:755-761.

19. Hangody L, Feczkó P, Bartha L, Bodó G, Kish G: Mosaicplasty for the treatment of articular defects of the knee and ankle. *Clin Orthop Relat Res* 2001;391:S328-S336.

20. Bobic V: Arthroscopic osteochondral autograft transplantation in anterior cruciate ligament reconstruction: A preliminary clinical study. *Knee Surg Sports Traumatol Arthrosc* 1996;3:262-264.

21. Gortz S, Bugbee WD: Allografts in articular cartilage repair. *J Bone Joint Surg Am* 2006;88:1374-1384.

22. Pearce SG, Hurtig MB, Clarnette R, Kalra M, Cowan B, Miniaci A: An investigation of 2 techniques for optimizing joint surface congruency using multiple cylindrical osteochondral autografts. *Arthroscopy* 2001;17:50-55.

23. Duchow J, Hess T, Kohn D: Primary stability of press-fit-implanted osteochondral grafts: Influence of graft size, repeated insertion, and harvesting technique. *Am J Sports Med* 2000;28:24-27.

24. Malda J, Woodfield TB, van der Vloodt F, et al: The effect of PEGT/PBT scaffold architecture on oxygen gradients in tissue engineered cartilaginous constructs. *Biomaterials* 2004;25:5773-5780.

25. Mikos AG, Bao Y, Cima LG, Ingber DE, Vacanti JP, Langer R: Preparation of poly(glycolic acid) bonded fiber structures for cell attachment and transplantation. *J Biomed Mater Res* 1993;27:183-189.

26. Muschler GF, Nakamoto C, Griffith LG: Engineering principles of clinical cell-based tissue engineering. *J Bone Joint Surg Am* 2004;86:1541-1558.

27. Bostman OM, Pihlajamaki HK: Adverse tissue reactions to bioabsorbable fixation devices. *Clin Orthop Relat Res* 2000;371:216-227.

28. Almarza AJ, Athanasiou KA: Seeding techniques and scaffolding choice for tissue engineering of the temporomandibular joint disk. *Tissue Eng* 2004;10:1787-1795.

29. Almarza AJ, Athanasiou KA: Design characteristics for the tissue engineering of cartilaginous tissues. *Ann Biomed Eng* 2004;32:2-17.

30. Almarza AJ, Athanasiou KA: Seeding techniques and scaffolding choice for tissue engineering of the temporomandibular joint disk. *Tissue Eng* 2004;10:1787-1795.

31. Cima LG, Vacanti JP, Vacanti C, Ingber D, Mooney D, Langer R: Tissue engineering by cell transplantation using degradable polymer substrates. *J Biomech Eng* 1991;113:143-151.

32. Cohen S, Bano MC, Cima LG, et al: Design of synthetic polymeric structures for cell transplantation and tissue engineering. *Clin Mater* 1993;13:3-10.

33. Freed LE, Grande DA, Lingbin Z, Emmanual J, Marquis JC, Langer R: Joint resurfacing using allograft chondrocytes and synthetic biodegradable polymer scaffolds. *J Biomed Mater Res* 1994;28:891-899.

34. Fuchs JR, Terada S, Hannouche D, Ochoa ER, Vacanti JP, Fauza DO: Engineered fetal cartilage: Structural and functional analysis in vitro. *J Pediatr Surg* 2002;37:1720-1725.

35. Grande DA, Halberstadt C, Naughton G, Schwartz R, Manji R: Evaluation of matrix scaffolds for tissue engineering of articular cartilage grafts. *J Biomed Mater Res* 1997;34:211-220.

36. Klompmaker J, Jansen HW, Veth RP, Nielsen HK, de Groot JH, Pennings AJ: Porous polymer implants for repair of full-thickness defects of articular cartilage: An experimental study in rabbit and dog. *Biomaterials* 1992;13:625-634.

37. Li YJ, Chung EH, Rodriguez RT, Firpo MT, Healy KE: Hydrogels as artificial matrices for human embryonic stem cell self-renewal. *J Biomed Mater Res A* 2006;79:1-5.

38. Behrens P, Bitter T, Kurz B, Russlies M: Matrix-associated autologous chondrocyte transplantation/implantation (MACT/MACI): 5-year follow-up. *Knee* 2006;13:194-202.

39. Marlovits S, Striessnig G, Kutscha-Lissberg F, et al: Early postoperative adherence of matrix-induced autologous chondrocyte implantation for the treatment of full-thickness cartilage defects of the femoral condyle. *Knee Surg Sports Traumatol Arthrosc* 2005;13:451-457.

40. Trattnig S, Pinker K, Krestan C, Plank C, Millington S, Marlovits S: Matrix-based autologous chondrocyte implantation for cartilage repair with HyalograftC: Two-year follow-up by magnetic resonance imaging. *Eur J Radiol* 2006;57:9-15.

41. van Susante JL, Buma P, Homminga GN, van den Berg WB, Veth RP: Chondrocyte-seeded hydroxyapatite for repair of large articular cartilage defects: A pilot study in the goat. *Biomaterials* 1998;19:2367-2374.

42. Vacanti CA, Langer R, Schloo B, Vacanti JP: Synthetic polymers seeded with chondrocytes provide a template for new cartilage formation. *Plast Reconstr Surg* 1991;88:753-759.

43. Mouw JK, Case ND, Guldberg RE, Plaas AH, Levenston ME: Variations in matrix composition and GAG fine structure among scaffolds for cartilage tissue engineering. *Osteoarthritis Cartilage* 2005;13:828-836.

44. Niederauer GG, Slivka MA, Leatherbury NC, et al: Evaluation of multiphase implants for repair of focal osteochondral defects in goats. *Biomaterials* 2000;21:2561-2574.

45. Slivka MA, Leatherbury NC, Kieswetter K, Niederauer GG: Porous, resorbable, fiber-reinforced scaffolds tailored for articular cartilage repair. *Tissue Eng* 2001;7:767-780.

46. Butnariu-Ephrat M, Robinson D, Mendes DG, Halperin N, Nevo Z: Resurfacing of goat articular cartilage by chondrocytes derived from bone marrow. *Clin Orthop Relat Res* 1996;330:234-243.

47. Jackson DW, Halbrecht J, Proctor C, Van Sickle D, Simon TM: Assessment of donor cell and matrix survival in fresh articular cartilage allografts in a goat model. *J Orthop Res* 1996;14:255-264.

48. Jackson DW, Lalor PA, Aberman HM, Simon TM: Spontaneous repair of full-thickness defects of articular cartilage in a goat model: A preliminary study. *J Bone Joint Surg Am* 2001;83-A:53-64.

49. Potter HG, Foo LF: Magnetic resonance imaging of articular cartilage: Trauma, degeneration, and repair. *Am J Sports Med* 2006;34:661-677.

50. Potter HG, Linklater JM, Allen AA, Hannafin JA, Haas SB: Magnetic resonance imaging of articular cartilage in the knee: An evaluation with use of fast-spin-echo imaging. *J Bone Joint Surg Am* 1998;80:1276-1284.

51. Bostman OM, Pihlajamaki HK: Late foreign-body reaction to an intraosseous bioabsorbable polylactic acid screw: A case report. *J Bone Joint Surg Am* 1998;80:1791-1794.

52. Burkart A, Imhoff AB, Roscher E: Foreign-body reaction to the bioabsorbable suretac device. *Arthroscopy* 2000;16:91-95.

53. Sassmannshausen G, Sukay M, Mair SD: Broken or dislodged poly-L-lactic acid bioabsorbable tacks in patients after SLAP lesion surgery. *Arthroscopy* 2006;22:615-619.

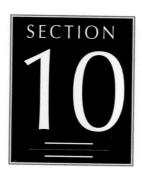

# SECTION 10

# Orthopaedic Medicine

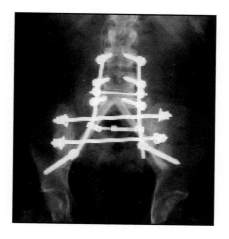

# Metabolic Bone Disease: A Review and Update

Henry J. Mankin, MD
Carole J. Mankin, MSLS

## Abstract

*Understanding the structure and formation of bone and the metabolic diseases that cause intrinsic biochemical alterations and ultimate damage to the skeletal system is an essential part of orthopaedic education and knowledge. Metabolic bone diseases such as rickets, osteomalacia, renal osteodystrophy, hyperparathyroidism, and osteoporosis often lead to subtle alterations in the patient's clinical status and to severe and disabling changes in the patient's bone structure. It is essential that orthopaedists recognize these conditions, provide a correct diagnosis, and use appropriate preventive and therapeutic treatments.*

**Instr Course Lect 2008;57:575-593.**

An understanding of the mechanisms of rickets, osteomalacia, renal osteodystrophy, osteoporosis, and hyperparathyroidism requires knowledge of how bones develop and become mineralized and of the methods involved in mineral exchanges with the body fluids.

## Bone Structure, Formation, Destruction, and Normal Metabolism

The organic structure of the bony tissue consists of type I collagen, which is closely cross-linked and relatively insoluble.[1-4] The collagen fibers define the shape and structural characteristics of the bone.[5] Impregnated within the collagen fibers are tiny crystals of an inorganic mineral, calcium hydroxyapatite ($Ca_{10}[PO_4][OH_2]$), with dimensions of $50 \times 100 \times 200$ Å.[6] Crystal deposition in collagen is mediated by osteonectin, bone sialoprotein, and tetranectin and is inhibited by osteopontin.[2,3,5,6] The crystals are in direct contact with the body's extracellular fluid and represent a highly reactive reservoir for free exchange with extracellular fluid and both rapid deposition and dissolution under circumstances of body fluid alterations.[3-9]

Bone is synthesized by osteoblasts, maintained by osteocytes, and destroyed by osteoclasts. Each of these cell types differs in origin, anatomic structure, and ability to alter the collagen configuration of the bone, thereby affecting its mineral content.[1,4,10] The osteoblast is a large cell with a prominent nucleus and a well-developed endoplasmic reticulum. Osteoblasts originate from osteoprogenitor cells, which are converted from stem cells under the influence of parathyroid hormone (PTH), transforming growth factor-beta (TGF-β), fibroblast growth factor (FGF), bone morphogenetic proteins (BMPs), insulin-like growth factors I and II, platelet-derived growth factor (PDGF), and prostaglandins.[3,10,11] The bone-producing cells acting under the influence of

osteoadherin, hyaluronan, osteonectin, osteopontin, and bone sialoprotein are capable of synthesizing type I collagen and organizing its structure into a bony segment.[7,10] The osteoblasts are laid down on the surface of a bone but synthesize osseous material at all margins and are soon surrounded by a bony structure that limits their contact with the extracellular fluids.[1] The cells, now known as osteocytes, develop multiple processes extending on all sides that reach from one cell to adjacent cells. The processes serve as a system for the transfer of nutrients from the adjacent blood supply.[1,4] The osteoclast is a multinucleated giant cell with centripetally located nuclei and site-specific ruffled border processes that destroy bone.[5,10,12,13] The osteoclast is formed from monocytes under the influence of receptor activator of nuclear factor-kappaB (RANK), which is activated by a ligand (RANKL) and is under the influence of c-Fos, osteocalcin, and other factors.[13] It is the only cell capable of destroying bone and is activated by PTH and 1,25-dihydroxyvitamin D and inhibited by calcitonin.

Four important rules describe the metabolism of bone in relation to calcium, phosphorus, and the body's mineral system.[4] (1) Calcium acid phosphate ($Ca^{++}HPO_4^{=}$) is not freely soluble in water; therefore, if either the calcium or phosphate concentrations or both exceed the critical solubility product, the material will be deposited as an insoluble calcium salt in soft tissues or other sites.[4,6,8] (2) Bone formation and destruction are closely coupled in maintaining bone health.[4,5,8,13] This coupling relationship is in part a function of and closely related to concentrations of TGF-β, BMPs, and insulin-like growth factors I and II.[3,5,10-12,14] (3) The nervous system is very responsive to the concentration of calcium in the extracellular fluid.[4] If calcium increases beyond the standard level, motor function, reflexes, and mental capacity will diminish and the patient will become paralyzed and unresponsive. Hypercalcemia can result in systolic cardiac arrest. If the calcium level diminishes, muscle and reflex activity increases and the patient develops central nervous system irritability and convulsive disorders; however, cardiac function slows and death occurs in diastole.[4,15] (4) Calcium in a lumen such as the gastrointestinal tract or the glomerulus cannot cross a cell boundary to enter the extracellular fluid without a transport system.[1,16,17] The body's transport system has two active components. The first component is PTH, which causes adenosine triphosphate to convert to adenosine monophosphate; this process opens up the cell membrane to calcium ions and also causes mitochondrions to release their calcium into the cell.[5,17] However, the calcium ions require a second system, which is activated by 1,25-dihydroxyvitamin D, to enter the extracellular fluid.[9,18-20] This material, calbindin or calcium-binding protein, which is synthesized in the kidney in situations of low serum calcium, low serum phosphate, and a high PTH level, activates messenger RNA to synthesize a calcium transport protein.[4,16] Calbindin

transports the calcium out of the cell and into the extracellular fluid. The system also works in the kidney to transport calcium out of the glomerulus by tubular reabsorption and back into the body's fluids, before urinary excretion.[21-23] The process is less clearly defined in the bone, where the action of low levels of PTH and 1,25-dihydroxyvitamin D appears to be responsible for a release of calcium from the calcium hydroxyapatite crystal by a process best described as crystallysis; however, if the PTH level rises significantly, the bone is subject to a gross destructive process caused by osteoclastic resorption.[17,24,25]

### Vitamin D Activities

In the absence of direct administration of vitamin D, there are two natural sources of the vitamin that require activation.[18,19] The first is known as provitamin D or ergosterol, a material absorbed from the gastrointestinal tract.[18,19] A second form of provitamin D, known as 7-dehydrocholesterol, is synthesized from cholesterol in the liver.[18,19] Both forms are lodged in the malpighian layer of the skin.[19] The two agents are activated by exposure to ultraviolet light at 315 nm. The two precursors become vitamins $D_2$ and $D_3$, respectively, and then become active as calcium transporters in the same manner as that of administered exogenous vitamin D.

Vitamins $D_2$ and $D_3$ pass through the liver and are acted on by microsomal P450 enzymes to become 25-hydroxyvitamin D.[26] This agent then enters the kidney. In the presence of low serum calcium, low phosphorus levels, and a high concentration of PTH, the 25-hydroxyvitamin D is converted to 1,25-dihydroxyvitamin D by exposure to oxygen, magnesium, re-

duced pyridine nucleotide, and 25-vitamin D-1-hydrolase.[18-20,26] The 1,25-dihydroxyvitamin D is the major actor in the calcium transport system from the gastrointestinal tract, the tubular reabsorption system in the glomerulus, and crystallysis in the bone. If there is no need for increased calcium transport (as determined by a high level of calcium, a high level of phosphate, or a low concentration of PTH), the 25-hydroxyvitamin D is converted to 24,25- or 25,26-dihydroxyvitamin D, both of which are relatively inactive.[4,19,20]

### The Role of PTH

PTH is an active component in the calcium and phosphorus metabolic system.[17,24] The lower the calcium concentration in the body fluids, the more PTH is synthesized and secreted. A high level of PTH is necessary to synthesize 1,25-dihydroxyvitamin D in the kidney. Together, PTH and 1,25-dihydroxyvitamin D are responsible for the transport of calcium across the distal duodenal and proximal jejunal gut cells. PTH working with 1,25-dihydroxyvitamin D is also responsible for increasing the tubular reabsorption of calcium from the kidney and is likely responsible for the process that releases calcium from the calcium hydroxyapatite crystals in bone.[4,19,20] PTH is also responsible for activating the osteoclasts to free and destroy the calcium hydroxyapatite crystal and to completely destroy the bone structure adjacent to the osteoclast cell to form a defect in the bone known as a Howship's lacuna.[2,20,25] PTH is associated with an increase in calcium concentration that may be sufficiently high to cause soft tissue and bony deposits of calcium salts (such as in renal osteodystrophy, nephrocalcinosis, and other disorders). However, the action of PTH on the system for the tubular reabsorption of phosphate (TRP) in the kidney is a major protective mechanism for preventing an abnormal rise in calcification.[17,23,24] In a healthy kidney, PTH will lower the percentage of TRP, causing a hyperphosphaturic state that results in hypophosphatemia and reduces the likelihood of abnormal calcium deposits, even in instances of a high level of serum calcium.[17,23,26]

Calcitonin is a material synthesized by the C cells of the thyroid gland in humans and is another agent that is active in the calcium control mechanisms related to vitamin D and PTH.[27-29] If sufficient calcitonin is present, the material acts to markedly decrease calcium reabsorption in the renal tubule and decreases the rate of bone destruction, principally by reducing the number of osteoclasts in bone and inhibiting their action.[28,29] Calcitonin acts on osteoclasts to enhance adenylate cyclase activity and stimulate cyclic adenosine monophosphate accumulation, which markedly interferes with osteoclastic destruction of bone.[28] In theory, calcitonin acts opposite to PTH; therefore, if it were present in sufficient concentration it would respond to an increased concentration of calcium, just as PTH responds to a lower concentration. Although the system is very active and competent in avian creatures (who daily lay eggs with a calcium carbonate shell), it works poorly in humans. Externally administered calcitonin can effectively treat patients with increased bone loss associated with certain types of tumors, osteoporosis, or Paget's disease, but the naturally produced material is ineffective in combating the complications as-

sociated with the pathologic increase in serum calcium in humans.[4,27,28]

### Phosphate Metabolism
Phosphate is prevalent in the human diet and only a few materials, such as aluminum, interfere with its absorption.[30-32] Phosphate is absorbed lower in the gastrointestinal tract than calcium. Although such agents as vitamin D have some effect on absorption, most ingested phosphate is absorbed.[4,21,30] There are few controls on phosphate in the extracellular space with the exception of the tubular reabsorption mechanism in the kidney, which is very sensitive to PTH.[31] The higher the PTH level, the lower the TRP level, leading to hyperphosphaturia and hypophosphatemia, both of which help to prevent deposition of calcified material in bones and soft tissues.[4,15,31,32]

## Rickets, Osteomalacia, and Renal Osteodystrophy
Rickets and osteomalacia are disorders of bone mineral metabolism, which occur as a result of insufficient amounts of available calcium, phosphorus, and/or vitamin D, all of which are required to maintain normal skeletal structure. Rickets occurs in childhood and affects both the bone structure and the epiphyseal cartilage. The adult form of the disease is known as osteomalacia. The term renal osteodystrophy describes the bone lesions associated with chronic renal disease, which are partly those of osteomalacia but are often associated with severe hyperparathyroidism, another cause of structural loss of bone from the skeleton.

### Rickets and Osteomalacia
Nutritional rickets and osteomalacia are the oldest and best known forms of hypocalcemic disorders. Several

causes for the syndromes are genetic, some are associated with other disorders, some are related to unusual dietary or drug-related syndromes, and some have an unknown cause.

Nutritional rickets was formerly the most common form of the disease and resulted from a diminished intake of vitamin D.[4,19,33-37] Most cases occurred in relation to dietary restrictions; however, other factors, including decreased stomach acidity, chelating agents such as phytate or oxalate in the diet, rapid transport of food through the gastrointestinal tract (dumping syndrome), chronic liver disease, aluminum toxicity (leading to phosphate loss), and chronic bowel disorders, have been implicated as causes of the disease.[1,4,9,30,33,34,38-40] If dietary vitamin D is insufficient, the synthesis of 1,25-dihydroxyvitamin D is decreased and leads to a diminished intestinal absorption of calcium.[6,8,9,15-17,21,24,26,34,40] As a result, the patient develops hypocalcemia, which causes a secondary hyperparathyroidism that brings the calcium level relatively close to normal.[4,41] The increased parathyroid activity causes the phosphate concentration to diminish as a result of decreased TRP and results in hyperphosphaturia and hypophosphatemia.[4,6,23,24,38,42,43] The bone changes are related to a decrease in the available calcium and phosphorus needed to synthesize calcium hydroxyapatite and a secondary hyperparathyroidism, which causes osteoclastic destruction of the existing bony structure.[4,5,12,17,24,40,44-46] These findings are characteristic for nutritional rickets or osteomalacia associated with an inadequate intake of vitamin D.

There are four forms of vitamin D-resistant rickets or osteomalacia, which result in similar changes to those that occur in the nutritional form of the disease. One form is a sex-linked genetic error with homologies to endopeptidases, which results in an error in phosphate reabsorption (increased TRP).[47] This increase in TRP causes hyperphosphaturia and hypophosphatemia syndromes and leads to a rachitic syndrome, which can be intractable, particularly if only vitamin D is used as treatment.[47,48] The syndrome will respond best to the administration of high concentrations of neutral phosphate; patients can be cured with this protocol even without the administration of increased amounts of vitamin D.[4]

Two other forms of vitamin D-resistant rickets are known as type 1 and type 2 dependent rickets, which are associated with two forms of failure of production or function of 1,25-dihydroxyvitamin D.[20,22,26,49-51] Type 1 dependent rickets or osteomalacia is characterized by a failure of the kidney to synthesize 1,25-dihydroxyvitamin D in sufficient quantities to prevent rachitic disease. In type 2 dependent disease, a sufficient amount of 1,25-dihydroxyvitamin D is synthesized, but the intestinal absorptive cells fail to recognize the material and the patient may become profoundly rachitic or osteomalacic. Both of these disorders are sometimes associated with alopecia.[49,51] Either type 1 or type 2 dependent disease can be effectively treated with exogenously administered 1,25-dihydroxyvitamin D.[51,52]

Another form of vitamin D-resistant rickets is related to the syndrome of renal tubular acidosis, which is characterized by a hyperchloremic, hyponatremic, hypocalcemic acidosis with alkaline urine. There are two forms of this disease: distal (classic), which represents a failure of hydrogen ion production in the distal tubule, and proximal, which is related to a bicarbonate wastage.[4,21,38,46] Either of these syndromes can be effectively treated by systemic alkalinization using oral agents to reverse the acidic state and restore the calcium concentration to normal.

Four additional causes of rickets and osteomalacia that are related to other conditions include two causes associated with genetic disorders. These include resistant rickets in patients with multiple sites of fibrous dysplasia, and a second type of resistant rickets in patients with type 1 neurofibromatosis.[4,35,53] A third form is an unusual disorder, known as oncologic osteomalacia, in which some cytokines produced by benign or malignant bone or soft-tissue tumors seem to interfere with the renal production of 1,25-dihydroxyvitamin D. This interference results in intractable rickets or osteomalacia.[54,55] The syndrome has recently been associated with FGF-23.[56] When the tumor is completely removed, the rickets and osteomalacia disappear; however, the conditions return shortly after the tumor recurs.

Another unusual cause of rachitic or osteomalacic syndrome is related to anticonvulsant medication. Patients with convulsive disorders are given an array of anticonvulsant medications, most of which interfere with microsomal P450 enzymes in the liver.[4,24,35,57] This interference results in a decrease in the synthesis of 25-hydroxyvitamin D, which leads to a reduction in the synthesis of 1,25-vitamin D and, as a result, a slowly developing rachitic syndrome. This syndrome is mild; however, diminished levels of serum calcium result in a more easily stimulated muscular, peripheral, and central nervous system, which increases the likelihood of convulsions and may lead to serious overuse of anticonvulsant agents.[36] The syndrome can be reversed by administration of sufficient amounts of vitamin D or more importantly, 1,25-hydroxyvitamin D.[52]

### Histologic Changes in the Bony and Epiphyseal Structures

Rachitic or osteomalacic disorders result in marked thinning of the cortices and diminished amounts of medullary bone.[3-5,31,33,35,58] The bony architecture is characterized by the presence of thinned segments (somewhat irregular in structure) and the presence of osteoid seams.[3,4,35] (Figure 1). The osteoid seams are thin layers of poorly calcified or uncalcified bone surrounding the calcified segment so that the staining characteristic with hematoxylin and eosin or other staining methods shows a striking alteration in coloration. Although osteoid seams are not specifically diagnostic of rickets or osteomalacia, they are usually so marked in extent and so uniformly present that they serve as a major histologic characteristic of the disease.[4,58] The presence of markedly increased concentrations of osteoid may be seen in transverse linear defects in the cortex, which is notable on histologic study and radiographs. These lytic areas are usually located in the concave sides of the long bones, the neck of the femur, pubic and ischial rami, the axillary border of the scapula, and the ribs. The lesions are known as Looser's lines, umbauzonen, or Milkman pseudofractures.[35,58] With increased parathyroid activity, osteoclasts increase in number and bone destruction (with some forms of rickets and osteomalacia) may dominate the histologic picture.[4,35,36,38,45]

Structural changes in the epiphyseal plates are quite remarkable and are virtually diagnostic for rick-

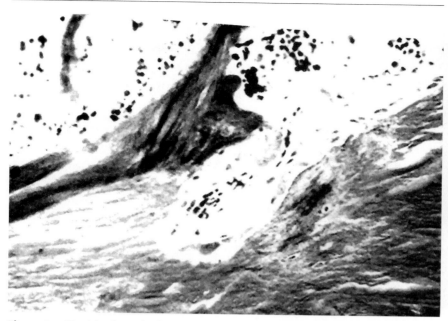

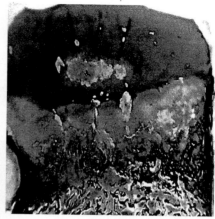

**Figure 2** Epiphysis and metaphysis of the humerus of a child with rickets who died. There is axial enlargement of the epiphyseal cartilage and irregular extension into the metaphysis. Bone formation is irregular (hematoxylin and eosin, ×30).

**Figure 1** The histologic findings in a bone segment from the femur of a patient with rickets. Note the irregularity of the bone structure but especially the osteoid seam, seen as a dark portion of the bone segment adjacent to the marrow space (hematoxylin and eosin, ×150).

ets in growing children. The resting and proliferative zones are relatively normal in appearance, but there is a marked increase in the size and the number of cells in the intermediate zone, with a profligate profusion of cell organization and structure. The zone of provisional calcification has very little calcific material within it, and the zone of primary spongiosa has small, irregular trabeculae with little bone and wide osteoid seams. The axial height of the epiphyseal cartilage is much larger than normally present, and it may extend far into the metaphysis of the underlying bone[4] (Figure 2). This characteristic is especially true for anatomic sites of rapid growth such as the distal femur, proximal tibia, and proximal radius, where the epiphyseal center is much longer and wider than normal. When structural changes occur in the ribs, marked enlargement of the costochondral

junction is produced with extension of the cartilage deep into the rib structure (Figure 3). This change results in the marked prominence of the junctions of the bone with cartilage at the rib ends, which is described clinically as the rachitic rosary.[3,4,35,36,45,58]

### Clinical Findings

By definition, rickets is a disease of childhood; however, it rarely occurs in infants younger than 6 months.[4,23,34,35,37,40] Rickets more frequently occurs in children from countries with cold climates or in those from impoverished families.[33,37,40] Children with nutritional rickets have a history of inadequate vitamin supplementation and diets limited in foods containing vitamin D or ergosterol.[37,40] These children are usually small for their age, are lethargic, apathetic, and irritable, and sometimes report severe bone pain associated with muscular hyperto-

nia. Back pain and spinal deformity may be a prominent finding. Physical examination shows short stature, prominence of the frontal bones, abdominal protrusion, and tender bones and joints.[4,33,37,40] In many patients age 2 years or older, the most striking features are bowing or knock-knee deformities of the lower extremities and forearms; prominence and tenderness of the epiphyseal portions of the distal femur, proximal tibia, and distal radius; multiple costochondral enlargements (the rachitic rosary), and back deformities[37,40] (Figure 4). Fractures are common. Laboratory studies usually show low levels of calcium and phosphate and a high concentration of PTH. Vitamin D levels are low, and the percentage of TRP is usually low.[4,37,40]

Most patients with adult osteomalacia are elderly persons with an inadequate dietary intake of calcium, vitamin D, or phosphate; people who have undergone complex abdominal surgery for ulcers or excessive weight; those with dumping

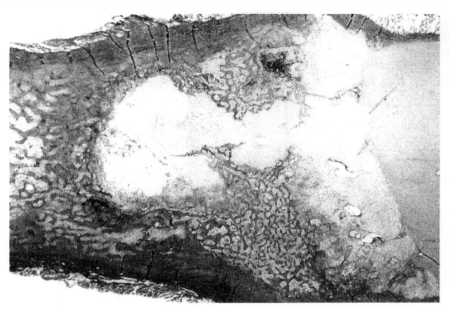

**Figure 3** Histologic findings in the costochondral junction of a patient with severe rickets. The epiphyseal cartilage extends far into the rib structure, and the bone is expanded, producing the characteristic known clinically as the rachitic rosary (hematoxylin and eosin, ×60).

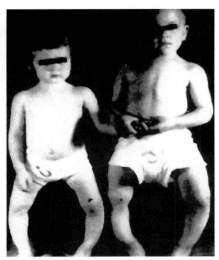

**Figure 4** Photograph of two children with severe untreated rickets who have bilateral bow legs (from the Jaffe Collection).

syndrome, Crohn's disease, or chronic ulcerative colitis; or patients who have undergone resections of large segments of the bowel.[4,8,33,35,36,39,46] Patients usually present with a fracture and are lethargic, irritable, and uncommunicative. They report bone pain and frequently have trouble with ambulation (particularly with stair climbing). Back pain and deformity are common; scoliosis, lordosis, kyphosis, and femoral neck fractures have been described.[4,33,59] The results of laboratory studies are similar to those of rachitic children.

### Imaging Studies

Radiographs or CT scans of the bones show thin cortices with indistinct structural characteristics for the medullary cavities (described as fuzzy texture).[4,33,35,45,58] In children with rickets, bowing or knock-knee deformities are common in the lower extremities, and the epiphyseal plates show an enormous increase in axial height and an increase in width to a lesser extent[4,19,34-37] (Figure 5). Fractures through Looser's lines are common, as are fractures in other sites.[4,37,45,58] Examination of the bones usually shows thin cortices and poorly structured medullary bone as well as many poorly healed and sometimes displaced fractures, particularly in the spine, pelvis, and ribs.[4,35,58]

### Treatment

Treatment of rickets and osteomalacia begins with an awareness of the diseases and the use of the patient's dietary history, physical findings, and laboratory and imaging studies to make the diagnosis. Suspicion of rickets is appropriate in children who are apathetic, are irritable, refuse to walk, and have bone tenderness and pain; this is especially true for those with a disadvantaged background. Adults with poor dietary habits, defective bone structure, and frequent instances of fracture with a history of minimal trauma should be carefully evaluated.[33-37,40] It is estimated that 15% to 20% of elderly patients with fractures of the hip that are allegedly related to osteoporosis also have some degree of osteomalacia.[4,59] Both of these groups should be carefully evaluated with imaging studies and with laboratory tests to determine levels of calcium, phosphorus, 25-hydroxyvitamin D, 1,25-hydroxyvitamin D, PTH, and urinary phosphate.[4,35]

Children with nutritional rickets can be effectively treated with vitamin D at 400 to 800 units per day; the same dose in adults is very effective in preventing the disease.[35,37,46] Children and adults with vitamin D-resistant rickets should be carefully evaluated and then treated with alkalinization for renal tubular acidosis, 1,25-dihydroxyvitamin D for type 1 and type 2 dependent disease, and phosphate for Albright's syndrome.[19,48,49,53]

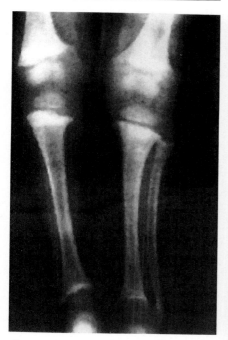

**Figure 5** Radiograph showing changes in the long bones in a child with severe rickets. Note the increase in the axial height of the epiphyseal plate, the irregularity of the bony contour, and cortical irregularity.

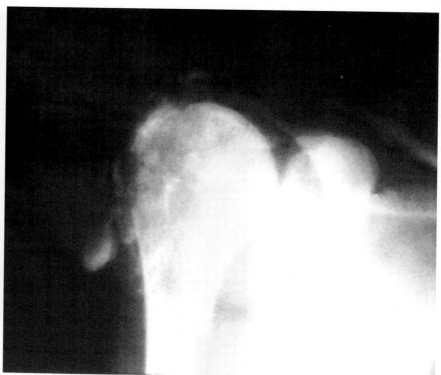

**Figure 6** Radiograph showing calcification in the deltoid in a patient with severe renal osteodystrophy. The increased PTH causes hypercalcemia in patients and increased phosphate, which is related to the renal failure.

## Renal Osteodystrophy

Renal osteodystrophy is a special form of rickets or osteomalacia that is principally caused by chronic renal failure. Although many of the characteristics of this disorder are similar to those of nutritional or vitamin D-resistant rickets or osteomalacia, some special factors exist in terms of the cause of the syndrome, its nature, and some of its complications.[60-62]

The cause of renal osteodystrophy is chronic renal failure with glomerular and tubular damage.[60,63-65] The renal failure causes a significant rise in blood urea nitrogen, creatinine, and phosphate, none of which can be excreted through the damaged kidney.[63-66] The injury to the renal tissue creates a reduced tubular mass, which makes it difficult or impossible for the kidney to synthesize 1,25-dihydroxyvitamin D.[4,60,65,66] This decrease in 1,25-dihydroxyvitamin D leads to a drop in serum calcium, which causes a marked increase in PTH and a resultant, sometimes severe, hyperparathyroidism.[60,63,65] The bones show changes consistent with rickets and osteomalacia and also evidence of hyperparathyroidism with considerable destruction of bone and release of calcium.[4,64] The rise in calcium prevents the symptoms of hypocalcemia, but is worrisome because of the high level of phosphate in the body fluids and the failure of PTH to lower the percentage of TRP. Rising levels of calcium and phosphate lead to deposition of calcific material in several sites, including the conjunctivae, the peripheral arteries and aorta, the skin, and connective tissue.[4,60,65,66] Calcification can occur in the shoulders, knees, or bursae[65,66] (Figure 6).

Histologic evaluation of the bones shows changes of osteomalacia in addition to marked alterations consistent with hyperparathyroidism, including bone destruction, lytic areas filled with osteoclasts, and fractures through Looser's lines. One other characteristic that is not clearly understood is the presence of areas of increased density within the bones.[4] These areas may affect the spine or the long bones and represent an increase in the number of trabeculae, which still show irregularity because of osteoclastic resorption and classic osteoid seams.[4]

Imaging studies show changes consistent with rickets or osteomalacia and also show findings consis-

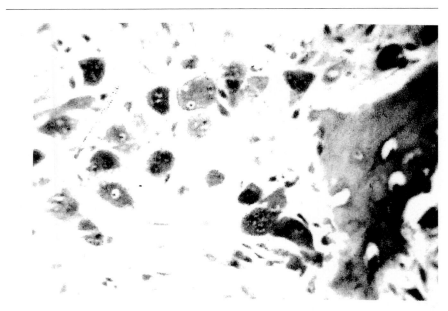

**Figure 7** Histologic findings of "osteoclast feeding frenzy" in a patient with hyperparathyroidism. The adjacent bone has been destroyed (hematoxylin and eosin, ×200).

tent with hyperparathyroidism with a marked decrease in cortical structure and lytic areas, described as brown tumors.[62,67] The spinal segments frequently show marked loss of medullary bone, and multiple fractures often are present. Sites of increased density in the bones should not be interpreted as healing. The most remarkable characteristic is the presence of calcification of the blood vessels, muscles, cartilage, and sometimes tendons.[4,62,67]

The treatment of renal osteodystrophy is dependent on the renal disorder and usually consists of dialysis, although a parathyroidectomy is occasionally required.[68] A new agent called cinacalcet, which blocks the actions of PTH in patients on dialysis, may be effective in reducing parathyroid disorders.[69]

## Primary Hyperparathyroidism

Hyperparathyroidism was for many years a mysterious condition of seemingly unknown cause that often resulted in severe renal, osseous,

cardiac, and neural symptomatology and sometimes death.[24,68,70,71]

### Etiology: Adenoma, Hyperplasia, and Carcinoma

Approximately 80% of patients with primary hyperparathyroidism have adenomas in a single gland.[69,70] These neoplasms are composed of clear cells and less commonly of oxyphil cells. The tumors are small in weight (0.5 to 5.0 g) and are not locally symptomatic. Parathyroid hyperplasia is less common, occurring in approximately 20% of the patients, and involves all four glands; it may histologically resemble an adenoma.[68,70] Carcinomas very rarely cause hyperparathyroidism (in fewer than 1% of patients) and may occur at any age. Carcinomas are locally invasive and may metastasize, usually to lymph nodes but occasionally to the lungs, liver, or bone.[68,70,72,73]

Primary hyperparathyroidism is rare in children and usually occurs in patients older than 35 years.[72,74]

The disease appears to be more common in women (especially postmenopausal women) than men.[75-77] Hyperparathyroidism may occur with two familial disorders, known as multiple endocrine neoplasia.[78-81]

### Clinical Findings

Regardless of whether the patient has primary or genetic disease and whether the lesion consists of an adenoma, hyperplasia, or carcinoma, clinical results are similar. Signals resulting from abnormal serum concentrations of calcium or phosphorus are ignored by the body.[4,68,72,73] PTH is produced in excessive concentration and acts as previously described to increase the calcium absorption in the gastrointestinal tract, increase the renal tubular reabsorption of calcium in the kidney, and increase the osteoclastic destruction of bone, all of which lead to an often extraordinary increase in the serum calcium[24,68,71,72] (Figure 7). In the presence of normal renal function, this process is associated with a decrease in the serum phosphorus related to the marked diminution in the TRP.[4,21,68,70]

The hypercalcemia that occurs in this syndrome sometimes causes profound changes in neuromuscular status that are characterized by lethargy, confusion, impaired mentation, depression, memory loss, and muscular weakness.[68,70,82,83] Bone changes are sometimes striking and consist of osteopenia observed on radiographs and with subperiosteal resorption of the tufts and digits of the hands and feet.[4,70,84] Fractures of long bones, clavicles, ribs, and the pelvis are common.[4,68,84] Because the disease appears to be more common in postmenopausal women, the findings may be confused with osteoporosis, except for the presence of erosions of the hand bones, the presence of a "salt and pepper skull," and especially brown tumors, which consist of lytic areas within the bones, sometimes with expansion of the cortex and pathologic fractures[4,68,76,84] (Figures 8 and 9). Renal manifestations are common and may include mild renal tubular acidosis, phosphaturia, aminoaciduria, and glycosuria.[73] Calcification of meniscal and articular cartilage and renal calculi frequently occurs and sometimes is the cause of the presenting complaint.[4,68,85,86] Patients with hyperparathyroidism often report gastrointestinal disorders, including loss of appetite, anorexia, nausea, vomiting, constipation, and sometimes peptic ulceration and pancreatitis.[24,68,70,,87] Occasionally, patients develop heart disorders that can result in death.[88,89]

## Laboratory Diagnosis

Some patients with hyperparathyroidism are asymptomatic and have serum calcium levels that are at times normal or only slightly elevated.[90-94] For these few patients, the only notable finding is the increase in the immunometric analysis for PTH and possibly hypophosphatemia. Most patients have hypercalcemia (as high as 16 mg/dL), often have profound hypophosphatemia, and usually have an increase in alkaline phosphatase.[72,95,96] Urinary findings usually show hypercalciuria, hyperphosphaturia, and mild hyperchloremic acidosis.[4,24,68,70,73,91] The most important study to assess the presence of the disease is measurement of PTH and calcium concentration in the serum.[68,70,73] The presence of a tumor in the neck may be identified with ultrasound, MRI, or, most recently, by a sestamibi or positron emission tomography scan.[75,96-99]

Bone markers frequently show

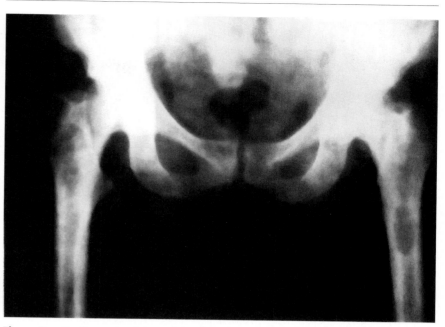

**Figure 8**    Radiograph of the pelvis of a patient with hyperparathyroidism showing thinning and irregularity of the cortices and the presence of lytic foci, known as brown tumors.

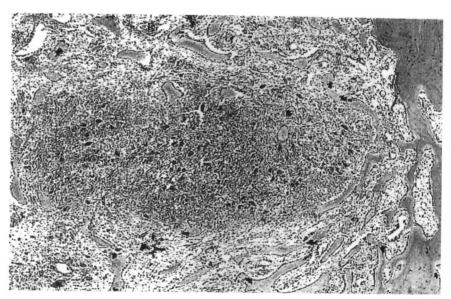

**Figure 9**    The histologic findings of a brown tumor. The cortical bone is poorly structured, and the central area of the medullary cavity has no bone but a large collection of monocytes and osteoclasts (hematoxylin and eosin, ×80).

an increase in alkaline phosphatase and a positive bone scan.[4,68,70,75] Osteocalcin may be elevated along with other markers suggestive of osteoporosis.[68,70] Bone densitometry will almost always show a low value on a dual energy x-ray absorptiometry (DEXA) scan.[72,75,77,91,94,96,100]

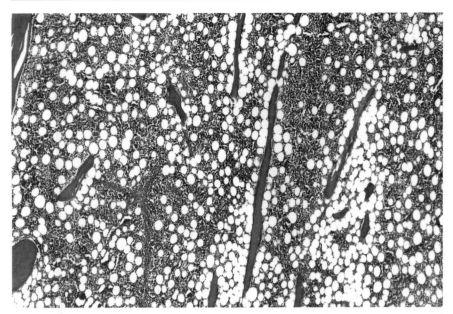

**Figure 10**    Histologic findings in the medullary bone of a patient with osteoporosis. The bone is normal in appearance, but the size of the segments is much smaller than normal (hematoxylin and eosin, ×60).

### Treatment

Every patient with hyperparathyroidism does not require treatment.[72,90-94] Most patients have mild disease.[72,90,92,93] Patients with very mild disease who have normal calcium levels, no overt bone lesions, and virtually no symptoms should have regular reevaluation. For patients suspected of having multiple endocrine neoplasias, a thorough evaluation for, evidence of tumors in other organs is essential. For patients with symptomatic disease and high calcium levels, the treatment may consist of several options. (1) Maintenance of fluid balance and control of renal and central nervous system disorders are essential. Body chemistries should be frequently evaluated to ensure that renal function is normal. Blood levels of calcium, phosphorus, blood urea nitrogen, creatinine, glucose, 25-hydroxyvitamin D, 1,25-dihydroxyvitamin D, PTH, thyroid-stimulating hormone, and liver function studies should be regularly measured.[92,95] (2) Surgical removal of a parathyroid adenoma can be curative.[100-103] Finding the affected gland by sestamibi scanning or positron emission tomography may be necessary to ensure that all hyperplastic or multiple adenomatous sites are present in the surgical field. Minimally invasive surgical techniques can be used for this procedure.[80,101,102,104,105] If necessary, a segment of a gland is implanted at another site to provide a source of PTH following resection of all four glands.[80,101] If there is concern about the possibility of a recurrence after surgery or the presence of a carcinoma, it is reasonable to use CT or ultrasound-guided needle biopsy before wide resection, and PET to determine if nodal or pulmonary disease is present.[97,103,106] Bone lesions sometimes require surgery, particularly if a fracture has occurred or if some type of deformity interferes with function. (3) Therapy with a medical agent can be administered. In the past, calcitonin, which is very effective in interfering with osteoclastic bone destruction, was the principal agent used to reduce potential damage from hypercalcemia and osteitis fibrosa cystica.[95,107] Estrogen therapy may also be useful for postmenopausal women with bone density disorders.[74] Bisphosphonates may be helpful in restoring strength to bone structure and avoiding pathologic fracture.[4,95] Recently, another group of drugs known as calcimimetics have been introduced.[69,108] Thus far, cinacalcet has been the most extensively used agent in this group of drugs and can markedly reduce an increased serum level of calcium in patients with either primary or secondary hyperparathyroidism.[69]

## Osteoporosis

Osteoporosis is one of the most serious current orthopaedic disorders and affects many patients, requiring hospital and rehabilitation services as well as treatment by physicians, nurses, and physiotherapists.

In patients with osteoporosis, the synthesis of bone is diminished and excessive destruction of bone is also likely to occur. These two factors cause bones to become thinner and more prone to fracture[4,109-112] (Figure 10). The loss of bone structure is asymptomatic. Patients do not report pain or disability until a fracture occurs so they are less likely to limit their activities or seek medical care, and physicians are less likely to consider the possibility of potentially serious bone disorders.[4,109,111,112]

### Etiology

Osteoporosis has many causes, including family history. The physician should inquire about the presence of the condition in the parents and grandparents of the patient.[4,109,111,112]

Generally, low body weight is more likely to be associated with osteoporosis than normal or increased weight.[111-113] Several studies have shown that osteoporosis is less likely to occur in patients who have osteoarthritis in multiple sites.[114] There is a high risk for osteoporosis in patients with eating disorders, in smokers, and in those who abuse alcohol (a group at great risk for fractures).[109-111,113,115] Other factors that increase the risk of osteoporosis include chronic physical disuse (such as in patients with extreme physical disability), long-term dietary calcium deficiency, chronic renal disease, diabetes mellitus, metastatic cancer, chronic hyperthyroidism or hypothyroidism, hypogonadism, corticosteroid use, rheumatoid arthritis, Gaucher's disease, Marfan syndrome, Turner's syndrome, osteogenesis imperfecta, homocystinuria, and many other disorders that are characterized by the presence of progressive and at times severe osteopenia.[4,109,110,116-119] However, all of the above cited factors account for fewer than 2% of the patients who present with osteoporosis. Most patients with the classic disease have what is now termed postmenopausal or senile osteoporosis.[4,111]

## Mechanism and Effect of Postmenopausal or Senile Osteoporosis

It is essential to understand the process of bone loss in patients with postmenopausal or senile osteoporosis. Bone continues to accrete in the skeleton until age 30 years. For a 10-year period bones remain stable—bone destruction and bone production are equivalent. At age 40 years, both males and females begin to have cortical and medullary bone loss of approximately 0.3% per year, which remains constant in men throughout life and

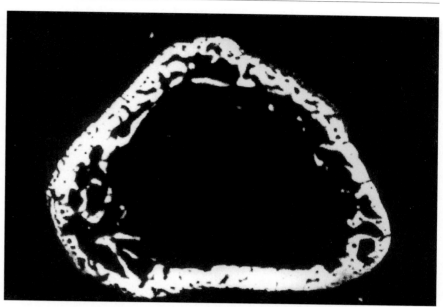

**Figure 11** Cross-sectional radiograph of a bone from a patient with severe osteoporosis. Note the very thin cortices and tiny fractures.

accounts for a loss of 3% of the bony tissue every 10 years. However, postmenopausal women have additional bone loss at 10 times that rate, accounting for a loss of 3% per year for the first 10 years after menopause. After losing 30% of their bone during those 10 years, bone loss returns to the standard rate of 0.3% per year.[4,109-111,115,120-122]

### Osteoporotic Fractures

The decline in bone structure caused by osteoporosis leads to fractures, which are known as fragility fractures or low-energy fractures (Figure 11).[109-111,120-122] Most fractures occur in the spine, wrist, hip, proximal humerus, and ankle and may be associated with alterations in physical stability either from neurologic disease or muscle wasting (Figure 12). Patients report a loss of balance and frequent falling.[123,124] Approximately 1.5 million osteoporotic fractures occur each year in the United States. Of these, 700,000 occur in the spine, 300,000 in

the hip, and 200,000 in the wrist.[109-111,115,125] Of greater concern is the fact that people with one fracture are five times more likely to have a second fracture in the same year; of greatest concern is the statistic that people with a hip fracture have a 20% chance of dying within 1 year.[109,115,121,126,127]

### Bone Mineral Density

Osteoporosis is best defined by determining bone mineral density (BMD), usually by a technique using DEXA.[111,125,128,129] The World Health Organization has defined normal BMD as equal to or less than 1 standard deviation (SD) below the mean for young, healthy individuals with no bone disease. A DEXA score of more than 1 SD but not more than 2.5 SD below normal is considered diagnostic of osteoporosis, whereas a score of more than 2.5 SD below normal represents severe osteoporosis with a very high risk of fracture.[111,125] Recently, ultrasound technology (quantitative ultrasound

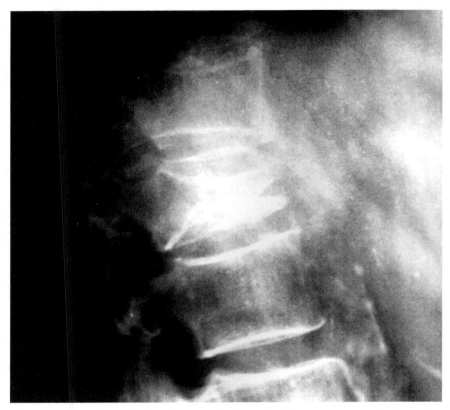

**Figure 12**  Radiograph showing a typical vertebral fracture in an elderly patient with severe osteoporosis.

or broadband ultrasound attenuation) has been introduced to determine BMD; however, there are limitations on how this technology can be applied, and there is concern regarding correlation to the "gold standard" BMD technologies.[130]

### Laboratory Studies

Laboratory studies for osteoporosis are more helpful in ruling out other disorders than for identifying postmenopausal or senile osteoporosis. Calcium, phosphorus, alkaline phosphatase, 25-hydroxyvitamin D, 1,25-dihydroxyvitamin D, and PTH levels are usually normal; if abnormal, osteomalacia or hyperparathyroidism should be suspected.[4] Thyroid function also should be normal; if abnormal, either hyperthyroidism

or hypothyroidism may be the cause.[117] Serum immunoelectrophoresis, hematocrit, and erythrocyte sedimentation rate are usually normal; if abnormal, myeloma, which occasionally presents as diffuse osteopenia, should be ruled out.[4] Some tests are helpful in assessing the extent of the disease. Homocysteine levels may be helpful in defining patients with a high risk for fracture.[111] Bone-specific alkaline phosphatase, osteocalcin, and N-terminal and C-terminal propeptides of type I collagen may indicate reduced bone formation.[128,131] Tartrate-resistant acid phosphatase may indicate bone resorption.[131] Urinary hydroxyproline and pyridine nucleotides may represent evidence of bone resorption, as may N

and C telopeptides of collagen cross-links (NTx and CTx).[128,131] These markers are of less value as diagnostic tools than as tools to assess the effectiveness of treatment.[4]

Imaging studies in patients with osteoporosis are sometimes helpful in defining the extent of the disease, identifying sites of stress fractures, and perhaps most importantly, ruling out other diseases such as other metabolic bone diseases, myeloma, lymphoma, or metastatic carcinoma.[4,110,120,121,132] Radiographs may show thin cortices and poorly defined medullary bone based on the tiny size of the trabecular structures. Vertebral segments are frequently affected and may show not only thin cortices but mild compression fractures of the anterior aspects of the segments that lead to a thoracic kyphotic appearance with a minimal lumbar lordosis (known as dowager's hump).[132] The presence of a clearly displayed Ward's triangle on radiographs of the hip may be indicative of osteoporosis and an impending fracture. Bone scans may be helpful to indicate the presence of impending or stress fractures. Stress fractures may be easier to identify on CT or MRI scans, and an MRI scan of the spine is very useful in assessing the presence of nerve or cord compression.[4,111]

### Treatment

The treatment of osteoporosis primarily depends on the age of the patient, the extent of the disease, and the needs for surgery, physiotherapy, or bracing to treat or prevent fractures.

### Prevention

Exercise is valuable for patients who are at risk for osteoporosis.[113,116,122,133] A young patient at risk for osteoporosis or an elderly patient with osteopenia should be encouraged to exercise daily by walking outdoors or on a treadmill or to use a stationary bicycle. Swimming is helpful but is less likely to facilitate increased bone structure because of the decreased weight bearing afforded by exercising in water. Bracing of the spine or lower extremities can be helpful.[111] The administration of calcium and vitamin D are essential for very young patients.[113,133-136] Adults should ingest at least 1,200 mg of calcium daily and a minimum of 800 units of vitamin D daily. Higher doses of both calcium and vitamin D can be given to elderly patients who have little exposure to sunlight.

The use of estrogen or progesterone or both for premenopausal or postmenopausal women is theoretically an excellent approach to prevention but has some serious potential adverse effects. These drugs probably stimulate osteoblastic activity and may decrease osteoclastic bone loss.[4,111,122,137] The incidence of heart disease, stroke, and breast and uterine cancer is considerably increased for patients who take estrogen, and the risk (especially for breast cancer) is far too great to warrant the use of this type of therapy.[137] Raloxifene has exhibited estrogen-like activity but is less likely to produce side effects similar to those of the hormone. It is, however, less effective than many other available agents.[111,138,139] Calcitonin, which acts to almost completely impede osteoclastic activity, may be valuable in the treatment of osteoporosis but has shown more benefit in treating spinal disease than hip disease; ideally, it should be taken by injection, making administration more difficult.[111,136,140,141] It is now possible to take calcitonin by nasal administration, which may make its use more tolerable.[140]

## Drugs That Decrease Bone Destruction

Bisphosphonates are drugs that interfere with bone resorption by altering the action of the osteoclast on the adjacent bone. Bisphosphonates are believed to induce caspase cleavage of mst-1 kinase during apoptosis.[142] Several drugs are currently available, but alendronate, risedronate, pamidronate, and zoledronate appear to be most useful in preventing bone resorption.

Alendronate is the most frequently used bisphosphonate. Several studies have shown increased BMD and decreased fracture risk with the use of 10 mg of alendronate daily or 70 mg weekly.[143-145] Alendronate may cause gastrointestinal complications, specifically esophagitis and gastritis.[145] The drug must be taken with water, in a standing position, and with no intake of food for approximately 1 hour. Complications and administration requirements make alendronate an unfavorable treatment for some patients. Under these circumstances the use of risedronate, which has a moderately diminished risk of adverse side effects, may be of some value.[146-148] Risedronate is administered in a similar manner as alendronate and is not quite as effective in reducing fracture risk or increasing BMD; however, risedronate may be a better treatment choice for older women.

Two drugs can be given intravenously and thus will reduce the possible effect on the gastrointestinal tract. Pamidronate is administered intravenously at approximately 2- to 3-month intervals and appears to be effective for treatment of osteoporosis, metastatic cancer, and myeloma.[149,150] In a study using pamidronate, BMD was increased and the number of fractures reduced. The most unusual bisphosphonate in terms of protocol is zoledronate, which very aggressively controls osteoclastic resorption of bone and has the most beneficial effect on BMD.[150,151] This drug is administered intravenously once yearly; its effect on the rate of fracture is still under investigation, but it has shown great promise.

## Drugs That Increase Bone Formation

Recombinant PTH (1-34) seems to aid in the management of osteoporosis by increasing bone formation. It is believed that the material activates adenyl cyclase and a number of phospholipases and thus increases the levels of cyclic adenosine monophosphate and calcium, and reduces osteoblast apoptosis.[152-154] The number of osteoclasts is also slightly increased, but the principal action affects bone production, which causes a marked increase in BMD at the recommended dosage. The drug is administered by daily subcutaneous injection and appears to be very effective in preventing fractures. It has been suggested that the use of PTH with bisphosphonates may be more effective than PTH alone, particularly for increasing BMD; this issue is still controversial.[155]

Two other agents are currently undergoing clinical trials. Strontium ranelate appears to stimulate bone formation; patients have been shown to have a lower fracture rate and increased BMD.[136,156] Also under study is low dose recombinant human growth hormone. This agent is administered nasally and may act by stimulating the production of insulin-like growth factor I.[139,157]

Issues concerning the use of all these agents involve questions regarding the duration of use and possible adverse side effects (especially in elderly patients).[146] Oral bisphosphonates may cause significant esophageal complications; recent reports suggest that patients may develop osteonecrosis of the jaw or temporary auditory or visual disorders.[158,159] PTH (1-34) and recombinant PTH may enhance the growth of malignant cells in tumors. The use of estrogen should be avoided; however, raloxifene may be safely used initially, but may in time have some estrogenic effects on the breast and uterus.[4,111,119,137,139]

### Surgical Treatment

Fractures of the wrist can usually be treated with immobilization or the insertion of bone substitute agents such as calcium sulfate, BMP-7, or demineralized bone matrix. Fractures of the spine are much more difficult to treat. If no root or cord complications occur, bracing is usually the only treatment used. Percutaneous kyphoplasty and the use of a balloon to expand the collapsed segment may be performed. Insertion of methylmethacrylate, with coralline or recombinant BMP-2, or a titanium mesh may correct the collapsed segment and diminish the symptoms.[159,160]

Fractures of the hip should usually be reduced and either fixed with appropriate hardware or, in cases of sufficient destruction, total hip replacement may be indicated.[110,121,126,151] The proximal humerus is generally less problematic to treat but may require immobilization, open reduction, or prosthetic replacement.

## Summary

Despite the advances in medicine over the past 50 or more years, metabolic bone disease continues to represent a major challenge for patients, their families, and physicians.

The diseases are sometimes difficult to diagnose. Treatment protocols for patients with rickets, osteomalacia, renal osteodystrophy, hyperparathyroidism, and osteoporosis are highly variable and sometimes difficult to apply. Orthopaedic surgeons treat patients with metabolic bone disease who have pain, deformities, and fractures, which can materially alter the life of the patient. It is essential that orthopaedic surgeons understand metabolic bone diseases and work to administer treatments to provide the best outcomes for patients with these sometimes devastating disorders.

## References

1. Bosk AL: Mineral-matrix interactions in bone and cartilage. *Clin Orthop Relat Res* 1992;281:244-274.

2. Glimcher MJ: The nature of the mineral component of bone and the mechanism of calcification, in Coe FL, Favus ME (eds): *Disorders of Bone and Mineral Metabolism.* New York, NY, Raven Press, 1992, pp 1265-1286.

3. Lian JB, Stein GS, Canalis E, Gehron Robey P, Boskey AL: Bone formation: Osteoblast lineage cells, growth factors, matrix proteins and the mineralization process, in Favus M (ed): *Primer on the Metabolic Bone Diseases and Disorders of Mineral Metabolism,* ed 4. Philadelphia, PA, Lippincott Williams and Wilkins, 1999, pp 14-29.

4. Mankin HJ: *Pathophysiology of Orthopaedic Disease.* Rosemont, IL, American Academy of Orthopaedic Surgeons, 2006.

5. Mundy GR: Bone remodeling, in Favus M (ed): *Primer on the Metabolic Bone Diseases and Disorders of Mineral Metabolism,* ed 4. Philadelphia, PA, Lippincott Williams and Wilkins, 1999, pp 30-38.

6. Boden SD, Kaplan FS: Calcium homeostasis. *Orthop Clin North Am* 1990;21:31-42.

7. Glimcher MJ: The nature of the mineral phase in bone, in Avioli LV, Krane SM (eds): *Metabolic Bone Diseases and Related Disorders,* ed 3. San Diego, CA, Academic Press, 1998, pp 23-95.

8. Broadus AE: Mineral balance and homeostasis, in Favus M (ed): *Primer on the Metabolic Bone Diseases and Disorders of Mineral Metabolism,* ed 4. Philadelphia, PA, Lippincott William and Wilkins, 1999, pp 74-80.

9. Lemann J Jr, Favus M: The intestinal absorption of calcium, magnesium, and phosphate, in Favus MJ (ed): *Primer on the Metabolic Bone Diseases and Disorders of Mineral Metabolism,* ed 4. Philadelphia, PA, Lippincott Williams and Wilkins, 1999, pp 63-66.

10. Katagiri T, Takahashi N: Regulatory mechanism of osteoblast and osteoclast differentiation. *Oral Dis* 2002;8:147-159.

11. Luo Q, Kang Q, Si W, et al: Connective tissue growth factor (CTGF) is regulated by Wnt and bone morphogenetic protein signaling in osteoblast differentiation of mesenchymal stem cells. *J Biol Chem* 2004;279:55958-55968.

12. Raisz LG: Mechanisms and regulation of bone resorption by osteoclastic cells, in Coe FL, Favus ME (eds): *Disorders of Bone and Mineral Metabolism.* New York, NY, Raven Press, 1992, pp 287-311.

13. Rodan GA: Introduction to bone biology. *Bone* 1992;13(suppl 1):S3-6.

14. Hoffmann A, Gross G: BMP signaling pathways in cartilage and bone formation. *Crit Rev Eukaryot Gene Expr* 2001;11:23-45.

15. Wasserman RH, Brindak ME, Buddle MM, et al: Recent studies on the biological actions of vitamin D on intestinal transport and the electrophysiology of peripheral nerve and cardiac muscle. *Prog Clin Biol Res* 1990;332:99-126.

16. Charles P: Calcium absorption and calcium bioavailability. *J Intern Med* 1992;231:161-168.

17. Jüppner H, Brown EM, Kronenburg HM: Parathyroid hormone, in Favus MJ (ed): *Primer on the Metabolic Bone Diseases and Disorders of Mineral Metabolism*, ed 4. Philadelphia, PA, Lippincott Williams and Wilkins, 1999, pp 80-87.

18. DeLuca HF: New concepts of vitamin D functions. *Ann NY Acad Sci* 1992;669:59-68.

19. Holick MF: Vitamin D: Photobiology, metabolism, mechanism of action, and clinical applications, in Favus MJ (ed): *Primer on the Metabolic Bone Diseases and Disorders of Mineral Metabolism*, ed 4. Philadelphia, PA, Lippincott Williams and Wilkins, 1999, pp 92-98.

20. Hollis BW, Clemens TL, Adams JS: Vitamin D metabolites, in Favus MJ (ed): *Primer on the Metabolic Bone Diseases and Disorders of Mineral Metabolism*, ed 4. Philadelphia, PA, Lippincott Williams and Wilkins, 1999, pp 124-127.

21. Bushinsky DA: Calcium, magnesium, and phosphorus: Renal handling and urinary excretion, in Favus MJ (ed): *Primer on the Metabolic Bone Diseases and Disorders of Mineral Metabolism*, ed 4. Philadelphia, PA, Lippincott Williams and Wilkins, 1999, pp 67-73.

22. Friedman PA, Gesek FA: Calcium transport in renal epithelial cells. *Am J Physiol* 1993;264:F181-F198.

23. Yanagawa N, Lee DB: Renal handling of calcium and phosphorus, in Coe FL, Favus ME (eds): *Disorders of Bone and Mineral Metabolism*. New York, NY, Raven Press, 1992, pp 3-40.

24. Bilezikian JP: Primary hyperparathyroidism, in Favus MJ (ed): *Primer on the Metabolic Bone Diseases and Disorders of Mineral Metabolism*, ed 4. Philadelphia, PA, Lippincott Williams and Wilkins, 1999, pp 187-191.

25. Strewler GJ, Nissenson RA: Parathyroid hormone-related protein, in Favus MJ (ed): *Primer on the Metabolic Bone Diseases and Disorders of Mineral Metabolism*, ed 4. Philadelphia, PA, Lippincott Williams and Wilkins, 1999, pp 88-91.

26. Kumar R: Vitamin D metabolism and mechanisms of transport. *J Am Soc Nephrol* 1990;1:30-42.

27. Care AD: The regulation of the secretion of calcitonin. *Bone Miner* 1992; 16:182-185.

28. Martin TJ, Findlay DM, Moseley JM, Sexton PM: Calcitonin, in Avioli LV, Krane SM (eds): *Metabolic Bone Disease and Clinically Related Disorders*. San Diego, CA, Academic Press, 1998, pp 96-123.

29. Matthews JL: Effect of calcitonin on bone cell ultrastructure. *Bone Miner* 1992;16:178-181.

30. Cross HS, Debiec H, Peterlik M: Mechanism and regulation of intestinal phosphate absorption. *Miner Electrolyte Metab* 1990;16:115-124.

31. Khosla S, Kleerekoper M: Biochemical markers of bone turnover, in Favus MJ (ed): *Primer on the Metabolic Bone Diseases and Disorders of Mineral Metabolism*, ed 4. Philadelphia, PA, Lippincott Williams and Wilkins, 1999, pp 128-133.

32. Kumar R: New insights into phosphate homeostasis: Fibroblast growth factor 23 and frizzled-related protein-4 are phosphaturic factors derived from tumors associated with osteomalacia. *Curr Opin Nephrol Hypertens* 2002;11: 547-553.

33. Klein GL: Nutritional rickets and osteomalacia, in Favus MJ (ed): *Primer on the Metabolic Bone Diseases and Disorders of Mineral Metabolism*, ed 4. Philadelphia, PA, Lippincott Williams and Wilkins, 1999, pp 315-318.

34. Ladhani S, Srinivasan L, Buchanan C, Allgrove J: Presentation of vitamin D deficiency. *Arch Dis Child* 2004;89: 781-784.

35. Mundy GR: Osteomalacia and rickets, in *Bone Remodeling and Its Disorders*, ed 2. London, England, Martin Dunitz, 1999, pp 200-207.

36. Reginato AJ, Coquia JA: Musculoskeletal manifestations of osteomalacia and rickets. *Best Pract Res Clin Rheumatol* 2003;17:1063-1080.

37. Weisberg P, Scanlon KS, Li R, Cogswell ME: Nutritional rickets among children in the United States: Review of cases reported between 1996 and 2003. *Am J Clin Nutr* 2004; 80:1697S-1705S.

38. Birge SJ, Avioli LV: Pathophysiology of calcium and phosphate absorptive disorders, in Avioli LV, Krane SM (eds): *Metabolic Bone Disease*, ed 2. Philadelphia, PA, WB Saunders, 1990, pp 196-221.

39. Carmichael KA, Fallon MD, Dalinka M, et al: Osteomalacia and osteitis fibrosa in a man ingesting aluminum hydroxide antacid. *Am J Med* 1984; 76:1137-1143.

40. Lemann J Jr: Intestinal absorption of calcium, magnesium and phosphorus, in Favus M (ed): *Primer on Metabolic Bone Diseases and Disorders of Mineral Metabolism*. Kelseyville, CA, American Society for Bone and Mineral Research, 1990, pp 37-41.

41. Segre GV: Secretion, metabolism and circulating heterogeneity of parathyroid hormone, in Favus M (ed): *Primer on Metabolic Bone Diseases and Disorders of Mineral Metabolism*. Kelseyville, CA, American Society for Bone and Mineral Research, 1990, pp 43-44.

42. Lemann J Jr : The urinary excretion of calcium, magnesium and phosphorus, in Favus M (ed): *Primer on Metabolic Bone Diseases and Disorders of Mineral Metabolism*. Kelseyville, CA, American Society for Bone and Mineral Research, 1990, pp 32-36.

43. Rizzoli R, Ferrari LS, Pizurki L, Caverzasio J, Bonjour JP: Actions of parathyroid hormone and parathyroid hormone-related protein. *J Endocrinol Invest* 1992;15(suppl 6):51-56.

44. Wharton B, Bishop N: Rickets. *Lancet* 2003;362:1389-1400.

45. States LJ: Imaging of rachitic bone. *Endocr Dev* 2003;6:80-92.

46. Bronner F: Current concepts of calcium absorption: An overview. *J Nutr* 1992;122(suppl 3):641-643.

47. Albright F, Butler AM, Bloomberg E: Rickets resistant to vitamin D

therapy. *Am J Dis Child* 1937;54: 529-547.

48. Glorieux FH: Hypophosphatemic vitamin D resistant rickets, in Favus MJ (ed): *Primer on the Metabolic Bone Diseases and Disorders of Mineral Metabolism*, ed 4. Philadelphia, PA, Lippincott Williams and Wilkins, 1999, pp 328-330.

49. Balsan S, Garabedian M, Liberman UA, et al: Rickets and alopecia with resistance to 1,25 dihydroxyvitamin D: Two different clinical syndrome with two different cellular defects. *J Clin Endocrinol Metab* 1983;57: 803-811.

50. Liberman UA, Marx SJ: Vitamin D dependent rickets, in Favus MJ (ed): *Primer on the Metabolic Bone Diseases and Disorders of Mineral Metabolism*, ed 4. Philadelphia, PA, Lippincott Williams and Wilkins, 1999, pp 323-327.

51. Sultan Al-Khenaizan, Vitale P: Vitamin D-dependent rickets type II with alopecia: Two case reports and review of the literature. *Int J Dermatol* 2003; 42:682-685.

52. Wu-Wong JR, Tian J, Goltzman D: Vitamin D analogs as therapeutic agents: A clinical study update. *Curr Opin Investig Drugs* 2004;5:320-326.

53. Chattopadhyay A, Bhansali A, Mohanty SK, Khandelwal N, Mathur SK, Dash RJ: Hypophosphatemic rickets and osteomalacia in polyostotic fibrous dysplasia. *J Pediatr Endocrinol* 2003;16:893-896.

54. Drezner MK: Tumor-induced osteomalacia, in Favus MJ (ed): *Primer on the Metabolic Bone Diseases and Disorders of Mineral Metabolism*, ed 4. Philadelphia, PA, Lippincott Williams and Wilkins, 1999, pp 331-336.

55. Shulman DI, Hahn G, Benator R, et al: Tumor-induced rickets: Usefulness of MR gradient echo recall imaging for tumor localization. *J Pediatr* 2004;144:381-385.

56. Fukumoto S, Yamashita T: Fibroblast growth factor-23 is the phosphaturic factor in tumor-induced osteomalacia and may be phosphatonin. *Curr Opin Nephrol Hypertens* 2002;11:385-389.

57. Pack AM, Gidal B, Vazquez B: Bone disease associated with analeptic drugs. *Cleve Clin J Med* 2004;71 (suppl 2):S42-S48.

58. Rauch F: The rachitic bone. *Endocr Dev* 2003;6:69-79.

59. Hordon LD, Peacock M: Vitamin D metabolism in women with femoral neck fracture. *Bone Miner* 1987;2: 413-426.

60. Goodman WG, Coburn JW, Slatopolsky E, Salusky IB: Renal osteodystrophy in adults and children, in Favus MJ (ed): *Primer on the Metabolic Bone Diseases and Disorders of Mineral Metabolism*, ed 4. Philadelphia, PA, Lippincott Williams and Wilkins, 1999, pp 347-366.

61. Moe SM: Management of renal osteodystrophy in peritoneal dialysis patients. *Perit Dial Int* 2004;24:209-216.

62. Roe S, Cassidy MJ: Diagnosis and monitoring of renal osteodystrophy. *Curr Opin Nephrol Hypertens* 2000;9: 675-681.

63. Cushner HM, Adams ND: Review: Renal osteodystrophy. Pathogenesis and treatment. *Am J Med Sci* 1986; 291:264-275.

64. Hoyland JA, Picton ML: Cellular mechanisms in renal osteodystrophy. *Kidney Int Suppl* 1999;73:S8-S13.

65. Slatopolsky E, Gonzalez E, Martin K: Pathogenesis and treatment of renal osteodystrophy. *Blood Purif* 2003;21: 318-326.

66. Sutton RA, Cameron EC: Renal osteodystrophy: Pathophysiology. *Semin Nephrol* 1992;12:91-100.

67. Ambrosoni P, Olaizola I, Heuguerot C, et al: The role of imaging techniques in the study of renal osteodystrophy. *Am J Med Sci* 2000; 320:90-95.

68. Potts JT Jr: Primary hyperparathyroidism, in Avioli LV, Krane SM (eds): *Metabolic Bone Disease*. San Diego, CA, Academic Press, 1998, pp 411-442.

69. Peacock M, Bilezikian JP, Klasse PS, et al: Cinacalcet hydrochloride maintains long-term normocalcemia in pa-

tients with primary hyperparathyroidism. *J Clin Endocrinol Metab* 2005; 90:135-141.

70. Mundy GR: *Bone Remodeling and Its Disorders*, ed 2. London, England, Martin Dunitz Ltd, 1999.

71. Silverberg SJ: Natural history of primary hyperparathyroidism. *Endocrinol Metab Clin North Am* 2000;29: 451-464.

72. Bilezikian JP, Silverberg SJ: Clinical spectrum of primary hyperparathyroidism. *Rev Endocr Metab Disord* 2000;1:237-245.

73. Silverberg SJ, Bilezikian JP: Primary hyperparathyroidism, in Becker KL, Bilezikian JP, Bremner W (eds): *Principals and Practice of Endocrinology and Metabolism*, ed 3. Philadelphia, PA, Lippincott, Williams and Wilkins, 2001, pp 564-573.

74. Joshua B, Feinmesser R, Ulanovski D, et al: Primary hyperparathyroidism in young adults. *Otolaryngol Head Neck Surg* 2004;131:628-632.

75. Adami S, Braga V, Squaranti R, et al: Bone measurements in asymptomatic primary hyperparathyroidism. *Bone* 1998;22:565-570.

76. Albertazzi P, Steel SA, Purdie DW: Hyperparathyroidism in elderly osteopenic women. *Maturitas* 2002;43: 245-249.

77. Sitges-Serra A, Girvent M, Pereira JA, et al: Bone mineral density in menopausal women with primary hyperparathyroidism before and after parathyroidectomy. *World J Surg* 2004;28: 1148-1152.

78. Brandi ML, Aurbach GD, Fitzpatrick LA, et al: Parathyroid mitogenic activity in plasma from patients with familial multiple endocrine neoplasia type 1. *N Engl J Med* 1986;314:1287-1293.

79. Brandi ML, Falchetti A: Genetics of primary hyperparathyroidism. *Urol Int* 2004;72(suppl 1):11-16.

80. Carling T, Udelsman R: Parathyroid surgery in familial hyperparathyroid disorders. *J Intern Med* 2005; 257:27-37.

81. Miedlich S, Krohn K, Lamesch P: Frequency of somatic MEN1 gene mutations in monoclonal parathyroid tumours of patients with primary hyperparathyroidism. *Eur J Endocrinol* 2000;143:47-54.

82. Joborn C, Hetta J, Johansson H, et al: Psychiatric morbidity in primary hyperparathyroidism. *World J Surg* 1988; 12:476-481.

83. Turken SA, Cafferty M, Silverberg SJ, et al: Neuromuscular involvement in mild, asymptomatic primary hyperparathyroidism. *Am J Med* 1989;87: 553-557.

84. Silverberg SJ, Shane E, de la Cruz L, et al: Skeletal disease in primary hyperparathyroidism. *J Clin Endocrinol Metab* 1989;4:283-291.

85. Dodds WJ, Steinbach HL: Primary hyperparathyroidism and articular cartilage calcification. *Am J Roentgenol Radium Ther Nucl Med* 1968;104: 884-892.

86. Rodman JS, Mahler RJ: Kidney stones as a manifestation of hypercalcemic disorders: Hyperparathyroidism and sarcoidosis. *Urol Clin North Am* 2000;27:275-285.

87. Bess MA, Edis AJ, van Heeridon JA: Hyperparathyroidism and pancreatitis: Chance or causal association. *JAMA* 1980;243:246-247.

88. Andersson P, Rydberg E, Willenheimer R: Primary hyperparathyroidism and heart disease: A review. *Eur Heart J* 2004;25:1776-1787.

89. Vestergaard P, Mollerup CL, Fokjaer VG, et al: Cardiovascular events before and after surgery for primary hyperparathyroidism. *World J Surg* 2003;27:216-222.

90. Bilezikian JP, Potts JT Jr: Asymptomatic primary hyperparathyroidism: New issues and new questions.Bridging the past with the future. *J Bone Miner Res* 2002;17(suppl 2): N57-N67.

91. Bilezikian JP, Silverberg SJ, Shane E, et al: Characterization and evaluation of asymptomatic primary hyperparathyroidism. *J Bone Miner Res* 1991;6 (suppl 2):S85-S89.

92. Bilezikian JP: Primary hyperparathyroidism: When to observe and when to operate. *Endocrinol Metab Clin North Am* 2000;29:465-478.

93. Clark OH, Wilkes W, Siperstein AE, Duh QY: Diagnosis and management of asymptomatic hyperparathyroidism: Safety, efficacy and deficiencies in our knowledge. *J Bone Miner Res* 1991;6(suppl 2):S135-S142.

94. Potts JT Jr: Clinical review 9: Management of asymptomatic hyperparathyroidism. *J Clin Endocrinol Metab* 1990;70:1489-1493.

95. Bilezikian JP: Management of acute hypercalcemia. *N Engl J Med* 1992; 326:1196-1203.

96. Valdemarsson S, Lindergaard B, Tibblen S, Bergenfelz A: Increased biochemical markers of bone formation and resorption in primary hyperparathyroidism, with special reference to patients with mild disease. *J Intern Med* 1998;243:115-122.

97. Catargi B, Raymond JM, Lfarge-Yensi V, et al: Localization of parathyroid tumors using endoscopic ultrasonography in primary hyperparathyroidism. *J Endocrinol Invest* 1999; 22:688-692.

98. De Feo ML, Colagrande S, Biagini C, et al: Parathyroid glands: Combination of (99m) Tc MIBI scintigraphy and US for demonstration of parathyroid glands and nodules. *Radiology* 2000;214:393-402.

99. Gotway MB, Higgins CB: MR imaging of the thyroid and parathyroid glands. *Magn Reson Imaging Clin N Am* 2000;8:163-182.

100. Gonnelli S, Montagnani A, Cepollaro C, et al: Quantitative ultrasound and bone mineral density in patients with primary hyperparathyroidism before and after surgical treatment. *Osteoporos Int* 2000;11: 255-260.

101. Eigelberger MS, Clark OH: Surgical approaches to primary hyperparathyroidism. *Endocrinol Metab Clin North Am* 2000;29:479-502.

102. Martin RC II, Greenwell D, Flynn MB: Initial neck exploration for untreated hyperparathyroidism. *Am Surg* 2000;66:269-272.

103. Walgenbach S, Hommel G, Junginger T: Outcome after surgery for primary hyperparathyroidism: Ten-year prospective follow-up study. *World J Surg* 2000;24:564-569.

104. Chen H, Sokoll LJ, Udelsman R: Outpatient minimally invasive parathyroidectomy: A combination of sestamibi-SPECT localization, cervical block anesthesia, and intraoperative parathyroid hormone assay. *Surgery* 1999;126:1016-1021.

105. Reeve TS, Babidge WJ, Parker RF, et al: Minimally invasive surgery for primary hyperparathyroidism: Systematic review. *Arch Surg* 2000;135: 481-487.

106. Shane E: Clinical review 122: Parathyroid carcinoma. *J Clin Endocrinol Metab* 2001;86:485-493.

107. Deftos LJ, Roos BA, Oates EL: Calcitonin, in Favus MJ (ed): *Primer on the Metabolic Bone Diseases and Disorders of Mineral Metabolism*, ed 4. Philadelphia, PA, Lippincott Williams and Wilkins, 1999, pp 99-103.

108. Joy MS, Kshirsagar A, Franceschini N: Calcimimetics and the treatment of primary and secondary hyperparathyroidism. *Ann Pharmacother* 2004;38:1871-1880.

109. Arden N, Cooper C: Present and future of osteoporosis: Epidemiology, in Meunier PJ (ed): *Osteoporosis: Diagnosis and Management*. St. Louis, MO, Mosby, 1998, pp 1-16.

110. Elliott ME: Osteoporotic fractures in older women. *Curr Womens Health Rep* 2002;2:356-365.

111. Lin JT, Lane JM: Osteoporosis: A review. *Clin Orthop Relat Res* 2004;425: 126-134.

112. Seeman E, Hopper JL, Bach LA, et al: Reduced bone mass in daughters of women with osteoporosis. *N Engl J Med* 1989;320:554-558.

113. Heaney RP: Non-pharmacological prevention of osteoporosis: Nutrition and exercise, in Meunier PJ (ed): *Osteoporosis: Diagnosis and Manage-*

*ment*. St. Louis, MO, Mosby, 1998, pp 161-164.

114. Dequeker J, Aerssens J, Luyten FP: Osteoarthritis and osteoporosis: Clinical and research evidence of inverse relationship. *Aging Clin Exp Res* 2003;15:426-439.

115. Cummings SR, Melton LJ: Epidemiology and outcomes of osteoporotic fractures. *Lancet* 2002;359:1761-1767.

116. Bassey EJ: Exercise in primary prevention of osteoporosis in women. *Ann Rheum Dis* 1995;54:861-862.

117. Greenspan SL, Greenspan FS: The effect of thyroid hormone on skeletal integrity. *Ann Intern Med* 1999;130:750-758.

118. Kemmler W, Luaber D, Weineck J, et al: Benefits of 2 years of intense exercise on bone density, physical fitness and blood lipids in early postmenopausal osteopenic women. *Arch Intern Med* 2004;164:1084-1091.

119. Mundy GR: Bone remodeling and mechanisms of bone loss in osteoporosis, in Meunier PJ (ed): *Osteoporosis: Diagnosis and Management*. St. Louis, MO, Mosby, 1998, pp 17-36.

120. Kado DM, Browner WS, Palermo L, et al: Vertebral fractures and mortality in older women: A prospective study. *Arch Intern Med* 1999;159:1215-1220.

121. Chao EY, Inoue N, Koo TK, Kim YH: Biomechanical considerations of fracture treatment and bone quality maintenance in elderly patients and patients with osteoporosis. *Clin Orthop Relat Res* 2004;425:12-25.

122. Kessel B: Hip fracture prevention in postmenopausal women. *Obstet Gynecol Surv* 2004;59:446-455.

123. Stevens JA, Olson S: Reducing falls and resulting hip fractures among older women. *MMWR Recomm Rep* 2000;49:3-12.

124. Westfall G, Littlefield R, Heaton A, Martin S: Methodology for identifying patients at high risk for osteoporotic fracture. *Clin Ther* 2001;23:1570-1588.

125. World Health Organization: Assessment of fracture risk and its application to screening for postmenopausal osteoporosis: Report of a WHO study group. *World Health Organ Tech Rep Ser* 1994;843:1-129.

126. Harrington JT, Broy SB, Derosa AM, et al: Hip fracture patients are not treated for osteoporosis: A call to action. *Arthritis Rheum* 2002;47:651-654.

127. Taillandier J, Langue F, Alemanni M, Taillander-Heriche E: Mortality and functional outcomes of pelvic insufficiency fractures in older patients. *Joint Bone Spine* 2003;70:287-289.

128. Ebeling PR, Atley LM, Guthrie JR, et al: Bone turnover markers and bone density across the menopausal transition. *J Clin Endocrinol Metab* 1996;81:3366-3371.

129. Jergas M, Genant HK: Contributions of bone mass measurements by densitometry in the definition and diagnosis of osteoporosis, in Meunier PJ (ed): *Osteoporosis: Diagnosis and Management*. St. Louis, MO, Mosby, 1998, pp 37-58.

130. Bauer DC, Palermo L, Black D, Cauley JA: Quantitative ultrasound and mortality: A prospective study. *Osteoporos Int* 2002;13:606-612.

131. Civatelli R: Biochemical markers of bone turnover, in Avioli LV (ed): *The Osteoporotic Syndrome: Detection, Prevention, and Treatment*, ed 4. San Diego, CA, Academic Press, 2000, pp 67-89.

132. Jeong GK, Bendo JA: Spinal disorders in the elderly. *Clin Orthop Relat Res* 2004;425:110-125.

133. Gardner MJ, Brophy RH, Dematrakopoulos D, et al: Interventions to improve osteoporosis treatment following hip fracture: A prospective randomized trial. *J Bone Joint Surg Am* 2005;87:3-7.

134. Chapuy MC, Arloltn ME, Duboeuf F, et al: Vitamin D3 and calcium to prevent hip fractures in the elderly women. *N Engl J Med* 1992;327:1637-1642.

135. Dawson-Hughes B: Calcium, vitamin D and bone metabolism, in Avioli LV (ed): *The Osteoporotic Syndrome: Detection, Prevention and Treatment*, ed 4. San Diego, CA, Academic Press, 2000, pp 91-99.

136. Reid IR, Ames RW, Evans MC, Gamble GD, Sharpe SJ: Long-term effects of calcium supplementation on bone loss and fractures in postmenopausal women: A randomized controlled study. *Am J Med* 1995;98:331-335.

137. Rossouw JE, Anderson GL, Prentice RL, et al: Risks and benefits of estrogen plus progestin in healthy postmenopausal women. *JAMA* 2002;288:321-333.

138. Maricic M, Adachi JD, Sarkar S, et al: Early effects of raloxifene on clinical vertebral fractures at 12 months in postmenopausal women with osteoporosis. *Arch Intern Med* 2002;162:1140-1143.

139. Rubin MR, Bilezikian JP: New anabolic therapies in osteoporosis. *Endocrinol Metab Clin North Am* 2003;32:285-307.

140. Chesnut CH III, Silverman S, Andriano K, et al: A randomized trial of nasal spray salmon calcitonin in postmenopausal women with established osteoporosis: The prevent recurrence of osteopenic fractures study: PROOF Study Group. *Am J Med* 2000;109:267-276.

141. Silverman SL: Calcitonin. *Endocrinol Metab Clin North Am* 2003;32:273-284.

142. Reszka AA, Halasy-Nagy JM, Masarachia PH, Rodan GA: Bisphosphonates act directly on the osteoclast to induce caspase cleavage of mst-1 kinase during apoptosis: A link between inhibition of the mevalonate pathway and regulation of an apoptosis-promoting kinase. *J Biol Chem* 1999;274:34967-34973.

143. Black DM, Cummings SR, Karpf DB, et al: Randomized trial of effect of alendronate on risk of fracture in women with existing vertebral fractures: Fracture Intervention Trial Research Group. *Lancet* 1996;348:1535-1541.

144. Koval KJ, Chen AL, Aharonoff GB, et al: Clinical pathway for hip fractures

in the elderly: The Hospital for Joint Diseases experience. *Clin Orthop Relat Res* 2004;425:72-81.

145. Rodan GA, Reszka AA: Osteoporosis and bisphosphonates. *J Bone Joint Surg Am* 2003;85:8-12.

146. Boonen S, McClung MR, Eastell R, et al: Safety and efficacy of risedronate in reducing fracture risk in osteoporotic women age 80 and older: Implications for the use of antiresorptive agents in the old and the oldest old. *J Am Geriatr Soc* 2004;52:1832-1839.

147. Cranney A, Waldegger L, Zytaruk N et al: Risedronate for the prevention and treatment of postmenopausal osteoporosis. *Cochrane Database Syst Rev* 2003;4:CD 004523.

148. Harris ST, Watts NF, Genant HK, et al: Effects of risedronate treatment on vertebral and non-vertebral fractures in women with postmenopausal osteoporosis: A randomized clinical trial. *JAMA* 1999;282:1344-1352.

149. Chan SS, Nery LM, McElduff A, et al: Intravenous pamidronate in the treatment and prevention of osteoporosis. *Intern Med J* 2004;34:162-166.

150. Sartori L, Adami S, Filipponi P, Crepaldi G: Injectable bisphosphonates in the treatment of postmenopausal osteoporosis. *Aging Clin Exp Res* 2003;15:271-283.

151. Reid IR, Brown JP, Burckhardt P, et al: Intravenous zoledronic acid in postmenopausal women with low bone mineral density. *N Engl J Med* 2002;346:653-661.

152. Brixen KT, Christensen PM, Ejersted C, Langdahl BL: Teriparatide (biosynthetic human parathyroid hormone 1-34): A new paradigm in the treatment of osteoporosis. *Basic Clin Pharmacol Toxicol* 2004;94:260-270.

153. Dempster DW, Cosman F, Kurland ES, et al: Effects of daily treatment with parathyroid hormone on bone microarchitecture and turnover in patients with osteoporosis. A paired biopsy study. *J Bone Miner Res* 2001;16:1846-1853.

154. Neer RM, Arnaud CD, Zanchetta JR, et al: Effect of parathyroid hormone (1-34) on fractures and bone mineral density in postmenopausal women with osteoporosis. *N Engl J Med* 2001;344:1434-1441.

155. Black DM, Greenspan XL, Ensrud KE, et al: The effects of parathyroid hormone and alendronate alone or in combination in postmenopausal osteoporosis. *N Engl J Med* 2003;349:1207-1215.

156. Doggrell SA: Present and future pharmacotherapy for osteoporosis. *Drugs Today (Barc)* 2003;39:633-657.

157. Landin-Wilhelmsen K, Nilsson A, Bosaeus I, Bengtson B: Growth hormone increases bone mineral content in postmenopausal osteoporosis: A randomized placebo-controlled trial. *J Bone Miner Res* 2003;18:393-405.

158. Ruggiero SL, Mehrotra B, Rosenberg TJ, Engroff SL: Osteonecrosis of the jaws associated with the use of bisphosphonates: A review of 63 cases. *J Oral Maxillofac Surg* 2004;62:527-534.

159. Coleman CI, Perkerson KA, Lewis A: Alendronate-induced auditory hallucinations and visual disturbances. *Pharmacotherapy* 2004;24:799-802.

160. Lieberman IH, Dudeney S, Reinhardt MK, Bell G: Initial outcome and efficacy of "kyphoplasty" in the treatment of painful osteoporotic vertebral compression fractures. *Spine* 2001;26:1631-1638.

# 48

# Osteoporosis: The Basics and Case-Based Advanced Treatment Update for the Orthopaedic Surgeon

*Barbara J. Campbell, MD

## Abstract

*When fragility fractures occur, urgent treatment is needed to reduce the risk of refracture. An extensive case-based review is used to provide an update on the basics of osteoporosis and the evaluation and treatment of patients with fragility fractures, with the goal of decreasing the risk of subsequent fracture. The pathophysiology of osteoporosis, mechanisms of action of optimal antifracture medications that will become a part of the pharmacologic armamentarium of every orthopaedic surgeon, and detailed evaluation and treatment information are presented to provide orthopaedic surgeons with the information needed to optimize the bone health of their patients.*

**Instr Course Lect 2008;57:595-636.**

Osteoporotic fractures are frequently a preventable consequence of malnutrition, a sedentary lifestyle, and hormonal loss, rather than an inevitable part of aging.[1] The first fragility fracture predictably heralds a downward spiral of disability and premature death. It is the most important risk factor for future fracture and is more predictive of refracture than low bone mineral density (BMD). The risk of another fracture is imminent and increases twofold to fourfold following the initial fracture[2-4] (Table 1).

Urgent treatment is needed to reduce refracture risk and can reduce fracture risk within months.[5,6] Forty percent of Caucasian women and 13% of Caucasian men older than 50 years will experience fragility fractures in their lifetimes[1,7,8] (Table 2). All other ethnic groups have a significant but slightly lower risk.[9,10] Fracture rates are rising exponentially as the population increases and ages; the worldwide incidence of hip fracture is projected to increase by 250% by 2050[1,8] (Figure 1).

Orthopaedic surgeons caring for patients with fragility fractures have a key role in reducing fracture risks by evaluating and recommending treatment to prevent a second fracture and can help patients of all ages optimize their bone health and quality of life.[11] Focused intervention by orthopaedic surgeons championing patient education and providing evaluation and treatment at the point of fracture care in the hospital and outpatient setting has been shown to greatly improve patient outcomes and is encouraged by the American Academy of Orthopaedic Surgeons (AAOS).[12-26]

This chapter will use case examples to provide an update on the basic pathophysiology of osteoporosis and the treatment of patients with fragility fractures to decrease the risk of subsequent fracture.

## Colles Fracture Case Presentation

BJC is a 55-year-old Caucasian woman who tripped over her dog and presented to the emergency department and then to the physician's office. She was diagnosed with a Colles fracture. BJC has a sedentary job, and this is her first fracture as an adult. The patient takes supplements of calcium with vitamin D three times daily. She reports that her mother had a humped back.

*Barbara J. Campbell, MD or the department with which she is affiliated has received miscellaneous nonincome support, commercially derived honoraria, or other nonresearch-related funding from Merck, GlaxoSmithKline, and Pfizer.*

## Table 1
### Relative Risks of Refracture in Males and Females Older Than 45 Years, According to Fracture Location*

| | Index Fracture | | | | |
| --- | --- | --- | --- | --- | --- |
| | **Hip** | **Wrist** | **Proximal Part of Humerus** | **Ankle** | **Any** |
| **Refracture** | **Relative Risk of Refracture (CI)** | | | | |
| Hip | 9.79 (9.07-10.55) | 3.22 (2.81-3.66) | 5.76 (4.94-6.68) | 1.30 (0.95-1.82) | 6.55 (6.17-6.94) |
| Wrist | 3.96 (3.59-4.36) | 4.63 (4.22-5.06) | 4.42 (3.83-5.08) | 2.03 (1.62-2.51) | 4.04 (3.79-4.29) |
| Proximal part of humerus | 6.50 (5.72-7.38) | 4.08 (3.46-4.79) | 7.91 (6.59-9.42) | 1.96 (1.32-2.81) | 5.23 (4.77-5.72) |
| Ankle | 1.74 (1.34-2.18) | 2.23 (1.81-2.74) | 2.20 (1.57-2.99) | 4.53 (3.57-5.66) | 2.41 (2.12-2.72) |
| Any | 5.76 (5.32-6.17) | 3.98 (3.52-4.42) | 4.87 (4.27-5.47) | 2.24 (1.89-2.59) | 3.89 (3.73-4.04) |

*Data are based on a large prospective study that evaluated refracture risk in 22,000 low-trauma fracture patients who were followed for more than 12 years. The risk of refracture after a prior fragility fracture is significant in both sexes after age 45 years, and the relative risk is actually somewhat higher in the younger groups.

CI = confidence interval

## Table 2
### Lifetime Risk of Fracture at Age 50 Years

| Type of Fracture | White Women (%) | White Men (%) |
| --- | --- | --- |
| Hip | 17.5 | 6.0 |
| Vertebra | 15.6 | 5.0 |
| Forearm | 16.0 | 2.5 |
| Any of the three types | 39.7 | 13.1 |

(Adapted with permission from Cummings SR, Melton LJ: Epidemiology and outcomes of osteoporotic fractures. *Lancet* 2002;359: 1761-1767.)

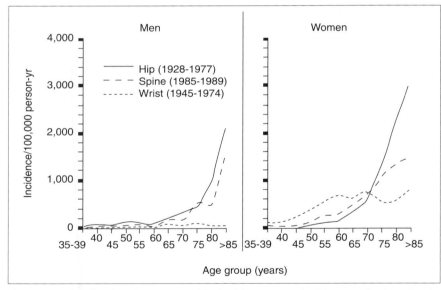

**Figure 1** Graphs showing age-specific incidence rates for hip, vertebral, and wrist fractures in men and women. (Adapted with permission from Cooper C, Atkinon EJ, O'Fallon WM, Melton LJ III: Incidence of clinically diagnosed vertebral fractures: A population-based study in Rochester, Minnestoa, 1985-1989. *J Bone Miner Res* 1992;7:221-227.)

### Does This Woman Have a Fragility Fracture?
Women older than 40 years and men older than 50 years who sustain a fracture when falling from a standing height or less are considered to have a fragility fracture.[27] It is imperative to recognize the ominous natural history of this common fracture and to address the underlying bone fragility. Distal radius fractures are frequently the first fragility fracture seen in a patient presenting to an orthopaedic surgeon.

### Does This Patient Have Osteoporosis?
The National Institutes of Health Consensus Statement of 2000 defines osteoporosis as a "skeletal disorder characterized by compromised bone strength, predisposing to fracture." Low BMD has been omitted from this definition because bone strength and fracture risk have many components in addition to BMD.[28,29] Because BJC has a fragility fracture, she has clinical "osteoporosis" and requires evaluation and treatment to decrease fracture risk.

### Incidence and Cost of Colles Fractures
The lifetime risk of a Colles fracture at age 50 years is 15% for women and 2.5% in men. There are approximately 250,000 distal forearm fractures per year in the United States, resulting in more than 20,000 hospital admissions and 530,000 office visits and requiring more outpatient

therapy than hip fractures. In the United States in 1995, direct health care costs for osteoporotic distal forearm fractures in patients older than 45 years was $385 million.[1,7,28,30]

### Increased Risk of Another Fracture in a Patient With a Colles Fracture

The risk of another fragility fracture at any site in postmenopausal women with a Colles fracture increases twofold to fivefold above the baseline risk and is even higher in men. The risk of another distal forearm fracture increases approximately threefold, the risk of subsequent vertebral fracture increases fivefold to tenfold, and the risk of future hip fracture is 1.5 to 3 times more likely. In patients with a Colles fracture who have a subsequent hip fracture, lag time from the wrist fracture to hip fracture is approximately 14 years and may be sooner in older patients.[1,31-33]

### Causes and Types of the Most Common Fragility Fractures

Most fragility fractures occur at sites high in trabecular bone such as the hip, vertebra, forearm, proximal humerus, and rib. These fractures are commonly associated with low BMD. However, even a fracture caused by significant trauma may indicate decreased bone strength and increased risk of future fractures. A significant number of patients with traumatic fractures have decreased BMD (osteoporosis or osteopenia).[32,34-36]

### Trabecular Bone: The Most Common Site of Fragility Fracture

Trabecular bone is the first area of the skeleton to show signs of osteoporosis and fracture because it has a much larger surface area avail-

able for cellular activity, making it more metabolically responsive to mechanisms of bone loss than cortical bone.[37] Cellular activity takes place at bone surfaces because the matrix is a hard tissue. Bone surfaces, completely covered with metabolically active cells in communication with buried osteocytes through the canalicular system that courses through the mineralized matrix, are exquisitely responsive to changes in physical and cellular stimuli. The typical adult skeleton is composed of 80% cortical and 20% trabecular bone. Eighty percent of the bone surface is devoted to ion exchange for calcium homeostasis and 20% to bone remodeling to maintain skeletal strength.[38-40]

The same cells and hormones that control fluxes of calcium also renew and repair the skeleton over time to maintain bone strength. Dietary calcium and hormonal and mechanical influences are critically important to prevent the gradual

dissolution of the aging skeleton in the interest of extracellular and serum calcium[38,39,41-43] (Table 3).

### Proper Response to a Patient With a Fragility Fracture

It is critical to optimize communication between all health care providers because the evaluation and treatment of underlying bone health issues is important for the best possible patient outcomes. Because of the low percentage of patients receiving evaluation and preventive treatment of poor bone health, it is desirable to put an automatic mechanism in place in the physician's office and hospital emergency department to notify primary care physicians about any patient with a fragility fracture and document this notification in the patient's chart. It is a pay-for-performance quality measure to communicate with the primary care provider to ensure coordination of bone health care after a fracture[2,44] (Table 4). Several health

---

**Table 3**
**Bone Active Hormones Have Dual Functions**

**Parathyroid Hormone (PTH)**

Calcium metabolism: controls extracellular calcium homeostasis, which is responsible for maintaining serum and extracellular fluid calcium levels for proper cellular functioning across three areas of extracellular exchange: gut, bone, and kidney. Decreases calcium loss from the kidney and increases calcium mobilization from bone surfaces to raise serum calcium.

Skeletal remodeling: controls and modulates cells active in the remodeling cycle. Physiologic role is to be a potent stimulator of osteoclast formation, increasing bone remodeling rate and overall resorption; intermittent pharmacologic doses increase osteoblast numbers and bone formation by increasing the size, activity, and working life of osteoblasts, strengthening remaining trabeculae, and bypassing local mechanostat limits.

**Vitamin D (1,25-dihydroxyvitamin $D_3$)**

Calcium metabolism: improves calcium absorption from the gut and stimulates bone resorption to raise serum calcium.

Skeletal remodeling: a potent stimulator of osteoclast activation and increased remodeling rate mediated by the osteoblast and the nuclear factor-kappaB (RANK) system.

**Calcitonin**

Calcium metabolism: complex actions on calcium balance in gut and kidney, decreases calcium mobilization from bone, lowering the overall level of serum calcium.

Skeletal remodeling: potent transient inhibitor of osteoclastic bone resorption acting through cyclic adenosine monophosphate, decreases osteoclast activation, and promotes osteoclast apoptosis.

**Other bone active hormones**

Estrogen, androgen, glucocorticoids, and thyroxine regulate production and action of several cytokines, which are involved in bone remodeling and mineral homeostasis.

---

**Table 4**
**2007 Physician Quality Reporting Initiative (PQRI): Physician Quality Measures Concerning Osteoporosis and Fracture Care**

| PQRI Number | Pay-for-Performance Measure* |
|---|---|
| 4 | Falls: screening for fall risk |
| 21 | Perioperative care: selection of prophylactic antibiotic, first- or second-generation cephalosporin |
| 22 | Perioperative care: discontinuation of prophylactic antibiotics |
| 23 | Perioperative care: venous thromboembolism prophylaxis |
| 24 | Osteoporosis: communication with the physician managing ongoing care after fracture |
| 39 | Screening or therapy for osteoporosis for women age 65 years and older |
| 40 | Osteoporosis: management following fracture: bone mineral density |
| 41 | Osteoporosis: pharmacologic therapy |
| 42 | Osteoporosis: counseling for vitamin D, calcium intake, and exercise |

*The pay-for-performance measures from the Centers for Medicare and Medicaid Services that apply to osteoporosis in general and also specifically to hip fractures.

care quality measures for osteoporosis have been defined by the Centers for Medicare and Medicaid Services (CMS).[44]

Patient education at all points of care improves treatment.[14,21] The patient should be informed that this fracture is commonly related to bone health disorders, and further evaluation and treatment is indicated because it can help prevent future fractures. Free patient education materials are available from the government and the AAOS.[45-47]

### Rationale for a BMD Test in a Patient With a Colles Fracture

A patient who sustains a fragility fracture meets all published guidelines for obtaining a definitive BMD test.[48] Patients younger than 66 years with Colles fractures have a lower BMD than expected for their age.[34,49-51]

BMD is a basic diagnostic test that is necessary in the long-term care of patients such as the woman in this case presentation. If not ordered at this point of care, the test often will not be done. If the orthopaedic surgeon lacks expertise in the area of bone evaluation and treatment, a clear and documented communication should be made to the primary care provider that a BMD test is indicated, and the bone health portion of the patient's care is being transferred to the primary care physician; this action should be documented in the patient's office chart. Ordering a BMD test as part of postfracture management of a patient and communicating with the primary care physician are pay-for-performance measures for the orthopaedic surgeon.[44]

In a patient with a fragility fracture, a BMD study is important as a baseline test that allows follow-up on the course of the patient's bone health, with or without treatment over time. Having both a fragility fracture and low BMD dramatically increases the risk of future fracture more than each one of these risk factors alone.[52,53] In patients without a fragility fracture, bone density is the most important and best measurable determinant of fracture risk.[54-56] Patient awareness of their BMD results has been shown to affect decisions to start treatment for fracture prevention. Providing the patient with handouts explaining BMD testing and fracture risks should be considered.[57]

### Measuring BMD in a Patient With a Fragility Fracture

BMD testing of the hip and spine with dual-energy x-ray absorptiometry (DXA) is the gold standard of bone density testing. DXA has high precision and accuracy, has less radiation exposure than a chest radiograph, measures sites of the most serious fractures, and is the best method to allow follow-up of individual patients through time.[58,59] Clinical trials that show fracture risk reduction with treatment have evaluated patients who were selected based on central DXA BMD levels at the hip and spine. Hip DXA is the most accurate site and method for diagnosis in older patients, although any skeletal site is useful for fracture prediction in elderly patients. Two to 3 years between DXA BMD testing is usually necessary to see any significant change with time and/or treatment.[60]

DXA provides vertebral fracture assessment, imaging the lateral thoracolumbar spine with less radiation and cost than standard radiographs. Seventy percent of vertebral fractures seen on radiographs are not clinically evident or have not been diagnosed. Any prevalent vertebral fracture greatly increases the risk of fragility fractures at all sites, provides useful information about bone quality, and increases fracture risk independent of BMD.[60] Vertebral fracture assessment can change the clinical classification and treatment of a patient.[53] Older women with increased thoracic kyphosis without prevalent vertebral body deformity also have a 1.7 times increased risk of symptomatic vertebral fracture in the future.[61]

## World Health Organization Classification of BMD Levels in Postmenopausal Women

A 1992 World Health Organization (WHO) study group developed diagnostic categories of BMD in postmenopausal women using T-scores, which are based on the relationship between forearm BMD in young white adult females and BMD in postmenopausal white females with prevalent hip fractures[62] (Figure 2). The T-score is defined as the number of standard deviations (SD) the patient's BMD is above or below the expected peak bone density at approximately age 30 years for someone of the same gender and ethnic group. A T-score of −1 or less defines osteopenia and −2.5 or less defines osteoporosis. In general, the same T-score designations are used in men. Each drop of 1 SD from mean peak bone mass confers an increase in fracture risk of approximately 1.5 to 2.5.[41] These BMD criteria are not directly applicable to younger patients.[60]

The Z-score is defined as the number of SDs the patient's bone density is above or below the expected bone density for their ethnic group, gender, and age. If the Z-score is below −1.0, secondary causes of bone loss are more likely to be found.[63] In the premenopausal period, the Z-score is used for diagnostic categories.

The WHO classification cannot be applied to BMD results obtained with other technologies and was not intended to be used as a guideline for treatment.[64] When WHO BMD criteria are used to assess fracture risk, age is a critical factor[34,65-70] Given the same BMD, the risk of fracture increases 8 to 10 times from age 45 to age 80 years[71] (Table 5). T-scores may eventually be abandoned in favor of an index that is

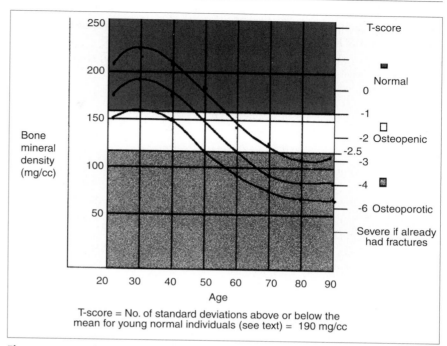

**Figure 2**    Graph showing the WHO definition of osteoporosis by BMD scores in postmenopausal women.

based on "absolute fracture risk." The WHO is working on a usable index for clinicians that will add major risk factors to those associated with BMD to calculate an absolute 10-year risk of fracture.[71-75]

## Clinical Risk Factors Predictive of Fractures

Risk factors for fracture can be associated with or may cause low bone mass, bone loss, or poor bone quality.[25] Major risk factors for osteoporotic fracture that are independent of BMD are advanced age, low body weight, smoking, previous fracture, positive family history, past or present corticosteroid use, and excessive alcohol intake. Rapid bone remodeling that can be identified by laboratory testing is also an independent risk factor for hip fracture.[76]

Fracture risk rises exponentially when low BMD is present in patients with these clinical risk fac-

tors.[33,53] A patient with normal or only slightly low BMD but with many clinical risk factors has a much greater risk of fracture than someone with low BMD but no other risk factors.[71] Having a previous fracture is a stronger predictor of future fracture risk than is low bone mass and is presumably related to bone quality and the risk for falls.[71] If only clinical risk factors are considered in predicting the risk for fracture in postmenopausal women, these factors predict 37% to 47% of radial fractures, 18% to 35% of vertebral fractures, and 17% to 27% of hip fractures. When low BMD is added to clinical risk factors, fracture prediction is significantly improved and vice versa.[1,32,48,49,53,65-68,77]

## Classification of BMD Based on DXA Results

In the case of the woman with a Colles fracture, the physician or-

**Table 5**
**Ten-Year Probability of Any Osteoporotic Fracture in Men and Women According to Age and Bone Mineral Density at the Femoral Neck**

| Age(years) | T-Score –0.5 | T-Score –1.0 | T-Score –1.5 | T-Score –2.0 | T-Score –2.5 | T-Score –3.0 | T-Score –4.0 |
|---|---|---|---|---|---|---|---|
| **Men** | | | | | | | |
| 50 | 3.4 | 4.2 | 5.1 | 6.3 | 7.7 | 9.4 | 14.0 |
| 55 | 3.7 | 4.6 | 5.7 | 7.0 | 8.6 | 10.6 | 16.0 |
| 60 | 4.4 | 5.4 | 6.5 | 7.9 | 9.5 | 11.5 | 16.7 |
| 65 | 5.1 | 6.2 | 7.4 | 8.8 | 10.4 | 12.4 | 17.4 |
| 70 | 6.1 | 7.4 | 9.0 | 10.9 | 13.1 | 15.7 | 22.4 |
| 75 | 7.8 | 9.6 | 11.8 | 14.4 | 17.5 | 21.2 | 30.4 |
| 80 | 9.2 | 11.1 | 13.3 | 15.8 | 18.7 | 22.2 | 30.3 |
| 85 | 8.8 | 10.4 | 12.2 | 14.3 | 16.7 | 19.5 | 26.1 |
| **Women** | | | | | | | |
| 50 | 4.7 | 5.9 | 7.4 | 9.2 | 11.3 | 14.1 | 21.3 |
| 55 | 5.3 | 6.7 | 8.5 | 10.7 | 13.4 | 16.8 | 26.0 |
| 60 | 6.5 | 8.2 | 10.4 | 13.0 | 16.2 | 20.2 | 30.0 |
| 65 | 8.0 | 10.0 | 12.6 | 15.6 | 19.3 | 23.9 | 35.5 |
| 70 | 9.0 | 11.5 | 14.6 | 18.3 | 22.8 | 28.4 | 42.3 |
| 75 | 9.1 | 11.8 | 15.2 | 19.4 | 24.5 | 30.8 | 46.2 |
| 80 | 9.9 | 12.7 | 16.2 | 20.5 | 25.5 | 31.8 | 46.4 |
| 85 | 9.4 | 12.0 | 15.3 | 19.1 | 23.8 | 29.4 | 42.7 |

(Adapted with permission from Kanis JA, Johnell O, Oden A, Dawson A, De Lact C, Jonsson B: Ten year probabilities of osteoporotic fractures according to BMD and diagnostic thresholds. *Osteoporos Int* 2001;12:989-995.)

dered a DXA BMD for the patient 1 month after the fracture. Results showed a T-score of –1.9 in the lumbar spine, +0.5 in the femoral neck, and +0.7 in the total femur. The physician must classify this patient's condition based on BMD and must determine if pharmacologic treatment is indicated.[62] Based on WHO BMD criteria, the patient is classified with osteopenia, with a diagnostic T-score of –1.9 at the spine. The International Society of Clinical Densitometrists recommends that the overall diagnosis of osteoporosis or osteopenia be made based on the BMD at the total hip, femoral neck, trochanter, one third radius, or spine, whichever T-score is lowest.[78] This patient is osteopenic based on BMD, but has documented bone fragility as evidenced by her recent fracture and is considered clinically "osteoporotic." The widely used National Osteoporosis Foundation (NOF) guidelines support pharmacologic therapy to reduce fracture risk in this patient with her determined risk factors and BMD.[48] Guidelines for treatment apply to patients with low BMD and also those with an existing (especially recent) low-impact traumatic fracture, regardless of BMD, if they have multiple risk factors for fracture. Postmenopausal and elderly patients with vertebral and hip fractures should be treated even if BMD testing is unavailable.[48,79] Although the risk of fracture and incidence of osteoporosis based on BMD (T-scores of –2.5 or worse) are increased in older patients, most patients with fragility fractures are not classified with osteoporosis based on BMD criteria. There are actually more fractures in middle-aged women because they represent a larger percentage of the population, even though their individual fracture risk is lower.[80,81] These younger individuals at risk for fracture are not well identified by BMD alone; clinical risk factors and rate of bone loss are helpful for fracture prediction[80,82,83] (Figure 3). BMD, although used as a proxy measurement of bone strength, explains less than one half of the observed fracture risks. Multiple other contributions to bone quality confer resistance to fracture.[84]

## Determinants of Bone Strength Other Than BMD

Factors other than BMD determine bone strength[85] (Figure 4). Bone can be dense but fragile, as seen in conditions such as osteopetrosis and Paget's disease.[38,86] Determinants of bone strength other than BMD are macroarchitecture, microarchitec-

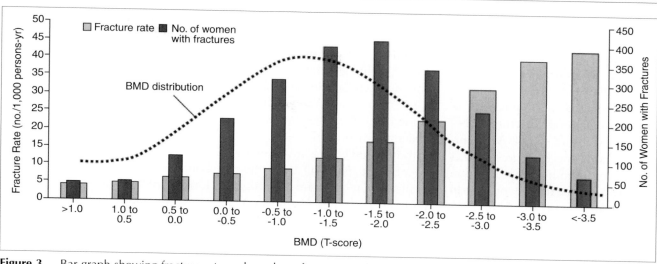

**Figure 3**    Bar graph showing fracture rate and number of women with fractures according to peripheral BMD. (Adapted with permission from Siris ES, Chen YT, Abbott TA, et al: Bone mineral density thresholds for pharmacological intervention to prevent fractures. *Arch Intern Med* 2004;164:1108-1110.)

ture, and bone material composition.[41,87]

Macroarchitectural factors such as bone shape, size, diameter, and cortical thickness contribute to fracture risk independent of BMD. Cortical diameter increases with age, caused by periosteal apposition and endosteal resorption. This increased diameter helps to maintain bone strength relative to torsional and bending loads as total mass is lost. Osteoporotic bone has increased cortical porosity and trabecularization of the endocortex leading to loss of cortical thickness and strength.[41] Small vertebral size is a risk factor independent of BMD for vertebral fractures.[88] Hip fracture risk doubles for every 1-SD increase in hip axis length, which varies by ethnic group.[41]

Microarchitectural factors that can weaken bone are loss of trabecular cross-bracing, excessive number of remodeling sites with deeper resorption pits, and trabecular plate thinning and perforation, which leads to loss of connectivity. A single horizontal trabecula confers a four-

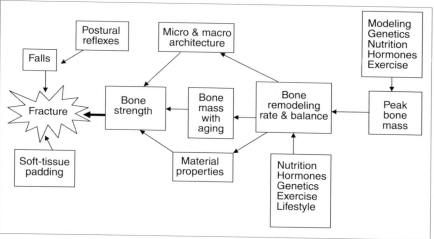

**Figure 4**    Lifetime factors contributing to bone strength and fracture risks. (Adapted with permission from Heany RP: Is the paradigm shifting? *Bone* 2003;33:457-465.)

fold increased load-bearing capacity and contributes importantly to skeletal strength. Damage accumulation and microfractures affect bone strength and resistance to fracture. Cement lines (a layer of woven weaker bone that marks the deepest site of bone resorption in a bone remodeling site) accumulate with age as a function of bone turnover and can propagate fracture lines.[41,52]

Bone material qualities related to

genetic defects and polymorphisms of the protein structure of type I collagen or crosslinking can predict fracture risk independent of BMD.[89-92] Progressive deterioration in the modulus of elasticity of bone occurs from repetitive loading with aging, and weakens bone. Human bone matrix is normally 60% mineralized with calcium hydroxyapatite crystals; undermineralization occurs in aged and osteoporotic bone, and a slight decrease in bone mineral content is associated with doubling the risks of breaking fragility. Overmineralization causes increased stiffness and also is detrimental to bone strength.[41]

New methods of noninvasive assessment of bone architecture are being developed and include MRI, micro CT, and image processing that can give morphometric information predictive of bone fragility, other than that provided by BMD.[41,93,94]

## Osteopenia and Postmenopausal Bone Loss

A patient with osteopenia, such as the patient with the Colles fracture, has not necessarily lost a large amount of bone since menopause. Low bone mass and fragility fracture can occur if a patient never acquires an optimal peak bone mass, has conditions causing abnormal bone, has progressive bone loss after peak acquisition, or with any combination of the three possibilities.[1,29] In this case example, it is unknown if this particular woman had a low peak bone mass or has lost significant bone since the onset of menopause; however, it is known that she has bone fragility.

## Peak Bone Mass

Peak bone mass is the maximal accumulation of bone size and strength that occurs in humans up to approximately age 30 years. Optimal peak bone accumulation is a major determinant of later skeletal health and provides protection against bone loss with aging, illness, bone-altering medications, and poor nutrition. Determinants of peak bone mass are choreographed by genetic, dietary, hormonal, and mechanical influences.[1,29,39,41,89,95-100] Approximately 80% of peak bone mass is genetically determined by multi-

ple genes, such as alleles for vitamin D receptor, estrogen receptors, collagen, and the low density lipoprotein-related protein 5 gene (*LRP-5*). In general, Asian and white women have lower peak bone mass than black and Hispanic women, and men have higher peak bone mass than women.[1]

Young adult bone is strong in ways independent of BMD by virtue of normal architecture and cortical size and thickness. Most fractures occur in children before attainment of peak bone mass, and in adults after the attainment of peak bone mass when bone is lost and quality diminishes. BMD is a bell curve at all ages; healthy women at the lower end of the bell curve may have thinner trabeculae but may have fracture resistance because of otherwise normal architecture. This explains the large discrepancy of fracture risk at a given BMD level at different ages.[1,101]

## Why Does Good Bone Go Bad?

Assuming that the woman in the case example had a normal peak BMD (T-score = 1 to –1 at age 30 years), how did she become osteopenic and sustain this fracture at age 55 years? Osteopenia and osteoporosis are an untoward consequence of a normal activity in bone—bone remodeling.[41]

The construction of the skeleton in childhood and adolescence is called modeling. Bone remodeling, the reconstruction of the skeleton after the end of growth, is the piecemeal removal of old bone and its replacement with new bone. This process continues throughout life, adjusting skeletal architecture to changes in mechanical load for optimal strength, removing apoptotic embedded osteocytes, repairing fatigue fractures and microdamage, opening marrow spaces for hemato-

poiesis, and maintaining calcium homeostasis by mobilizing calcium as needed.[41]

Bone remodeling occurs in discrete units of the skeleton called basic multicellular units (BMU), each approximately 0.5 mL in size, numbering 3 to 4 million in the adult human skeleton. Remodeling proceeds through a stereotyped sequence of bone resorption followed by bone formation[1,38] (Figure 5). In human bone, the entire sequence takes approximately 4 months.[102] In bone remodeling in the normal young adult, bone resorption is coupled to and followed by equal amounts of bone formation. Subsequent full mineralization of matrix can take up to 8 months. Cancellous bone is remodeled at a rate of approximately 30% per year and cortical bone at a rate of approximately 3% per year. Approximately 10% of the adult human skeleton is remodeled or "turned over" each year, replacing the entire skeleton every 10 years.[103,104]

Loss of bone mass and quality after attainment of peak bone mass is usually related to fast rates of bone remodeling with excessive numbers of remodeling sites and an imbalance in resorption and formation at each site. Loss of gonadal hormones from any etiology at any age in either sex induces a rapid remodeling state with accelerated bone loss[99] (Figure 6). Increased activation of BMUs and deeper resorption pits are mediated through increased levels of cytokines.[39,95,99] Osteoblast life span and function appear to decline beginning in middle age. Calcium and vitamin D deficiency cause a secondary hyperparathyroidism of aging, which contributes to bone loss. Small changes in BMU balance are magnified across the skeleton by the rapid remodeling rate. Decreasing bone remodeling is an effective strategy to help maintain the skeleton as an individual ages[41] (Figure 7).

## Rates of Bone Loss With Aging in Men and Women

After age 30 years, bone mass plateaus until approximately age 40 years. Women then lose approximately 0.3% to 0.5% of their cortical bone per year and approximately 1.2% of trabecular bone per year. At menopause, bone loss accelerates to 2% to 3% per year for 8 to 10 years, then slows again to a rate of loss of 0.3% to 0.5% per year over the long term. Women can lose up to 40% of trabecular bone mass and 10% of cortical bone in the first 10 years after menopause.[38,41] Some women have another acceleration of bone loss with rapid remodeling in their seventh decade of life and beyond.[103]

Men lose approximately 0.3% to 0.4% of cortical bone and 0.7% to 1.2% of trabecular bone per year after age 40 years, and possibly more after age 50 years. Because there is not an acute loss of gonadal hormones in men in middle age, they do not have rapid bone remodeling and the accelerated bone loss that occurs in women. Slow thinning of the trabeculae and bone loss caused by the imbalance of resorption and formation occurs with age, but the slower remodeling does not cause the degree of architectural loss as that which occurs in women. The thicker cortex and larger long-bone diameter of men also contribute to preserving resistance to fracture with aging.[38,41]

## Control of the Balance Between Bone Formation and Resorption

Bone active hormones and communication between the major cellular components of bone act to control bone remodeling and calcium ho-

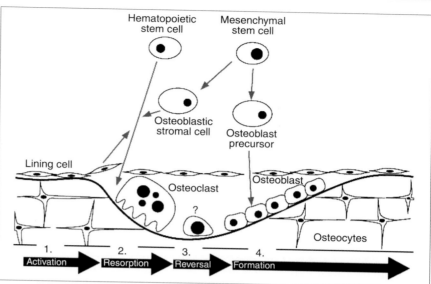

**Figure 5**    The steps in bone remodeling. **1.** Activation: Osteoclasts are most likely activated by soluble signal proteins released from surface osteocytes. Lining cells retract, exposing osteoid, facilitated by the release of a latent collagenase from osteoblasts. This process is controlled by PTH. PTH triggers osteoblasts to make interleukin-6 and RANKL to stimulate osteoclast differentiation and proliferation. Activation is increased by PTH and thyroid hormone and decreased by calcitonin and estrogen. **2.** Resorption: Osteoclasts insinuate an arm onto the exposed bone surface and attach, forming the ruffled border, and resorption progresses. PTH, thyroid hormone, and calcitriol can increase resorption depth; calcitonin, bisphosphonates, and fluoride can decrease it. **3.** Reversal: Once resorption is completed, the osteoclasts disintegrate, and the cavity is invaded by osteoblasts, attracted by local growth factors released from degraded bone. Lysomal enzymes left on the resorbing surface induce osteoblast attachment. **4.** Formation: Osteoblasts begin forming osteoid (90% type I collagen), which is then mineralized. Formation can be increased by phosphate, vitamin D, and intermittent PTH and decreased by cortisol and aging factors. (Adapted from US Department of Health and Human Services: The basics of bone in health and disease, in *Bone Health and Osteoporosis: A Report of the Surgeon General*. Rockville, MD, US Department of Health and Human Services, Office of the Surgeon General, 2004, pp 17-38.)

meostasis. Bone cells originate in the marrow from two different stem cell lines[39] (Figure 8). Osteoblasts arise from mesenchymal stem cells in bone marrow or pericyte-mesenchymal cells adherent to the endothelial layer of vessels; these same mesenchymal cells also can differentiate into fibroblasts, chondrocytes, adipocytes, or muscle cells. Osteoclasts develop from the hematopoietic stem cells that inhabit a specialized niche in bone marrow near osteoblasts. The osteoclast dif-

ferentiates from the promonocyte line, which produces monocytes, macrophages, and giant cells.[95]

The death of buried osteocytes, microcracks in bone, and other microenvironmental stimuli appear to initiate BMU formation by communication with bone surface lining cells, starting a cascade of osteoclast differentiation at the site of damage. Factors released during degradation of bone appear to attract osteoblasts to the site of bone resorption, thus the osteocyte has a role in initiating

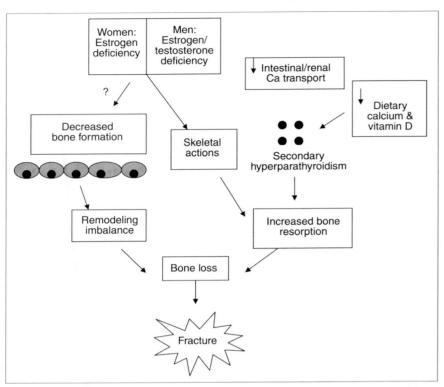

**Figure 6** Pathogenesis of osteoporosis in aging women and men. (Adapted from US Department of Health and Human Services: Diseases of bone, in *Bone Health and Osteoporosis: A Report of the Surgeon General*. Rockville, MD, US Department of Health and Human Services, Office of the Surgeon General, 2004, pp 40-65.)

local remodeling and its control.[41,105,106]

Calciotropic proresorptive factors and anabolic antiresorptive factors act through similar pathways at the root of the molecular mechanism of the coupling of osteoclastic bone resorption and osteoblastic bone formation. Coupling of resorption and formation appears to be controlled by three proteins involved in the tumor necrosis factor (TNF) signaling pathway. Two of these proteins, receptor activator of nuclear factor-kappaB (RANK), and RANK-ligand (RANKL) are membrane-bound cytokine-like molecules. RANKL is expressed on mesenchymal-derived bone marrow stromal cells, osteoblasts, and synovial fibroblasts. RANK is found on hematopoietic

stem cell-derived preosteoclasts and multinucleated osteoclasts. RANK binds with RANKL and with macrophage colony-stimulating factor, triggering the activation, final differentiation, functioning, and survival of the mature osteoclasts[1,107] (Figure 9).

Osteoprotegerin (OPG), a secreted glycoprotein from osteoblasts and mesenchymal stromal cells, is a potent inhibitor of osteoclastogenesis that binds to RANKL as a decoy, blocking RANK/RANKL interaction. Overexpression of OPG causes osteopetrosis, and underexpression causes severe osteoporosis in mice.

The loss of gonadal hormones and secondary hyperparathyroidism upregulates RANKL, causing increased bone loss, whereas gonadal

hormones and adequate calcium levels act to downregulate RANKL and increase OPG, preventing bone loss.[107]

The control of bone turnover and balance and coupling of formation and resorption appears to hinge on a bone morphogenetic protein, osteoblast specific transcription factor (*Cbfa1*), and RANKL gene cascade.[39,95] To treat osteoporosis, newer pharmacologic agents are being developed that directly affect this pathway. Denosumab, a fully human monoclonal antibody that binds to RANKL and inhibits osteoclastogenesis, is presently undergoing clinical trials.[108]

The RANK/RANKL/OPG circuit also regulates several other biologic systems.[106] RANKL is expressed on hematopoietic stem cell–derived activated T lymphocytes, and dendritic (macrophage-related) cells, which are involved in immunomodulation, inflammation, and vascular endothelial function.[106]

A better understanding of the regulation of osteoblast proliferation and function is emerging and will likely lead to new treatments focused on uncoupling bone turnover in favor of formation. Two major signals for osteoblast differentiation are bone morphogenetic proteins and *Wnt* (a homolog of the wingless gene in the fruit fly). The *LRP-5* gene codes for cell surface receptors that are important to many biologic processes, specifically bone formation and vision in humans. Inactivation of the gene produces a rare genetic disorder causing low bone mass and vision disorders. *LRP-5* is a homolog to the fruit-fly arrow gene and acts as a coreceptor for Wnt proteins. The Wnt pathway can be antagonized by secreted proteins from the Dickkopf (Dkk) family that bind to LRP-5 and directly prevent Wnt binding. Insulin-like growth factor, induced by PTH and growth hormone, is a systemic and local factor that contributes to osteoblast function. PTH appears to downregulate antagonists of Wnt, possibly explaining its anabolic effects on bone.[98,109-114]

### Types of Osteoporosis

Osteoporosis is categorized into two major types: primary and secondary. Primary osteoporosis is further divided into types I and II. Type I is postmenopausal osteoporosis caused by the abrupt reduction of gonadal hormones with accelerated loss of trabecular bone. Type II is senile osteoporosis, manifested by a slow, continuous loss throughout life of primarily cortical and trabecular bone, which is associated with age-related secondary hyperparathyroidism and the age-related decreases in bone formation. There is a significant overlap between type I and type II primary osteoporosis. Estrogen deficiency causes primary osteoporosis in postmenopausal women and contributes to bone loss in aging men.[99] Primary osteoporosis can occur in both genders at all ages but most often occurs in postmenopausal women and in men later in life. In aging men, estrogen and testosterone are probably equally important in determining bone mass.[99,115-117]

Postmenopausal women with or without osteoporosis have similar postmenopausal estrogen levels, but osteoporotic women have higher rates of bone turnover and seem to have a genetically determined hypersensitive bone response to estrogen loss.[118]

If no other reason for bone fragility is found, the woman in the case example appears to have primary type I postmenopausal osteoporosis, caused by a loss of the restraining ef-

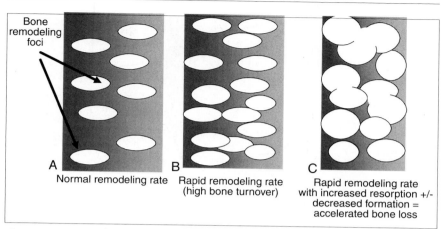

**Figure 7**    Bone remodeling and the pathogenesis of osteoporosis. **A,** Normal young bone remodeling: coupling between formation and resorption. Bone loss is equal to bone formation, maintaining normal bone mass. **B,** Rapid bone remodeling (high bone turnover). An increased number of remodeling sites is seen with increased activation frequency. If bone formation equals bone resorption at any given time, there is increased porosity of bone. This bone loss is theoretically reversible bone loss because as the remodeling cycle progresses at each site, these cavities can fill back up with bone, leading to no net bone loss. **C,** Rapid bone remodeling with either decreased formation, increased resorption, or both. The sizes of the cavities are larger than normal and are not fully filled at each cycle. There is irreversible bone loss when these cavities coalesce, perforating the trabecular plates and causing loss of structural elements. The risk of perforation increases with increased resorption depth, increased activation frequency, and decreased bone formation.

fects of estrogen on bone turnover. Secondary osteoporosis is by definition related to normal aging or hormone loss and can be caused by medication, illness, or genetic defects.[119]

### Laboratory Investigation to Determine a Secondary Cause of Osteoporosis

There is good evidence that most patients with fragility fractures have underlying secondary factors that contribute to their poor bone health [5,120,121] (Table 6). Fracture patients have established bone fragility and should be evaluated for treatable conditions to improve and protect their bone health.[1,2,5]

Up to 50% of perimenopausal women have some secondary cause that contributes to bone loss, most commonly osteomalacia, early ova-

rian failure, corticosteroid use, or excessive thyroid hormone replacement. A variety of secondary causes of bone loss (commonly osteomalacia) are present in 20% of older patients; marrow disorders or tumors also should be considered.[119,122]

Approximately 40% of men are considered to have true secondary osteoporosis, 30% have idiopathic osteoporosis, and 30% have age-related primary type bone loss and/or have hypogonadism. Secondary causes of osteoporosis are associated with medication usage (especially glucocorticoid use) or alcoholism. Idiopathic male osteoporosis can be related to low peak bone mass or other genetic factors, especially aromatase abnormalities affecting estrogen metabolism in younger men.[123,124]

Laboratory evaluation for sec-

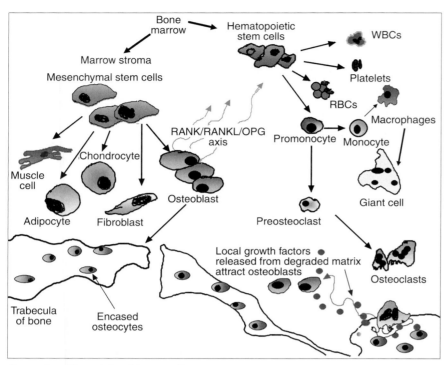

**Figure 8**   The origin of bone cells.

ondary contributing factors for bone fragility usually includes determination of 25-hydroxyvitamin D level, which best indicates vitamin status in the body; a complete blood count; determination of the erythrocyte sedimentation rate; a comprehensive chemistry panel; a thyroid-stimulating hormone test in patients receiving thyroid hormone replacement or if the test is clinically indicated; determination of serum PTH level; and a 24-hour urine calcium test. Omitting the 24-hour urine calcium test is the least cost-effective testing strategy because abnormal results can indicate hyperparathyroidism, vitamin D deficiency, excessive thyroid hormone replacement, Cushing disease, and hypocalcemic hypercalciuria. A serum PTH analysis is useful because patients with mild primary or secondary hyperparathyroidism do not always have elevated serum calcium levels.

Abnormal laboratory findings and/or the patient's history, medications, and physical examination may lead to more extensive laboratory testing or referral to another specialist.[119-122,125-127]

### Laboratory Tests to Evaluate the Rate of Bone Loss

Biochemical markers of bone formation or resorption in blood serum and urine are elevated by increased rates of bone remodeling, one of the leading causes of bone loss. Because of the coupling of bone resorption and bone formation, elevation of either marker represents increased bone remodeling. An elevation in bone remodeling markers predicts the future decline of BMD, is a risk factor for fracture that is independent of BMD, and can signal secondary causes of bone loss. Patients with rapid bone remodeling should be evaluated for secondary causes of bone loss even if

BMD is normal.[128] Significant increases in markers are seen in patients with hyperparathyroidism, hyperthyroidism, Paget's disease, myeloma, and metastatic cancer.[29]

Breakdown products of bone-specific type I collagen crosslinks, urine N-telopeptide of type I collagen (NTX), are released into the bloodstream and excreted unchanged in the urine. The level of this marker, obtained from a urine sample and expressed as an N-telopeptide/creatinine ratio (nM BCE/mM creatinine), is indicative of the rate of bone resorption and bone remodeling and is a widely available test. Many other markers of bone resorption and formation are used in research studies.[29]

A second-morning, spot urine NTX test is a responsive marker to increases in bone remodeling from any source. Therapy that is effective in slowing bone loss will decrease elevated bone marker levels to normal levels. The normal level has a wide range of values, but anything greater than 39 nM BCE/mM indicates significant ongoing bone loss[129] (Table 7). A 24-hour urine NTX test also can be obtained to correct for the 24-hour daily variation in this biomarker (the same guidelines for interpreting rate of bone loss with NTX are used).[129-131]

Bone markers show a response within 3 months of beginnng antiresorptive therapy and can be used to monitor therapy and compliance, giving patients some tangible proof that treatment is working before the 12 to 24 months needed for significant BMD changes to occur. Patients who do not respond to therapy, noncompliant patients, and those who are not taking their medications correctly can be detected with bone markers.[132,133]

The use of bone markers in clinical practice is debated because they cannot be used to diagnose osteoporosis, and treatment recommendations are not presently based on bone marker levels.[19,134] However, within-person variability does not preclude their use in the evaluation of individual patients. Serum cholesterol shows similar variability but is widely used to assess clinical risk with an end point of cardiovascular events.[135]

In the future, bone markers may assist the clinician in choosing the most efficacious treatment for a given patient. In the case example, BJC has an elevated NTX of 50, and no obvious causes for her bone fragility except postmenopausal high bone turnover.[136]

## Nonpharmacologic Recommendations to Decrease Fracture Risk

Adequate calcium and vitamin D intake, weight-bearing exercise, maintenance of a healthy weight, and cessation of smoking are global recommendations for all patients to decrease the risk of fracture[1,137,138] (Table 8). Effective smoking cessation medications rather than nicotine replacements are now approved by the US Food and Drug Administration (FDA) and can be used while patients are hospitalized and after discharge to improve bone health and decrease fracture risk.[139,140]

Optimal calcium and vitamin D intake permits accumulation of maximal peak bone mass and is necessary for preserving the aging skeleton. Approximately 350 mg of calcium is lost daily from the gastrointestinal tract and kidneys. Over time, a negative calcium balance equivalent to the calcium in one fourth of a glass of milk per day can cause low-grade secondary hyperparathyroidism with bone loss and osteoporosis.[141,142]

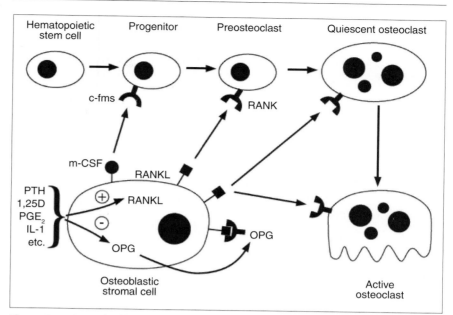

**Figure 9**    Control of bone resorption by the RANK/RANKL/OPG axis. RANKL is expressed on mesenchymal-derived bone marrow stromal cells, osteoblasts, synovial fibroblasts, and hematopoietic stem cell-derived activated T lymphocytes and dendritic cells. RANKL then binds to membrane-bound receptor RANK, found on hematopoietic stem cell-derived preosteoclast and multinucleated osteoclasts triggering the activation, final differentiation, functioning, and survival of the mature osteoclasts. OPG is a decoy molecule produced by osteoblasts that binds to RANKL and prevents it from activating RANK receptor sites on osteoclasts and their progenitors, blocking activation. PTH = parathyroid hormone; 1,25D = 1,25-dihydroxyvitamin D; $PGE_2$ = prostaglandin $E_2$, IL-1 = interleukin-1, OPG = osteoprotegerin, m-CSF = macrophage colony-stimulating factor; c-fms = mouse colony-stimulating factor 1 receptor. (Adapted from US Department of Health and Human Services: The basics of bone in health and disease, in *Bone Health and Osteoporosis: A Report of the Surgeon General*. Rockville, MD, US Department of Health and Human Services, Office of the Surgeon General, 2004, pp 17-38.)

The case example patient may be obtaining adequate calcium from supplements, but it is unlikely that she is taking adequate vitamin D.[143] Less than 50% of the adult population meets established requirements for calcium and vitamin D intake, even patients receiving pharmacologic treatment for osteoporosis. People living at higher latitudes, institutionalized patients, those who use sunscreen consistently, and darker-skinned people are at high risk for suboptimal vitamin D levels.[144] Excess calcium intake is unlikely with current diets that usually provide less than one half of the recommended daily calcium intake. Optimal vitamin D intake requires adequate sun exposure or supplements.

Orthopaedic surgeons can recommend optimal calcium and vitamin D intake to patients with fragility fractures and to all orthopaedic patients; counseling regarding calcium and vitamin D requirements is a pay-for-performance measure.[24,44] Information handouts on self-assessment of present calcium and vitamin D intake, optimal intake amounts, and sources in food or supplements can be given to patients.[145,146]

**Table 6**
**Laboratory Testing for Secondary Causes of Osteoporosis**

| Laboratory Test | Test Result | Possible Diagnoses | Treatment |
|---|---|---|---|
| Serum calcium | Low | Malabsorption, low albumin, low vitamin D | Improve nutrition, protein, calcium, and vitamin D intake |
| | High | Hyperparathyroidism, malignancy, risk kidney stones | Refer to specialist: bisphosphonates can lower serum calcium and protect the skeleton |
| Alkaline phosphatase | Increased | Osteomalacia, malignancy, liver disease, Paget's disease | Further evaluation; avoid teriparatide |
| Creatinine clearance or GFR | < 30 mL/min/24 h | Renal failure | Bisphosphonates and teriparatide not recommended; refer to renal specialist |
| SPEP | Abnormal | Myeloma | Further studies and referral needed |
| Serum PTH | Elevated | Primary or secondary hyperparathyroidism | Endocrinology of renal referral; do not use teriparatide |
| 25-hydroxyvitamin D | ≥ 35 ng/mL < 100 | Optimal range | Maintain daily vitamin D intake at approximately 1,000 IU/day up to 2,000 IU |
| | < 31 ng/mL | Causes secondary hyperparathyroidism | Daily intake as above; sliding scale of 50,000 IU/week vitamin D |
| 24-hour urine calcium | Hypercalciuria | Renal or idiopathic hyperparathyroidism | May improve with thiazides; treat hyperparathyroidism |
| | Hypocalciuria | Relative calcium malabsorption with normal vitamin D | May improve with increased calcium supplementation |
| | | Low vitamin D | Optimize vitamin D levels |
| | | Celiac sprue: urine calcium is < 100 mg/24 h | Further evaluation; treat with low gluten diet |
| TSH (0.46-4.68) | < 0.465 | Hyperthyroidism: causes increased bone loss | Evaluate and treat causes of hyperthyroidism |
| | < 0.1 on thyroid | Excess thyroid replacement causes bone loss | If iatrogenic, lower the dose of thyroid medication replacement to normalize TSH |
| CBC | Abnormal | Marrow disorder, malignancy | Further evaluation, SPEP, urine PEP, referral, and treatment |
| Erythrocyte sedimentation rate | Elevated | Anemia: various causes, marrow tumors, inflammatory conditions | Iron studies, vitamin $B_{12}$, folate, further evaluation and studies, referral if needed for treatment of renal bone fragility |
| Urine NTX | > 39 nM BEC/mM creatinine | Excessive bone turnover: Cushing disease, Paget's disease, tumors | Evaluate carefully for secondary bone loss and treat to slow bone loss |

GFR = glomerular filtration rate, SPEP = serum protein electrophoresis, PEP = protein electrophoresis, PTH = parathyroid hormone, IU = international unit, TSH = thyroid-stimulating hormone, CBC = complete blood count, NTX = urine N-telopeptide of type I collagen

## Optimal Calcium Intake

The general consensus is that 1,200 to 1,500 mg daily of elemental calcium through diet or supplements is ideal in people older than 50 years.[1,147] The safe upper limit for total calcium is 2,500 mg daily but more than 2,000 mg per day can cause renal impairment and kidney stones. A high intake of supplements, but not dietary calcium, may increase the risk of stones. No studies have shown that restrict-ing calcium intake reduces the risk for kidney stones. The risk of kidney stones from calcium supplementation is probably reduced by consuming calcium with meals.[148] Calcium carbonate is usually recommended for supplementation, although calcium citrate should be considered for those who cannot tolerate calcium carbonate or are likely to have decreased gastric acid.[1] Long-term use of gastric acid-lowering medication has been shown to increase the risk of hip fracture, possibly by decreasing calcium carbonate absorption from the stomach; calcium citrate, which does not require gastric acid for absorption, may be a better nondairy calcium source for these patients.[149]

## Sources, Metabolism, and Functions of Vitamin D

The main source of vitamin D in humans is provided by the action of ultraviolet band sunlight on skin cells to form previtamin $D_3$ or from supplements, such as vitamin $D_2$. Fifteen minutes of sun exposure in lower latitude sunlight produces 10,000 international units (IU) of vitamin D in human skin.[150] Vitamin $D_3$ from the sun or diet is activated by the liver to 25-hydroxyvitamin D and then by the kidney to 1,25-dihydroxyvitamin D. The active hormonal form, 1,25-dihydroxyvitamin D (calcitriol), has three major sites of action: the small intestine (increasing calcium absorption), the osteoblast (altering RANKL/OPG ratios and PTH levels to mobilize bone calcium when needed), and the kidney (decreasing calcium loss in urine). All of these actions are aimed at maintaining cellular, extracellular, and serum calcium levels in the body for normal mineralization of matrix and cellular function. The synthesis of many bone matrix proteins produced by osteoblasts is modulated by 1,25-dihydroxyvitamin D at the transcription level, increasing osteoid production.[150]

Vitamin D is more than a bone-active hormone. The activated form, 1,25-dihydroxyvitamin D, is important to skeletal muscle function, which prevents falls and also increases myocardial contractility. It is active in insulin metabolism and has a role in diabetes prevention and control. 1,25-dihydroxyvitamin D inhibits synthesis of renin, influencing the renin-angiotensin pathway, and plays a role in preventing and controlling high blood pressure.[150-154] Patients with renal failure, who cannot normally metabolize 25-hydroxyvitamin D through the kidney to 1,25-dihydroxyvitamin D, need supplementation with both forms of vitamin D (cholecalciferol and calcitriol) to benefit from these extraosseous effects.

**Table 7**
**Urinary N-Telopeptide of Type I Collagen (NTX) Can Monitor Therapeutic Effect of Treatment and Predicts Response of Bone Mineral Density**

Relative Risk of Bone Loss With Levels of Elevation of Urine N-Telopeptide

| Baseline NTX (nM BCE/mM creatinine) | Relative risk of significant bone loss on follow-up DXA | 95% CI |
|---|---|---|
| 18-38 | 1.4 | 0.8-2.5 |
| 38-51 | 2.5 | 1.0-6.1 |
| 51-67 | 3.8 | 1.6-9.1 |
| 67-188 | 17.3 | 2.5-118.5 |

DXA = dual-energy x-ray absorptiometry, CI = confidence interval, BCE = bone collagen equivalent

(Adapted with permission from Chesnut CH III, Bell NH, Clark GS, et al: Hormone replacement therapy in postmenopausal women: Urinary N-telopeptide of type I collagen monitors therapeutic effect and predicts response of bone mineral density. *Am J Med* 1997;102:29-37.)

**Table 8**
**Nonpharmacologic Recommendations for Preventing Osteoporotic Fractures**

| Intervention | Objective |
|---|---|
| Balanced diet, adequate calories<br>Calcium: 1,200 mg/day<br>Vitamin D: approximately 1,000 IU/day | Maintain weight<br>Essential to bone health<br>Substrate for bone formation |
| Exercise<br>  Weight bearing<br>  Muscle strengthening | Maintain bone mass in adults<br>Decrease fall risk<br>Improve balance |
| Smoking cessation | Eliminates suppression of bone formation |
| Avoid excess alcohol | Eliminate detrimental effects on BMD and decrease fall risk |
| Optimize vision<br>Home safety measures<br>Avoid medications that can cause falling | Reduce falls |

Some of the 25-hydroxyvitamin D from the liver bypasses the kidney and is taken into cells of the colon, prostate, breast, and pancreatic and immune systems and activated intracellularly to 1,25-dihydroxyvitamin D. This intracellular 1,25-dihydroxyvitamin D appears to inhibit cell proliferation and promote maturation, significantly decreasing cancer risk. 1,25-dihydroxyvitamin D is also a potent modulator of immune function, decreasing the risk of infections and autoimmune diseases such as type 1 diabetes, multiple sclerosis, and rheumatoid arthritis. Risk of osteoarthritis also is decreased by optimal vitamin D levels.[151-155]

A serum level more than 32 ng/mL (equals approximately 77 nmol/L) of 25-hydroxyvitamin D is needed to maintain serum calcium without provoking secondary hyperparathyroidism. Levels from 35 to 55 ng/mL are considered optimal, but levels of 80 to 100 ng/mL can occur in people with frequent sun exposure or tanning and are considered normal. Levels of 35 ng/mL or more not only prevent clinical rickets or osteomalacia but also confer the previously noted nonskeletal benefits.[141,156,157] 1,25-dihydroxyvitamin D levels are tightly controlled by the body and generally do not reflect overall vitamin D stores (Figure 10).

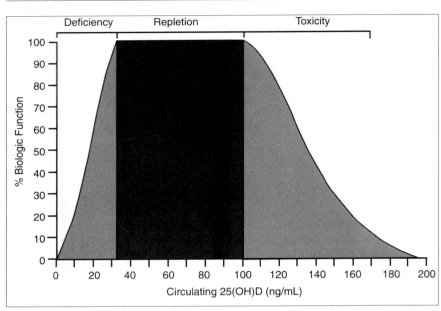

**Figure 10** Stages of nutritional vitamin D status. (Reproduced with permission from Hollis BW: Circulating 25-hydroxyvitamin D levels indicative of vitamin D sufficiency: Implications for establishing a new effective dietary intake recommendation for vitamin D. *J Nutr* 2005;135:317-322.)

Daily doses of vitamin D needed to maintain these serum levels are far higher than the 400 to 600 IU of vitamin D currently recommended by the National Academy of Sciences for adults older than 50 years. The older NOF recommendation of 800 IU per day for those at risk of deficiency, such as elderly, chronically ill, homebound, or institutionalized individuals, cannot improve serum levels to optimal levels if they are very low to begin with. The NOF has recently increased the daily recommendation to 1,000 IU of vitamin D daily.[158] Vitamin $D_2$ (ergocalciferol) is approximately 30% less bioactive than $D_3$ (cholecalciferol) but is preferable for vegetarians. Vitamin $D_3$ is available as over-the-counter capsules in doses up to 1,000 IU. In the United States, it is difficult to obtain the 50,000 IU capsule of vitamin $D_3$ used to treat deficiency.[142]

Optimal daily intake of vitamin D is likely to be at least 1,000 IU of over-the-counter vitamin D (cholecalciferol) in vitamin D-replete adults. A safe upper limit of 2,000 IU per day of over-the-counter vitamin D has been set by the National Academy of Science.[158] Toxicity is possible with excessive doses of over-the-counter vitamin D but is more likely with activated forms of vitamin D, such as calcitriol, which are prescribed for treating specific metabolic bone diseases other than postmenopausal or age-related bone loss.[142,159]

After testing, the woman with the Colles fracture in the case presentation is found to have a 10 ng/mL level of 25-hydroxyvitamin D. This level is considered a severe deficiency and can have multiple negative effects on the patient's health. Once a patient is deficient in vitamin D, it takes much higher doses to return the serum level to the optimal level.[141,156] If the serum level is less than 35 ng/mL, 50,000 IU of oral vitamin D can be given weekly in addition to the daily recommended dose of 1,000 IU of vitamin $D_3$, using a sliding scale of up to 12 weeks. In a patient with a fragility fracture, the serum level should be rechecked in 3 months to verify that the serum level is improved; if inadequate improvement is found (level is < 32 ng/mL), weekly loading doses of oral vitamin D (50,000 IU) should be given for another few weeks as necessary to improve the level to the optimal range. This loading dose may occasionally need to be repeated or even continued once monthly in institutionalized or resistant patients.[157,159,160]

Using these guidelines, overdosing a patient with ergocalciferol ($D_2$) or cholecalciferol ($D_3$) is unlikely. Serum calcium monitoring is not necessary if it was normal to begin with. If an ionized or direct serum calcium is truly elevated, the patient usually should be referred to an endocrinologist or some other specialist with expertise in treating more complicated metabolic bone disease.[159] Some researchers and clinicians recommend that yearly 25-hydroxyvitamin D levels be included in preventive medical evaluations by primary care physicians because of the high prevalence of deficiency and benefits of optimal vitamin D levels on multiple health outcomes.[155,159,161]

### The Role of Optimal Calcium and Vitamin D Intake in Fracture Risk Reduction

The results of studies on the roles of calcium and vitamin D alone in fracture risk reduction are conflicting. The large randomized Women's Health Initiative study did not show fracture risk reduction with calcium and vitamin D intake; however, dosing was at lower levels than currently recommended, and patient noncompliance was a factor.[162-164] Women who were compliant (took at least 80% of their study medications) had a 29% reduction in hip fracture, and subgroup analyses of older women with a higher absolute risk of fracture showed a significantly decreased risk of hip fracture.[164] Many studies and meta-analyses have noted fracture reduction in vertebral and hip fractures of up to 25% with calcium and vitamin D supplementation in more optimal doses, especially in groups at high risk for deficiency. Daily doses of 1,200 mg of calcium and more than 800 IU of vitamin D appear to be needed to achieve reduction in fracture risk.[165-168]

The case study patient meets NOF guidelines as well as multiple other guidelines for pharmacologic intervention.[44,79] Her fracture history, BMD, and risk factors contribute to a significant risk of further fractures. There is compelling evidence that treating patients with fragility fractures is a cost-effective intervention and decreases future fracture risk for the individual patient.[2,3,5,6] The pharmacologic treatment goal in a patient with a fragility fracture is to decrease fracture risk by 50%. No treatment of osteoporosis will prevent all future fractures. Using the best available agents can reduce fracture risk by approximately 50%. All patients treated for fracture reduction need to be calcium and vitamin D replete for other pharmacologic agents to be maximally effective.[3,169]

### FDA-Approved Pharmacologic Agents for Osteoporosis

There are two types of agents for the treatment of osteoporosis[170] (Figure 11). Antiresorptive agents

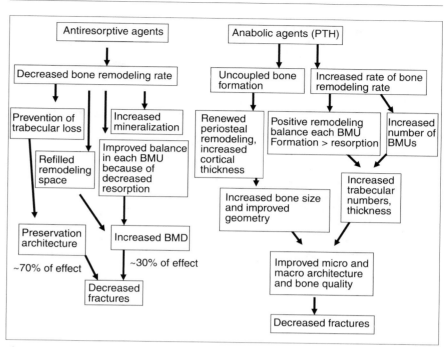

**Figure 11**    Mechanism of fracture reduction by antiresorptive and anabolic agents.

primarily decrease bone resorption and therefore also decrease overall bone remodeling and bone loss. Bone-forming agents act primarily to increase bone formation more than resorption.[170] Antiresorptive agents are first-line medications for the prevention and treatment of osteoporosis.[41] FDA-approved antiresorptive agents for the treatment of osteoporosis are bisphosphonates, including alendronate, risedronate, ibandronate, raloxifene, and calcitonin.[48,171] Estrogen is no longer FDA approved for the treatment of osteoporosis[136,172] (Table 9).

Formation agents presently only are approved in patients with severe osteoporosis and may not be covered by insurance unless patients are intolerant to other medications or have been unsuccessfully treated with antiresorptive agents. The first clinically available formation agent, teriparatide (human recombinant 1-34 PTH), was approved by the

FDA in 2002 for the treatment of severe osteoporosis in postmenopausal women with a high risk of fracture and in men with primary or hypogonadal osteoporosis. Toxicities of all available agents for treating osteoporosis are generally less than those of nonsteroidal anti-inflammatory drugs or antibiotics, which are commonly used in the treatment of musculoskeletal disorders.[173,174]

Antiresorptive agents decrease the birth rate (activation rate) of new remodeling sites and also decrease the amount of resorption at each site. These actions allow time for better mineralization, prevent further loss of architecture, and reduce bone loss. Antiresorptive agents have limited bone-building action. They can reduce fracture risk up to approximately 50% for vertebral fractures, and the more potent agents can reduce the risk of non-vertebral fractures by approximately

**Table 9**
**Osteoporosis Medications Approved by the Food and Drug Administration for Treatment: Dosing, Fracture Reduction, Side Effects, and Contraindications**

| Drugs | Route and Dose | Fracture Risk Reduction | Side Effects | Major Contraindications |
|---|---|---|---|---|
| Antiresorptive Agents Bisphosphonates Alendronate | Oral 70 mg weekly ± vitamin D | Vertebral Nonvertebral Hip | Common: esophagitis myalgias Rare: severe bone and muscle pain ocular inflammation may cause osteonecrosis of the jaw | Allergy Severe esophageal problems: stricture, poor motility Inability to sit upright 30 to 60 minutes Creatinine clearance < 30 mL/min/24 h |
| Risedronate | Oral 35 mg weekly | Vertebral Nonvertebral Hip | | |
| Ibandronate | Oral 150 mg monthly | Vertebral | | |
| Ibandronate | Intravenous 3 mg every 3 months | Vertebral | UGI similar to placebo Flulike symptoms | Low serum calcium Renal failure |
| Zolendronate | Intravenous 5 mg yearly | Vertebral Nonvertebral Hip | UGI similar to placebo Flulike symptoms | Allergy |
| SERM Raloxifene | Oral 60 mg daily | Vertebral only | Hot flashes, nausea, leg cramps, deep venous thrombosis Increase in stroke mortality, not incidence | Previous venous thrombosis Allergy |
| Calcitonin | Nasal spray 200 IU daily | Vertebral only | Rhinitis | Allergy |
| Anabolic drugs PTH (1-34) (teriparatide) | Subcutaneous 20 µg daily | Vertebral Nonvertebral | Mild transient hypercalcemia or hypercalciuria Nausea Dizziness Leg cramps | Hypersensitivity Creatinine clearance < 35mL/min/24 h Patients with increased risk of osteosarcoma (such as children and those with Paget's disease, previous radiation, or an unexplained increase in alkaline phosphatase levels) |

SERM = selective estrogen receptor modulators, PTH = parathyroid hormone, UGI = upper gastrointestinal
(Data from Rosen CJ: Postmenopaursal osteoporosis. *N Engl J Med* 2005;353:595-598.)

50%. Significant fracture risk reduction occurs at 3 to 6 months after initiation of treatment and precedes the 1- to 2-year period needed to see a significant increase in BMD[5,6,169,175-192] (Table 10).

For the woman in the case study who already had a fragility fracture, bisphosphonates is the best evidence-based pharmacologic treatment. Bisphosphonates are the most efficacious antiresorptive agents for fracture reduction and the only antiresorptive agents that reduce the risk of hip fracture. They have a more

than 90% responder rate.[6] The oral bisphosphonates (alendronate, risedronate and ibandronate) can reduce vertebral fracture risk by more than 50%. Alendronate and risedronate also can reduce the risk of new nonvertebral fractures by approximately 50%.[178,179] Alendronate has a specific FDA indication for hip fracture prevention.[3,169,179-186]

There is some emerging evidence that less than weekly dosing can improve compliance.[187,188] The best fracture reduction outcomes have been achieved with daily bisphosphonate

administration using newer bisphosphonates or in dosing regimens studied with noninferiority BMD trials (studies in which different dosing schedules only had to show the same or better BMD improvement compared with the daily or original doses).[184,185,189,190]

Bisphosphonates target bone specifically, have excellent risk-benefit profiles, provide fracture risk reduction within months, and maintain this reduction in risk for 7 to 10 years.[189,190] They do not significantly inhibit fracture healing at

**Table 10**
**Estimated Fracture Reduction Rates With Treatment Medications (Not Head-to-Head Trials)**

| | Teriparatide Neer et al [263] (2001) | Alendronate Black et al[175] (1996) | Risedronate Harris et al[176] (1999) Reginster et al[177] (2000) McClung et al[178] (2001) | | Oral Ibandronate Chesnut et al[180] (2004) | Intravenous Ibandronate Recker et al[191] (2004) | Intravenous Zolendronate Black et al[192] (2007) |
|---|---|---|---|---|---|---|---|
| **New Vertebral Fractures** | | | | | | | |
| Relative risk (95% CI) | 0.4 | 0.5 | 0.6 | 0.5 | 0.49 | No fracture data | 0.3 |
| Placebo fracture rate | 14% | 15% | 16% | 29% | 9.6% | | 10.9% |
| Absolute risk reduction | 9% | 7% | 5% | 11% | 4.9% | | |
| **New Nonvertebral Fractures** | | | | | | | |
| Relative risk (95% CI) | 0.5 | 0.8 | 0.6 | 0.7 | 1.0 | No fracture data | 0.75 (hip 0.59) |
| Placebo rate | 6% | 15% | 8% | 51% | 8.2% | | 9% (hip 2.5%) |
| Absolute risk reduction | 3% | 3% | 3% | 15% | 0% | Noninferiority BMD versus oral daily dose data | 3% (hip approximately 4%) |

CI = confidence interval

doses used to treat osteoporosis, may protect against total joint loosening, and have antitumor effects in bone.[193-196]

Selective estrogen receptor modulators are nonhormonal agents that bind to estrogen receptors and prevent bone loss without increasing the risk of breast and uterine cancer as seen with estrogen use. Raloxifene can reduce the risk of vertebral fracture approximately 40% but does not decrease nonvertebral fracture risk; it does significantly decrease the risk of invasive breast cancer and is FDA approved for this indication.[6,172]

Estrogen and hormone replacement therapy (HRT), although efficacious antiresorptive agents, are no longer approved for the treatment of osteoporosis. HRT can reduce the risk of clinical vertebral and hip fractures by 34% but increases the risk of myocardial infarction, stroke, invasive breast cancer, pulmonary emboli, deep venous thrombosis, gallbladder disease, and dementia.[197-199] HRT is no longer recommended for long-term

use in the prevention of chronic disease, but it is still approved for the reduction of postmenopausal symptoms at the lowest dose and shortest duration possible. Approximately 20% of women using HRT do not have slowing of bone loss and are considered nonresponders. Women who continue HRT for menopausal symptom relief should be evaluated to ensure that they are adequately protected against bone loss. Many postmenopausal women who stopped estrogen replacement therapy in 2002 when the risks of use were reported are now at increased fracture risk if they did not receive approved antiresorptive agents when indicated.[200]

Both estrogen and selective estrogen receptor modulators increase the relative risk of venous thrombosis by 44% and fatal stroke by 49%.[172,197,201] Orthopaedic surgeons should consider stopping estrogen and raloxifene therapy in patients scheduled to undergo major orthopaedic procedures because both agents increase the risk of thrombotic events.[202,203]

Calcitonin is the weakest FDA-approved antiresorptive agent. It decreases vertebral fracture risk approximately 30% and does not afford protection against nonvertebral fractures. It has useful analgesic properties in acute vertebral fractures.[6]

## The Effects of Bisphosphonates on Bone

Bisphosphonates are pyrophosphate analogs that bind to exposed mineral surfaces of bone and are incorporated into newly formed matrix. When these molecules are phagocytized by osteoclasts, they interfere with osteoclast activation and function by interrupting the mevalonate pathway for cholesterol biosynthesis, preventing formation of the ruffled border. Statins act on a similar pathway. The newer, potent nitrogen-containing bisphosphonates (amino-bisphosphonates) currently approved for use in postmenopausal osteoporosis act by inhibiting the protein prenylation action of an enzyme, farnesyl pyrophosphate synthetase, and disrupt the biosynthesis of downstream small proteins necessary for osteoclast function. The actions of bisphosphonates affect cytoskeletal organization and vesicular fusion, and cause osteoclast apoptosis. Simpler, non–nitrogen-containing bisphosphonates (such as clodronate and etidronate) do not inhibit protein prenylation but may act by inhibiting enzymes in the adenosine triphosphate pathway, forming cytotoxic metabolites. Understanding the subtle differences between individual bisphosphonates may help to improve clinical efficacy in the future.[204,205]

Bisphosphonates decrease the remodeling rate and the depth of resorption cavities. Because resorption and formation are coupled, formation at the tissue level, but not at the cellular level, is also decreased. Aminobisphosphonates, unlike first-generation bisphosphonates, inhibit osteoclast resorption at doses that do not impair mineralization. Bisphosphonates also improve osteoblast and osteocyte preservation by decreasing apoptosis. Biopsy data have shown normal bone histology and strength. Bisphosphonates have a long half-life in bone: 10 years for alendronate, 1 year for risedronate, and approximately 1.5 years for ibandronate. This finding explains their sustained effects of decreasing bone remodeling months to years after the agents are stopped—they are slowly released from newly remodeled bone mineral over time and continue to cause decreased remodeling until they are gradually eliminated from the body.[204,205]

## Bisphosphonate Dosing, Contraindications, and Adverse Side Effects

Oral bisphosphonates must be taken on an empty stomach because they are so poorly absorbed; if taken with anything except water, they will not be absorbed at all. These medications can be a direct irritant to the esophagus if the pill gets caught in the esophagus or if high concentrations are splashed into the esophagus by reflux; this can cause esophageal erosions.[206] The dosing regimen requires 30 to 60 minutes of maintaining an upright posture to prevent reflux of bisphosphonate material into the esophagus.[174]

Major contraindications to bisphosphonate therapy are hypersensitivity to the drug; severe esophageal problems, especially stricture or motility disorders; and inability of a patient sit upright for 30 to 60 minutes. Bisphosphonates are not approved by the FDA for premenopausal women, pregnant women (category C drug), and children. Bisphosphonates are not contraindicated in patients with occasional reflux or in those with gastroesophageal reflux disease if symptoms are well controlled with medication. Administration of these medications in patients with Barrett's esophagus without stricture or motility problems may be safe; however, the treatment decision generally should be made by the primary care physician and/or gastrointestinal specialist. If the patient has a high fracture risk and cannot tolerate oral bisphosphonates, intravenous bisphosphonates or formation agents may be recommended; calcitonin is not the best option in these high-risk patients.

Hypocalcemia that is not simply related to low albumin is a contraindication to the use of bisphosphonates. Direct or ionized serum calcium can be checked to determine if the patient has true hypocalcemia of clinical significance. If the ionized calcium is low, it is frequently related to severe calcium and vitamin D deficiency and should be corrected before starting bisphosphonate therapy. Calcium and vitamin D supplementation should be given to all patients with a fragility fracture.

Severe renal insufficiency, with a creatinine clearance of less than 30 mL/min, is considered a contraindication for bisphosphonate therapy. Bisphosphonates are excreted by the kidney but are not nephrotoxic.[204,205]

Adverse side effects of oral bisphosphonates are generally gastrointestinal. Rare serious esophagitis has been reported. Gastrointestinal disturbances such as heartburn, esophageal irritation, abdominal pain, and diarrhea are common and similar in incidence to those of a control group using a placebo. Similar gastrointestinal precautions are applicable to all oral bisphosphonates.[206,207]

Rare musculoskeletal side effects include severe bone, joint, and/or muscle pain that can begin an average of 3 months after the onset of therapy (range, 1 day to 52 months). Most patients improve when the drug is stopped, but 30% of patients can have persistent, disabling pain. In some patients, the pain can reoccur after trying the medication again.[208] Ocular inflammation is rare in patients treated with bisphosphonates. Blurred vision, eye pain, and inflammation of the conjunctiva, uvea, and sclera have been reported with alendronate and risedronate use and may occasionally resolve only after stopping the medication.[209]

The rare occurrence of osteonecrosis of the jaw also has been reported in patients taking bisphosphonates for postmenopausal osteoporosis. Most instances of this disorder have occurred in patients treated with high-dose intravenous bisphosphonate therapy for cancer who are also being treated with chemotherapy and corticosteroids; however, nonhealing necrotic bone areas in the jaw have been reported in some women without cancer (< 1/300,000) who were taking oral bisphosphonates for osteoporosis. Osteonecrosis of the jaw occurs most commonly in patients after oral surgery or tooth extraction.[196] The reasons that osteonecrosis may occur in membranous bone in the oral cavity and not elsewhere from bisphosphonate use are related to anatomy, circulation, trauma, and oral flora.[210] The jaw remodeling rate is 10 times faster than that of the long bones. The risk of osteonecrosis of the jaw appears to increase after 3 years and with more potent bisphosphonates. Examining bone remodeling rates may help predict who is at highest risk.[211]

Patients should be informed about the low risk of osteonecrosis of the jaw at the doses used to treat postmenopausal osteoporosis. If they need oral surgery or tooth extraction, bisphosphonate therapy can be postponed or stopped until the jaw has healed, although there is no good evidence that this precaution is necessary. Patients at high risk of fracture who are concerned about the risk of osteonecrosis should be informed about the low risk of osteonecrosis of the jaw versus the risk of refracture and the morbidity and mortality of osteoporosis.[196,210,212-216]

Handouts explaining the risks and benefits of osteoporosis medications are available. Management of osteoporosis after a fragility fracture and treatment with appropriate medications to decrease fracture risk are pay-for-performance measures.[44]

## Duration of Bisphosphonate Therapy

Use of oral bisphosphonates for osteoporosis appears to be safe and effective for 7 to 10 years.[189,190,217] There are concerns that the decreased remodeling rate may eventually cause hypermineralization with increased stiffness and/or cause accumulation of microdamage, leading to increased fracture risk. However, at the usual doses for treating osteoporosis, bisphosphonates do not appear to decrease the remodeling rate below that of young, normal individuals.[218-220] BMD gained during bisphosphonate therapy and continued fracture risk reduction are frequently sustained after withdrawal for 1 to 2 years (more so in older patients).[221,222] This advantage is in contrast to the rapid rate of bone loss that occurs after the cessation of estrogen.[223]

## Vertebral Fracture Case Presentation

BJC, a 65-year-old Caucasian women, is admitted to the hospital with severe midback pain after picking up a gallon of milk. The orthopaedic surgeon treated this patient 10 years ago when she sustained a Colles fracture. At that time, she was started on therapy with antiresorptive agents but did not continue the medication and was lost to follow-up after her wrist fracture healed. The patient's family doctor consult the orthopaedic surgeon for treatment and pain management recommendations for BJC. The patient has lost 4 inches in height, and her admission spine radiographs show a 20% anterior vertebral wedge at L1. On physical examination, she has thoracic kyphosis, a flattened lumbar lordosis, increased cervical lordosis, and a protuberant abdomen.

The orthopaedic surgeon must determine if this patient has a vertebral compression fracture. The dowager's hump, an iconic portrait of osteoporosis, is difficult to miss but frequently is not addressed. Radiology reports do not mention 50% of prevalent vertebral fractures. If reported as an incidental finding on the chest radiograph of hospitalized patients, the information reaches the discharge summary only 10% of the time, and bone fragility is diagnosed and treated in an even smaller percentage of patients.[224]

There is presently no consensus for the radiographic diagnosis of vertebral fractures. Radiographic diagnosis is complicated by variations in technique, difficulty in distinguishing nonfracture deformity from fracture, and dynamic changes in fractured vertebra over time.[225] Radiographic assessment of vertebral deformities may be done by semiquantitative visual or quantitative (morphometric) techniques. A vertebral height loss of even 15% may be clinically significant and predictive of future fracture.[226]

Until a consensus is reached for the radiographic diagnosis of vertebral fracture, the visual inspection technique of Genant and associates[227] that classifies fractures according to estimated loss of vertebral body height on lateral spine imaging is useful. This semiquantitative visual assessment considers loss of vertebral height in the range of 0% to less than 20% as normal, 20% to 25% as mild, more than 25% to 40% as moderate; and more than 40% as severe. Vertebral fragility fractures can be wedged, biconcave (cod-fished), or crushed (vertebra plana).

The multiple etiologies of back pain can make it difficult to verify that this radiographic vertebral wedge is the cause of the patient's acute pain, but given her history and examination, osteoporotic fracture should be strongly suspected in the differential diagnosis. Vertebral fractures frequently occur with minimal to no obvious trauma during activities of daily living such as bending or lifting; however, 25% to 50% are related to falls.[8]

Bone scans can confirm an acute fracture site, especially when the patient has vertebral wedging at multiple levels or other deformities, but their use is limited by the 7 to 10 days it may take to see a positive scan in an elderly patient. An MRI scan allows immediate location of any acute process and also may identify marrow disorders or tumors.[228]

All patients with a fragility fracture need a basic laboratory evaluation as has been previously discussed. Additional studies are indicated for possible marrow disorders or malignancy. Serum and urine electrophoreses are useful, and vertebral biopsy or bone marrow biopsy is done if indicated. Urine NTX and 24-hour urine calcium levels can be elevated by fractures and bed rest and may not reflect prefracture levels, but can provide useful information if levels are significantly abnormal.

Hospitalized patients with fragility fractures have a high incidence of low 25-hydroxyvitamin D levels. If the serum calcium does not have a high reading on admission, it is reasonable to start daily calcium and vitamin D supplementation and to give 50,000 IU of oral vitamin D weekly until the vitamin D level is available.[143,157]

Treatment is more urgent than BMD testing in patients with osteoporotic vertebral fractures. BMD testing is useful and can be ordered at discharge as an outpatient test because it is not presently covered under diagnostic-related groups (DRGs) used by Medicare to determine payment to hospitals. Treatment should be started even without access to BMD information in patients with hip and spine fractures, after basic laboratory investigation is available, and before completion of an extensive workup for secondary causes of osteoporosis if the patient has no contraindications to treatment.

## Incidence and Cost of Vertebral Fractures

Vertebral fractures are the most common type of osteoporotic fracture, with more than 700,000 new vertebral fractures per year in the United States.[1] Vertebral fracture incidence increases at approximately age 50 to 55 years and increases exponentially at approximately age 60 years. Lifetime risk of vertebral fracture is 15.6% in Caucasian women and 5% in Caucasian men. Lifetime risk for nonwhites is less for all fracture types, except for vertebral fractures in Asians, who have as high a risk as that of Caucasians.[8,229] Prevalence increases with age for both sexes, although the gradient is steeper for females.[230] Direct health care cost associated with spine fractures was $746 million in 1995.[1]

One or two painless vertebral deformities in younger men are often traumatic in origin, whereas three or more vertebral fractures, especially in older men, are more likely related to osteoporosis. Men with symptomatic vertebral fractures have low BMD and increased refracture risk.[231]

## Morbidity and Mortality Associated With Vertebral Compression Fractures

Clinical consequences of silent or symptomatic vertebral compression fractures can include acute and chronic back pain with fatigue discomfort in the midkyphos; pain from compensatory curves and arthritis around the main deformity or caused by the ribs impinging on the iliac crests; progressive height loss; acute or gradually increasing spinal deformity; reduced pulmonary function that worsens with each added vertebral compression fracture; poor balance with increased risk of a fall; anxiety, depression, and decreased self-esteem; weight loss, malnutrition, and early satiety; sleep disturbance and difficulties in finding clothing that fits properly. The morbidity of vertebral fractures is similar to that of hip fracture in adversely affecting the activities of daily living.[1] Inactivity accelerates bone loss and muscle deconditioning.[232-234] Spine fractures are associated with a 20% reduction in quality of life in the first 12 months and 15% after 2 years.[235]

The intense pain of acute fractures may last 4 to 6 weeks but can continue for months.[236] Chronic pain frequently follows, especially with multiple compression fractures and progressive collapse or motion at the fracture site. The greater the deformity, the greater the likelihood of developing chronic pain and disability. Lumbar spine fractures are more likely to cause back pain than those in the thoracic spine. Most vertebral compression fractures occur at the thoracolumbar junction, where stresses for fracture are greatest. If a fracture is at T4 or above, it is more likely to be pathologic.[232]

In 1995, spine fractures that were conservatively treated accounted for 8% of hospitalizations, 3% of residents requiring nursing home care, and 3% of physician visits; 4% of emergency department visits were for osteoporotic fracture.[1] Osteoporotic vertebral compression fractures are associated with a 30% age-adjusted increase in mortality.[237] Most deaths after spine fracture occur long after from underlying medical conditions that contributed to the osteoporosis.[1,238-240]

### Risks of Another Fracture in a Patient With a Vertebral Fracture

After one vertebral compression fracture, the risk of a subsequent fracture is increased fivefold; one in five women with a vertebral fracture will have another fracture within 1 year. After two or more vertebral compression fractures, the risk of a subsequent fracture increases twelvefold.[241,242] With prevalent vertebral fracture, vertebral fracture risk and severity increases.[242]

Preexisting vertebral fractures predict future fractures independent of BMD but are even more predictive when combined with low BMD. Low bone mass (< 33rd percentile) combined with two or more previous vertebral compression fractures results in a 75-fold increased risk of subsequent vertebral compression fracture.[53,229] Refractures are especially frequent in areas adjacent to the previously fractured levels.[8,243] One vertebral fracture increases the risk of subsequent hip fracture twofold.[54]

### Pharmacologic Treatment

The usual nonpharmacologic recommendations should be followed.[1,2] Pharmacologic intervention can greatly reduce the risk of additional fragility fractures. BMD changes and fracture risk reduction in the spine are used by the FDA as the standard for approving osteoporosis medication because the vertebra is the most measurable, representative, and responsive bone

in the body to the treatment of bone loss.[6,171] Small gains in BMD of the vertebrae result in large gains in vertebral strength because the strength of a trabecular strut is proportional to the square of its radius.[243] The selection of therapy should be based on the level of fracture risk, comorbid conditions, patient preferences, the physician's skill, and economic factors; however, pharmacologic intervention should start in the hospital or be arranged to begin as soon as possible after the patient's discharge.

The bisphosphonates are the most effective antiresorptive therapy currently available for secondary reduction of fractures in patients with fragility fractures.[6] They reduce vertebral fracture risk up to 50% within 6 months to 1 year and the risk of multiple vertebral fractures up to 80%. Spine BMD increases about 12% in 10 years.[169,189]

The patient in the case presentation cannot take oral bisphosphonates because of significant upper gastrointestinal contraindications and has difficulty sitting upright in the hospital because of the acute spine fracture; therefore, intravenous bisphosphonates should be considered. Intravenous ibandronate and intravenous zolendronate are FDA-approved intravenous bisphosphonates for postmenopausal osteoporosis, although many other intravenous bisphosphonates are approved for treating hypercalcemia and malignant bone involvement. Intravenous bisphosphonates are generally believed to be safe for patients who cannot tolerate or should not use oral bisphosphonates; they usually do not cause upper gastrointestinal effects, although dyspepsia, abdominal pain, and diarrhea (conditions similar to those of patients receiving a placebo) have

been reported. Low serum calcium, renal failure, and hypersensitivity to the drug are major contraindications for use. Approximately 50% of an intravenous ibandronate dose binds to bone, and the remainder is excreted unchanged in the urine.[244] Ibandronate is approximately 10 times more potent than alendronate in inhibiting bone resorption.[245]

Intravenous ibandronate is approved by the FDA for use once every 3 months in patients with postmenopausal osteoporosis. It can be administered in the outpatient setting in a medical office, in a hospital short-procedure unit, or by a company that provides infusion in the patient's home. Dosing is 3 mg every 3 months administered over 15 to 30 seconds. This is a much shorter infusion time than is needed with other intravenous bisphosphonates. It is recommended that serum creatinine be checked before the first dose and then just before subsequent doses, although renal toxicity is generally rare. Treatment should be withheld if renal deterioration occurs. BMD increases approximately 5% at the spine and 2.5% at the hip in 1 year, which is similar or slightly better than the 2.5% increase expected with oral daily ibandronate. Studies show that markers of bone turnover decrease 50% in all the compared groups.[245-247] Good fracture reduction data are not yet available for intravenous ibandronate; oral bisphosphonates with proven long-term significant fracture reduction are preferred if they can be tolerated by the patient.[191,248,249]

Patients should be given supplemental calcium and vitamin D therapy. Intravenous bisphosphonates should not be used for patients with true low ionized serum calcium or poor calcium/vitamin D status because it could result in a further drop in serum calcium.[244] Acute phase reaction-like events can occur (flulike symptoms) with joint and muscle pain and fever, usually with the first dose; anecdotal information suggests that pretreatment with acetaminophen may improve symptoms.[244]

Intravenous zolendronate given at 5 mg yearly has been shown to reduce vertebral fracture risk approximately 70% and hip fracture risk by approximately 50% at 1 year after treatment begins and has shown continuing risk reduction through 3 years in women with postmenopausal osteoporosis. If given within 3 months of an osteoporotic hip fracture, it can provide a 35% risk reduction in new fractures and a 28% decrease in mortality compared with placebo.[250] An increased risk of atrial fibrillation was seen in this study but generally occurred more than 30 days after the bisphosphonate was administered and was not believed to be causal; this risk will be closely monitored after the product is marketed.[192,251] Zolendronate is more potent than ibandronate in decreasing bone resorption.[245]

Other evidence-based pharmacologic options are available for treating severe osteoporosis in patients such as in the case presentation patient, who is at high risk for further fractures. Many patients with severe osteoporosis continue to have fractures in spite of the 50% decreased risk with optimal bisphosphonate therapy. The answer to further fracture reduction appears to lie with formation agents, such as teriparatide.[252,253]

Chronic hyperparathyroidism increases bone remodeling with resorption greater than formation, leading to net bone loss. This loss can be slowed with antiresorptive

agents. The bone loss in primary hyperparathyroidism does not cause the same degree of loss of bone architecture that is seen in hypogonadism because tunneling rather than perforation of trabeculae occurs.[254]

Intermittent administration of pharmacologic PTH has a very different effect. It increases bone mass and strength dramatically by increasing the numbers, life span, and function of osteoblasts, which increases bone formation. It uncouples bone formation from resorption, promoting bone deposition on surfaces not preexcavated by osteoclasts. The result is a reconstruction of the skeleton with increased trabecular thickness, reconnected trabeculae, and increased cortical thickness without increased cortical porosity. After 18 months of intermittent 1-34 PTH (teriparatide) use, remodeling returns to a more equal balance.[255-257] Bone formation markers such as bone-specific alkaline phosphatase are markedly elevated for the first few months, then bone resorption markers also increase and overall turnover markers are elevated for 18 to 24 months. After 18 months, the markers decline to baseline levels despite ongoing PTH administration.[252,258] Intermittent PTH appears to promote fracture healing in animal studies.[105,259-261]

## BMD Results and Fracture Reduction With PTH Therapy Alone

Weekly doses of subcutaneous PTH in postmenopausal women increased spine BMD 5% to 8% in 48 months with no change in cortical thickness and good dose response.[262] In postmenopausal women with severe osteoporosis treated with daily subcutaneous

doses of 1-34 PTH (teriparatide), spine BMD increased 10% to 14%, and total hip BMD increased 2.6% to 4% over a 1- to 3-year period compared with a placebo; the responder rate was 96%. Maximal BMD increases occur during the first 18 months of therapy. The risk of vertebral fracture decreased by 65% and nonvertebral fractures by 50% over 21 months, with fracture reduction evident at 6 months.[263] Administration of daily subcutaneous 1-34 PTH (teriparatide, 40 $\mu$g/day) for 14 months provided a significant reduction in nonvertebral fractures compared with alendronate (10 mg/day); 4.1% of patients in the PTH group had nonvertebral fractures compared with 13.7% in the alendronate group.[264]

Men with idiopathic osteoporosis with low bone turnover who were treated daily with subcutaneous PTH for 18 months had a 13.5% increase in BMD of the spine and a 2.9% increase at the hip with an overall increased bone turnover rate.[265]

Multiple studies with subcutaneous PTH in men and women with severe osteoporosis have shown consistent, significant reductions in vertebral and nonvertebral fractures, although not specifically in hip fractures.[262-268] BMD increases with PTH are of significantly greater magnitude compared with those seen with bisphosphonates and occur in a shorter period of time. Gains in BMD can be lost if an antiresorptive agent is not used long term following PTH treatment.[254,269,270]

PTH or bisphosphonates are both excellent choices for patients with prior fractures and who are clinically osteoporotic. Patients with high bone turnover before treatment have more robust increases in

BMD with antiresorptive and bone formation agents.[134,271] Patients with low-turnover osteoporosis seem to be especially good candidates for formation agents; however, pretreatment bone turnover levels do not clearly correlate with fracture risk reduction with antiresorptive or bone formation agents. Fracture risk reduction seems largely independent of age, initial BMD, prevalent fractures at baseline, and pretreatment bone turnover with both types of medications.[6,268,272,273]

### PTH Therapy for Patients Who Have Been Treated With Antiresorptive Agents

Pretreatment or cotreatment with antiresorptive agents can blunt the osteogenic response of PTH, more so with potent antiresorptive agents such as bisphosphonates.[266,269,274-276] Pretreatment and combination therapy with weaker, shorter-acting antiresorptive agents such as estrogen, calcitonin, and raloxifene does not materially blunt the bone-forming effects of PTH and can allow continuous improvement in vertebral (13%) and hip (4%) BMD over a 3-year period, with a significant decrease (75% to 100%) in the rate of vertebral fractures compared with a 30% decrease in risk with the weak antiresorptive agent alone.[273,274]

One year of pretreatment or ongoing concomitant treatment with alendronate of postmenopausal osteoporotic women treated with PTH (teriparatide) blunted the gains in BMD compared with gains with PTH alone; however, gains were still significantly greater than with alendronate alone.[277]

Based on bone markers, giving PTH (teriparatide) cyclically (3 months on, 3 months off) seems to promote the bone formation burst seen in the first few weeks of PTH use. After the 3 months without PTH, each subsequent cycle stimulated bone formation similar to that seen in the initial course of treatment, unlike the gradual plateau in formation markers seen with continuous PTH therapy over 18 months.[277] Using shorter-acting and weaker antiresorptive agents concomitant with cyclical PTH may further improve the results by not blunting the next formation cycle but damping down bone resorption.[262,276,277] Because of the high cost of subcutaneous PTH, future protocols in patients with severe osteoporosis may involve using cycles of intermittent doses of PTH followed by weak, short-acting antiresorptive agents until the patient is above the fracture threshold, and then returning to long-term use of more potent antiresorptive agents.[252,262,276-279]

### Indications and Dosage for PTH

A daily 20-$\mu$g subcutaneous injection of 1-34 PTH (teriparatide) is approved by the FDA for patients with severe osteoporosis, previous osteoporotic fracture, multiple risk factors for fracture, or intolerance to therapy or in whom osteoporosis therapy has failed. It is presently approved for only 2 years of use.

Laboratory evaluation to rule out contraindications to teriparatide should include the usual tests to investigate causes of secondary osteoporosis, specifically tests for serum calcium, phosphorus, creatinine, alkaline phosphatase, albumin, 25-hydroxyvitamin D level, 24-hour urine calcium and creatinine clearance, and serum PTH level. The patient should be treated for osteomalacia, and calcium and vitamin D status should be optimized when using teriparatide. There are no FDA guidelines requiring reevaluation of serum calcium after starting teriparatide therapy, although a 1-month check is reasonable. If serum calcium is persistently high on teriparatide with no other explanation, then a decrease in calcium and vitamin D intake is recommended.[136]

### Contraindications to PTH (Teriparatide)

PTH (teriparatide) is contraindicated in patients who are allergic to teriparatide, in women who are pregnant or nursing, and in patients with an increased risk of osteosarcoma. Because osteosarcoma developed in 26% of rats treated throughout their lives with teriparatide with doses 3 to 60 times above those approved for humans, the FDA requires a black-box warning for teriparatide concerning the possible risk of osteosarcoma; this complication did not occur in primate species studied.[280] PTH can activate certain kinases that are known to be strong tumor promoters.[254] At this time, it is believed that the increased risk of osteosarcoma in rats is related to species, dose, and duration of use. There are also rare reports of osteosarcoma in patients with hyperparathyroidism.[281]

Because of the issue of potential teratogenicity, the use of teriparatide is not FDA approved in patients who have conditions associated with an increased risk of osteosarcoma, and its use is limited to 2 years, with a recommendation for use only in those patients with severe osteoporosis. Patients with Paget's disease, unexplained elevation of alkaline phosphatase, open growth plates, or previous radiation therapy involving the bone should not be given teriparatide.

Teriparatide is not indicated in patients with poor renal function (creatinine clearance < 35 mL/min/24 h) or for metabolic bone diseases other than osteoporosis (such as hyperparathyroidism, renal osteodystrophy, hypercalcemia of unknown etiology, hypercalciuria, or renal stones). It is not indicated in patients who may have secondary hyperparathyroidism related to renal failure and is not recommended for patients diagnosed with cancer or metastatic cancer to bone.

There is a theoretic concern that PTH, by increasing bone remodeling, could open up spaces in which bone metastases could grow. Cancers release cytokines that stimulate the RANK system in much the same way as PTH increases local osteoclastic activity.

Bisphosphonates may be used in patients with a history of cancer because they seemingly offer some protection from the growth of bone metastases, mainly by decreasing turnover and restricting resorption pits that tumor cells could occupy. Bisphosphonates reduce the local release of factors that stimulate tumor growth and seem to have antitumor and some antiangiogenesis properties in bone.[196]

### Adverse Effects of Teriparatide

Mild and transient hypercalcemia and hypercalciuria are the most common adverse effects of PTH treatment. Nausea, dizziness, and leg cramps can occur. Teriparatide is generally well tolerated and safe, even in elderly patients.[282-286]

### Nonsurgical Treatments for Severe Vertebral Fracture Pain

Conventional therapy for acute vertebral fractures includes initial bed rest, attempted mobilization of the patient with external back bracing if needed, physical therapy, calcium and vitamin D supplementation, narcotic analgesics, nutritional and psychosocial support, and medication to reduce refracture risk. Despite these measures, patients may continue to have severe pain.[287] Narcotics may help alleviate pain but cause many adverse events in frail, elderly patients.

Intranasal calcitonin, more so than injectable calcitonin, has useful analgesic properties that appear to directly affect the central nervous system. Calcitonin can decrease the pain of acute vertebral fractures within 1 week of starting therapy, can be used short-term for this purpose, and can be given concomitantly with bisphosphonates or PTH.[288,289]

Multiple studies have shown that intravenous bisphosphonates can provide rapid relief from the pain of bony metastases and also appear to relieve pain in patients with acute vertebral fractures. Intravenous pamidronate at a dose of 30 mg per day for 3 days has shown significant reduction in acute osteoporotic vertebral compression fracture pain compared with a placebo; however, it is not approved by the FDA for use in postmenopausal osteoporosis.[290] Acetaminophen (1,000 mg three times daily) given with intravenous bisphosphonates seems to decrease flu-like symptoms and provides added pain relief.[290] Multiple studies also show that subcutaneous teriparatide seems to improve chronic and acute back pain 30% to 40% more than oral bisphosphonates.[291]

### Emerging Treatments for Osteoporotic Fractures

Relieving pain and mobilizing the patient have been the standard of care for the treatment of disabling osteoporotic fractures. Conservative medical management for vertebral compression fractures that is not effective in mobilizing the patient can increase bone loss and the risk of further fractures, and many patients continue to experience severe chronic pain.[292] Open reduction and stabilization of osteoporotic spine fractures is only indicated for severe instability or neurologic deficit, not just for pain relief.[228]

Rapid pain relief and mobilization of patients with vertebral fractures can be provided by two minimally invasive procedures: vertebroplasty and kyphoplasty.[293] These percutaneous techniques introduce methylmethacrylate into the fractured vertebral body under fluoroscopy to stabilize it, resulting in almost immediate pain relief and return of function. Both techniques have shown more than 90% good to excellent pain relief within the first 24 hours of the procedure and maintenance of improvement with time. Another advantage of these procedures is that a biopsy can be done at the same time to assist in diagnosing underlying pathology.[294]

Complication rates related to the initial procedure are approximately 1%; however, vertebroplasty and kyphoplasty have a significant and sometimes rapid refracture rate approaching 20%. Although there is concern that the change in stiffness of the injected vertebral body and increased activity in these patients (because of pain relief) may increase the risk of another vertebral fracture, these rates are similar to recurrence rates seen in the natural history of reoccurrence of vertebral fractures in women with osteoporosis.[169,228,242,295-297] Studies are needed to assess the long-term effects of bone cement in vertebrae.

Although rare, serious risks of these procedures have been well documented and include transient or permanent neurologic deficit, epidural cement embolism, and pulmonary cement embolism.[287,298,299] Clinically asymptomatic cement leakage of approximately 13% occurs in both procedures, more so with vertebroplasty. These procedures should be performed with a spine surgeon available to provide consultation because of the risk of devastating neurologic consequences, although rare.[300]

It is unknown whether vertebroplasty and kyphoplasty can improve long-term outcomes in patients compared with those treated with conventional medical therapy. These procedures may prove to be safe and efficacious enough to consider immediately after painful vertebral fractures. Most clinical studies of these procedures do not report aggressive evaluation and treatment of the underlying osteoporosis in their protocols. The combination of surgical treatment with pharmacologic intervention and nutrition may greatly improve outcomes.[293,301]

## Hip Fracture Case Presentation

BJC, an 80-year-old woman, is admitted to the hospital with left hip pain and deformity after a fall at home. The treating physician has previously treated BJC for a Colles fracture and a spine fracture. She is seen in the emergency department and a displaced intertrochanteric hip fracture is diagnosed; the orthopaedic surgeon will provide definitive care.

### Incidence and Cost of Hip Fractures

There are more than 300,000 patients with hip fractures yearly in the United States, with a median patient age of 80 years. Lifetime risk of hip fracture in Caucasian women older than 50 years is approximately

17.5% and in Caucasian men it is approximately 6%. The hip fracture rate increases exponentially in patients older than 80 years. The incidence of hip fracture in Caucasian women older than 85 years is more than the incidence of stroke, breast cancer, and diabetes and equals the combined risk of breast, uterine, and ovarian cancer.[302] Women sustain 80% of all hip fractures because of their longer life spans compared with men. Other ethnic groups have lower but very significant risk.[1,10]

Hip fractures lead to more than one half of the total hospitalizations for osteoporotic fracture in the United States and cost more than $16 billion per year, representing more than 90% of the health budget for osteoporosis.[1,30]

### Morbidity and Mortality of Hip Fractures

Hip fractures are the most devastating osteoporotic fracture. Only 25% of patients with a hip fracture return to prefracture activities.[303] More than 20% of these patients are disabled by their fracture and require long-term nursing home care. Women fare worse than men—50% lose the ability to walk independently, and 50% are institutionalized.[1,30] When questioned, most patients report that they prefer death to nursing home placement.[304]

The adjusted rate of mortality is increased by 31% in men and 17% in women following a hip fracture, with most of this excess mortality occurring within the first 6 months after the fracture. Twenty percent of patients older than 65 years die within 1 year. Nearly 65,000 American women die from complications of hip fracture each year, 4% during their hospitalization and 10% to 24% in the first year after fracture.[17] Prospective studies of women older

than 65 years have shown that each SD of bone loss at the hip is associated with a 30% increase in total mortality. Mortality rates are higher in men than in women, and rates are higher in blacks than in whites.[305,306]

### The Risk of Other Fractures in Patients With Hip Fracture

Accelerated bone loss occurs following a hip fracture, with a decrease of 4% to 5% BMD at the uninjured femur and a 2.4% loss of BMD at the lumbar spine in the first year.[138,292] After the first hip fracture, there is an 11% increased risk of fracturing the contralateral hip during the patient's remaining lifetime; 30% of patients fracture the contralateral hip. There is a 2.4 relative risk of another fracture at any site and a 2.5 relative risk of vertebral fracture. Refractures can occur soon after the initial fracture, and timely treatment to decrease fracture risk is indicated.[3,54,137]

### Incidence of Secondary Osteoporosis in Patients With Hip Fracture

Up to 89% of patients with a hip fracture have low vitamin D levels (< 30 ng/mL).[145] There is an age-related decrease in renal 1-α-hydroxylase activity in the kidney and, therefore, less 1,25-dihydroxyvitamin D production that causes increased urinary calcium loss and less calcium absorption by the gut. This stimulates a secondary hyperparathyroidism that increases the bone remodeling rate and bone resorption to maintain the calcium level. The increased bone resorption and rapid remodeling rate, combined with an age-related decreased bone formation rate, causes net bone loss at each BMU and also at the tissue level.[41] Adequate vitamin D levels not only help prevent osteoporosis but also decrease the risk of a fall by effects on muscle.[152] Secondary causes of osteoporosis in older patient groups should be determined and treated.[119,121,125,127]

### Exercise Programs: Effects on Bone Strength and Fall Risk in Elderly Patients

Although exercise does not increase bone mass in elderly patients, low-impact exercise and light weight training can slow bone loss and decrease the risk of falling.[1] Because a fall is the injury mechanism in 95% of patients with a hip fracture, reducing the risk of a fall is essential at all levels of care, in and out of the hospital.[29] The risk of falling increases with age: 24% of women older than 50 years and 48% older than 85 years report falling each year. Men fall less frequently, with 16% of men older than 50 years and 35% older than 85 years falling each year.[1,307]

Exercises that are safe for osteoporotic patients include spinal extension, walking, isometric abdominals, water exercises, weight bearing of any type for 4 to 6 hours a day, and exercise with light, free weights. Newer studies are delineating the amount of mechanical strain needed to influence bone remodeling; however, it is difficult to quantitate the benefits of exercise on fracture risk.[308-310]

Balance training and tai chi have been shown to decrease falls 47% and cut the risk of hip fracture approximately 25%. Prospective studies have shown that men who participate in vigorous physical exercise tend to have a lower risk of hip fracture.[307,311-316]

Hip protectors have been shown to decrease hip fractures from falls onto the trochanter, but compliance in using the protectors is poor. It is difficult to prove that hip protectors are effective, but many studies have shown some benefit. Randomized trials using the opposite hip as a control have not shown significant fracture reduction.[317-319]

A systematic review found that there is some evidence that multifaceted interventions in the hospital can reduce the number of falls, and hip protectors for patients in nursing care facilities can decrease the risk of hip fractures.[320] The AAOS provides brochures and handouts detailing recommendations for fall risk reduction for patients.

### Patient Recognition of Osteoporosis

It cannot be assumed that the woman in the case presentation is aware that she has osteoporosis. Patients such as BJC with fractures caused by minimal trauma are frequently unaware, do not remember being told, or were not told that they have poor bone health. Many patients do not understand the connection between fractures and low bone density, osteoporosis, and the risk of future fractures. Most orthopaedic surgeons do not discuss osteoporosis with their patients.[27]

The diagnosis of osteoporosis brings to mind disability and nursing home placement and may be as frightening to patients as a diagnosis of Alzheimer's disease. When confronted with a diagnosis of osteoporosis, many patients argue that they do not have osteoporosis and believe that their fracture was to be expected because they had an injury, no matter how trivial. Studies based on the results of fracture awareness questionnaires showed that 73% of patients hospitalized for a fragility fracture believed their fractures were not related to osteoporosis and declined evaluation and treatment.[12,21,27]

It is important to communicate in simple language with patients and their families that their bones are more fragile than when they were younger, that one fracture leads to another, and most importantly, that good treatment is available at any age to decrease fracture risk, morbidity, and mortality.[45-47] Patient education provided to the hospitalized patient has been shown to improve the evaluation and treatment rates of fracture patients.[21,22]

### Likelihood That a Patient With a Hip Fracture Will Receive Evidence-Based Care

There is approximately a 50% chance of a patient getting the correct care at the correct time in the US health care system; the chances are worse for hip fracture patients such as BJC who have less than a 30% chance of receiving evidence-based care.[17,25,321] The orthopaedic literature documents low rates of bone health evaluation and treatment in patients with hip fracture.[2,17] Fewer than 25% of these patients are given calcium and vitamin D supplements in the hospital or at discharge, ever get a bone density test, or receive treatment with effective antiresorptive or anabolic drugs to significantly decrease the risk of refracture.[2,3,17]

There are many barriers to treating the underlying bone fragility of patients with hip fractures.[14,44] Although orthopaedic surgeons cannot make improvements in the care of these patients without hospital support and multidisciplinary physician involvement, many steps can be taken to improve the bone health of these patients.[12,14,21]

Standing admission and discharge orders can be instituted to assist all those involved in delivering care (Figure 12). These orders need

## Fragility Fracture Admission Protocol Orders

**Attending physician: your signature is required at the bottom of this form.**
**Nursing staff: your signature is required after the osteoporosis nursing intake portion.**
Calcium and vitamin D supplementation and pharmacologic intervention for fragility fractures
to start on admission or as soon as possible.

<u>**Nursing staff to check any applicable boxes**</u>
**Does this patient have contraindications to bisphosphonates? These are**

- ☐ Hypersensitivity to these drugs (alendronate, risedronate, ibandronate, pamidronate, zolendronate)
- ☐ Not approved in premenopause, pregnancy, or for children
- ☐ Severe esophageal problems, especially stricture or achalasia (for oral meds)
- ☐ Inability to sit upright for 30-60 minutes after taking the medication (oral meds)
- ☐ Low serum calcium (alert physician)
- ☐ Creatinine clearance or GFR < 30 mL/min
- ☐ Severe or frequent reflux or heartburn not controlled (for oral meds)

**Contraindications to Forteo?**

- ☐ Allergy to teriparatide
- ☐ Creatinine clearance or GFR < 30 mL/min
- ☐ Women who are pregnant or nursing
- ☐ Conditions/patients with increased risk of osteosarcoma: Paget's disease, children, unexplained elevated alkaline phosphatase, previous radiation to bone
- ☐ History of malignancy

**<u>RN signature:</u>** _____ **date/time**

## <u>Physician orders:</u>

- ☐ Nursing and Dietary to provide education about calcium and vitamin D intake and importance to patient and/or family
- ☐ One oral multivitamin daily. If npo, give IV multivitamin until can take po, then continue orally
- ☐ Vitamin D 1,000 units daily po
- ☐ Serum 25 OH vitamin D level
- ☐ Vitamin D 50,000 units po weekly unless serum calcium is elevated on admission (alert physician)
- ☐ Start 1,200 mg of elemental calcium po daily in divided doses, when taking po

**Pharmacologic medications** (see contraindications above)

- ☐ <u>Patient cannot be started on pharmacologic treatment at this time</u>
  - ○ Osteoporosis meds contraindicated presently
  - ○ Patient and/or power of attorney refusal
  - ○ Socioeconomic issues
- ☐ Start oral bisphosphonates as soon as taking good po, has resumed usual diet, and can sit up for 30-60 minutes after dose
  - ○ Alendronate (Fosomax) 70 mg once a week po (sit up at least 30 minutes)
  - ○ Risedraonate (Actonel) 35 mg once a week (sit up at least 30 minutes)
  - ○ Ibandronate (Boniva) 150 mg once a month (sit up at least 60 minutes)
- ☐ Miacalcin nasal spray: one spray alternating nostrils daily (for analgesia, no nonvertebral fracture reduction; can add to other antifracture meds)

**If patient cannot take oral bisphosphonates or oral medications but no other contraindications to bisphosphonates, consider IV bisphosphonates or Forteo subcutaneously for severe osteoporosis**

- ☐ Start IV bisphosphonates (must be calcium and vitamin D replete)
  - ○ Ibandronate (Boniva) IV 3 mg every 3 months to start when vitamin D level is therapeutic (> 30)
  - ○ Zolendronate (Reclast) IV 5 mg (once a year) when vitamin D level is therapeutic
- ☐ Start Forteo 20 μg subcutaneously once daily

**<u>Physician signature:</u>** _____ **date/time**
FAX COPY TO PHYSICIANS' OFFICES

**Figure 12**     Example of a fragility fracture admission protocol order.

to specifically target patient and family education; laboratory evaluation beyond usual admission orders to assess secondary causes of poor bone quality; automatic dietary consultations to assist with calcium, vitamin D, and nutritional supplementation on admission and after discharge; occupational and physical therapy fall prevention strategies (both inpatient and at discharge); nursing documentation of an admission fracture risk assessment to assist in the patient care plan; treatment with antiresorptive or anabolic agents (if not contraindicated) while in the hospital and continued at discharge; BMD testing to be performed in the hospital or within 3 months of discharge, with reports to be sent to all caregivers; and automatic postdischarge referral to the primary care physician with the discharge summary and laboratory results from the hospital.[2,12,14,20,21]

The hospital nursing staff should provide the patient with educational materials. Many free materials are available online.[46,47,322] The hospital laboratory can assist in establishing standing orders for additional bone-related admission's tests.[40] Hospital management of hip fracture patients should include attention to nutrition, especially protein. The patient's diet should be evaluated, and increased protein intake should be considered for elderly patients recovering from a hip fracture.[323,324] The best predictor of mortality in elderly patients with hip fractures is a low serum albumin on admission.[243,320,325]

If pharmacologic treatment is not started, the reason for this should be documented in the patient's chart.[44] Excellent care of the hip fracture patient is often difficult to arrange, and multiple caregivers must be enlisted to help. The orthopaedic surgeon, who best understands the consequences of the fracture, should work to facilitate adequate communication between specialists so that delegation of care does not lead to poor overall care.[44]

## Summary

There are adequate evidence-based measures for orthopaedic surgeons to use to decrease fracture risk and optimize care in patients with fragility fractures. Better global care of these patients involves quality of care and patient advocacy and safety.[26] Poor bone health is asymptomatic until the first fracture. BMD predicts fracture better than blood pressure predicts stroke and cholesterol levels predict myocardial infarction. Studies confirm the predictive value of peripheral screening of BMD starting at approximately age 50 years, with studies such as a peripheral DXA of the wrist.[56] Studies showed that younger (age 50 to 60 years) postmenopausal women with osteopenia had increased fracture rates (1.8 times) of those without osteopenia; many fractures occurred within 1 year of testing.[74,82] The Surgeon General's report suggests more widespread use of peripheral screening by physicians for patients not covered for central DXA BMD testing to help prevent the first fracture.[1]

Recently reported modest declines in hip fracture rates will not compensate for the large increase of absolute numbers of hip fractures projected because of the aging population. By 2020, 50% of Americans older than 50 years are expected to have osteoporosis of the hip. A dramatic decrease in hip fracture rates is needed to reduce the number of hip fractures in the next 15 years.[326] The goals of the "Healthy People 2010" initiative are to decrease hip fracture rates by 50% in women and by 20% in men.[1]

Orthopaedic surgeons can use the American Heart Association's "Get With the Guidelines" campaign to improve aspirin and β-blocker use after myocardial infarction as a model of a systematic approach that can change the national paradigm. That campaign reduced expected mortality in the United States by more than 25% between 1970 and 2000.[327]

The American Orthopaedic Association's "Own the Bone" initiative established the systems level framework needed to help orthopaedic surgeons improve bone health in their patients.[25] However, compliance with medication usage is the weakest link in treating patients with many chronic diseases, and there is no guarantee that the patient will continue to comply with the medication or risk reduction program.[326-333] It also may be difficult to adhere to clinical practice guidelines when treating older patients with significant comorbidities that can result in conflicting recommendations.[334]

The elderly patient with osteoporosis continues to lose bone until the end of life, with an increasing fracture risk. In studies of elderly nursing home populations, calcium and vitamin D supplements decreased the risk of fracture by 27% in 3 years.[165] An antiresorptive or a bone formation agent should also be used in patients with such a high risk of refracture. It is clear that bone loss cannot be completely reversed, but fracture risk can be decreased by intervening to slow bone loss and/or build new bone. Because treatment with antiresorptive or bone formation agents can decrease fracture risk 50% in less than 1 year of treatment, it is cost effective to treat even the very elderly osteoporotic patients.[6,268,335] It is urgent to initiate evaluation and treatment of the bone health of fracture patients and to communicate to them, and to their other care providers, the dire consequences of further fractures.

# References

1. US Department of Health and Human Services Website. Bone Health and Osteoporosis: A report of the Surgeon General. Available at http://www.surgeongeneral.gov/library/bonehealth/. Accessed December 4, 2007.

2. Robinson CM, Royds M, Abraham A, McQueen MM, Court-Brown CM, Christie J: Refractures in patients at least forty-five years old: A prospective analysis of twenty-two thousand and sixty patients. *J Bone Joint Surg Am* 2002;84-A:1528-1533.

3. Klotzbuecher CM, Ross PD, Landsman PB, Abbott TA III, Berger M: Patients with prior fractures have an increased risk of future fractures: A summary of the literature and statistical synthesis. *J Bone Miner Res* 2000;15:721-739.

4. Haentjens P, Autier P, Collins J, Velkeniers B, Vanderschueren D, Boonen S: Colles fracture, spine fracture, and subsequent risk of hip fracture in men and women: A meta-analysis. *J Bone Joint Surg Am* 2003;85-A:1936-1943.

5. Bouxsein ML, Kaufman J, Tosi L, Cummings S, Lane J, Johnell O: Recommendations for optimal care of the fragility fracture patient to reduce the risk of future fracture. *J Am Acad Orthop Surg* 2004;12:385-395.

6. Cranney A, Guyatt G, Griffith L, et al: Meta-analyses of therapies for postmenopausal osteoporosis: IX. Summary of meta-analyses of therapies for postmenopausal osteoporosis. *Endocr Rev* 2002;23:570-578.

7. Cummings SR, Melton LJ: Epidemiology and outcomes of osteoporotic fractures. *Lancet* 2002;359:1761-1767.

8. Cooper C, Atkinson EJ, O'Fallon WM, Melton LJ III: Incidence of clinically diagnosed vertebral fractures: A population-based study in Rochester, Minnesota, 1985-1989. *J Bone Miner Res* 1992;7:221-227.

9. Melton LJ III: The prevalence of osteoporosis: Gender and racial comparison. *Calcif Tissue Int* 2001;69:179-181.

10. Barrett-Connor E, Siris ES, Wehren LE, et al: Osteoporosis and fracture risk in women of different ethnic groups. *J Bone Miner Res* 2005;20:185-194

11. Rosier RN: Expanding the role of the orthopaedic surgeon in the treatment of osteoporosis. *Clin Orthop Relat Res* 2001;385:57-67.

12. Gardner MJ, Brophy RH, Demetrakopoulos D, et al: Interventions to improve osteoporosis treatment following hip fracture: A prospective, randomized trial. *J Bone Joint Surg Am* 2005;87:3-7.

13. Chevalley T, Hoffmeyer P, Bonjour JP, Rizzoli R: An osteoporosis clinical pathway for the medical management of patients with low-trauma fracture. *Osteoporos Int* 2002;13:450-455.

14. Kaufman JD, Bolander ME, Bunta AD, Edwards BJ, Fitzpatrick LA, Simonelli C: Barriers and solutions to osteoporosis care in patients with a hip fracture. *J Bone Joint Surg Am* 2003;85:1837-1843.

15. McLellan AR, Gallacher SJ, Fraser M, McQuillian C: The fracture liaison service: Success of a program for the evaluation and management of patients with osteoporotic fracture. *Osteoporos Int* 2003;14:1028-1034.

16. Skedros JG: The orthopaedic surgeon's role in diagnosing and treating patients with osteoporotic fractures: Standing discharge orders may be the solution for timely medical care. *Osteoporos Int* 2004;15:405-410.

17. Dreinhofer KE, Feron JM, Herrera A, et al: Orthopaedic surgeons and fragility fractures: A survey by the Bone and Joint Decade and the International Osteoporosis Foundation.

*J Bone Joint Surg Br* 2004;86:958-961.

18. Sidwell AI, Wilkinson TJ, Hanger HC: Secondary prevention of fractures in older people: Evaluation of a program for the investigation and treatment of osteoporosis. *Intern Med J* 2004;34:129-132.

19. Harrington JT, Deal CL: Successes and failures in improving osteoporosis care after fragility fracture: Results of a multiple-site clinical improvement project. *Arthritis Rheum* 2006;55:724-728.

20. Edwards BJ, Bunta AD, Madison L, et al: An osteoporosis intervention program increases the rates of diagnosis and treatment for osteoporosis at the time to minimal trauma fractures. *Jt Comm J Qual Patient Saf* 2005;31:267-274.

21. Bogoch ER, Elliot-Gibson V, Beaton DE, Jamal SA, Josse RG, Murray TM: Effective initiation of osteoporosis diagnosis and treatment for patients with a fragility fracture in an orthopaedic environment. *J Bone Joint Surg Am* 2006;88:25-34.

22. Tosi LL, Lane JM: Osteoporosis prevention and the orthopaedic surgeon: When fracture care is not enough. *J Bone Joint Surg Am* 1998;80:1567-1569.

23. American Academy of Orthopaedic Surgeons Website. Position statement: Osteoporosis as a national public health priority. A joint position statement of the American Academy of Orthopaedic Surgeons and the National Osteoporosis Foundation. Available at: http://www.aaos.org/about/papers/position/1113.asp. Accessed December 4, 2007.

24. American Academy of Orthopaedic Surgeons Website Position statement. Recommendations for enhancing the care of patients with fragility fractures. Available at: http://www.aaos.org/about/papers/position/1159. Accessed December 4, 2007.

25. American Orthopaedic Association: Leadership in orthopaedics: Taking a stand to own the bone: American Orthopaedic Association position paper.

*J Bone Joint Surg Am* 2005;87:1389-1391.

26. Tosi LL, Kyle RF: Fragility fractures: The fall and decline of bone health. Commentary on "Interventions to improve osteoporosis treatment following hip fracture" by Gardner et al. *J Bone Joint Surg Am* 2005;87:1-2.

27. Edwards BJ, Iris M, Ferkel E, Feinglass J: Postmenopausal women with minimal trauma fractures are unapprised of the existence of low bone mass or osteoporosis. *Maturitas* 2006; 53:260-266.

28. Riggs BL, Melton LJ III: The worldwide problem of osteoporosis: Insights afforded by epidemiology. *Bone* 1995;17(suppl 5):505S-511S.

29. NIH Consensus Development Panel on Osteoporosis Prevention: Osteoporosis prevention, diagnosis, and therapy. *JAMA* 2001;285:785-795.

30. Ray NF, Chan JK, Thamer M, Melton LJ III: Medical expenditures for the treatment of osteoporotic fractures in the United States in 1995: Report from the National Osteoporosis Foundation. *J Bone Miner Res* 1997;12:24-35.

31. Cuddihy MT, Gabriel SE, Crowson CS, et al: Osteoporosis intervention following radius fractures: A missed opportunity. *Arch Intern Med* 2002; 162:421-426.

32. Wigderowitz CA, Rowley DI, Mole PA, Paterson CR, Abel EW: Bone mineral density of the radius in patients with Colles' fracture. *J Bone Joint Surg Br* 2000;82:87-89.

33. Eastell R, Reid DM, Compston J, et al: Secondary prevention of osteoporosis: When should a nonvertebral fracture be a trigger for action? *QJM* 2001;94:575-597.

34. Kanis JA, Johnell O, De Laet C, et al: A meta-analysis of previous fracture and subsequent fracture risk. *Bone* 2004;35:375-382.

35. Sanders KM, Pasco JA, Ugoni AM, et al: The exclusion of high trauma fractures may underestimate the prevalence of bone fragility fractures in the community: The Geelong Osteoporosis Study. *J Bone Miner Res* 1998;13:1337-1342.

36. Collinge C, Gehrig L: Assessment for osteoporosis in hospitalized orthopaedic trauma patients: An opportunity to intervene. *J Orthop Trauma*, in press.

37. Favus MJ: *Primer on the Metabolic Bone Diseases and Disorders of Mineral Metabolism*, ed 5. Philadelphia, PA, Lippincott Williams and Wilkins, 2003.

38. Broadus AE: Mineral balance and homeostasis, in Favus MJ, Christakos S (eds): *Primer on the Metabolic Bone Diseases and Disorders of Mineral Metabolism*, ed 3. Philadelphia, PA, Lippincott-Raven, 1996, pp 57-63.

39. Manolagas SC: Birth and death of bone cells: Basic regulatory mechanisms and implications for the pathogenesis and treatment of osteoporosis. *Endocr Rev* 2000;21:115-137.

40. Lin JT, Lane JM: Osteoporosis: A review. *Clin Orthop Relat Res* 2004;425: 126-134.

41. Seeman E, Delmas PD: Bone quality: The material and structural basis of bone strength and fragility. *N Engl J Med* 2006;354:2250-2261.

42. Holick MF, Krane SM, Potts JT: Calcium, phosphorus, and bone metabolism: Calcium regulating hormones, in *Harrison's Principles of Internal Medicine*, ed 14. New York, NY, McGraw-Hill, 1998, pp 2214-2227.

43. Hase H, Ando T, Eldeiry L, et al: TNF-alpha mediates the skeletal effects of thyroid-stimulating hormone. *Proc Natl Acad Sci USA* 2006;103: 12849-12854.

44. Centers for Medicare and Medicaid Services Website: Physician Voluntary Reporting Program (PVRP). Guidelines concerning osteoporosis. Available at: http://www.cms.hhs.gov/PQRI/Downloads/PVRPQualityMeasuresList.pdf. Accessed December 4, 2007.

45. The Joint Commission Website: What did the doctor say? Improving health literacy to protect patient safety. Available at: http://www.jointcommission.org/NewsRoom/PressKits/Health_Literacy/. Accessed January 7, 2008.

46. National Institute of Health Website. Once is enough: A guide to preventing future fractures. Available at: http://www.niams.nih.gov/Health_Info/Bone/Osteoporosis/Fracture/preventing_fracture.pdf. Accessed December 4, 2007.

47. National Osteoporosis Foundation Website. Osteoporosis: What is it? Available at: http://www.nof.org/osteoporosis/index.htm. Accessed December 4, 2007.

48. National Osteoporosis Foundation Website. Physician's guide to prevention and treatment of osteoporosis. Available at: http://www.nof.org/physguide/index.asp. Accessed December 4, 2007.

49. Dolan P, Torgerson DJ: The cost of treating osteoporotic fractures in the United Kingdom female population. *Osteoporosis Int* 1998;8:611-617.

50. Ribot C, Tremollieres F, Pouilles JM: Can we detect women with low bone mass using clinical risk factors? *Am J Med* 1995;98(2A):52S-55S.

51. Earnshaw SA, Cawte SA, Worley A, Hosking DJ: Colles' fracture of the wrist as an indicator of underlying osteoporosis in postmenopausal women: A prospective study of bone mineral density and bone turnover rate. *Osteoporos Int* 1998;8:53-60.

52. Marcus R: Clinical review 76: The nature of osteoporosis. *J Clin Endocrinol Metab* 1996;81:1-5.

53. Ross PD, Davis JW, Epstein RS, Wasnich RD: Pre-existing fractures and bone mass predict vertebral fracture incidence in women. *Ann Intern Med* 1991;114:919-923.

54. Marshall D, Johnell O, Wedel H: Meta-analysis of how well measures of bone mineral density predict occurrence of osteoporotic fractures. *BMJ* 1996;312:1254-1259.

55. Melton LJ III, Orwoll ES, Wasnich RD: Does bone density predict fractures comparably in men and

women? *Osteoporos Int* 2001;12: 707-709.

56. Abrahamsen B, Vestergaard P, Rud B, et al: Ten-year absolute risk of osteoporotic fractures according to BMD T score at menopause: The Danish Osteoporosis Prevention Study. *J Bone Miner Res* 2006;21: 796-800.

57. Bone and Joint Decade Website. Are you fit to a T? Available at: http://www.usbjd.org/projects/Fit2aT_op.cfm?dirID=224. Accessed December 4, 2007.

58. Genant HK, Engelke K, Fuerst T, et al: Noninvasive assessment of bone mineral and structure: State of the art. *J Bone Miner Res* 1996;11:707-730.

59. Miller PD, Zapalowski C, Kulak CA, Bilezikian JP: Bone densitometry: The best way to detect osteoporosis and to monitor therapy. *J Clin Endocrinol Metab* 1999;84:1867-1871.

60. Lewiecki EM, Kendler DL, Kiebzak GM, et al: Special report on the official positions of the International Society for Clinical Densitometry. *Osteoporos Int* 2004;15:779-784.

61. Huang MH, Barrett-Connor E, Greendale GA, Kado DM: Hyperkyphotic posture and risk of future osteoporotic fractures: The Rancho Bernardo study. *J Bone Miner Res* 2006;21:419-423.

62. WHO Study Group: Assessment of fracture risk and its application to screening for postmenopausal osteoporosis, in *Report of a WHO Study Group: WHO Technical Series 843*. Geneva, Switzerland, World Health Organization, 1994, pp 1-129.

63. Mauck KF, Clarke BL: Diagnosis, screening, prevention, and treatment of osteoporosis. *Mayo Clin Proc* 2006; 81:662-672.

64. Faulkner KG, von Stetten E, Miller P: Discordance in patient classification using T-scores. *J Clin Densitom* 1999; 2:343-350.

65. De Laet C, Kanis JA, Oden A, et al: Body mass index as a predictor of fracture risk: A meta-analysis. *Osteoporos Int* 2005;16:1330-1338.

66. Kanis JA, Johnell O, Oden A, et al: Smoking and fracture risk: A meta-analysis. *Osteoporos Int* 2005;16: 155-162.

67. Kanis JA, Johansson H, Oden A, et al: A family history of fracture and fracture risk: A meta-analysis. *Bone* 2004; 35:1029-1037.

68. Kanis JA, Johansson H, Oden A, et al: A meta-analysis of prior corticosteroid use and fracture risk. *J Bone Miner Res* 2004;19:893-899.

69. Kanis JA, Johansson H, Johnell O, et al: Alcohol intake as a risk factor for fracture. *Osteoporos Int* 2005;16: 737-742.

70. Johnell O, Kanis JA, Oden A, et al: Predictive value of BMD for hip and other fractures. *J Bone Miner Res* 2005; 20:1185-1194.

71. Cummings SR, Nevitt MC, Browner WS, et al: Risk factors for hip fracture in white women: Study of Osteoporotic Fractures Research Group. *N Engl J Med* 1995;332:767-773.

72. Silverman SL: Selecting patients for osteoporosis therapy. *Curr Osteoporos Rep* 2006;4:91-95.

73. Delmas PD: Do we need to change the WHO definition of osteoporosis? *Osteoporos Int* 2000;11:189-191.

74. Siris ES, Genant HK, Laster AJ, Chen P, Misurski DA, Krege JH: Enhanced prediction of fracture risk combining vertebral fracture status and BMD. *Osteoporos Int* 2007;18:761-770.

75. Kanis JA, Johnell O, Oden A, et al: Ten year probabilities of osteoporotic fractures according to BMD and diagnostic thresholds. *Osteoporos Int* 2001;12:989-995.

76. Ganero P, Hausherr E, Chapuy MC, et al: Markers of bone resorption predict hip fracture in elderly women: The EPIDOS Prospective Study. *J Bone Miner Res* 1996;11:1531-1538.

77. Kanis JA, Borgstrom F, De Laet C, et al: Assessment of fracture risk. *Osteoporos Int* 2005;16:581-589.

78. Leib ES, Lewiecki EM, Binkley N, Hamdy RC, International Society for Clinical Densitometry: Official positions of the International Society for Clinical Densitometry. *J Clin Densitom* 2004;7:1-6.

79. Lewiecki EM: Review of guidelines for bone mineral density testing and treatment of osteoporosis. *Curr Osteoporos Rep* 2005;3:75-83.

80. Siris ES, Chen YT, Abbott TA, et al: Bone mineral density thresholds for pharmacological intervention to prevent fractures. *Arch Intern Med* 2004; 164:1108-1112.

81. Wainwright SA, Phipps KR, Stone JV, et al: A large proportion of fractures in postmenopausal women occur with baseline bone mineral density T-score > -2.5. *J Bone Miner Res* 2001; 16(suppl 1):S155.

82. Siris ES, Brenneman SK, Miller PD, et al: Predictive value of low BMD for 1-year fracture outcomes is similar for postmenopausal women ages 50-64 and 65 and older: Results from the National Osteoporosis Risk Assessment (NORA). *J Bone Miner Res* 2004;19:1215-1220.

83. Sornay-Rendu E, Munoz F, Ganero P, Duboeuf F, Delmas PD: Identification of osteopenic women at high risk of fracture: The OFELY study. *J Bone Miner Res* 2005;20: 1813-1819.

84. Weinstein RS: True strength. *J Bone Miner Res* 2000;15:621-625.

85. Heaney RP: Is the paradigm shifting? *Bone* 2003;33:457-465.

86. Lazner F, Gowen M, Pavasovic D, Kola I: Osteopetrosis and osteoporosis: Two sides of the same coin. *Hum Mol Genet* 1999;8:1839-1846.

87. Nelson DA, Megyesi MS: Sex and ethnic differences in bone architecture. *Curr Osteoporos Rep* 2004;2: 65-69.

88. Ruyssen-Witrand A, Gossec L, Kolta S, Dougados M, Roux C: Vertebral dimensions as risk factor of vertebral fracture in osteoporotic patients: A systematic literature review. *Osteoporos Int* 2007;18:1271-1278.

89. Ralston SH, de Crombrugghe B: Review: Genetic regulation of bone

mass and susceptibility to osteoporosis. *Genes Dev* 2006;20:2492-2506.

90. Tabensky A, Duan Y, Edmonds J, Seeman E: The contribution of reduced peak accrual of bone and age-related bone loss to osteoporosis at the spine and hip: Insights from the daughters of women with vertebral or hip fractures. *J Bone Miner Res* 2001; 16:1101-1107.

91. Nguyen TV, Eisman JA: Genetics of fracture: Challenges and opportunities. *J Bone Miner Res* 2000;15:1253-1256.

92. Byers PH: Disorders of collagen biosynthesis and structure, in Scriver CR, Beardet AL, Sly WA, Valle D, Childs B, Vogelstei B (eds): *The Metabolic and Molecular Bases of Inherited Disease*, ed 8. New York, NY, McGraw-Hill, 2001, pp 5241-5285.

93. Carballido-Gamio J, Phan C, Link TM, Majumdar S: Characterization of trabecular bone structure from high-resolution magnetic resonance images using fuzzy logic. *Magn Reson Imaging* 2006;24:1023-1029.

94. Boutroy S, Bouxsein ML, Munoz F, Delmas PD: In vivo assessment of trabecular bone microarchitecture by high-resolution peripheral quantitative computed tomography. *J Clin Endocrinol Metab* 2005;90:6508-6515.

95. Manolagas SC, Jilka RL: Bone marrow, cytokines, and bone remodeling: Emerging insights into the pathophysiology of osteoporosis. *N Engl J Med* 1995;332:305-311.

96. Garnero P, Munoz F, Borel O, Sornay-Rendu E, Delmas PD: Vitamin D receptor gene polymorphisms are associated with the risk of fractures in postmenopausal women, independently of bone mineral density. *J Clin Endocrinol Metab* 2005;90:4829-4835.

97. Langdahl BL, Gravholt CH, Brixen K, Eriksen EF: Polymorphisms in the vitamin D receptor gene and bone mass, bone turnover and osteoporotic fractures. *Eur J Clin Invest* 2000;30:608-617.

98. Boyden LM, Mao J, Belsky J, et al: High bone density due to a mutation in LDL-receptor-related protein 5. *N Engl J Med* 2002;346:1513-1521.

99. Riggs BL, Khosla S, Melton LJ III: A unitary model for involutional osteoporosis: Estrogen deficiency causes both type I and type II osteoporosis in postmenopausal women and contributes to bone loss in aging men. *J Bone Miner Res* 1998;13: 763-773.

100. Ducy P, Amling M, Takeda S, et al: Leptin inhibits bone formation through a hypothalamic relay: A central control of bone mass. *Cell* 2000; 100:197-207.

101. Sambrook P, Cooper C: Seminar: Osteoporosis. *Lancet* 2006;367:2010-2018.

102. Rosen CJ: Restoring aging bones. *Sci Am* 2003;288:70-77.

103. Rosen CJ, Kiel DP: Age-related osteoporosis, in Murray E, Favus J (eds): *Primer on the Metabolic Bone Diseases and Disorders of Mineral Metabolism*, ed 5. Washington DC, American Society for Bone and Mineral Research, 2003.

104. Eastell R: Treatment of postmenopausal osteoporosis. *N Engl J Med* 1998;338:736-746.

105. Whitfield JF: How to grow bone to treat osteoporosis and mend fractures. *Curr Osteoporos Rep* 2003;1:32-40.

106. Hofbauer LC, Schoppet M: Clinical implications of the osteoprotegerin/RANKL/RANK system for bone and vascular diseases. *JAMA* 2004;292: 490-495.

107. Boyle WJ, Simonet WS, Lacey DL: Osteoclast differentiation and activation. *Nature* 2003;423:337-342.

108. McClung MR, Lewiecki EM, Cohen SB, et al: Denosumab in postmenopausal women with low bone mineral density. *N Engl J Med* 2006;354: 821-831.

109. Braidman I, Baris C, Wood L, et al: Preliminary evidence for impaired estrogen receptor-alpha protein expression in osteoblasts and osteocytes from men with idiopathic osteoporosis. *Bone* 2000;26:423-427.

110. Russell RG, Espina B, Hulley P: Bone biology and the pathogenesis of osteoporosis. *Curr Opin Rheumatol* 2006; 18(suppl 1):S3-S10.

111. Patel MS, Karsenty G: Regulation of bone formation and vision by LRP5. *N Engl J Med* 2002;346:1572-1574.

112. Johnson ML: The high bone mass family: The role of Wnt/Lrp5 signaling in the regulation of bone mass. *J Musculoskelet Neuronal Interact* 2004;4: 135-138.

113. Serhan CN: Clues for new therapeutics in osteoporosis. *N Engl J Med* 2004;350:1902-1903.

114. Canalis E, Giustina A, Bilezikian JP: Mechanisms of anabolic therapies for osteoporosis. *N Engl J Med* 2007;357: 905-916.

115. Falahati-Nini A, Riggs BL, Atkinson EJ, O'Fallon WM, Eastell R, Khosla S: Relative contributions of testosterone and estrogen in regulating bone resorption and formation in normal elderly men. *J Clin Invest* 2000;106:1553-1560.

116. Weitzman MN, Pacifici R: Estrogen deficiency and bone loss: An inflammatory tale. *J Clin Invest* 2006;116: 1186-1194.

117. Amin S, Zhang Y, Sawin CT, et al: Association of hypogonadism and estradiol levels with bone mineral density in elderly men from the Framingham study. *Ann Intern Med* 2000;133: 951-963.

118. Riggs BL, Khosla S, Atkinson EJ, Dunstan CR, Melton LJ III: Evidence that type I osteoporosis results from enhanced responsiveness of bone to estrogen deficiency. *Osteoporos Int* 2003;14:728-733.

119. Templeton K: Secondary osteoporosis. *J Am Acad Orthop Surg* 2005;13: 475-486.

120. American Medical Association: Managing osteoporosis, in *Part Four: Detection and Clinical Issues in Testing*. Chicago, IL, American Medical Association, 1999.

121. Crandall C: Laboratory work up for

osteoporosis: Which tests are most cost effective? *Postgrad Med* 2003;114: 41-44.

122. American Medical Association: Managing osteoporosis, in *Part One: Update in Patient Management*. Chicago, IL, American Medical Association, 2001.

123. Compston J: Secondary causes of osteoporosis in men. *Calcif Tissue Int* 2001;69:193-195.

124. Wright VJ: Osteoporosis in men. *J Am Acad Orthop Surg* 2006;14:347-353.

125. Wagman RB, Marcus R: Beyond bone mineral density: Navigating the laboratory assessment of patients with osteoporosis. *J Clin Endocrinol Metab* 2002;87:4429-4430.

126. Bauer DC, Ettinger B, Nevitt MC, Stone KL: Risk for fracture in women with low serum levels of thyroid-stimulating hormone. *Ann Intern Med* 2001;134:561-568.

127. Dawson-Hughes B: Bone loss accompanying medical therapies. *N Engl J Med* 2001;345:989-991.

128. Adachi JD: The correlation of bone mineral density and biochemical markers to fracture risk. *Calcif Tissue Int* 1996;59:16-19.

129. Chesnut CH III, Bell NH, Clark GS, et al: Hormone replacement therapy in postmenopausal women: Urinary N-telopeptide of type I collagen monitors therapeutic effect and predicts response of bone mineral density. *Am J Med* 1997;102:29-37.

130. Looker AC, Bauer DC, Chesnut CH III, et al: Clinical use of biochemical markers of bone remodeling: Current status and future directions. *Osteoporos Int* 2000;11:467-480.

131. Bauer DC, Sklarin PM, Stone KL, et al: Biochemical markers of bone turnover and prediction of hip bone loss in older women: The study of osteoporotic fractures. *J Bone Miner Res* 1999;14:1404-1410.

132. Delmas PD, Hardy P, Garnero P, Dain M: Monitoring individual response to hormone replacement therapy with bone markers. *Bone* 2000;26:553-560.

133. Garnero P, Delmas PD: Clinical usefulness of markers of bone remodeling in osteoporosis, in Meunier PJ (ed): *Osteoporosis: Diagnosis and Management*. London, England, Martin Dunitz, 1998, pp 79-101.

134. Bauer DC, Garnero P, Hochberg MC, et al: Pretreatment levels of bone turnover and the antifracture efficacy of alendronate: The fracture intervention trial. *J Bone Miner Res* 2006; 21:292-299.

135. Riggs BL: Are biochemical markers for bone turnover clinically useful for monitoring therapy in individual osteoporotic patients? *Bone* 2000;26: 551-552.

136. Rosen CJ: Clinical practice: Postmenopausal osteoporosis. *N Engl J Med* 2005;353:595-603.

137. Chapurlat RD, Bauer DC, Nevitt M, Stone K, Cummings SR: Incidence and risk factors for a second hip fracture in elderly women: The study of osteoporotic fractures. *Osteoporos Int* 2003;14:130-136.

138. Colon-Emeric C, Kuchibhatla M, Pieper C, et al: The contribution of hip fracture to risk of subsequent fractures: Data from two longitudinal studies. *Osteoporos Int* 2003;14: 879-883.

139. Oncken C, Gonzales D, Nides M, et al: Efficacy and safety of the novel selective nicotinic acetylcholine receptorpartial agonist, varenicline, for smoking cessation. *Arch Intern Med* 2006;166:1571-1577.

140. Nides M, Oncken C, Gonzales D, et al: Smoking cessation with varenicline, a selective alpha4beta2 nicotinic receptorpartial agonist: Results from a 7-week, randomized, placebo- and bupropion-controlled trial with 1-year follow-up. *Arch Intern Med* 2006;166:1561-1568.

141. Heaney RP: Functional indices of vitamin D status and ramifications of vitamin D deficiency. *Am J Clin Nutr* 2004;80(suppl 6):1706S-1709S.

142. Holick MF: Vitamin D requirements for humans of all ages: New increased

requirements for women and men 50 years and older. *Osteoporos Int* 1998; 8:S24-S29.

143. Simonelli C, Weiss TW, Morancey J, Swanson L, Chen YT: Prevalence of vitamin D inadequacy in a minimal trauma fracture population. *Curr Med Res Opin* 2005;21:1069-1074.

144. Holick MF, Siris ES, Binkley N, et al: Prevalence of vitamin D inadequacy among postmenopausal North American women receiving osteoporosis therapy. *J Clin Endocrinol Metab* 2005;90:3215-3224.

145. Greer FR, Krebs NF, American Academy of Pediatrics Committee on Nutrition: Optimizing bone health and calcium intakes of infants, children, and adolescents. *Pediatrics* 2006;117: 578-585.

146. NIAMS National Institute of Arthritis and Musculoskeletal and Skin Diseases Website: Calcium intake tools. Available at: http://www.niams.nih. gov/Health_Info/Bone/Bone_Health/ Nutrition/calcium_intake.asp. Accessed January 8, 2008.

147. National Academy of Sciences: *Dietary Reference Intakes for Calcium, Phosphorus, Magnesium, Vitamin D, and Fluoride*. Washington, DC, Institute of Medicine, National Academy Press, 1997.

148. Curhan GC, Willett WC, Speizer FE, Spiegelman D, Stampfer MJ: Comparison of dietary calcium with supplemental calcium and other nutrients as factors affecting the risk for kidney stones in women. *Ann Intern Med* 1997;126:497-504.

149. Yang YX, Lewis JD, Epstein S, Metz DC: Long-term proton pump inhibitor therapy and the risk of hip fracture. *JAMA* 2006;296:2947-2953.

150. Holick MF: Vitamin D: A millenium perspective. *J Cell Biochem* 2003;88: 296-307.

151. Holick MF: Vitamin D: Importance in the prevention of cancers, type 1 diabetes, heart disease, and osteoporosis. *Am J Clin Nutr* 2004;79: 362-371.

152. Bischoff-Ferrari    HA,    Dawson-

Hughes B, Willett WC, et al: Effect of vitamin D on falls: A meta-analysis. *JAMA* 2004;291:1999-2006.

153. Need AG, O'Loughlin PD, Horowitz M, Nordin BE: Relationship between fasting serum glucose, age, body mass index, and serum 25 hydroxyvitamin D in postmenopausal women. *Clin Endocrinol (Oxf)* 2005;62: 738-741.

154. Holick MF: Vitamin D for health and in chronic kidney disease. *Semin Dial* 2005;18:266-275.

155. Bischoff-Ferrari HA, Giovannucci E, Willett WC, Dietrich T, Dawson-Hughes B: Estimation of optimal serum concentrations of 25-hydroxyvitamin D for multiple health outcomes. *Am J Clin Nutr* 2006;84: 18-28.

156. Hollis BW: Circulating 25-hydroxyvitamin D levels indicative of vitamin D sufficiency: Implications for establishing a new effective dietary intake recommendation for vitamin D. *J Nutr* 2005;135:317-322.

157. Rao DS, Alqurashi S: Management of vitamin D depletion in postmenopausal women. *Curr Osteoporos Rep* 2003;1:110-115.

158. National Osteoporosis Foundation Website. National Osteoporosis Foundation's Updated Recommendations for Calcium and Vitamin D Intake. Available at: http://www.nof.org/prevention/calcium_and_VitaminD.htm. Accessed December 4, 2007.

159. Holick MF: Vitamin D deficiency. *N Engl J Med* 2007;357:266-281.

160. Powell HS, Greenberg D: Tackling vitamin D deficiency. *Postgrad Med* 2006;119:25-30.

161. Aloia JF, Talwar SA, Pollack S, Feuerman M, Yeh JK: Optimal vitamin D status and serum parathyroid hormone concentrations in African American women. *Am J Clin Nutr* 2006;84:602-609.

162. Grant AM, Avenell A, Campbell MK, et al: Oral vitamin D3 and calcium for secondary prevention of low-trauma fractures in elderly people (Ran-domised evaluation of calcium or vitamin D, RECORD): A randomised placebo-controlled trial. *Lancet* 2005; 365:1621-1628.

163. Porthouse J, Cockayne S, King C, et al: Randomised controlled trial of calcium and supplementation with cholecalciferol (vitamin D3) for prevention of fractures in primary care. *BMJ* 2005;330:1003.

164. Jackson RD, LaCroix AZ, Gass M, et al: Calcium plus vitamin D supplementation and the risk of fractures. *N Engl J Med* 2006;354:1102.

165. Chapuy MC, Arlot ME, Duboeuf F, et al: Vitamin D3 and calcium to prevent hip fractures in the elderly women. *N Engl J Med* 1992;327:1637-1642.

166. Trivedi DP, Doll R, Khaw KT: Effect of four monthly oral vitamin D3 (cholecalciferol) supplementation on fractures and mortality in men and women living in the community: Randomized double blind controlled trial. *BMJ* 2003;326:469.

167. Bischoff-Ferrari HA, Willett WC, Wong JB, Giovannucci E, Dietrich T, Dawson-Hughes B: Fracture prevention with vitamin D supplementation: A meta-analysis of randomized controlled trials. *JAMA* 2005;293: 2257-2264.

168. Tang BM, Eslick GD, Nowson C, Smith C, Bensoussan A: Use of calcium or calcium in combination with vitamin D supplementation to prevent fractures and bone loss in people aged 50 years and older: A meta-analysis. *Lancet* 2007;370:657-666.

169. Marcus R, Wong M, Heath H III, Stock JL: Antiresorptive treatment of postmenopausal osteoporosis: Comparison of study designs and outcomes in large clinical trials with fracture as an endpoint. *Endocr Rev* 2002; 23:16-37.

170. Riggs BL, Parfitt AM: Drugs used to treat osteoporosis: The critical need for a uniform nomenclature based on their action on bone remodeling. *J Bone Miner Res* 2005;20:177-184.

171. FDA Division of Metabolism and En-docrine Drug Products. Guidelines for Preclinical and Clinical Evaluation of Agents Used in the Prevention and Treatment of Postmenopausal Osteoporosis. Available at: http://www.fda.gov/ohrms/dockets/dockets/98p0311/Tab0026.pdf. Accessed January 8, 2008.

172. Barrett-Connor E, Mosca L, Collins P, et al: Effects of raloxifene on cardiovascular events and breast cancer in postmenopausal women. *N Engl J Med* 2006;355:125-137.

173. Naesdal J, Brown K: NSAID-associated adverse effects and acid control aids to prevent them: A review of current treatment options. *Drug Saf* 2006;29:119-132.

174. Miller MA, Hyland M, Ofner-Agostini M, et al: Morbidity, mortality, and healthcare burden of nosocomial Clostridium difficile-associated diarrhea in Canadian hospitals. *Infect Control Hosp Epidemiol* 2002;23: 137-140.

175. Black DM, Cummings SR, Karpf DB, et al: Randomised trial of effect of alendronate on risk of fracture in women with existing vertebral fractures: Fracture Intervention Trial Research Group. *Lancet* 1996;348:1535-1541.

176. Harris ST, Watts NB, Genant HK, et al: Effects of risedronate treatment on vertebral and nonvertebral fractures in women with postmenopausal osteoporosis: A randomized controlled trial: Vertebral Efficacy With Risedronate Therapy (VERT) Study Group. *JAMA* 1999;282:1344-1352.

177. Reginster J, Minne HW, Sorensen OH, et al: Randomized trial of the effects of risedronate on vertebral fractures in women with established postmenopausal osteoporosis: Vertebral Efficacy with Risedronate Therapy (VERT) Study Group. *Osteoporos Int* 2000;11:83-91.

178. McClung MR, Geusens P, Miller PD, et al: Effect of risedronate on the risk of hip fracture in elderly women: Hip Intervention Program Study Group. *N Engl J Med* 2001;344: 333-340.

179. Cranney A, Wells G, Willan A, et al: Meta-analyses of therapies for post-menopausal osteoporosis: II. Meta-analysis of alendronate for the treatment of postmenopausal women. *Endocr Rev* 2002;23:508-516.

180. Chesnut III CH, Skag A, Christiansen C, et al: Effects of oral ibandronate administered daily or intermittently on fracture risk in postmenopausal osteoporosis. *J Bone Miner Res* 2004;19:1241-1249.

181. Delmas PD, Recker RR, Chesnut CH III, et al: Daily and intermittent oral ibandronate normalize bone turnover and provide significant reduction in vertebral fracture risk: Results from the BONE study. *Osteoporos Int* 2004;15:792-798.

182. Chestnut CH III, Ettinger MP, Miller PD, et al: Ibandronate produces significant, similar antifracture efficacy in North American and European women: New clinical findings from BONE. *Curr Med Res Opin* 2005;21:391-401.

183. Bauss F, Russell RG: Effects of ibandronate on bone quality: Preclinical studies. *Bone* 2007;40:265-273.

184. Reginster JY, Adami S, Lakatos P, et al: Efficacy and tolerability of once-monthly oral ibandronate in postmenopausal osteoporosis: 2 year results from the MOBILE study. *Ann Rheum Dis* 2006;65:654-661.

185. Alendronate (Fosamax) and risedronate (Actonel) revisited. *Med Lett Drugs Ther* 2005;47:33-35.

186. Ibandronate (Boniva): A new oral bisphosphonate. *Med Lett Drugs Ther* 2005;47:35.

187. Cooper A, Drake J, Brankin E, The PERSIST Investigators: Treatment persistence with once-monthly ibandronate and patient support vs once-weekly alendronate: Results from the PERSIST study. *Int J Clin Pract* 2006;60:896-905.

188. Emkey R, Koltun W, Beusterien K, et al: Patient preference for once-monthly ibandronate versus once-weekly alendronate in a randomized, open-label, cross-over trial: The Boniva Alendronate Trial in Osteoporosis (BALTO). *Curr Med Res Opin* 2005;21:1895-1903.

189. Bone HG, Hosking D, Devogelaer JP, et al: Ten years' experience with alendronate for osteoporosis in postmenopausal women. *N Engl J Med* 2004;350:1189-1199.

190. Mellstrom DD, Sorensen OH, Goemaere S, Roux C, Johnson TD, Chines AA: Seven years of treatment with risedronate in women with postmenopausal osteoporosis. *Calcif Tissue Int* 2004;75:462-468.

191. Recker R, Stakkestad JA, Chesnut CH III, et al: Insufficiently dosed intravenous ibandronate injections are associated with suboptimal antifracture efficacy in postmenopausal osteoporosis. *Bone* 2004;34:890-899.

192. Black DM, Delmas PD, Eastell R, et al: Once-yearly zoledronic acid for treatment of postmenopausal osteoporosis. *N Engl J Med* 2007;356:1809-1822.

193. Cao Y, Mori S, Mashiba T, et al: Raloxifene, estrogen, and alendronate affect the processes of fracture repair differently in ovariectomized rats. *J Bone Miner Res* 2002;17:2237-2246.

194. Bhandari M, Bajammal S, Guyatt GH, et al: Effect of bisphosphonates on periprosthetic bone mineral density after total joint arthroplasty: A meta-analysis. *J Bone Joint Surg Am* 2005;87:293-301.

195. Dan D, Germann D, Burki H, et al: Bone loss after total hip arthroplasty. *Rheumatol Int* 2006;26:792-798.

196. Durie BG, Katz M, Crowley J: Osteonecrosis of the jaw and bisphosphonates. *N Engl J Med* 2005;353:99-102.

197. Rossouw JE, Anderson GL, Prentice RL, et al: Risks and benefits of estrogen plus progestin in healthy postmenopausal women: Principal results from the Women's Health Initiative randomized controlled trial. *JAMA* 2002;288:321-333.

198. Shumaker SA, Legault C, Rapp SR, et al: Estrogen plus progestin and the incidence of dementia and mild cognitive impairment in postmenopausal women: The Women's Health Initiative Memory Study: A randomized controlled trial. *JAMA* 2003;289:2651-2662.

199. Torgerson DJ, Bell-Syer SE: Hormone replacement therapy and prevention of nonvertebral fractures: A meta-analysis of randomized trials. *JAMA* 2001;285:2891-2897.

200. Yates J, Barrett-Connor E, Barlas S, Chen YT, Miller PD, Siris ES: Rapid loss of hip fracture protection after estrogen cessation: Evidence from the National Osteoporosis Risk Assessment. *Obstet Gynecol* 2004;103:440-446.

201. Stefanick ML: Risk-benefit profiles of raloxifene for women. *N Engl J Med* 2006;355:190-192.

202. Brinker A, Beitz J: Spontaneous reports of pulmonary embolism in association with raloxifene. *Obstet Gynecol* 2001;98:1151.

203. Cranney A, Adachi JD: Benefit-risk assessment of raloxifene in postmenopausal osteoporosis. *Drug Saf* 2005;28:721-730.

204. Roelofs AJ, Thompson K, Gordon S, Rogers MJ: Molecular mechanisms of action of bisphosphonates: Current status. *Clin Cancer Res* 2006;12:6222s-6230s.

205. Russell RG: Bisphosphonates: Mode of action and pharmacology. *Pediatrics* 2007;119(suppl 2):S150-S162.

206. Bauer DC, Black D, Ensrud K, et al: Upper gastrointestinal tract safety profile of alendronate: The fracture intervention trial. *Arch Intern Med* 2000;160:517-525.

207. Lowe CE, Depew WT, Vanner SJ, Paterson WG, Meddings JB: Upper gastrointestinal toxicity of alendronate. *Am J Gastroenterol* 2000;95:634-640.

208. Wysowski DK, Chang JT: Alendronate and risedronate: Reports of severe bone, joint, and muscle pain. *Arch Intern Med* 2005;165:346-347.

209. Fraunfelder FW, Fraunfelder FT: Bisphosphonates and ocular inflamma-

tion. *N Engl J Med* 2003;348:1187-1188.

210. Somerman MJ, McCauley LK: Bisphosphonates: Sacrificing the jaw to save the skeleton? *BoneKEy-Osteovision* 2006;3:12-18.

211. Marx RE, Cillo JE Jr, Ulloa JJ: Oral bisphosphonate-induced osteonecrosis: Risk factors, predictions of risk using serum CTX testing, prevention, and treatment. *J Oral Maxillofac Surg* 2007;65:2397-2410.

212. Woo SB, Hellstein JW, Kalmar JR: Bisphosphonates and osteonecrosis of the jaws. *Ann Intern Med* 2006;144:753-761.

213. Koka S, Clarke BL, Amin S, Gertz M, Ruggiero SL: Oral bisphosphonate therapy and osteonecrosis of the jaw: What to tell the concerned patient. *Int J Prosthodont* 2007;20:115-122.

214. Advisory Task Force on Bisphosphonate-Related Osteonecrosis of the Jaws, American Association of Oral and Maxillofacial Surgeons: American Association of Oral and Maxillofacial Surgeons position paper on bisphosphonate-related osteonecrosis of the jaws. *J Oral Maxillofac Surg* 2007;65:369-376.

215. Bilezikian JP: Osteonecrosis of the jaw: Do bisphosphonates pose a risk? *N Engl J Med* 2006;355:2278-2281.

216. Aspenberg P: Osteonecrosis: What does it mean? One condition partly caused by bisphosphonates: Or another one, preferably treated with them? *Acta Orthop* 2006;77:693-694.

217. Rizzoli R: Long-term outcome of weekly bisphosphonates. *Clin Orthop Relat Res* 2006;443:61-65.

218. Cosman F, Cummings S, Lindsay R: How long should patients with osteoporosis be treated with bisphosphonates? *J Womens Health Gend Based Med* 2000;9:81-84.

219. Odvina CV, Zerwekh JE, Rao DS, Maalouf N, Gottschalk FA, Pak CY: Severely suppressed bone turnover: A potential complication of alendronate therapy. *J Clin Endocrinol Metab* 2005;90:1294-1301.

220. Mathoo JM, Cranney A, Papaioannou A, Adachi JD: Rational use of oral bisphosphonates for the treatment of osteoporosis. *Curr Osteoporos Rep* 2004;2:17-23.

221. Black DM, Schwartz AV, Ensrud KE, et al: Effects of continuing or stopping alendronate after 5 years of treatment: The Fracture Intervention Trial Long-term Extension (FLEX): A randomized trial. *JAMA* 2006;296:2927-2938.

222. Ravn P, Weiss SR, Rodriguez-Portales JA, et al: Alendronate in early postmenopausal women: Effects on bone mass during long-term treatment and after withdrawal: Alendronate Osteoporosis Prevention Study Group. *J Clin Endocrinol Metab* 2000;85:1492-1497.

223. Greenspan SL, Emkey RD, Bone HG, et al: Significant differential effects of alendronate, estrogen, or combination therapy on the rate of bone loss after discontinuation of treatment of postmenopausal osteoporosis: A randomized, double-blind, placebo-controlled trial. *Ann Intern Med* 2002;137:875-883.

224. Gehlbach SH, Bigelow C, Heimisdottir M, May S, Walker M, Kirkwood JR: Recognition of vertebral fracture in a clinical setting. *Osteoporos Int* 2000;11:577-582.

225. Boszczyk B, Bierschneider M, Potulski M, Robert B, Vastmans J, Jaksche H: Extended kyphoplasty indications for stabilization of osteoporotic vertebral compression fractures. *Unfallchirurg* 2002;105:952-957.

226. Nevitt MC, Ettinger B, Black D, et al: The association of radiographically detected vertebral fractures with back pain and function: A prospective study. *Ann Intern Med* 1998;128:793-800.

227. Genant HK, Wu CY, van Kuijk C, Nevitt MC: Vertebral fracture assessment using a semiquantitative technique. *J Bone Miner Res* 1993;8:1137-1148.

228. Manson NA, Phillips FM: Minimally invasive techniques for the treatment

of osteoporotic vertebral fractures. *J Bone Joint Surg Am* 2006;88:1862-1872.

229. Melton LJ III, Kan SH, Frye MA, Wahner HW, O'Fallon WM, Riggs BL: Epidemiology of vertebral fractures in women. *Am J Epidemiol* 1989;129:1000-1011.

230. O'Neill TW, Felsenberg D, Varlow J, Cooper C, Kanis JA, Silman AJ: The prevalence of vertebral deformity in european men and women: The European Vertebral Osteoporosis Study. *J Bone Miner Res* 1996;11:1010-1018.

231. Ismail AA, O'Neill TW, Cooper C, Silman AJ: Risk factors for vertebral deformities in men: Relationship to number of vertebral deformities: European Vertebral Osteoporosis Study Group. *J Bone Miner Res* 2000;15:278-283.

232. Cockerill W, Ismail AA, Cooper C, et al: Does location of vertebral deformity within the spine influence back pain and disability?: European Vertebral Osteoporosis Study (EVOS) Group. *Ann Rheum Dis* 2000;59:368-371.

233. Cortet B, Houvenagel E, Puisieux F, Roches E, Garnier P, Delcambre B: Spinal curvatures and quality of life in women with vertebral fractures secondary to osteoporosis. *Spine* 1999;24:1921-1925.

234. Schlaich C, Minne HW, Bruckner T, et al: Reduced pulmonary function in patients with spinal osteoporotic fractures. *Osteoporos Int* 1998;8:261-267.

235. Tosteson AN, Gabriel SE, Grove MR, Moncur MM, Kneeland TS, Melton LJ III: Impact of hip and vertebral fractures on quality-adjusted life years. *Osteoporos Int* 2001;12:1042-1049.

236. Ross PD: Clinical consequences of vertebral fractures. *Am J Med* 1997;103:30S-42S.

237. Melton LJ III: Adverse outcomes of osteoporotic fractures in the general population. *J Bone Miner Res* 2003;18:1139-1141.

238. Cauley JA, Thompson DE, Ensrud KC, Scott JC, Black D: Risk of mor-

tality following clinical fractures. *Osteoporos Int* 2000;11:556-561.

239. Kado DM, Browner WS, Palermo L, Nevitamint MC, Genant HK, Cummings SR: Vertebral fractures and mortality in older women: A prospective study. *Arch Intern Med* 1999;159:1215-1220.

240. Cooper C, Atkinson EJ, Jacobsen SJ, et al: Population-based study of survival after osteoporotic fractures. *Am J Epidemiol* 1993;137:1001-1005.

241. Davis JW, Grove JS, Wasnich RD, Ross PD: Spatial relationships between prevalent and incident spine fractures. *Bone* 1999;24:261-264.

242. Lindsay R, Silverman SL, Cooper C, et al: Risk of new vertebral fracture in the year following a fracture. *JAMA* 2001;285:320-323.

243. Heaney RP: Pathophysiology of osteoporosis. *Endocrinol Metab Clin North Am* 1998;27:255-265.

244. Intravenous ibandronate (Boniva). *Med Lett Drugs Ther* 2006;48:68-69.

245. Dempster DW, Bolognese MA: Ibandronate: The evolution of a once-a-month oral therapy for postmenopausal osteoporosis. *J Clin Densitom* 2006;9:58-65.

246. Delmas PD, Adami S, Strugala C, et al: Intravenous ibandronate injections in postmenopausal women with osteoporosis: One-year results from the dosing intravenous administration study. *Arthritis Rheum* 2006;54:1838-1846.

247. Bone HG, Schurr W: Intravenous bisphosphonate therapy for osteoporosis: Where do we stand? *Curr Osteoporos Rep* 2004;2:24-30.

248. Adami S, Felsenberg D, Christiansen C, et al: Efficacy and safety of ibandronate given by intravenous injection once every 3 months. *Bone* 2004;34:881-889.

249. Croom KF, Scott LJ: Intravenous ibandronate: In the treatment of osteoporosis. *Drugs* 2006;66:1593-1601.

250. Lyles KW, Colón-Emeric CS, Magaziner JS, et al: Zolendronic acid and clincal fracture and mortality after hip fracture. *N Engl J Med* 2007;357:1799-1809.

251. Cummings SR, Schwartz AV, Black DM: Alendronate and atrial fibrillation. *N Engl J Med* 2007;356:1895-1896.

252. Cosman F: Anabolic therapy for osteoporosis: Parathyroid hormone. *Curr Rheumatol Rep* 2006;8:63-69.

253. Rittmaster RS, Bolognese M, Ettinger MP, et al: Enhancement of bone mass in osteoporotic women with parathyroid hormone followed by alendronate. *J Clin Endocrinol Metab* 2000;85:2129-2134.

254. Whitfield JF, Morley P, Willick GE: The bone-building action of the parathyroid hormone: Implications for the treatment of osteoporosis. *Drugs Aging* 1999;15:117-129.

255. Dempster DW, Cosman F, Kurland ES, et al: Effects of daily treatment with parathyroid hormone on bone microarchitecture and turnover in patients with osteoporosis: A paired biopsy study. *J Bone Miner Res* 2001;16:1846-1853.

256. Arlot M, Meunier PJ, Boivin G, et al: Differential effects of teriparatide and alendronate on bone remodeling in postmenopausal women assessed by histomorphometric parameters. *J Bone Miner Res* 2005;20:1244-1253.

257. Mierke DF, Pellegrini M: Parathyroid hormone and parathyroid hormone-related protein: Model systems for the development of an osteoporosis therapy. *Curr Pharm Des* 1999;5:21-36.

258. Kurland ES, Cosman F, McMahon DJ, Rosen CJ, Lindsay R, Bilezikian JP: Parathyroid hormone as a therapy for idiopathic osteoporosis in men: Effects on bone mineral density and bone markers. *J Clin Endocrinol Metab* 2000;85:3069-3076.

259. Alkhiary YM, Gerstenfeld LC, Krall E, et al: Enhancement of experimental fracture-healing by systemic administration of recombinant human parathyroid hormone (PTH 1-34). *J Bone Joint Surg Am* 2005;87:731-741.

260. Manabe T, Mori S, Mashiba T, et al: Human parathyroid hormone (1-34) accelerates natural fracture healing process in the femoral osteotomy model of cynomolgus monkeys. *Bone* 2007;40:1475-1482.

261. Tsiridis E, Morgan EF, Bancroft JM, et al: Effects of OP-1 and PTH in a new experimental model for the study of metaphyseal bone healing. *J Orthop Res* 2007;25:1193-1203.

262. Fujita T, Inoue T, Morii H, et al: Effect of an intermittent weekly dose of human parathyroid hormone (1-34) on osteoporosis: A randomized double-masked prospective study using three dose levels. *Osteoporos Int* 1999;9:296-306.

263. Neer RM, Arnaud CD, Zanchetta JR, et al: Effect of parathyroid hormone (1-34) on fractures and bone mineral density in postmenopausal women with osteoporosis. *N Engl J Med* 2001;344:1434-1441.

264. Body JJ, Gaich GA, Scheele WH, et al: A randomized double-blind trial to compare the efficacy of teriparatide (recombinant human parathyroid hormone [1-34]) with alendronate in postmenopausal women with osteoporosis. *J Clin Endocrinol Metab* 2002;87:4528-4535.

265. Bilezikian JP, Kurland ES: Therapy of male osteoporosis with parathyroid hormone. *Calcif Tissue Int* 2001;69:248-251.

266. Lindsay R, Nieves J, Formica C, et al: Randomised controlled study of effect of parathyroid hormone on vertebral-bone mass and fracture incidence among postmenopausal women on estrogen with osteoporosis. *Lancet* 1997;350:550-555.

267. Genant HK, Siris E, Crans GG, Desaiah D, Krege JH: Reduction in vertebral fracture risk in teriparatide-treated postmenopausal women as assessed by spinal deformity index. *Bone* 2005;37:170-174.

268. Cranney A, Papaioannou A, Zytaruk N, et al: Parathyroid hormone for the treatment of osteoporosis: A systematic review. *CMAJ* 2006;175:52-59.

269. Black DM, Greenspan SL, Ensrud

KE, et al: The effects of parathyroid hormone and alendronate alone or in combination in postmenopausal osteoporosis. *N Engl J Med* 2003;349: 1207-1215.

270. Hodsman A, Scientific Advisory Council of Osteoporosis Canada, Papaioannou A, Clinical Guidelines Committee, Cranney A, Writing Group on the Systematic Review of Parathyroid Hormone for the Treatment of Osteoporosis: Clinical practice guidelines for the use of parathyroid hormone in the treatment of osteoporosis. *CMAJ* 2006;175:48.

271. Bauer DC, Garnero P, Bilezikian JP, et al: Short-term changes in bone turnover markers and bone mineral density response to parathyroid hormone in postmenopausal women with osteoporosis. *J Clin Endocrinol Metab* 2006;91:1370-1375.

272. Delmas PD, Licata AA, Reginster JY, et al: Fracture risk reduction during treatment with teriparatide is independent of pretreatment bone turnover. *Bone* 2006;39:237-243.

273. Hodsman AB, Bauer DC, Dempster DW, et al: Parathyroid hormone and teriparatide for the treatment of osteoporosis: A review of the evidence and suggested guidelines for its use. *Endocr Rev* 2005;26:688-703

274. Cosman F, Nieves J, Woelfert L, et al: Parathyroid hormone added to established hormone therapy: Effects on vertebral fracture and maintenance of bone mass after parathyroid hormone withdrawal. *J Bone Miner Res* 2001;16: 925-931.

275. Finkelstein JS, Hayes A, Hunzelman JL, Wyland JJ, Lee H, Neer RM: The effects of parathyroid hormone, alendronate, or both in men with osteoporosis. *N Engl J Med* 2003;349: 1216-1226.

276. Deal C, Omizo M, Schwartz EN, et al: Combination teriparatide and raloxifene therapy for postmenopausal osteoporosis: Results from a 6-month double-blind placebo-controlled trial. *J Bone Miner Res* 2005;20:1905-1911.

277. Cosman F, Nieves J, Zion M,

Woelfert L, Luckey M, Lindsay R: Daily and cyclic parathyroid hormone in women receiving alendronate. *N Engl J Med* 2005;353:566-575.

278. Heaney RP, Recker RR: Combination and sequential therapy for osteoporosis. *N Engl J Med* 2005;353: 624-625.

279. Liu H, Michaud K, Nayak S, Karpf DB, Owens DK, Garber AM: The cost-effectiveness of therapy with teriparatide and alendronate in women with severe osteoporosis. *Arch Intern Med* 2006;166:1209-1217.

280. Harper KD, Krege JH, Marcus R, Mitlak BH: Osteosarcoma and teriparatide? *J Bone Miner Res* 2007;22:334.

281. Jutte PC, Rosso R, de Paolis M, et al: Osteosarcoma associated with hyperparathyroidism. *Skeletal Radiol* 2004; 33:473-476.

282. Boonen S, Marin F, Mellstrom D, et al: Safety and efficacy of teriparatide in elderly women with established osteoporosis: Bone anabolic therapy from a geriatric perspective. *J Am Geriatr Soc* 2006;54:782-789.

283. Gold DT, Pantos BS, Masica DN, Misurski DA, Marcus R: Initial experience with teriparatide in the United States. *Curr Med Res Opin* 2006;22: 703-708.

284. Arden NK, Earl S, Fisher DJ, Cooper C, Carruthers S, Goater M: Persistence with teriparatide in patients with osteoporosis: The UK experience. *Osteoporos Int* 2006;17:1626-1629.

285. Tashjian AH Jr, Gagel RF: Teriparatide (human PTH [1-34]): 2.5 years of experience on the use and safety of the drug for the treatment of osteoporosis. *J Bone Miner Res* 2006; 21:354-365.

286. Tashjian AH Jr, Gagel RF: Teriparatide (human PTH[1-34]): 2.5 years of experience on the use and safety of the drug for the treatment of osteoporosis. *J Bone Miner Res* 2007;22:334.

287. Lane JM, Johnson CE, Khan SN, Girardi FP, Cammisa FP Jr: Minimally

invasive options for the treatment of osteoporotic vertebral compression fractures. *Orthop Clin North Am* 2002; 33:431-438.

288. Reginster JY, Deroisy R, Lecart MP, et al: A double-blind, placebo-controlled, dose-finding trial of intermittent nasal salmon calcitonin for prevention of postmenopausal lumbar spine bone loss. *Am J Med* 1995; 98:452-458.

289. Lyritis GP, Ioannidis GV, Karachalios T, et al: Analgesic effect of salmon calcitonin suppositories in patients with acute pain due to recent osteoporotic vertebral crush fractures: A prospective double-blind, randomized, placebo controlled clinical study. *Clin J Pain* 1999;15:284-289.

290. Armingeat T, Brondino R, Pham T, Legre V, Lafforgue P: Intravenous pamidronate for pain relief in recent osteoporotic vertebral compression fracture: A randomized double-blind controlled study. *Osteoporos Int* 2006; 17:1659-1665.

291. Nevitt MC, Chen P, Dore RK, et al: Reduced risk of back pain following teriparatide treatment: A meta-analysis. *Osteoporos Int* 2006;17: 273-280.

292. Karlsson M, Nilsson JA, Redlund-Johnell I, Johnell O, Obrant KJ: Changes of BMD and soft tissue after hip fracture. *Bone* 1996;18:19-22.

293. Lewiecki EM: Vertebroplasty and kyphoplasty in 2001. *J Clin Densitom* 2001;4:185-187.

294. Togawa D, Lieberman IH, Bauer TW, Reinhardt MK, Kayanja MM: Histological evaluation of biopsies obtained from vertebral compression fractures: Unsuspected myeloma and osteomalacia. *Spine* 2005;30:781-786.

295. Hardouin P, Fayada P, Leclet H, Chopin D: Kyphoplasty. *Joint Bone Spine* 2002;69:256-261.

296. Syed MI, Patel NA, Jan S, Harron MS, Morar K, Shaikh A: New symptomatic vertebral compression fractures within a year following vertebroplasty in osteoporotic women. *AJNR Am J Neuroradiol* 2005;26: 1601-1604.

297. Keller TS, Kosmopoulos V, Lieberman IH: Vertebroplasty and kyphoplasty affect vertebral motion segment stiffness and stress distributions: A microstructural finite-element study. *Spine* 2005;30:1258-1265.

298. Bai B, Jazrawi LM, Kummer FJ, Spivak JM: The use of an injectable, biodegradable calcium phosphate bone substitute for the prophylactic augmentation of osteoporotic vertebrae and the management of vertebral compression fractures. *Spine* 1999;24:1521-1526.

299. Garfin SR, Yuan HA, Reiley MA: New technologies in spine: Kyphoplasty and vertebroplasty for the treatment of painful osteoporotic compression fractures. *Spine* 2001;26:1511-1515.

300. Phillips FM, Todd Wetzel F, Lieberman I, Campbell-Hupp M: An in vivo comparison of the potential for extravertebral cement leak after vertebroplasty and kyphoplasty. *Spine* 2002;27:2173-2178.

301. Pflugmacher R, Schroeder RJ, Klostermann CK: Incidence of adjacent vertebral fractures in patients treated with balloon kyphoplasty: Two years' prospective follow-up. *Acta Radiol* 2006;47:830-840.

302. Oden A, Dawson A, Dere W, Johnell O, Jonsson B, Kanis JA: Lifetime risk of hip fractures is underestimated. *Osteoporos Int* 1998;8:599-603.

303. Magaziner J, Fredman L, Hawkes W, et al: Changes in functional status attributable to hip fracture: A comparison of hip fracture patients to community-dwelling aged. *Am J Epidemiol* 2003;157:1023-1031.

304. Salkeld G, Cameron ID, Cumming RG, et al: Quality of life related to fear of falling and hip fracture in older women: A time trade off study. *BMJ* 2000;320:341-346.

305. Leibson CL, Tosteson AN, Gabriel SE, Ransom JE, Melton LJ: Mortality, disability, and nursing home use for persons with and without hip fracture: A population-based study. *J Am Geriatr Soc* 2002;50:1644-1650.

306. Richmond J, Aharonoff GB, Zuckerman JD, Koval KJ: Mortality risk after hip fracture: 2003. *J Orthop Trauma* 2003;17(suppl 8):S2-S5.

307. Gillespie WJ, Gillespie LD, Handoll HH, Madhok R: The Cochrane Musculoskeletal Injuries Group. *Acta Orthop Scand Suppl* 2002;73:15-19.

308. Shipp KM: Exercise for people with osteoporosis: Translating the science into clinical practice. *Curr Osteoporos Rep* 2006;4:129-133.

309. Gilsanz V, Wren TA, Sanchez M, Dorey F, Judex S, Rubin C: Low-level, high-frequency mechanical signals enhance musculoskeletal development of young women with low BMD. *J Bone Miner Res* 2006;21:1464-1474.

310. Bonaiuti D, Shea B, Iovine R, et al: Exercise for preventing and treating osteoporosis in postmenopausal women. *Cochrane Database Syst Rev* 2002;3:CD000333.

311. Nordstrom A, Karlsson C, Nyquist F, Olsson T, Nordstrom P, Karlsson M: Bone loss and fracture risk after reduced physical activity. *J Bone Miner Res* 2005;20:202-207

312. Kujala UM: Physical activity and osteoporotic hip fracture risk in men. *Arch Intern Med* 2000;160:705-708.

313. Kerschan-Schindl K, Uher E, Kainberger F, Kaider A, Ghanem AH, Preisinger E: Long-term home exercise program: Effect in women at high risk of fracture. *Arch Phys Med Rehabil* 2000;81:319-323.

314. Lin JT, Lane JM: Rehabilitation of the older adult with an osteoporosis-related fracture. *Clin Geriatr Med* 2006;22:435-447.

315. Tinetti ME, Baker DI, McAvay G, et al: A multifactorial intervention to reduce the risk of falling among elderly people living in the community. *N Engl J Med* 1994;331:821-827.

316. Qin L, Au S, Choy W, et al: Regular Tai Chi Chuan exercise may retard bone loss in postmenopausal women: A case-control study. *Arch Phys Med Rehabil* 2002;83:1355-1359.

317. Parker MJ, Gillespie LD, Gillespie WJ: Hip protectors for preventing hip fractures in the elderly. *Cochrane Database Syst Rev* 2001;2:CD001255.

318. Kiel DP, Magaziner J, Zimmerman S, et al: Efficacy of a hip protector to prevent hip fracture in nursing home residents: The HIP PRO randomized controlled trial. *JAMA* 2007;298:413-422.

319. Kannus P, Parkkari J: Hip protectors for preventing hip fracture. *JAMA* 2007;298:413-422.

320. Oliver D, Connelly JB, Victor CR, et al: Strategies to prevent falls and fractures in hospitals and care homes and effect of cognitive impairment: Systematic review and meta-analyses. *BMJ* 2007;334:82.

321. McGlynn EA, Asch SM, Adams J, et al: The quality of health care delivered to adults in the United States. *N Engl J Med* 2003;348:2635-2645.

322. National Institute of Arthritis and Musculoskeletal and Skin Diseases Website. The NIH Osteoporosis and Related Bone Diseases–National Resource Center. Available at: http://www.niams.nih.gov/bone. Accessed December 4, 2007.

323. Rizzoli R, Bonjour JP: Dietary protein and bone health. *J Bone Miner Res* 2004;19:527-531.

324. Promislow JH, Goodman-Gruen D, Slymen DJ, Barrett-Connor E: Protein consumption and bone mineral density in the elderly: The Rancho Bernardo Study. *Am J Epidemiol* 2002;155:636-644.

325. Avenell A, Handoll HH: Nutritional supplementation for hip fracture aftercare in the elderly. *Cochrane Database Syst Rev* 2005;2:CD001880.

326. Kuehn BM: Better osteoporosis management a priority: Impact predicted to soar with aging population. *JAMA* 2005;293:2453-2458.

327. Fox KA, Steg PG, Eagle KA, et al: Decline in rates of death and heart failure in acute coronary syndromes, 1999-2006. *JAMA* 2007;297:1892-1900.

328. Penning-van Beest FJ, Goettsch WG,

Erkens JA, Herings RM: Determinants of persistence with bisphosphonates: A study in women with postmenopausal osteoporosis. *Clin Ther* 2006;28:236-242.

329. Siris ES, Harris ST, Rosen CJ, et al: Adherence to bisphosphonate therapy and fracture rates in osteoporotic women: Relationship to vertebral and nonvertebral fractures from 2 US claims databases. *Mayo Clin Proc* 2006; 81:1013-1022.

330. Brookhart MA, Avorn J, Katz JN, et al: Gaps in treatment among users of osteoporosis medications: The dynamics of noncompliance. *Am J Med* 2007;120:251-256.

331. Compston JE, Seeman E: Compliance with osteoporosis therapy is the weakest link. *Lancet* 2006;368: 973-974.

332. Solomon DH, Avorn J, Katz JN, et al: Compliance with osteoporosis medications. *Arch Intern Med* 2005;165: 2414-2419.

333. van den Boogaard CH, Breekveldt-Postma NS, Borggreve SE, Goettsch WG, Herings RM: Persistent bisphosphonate use and the risk of osteoporotic fractures in clinical practice: A database analysis study. *Curr Med Res Opin* 2006;22:1757-1764.

334. Boyd CM, Darer J, Boult C, Fried LP, Boult L, Wu AW: Clinical practice guidelines and quality of care for older patients with multiple comorbid diseases: Implications for pay for performance. *JAMA* 2006;295:34.

335. Greenspan SL, Schneider DL, McClung MR, et al: Alendronate improves bone mineral density in elderly women with osteoporosis residing in long-term care facilities: A randomized, double-blind, placebo-controlled trial. *Ann Intern Med* 2002; 136:742-746.

# Venous Thromboembolic Disease After Total Hip and Knee Arthroplasty: Current Perspectives in a Regulated Environment

Vincent D. Pellegrini, Jr, MD
Nigel E. Sharrock, MD, ChB
Guy D. Paiement, MD
Rhys Morris, PhD
David J. Warwick, MD, FRCS (Orth), EDipHS

## Abstract

*Venous thromboembolic disease is the single most common reason for readmission to the hospital following total hip and total knee arthroplasty and remains a genuine threat to the life of the patient. Nevertheless, advances in surgical procedure, anesthetic management, and postoperative convalescence have altered the risks of venous thromboembolism after total joint arthroplasty in the lower extremity. Regional anesthetic techniques reduce the prevalence of venographic thrombosis by approximately 50%, and intraoperative monitoring has identified preparation of the femoral canal as the sentinel event that activates the coagulation cascade by the intravasation of marrow fat into the systemic circulation. Prevention of venographic thrombosis is most efficacious by administering fractionated heparin followed by warfarin; warfarin (international normalized ratio 2.0) appears to have a greater safety margin than fractionated heparin based on clinically meaningful bleeding events. Prevention of readmission events, proximal thrombosis, or pulmonary embolism has been demonstrated by using low-intensity warfarin. Aspirin, when used in conjunction with hypotensive epidural anesthesia after hip arthroplasty and regional anesthesia after knee arthroplasty, combined with pneumatic compression devices, also has been suggested to prevent clinical venous thromboembolism, as measured by readmission events. Oral thrombin inhibitors hold promise, but instances of liver toxicity have precluded approval in North America to date. Mechanical compression devices enhance venous flow and increase fibrinolytic activity in the lower extremity; clinical trials demonstrate efficacy in reducing venographic thrombosis alone after total knee arthroplasty and in combination with other chemoprophylactic agents after total hip arthroplasty. Extended chemoprophylaxis for 3 to 6 weeks after surgery is prudent in view of the protracted risk of thrombogenesis and the late occurrence of readmission for venous thrombosis and pulmonary embolism.*

**Instr Course Lect 2008;57:637-661.**

Total joint arthroplasty in the lower extremity is an operation with a strong propensity for thromboembolic complications with potentially life-threatening consequences. In a study of 7,959 total hip arthroplasties (THAs) from 1962 to 1973, the overall prevalence of pulmonary embolism (PE) was reported as 7.89%, with fatal embolisms in 1.04% of patients.[1,2] Charnley[3] stated, "The possibility of fatal pulmonary embolism after total hip replacement is a hip surgeon's constant worry ... no matter how rare this might be." In the early 1970s, Coventry and associates[4] identified an overall prevalence of PE in 2.2% of patients in a study of 2,012 consecutive THAs; in a subset of patients who received no prophylactic anticoagulation, the prevalence of fatal PE was 3.4%. At that time, the average duration of surgery was 2.4 hours, blood loss was 1,650 mL, and 1,144 mL blood was transfused. Prophylactic anticoagulation with warfarin was started 5 days after surgery. On average, patients remained at bed rest for 1 week before walking and were discharged 3 weeks after surgery. In 1984, Insall[5] suggested that every orthopaedic surgeon should try to prevent thrombophlebitis and PE when performing total knee arthroplasty (TKA). In a 1984 study, Stulberg and associates[6] reported an 84% prevalence of deep venous thrombosis (DVT) in patients who did not receive venous thromboembolic disease (VTED) prophylaxis, no fatal PEs, and a clinically evident PE rate of 1.7%. The authors concluded that a positive venogram had clinical significance, although it was not associated with local symptoms. Although symptomatic and sometimes fatal PE is less common following TKA than after THA, the residual prevalence of DVT is even greater than after THA and has been far more refractory to pharmacologic prophylaxis.

## Prevalence

The National Institutes of Health Consensus Conference in 1986 further raised the general awareness of the high risk of DVT and PE and stratified patient risks by types of surgery.[7] Based on data available at that time, orthopaedic surgery of the lower extremity, including TKA, THA, and hip fracture, were determined to present the highest risk for VTED without prophylaxis. Prophylaxis was recommended for these patient groups; the agents and time frames of prophylaxis varied. One of the last clinical trials using a placebo control for thrombosis was performed in Canada in the 1980s. The authors reported a 49% rate of total DVT (77 of 158 patients) and a 27% rate for proximal DVT (42 of 158 patients) after THA.[8] It is unlikely that the US Food and Drug Administration will approve any further thrombosis studies using placebo controls for patients undergoing TKA, THA, or hip fracture surgery.

The clinical management of arthroplasty patients has changed from this historical benchmark; some would contend that a concomitant reduction in the prevalence of VTED has been one benefit of an expedited convalescence and improved anesthetic management.[9,10] Despite an apparent reduction in fatal VTED coinciding with more widespread use of routine anti-

coagulant prophylaxis and faster rehabilitation, DVT remains the most common reason for emergency readmission following total joint arthroplasty.[11] In one study of 1,638 total joint arthroplasties managed with routine surveillance venography and warfarin treatment of all DVTs, the overall 6-month readmission rate was 1.3% (22 of 1,638 arthroplasties). Of greater interest, readmission for venous thromboembolic events after THA (1.8%; 19 of 1,079 arthroplasties) occurred more than three times as frequently after TKA (0.54%; 3 of 559 arthroplasties; $P = 0.04$). The overall 6-month mortality rate was 0.79%, with two fatal PEs (0.12%) accounting for 15% of deaths from all causes.[12]

It is essential to recognize that thromboembolic disease following THA and TKA is manifest clinically as two very different conditions.[13,14] Prior to acceptance of routine prophylaxis, proximal (femoral and popliteal) DVT accounted for 50% to 60% of all observed deep vein thrombi after THA. Presently, with the use of warfarin or fractionated heparin prophylaxis after THA, more than 90% of deep thrombi occur in the calf, and 10% or less are found in the thigh. Nearly all proximal thrombi are segmental in nature, frequently occur in the region of the femoral vein near the lesser trochanter, and do not communicate with more distal thrombi in the calf. The situation following TKA is considerably different. Approximately 90% of all DVT after knee replacement occurs primarily in the calf veins, with proximal thrombosis occurring infrequently and accounting for less than 10% of all thrombi. When present, proximal thrombosis after TKA is nearly always contiguous with more distal disease in the

calf and rarely extends more proximally than the popliteal vein. Unlike the situation following THA, this regional distribution of DVT after knee replacement has remained unchanged with warfarin or other anticoagulant prophylaxis. The prevalence of DVT after knee replacement with warfarin prophylaxis remains 35% to 55%. Although this represents an improvement from the 80% to 90% rates observed after TKA before routine prophylaxis, this residual rate remains far more refractory to prophylactic anticoagulation than the comparable situation following THA.

In the setting of both hip and knee replacement, a systemic diathesis is evident; bilateral venogram trials have shown a 10% to 15% prevalence of DVT in the nonsurgical limb following each procedure. It is unclear whether using a tourniquet during knee replacement aggravates this clotting propensity by causing stasis in the leg or if the stimulation of endothelial cell-mediated fibrinolysis mitigates this effect and actually results in a lower prevalence of thrombosis than would be observed without tourniquet use.

Two caveats that differentiate management of VTED about the knee and hip deserve special mention. With respect to bleeding complications of anticoagulant prophylaxis, the skin envelope surrounding the knee is much less forgiving than that around the hip; therefore, a wound hematoma is less well tolerated after knee replacement than following comparable surgery about the hip. It is also important to acknowledge that calf thrombosis is generally a less feared complication than proximal DVT because of a lower risk of direct embolization; however, calf clots propagate to the thigh in 17% to 25% of patients postoperatively and present a greater risk of embolization. Accordingly, there is a risk of undertreating this condition if the literature from ambulatory medical patients is used to guide treatment.

## Pathophysiology and Prevention

During the past decade, substantial advances have been made in understanding the pathophysiology and prevention of VTED, largely associated with THA.[15] The prevalence of fatal PE with contemporary surgical techniques in the absence of anticoagulant prophylaxis was reported to be 0.5% following 1,162 THAs performed in the United Kingdom.[16] In North America, several studies have reported that warfarin prophylaxis and the collective use of predonated autologous blood, expeditious surgery, and early mobilization have lowered the rate of fatal PE to less than 0.1%.[17-19] An increased awareness of the intense activation of the clotting cascade that occurs during surgery and persists for more than 24 hours has recently underscored the importance of intraoperative events.[20,21] It has been established that activation of the clotting cascade occurs during instrumentation of the medullary canal in hip arthroplasty;[20] a similar phenomenon with intramedullary instrumentation of the distal femur during knee replacement can logically be expected. The problem is compounded by stasis in the lower extremity caused by obstruction of femoral venous flow, either while the lower extremity is kept in an extreme position to provide adequate exposure for femoral preparation and hip component insertion or with the leg folded upon itself to gain exposure of the proximal tibia during knee replacement.[22-24] This kinking of the femoral or popliteal veins can produce endothelial injury, providing the nidus for the formation and propagation of clots. Whether caused by prosthetic joint arthroplasty, during intramedullary fracture fixation, or by a fracture resulting from a vehicular crash, disturbance of the intramedullary canal with intravasation of marrow fat remains the most potent stimulus of the clotting cascade and results in a unique propensity for VTED in the orthopaedic patient population.

Notwithstanding the magnitude of this physiologic insult, in recent years the sociopolitical spotlight has focused on prevention of venous thromboembolism. Under such scrutiny, the orthopaedic community has focused the emphasis of prophylaxis on prevention of clinical events rather than reduction in venographic disease in an effort to balance the risks of bleeding with the positive benefits of anticoagulation. The Joint Commission, the National Quality Forum, and the Centers for Medicare and Medicaid Services have joined forces to shepherd the establishment of voluntary consensus standards for VTED prophylaxis and treatment. It is likely that these consensus standards will serve as another benchmark for a federal pay-for-performance initiative. Hospital performance on these measures will become a matter of public record via reporting at the Health and Human Services Website. The orthopaedic community has been preoccupied with VTED risk and the possibility of fatal PE complications after total joint arthroplasty. However, the orthopaedic surgeon is equally conscious of the delicate balance that accompanies the use of potent anticoagulants with their associated risk of bleeding in the perioperative period that can lead to stiffness, wound breakdown, infection, and even loss of the prosthetic device. The current reference standard for prophylaxis is the guidelines of the American College of Chest Physicians (ACCP), despite a widely held belief that these recommendations overemphasize the use of potent anticoagulants with little appreciation for their associated bleeding complications. The most recent ACCP guidelines,[25] published in 2004, recommend the use of warfarin (international normalized ratio [INR] 2 to 3), low-molecular-weight heparin (LMWH), or fondaparinux as suitable prophylaxis after THA, TKA, and hip fracture for a duration of at least 10 days, with THA and hip fracture patients suggested to receive prophylaxis for 28 to 35 days (Table 1). For the first time since their initial publication, the ACCP guidelines recommended against specific practices—administering aspirin as a prophylactic agent in any

**Table 1**
**ACCP 2004 Recommendations for LMWH**

**Elective hip replacement**

Duration: 28 to 35 days

Usual dose: 12 hours before surgery or 12 to 24 hours after surgery

One half dose 4 to 6 hours after surgery; usual dose the next day

**Elective knee replacement**

Duration: 10 days

Usual dose: 12 hours before surgery or 12 to 24 hours after surgery

One half dose 4 to 6 hours after surgery; usual dose the next day

**Hip fracture surgery**

Duration: 28 to 35 days

Usual dose: 12 hours before surgery or 12 to 24 hours after surgery

One half dose 4 to 6 hours after surgery; usual dose the next day

ACCP = American College of Chest Physicians, LMWH = low molecular weight heparin setting or using Doppler screening for DVT in asymptomatic patients at the time of hospital discharge. The American Academy of Orthopaedic Surgeons is preparing to issue its own guidelines for appropriate VTED prophylaxis related to THA and TKA. These guidelines are likely to include a strong caution with respect to anticoagulant-associated bleeding and will recommend a considered balance between the opposing issues of fatal PE and bleeding. Never before have medical and social forces been so focused on the issue of VTED, and never before has it been so critical for the orthopaedic practitioner to have an appreciation of what is considered appropriate management of this often silent but occasionally fatal disease.

## Thrombogenic Events and Effects of Regional Anesthesia

### Intraoperative Thrombogenesis

Thrombi initially form intraoperatively during THA. There is minimal activation of thrombogenesis during initial surgical exposure, preparation of the acetabulum, or impaction of the cup.[20] However, with reaming of the femur and insertion of the cemented femoral component, significant activation of thrombogenesis is noted and is most prominent when cemented rather than noncemented femoral components are inserted. Kinking and obstruction of the femoral vessels occurs during insertion of the femoral component and provides the setting for the initiation of femoral venous thrombosis. Efforts to reduce the degree or duration of femoral venous occlusion (such as quick surgery, intermittent relocation of the hip to unkink the vessels, or intraoperative use of pneumatic compression devices) may modify the risk of DVT formation.[15]

Thrombi form primarily in the femoral vein but may also form in calf or pelvic vessels following THA. Isolated femoral DVT is caused by intraoperative factors. DVT also form in the iliac vessels, which are assessed by MRI.[26] The rate of DVT may be reduced by pneumatic compression devices but not with intraoperative heparin, suggesting that thrombi also form in the postoperative period.

Thrombosis also begins intraoperatively during TKA. This process occurs during both general and epidural anesthesia and with or without the use of a tourniquet.[27,28] Evidence for intraoperative genesis of DVT has been collected using markers of thrombosis, transesophageal echocardiography, and aspirating thrombi from femoral vessels following tourniquet deflation.[29] In 70% of patients in whom DVT develops, there is venographic evidence of DVT by 24 hours following surgery.[30]

These data suggest that interventions to reduce the risk of DVT should begin during surgery if possible. Modalities such as intraoperative heparin, pneumatic compression boots placed during or immediately following surgery, and initiation of LMWH shortly after surgery is recommended. However, initiating anticoagulation too soon after surgery may increase the risk of perioperative bleeding.

### Postoperative Thrombogenesis

Following surgery, the risk of thrombogenesis persists for several weeks, and readmission for thromboembolic events typically occurs as late as 3 months after surgery. There is an ongoing process of clot formation and clot lysis (caused by fibrinolysis). For this reason, administration of anticoagulants for 4 to 6 weeks following surgery is reasonable and generally recommended. The choice of anticoagulation may depend on the modulation of intraoperative risk and the patient profile.

### Effects of Anesthesia

Randomized trials have shown that regional anesthesia (spinal or epidural) reduces the risk of DVT (proximal and distal) and PE following hip surgery by 40% to 50%.[31] The mechanism is unknown but may be secondary to reduced intraoperative blood loss, increased fibrinolysis, or enhanced lower extremity blood flow with regional anesthesia.[32] In patients receiving LMWH, regional anesthesia reduces the risk of DVT compared with general anesthesia.[33] However, in a trial of fondaparinux in which DVT rates were approximately 7%, there was no demonstrable difference between regional and general anesthesia.[34]

Following TKA, epidural anesthesia reduces the risk of calf DVT by approximately 20%, and the rate of proximal DVT is reduced by 50% or more.[35] Intraoperative thrombogenesis and fibrinolysis are not affected by anesthesia; this finding suggests that the mechanism of action whereby regional anesthesia reduces rates of DVT is probably caused by enhanced blood flow immediately following surgery.[27] By combining epidural anesthesia and pneumatic compression, low rates of DVT can be achieved with minimal risk of bleeding.[36]

### Blood Flow

Maintenance of lower extremity blood flow is critical to avoid venous stasis. Lower extremity blood flow is diminished following general anesthesia, whereas it is maintained with epidural anesthesia.[37] The technique of hypotensive epidural anesthesia increases lower extremity blood flow more than epidural anesthesia alone.[38] Enhanced blood flow in the immediate postoperative period with epidural anesthesia may be important as a bridging technique before pneumatic compression devices are instituted.

### Anesthesia and Multimodal Thromboprophylaxis

By combining regional anesthesia with other modalities (so-called multimodal or stacked therapy), further reduction in the risk of DVT can be achieved. For example, intraoperative heparin reduces DVT following THA, and pneumatic compression reduces the risk of DVT following TKA in patients receiving epidural anesthesia.[36,39]

In an attempt to assess the ultimate effectiveness of multimodal thromboprophylaxis, an extensive review of the literature from 1998 to 2006 that included 6-week or 3-month follow-up for all-cause mortality was performed. Multimodal prophylaxis was defined as a protocol using regional anesthesia (epidural or spinal) with or without intraoperative heparin during surgery; and pneumatic compression and aspirin after surgery. This protocol was compared with studies using warfarin or more recently introduced anticoagulants such as LMWH, ximelagatran, or fondaparinux. Only studies published in the years from 1998 to 2006 were included to restrict this review to current clinical practice protocols. Both randomized trials and consecutive cohorts were included in the review if 6-week or 3-month mortality rates were provided. Twenty publications were identified: 10 using LMWH, ximelagatran, or fondaparinux (group A; 12,291 patients); 6 studies with a protocol using regional anes-

thesia (epidural or spinal), with or without intraoperative heparin, pneumatic compression, and aspirin (group B; 7,193 patients); and 4 using warfarin (group C; 4,370 patients). The rate of clinical nonfatal PE was significantly higher in group A than in group B (0.65% versus 0.35%; $P = 0.008$). Overall mortality was significantly higher in group A than in group B (0.47% versus 0.19%; $P = 0.003$). Nonfatal PE and mortality rates for group C were 0.5% and 0.41%, respectively.

These data suggest that multimodal thromboprophylaxis is an effective strategy to reduce clinical events and can be safely used in lieu of more potent anticoagulants that expose patients to the risk of bleeding. It is not clear from this review whether using more potent anticoagulants confers any benefit in overall mortality following total joint arthroplasty.

### Anticoagulants and Regional Anesthesia

Following the introduction of LMWH, instances of epidural hematoma causing paraplegia were reported in patients receiving epidural/spinal anesthesia.[40] The resulting recommendation from the American Society of Regional Anesthesia warned against using regional anesthesia in patients who had received LMWH, removing epidural catheters in patients receiving LMWH, and catheter removal in patients with a prolonged INR from warfarin. The warning concerning the use of regional anesthesia has an objective basis, but the other two warnings are more debatable and have witnessed considerable variability in perioperative management.

Elderly patients often have unrecognized renal dysfunction; 40% of LMWH is cleared by the kidney.

Epidural hematomas developed most often in elderly women—the group most at risk for subclinical unrecognized renal dysfunction. For these patients, the dose of LMWH should be reduced to minimize the risk of bleeding.

### A Place for Warfarin Prophylaxis?

Over the past three decades, interrupted only by a transient surge in the popularity of fractionated heparins, warfarin has enjoyed increasing favor and is arguably the most commonly used single agent in North America for prophylaxis of VTED following total joint arthroplasty. Current warfarin prophylaxis following THA has resulted in venographically documented DVT in 9% to 26% of patients, with proximal thrombosis rates of approximately 2% to 5%.[19,41-44] Comparable rates after knee replacement with warfarin prophylaxis reveal a persistent overall prevalence of DVT of 35% to 55%, with proximal thrombosis rates of 2% to 14%. Warfarin has shown a peculiar propensity for reducing proximal DVT compared with distal calf thrombosis after THA; this situation is well illustrated by several studies comparing warfarin with pneumatic compression devices.[8,36,45] In at least three studies specifically concerned with THA, the overall rate of DVT was not significantly different between patients treated with pneumatic compression sleeves and those treated with warfarin. There was a complementary decrease in distal DVT and a worrisome increase in proximal DVT with pneumatic sleeves compared with warfarin, suggesting relative inefficacy of thigh-high pneumatic compression sleeves when used alone to prevent proximal thrombosis after THA.[19,42,46-48]

Consistent with most reports on the effects of regional anesthesia on the prevalence of DVT,[49-52] recent evidence suggests that 48 hours of continuous epidural anesthesia or analgesia along with warfarin is associated with a 50% reduction in DVT compared with warfarin in combination with general anesthesia.[41] In 322 consecutive patients undergoing THA, warfarin was used to prolong the INR to 2.0 to 2.5, and an epidural catheter was placed preoperatively and maintained for 36 to 48 hours.[41] The overall prevalence of venographic DVT was 8.9% (23 of 258 thrombi), with 17 calf (6.6%) and 6 proximal (2.3%) thrombi; all proximal thrombi were contiguous popliteal extensions of thrombosis in the calf, and there were no segmental femoral vein thrombi. There were no wound hematomas requiring revision or other morbid bleeding events. Accordingly, the prevalence of DVT with combined warfarin and epidural anesthesia compared favorably with published results with any pharmacologic regimen, including fractionated heparin, without the associated bleeding complications.

Early warfarin studies reported bleeding rates of 8% to 12%, with occasional life-threatening events.[53] More recent recommendations favoring reduced-intensity anticoagulation with a prothrombin time ratio of 1.3 to 1.5 times controls, or an INR of 2.0 to 2.5, are predicated on a lower rate of bleeding in the postoperative period with warfarin.[54-56] Contemporary bleeding rates with reduced intensity warfarin anticoagulation range from 1.2% to 3.7%.[17,19,57,58] Nonwound-related bleeding complications in orthopaedic patients on anticoagulant therapy have predominantly in-volved the gastrointestinal and genitourinary tracts. Similarly, medical patients newly started on outpatient warfarin have experienced a major bleeding rate of 3% in the first month following discharge, with an incremental rate of 0.8% per month for each subsequent month on anticoagulant therapy.[59-61] In a meta-analysis of methods used for the prevention of DVT after hip replacement, Imperiale and Speroff[62] identified a sixfold greater risk of "clinically important" bleeding associated with LMWH than with controls and a 50% greater risk than with warfarin.

In a prospective controlled trial with dalteparin versus warfarin in 580 patients undergoing THA, overall rates of major bleeding events were not significantly different between the groups (2.2% with dalteparin versus 1.4% with warfarin; $P$ = not significant). More patients treated with dalteparin required red cell transfusion (48% versus 31%; $P$ = 0.001), and bleeding complications on the surgical side were four times more frequent in the dalteparin group (4.4% versus 1%; $P$ = 0.03).[43] One patient treated with dalteparin experienced transient thrombocytopenia and required revision surgery for evacuation of a draining hematoma. Colwell and associates[63] compared clinically evident VTED after THA between groups receiving either adjusted dose warfarin (1,494 patients) or 30 mg enoxaparin prophylaxis every 12 hours (1,517 patients). Pharmacologic prophylaxis was administered for an average of 6.5 days in each group, and venous thromboembolism events were monitored for 3 months following hospital discharge. At final follow-up, confirmed venous thromboembolism was noted in 3.6% of patients taking enoxaparin and 3.8% of those taking warfarin. Thromboembolic events were more common in the hospital in the warfarin group (1.1%) than in the enoxaparin group (0.3%), and more frequent following hospital discharge in the enoxaparin group (3.3%) than in the group taking warfarin (2.7%). Clinically important bleeding occurred in 20 patients (1.3%) treated with enoxaparin and 8 patients (0.5%) treated with warfarin. Analysis of adverse bleeding events showed that 78% of enoxaparin patients with a notable bleed had either received the initial enoxaparin dose within 12 hours of surgery or had the drug administered twice daily rather than on a once daily schedule. It has become increasingly evident that bleeding complications (especially those related to the surgical wound) associated with the use of fractionated heparin at a dose sufficient to significantly reduce the prevalence of DVT occur at rates considerably greater than those observed with low-dose warfarin regimens.

More recently, the issues of duration of prophylaxis after hospital discharge and routine surveillance screening for DVT have come to prominence. An accurate knowledge of the presence or absence of DVT at the time of hospital discharge can more specifically direct outpatient prophylaxis and limit extended anticoagulant exposure to only those patients with known DVT. A prospective longitudinal outcome study of 3,293 patients followed for 6 months after discharge following THA or TKA was conducted from 1984 to 2003.[64,65] Contrast venography was used for routine surveillance before hospital discharge, and all patients with negative venograms were discharged without any further prophylaxis. Patients with documented venous thromboembolism were treated with low-intensity warfarin (INR 2.0). Calf clots were treated for 6 weeks, thigh clots for 12 weeks, and PE for 3 months. For the first decade of the study, patients not completing venography were discharged without any further anticoagulant prophylaxis. Because of observed readmissions for embolic events in this group, during the second decade of the study all patients who failed to complete venography at discharge were presumed to have an undiagnosed calf thrombosis and received low-intensity warfarin for 6 weeks after discharge. Readmissions for venous thromboembolism, DVT, PE, or bleeding complications were audited at 6 months after surgery by either direct patient contact or communication with the primary care physician. Of 1,842 venograms, the prevalence of DVT was 17% (175 of 1,032) after THA and 42.3% (343 of 810) after TKA. Overall readmission for venous thromboembolism occurred after 1.6% of THAs (32 of 1,972; 14 PEs and 18 DVTs)[64] compared with 0.6% of TKAs (8 of 1,321; 3 PEs and 5 DVTs; $P = 0.009$).[65] Readmission occurred after 2.2% of THAs with negative venography (19 of 880) and no further anticoagulation, compared with 0.28% of THA patients (1 of 360; $P = 0.013$) treated with outpatient warfarin therapy.[64] Six weeks of warfarin therapy eliminated PE (0 of 844 versus 17 of 2,449; $P = 0.01$) and significantly reduced venous thromboembolism-related readmission in the combined THA and TKA populations (2 of 844 = 0.2% versus 38 of 2,449 = 1.6%; $P = 0.0015$). Three bleeding events (3 of 3,292 = 0.1%) resulted in one death (intracranial bleed in one patient treated with warfarin) and

two revisions (hematoma in two patients treated with fractionated heparin). Routine surveillance, even with contrast venography, was a poor predictor of the need for continued anticoagulant prophylaxis after discharge. Extended warfarin therapy as a method of secondary prophylaxis eliminated PE-related deaths and reduced venous thromboembolism-related readmission following THA or TKA.

Low-intensity warfarin is a time-honored method of prophylaxis with contemporary bleeding rates of less than 1% and a residual overall DVT frequency of less than 10% in conjunction with sustained epidural anesthesia.[66] Optimal use of warfarin should begin the evening before surgery in view of its 24- to 48-hour latency to onset of anticoagulant effect; the combination of preoperative warfarin and epidural anesthesia is safe to use in standard practice. Warfarin prophylaxis is used for 6 weeks following THA and TKA without routine screening. It is believed that warfarin combines the best profile of safety and demonstrated efficacy for prophylaxis of clinical thromboembolic events after THA and TKA. Warfarin is highly effective in preventing venous thromboembolism-related morbidity and mortality as judged by late readmission and death, even in patients on primary warfarin prophylaxis in whom thrombi form.

## A Role for Aspirin?

Although aspirin is widely used as an antiplatelet agent to prevent arterial tree embolic events, there is a paucity of quality data concerning its efficacy in preventing DVT. In 1986 the National Institutes of Health Consensus Conference declared aspirin to be ineffective in preventing

DVT after total joint arthroplasty.[7] Only when used in conjunction with hypotensive epidural anesthesia, intraoperative heparin, and pneumatic compression devices has aspirin demonstrated any efficacy in the reduction of DVT after THA; in these instances it was unclear whether aspirin was actually the effective agent.[32,67] However, because bleeding events become more apparent with the use of fractionated heparin, aspirin had a resurgence in popularity as a prophylactic agent during the 1990s. This resurgence in popularity did not result from any demonstrated efficacy in preventing DVT but was the result of aspirin's better safety profile regarding the avoidance of bleeding compared with newer agents.

Two studies are frequently cited in an attempt to lend credence to the use of aspirin as a prophylactic agent. The Antiplatelet Trialists' Collaboration[68] assessed the efficacy of aspirin among other antiplatelet drugs in preventing DVT in 8,400 general surgical and orthopaedic patients included in 53 published studies. In this overall group, DVT was reduced from 34.8% to 26% ($P < 0.00001$), and PE was reduced from 2.7% to 1.0% ($P < 0.00001$). If specific orthopaedic trials are considered using aspirin with a venogram end point, then only one TKA study of 24 patients and one THA study of 60 patients provide sufficient data to allow any meaningful conclusions in the orthopaedic population. The Pulmonary Embolism Prevention Trial evaluated the use of 160 mg of aspirin compared with placebo in the prevention of clinical morbidity and mortality from DVT and PE for 35 days after surgery in 13,356 hip fracture and 4,088 elective arthroplasty patients.[69] Overall thromboembolic events (DVT and PE) were reduced in these 17,444 patients from 2.3% to 1.6% with the use of aspirin ($P = 0.0003$). The use of concomitant anticoagulants, such as fractionated heparin, did not preclude entry into the study and there was no stratification by type of anesthetic used during surgery. Accordingly, 44% of hip fracture patients received either fractionated (26%) or unfractionated (18%) heparin in addition to aspirin prophylaxis and one third of patients had a regional anesthetic. In the hip fracture group, DVT was reduced from 1.5% to 1.0% ($P = 0.03$), and clinical PE was reduced from 1.2% to 0.7% ($P = 0.002$) in patients receiving aspirin. In the elective arthroplasty group (2,648 THAs and 1,440 TKAs; not segregated), 37% of patients received either fractionated (35%) or unfractionated (2%) heparin in addition to aspirin. No significant differences were observed in this cohort. DVT was evident in 0.7% of patients in the aspirin groups and 0.9% in the placebo groups and PE occurred in 0.4% of patients in both groups. Revision surgery for evacuation of a hematoma was necessary in 0.8% and 0.4% in the aspirin and placebo groups, respectively ($P = 0.1$). These two studies provide little evidence for using aspirin as thromboembolism prophylaxis after total joint arthroplasty.

More recently, with an emphasis on clinical thromboembolic events, one THA and one TKA study using aspirin have provided more information on this controversial subject.[70,71] In 1,947 patients undergoing THA with a multimodal approach (hypotensive epidural anesthesia, intraoperative unfractionated heparin during femoral canal preparation, and pneumatic compression) to prophylaxis for venous throm-

boembolism, 82% of patients received aspirin (325 mg twice a day), and 18% received warfarin (INR 2.0) for 6 weeks after surgery based on stratified VTED risks.[70] Patients who were determined to be at greater risk for DVT and/or PE were given warfarin rather than aspirin following surgery. At 3-month follow-up, no fatal PEs were reported, and there was a 3.2% readmission rate for nonfatal PE (0.6%) and proximal DVT (2.6%). Meaningful bleeding occurred in four patients (0.2%), including three wound hematomas and one patient with hematuria. Similarly, in a study of 3,473 consecutive patients undergoing TKA, 95% were treated with a regional anesthetic, and all but 71 patients received aspirin (325 mg twice a day for 6 weeks) as VTED prophylaxis.[71] Those patients not receiving aspirin were deemed to be at increased risk and received warfarin for venous thromboembolic prophylaxis. At only 6-week follow-up, fatal PE approximated 0.1% and readmission for nonfatal PE or proximal DVT occurred in 0.5% of patients; 8 patients (0.5%) required aspiration of the knee for a postoperative hematoma. Although both of these studies stratified the risk of venous thromboembolism using warfarin prophylaxis for high-risk patients and are, therefore, not true tests of the prophylactic efficacy of aspirin, they do suggest some role for aspirin in conjunction with regional anesthesia in preventing clinical thromboembolic events for most patients undergoing THA and TKA.

## Newer Pharmacologic Prophylaxis

LMWHs have been in use for a few years. Fondaparinux, a synthetic pentasaccharide, has been recently

approved by the Food and Drug Administration. Various oral thrombin inhibitors are currently in phase II and III clinical trials. One of those oral thrombin inhibitors, ximelagatran, is presented as a prototype for this new class of drugs. Some of these drugs interact at multiple points in the coagulation cascade, but each new compound is primarily targeted to affect a specific step (Figure 1).

### Low-Molecular-Weight Heparin
#### Pharmacology

Two observations prompted the development of LMWH. In animal models, LMWH produced less bleeding than unfractionated (standard) heparin for the same antithrombotic effect, and LMWH does not prolong the partial thromboplastin time while retaining its antifactor X activity.

Heparin is a mixture of glycosaminoglycans of a molecular weight ranging from 3 kDa to 40 kDa. Commercial unfractionated heparin preparations have an average molecular weight of 12 kDa to 15 kDa. These molecules occur naturally in various mammalian tissues, including the liver, lungs, and intestines. Commercial preparations have a porcine or bovine origin. Dosages are expressed in heparin units (the quantity of heparin required to keep 1 mL of cat blood in a liquid state for 24 hours at 0°C; this quantity is equivalent to approximately 0.002 mg of pure heparin). LMWH preparations are not homogenous drugs; their average molecular weight is approximately 5,000 Da and ranges from 3 kDa to 15 kDa. There are currently many different LMWHs; they are prepared by different processes and are not pharmacologically identical. It is not known if they are clinically distinctive because no large trials have compared these

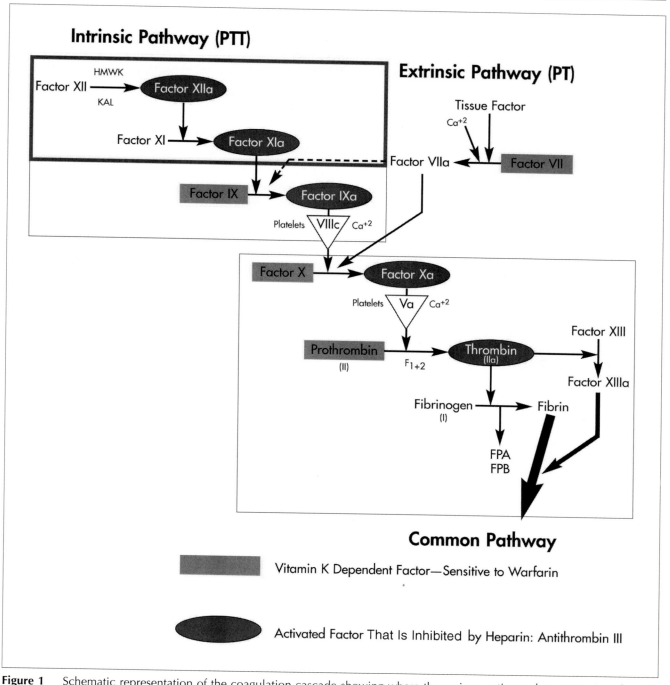

**Figure 1** Schematic representation of the coagulation cascade showing where the various anticoagulant agents act along its course. PTT = partial thromboplastin time, PT = prothrombin time, HMWK = high-molecular-weight kininogen; KAL = kallikrein, FPA = fibrinopeptide A, FPB = fibrinopeptide B. (Reproduced with permission from Stead RB: Regulation of hemostasis, in Goldhaber SZ (ed): *Pulmonary Embolism and Deep Venous Thromboembolism*. Philadelphia, PA, WB Saunders, 1985, p 32.)

drugs. The potential advantages of LMWH compared with unfractionated heparin include a more predictable and rapid dose response, a longer half-life, and a lesser hemorrhagic effect for the same antithrombotic efficacy. Important facts concerning LMWHs are summarized in Table 2.

*Clinical Studies*
In trials with unfractionated heparin in THA using venography as a diagnostic end point, LMWH has pro-

## Table 2
**Summary of Important Facts Concerning LMWH in Orthopaedic Surgery**

Preparation of heparin of animal origin

Average molecular weight: approximately 5 kDa

Peak plasma concentration: 0.5 to 1.5 hours

Bioavailability: 80% to 90% after subcutaneous injection

Renal excretion: approximately 80%

Half-life: 4 to 5 hours

Once or twice a day fixed dosage

Twice a day, may be more effective

Low potential for drug interaction

No anticoagulation monitoring

No drug level monitoring

Lower risk of heparin-induced thrombocytopenia (0.2%) than unfractionated heparin but risk not absent

Platelet monitoring recommended

Superior to unfractionated heparin in preventing thromboembolism as measured by venography in joint arthroplasty patients and patients with multiple injuries with long-bone fractures

Major bleeding rate is similar to warfarin

Overall bleeding rate may be higher than warfarin, especially in knee replacement patients

More effective than warfarin in knee replacement (based on venographic data)

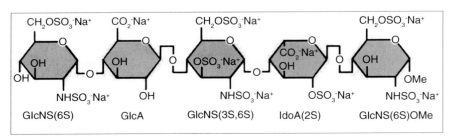

**Figure 2** Chemical structure of fondaparinux.

duced a lower venographic DVT rate, lower symptomatic PE rate, and a lower rate of major bleeding.[25] However, studies have neither demonstrated a significant advantage in favor of LMWH nor any difference in bleeding complications when compared with warfarin (INR 2.0 to 3.0) in THA patients.[72]

LMWH (enoxaparin) also has been compared with unfractionated heparin (5,000 international units subcutaneously) given twice daily in multiple-trauma patients (injury severity score > 9; likely survival > 7 days).[73] Patients with intracranial bleeding, uncontrolled hemorrhage, coagulopathy, or contrast al-

lergy were excluded from this randomized, double-blind study. Patients were stratified for the presence of lower extremity fractures. Bilateral venography was performed on 265 patients (129 treated with enoxaparin, 136 treated with heparin) on or before day 14. There were no fatal PEs in either group, and the overall DVT rate was 44% with regular heparin and 31% with LMWH ($P = 0.014$). The rates of proximal DVT were 15% for patients treated with unfractionated heparin and 6% for LMWH ($P = 0.017$), respectively. There were only six major bleeding events (1.7%). In patients who underwent knee replacement, venographic DVT rates were lower with LMWH than with warfarin, but bleeding complications were more common with LMWH.[25]

Heparin-induced thrombocytopenia is an uncommon but potentially devastating complication encountered in patients treated with heparins. The incidence of this complication is estimated to be 0.2% in patients on LMWH prophylaxis compared with 2.6% in patients on unfractionated heparin.[74] The ACCP recommends a baseline and repeat platelet count within 24 hours of starting prophylaxis.[75]

LMWHs are heparin preparations of smaller and more uniform molecular weight than standard unfractionated heparin. They have excel-

lent bioavailability of up to 90% after subcutaneous injection. Peak plasma concentration is reached within 90 minutes and the drug is excreted by the kidneys. The half-life of LMWH is 4 to 6 hours and it is given on a fixed dosage once or twice a day without monitoring. There is a low risk (0.2%) for heparin-induced thrombocytopenia. Although its efficacy as VTED prophylaxis in orthopaedic patients is undeniable, the safety of LMWH is still debated.

### Activated Factor X Inhibitors: Fondaparinux
#### Pharmacology
Fondaparinux is a completely synthetic pentasaccharide analog of the antithrombin binding site found on heparin molecules (Figure 2). It has a high affinity for antithrombin and, once bound to it, triggers a conformational change that increases affinity and reactivity of the resulting molecule with factor Xa. Once the antithrombin and factor Xa complex is formed, fondaparinux dissociates and can activate more antithrombin molecules. Fondaparinux has no effect on routine coagulation tests but may be monitored by chromogenic antifactor Xa assay. A second generation pentasaccharide, idraparinux, is in development; it is more negatively charged and has a greater affinity for antithrombin. With a half-life of 80 hours, once-a-week subcutaneous dosing is theoretically feasible.

**Table 3**
**Comparison of Important Characteristics of Fondaparinux and LMWH**

| Characteristic | Fondaparinux | LMWH |
|---|---|---|
| Target | Factor Xa | Factor Xa and thrombin |
| Route | Subcutaneous | Subcutaneous |
| Half-life | 17 hours | 4 to 6 hours |
| Endothelial cell binding | None | Some |
| Protein binding | None | Some |
| Clearance | Renal | Renal |
| Heparin-induced thrombocytopenia | Case reports? | 0.2% |
| Antidote | None | Partial-protamine sulfate |

LMWH = low-molecular-weight heparin

**Table 4**
**Comparison of Fondaparinux and Enoxaparin: Efficacy***

| Patient Population | Risk Reduction | 95% CI |
|---|---|---|
| Hip fractures | 62% | 45% to 73% |
| Hip arthroplasty: Europe | 58% | 38% to 73% |
| Hip arthroplasty: North America | 28% | 52% to 108% |
| Knee arthroplasty: North America | 63% | 45% to 76% |

*All studies, relative reductions compared to enoxaparin. Efficacy measured by venography.
CI = confidence interval

**Table 5**
**Comparison of Fondaparinux and Enoxaparin: Safety***

| | Fondaparinux | Enoxaparin | P Value |
|---|---|---|---|
| Sample size | 3,616 | 3,956 | |
| Major bleeding | 96 (2.7%) | 75 (1.9%) | NS |
| Bleeding index > 2 | 84 (2.3%) | 63 (1.6%) | < 0.05 |

*All studies compared to enoxaparin. Safety measured by bleeding. Bleeding index was higher in knee replacement patients treated with fondaparinux.
NS = not significant

**Table 6**
**ACCP Recommendations for Fondaparinux***

**Elective hip replacement**
Duration: 28 to 35 days
Dose: 2.5 mg subcutaneously daily

**Elective knee replacement**
Duration: 10 days
Dose: 2.5 mg subcutaneously daily

**Hip fracture surgery**
Duration: 28 to 35 days
Dose: 2.5 mg subcutaneously daily

*Clinical studies have found this medication especially effective in hip fracture patients. There is no definitive explanation for this observation. Bleeding complications are significantly higher if the medication is started within 8 hours after surgery.
ACCP = American College of Chest Physicians

**Table 7**
**Summary of Important Facts Concerning Fondaparinux for Orthopaedic Surgery**

Activated factor X inhibitor

Synthetic analog of the antithrombin-binding pentasaccharide found in heparin molecules

Average molecular weight: approximately 500 Da

Peak plasma concentration: 0.5 to 1.5 hours

Bioavailability: approximately 100% after subcutaneous injection

Renal excretion: approximately 100%

Renal insufficiency can be a complication

Half-life: 17 hours

Once a day fixed dosage

Low potential for drug interaction

No anticoagulation monitoring

No drug levels monitoring

No theoretic risk of heparin-induced thrombocytopenia

Platelets monitoring not recommended

Superior to enoxaparin in preventing venous thromboembolism as measured by venography in joint arthroplasty and hip fracture patients

Major bleeding rate is similar to enoxaparin

Overall bleeding rate may be higher than enoxaparin in knee replacement patients

Drug should not be started less than 8 hours after skin closure

Table 3 compares important characteristics of fondaparinux and LMWH.

### Clinical Studies
Fondaparinux has been compared to LMWH in clinical trials involving hip replacement, hip fracture, and knee replacement patients (Table 4). In all three groups, fondaparinux had a lower rate of venographic DVT when compared to enoxaparin. Bleeding parameters were not significantly different, except that the bleeding index was observed to be higher for fondaparinux in knee replacement patients[76-79] (Table 5). The 2004 ACCP recommendations for fondaparinux are described in Table 6, and the major characteristics of the drug are described in Table 7.

### Oral Thrombin Inhibitors
#### Pharmacology
Thrombin is the crucial enzyme that transforms fibrinogen into fibrin.

**Table 8**
**Summary of North American Clinical Trials Comparing Ximelagatran With Warfarin in Knee Replacement Patients**

|  | Exult A | Exult B |
|---|---|---|
| Design | Randomized double-blind | Randomized double-blind |
| Control | Warfarin (INR 2.5) evening after surgery | Warfarin (INR 2.5) evening after surgery |
| Treatment | Ximelagatran 12 hours after surgery for 7 to 12 days 24 mg orally bid 36 mg orally bid | Ximelagatran morning after surgery for 7 to 12 days 36 mg orally bid |
| Sample size | Control, n = 608 24 mg, n = 614 36 mg, n = 629 | Control, n = 1,148 36 mg, n = 1,151 |
| Total venous thromboembolism | Control 27.6% 24 mg 24.9% ($P < 0.05$) 36 mg 20.3% ($P < 0.05$) | Control 31.9% 36 mg 22.5% ($P < 0.05$) |
| Major venous thromboembolism | Control 4.1% 24 mg 2.5% NS 36 mg 2.7% NS | Control 4.1% 36 mg 3.9% NS |
| Fatal or major bleeding | Control 0.7% 24 mg 36 mg | Control 0.4% 36 mg 1.0% NS |

NS = not significant

Thrombin exerts many other effects, including a strong positive feedback on activation of factors V and VII, further platelet activation, and promotion of clot dissolution and healing. Many anticoagulant drugs targeting thrombin are currently approved for use in Europe or are in advanced stages of clinical testing in North America and Australia.

The best known and clinically tested thrombin-inhibiting drug is ximelagatran, an oral prodrug of melagatran.[80,81] Melagatran is a dipeptide originally synthesized in 1985 to specifically target thrombin. It is a parenteral agent with very low oral bioavailability. Ximelagatran is the oral form of melagatran; it is rapidly absorbed by the gastrointestinal tract and has minimal food or drug interactions. Once absorbed, it is rapidly converted to melagatran in the liver, with peak plasma concentrations reached within 1.5 to 2.5 hours after intake. Melagatran does not substantially bind to plasma proteins and is not metabolized; 80% of the drug is excreted by the kidneys within 24 hours. Half-life is a short 1.5 to 2 hours in young healthy volunteers but longer (4 to 5 hours) in the typical 70-year-old patient. There is no meaningful accumulation with repeat dosing in either age group. Severe renal impairment will prolong the plasma half-life of melagatran, but the impact of renal impairment on dosing and adverse effects have not been extensively studied.

More than 17,000 patients have received the drug in clinical studies worldwide. No interactions with concomitant medications have been reported, except for one healthy volunteer in whom concomitant administration of erythromycin increased peak melagatran plasma concentrations twofold.

### Clinical Studies

Clinical trials have been conducted in North America comparing ximel-agatran with warfarin in knee replacement patients[80,81] (Table 8). Equivalent efficacy and safety were demonstrated, and ximelagatran required no monitoring. Concerns regarding hepatotoxicity with long-term use of ximelagatran have prevented its approval in the United States.

## Mechanical Prophylaxis
### Introduction

Mechanical compression of veins has been used to prevent thrombosis since at least the early 20th century. Virchow[82] established stasis as one of the three causes of venous thromboembolism and encouraged the development of several techniques to assist the removal of blood from the deep veins of immobile patients. Early weight bearing alone can reduce the frequency of thrombosis after hip replacement.[83,84] Although the availability of LMWHs has established pharmacologic prophylaxis in a wide range of surgical and medical specialties, the different physiologic basis of the effects of mechanical methods has ensured continued growth in their use, both as sole methods of prophylaxis and in combination with anticoagulants. The variety of available mechanical systems makes it difficult to select the appropriate prophylactic system. It is essential to understand the clinical and physiologic evidence that supports these techniques and their relative efficacies to ensure optimal protection from DVT.

### Mechanical Principles and Physiologic Actions

The objective of mechanical prophylaxis is to substitute the action of the muscle pumps of the leg that are normally activated during ambulation. There are four types of mechanical prophylaxis: graduated compression stockings, intermittent pneumatic compression, electrical stimulation, and exercise devices; each type has its own principles of action.

### Graduated Compression Stockings

Graduated compression stockings apply a constant pressure to the limb, graduated from approximately 18 mm Hg at the ankle to 14 mm Hg in the upper calf; thigh-length stockings provide a pressure of 8 mm Hg at the upper thigh.[85] This broad pressure gradient encourages blood flow toward the heart. It was theorized that the graduated pressure applied to the deep veins reduced their caliber, and that the constant venous outflow increased venous velocity through the veins and reduced stasis. The evidence of early Doppler ultrasound and radioisotope techniques appeared to confirm this mechanism.[86-90] However, more recent investigation with modern Doppler ultrasound has not shown such consistent velocity increases, and it may be that a major action of stockings in preventing thromboembolism is to prevent venous distension and pooling of blood.[91-94]

### Intermittent Pneumatic Compression

Intermittent pneumatic compression involves applying cuffs to the limb that are automatically inflated and deflated by a pump. Systems for DVT prevention typically consist of bilateral thigh and calf, calf only, or foot cuffs. Thigh- and calf-length cuffs are normally inflated to approximately 40 mm Hg in cycles of approximately 12 seconds every minute, although some systems offer more rapid inflation and higher pressures. Foot compression was developed to mimic the action of the compression of the plantar venous plexus during ambulation.[95] Compression is applied rapidly to the sole of the foot for approximately 3 seconds every 20 seconds, and the pressure required to empty the plexus is higher, typically 130 mm Hg.

There are different methods of applying pneumatic compression to a limb. Pressure can be applied with an air bladder that entirely surrounds the limb circumference. These may be large boot-type cuffs that zip up the front or wrap-around garments similar to sphygmomanometer cuffs. Although these devices apply pressure evenly over the surface of the limb, the large volume of air within the bladder either leads to slow inflation rates or requires the use of powerful pumps. In DVT prophylaxis, intermittent compression would require continuous use while a patient is immobile; therefore, systems have been developed with smaller, quieter pumps that inflate rapidly enough to increase venous velocity. This rapid inflation has been achieved by devising noncircumferential or asymmetric cuff designs. Such garments have a small air bladder that is placed at the rear of the limb and nonstretchable material to cover the rest of the limb. Theoretic analysis has suggested that this pattern of compression may be more efficient at compressing veins.[96]

Compression can be applied to the entire limb simultaneously (uniform compression), or the garment can be divided into several independent air bladders to apply compression to different parts of the limb in a distal-to-proximal sequence (sequential compression). A further refinement is to apply a gradient of pressure across the bladders, in a method similar to graduated compression stockings (graded sequential compression). The most distal chamber inflates first to a lower pressure, the next to a slightly higher pressure, and so on. Although systems for edema reduction may contain 12 or more bladders, DVT-prevention garments typically use no more than 3 bladders.

Intermittent compression is known to compress deep veins completely at 40 mm Hg. This results in a pulse of venous blood that travels proximally, and can easily be detected with Doppler ultrasound at the posterior tibial (in foot compression), popliteal, and common femoral veins. A major difference with stockings is that intermittent compression is a distinctly active treatment. The pulse is typically characterized by its peak velocity or the percentage augmentation in velocity over a resting velocity, if this can be detected. The type of compression (uniform/graded sequential, foot/calf) and the inflation rate and pressure will affect the velocity profile produced and the peak velocity. At the femoral vein the maximum velocity typically will be 35 to 60 m/s, corresponding to augmentation of flow of 50% to 250% when 40 mm Hg pressure is applied.[97] The more rapid the compression and higher the pressure, the greater the peak velocity; however, this may be less well tolerated by the patient. After knee replacement surgery, there is a wide variation in peak venous velocity with different mechanical devices, with rapid asymmetric compression producing a 6.9% DVT rate compared with 15% for sequential compression.[98,99] In a comparison between the foot pump and intermittent pneumatic compression in 124 patients with major trauma, the former device seemed less effective at reducing ultrasound-demonstrated DVT (25%) than the latter (6.5%; $P = 0.009$).[100]

### Foot Pumps

Foot pumps provide intermittent compression that substitutes for the natural expulsion of blood from the plantar venous plexus in the sole of the foot when the patient cannot bear weight.[101] A bladder envelops the sole and is compressed for 1 second every 20 seconds at 130 mm Hg. The mechanism requires preload of the plantar veins, so the foot must be slightly dependent or at least straight but not elevated.[100,102]

### Electrical Stimulation

Electrical stimulation for DVT prophylaxis has been used sporadically but can be quite uncomfortable if not painful for a conscious patient.[103,104] For this reason it is mainly used intraoperatively, rather than in the recovery period when there is a substantial risk of thromboembolism. Active mechanical manipulation of the limbs by strapping the feet to electrically driven pedals also was used with some success but was not demonstrated to be more practical than other methods.[105,106] Mechanical exercise devices that encourage the activation of the muscle pumps by the user (such as treadles, air cushions, and rollers) are unrealistic for hospitalized patients but have achieved some popularity in long-distance travelers.[107] Although these devices are effective in preventing stasis if they encourage plantar flexion, which effectively empties deep veins, the necessity of conscious effort by the user renders them useless during sleep periods when travelers may be at higher risk.

In orthopaedic surgery, only stockings and intermittent pneumatic compression have become established as mechanical prophylaxis devices. Although various types of devices are used, foot intermittent compression is more popular than in other types of surgery.

### Hematologic Effects

The rationale behind mechanical prophylaxis is primarily to prevent venous stasis; therefore, devices have been validated and optimized according to their hemodynamic effects. Early in the investigation of intermittent pneumatic compression for DVT prevention, experimental data suggested that the period of vein compression may have an important role beyond the increase in blood flow seen during initial compression. Euglobulin clot lysis time was shown to increase in patients using intermittent compression, whereas reductions (fibrinolytic shutdown) were normal during and after surgery.[108] It was subsequently shown that intermittent compression of the arm reduced DVT incidence in the legs in surgical patients, clearly suggesting that the compression was producing a global increase in fibrinolytic activity.[109]

Most subsequent studies have confirmed this effect, and it is now generally accepted that intermittent compression affects blood coagulability.[110,111] There is insufficient evidence to prove which property of the therapy is producing the hematologic effect; however, a recent study has shown that rapid inflation and deflation has a lesser effect on fibrinolytic activity in healthy volunteers than a slower cycle.[112] This may support the notion that the compression of the vein itself is involved, and the duration of compression must reach a threshold for effect. The specific components of the fibrinolytic process that are affected are also unknown; however, there is some evidence of reductions in the antigen-to-tissue plasminogen activator and increases in plasminogen activator-inhibitor activity over that which would otherwise be expected.[111,113]

Whereas older research concentrated on fibrinolytic effects, there are published indications of changes in procoagulant activation with intermittent compression. Reductions in factor VIIa activity and increases in tissue factor pathway inhibitor have been noted,[114] which suggest that mechanical prophylaxis may not only help to break up nascent thrombi but may also inhibit their formation. Tentative evidence also shows increased prostaglandin and nitric oxide production with such systems, which would inhibit platelet aggregation.[115,116]

Comparatively little research into the hematologic effects of graduated compression stockings has taken place. Unpublished research by one of the authors (DJW) suggests that there may be some effects, including reduction in factor VIIa and tissue factor pathway inhibitor, but no significant change in fibrinolytic potential. Stockings with a 45° reverse Trendelenburg position have been shown to increase tissue factor pathway inhibitor, whereas another study showed no changes in factor VIII with either stockings or intermittent compression.[117,118]

### Clinical Evidence

The clinical evidence in support of mechanical prophylaxis is extensive, and there is little doubt that both stockings and intermittent compression are effective in the prevention of venous thromboembolism.

### Graduated Compression Stockings

Elastic stockings were shown to be clinically effective in preventing PE as early as 1952, but subsequent research was less supportive.[119] At that time, elastic tubular bandages and stockings were used to provide uniform pressure; however, it was soon determined that they did not provide adequate prophylaxis.[120] Subsequent use of graduated compression stockings has been more successful in general, orthopaedic, gynecologic, and other surgeries.[85] This suggests that the correct pressure profile is vital to ensure the protective effect.

Several brands of compression stockings are now available and are similar in design and pressure profile, with both calf- and thigh-length options. There is little good clinical evidence to support the use of one type over another, but many patients find thigh-length stockings difficult to wear and maintain in position. For this reason, recent reviews have tended to advocate calf-length stockings.[121-123]

Although debate will continue on the appropriate length of stocking to use, the need to determine correct fit is often neglected. Graduated compression stockings are designed to have an ideal pressure gradient; therefore, different lengths and sizes are produced for different limb geometries to ensure a close approximation to that ideal. If an incorrect size is used, there is a real possibility of the stocking either being too loose and not providing adequate compression and protection or being too tight. If a stocking is too tight at the proximal end, it can cause a reverse gradient in which pressure is highest at the proximal end; this gradient does not favor blood flow out of the limb. This circumstance has been reported to cause ischemia and is believed to have been the reason for the failure of uniform compression stockings in early clinical trials.[85,124]

Pressure interface measurement with three leading brands of thigh-length stockings in volunteers has shown that less than 30% of readings were within 20% of the ideal profile, and 70% of readings showed a reversed pressure gradient. In the sitting position, pressures of more than 28 mm Hg were measured at the popliteal fossa, whereas the ideal is 8 mm Hg.[125] Although these results would reinforce the choice of calf-length stockings, a follow-up study of calf-length stockings in orthopaedic patients showed 98% of stockings failed to be within 20% of the ideal pressure, and 54% produced a reverse gradient. The incidence of DVT in those with a reverse pressure gradient was significantly higher compared with patients using stockings without a reverse pressure gradient (25.6% versus 6.1%, respectively).[126] The potential general effectiveness of compression stockings is severely inhibited by the reverse pressure gradient and garter effects. The implication is that the regular measurement and monitoring of limb size, the correct choice of stockings, and the correct application and wearing of stockings is vital to ensure adequate prophylaxis. In a typical hospital situation, the effectiveness in thromboprophylaxis may not match that of published reports if the rigorous protocols of published studies are not fully followed.

### Intermittent Pneumatic Compression

Although intermittent pneumatic compression has been used to prevent DVT since the 1920s in Germany and the United States, the first clinical trials were performed by two groups of investigators in London in the 1970s.[127,128] As is the case with graduated compression stockings, many reports have established the effectiveness of intermittent pneumatic compression in a wide range of surgical and medical specialties.[129] Because intermittent compression systems have more designs and functions than stockings, it is more difficult to compare study results. There is a substantial amount of evidence that all the major types, including thigh-length, calf, foot, uniform and graded sequential, and circumferential and asymmetric, are effective for use in orthopaedic surgery. Each type, no matter what the compression time and pressure, is designed to compress the deep veins.

There are relatively few reports of adverse events with intermittent compression. There have been some instances of peroneal nerve palsy; therefore, most garment designs in the past two decades have ensured that the region of the popliteal fossa is not compressed.[130,131] Compartment syndrome in patients in the lithotomy position has been shown to be caused by the position rather that the intermittent compression, which may reduce intracompartmental pressure.[132] There are no substantial fitting difficulties with intermittent compression devices because the devices self-regulate pressures, and the cuffs are typically fastened with Velcro, which can be adjusted as necessary. Treatment protocol is a more important issue. For maximum effectiveness, intermittent compression should be used whenever a patient is immobile; ideally before, during, and after surgery. Once a patient can ambulate, the calf muscle pump will be far more efficient at preventing venous stasis. Although early ambulation has become more common after surgery, the restricted mobility of orthopaedic patients and their high-risk status elevate the importance of compression systems that can be used throughout the hospital stay. The orthopaedic literature shows that

**Table 9**
**Knee Replacement and Intermittent Pneumatic Compression**

| Author | Date | Number | DVT | % |
|---|---|---|---|---|
| Hull et al[136] | 1979 | 29 | 2 | 6 |
| McKenna et al[137] | 1980 | 10 | 1 | 10 |
| Lynch et al[138] | 1990 | 307 | 31 | 11 |
| Haas et al[135] | 1990 | 36 | 8 | 22 |

Combined deep venous thrombosis (DVT) rate - 11%; 95% confidence interval 8% to 14%

**Table 10**
**Hip Replacement and Intermittent Pneumatic Compression (IPC)\***

| Author | Control | Number | DVT % Control | DVT % IPC |
|---|---|---|---|---|
| Hartman et al[139] (1982) | Nil | 104 | 19 | 9 |
| Gallus et al[140] (1983) | Nil | 90 | 53 | 35 |
| Paiement et al[47] (1987) | Warfarin | 158 | 17 | 13 |
| Hull et al[8] (1990) | Nil | 310 | 49 | 24 |
| Bailey et al[141] (1991) | Warfarin | 97 | 27 | 6 |
| Kaempffe et al[142] (1991) | Warfarin | 40 | 24 | 16 |
| Francis[42] (1992) | Warfarin | 201 | 31 | 27 |

\*All studies show significant risk reduction. DVT = deep venous thrombosis

intermittent pneumatic compression does significantly reduce DVT after THA and TKA[8,42,47,133-142] (Tables 9 and 10).

## Foot Pumps

A preference for foot compression in orthopaedic surgery has developed since its introduction in the late 1980s.[101] Foot pumps are perceived as being less obtrusive during surgery, particularly TKA. If feasible, calf compression may be considered because the lower pressure may yield better patient compliance, and the garments may be detached from the pumps during periods of mobility without their complete removal. Foot pumps are fairly effective after TKA and quite possibly equivalent to LMWH after THA[143-153] (Tables 11 and 12).

## Published Meta-Analyses

Meta-analyses of the effectiveness of mechanical compression in DVT prevention have been published for specific surgical modalities, with a few for general use. Cochrane reviews are available for the general use of graduated compression stockings, general prophylaxis in hip fracture and colorectal surgery, and physical methods in stroke.[154-157] Nine randomized controlled trials of groups treated with stockings only compared with control groups showed a 13% incidence of DVT in the stocking group compared with 27% for controls.[154] The rate of DVT in the control group (composed of patients primarily from general surgery) was low compared with that expected for orthopaedic surgery patients. In a review of other types of prophylaxis, seven trials yielded a DVT rate of only 2% compared with 15% for controls, clearly indicating that using stockings as the sole method of prophylaxis can produce suboptimal results. An earlier review of 15 trials

broadly concurred with these findings and concluded that stockings reduce the incidence of DVT by 64% in general surgical patients and 57% in THA patients compared with controls.[158]

Vanek[129] conducted a systematic review comparing intermittent compression with other modalities and showed that intermittent compression reduced the relative risk of DVT by 62% compared with placebo, 47% compared with stockings, and 48% compared with minidose heparin. At the time of Vanek's review, there were insufficient studies comparing intermittent compression with LMWH. The analysis comprised direct comparisons between methods, rather than compiling separate incidences for each method, because differences (such as protocol, type of surgery, and patient groups) can affect comparisons across studies. This is probably why the risk reduction compared with placebo is similar to that for stockings in the previous analysis, while also showing intermittent compression to be more effective than stockings. In major orthopaedic surgery the relative risk reduction was found to be 69% relative to placebo and 29% compared with warfarin.

The most recent meta-analysis through the United Kingdom National Health Service Health Technology Assessment process[159] reviewed 17 graduated compression stocking trials, 22 intermittent pneumatic compresssion trials, and 3 foot pump trials. Of these, 14 trials were in hip and knee surgery. The review reported a 72% odds reduction for mechanical methods when used alone.

Meta-analyses specific to orthopaedic surgery have compared intermittent compression with pharmacological prophylaxis. In THA,

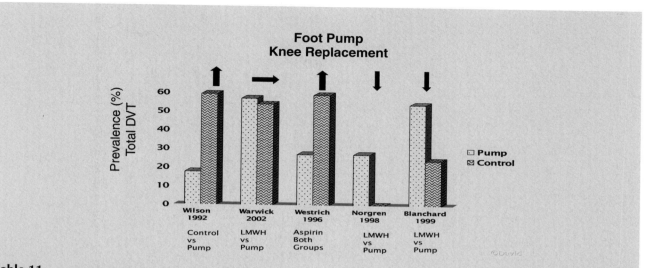

### Table 11
### Compression as a Prophylaxis After Knee Replacement

| Author | Center | Control | Control (n) | DVT % (Total/Proximal) | Foot Pump (n) | DVT % (Total/Proximal) |
|---|---|---|---|---|---|---|
| Wilson et al[143] | London | Nil | 32 | 69/19 | 28 | 50/0 |
| Warwick et al[144] | Bristol | Nil | 89 | 54/0 | 99 | 57/4 |
| Westrich et al[145] | New York | Nil | 83 | 59/14 | 81 | 27/0 |
| Norgren et al[146] | Lund | LMWH | 15 | 0/0 | 15 | 27/0 |
| Blanchard et al[147] | Lausanne | LMWH | 60 | 27/3 | 48 | 65/6 |

DVT = deep venous thrombosis, LMWH = low-molecular-weight heparin

Freedman and associates[72] showed that intermittent compression produced a DVT incidence comparable with that of LMWH (21% and 18%, respectively overall, placebo 49%). In TKA patients, Westrich and associates[160] found intermittent compression and LMWH to be comparable (17% and 29%, respectively) and significantly better than warfarin or aspirin. Other orthopaedic meta-analyses have reached similar conclusions, including one in which stockings and intermittent compression were included together.[62,161] In hip fracture patients, the Cochrane review also showed the effectiveness of intermittent compression while commenting on the paucity of good quality trials.

### Consensus Recommendations
Both the ACCP and the Institute of Clinical Systems Improvement (ICSI) have published consensus recommendations regarding DVT prevention. The ACCP guidelines are in regard to specific surgical specialties,[25] and the ICSI guidelines are more general.[162] Both groups place most types of orthopaedic surgery in their highest risk categories.

For elective THA, the ACCP recommends the administration of LMWH, fondaparinux, or adjusted-dose warfarin. Intermittent pneumatic compression or graduated compression stockings are recommended only as an adjuvant. For TKA, recommendations are similar, noting that intermittent compression can be used as an alternative to anticoagulants in patients in whom the latter are contraindicated. In patients with hip fracture, mechanical methods are suggested if anticoagulants are contraindicated; however, in TKA patients, only early mobilization is recommended.

In the ICSI very high risk category, mechanical methods are recommended in combination with LMWH or adjusted-dose warfarin. ICSI also recommends elastic stockings for all patients and intermittent pneumatic compression for immobile patients.

The International Consensus Statement[163] recommends intermittent pneumatic compression or foot pumps as an alternative to chemical methods for those hip surgery patients in whom bleeding is a concern. These methods are to be used as long as tolerated and should then be replaced with prolonged LMWH or pentasaccharide therapy. After knee replacement, intermittent pneumatic compression or foot

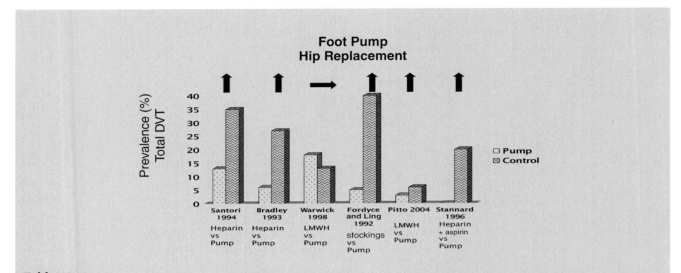

Table 12
**Foot Pump Compression as a Prophylaxis After Hip Replacement**

| Author | Test | Control Type | N | DVT % (Total/Proximal) | Foot Pump (N) | DVT % (Total/Proximal) |
|---|---|---|---|---|---|---|
| Santori et al[148] | US | Heparin | 65 | 35/20 | 67 | 13/3 |
| Bradley et al[149] | VG | Heparin | 44 | 27/25 | 30 | 7/7 |
| Warwick et al[150] | VG | LMWH | 138 | /17 | 136 | /9 |
| Fordyce and Ling[151] | VG | Stockings | 40 | 40/32 | 39 | 5/2 |
| Pitto et al[152] | US | LMWH | 100 | 6/2 | 100 | 3/3 |
| Stannard et al[153] | US | Heparin + aspirin | 25 | 20 | 25 | 0/0 |

DVT = deep venous thrombosis, VG = venography, US = ultrasound, LMWH = low-molecular-weight heparin

pumps are considered an alternative to chemical methods, but more studies are recommended.

## Combinations of Mechanical Methods
Because graduated compression stockings and intermittent pneumatic compression act on the limbs in different ways, the combined use of the two methods has been suggested for optimal DVT prevention; however, clinical evidence is weak. One report has shown that bilateral use of intermittent compression with unilateral application of a stocking in surgical patients results in a significantly greater incidence of DVT in the limb without the stocking.[164] A previous study in patients undergoing abdominal surgery had shown no additional benefits with stocking use.[165] Thigh-length stockings have made no hemodynamic difference to thigh-length intermittent compression. By reducing the capacity of veins to store blood, stockings have reduced the peak velocities produced by intermittent compression of the feet.[91,166] The simultaneous use of stockings and foot pumps probably reduces efficacy by reducing the preload required for effective expulsion of blood.[166] Similarly, the addition of graduated stockings to intermittent pneumatic compression does not improve peak venous velocity.[167]

## Combination With Anticoagulants
Meta-analysis of graduated compression stockings has shown that their use with other prophylactic techniques, principally anticoagulants, is more effective than stockings alone; therefore, combined use is recommended.[154] Anticoagulants are commonly used with intermittent compression, but the substantial research data are sparse. One meta-analysis[159] reviewed 12 studies (6 orthopaedic) with combined chemical and mechanical methods (8 graduated compression stocking, 3 intermittent pneumatic compression, 1 foot pump). The study demonstrated a 53% further reduction when mechanical methods were used as an adjunct to chemical methods. Aspirin in THA has been shown to be more effective when combined with compression of the

feet (27% DVT combined; 59% DVT aspirin alone), although the aspirin itself appeared to have little effect.[145] Silbersack and associates[168] in a randomized trial of 131 arthroplasty patients found a 40% DVT rate (determined by ultrasound) in TKA patients and 14% in THA patients with combined LMWH and graduated compression stocking prophylaxis compared with 0% for both groups with combined LMWH and intermittent pneumatic compression; however, there was 25% noncompliance. In a study by Fuchs and associates[169] of 227 trauma patients, a DVT rate of 25% was reported in patients treated with LMWH compared with 3.5% in those treated with both LMWH and a passive motion device. Bradley and associates[149] showed that the addition of a foot pump to LMWH reduced the venographic DVT rate from 27% to 6%. There appears to be an advantage to combining mechanical and chemical methods, but further work is needed to establish the safest and most effective combination.

### Drawbacks of Mechanical Methods

The primary drawback of mechanical methods is compliance. Graduated compression stockings can be uncomfortable, particularly if they are too tight proximally or roll down. Intermittent pneumatic compression bladders enclose the leg, and some types may cause feelings of claustrophobia and may be uncomfortably hot. Foot pumps are less enclosing but apply higher pressures with rapid inflation. The noise of the mechanical compressor can be irritating to the patient and to other patients in close proximity. Foot cuffs need to be removed for ambulation, and others disconnected from pumps, involving extra work for the therapist or nurse.

The patient may risk a hip dislocation following arthroplasty if the leg is flexed to remove the device or stockings. These devices can be relatively expensive considering the cost of the disposable sleeves and, in some instances, the capital cost of a pump.

### Future Directions

Mechanical prophylaxis is now well enough established in orthopaedic surgery such that the research focus has shifted from proving efficacy to improving prophylaxis. For both graduated compression stockings and intermittent pneumatic compression, there is great potential for better tailoring of the pressure, pressure profile, and compression sequence to individual physiology. Clinical proof of the better efficacy of one system over another can be difficult when resulting DVT rates are low. Thousands of patients may need to be recruited to studies to achieve statistical significance; low statistical power is a weakness of many published trials. Research using computer modeling of tissue deformation and fluid flow may provide a more viable method of optimizing the design of mechanical devices.

The efficient and effective overlap of mechanical methods with chemical methods needs further research. The most suitable protocol may involve mechanical methods during and immediately after surgery to avoid surgical and neuraxial bleeding, followed by additional chemical methods for a period to provide maximum efficacy, followed by an extended period of oral chemical prophylaxis to provide protection against thrombosis after hospital discharge. This strategy has already been described in the trauma setting with encouraging results.[170]

### Summary

Venous thromboembolism remains a life-threatening condition for patients undergoing lower extremity arthroplasty and continues to demand the attention of the orthopaedic surgeon. Regional anesthesia, expeditious surgery, and accelerated rehabilitation seem to have lessened the risk of fatal PE, but prophylaxis for all patients, extended for a period of weeks after surgery is appropriate. Increasing regulatory intervention requires the continued vigilance of the orthopaedic surgeon to maintain current practices in keeping with approved guidelines.

### References

1. Johnson R, Carmichael JH, Almond HGA, Loynes RP: Deep venous thrombosis following Charnley arthroplasty. *Clin Orthop Relat Res* 1978; 132:24-30.

2. Johnson R, Green JR, Charnley J: Pulmonary embolism and its prophylaxis following the Charnley total hip replacement. *Clin Orthop Relat Res* 1977;127:123-132.

3. Charnley J: *Low Friction Arthroplasty of the Hip: Theory and Practice.* Berlin, Germany, Springer-Verlag, 1979.

4. Coventry MB, Beckenbaugh RD, Nolan DR, Ilstrup DM: 2,012 total hip arthroplasties: A study of postoperative course and early complications. *J Bone Joint Surg Am* 1974;56: 273-284.

5. Insall JN: *Surgery of the Knee.* New York, NY, Churchill Livingstone, 1984, pp 646-647.

6. Stulberg BN, Insall JN, Williams GW, Ghelman B: Deep-vein thrombosis following total knee replacement: An analysis of six hundred and thirty-eight arthroplasties. *J Bone Joint Surg Am* 1984;66:194-201.

7. Prevention of venous thrombosis and pulmonary embolism: NIH Consensus Development. *JAMA* 1986;256: 744-749.

8. Hull RD, Raskob GE, Gent M, et al: Effectiveness of intermittent pneumatic leg compression for preventing deep vein thrombosis after total hip replacement. *JAMA* 1990;263:2313-2317.

9. Seagroatt V, Tan HS, Goldacre M, Bulstrode C, Nugent I, Gill L: Elective total hip replacement prevalence, emergency readmission rate, and post-operative mortality. *BMJ* 1991;303:1431-1435.

10. Sharrock NE, Cazan MG, Hargett MJL, Williams-Russo P, Wilson PD Jr: Changes in mortality after total hip and knee arthroplasty over a ten-year period. *Anesth Analg* 1995;80:242-248.

11. Pellegrini VD Jr: Prevention of thromboembolic disease in patients after total joint arthroplasty by selective posthospitalization treatment, in Fitzgerald RH (ed): *Seminars in Arthroplasty*, Philadelphia, PA, WB Saunders, 1997, pp 248-257.

12. Pellegrini VD Jr, Clement D, Lush-Ehmann C, et al: The natural history of thromboembolic disease after total joint arthroplasty: The case for routine surveillance as a contemporary management strategy. *Orthop Trans* 1994;18.

13. Hull RD, Raskob GE: Current concepts review: Prophylaxis of venous thromboembolic disease following hip and knee operation. *J Bone Joint Surg Am* 1986;68:146-150.

14. Lotke PA, Palevsky H, Keenan HM, et al: Equivalence of aspirin and warfarin as prophylaxis for thromboembolic disease after total joint arthroplasty. *Clin Orthop Relat Res* 1996;324:251-258.

15. Salvati EA, Pellegrini VD, Sharrock NE, et al: Recent advances in venous thromboembolic prophylaxis during and after total hip replacement. *J Bone Joint Surg Am* 2000;82:252-270.

16. Warwick D, Williams MH, Bannister GC: Death and thromboembolic disease after total hip replacement: A series of 1162 cases with no routine chemical prophylaxis. *J Bone Joint Surg Br* 1995;77:6-10.

17. Amstutz HC, Friscia DA, Dorey F, Carney B: Warfarin prophylaxis to prevent mortality from pulmonary embolism after total hip replacement. *J Bone Joint Surg Am* 1989;71:321-326.

18. Lieberman JR, Wollaeger J, Dorey F, et al: The efficacy of prophylaxis with low-dose warfarin for prevention of pulmonary embolism following total hip arthroplasty. *J Bone Joint Surg Am* 1997;79:319-325.

19. Pellegrini VD Jr, Clement D, Lush-Ehmann C, Keller GS, Evarts CM: The natural history of thromboembolic disease following hospital discharge after total hip arthroplasty. *Clin Orthop Relat Res* 1996;333:27-40.

20. Sharrock NE, Go G, Harpel PC, Ranawat CS, Sculco TP, Salvati EA: Thrombogenesis during total hip replacement. *Clin Orthop Relat Res* 1995;319:16-27.

21. Sharrock NE, Go G, Salvati EA, Sculco TP, Harpel PC: Abstract: The effect of intraoperative heparin on markers of thrombosis during hybrid total hip arthroplasty. *Thromb Haemost* 1997;608(suppl):2477.

22. Binns M, Pho R: Femoral vein occlusion during hip arthroplasty. *Clin Orthop Relat Res* 1990;255:168-172.

23. Planès A, Vochelle N, Fagola M: Total hip replacement and deep vein thrombosis: A venographic and necropsy study. *J Bone Joint Surg Br* 1990;72:9-13.

24. Stamatakis JD, Kakkar VV, Sager S, Lawrence D, Nairn D, Bentley PG: Femoral vein thrombosis and total hip replacement. *BMJ* 1977;2:223-225.

25. Geerts WH, Pineo GF, Heit JA, et al: Prevention of thromboembolism: The seventh ACCP conference on antithrombotic and thrombolytic therapy. *Chest* 2004;126:338S-400S.

26. Ryan MG, Westrich GH, Potter HG, et al: Effect of mechanical compression on the prevalence of proximal deep venous thrombosis as assessed by magnetic resonance venography. *J Bone Joint Surg Am* 2002;84:1998-2004.

27. Sharrock NE, Go G, Williams-Russo P, Haas SB, Harpel PC: Comparison of extradural and general anaesthesia on the fibrinolytic response to total knee arthroplasty. *Br J Anaesth* 1997;79:29-34.

28. Aglietti P, Baldini A, Vena LM, Abbate R, Fedi S, Falciani M: Effect of tourniquet use on activation of coagulation in total knee replacement. *Clin Orthop Relat Res* 2000;371:169-177.

29. Berman AT, Parmet JL, Harding SP, et al: Emboli observed with use of transesophageal echocardiography immediately after tourniquet release during total knee arthroplasty with cement. *J Bone Joint Surg Am* 1998;80:389-396.

30. Maynard MJ, Sculco TP, Ghelman B: Progression and regression of deep vein thrombosis after total knee arthroplasty. *Clin Orthop Relat Res* 1991;273:125-130.

31. Rodgers A, Walker N, Schug S, et al: Reduction of postoperative mortality and morbidity with epidural or spinal anaesthesia: Results from overview of randomised trials. *BMJ* 2000;321:1493-1497.

32. Lieberman JR, Huo MH, Hanway J, Salvati EA, Sculco TP, Sharrock NE: The prevalence of deep venous thrombosis after total hip arthroplasty with hypotensive epidural anesthesia. *J Bone Joint Surg Am* 1994;76:341-348.

33. Eriksson BI, Wille-Jorgensen P, Kalebo P, et al: A comparison of recombinant hirudin with a low-molecular-weight heparin to prevent thromboembolic complications after total hip replacement. *N Engl J Med* 1997;337:1329-1335.

34. Chelly JE, Sullivan E, Hantler CB: Regional anesthesia in the anticoagulated patient: Lessons from the fondaparinux database, in *American Society of Anesthesiologists*. San Francisco, CA, 2003.

35. Sharrock NE, Haas SB, Hargett MJ, Urquhart B, Insall JN, Scuderi G: Effects of epidural anesthesia on the incidence of deep-vein thrombosis after

total knee arthroplasty. *J Bone Joint Surg Am* 1991;73:502-506.

36. Westrich GH, Sculco TP: Prophylaxis against deep venous thrombosis after total knee arthroplasty: Pneumatic plantar compression and aspirin compared with aspirin alone. *J Bone Joint Surg Am* 1996;78:826-834.

37. Knaggs AL, Delis KT, Mason P, Macleod K: Perioperative lower limb venous haemodynamics in patients under general anaesthesia. *Br J Anaesth* 2005;94:292-295.

38. Bading B, Blank S, Sculco TP, Pickering TG, Sharrock NE: Augmentation of calf blood flow by epinephrine infusion during lumbar epidural anesthesia. *Anesth Analg* 1994;78:1119-1124.

39. DiGiovanni CW, Restrepo A, González Della Valle AG, et al: The safety and efficacy of intraoperative heparin in total hip arthroplasty. *Clin Orthop Relat Res* 2000;379:178-185.

40. Horlocker TT, Wedel DJ, Benzon H, et al: Regional anesthesia in the anticoagulated patient: Defining the risks (the second ASRA Consensus Conference on Neuraxial Anesthesia and Anticoagulation). *Reg Anesth Pain Med* 2003;28:172-197.

41. Dalldorf PG, Perkins FM, Totterman S, Pellegrini VD Jr: Deep venous thrombosis following total hip arthroplasty: Effects of prolonged postoperative epidural anesthesia. *J Arthroplasty* 1994;9:611-616.

42. Francis CW, Pellegrini VD Jr, Marder VJ, et al: Comparison of warfarin and external pneumatic compression in prevention of venous thrombosis after total hip replacement. *JAMA* 1992;267:2911-2915.

43. Francis CW, Pellegrini VD Jr, Totterman S, et al: Prevention of deep-vein thrombosis after total hip arthroplasty: Comparison of warfarin and dalteparin. *J Bone Joint Surg Am* 1997;79:1365-1372.

44. Hull R, Raskob GE, Pineo G, et al: A comparison of subcutaneous low-molecular-weight heparin with warfarin sodium for prophylaxis against

deep-vein thrombosis after hip or knee implantation. *N Engl J Med* 1993;329:1370-1376.

45. Woolson ST: Intermittent pneumatic compression prophylaxis for proximal deep venous thrombosis after total hip replacement. *J Bone Joint Surg Am* 1996;78:1735-1740.

46. Kaempffe FA, Lifeso RM, Meinking C: Intermittent pneumatic compression versus coumadin. *Clin Orthop Relat Res* 1991;269:89-97.

47. Paiement G, Wessinger SJ, Waltman AC, Harris WH: Low-dose warfarin versus external pneumatic compression for prophylaxis against venous thromboembolism following total hip replacement. *J Arthroplasty* 1987;2:23-26.

48. Paiement GD, Beisaw N, Lotke P, Elia E, Wessinger S, Harris W: Advances in the prevention of venous thromboembolic disease after hip and knee operation. *Orthop Rev* 1989;18:1-20.

49. Modig J: Beneficial effects on intraoperative and postoperative blood loss in total hip replacement when performed under lumbar epidural anesthesia: An explanatory study. *Acta Chir Scand Suppl* 1989;550:95-100.

50. Modig J: Influence of regional anesthesia, local anesthetics and sympathicomimetics on the pathophysiology of deep vein thrombosis. *Acta Chir Scand Suppl* 1989;550:119-124.

51. Modig J, Borg T, Karlström G, Maripuu E, Sahlstedt B: Thromboembolism after total hip replacement: Role of epidural and general anesthesia. *Anesth Analg* 1983;62:174-180.

52. Modig J, Maripuu E, Sahlstedt B: Thromboembolism following total hip replacement: A prospective investigation of 94 patients with emphasis on the efficacy of lumbar epidural anesthesia in prophylaxis. *Reg Anesth* 1986;11:72-79.

53. Dearborn JT, Harris WH: Postoperative mortality after total hip arthroplasty: An analysis of deaths after two thousand seven hundred thirty-six

procedures. *J Bone Joint Surg Am* 1998;80:1291-1294.

54. Hirsch J: Therapeutic range for the control of oral anticoagulant therapy. *Arch Intern Med* 1985;145:1187-1188.

55. Hirsh J: Oral anticoagulant drugs. *N Engl J Med* 1991;324:1865-1875.

56. Hirsh J, Levine MN: The optimal intensity of oral anticoagulant therapy. *JAMA* 1987;258:2723-2726.

57. Paiement GD, Wessinger SJ, Hughes R, Harris W: Routine use of adjusted low-dose warfarin to prevent venous thromboembolism after total hip replacement. *J Bone Joint Surg Am* 1993;75:893-898.

58. Reis SE, Hirsch D, Wilson M, Donovan D, Goldhaber S: Program for the prevention of venous thromboembolism in high risk orthopaedic patients. *J Arthroplasty* 1991;6:S11-S16.

59. Landefeld CS, Cook EF, Flatley M, Weisberg M, Goldman L: Identification and preliminary validation of predictors of major bleeding in hospitalized patients starting anticoagulant therapy. *Am J Med* 1987;82:703-713.

60. Landefeld CS, Goldman L: Major bleeding in outpatients treated with warfarin: Incidence and prediction by factors known at the start of outpatient therapy. *Am J Med* 1989;87:144-152.

61. Landefeld CS, Rosenblatt MW, Goldman L: Bleeding in outpatients treated with warfarin: Relation to the prothrombin time and important remediable lesions. *Am J Med* 1989;87:153-159.

62. Imperiale TF, Speroff T: A meta-analysis of methods to prevent venous thromboembolism following total hip replacement. *JAMA* 1994;271:1780-1785.

63. Colwell CW Jr, Collis D, Paulson R, et al: Enoxaparin versus warfarin: Hospital management for prevention of deep venous thrombosis following total hip arthroplasty with inpatient and three month evaluation. *Orthop Trans* 1997;21:125.

64. Pellegrini VD Jr, Donaldson CT, Farber DC, Lehman EB, Evarts CM: The John Charnley Award: Prevention of readmission for venous thromboembolic disease after total hip arthroplasty. *Clin Orthop Relat Res* 2005;441:56-62.

65. Pellegrini VD Jr, Donaldson CT, Farber DC, Lehman EB, Evarts CM: The Mark Coventry Award: Prevention of readmission for venous thromboembolic disease after total knee arthroplasty. *Clin Orthop Relat Res* 2006;452:21-27.

66. Francis CW, Marder VJ, Evarts CM, Yaukoolbodi S: Two-step warfarin therapy: Prevention of postoperative venous thrombosis without excessive bleeding. *JAMA* 1983;249:374-378.

67. Westrich GH, Farrell C, Bono JV, Ranawat CS, Salvati EA, Sculco TP: Incidence of venous thromboembolism following total hip arthroplasty: A specific hypotensive epidural anesthesia protocol. *J Arthroplasty* 1999;14:456-463.

68. Collaborative overview of randomized trials of antiplatelet therapy: III. Reduction in venous thrombosis and pulmonary embolism by antiplatelet prophylaxis among surgical and medical patients: Antiplatelet Trialists' Collaboration. *BMJ* 1994;308:235-246.

69. Prevention of pulmonary embolism and deep venous thrombosis with low dose aspirin: Pulmonary Embolism Prevention (PEP) Trial. *Lancet* 2000;355:1295-1302.

70. González Della Valle A, Serota A, Go G, et al: Venous thromboembolism is rare with a multimodal prophylaxis protocol after total hip arthroplasty. *Clin Orthop Relat Res* 2006;444:146-153.

71. Lotke PA, Lonner JH: The benefit of aspirin chemoprophylaxis for thromboembolism after total knee arthroplasty. *Clin Orthop Relat Res* 2006;452:175-180.

72. Freedman KB, Brookenthal KR, Fitzgerald RH, Williams S, Lonner JH: A meta-analysis of thromboembolism prophylaxis following elective total hip arthroplasty. *J Bone Joint Surg Am* 2000;82:929-938.

73. Geerts WH, Jay RM, Code KI, et al: A comparison of low dose heparin and low molecular weight heparin as prophylaxis against venous thromboembolism after major trauma. *N Engl J Med* 1996;335:701-707.

74. Martel N, Lee J, Wells PS: Risk for heparin-induced thrombocytopenia with unfractionated and low molecular weight heparin thromboprophylaxis: A meta-analysis. *Blood* 2005;106:2710-2715.

75. Warkentin TE, Greinacher A: Heparin-induced thrombocytopenia recognition, treatment, and prevention: The seventh ACCP conference on antithrombotic and thrombolytic therapy. *Chest* 2004;126:311S-337S.

76. Lassen MR, Bauer KA, Eriksson BI, et al: Postoperative fondaparinux versus preoperative enoxaparin for prevention of venous thromboembolism in elective hip replacement surgery: A randomized double blind trial. *Lancet* 2002;359:1715-1720.

77. Turpie AG, Bauer KA, Eriksson BI, et al: Postoperative fondaparinux versus postoperative enoxaparin for prevention of venous thromboembolism in elective hip replacement surgery: A randomized double blind trial. *Lancet* 2002;359:1721-1726.

78. Bauer KA, Eriksson BI, Lassen MR, et al: Fondaparinux compared with enoxaparin for prevention of venous thromboembolism after elective major knee surgery. *N Engl J Med* 2001;345:1305-1310.

79. Lassen MR, Bauer KA, Eriksson BI, et al: Postoperative fondaparinux versus preoperative enoxaparin for prevention of venous thromboembolism in hip fracture surgery. *N Engl J Med* 2001;345:1298-1304.

80. Francis CW, Berkowitz SD, Comp PC, et al: Oral direct thrombin inhibitor ximelagatran compared with warfarin for the prevention of venous thromboembolism after total knee replacement. *N Engl J Med* 2003;349:1703-1712.

81. Colwell CW, Berkowitz SD, Comp PC, et al: Oral direct thrombin inhibitor ximelagatran compared with warfarin for the prevention of venous thromboembolism after total knee replacement. *J Bone Joint Surg Am* 2005;87:2169-2177.

82. Virchow RL: Die Verstopfung den Lungenarterie und ihre Flogen. *Beitr Exper Path Physiol* 1846;2:227-380.

83. Buehler KO, D'Lima DD, Petersilge WJ, Colwell CW, Walker RH: Late deep venous thrombosis and delayed weight bearing after total hip arthroplasty. *Clin Orthop Relat Res* 1999;361:123-130.

84. Lassen MR, Borris LC: Mobilisation after hip surgery and efficacy of thromboprophylaxis. *Lancet* 1991;337:618.

85. Jeffery PC, Nicolaides AN: Graduated compression stockings in the prevention of postoperative deep vein thrombosis. *Br J Surg* 1990;77:380-383.

86. Meyerowitz BR, Nelson R: Measurement of the velocity of blood in lower limb veins with and without compression. *Surgery* 1964;56:481-486.

87. Makin GS, Mayes FB, Holroyd AM: Studies on the effect of tubigrip on flow in the deep veins of the calf. *Br J Surg* 1969;56:369-372.

88. Lawrence D, Kakkar VV: Graduated, static, external compression of the lower limb: A physiological assessment. *Br J Surg* 1980;67:119-121.

89. Sigel B, Edelstein AL, Felix WR Jr, Memhardt CR: Compression of the deep venous system of the lower leg during inactive recumbency. *Arch Surg* 1973;106:38-43.

90. Sigel B, Edelstein AL, Savitch L, Hasty JH, Felix WR Jr: Type of compression for reducing venous stasis: A study of lower extremities during inactive recumbency. *Arch Surg* 1975;110:171-175.

91. Keith SL, McLaughlin DJ, Anderson FA Jr, et al: Do graduated compression stockings and pneumatic boots have an additive effect on the peak velocity of venous blood flow? *Arch Surg* 1992;127:727-730.

92. Mayberry JC, Moneta GL, de Frang RD, Porter JM: The influence of elastic compression stockings on deep venous hemodynamics. *J Vasc Surg* 1991;13:91-99.

93. Macklon NS, Greer IA: Technical note: Compression stockings and posture. A comparative study of their effects on the proximal deep veins of the leg at rest. *Br J Radiol* 1995;68: 515-518.

94. Coleridge-Smith PD, Hasty JH, Scurr JH: Deep vein thrombosis: Effect of graduated compression stockings on distension of the deep veins of the calf. *Br J Surg* 1991;78: 724-726.

95. Gardner AM, Fox RH: The venous footpump: Influence on tissue perfusion and prevention of venous thrombosis. *Ann Rheum Dis* 1992;51: 1173-1178.

96. Dai G, Gertler JP, Kamm RD: The effects of external compression on venous blood flow and tissue deformation in the lower leg. *J Biomech Eng* 1999;121:557-564.

97. Morris RJ, Woodcock JP: Evidence-based compression: Prevention of stasis and deep vein thrombosis. *Ann Surg* 2004;239:162-171.

98. Westrich GH, Specht LM, Sharrock NE, et al: Venous haemodynamics after total knee arthroplasty: Evaluation of active dorsal to plantar flexion and several mechanical devices. *J Bone Joint Surg Br* 1998;80:1057-1106.

99. Lachiewicz PF, Kelley SS, Haden LR: Two mechanical devices for prophylaxis after total knee arthroplasty. *J Bone Joint Surg Br* 2004;86: 1137-1141.

100. Elliott CG, Dudney TM, Egger M, et al: Calf-thigh sequential pneumatic compression compared with plantar venous pneumatic compression to prevent deep-vein thrombosis after non-lower extremity trauma. *J Trauma* 1999;47:25-31.

101. Gardner AM, Fox RH: *The Return of Blood to the Heart: Venous Pumps in Health and Disease.* London, UK, John Libby, 2001.

102. Pitto RP, Hamer H, Kuhle JW, Radespiel-Tröger M, Pietsch M: Haemodynamics of the lower extremity with pneumatic foot compression. *Biomed Tech (Berl)* 2001;46:124-128.

103. Browse NL, Negus D: Prevention of postoperative leg vein thrombosis by electrical muscle stimulation: An evaluation with 125I-labelled fibrinogen. *BMJ* 1970;3:615-618.

104. Faghri PD, Van Meerdervort HF, Glaser RM, Figoni SF: Electrical stimulation-induced contraction to reduce blood stasis during arthroplasty. *IEEE Trans Rehabil Eng* 1997;5: 62-69.

105. Roberts VC, Sabri S, Pietroni MC, Gurewich V, Cotton LT: Passive flexion and femoral vein flow: A study using a motorized foot mover. *BMJ* 1971;3:78-81.

106. Sabri S, Roberts VC, Cotton LT: Prevention of early postoperative deep vein thrombosis by passive exercise of leg during surgery. *BMJ* 1971;3: 82-83.

107. Caruana MF, Brightwell RE, Huguet EL, Whitear P, Hodgkinson DW, Osman IS: Calf exercise in the seated position using a new dynamic biped device increases femoral vein peak velocity up to eight-fold. *Phlebology* 2003;18:70-72.

108. Allenby F: Diagnosis, prevention and management of thromboembolism: Biological effects of intermittent compression of the calf. *Proc R Soc Med* 1974;67:706.

109. Knight MT, Dawson R: Effect of intermittent compression of the arms on deep venous thrombosis in the legs. *Lancet* 1976;2:1265-1268.

110. Jacobs DG, Piotrowski JJ, Hoppensteadt DA, Salvator AE, Fareed J: Hemodynamic and fibrinolytic consequences of intermittent pneumatic compression: Preliminary results. *J Trauma* 1996;40:710-716.

111. Comerota AJ, Chouhan V, Harada RN, et al: The fibrinolytic effects of intermittent pneumatic compression: Mechanism of enhanced fibrinolysis. *Ann Surg* 1997;226:306-313.

112. Morris RJ, Giddings JC, Ralis HM, et al: The influence of inflation rate on the hematologic and hemodynamic effects of intermittent pneumatic calf compression for deep vein thrombosis prophylaxis. *J Vasc Surg* 2006;44:1039-1045.

113. Kessler CM, Hirsch DR, Jacobs H, MacDougall R, Goldhaber SZ: Intermittent pneumatic compression in chronic venous insufficiency favorably affects fibrinolytic potential and platelet activation. *Blood Coagul Fibrinolysis* 1996;7:437-446.

114. Giddings JC, Morris RJ, Ralis HM, Jennings GM, Davies DA, Woodcock JP: Systemic haemostasis after intermittent pneumatic compression: Clues for the investigation of DVT prophylaxis and travelers thrombosis. *Clin Lab Haematol* 2004;26:269-273.

115. Guyton DP, Khayat A, Husni EA, Schreiber H: Elevated levels of 6-keto-prostaglandin-F1α from a lower extremity during external pneumatic compression. *Surg Gynecol Obstet* 1988;166:338-342.

116. Dai G, Tsukurov O, Chen M, Gertler JP, Kamm RD: Endothelial nitric oxide production during in vitro simulation of external limb compression. *Am J Physiol Heart Circ Physiol* 2002; 282:H2066-H2075.

117. Arcelus JI, Caprini JA, Hoffman KN, Traverso CI, Hoppensteadt D, Fareed J: Modifications of plasma levels of tissue factor pathway inhibitor and endothelin-1 induced by a reverse Trendelenburg position. Influence of elastic compression: Preliminary results. *J Vasc Surg* 1995;22:568-572.

118. Ljungnér H, Bergqvist D, Nilsson IM: Effect of intermittent pneumatic and graduated static compression on factor VIII and the fibrinolytic system. *Acta Chir Scand* 1981;147: 657-661.

119. Wilkins RW, Mixter G Jr, Stanton JR, Litter J: Elastic stockings in prevention of pulmonary embolism: Preliminary report. *N Engl J Med* 1952; 246:360-364.

120. Rosengarten DS, Laird J, Jeyasingh K, Martin P: The failure of compression stockings (Tubigrip) to prevent deep venous thrombosis after operation. *Br J Surg* 1970;57:296-299.

121. Byrne B: Deep vein thrombosis prophylaxis: The effectiveness and implications of using below-knee or thigh-length graduated compression stockings. *J Vasc Nurs* 2002;20: 53-59.

122. Hameed MF, Browse DJ, Immelman EJ, Goldberg PA: Should knee-length replace thigh-length graduated compression stockings in the prevention of deep-vein thrombosis? *S Afr J Surg* 2002;40:15-16.

123. Ingram JE: A review of thigh-length vs knee-length antiembolism stockings. *Br J Nurs* 2003;12:845-851.

124. Merrett ND, Hanel KC: Ischaemic complications of graduated compression stockings in the treatment of deep venous thrombosis. *Postgrad Med J* 1993;69:232-234.

125. Wildin CJ, Hui AC, Esler CN, Gregg PJ: In vivo pressure profiles of thigh-length graduated compression stockings. *Br J Surg* 1998;85:1228-1231.

126. Best AJ, Williams S, Crozier A, Bhatt R, Gregg PJ, Hui AC: Graded compression stockings in elective orthopaedic surgery: An assessment of the in vivo performance of commercially available stockings in patients having hip and knee arthroplasty. *J Bone Joint Surg Br* 2000;82:116-118.

127. Hills NH, Pflug JJ, Jeyasingh K, Boardman L, Calnan JS: Prevention of deep vein thrombosis by intermittent pneumatic compression of calf. *BMJ* 1972;1:131-135.

128. Cotton LT: Intermittent compression of the legs during operation as a method of prevention of deep vein thrombosis. *Proc R Soc Med* 1974; 67:708.

129. Vanek VW: Meta-analysis of effectiveness of intermittent pneumatic compression devices with a comparison of thigh-high to knee-high sleeves. *Am Surg* 1998;64:1050-1058.

130. Pittman GR: Peroneal nerve palsy following sequential pneumatic compression. *JAMA* 1989;261:2201-2202.

131. McGrory BJ, Burke DW: Peroneal nerve palsy following intermittent sequential pneumatic compression. *Orthopedics* 2000;23:1103-1105.

132. Pfeffer SD, Halliwill JR, Warner MA: Effects of lithotomy position and external compression on lower leg muscle compartment pressure. *Anesthesiology* 2001;95:632-636.

133. Gallus A, Raman K, Darby T: Venous thrombosis after elective hip replacement: The influence of preventive intermittent calf compression and of surgical technique. *Br J Surg* 1983;70: 17-19.

134. Hartman JT, Pugh JL, Smith RD, Robertson WW, Yost RP, Janssen HF: Cyclic sequential compression of the lower limb in prevention of deep vein thrombosis. *J Bone Joint Surg Am* 1982;64:1059-1062.

135. Haas SB, Insall JN, Scuderi GR, Windsor RE, Ghelman B: Pneumatic sequential compression boots compared with aspirin prophylaxis of deep vein thrombosis after total knee arthroplasty. *J Bone Joint Surg Am* 1990;72:27-31.

136. Hull R, Delmore TJ, Hirsh J, et al: Effectiveness of intermittent pulsatile elastic stockings for the prevention of calf and thigh vein thrombosis in patients undergoing elective knee replacement. *Thromb Res* 1979;16: 37-45.

137. McKenna R, Galante J, Bachmann F, Wallace DL, Kaushal SP, Meredith P: Prevention of venous thromboembolism after total knee replacement by high-dose aspirin or intermittent calf and thigh compression. *B Med J* 1980; 280:514-517.

138. Lynch JA, Baker PL, Polly RE, et al: Mechanical measures in the prophylaxis of post-operative thromboembolism in total knee arthroplasty. *Clin Orthop Relat Res* 1990;260:24-29.

139. Hartman JT, Pugh JL, Smith RD, Robertson WW, Yost RP, Janssen HF: Cyclic sequential compression of the lower limb in prevention of deep vein thrombosis. *J Bone Joint Surg Am* 1982;64:1059-1062.

140. Gallus A, Raman K, Darby T: Venous thrombosis after elective hip replacement: The influence of preventive intermittent calf compression and of surgical technique. *Br J Surg* 1983;70: 17-19.

141. Bailey JP, Kruger MP, Solano FX, Zajko AB, Rubash HE: Prospective randomised trial of sequential compression devices versus low-dose warfarin for deep venous thrombosis prophylaxis in hip arthroplasty. *J Arthroplasty* 1991;6:S29-S34.

142. Kaempffe FA, Lifeso RM, Meinking C: Intermittent pneumatic compression versus comadin: Prevention of deep vein thrombosis in lower extremity total joint arthroplasty. *Clin Orthop Relat Res* 1991;269:89-97.

143. Wilson NV, Das SK, Kakkar VV, et al: Thromboembolic prophylaxis in total knee replacement. *J Bone Joint Surg Br* 1992;74:50-52.

144. Warwick D, Harrison J, Whitehouse S, Mitchelmore A, Thornton M: A randomized comparison of a foot pump and low molecular weight heparin in the prevention of deep vein thrombosis after total knee replacement. *J Bone Joint Surg Br* 2002;84: 344-350.

145. Westrich GH, Sculco TP: Prophylaxis against deep venous thrombosis after total knee arthroplasty: Pneumatic plantar compression and aspirin compared with aspirin alone. *J Bone Joint Surg Am* 1996;78:826-834.

146. Norgren L, Toksvig-Larsen S, Magyar G, Lindstrand A, Albrechtsson U: Prevention of deep vein thrombosis in knee arthroplasty: Preliminary results from a randomised controlled study of low molecular weight heparin vs foot pump compression. *Int Angiol* 1998;17:93-96.

147. Blanchard J, Meuwly JY, Leyvraz PF, et al: Prevention of deep vein thrombosis after total knee replacement: Randomised comparison between a low molecular weight heparin (na-

droparin) and mechanical prophylaxis with a foot-pump system. *J Bone Joint Surg Br* 1999;81:654-659.

148. Santori FS, Vitullo A, Stopponi M, Santori N, Ghera S: Prophylaxis against deep venous thrombosis in total hip replacement. *J Bone Joint Surg Br* 1994;76:579-583.

149. Bradley JG, Krugener GH, Jager HJ: The effectiveness of intermittent plantar venous compression in the prevention of deep venous thrombosis after total hip arthroplasty. *J Arthroplasty* 1993;8:57-60.

150. Warwick D, Harrison J, Glew D, Mitchelmore A, Peters T, Donovan J: Comparison of the use of a foot pump with the use of low molecular weight heparin for the prevention of deep vein thrombosis after total hip replacement. *J Bone Joint Surg Am* 1998;80:1158-1166.

151. Fordyce MJ, Ling RS: A venous foot pump reduces thrombosis after hip replacement. *J Bone Joint Surg Br* 1992;74:45-49.

152. Pitto RP, Hamer H, Heiss-Dunlop W, Kuehle J: Mechanical prophylaxis of deep-vein thrombosis after total hip replacement: A randomized clinical trial. *J Bone Joint Surg Br* 2004;86: 639-642.

153. Stannard JP, Harris RM, Bucknell AL, Cossi A, Ward J, Arington ED: Prophylaxis of deep venous thrombosis after total hip arthroplasty by using intermittent compression of the plantar venous plexus. *Am J Orthop* 1996; 25:127-134.

154. Amaragiri SV, Lees TA: Elastic compression stockings for prevention of deep vein thrombosis. *Cochrane Database Syst Rev* 2000;3:CD001484.

155. Handoll HH, Farrar MJ, McBirnie J, Tytherleigh-Strong G, Milne AA, Gillespie WJ: Heparin, low molecular weight heparin and physical methods for preventing deep vein thrombosis and pulmonary embolism following

surgery for hip fractures. *Cochrane Database Syst Rev* 2002;4:CD000305.

156. Wille-Jørgensen P, Rasmussen M, Andersen B, Borly L: Heparins and mechanical methods for thromboprophylaxis in colorectal surgery. *Cochrane Database Syst Rev* 2003;4: CD001217.

157. Mazzone C, Chiodo GF, Sandercock P, Miccio M, Salvi R: Physical methods for preventing deep vein thrombosis in stroke. *Cochrane Database Syst Rev* 2004;4:CD001922.

158. Agu O, Hamilton G, Baker D: Graduated compression stockings in the prevention of venous thromboembolism. *Br J Surg* 1999;86:992-1004.

159. Roderick P, Ferris G, Wilson K, et al: Towards evidence based guidelines for the prevention of venous thromboembolism: Systematic review of mechanical methods, oral anticoagulation, dextran and regional anesthesia as thromboprophylaxis. *Health Technol Assess* 2005;9:1-78.

160. Westrich GH, Haas SB, Mosca P, Peterson M: Meta-analysis of thromboembolic prophylaxis after total knee arthroplasty. *J Bone Joint Surg Br* 2000;82:795-800.

161. Brookenthal KR, Freedman KB, Lotke PA, Fitzgerald RH, Lonner JH: A meta-analysis of thromboembolic prophylaxis in total knee arthroplasty. *J Arthroplasty* 2001;16:293-300.

162. .Institute of Clinical Systems Improvement (ICSI): *Venous Thromboembolism Prophylaxis.* Bloomington, MN, Institute of Clinical Systems Improvement, 2006.

163. Cardiovascular Disease Educational and Research Trust, Cyprus Cardiovascular Disease Educational and Research Trust, European Venous Forum, International Surgical Thrombosis Forum, International Union of Angiology, Union Internationale de

Phlébologie: Prevention and treatment of venous thromboembolism, International Consensus Statement. *Int Angiol* 2006;25:101-161.

164. Scurr JH, Coleridge-Smith PD, Hasty JH: Regimen for improved effectiveness of intermittent pneumatic compression in deep venous thrombosis prophylaxis. *Surgery* 1987;102: 816-820.

165. Mellbring G, Palmer K: Prophylaxis of deep vein thrombosis after major abdominal surgery: Comparison between dihydroergotamine-heparin and intermittent pneumatic calf compression and evaluation of added graduated static compression. *Acta Chir Scand* 1986;152:597-600.

166. Warwick DJ, Pandit H, Shewale S, Sulkin T: Venous impulse foot pumps: Should graduated compression stockings be used? *J Arthroplasty* 2002;17:446-448.

167. Keith SL, McLaughlin DJ, Anderson FA Jr, et al: Do graduated compression stockings and pneumatic boots have an additive effect on the peak velocity of venous blood flow? *Arch Surg* 1992;127:727-730.

168. Silbersack Y, Taute BM, Hein W, Podhaisky H: Prevention of deep vein thrombosis after total hip and knee replacement. *J Bone Joint Surg Br* 2004;86:809-812.

169. Fuchs S, Heyse T, Rudolfsky G, Gosheger G, Chylarecki C: Continuous passive motion in the prevention of deep vein thrombosis. *J Bone Joint Surg Br* 2005;87:1117-1122.

170. Stannard JP, Lopez RR, Volgas DA, et al: Prophylaxis against deep-vein thrombosis following trauma: A prospective randomized comparison of mechanical and pharmacologic prophylaxis. *J Bone Joint Surg Am* 2006;88: 261-266.

# Controversies in Lower Extremity Amputation

Michael S. Pinzur, MD
Frank Gottschalk, MB.BCh, FRCSEd
Marco Antonio Guedes de Souza Pinto, MD
*Douglas G. Smith, MD

## Abstract

*Using the experience gained from taking care of World War II veterans with amputations, Ernest Burgess taught that amputation surgery is reconstructive surgery. It is the first step in the rehabilitation process for patients with an amputation and should be thought of in this way. An amputation is often a more appropriate option than limb salvage, irrespective of the underlying cause. The decision making and selection of the amputation level must be based on realistic expectations with regard to functional outcome and must be adapted to both the disease process being treated and the unique needs of the patient. Sometimes the amputation is done as a life-saving procedure in a patient who is not expected to walk, but more often it is done for a patient who should be able to return to a full, active life. When considering amputation, the physician should establish reasonable goals when confronted with the question of limb salvage versus amputation, understand the roles of the soft-tissue envelope and osseous platform in the creation of a residual limb, understand the method of weight bearing within a prosthetic socket, and determine whether a bone bridge is a positive addition to a transtibial amputation.*

**Instr Course Lect 2008;57:663-672.**

The Lower Extremity Assessment Project (LEAP) has provided objective outcome data on patients with mutilating limb injuries.[1] Five hundred sixty-nine consecutive patients with mutilating limb injuries treated at eight academic trauma centers provided objective observational outcome data relative to limb salvage and amputation. One hundred forty-nine patients underwent lower-extremity amputation during the course of their care. This ongoing study is providing a realistic understanding of the less-than-favorable results associated with both limb salvage and amputation. Much of what has been learned from LEAP can be applied to the care of patients with a nontraumatic amputation.

A reasonable functional goal should be established before an extremity amputation is performed. The goals for a young individual who is going to reenter the workforce after a traumatic amputation are very different from those for an elderly debilitated patient with diabetes who has a limited life expectancy. Before surgery is performed, four issues need to be addressed, so as to create a needs assessment:

1. If the limb is salvaged, will the functional outcome be better than it would be after an amputation and fitting of a prosthetic limb? This question needs to be addressed regardless of whether the patient has a mutilating limb injury, a diabetic foot infection, a tumor, or a congenital anomaly.

2. What is a realistic expectation following treatment? The realistic expected functional outcome is the average functional outcome for patients with the same comorbidities and level of amputation; it is not the best possible outcome.

3. What is the cost of care? This cost goes beyond resource consumption. Can the patient and his or her family afford the multiple operations and the time off from work necessary to accomplish limb sal-

*Douglas G. Smith, MD or the department with which he is affiliated has received research or institutional support from Otto Bock.*

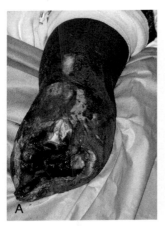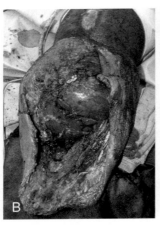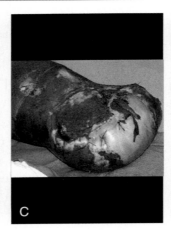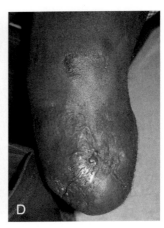

**Figure 1** **A,** Photograph taken at the time that a young, active male patient first returned to the operating room following a traumatic amputation. **B,** The remaining gastrocnemius muscle was used to create a cushioned soft-tissue envelope. The skin was degloved and did not survive. **C,** Following the use of vacuum-assisted wound management, there was an adequate base for split-thickness skin grafting. **D,** The residual limb 18 months following the injury. A silicone suspension liner within the prosthetic socket was used to compensate for the split-thickness skin graft over the residual anterior aspect of the tibia.

vage, or are they best served by amputation and fitting of a prosthetic limb?

4. What are the risks? Limb-salvage surgery for any diagnosis is riskier than an amputation. When a patient has had an infection in an ischemic limb, the risk of recurrent infection and sepsis is far lower when the limb is removed than when it is retained.

Once these issues have been addressed, the patient and the surgical team generally have sufficient data to support the decision-making process.

When performing an amputation as a reconstructive effort after trauma, infection, tumor, or vascular insufficiency, one should strive to create optimal residual limb length without osseous prominences; reasonable function in the joint proximal to the level of the amputation to enhance prosthetic function; and a durable soft-tissue envelope. Although new prosthetic technology allows compensation for a suboptimal soft-tissue envelope, it is well

accepted that amputees fare better with a durable soft-tissue envelope and fare worse when the skin is adherent to bone or there is a split-thickness skin graft in areas of high pressure or shear.[2,3] Therefore, muscles should be secured to bone to prevent retraction. When possible, full-thickness myocutaneous flaps should be used, with muscle cushioning in areas of high pressure and shear (Figure 1).

## Disarticulation Compared With Transosseous Amputation

The more distal the level of lower extremity amputation, the better the walking independence and functional outcome, unless the quality of the residual limb creates so much discomfort that it negates the potential benefits of limb-length retention. Therefore, the amputation should be done at the most distal level that will result in a functional residual limb. Efforts to create a functional residual limb should take into account the method of weight

bearing (load transfer) and the tissues available to create a soft-tissue envelope.

The best residual limb cannot duplicate the unique weight-bearing properties of a normal foot. The foot has multiple bones and articulations that function as a shock absorber at heel strike, a stable platform during stance phase, and a "starting block" for stability at push-off. The multiple bones and joints allow positioning of the durable plantar soft-tissue envelope in an optimal orientation for accepting load. An amputee has, in place of a foot, a residual limb that must tolerate weight bearing (load transfer) with the socket of a prosthesis.

When the amputation is through a joint (disarticulation), the load transfer can be accomplished directly; that is, there is end-bearing. When the amputation is done through the bone (transosseous), the load transfer must be accomplished indirectly by the entire residual limb, through a total-contact socket of the prosthesis, as weight bearing on the end of the residual limb is too painful. Disarticulation allows dissipation of the load over a large surface area of less stiff metaphyseal bone. With a well-constructed soft-tissue envelope to cushion the residual osseous platform, the direct-transfer prosthetic socket need only suspend the prosthesis. This differs from transosseous amputation at the transtibial or transfemoral level, where the surface area of the end of the bone is small and the diaphyseal bone is less resilient. The end of the bone must be "unweighted" by dissipating the load over the entire surface of the residual limb. This indirect load transfer requires a durable and mobile soft-tissue envelope that can tolerate the shearing forces associated with weight bearing. The socket fit becomes crucial. When a patient loses weight, the residual limb tends to bottom out, and painful end-bearing or tissue breakdown develops. Patients who gain weight are not able to fit the limb into the prosthesis. The choice of disarticulation or transosseous amputation must be individualized for each patient.

## Transtibial (Below-the-Knee) Amputation

The standard transtibial prosthetic socket is fabricated with the knee in approximately 10° of flexion, to unload the distal part of the tibia and optimally distribute the load. Load transfer is accomplished by distributing the load over the entire surface area of the residual limb, with a concentration over the anteromedial and anterolateral areas of the tibial metaphysis.

Mutilating limb injuries frequently disrupt the interosseous membrane, disengaging the relationship between the tibia and fibula.

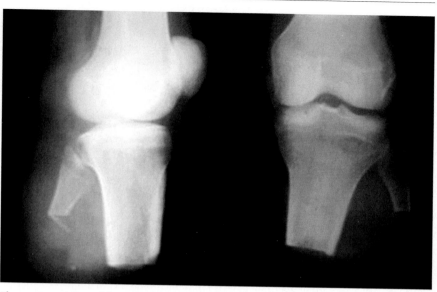

**Figure 2**    AP and lateral plain radiographs of a patient with an unstable fibula caused by disruption of the interosseous membrane by a transtibial amputation. The short, unstable fibula is not able to serve as an efficient platform for weight bearing. The abducted residual distal part of the fibula also creates an osseous prominence that interferes with prosthetic limb fitting. (Reprinted with permission from Pinzur MS, Pinto MA, Schon LC, Smith DG: Controversies in amputation surgery. *Instr Course Lect* 2003;52:448.)

This loss of integrity of the interosseous membrane prevents the fibula from participating in normal load transfer. In other situations, the residual fibula may become unstable following transtibial amputation because of loss of the integrity of the interosseous membrane or as a result of loss of the integrity of the proximal tibiofibular joint even without an obvious traumatic disruption.

Individuals with instability of the residual fibula following transtibial amputation can have pain because of several causes. When the residual limb is compressed within the prosthetic socket, the residual fibula may angulate toward the tibia with prolonged weight bearing. The result is a conical, pointed residual limb, which tends to bottom out during prolonged weight bearing. The conical residual limb acts as a wedge, leading to painful end-bearing and soft-tissue breakdown over the terminal tibia. When the residual limb is short, or the interosseous membrane has been disrupted, the residual fibula can be abducted as a result of unopposed action of the biceps femoris muscle[4,5] (Figure 2). These alterations of the load-bearing platform become accentuated in younger, more active amputees, with higher demand, or with prolonged activities.[6,7]

During World War I, Ertl[8] proposed the creation of an osteoperiosteal tube, derived mostly from tibial periosteum, and affixing it to the fibula to create a stable residual limb. Following World War II, his concept was successfully introduced in the United States by Loon,[4] Deffer,[9] and others.[10] Arthrodesis, or bone bridging, of the distal parts of the tibia and fibula has recently become a controversial topic, with

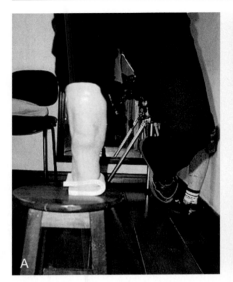
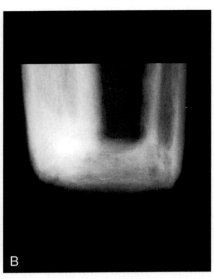

**Figure 3**    **A,** This patient was able to stand directly on the residual limb because he had a stable platform for weight bearing following the creation of an Ertl bone bridge between the distal parts of the tibia and fibula. (Reprinted with permission from Pinzur MS, Pinto MA, Schon LC, Smith DG: Controversies in amputation surgery. *Instr Course Lect* 2003;52:449.) **B,** Radiograph obtained 1 year following the creation of the bone bridge.

both ardent supporters and strong detractors. Recent investigations suggest that the technique may provide a potential benefit for an active amputee by creating a stable platform with an enhanced surface area for load transfer[5,11,12] (Figure 3). Most supporters suggest that the technique should be reserved for younger, more active amputees who will benefit from the potentially enhanced functional residual limb and are more able to tolerate the increased morbidity risk associated with the additional surgery necessary to obtain the bone bridge.

The surgery can also be performed as a late reconstruction for active amputees with residual limb pain that appears to be associated with an unstable or disengaged residual fibula. These patients may have a conical end-bearing residual limb, usually with pain at the end of the residual limb and occasionally with tissue breakdown. Others may have pain along a prominent or unstable fibula. On examination, the fibula usually can be felt to be unstable.

The operation involves use of a long posterior myocutaneous flap. For the average 6-ft (1.8 m)-tall patient, the optimal residual tibial length should be a minimum of 10 to 12 cm to create an adequate weight-bearing platform, but it should not be longer than 15 to 18 cm. (An excessively long residual limb requires the prosthetic socket to be put into full extension. This leads to increased distal pressure, increased end-bearing, and more stump failures.) The fibula is divided 4 cm distal to the tibia to allow the creation of the bone bridge. Care is taken to maintain as many muscular attachments to the distal aspect of the fibula as possible. One centimeter of the fibula is removed at the level of the distal tibial cut to allow rotation of the vascularized bone. A notch is made in the lateral cortex of the residual tibia to accept the rotated fibu-

lar segment. Stability can be obtained by suturing the fibular segment through drill holes or with screw fixation (Figure 3, *B*).

The transferred fibular segment used between the distal parts of the fibula and tibia can be supplemented with a vascularized periosteal sleeve taken from the tibia, as described by Ertl.[8] The periosteum on the anterior surface of the tibia, which is quite thick, is raised from the tibia distal to the level of the tibial transection. When the periosteum is raised, it is important to keep it attached proximally and to take a thin slice of cortical bone with it. This almost guarantees that the periosteum obtained has maintained its vascular supply. A 1-in (2.5-cm) osteotome is used to raise the periosteum and the thin slice of cortical bone. The periosteal sleeve is sutured over the rotated fibular segment. The periosteal graft alone has also been used in place of the fibula, but we have no experience with that technique and do not recommend it.

The anterior aspect of the distal surface of the tibia is beveled, and a durable, full-thickness myocutaneous flap is repaired to the anterior aspect of the tibia through drill holes or by suturing the posterior gastrocnemius fascia to the anterior periosteum of the residual tibia and the anterior compartment fascia.

When the surgery is performed as a late reconstruction or if there is no distal part of the fibula with which to create the bone bridge, a tricortical iliac crest bone graft is wedged between the terminal residual tibia and fibula after the inner surfaces of both have been prepared with a burr (Figure 4).

### Postoperative Care

A rigid plaster dressing is applied to protect the residual limb and to con-

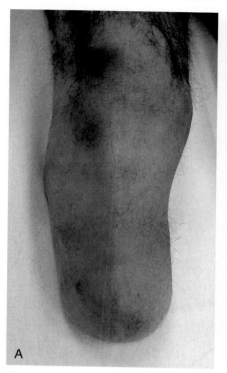
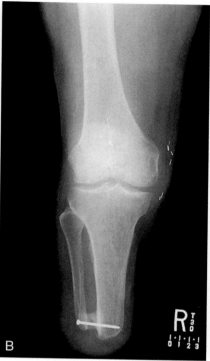
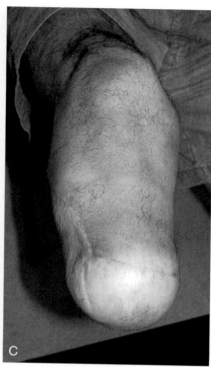

**Figure 4**    **A,** An active patient with a transtibial amputation reported pain in the distal part of the residual limb after prolonged activity. The conical shape of the residual limb allowed it to wedge into the prosthetic socket, creating painful end-bearing. **B,** Radiograph obtained 1 year after a successful bone bridge procedure with a tricortical iliac crest bone graft placed between the fibula and tibia. **C,** The more square shape of the residual limb created an excellent platform for load transmission. The residual limb no longer bottomed out in the prosthesis, providing better comfort with weight bearing.

trol postoperative swelling. Another option is to use elastic bandages for a compressive dressing, but these need to be put on carefully so as not to produce a pressure sore. This is especially important when a patient has a peripheral neuropathy. Our experience has been that if the patient has pain at the end of the stump or in the stump shortly after surgery, it is caused by a local problem and the dressing needs to be changed, but pain that seems to be in the distal, amputated part of the limb is the so-called phantom limb phenomenon. Phantom sensation is a normal response after an amputation that usually resolves. Telling the patient before the surgery that they will have phantom sensations tends to de-

crease anxiety about this phenomenon.

Weight bearing with a temporary prosthesis is initiated when the residual limb appears capable of tolerating weight bearing. Pain with weight bearing lasts longer for patients who have had a bone bridge reconstruction than it does for those without a bone bridge. The pain may last for 6 to 9 months and seems to resolve as the bone bridge heals. It is assumed that the site of healing between the fibula and tibia remains tender until the bone becomes solid. The pain should be treated nonsurgically unless there is a sign of inadequate placement of the graft or sutures. Usually, the patient can be fitted for a prosthesis, but he or she

may not be able to bear full weight until the tenderness resolves.

### Skin Flap for Transtibial (Below-the-Knee) Amputation
Load transfer following transtibial amputation appears to be enhanced when the residual limb has a large osseous surface area covered with a durable soft-tissue envelope composed of a well-cushioned mobile muscle mass and full-thickness skin. This desired result is best achieved through use of a long posterior myofasciocutaneous flap. Despite the fact that the standard posterior flap for transtibial amputation is satisfactory for most patients, retraction of the flap over time can lead to a troublesome pressure point overlying the anterior aspect of

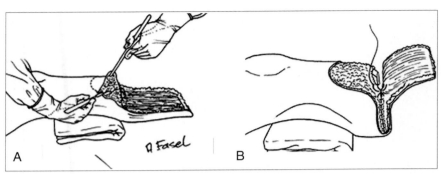

**Figure 5**   Artist's drawings of the extended posterior myocutaneous flap. **A,** The long posterior flap is several centimeters longer than the traditional posterior flap. **B,** A corresponding amount of proximal skin is removed to advance the suture line proximal to the anterior aspect of the distal tibial region. (Reprinted with permission from Assal M, Blanck R, Smith DG: Extended posterior flap for transtibial amputation. *Orthopaedics* 2005;28:544.)

the distal part of the residual tibia. The standard transtibial amputation technique, popularized by Burgess and associates,[13] often places the surgical incision directly over that portion of the residual tibia. This raises the potential for adherent scarring of the skin to that part of the tibia or for inadequate cushioning of this region during weight bearing. When the anterior aspect of the distal part of the residual tibia is not sufficiently padded, there is an increased likelihood of localized discomfort, blistering, or tissue breakdown associated with the normal pistoning that occurs between the residual limb and the prosthetic socket during normal walking. An extended posterior flap appears to prevent these potential morbidities by providing improved cushioning and comfort even for individuals who are capable of only limited activity.[14] The encouraging results of this relatively simple modification support the well-accepted notion that an optimal residual limb should be composed of a sufficient osseous platform and a durable and cushioned soft-tissue envelope.[11]

The extended posterior flap is created by increasing the length of the standard posterior flap by several centimeters (Figure 5). The posterior myocutaneous flap is created and the osseous cuts are performed in the traditional manner. The myocutaneous flap is generally created from the gastrocnemius muscle and overlying skin, with removal of the soleus muscle belly in all but very thin patients. Care is taken in the handling of the transected nerves to avoid the development of sensitive, painful neuromas. It is advised to avoid clamping of the nerves before transection to avoid the pain so frequently encountered following crushing injuries. The nerves should be dissected proximal to the level of the bone transection, with use of gentle traction with a sponge, and then they are transected with a fresh scalpel blade. This allows the inevitable terminal neuroma to be cushioned within bulky muscle. To avoid a bulbous stump, the posterior and lateral compartment muscles (except the gastrocnemius) should be transected at the level of the transected tibia. Anterior skin is removed to allow proximal attachment of the muscle flap and proximal placement of the wound scar. A myodesis of the

posterior muscle flap to the tibia can be performed through drill holes. The posterior gastrocnemius fascia is secured to the transected anterior compartment fascia and tibial periosteum with horizontal mattress sutures (Figure 6). A rigid plaster dressing is applied, and prosthetic fitting is initiated when the residual limb appears capable of weight bearing.

## Transfemoral (Above-the-Knee) Amputation

Transfemoral amputation is performed less frequently than in the past, but it is still necessary in some patients with severe vascular disease, a neoplasm, infection, or trauma in whom reconstruction at a more distal level is not feasible.[15,16] The energy expenditure for walking, even on a level surface, by an individual with a transfemoral amputation has been shown to be as much as 65% greater than that for similar, able-bodied individuals.[17,18] Energy expenditure can be minimized by a properly performed above-the-knee amputation.

The anatomic alignment of the lower limb has been well defined. The mechanical axis lies on a line from the center of the femoral head through the center of the knee to the center of the ankle. In normal two-limbed stance, this axis measures 3° from the vertical axis and the femoral shaft axis measures 9° from the vertical axis.[19] The femur is normally oriented in relative adduction, which allows the hip stabilizers (the gluteus medius and minimus) and abductors (the gluteus medius and the tensor fasciae latae) to act on it to reduce the lateral motion of the center of mass of the body, producing an energy-efficient gait (Figure 7).

In most individuals who have undergone a transfemoral amputation, the mechanical and anatomic align-

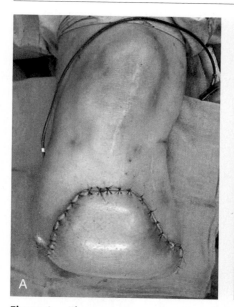 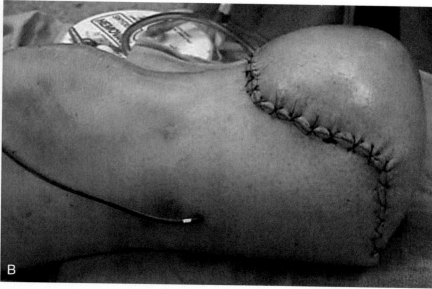

**Figure 6**    The appearance of an extended posterior flap immediately after closure. The bulbous end will shrink and smooth contours will develop with time. **A**, AP view. **B**, Lateral view.

ment is altered as a result of disruption of the adductor magnus insertion at the adductor tubercle and the distal part of the linea aspera.[20] This allows the residual femur to drift into abduction as a result of the unopposed action of the hip abductors. Many patients who have undergone a transfemoral amputation encounter difficulties with prosthetic fitting due to inadequate muscle stabilization at the time of the amputation.[21] The unstable femur disrupts the relationship between the anatomic and mechanical axes of the limb. The abductor lurch, so common after transfemoral amputation, is a consequence of the unopposed action of the intact hip abductors. This dynamic deformity overcomes the capacity of even modern prostheses to compensate.

Traditional transfemoral amputation is done by suturing the femur flexors to the extensors—that is, creating a myoplasty—while ignoring the adductors that contribute to stability of the residual femur.[22] When

the adductors are not anchored to bone, the hip abductors are able to act unopposed, producing a dynamic flexion-abduction deformity. This deformity prepositions the femur in an orientation that is not conducive to efficient walking.[23,24] The retracted adductor muscles lead to a poorly cushioning soft-tissue envelope, further complicating prosthetic fitting.[25]

The cross-sectional area of the adductor magnus is three to four times larger than that of the adductor longus and brevis combined. It has a moment arm with the best mechanical advantage. Transection of the adductor magnus at the time of amputation leads to substantial loss of cross-sectional area, a reduction in the effective moment arm, and loss of up to 70% of the adductor pull.[20,25] This results in overall weakness of the adductor force of the thigh and subsequent abduction of the residual femur (Figure 7). The decrease in overall limb strength is due to (1) a reduction in muscle mass at the time

of the amputation, (2) inadequate mechanical fixation of the remaining muscles, and (3) atrophy of the remaining muscles.[26,27]

MRI has demonstrated a 40% to 60% decrease in muscle bulk after a traumatic transfemoral amputation. Most of the atrophy is in the adductor and hamstring muscles, whereas the intact hip abductors and flexors show smaller changes, ranging from 0% to 30%.[28,29] As much as 70% atrophy of the adductor magnus has been found. The amount of atrophy correlates with the length of the residual limb, and this atrophy is most likely due to loss of the muscle insertion.

Electromyographic studies of residual limbs following transfemoral amputation have revealed normal muscle phasic activity; however, the active period of the retained muscles appears to be prolonged.[29] The electrical activity of sectioned muscles varies, depending on whether the muscles have been reanchored and on the length of the residual fe-

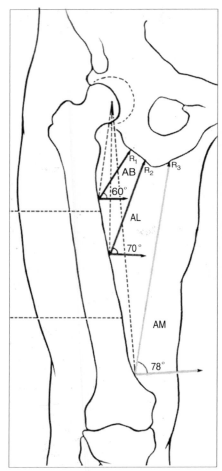

**Figure 7** Diagram of the resultant forces of the adductor muscles. The relative insertion sites of the abductors are indicated. The shorter the residual femur, the weaker the limb. AB = adductor brevis muscle, AL = adductor longus muscle, AM = adductor magnus muscle.

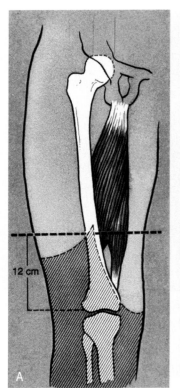
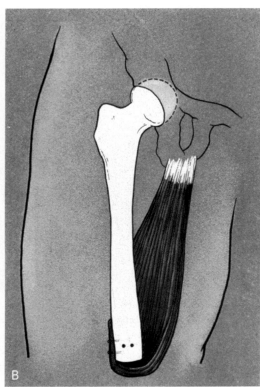

**Figure 8** Adductor myodesis method of transfemoral amputation. **A,** Skin flaps and proposed bone cut. The osseous transection is optimally created at 5 in (12.5 cm) proximal to the knee joint, but it can be more proximal if necessary. **B,** The adductor magnus tendon is secured to the residual femur through drill holes in the lateral cortex. (Reprinted with permission from Gottschalk F: Transfemoral amputation: Surgical management, in Smith DG, Michael JW, Bowker JH (eds): *Atlas of Amputations and Limb Deficiencies*, ed 3. Rosemont, IL, American Academy of Orthopaedic Surgeons, 2004, p 537-538.)

mur. Furthermore, asymmetric gait has been related to residual limb length, and lateral bending of the trunk has been correlated directly with atrophy of the hip stabilizing muscles.[30]

All of these findings indicate the need to preserve the hip adductors and hamstrings. Preservation of a functional adductor magnus helps to maintain the muscle balance between the adductors and abductors by allowing the adductor magnus to maintain its power and retain the mechanical advantage for positioning the femur. Preservation is best accomplished with a myodesis. The patient is positioned supine with a sandbag under the buttocks to avoid performing the myodesis with the hip in a flexed position and thus producing an iatrogenic hip flexion contracture. A tourniquet is generally not necessary for patients with peripheral vascular disease. Depending on the size of the patient, a standard, or a sterile, tourniquet can be used when the transfemoral amputation is being performed because of a traumatic injury or a tumor and normal femoral vessels can be expected.

Equal anterior and posterior flaps should be avoided, as such flaps place the suture line under the end of the residual limb, making prosthetic fitting more difficult and adequate muscular padding less likely. A long medial-based myofasciocutaneous flap is dependent on the vascular supply from the obturator artery, which generally has less severe vascular disease and is thus preferred[31] (Figure 8). The flap configuration may need to be modified, to preserve residual limb length, when an amputation is done after trauma or because of neoplastic disease. The tendon of the adductor magnus is detached. The femoral vessels are identified in Hunter's canal and are ligated. The major nerves should be dissected 2 to 4 cm proximal to the proposed bone cut, gently retracted, and sectioned with a new sharp blade. The quadriceps is detached just proximal to the patella, with retention of some of its tendinous portion. The smaller muscles, including the sartorius and gracilis and the more posterior group of hamstrings (biceps femoris, semitendinosus, and semimembranosus) should be transected 2 to 2.5 cm longer than the proposed bone cut to facilitate the anchoring of those muscles in bone.

The femur is then transected with an oscillating power saw 12 to 14 cm proximal to the knee joint to allow sufficient space for the prosthetic knee joint. Drill holes are made in the distal end of the femur to anchor the transected muscles. The adductor magnus is attached to the lateral cortex of the femur while the femur is held in maximum adduction. This allows appropriate tensioning of the anchored muscle. The hip is positioned in extension for reattachment of the quadriceps to the posterior part of the femur, and the remaining hamstrings are anchored to the posterior area of the adductor magnus or the quadriceps.[32]

### Postoperative Care

A soft compression dressing with a mini-spica wrap above the pelvis is used in the early postoperative period. Because the residual limb is relatively short, it is difficult to maintain a rigid plaster dressing. Range of motion exercises and early walking are encouraged. Preparatory prosthetic fitting can be initiated as soon as the residual limb appears capable of accepting the load associated with weight bearing. This varies with individual patients and the experience of the rehabilitation team.

### Summary

An amputation should be considered the first step in the rehabilitation of a patient for whom reconstruction of a functional limb is not possible. Care should be taken to create a residual limb that can optimally interact with a prosthetic socket to create a residual limb-prosthetic socket relationship capable of substituting for the highly adaptive end organ of weight bearing. A well-motivated patient in whom the amputation is done well and who is taught how to use the prosthesis will be able to return to most activities.

### References

1. Bosse MJ, MacKenzie EJ, Kellam JF, et al: An analysis of outcomes of reconstruction or amputation after leg-threatening injuries. *N Engl J Med* 2002;347:1924-1931.

2. Gottschalk F: Transfemoral amputation: Biomechanics and surgery. *Clin Orthop Relat Res* 1999;361:15-22.

3. Pinzur MS: New concepts in lower-limb amputation and prosthetic management. *Instr Course Lect* 1990;39:361-366.

4. Loon HE. Below-knee amputation surgery. *Artif Limbs.* 1962;6:86-99.

5. Pinto MA, Harris WW: Fibular segment bone bridging in trans-tibial amputation. *Prosthet Orthot Int* 2004;28:220-224.

6. Hoaglund FT, Jergesen HE, Wilson L, Lamoreux LW, Roberts R: Evaluation of problems and needs of veteran lower-limb amputees in the San Francisco Bay Area during the period 1977-1980. *J Rehabil R D* 1983;20:57-71.

7. Legro MW, Reiber GD, Smith DG, del Aguila M, Larsen J, Boone D: Prosthesis evaluation questionnaire for persons with lower limb amputations: Assessing prosthesis-related quality of life. *Arch Phys Med Rehabil* 1998;79:931-938.

8. Ertl J: Uber amputationsstumpfe. *Chirurg* 1949;20:218-224.

9. Deffer PA. Ertl osteoplasty at Valley Forge General Hospital (interview). Committee on Prosthetic-Orthotic Education. Newsletter Amputee Clinics 1969;1.

10. Murdoch G (ed): Prosthetic and orthotic practice, based on a conference held in Dundee, June, 1969. London, UK, Edward Arnold, 1970, pp 52-56.

11. Pinzur MS, Pinto MA, Saltzman M, Batista F, Gottschalk F, Juknelis D: Health-related quality of life in patients with transtibial amputation and reconstruction with bone bridging of the distal tibia and fibula. *Foot Ankle Int* 2006;27:907-912.

12. Pinzur MS, Pinto MA, Schon LC, Smith DG: Controversies in amputation surgery. *Instr Course Lect* 2003;52:445-451.

13. Burgess EM, Romano RL, Zettl JH, Prosthetic Research Study: The management of lower-extremity amputations: Surgery, immediate postsurgical prosthetic fitting, patient care. Washington, DC, US Government Printing Office, 1969. Available at: http://www.prs-research.org/htmPages/Reference/BibRefs.html#text. Accessed March 13, 2007.

14. Assal M, Blanck R, Smith DG: Extended posterior flap for transtibial amputation. *Orthopedics* 2005;28:542-546.

15. Van Niekerk LJ, Stewart CP, Jain AS: Major lower limb amputation following failed infrainguinal vascular bypass surgery: A prospective study on amputation levels and stump complications. *Prosthet Orthot Int* 2001;25:29-33.

16. Jensen JS, Mandrup-Poulsen T, Kras-

nik M: Wound healing complications following major amputations of the lower limb. *Prosthet Orthot Int* 1982; 6:105-107.

17. Volpicelli LJ, Chambers RB, Wagner FW Jr: Ambulation levels of bilateral lower-extremity amputees: Analysis of one hundred and three cases. *J Bone Joint Surg Am* 1983;65: 599-605.

18. Gonzalez EG, Corcoran PJ, Reyes RL: Energy expenditure in below-knee amputees: Correlation with stump length. *Arch Phys Med Rehabil* 1974;55:111-119.

19. Long IA: Normal shape-normal alignment (NSNA) above-knee prosthesis. *Clin Prosthet Orthot* 1985; 9:9-14.

20. Gottschalk FA, Kourosh S, Stills M, McClellan B, Roberts J: Does socket configuration influence the position of the femur in above-knee amputation? *J Prosthet Orthot* 1990;2:94-102.

21. Waters RL, Perry J, Antonelli D, Hislop H: Energy cost of walking of amputees: The influence of level of amputation. *J Bone Joint Surg Am* 1976; 58:42-46.

22. Hagberg K, Branemark R: Consequences of non-vascular transfemoral amputation: A survey of quality of life, prosthetic use and problems. *Prosthet Orthot Int* 2001;25: 186-194.

23. Barnes RW, Cox B: *Amputations: An Illustrated Manual*. Philadelphia, PA, Hanley and Belfus, 2000, pp 103-117.

24. Sabolich J: Contoured adducted trochanteric-controlled alignment method (CAT-CAM): Introduction and basic principles. *Clin Prosthet Orthot* 1985;9:15-26.

25. Hungerford DS, Krackow KA, Kenna RV (eds): *Total Knee Arthroplasty: A Comprehensive Approach*. Baltimore, MD, Williams and Wilkins, 1984, pp 34-39.

26. Gottschalk FA, Stills M: The biomechanics of trans-femoral amputation. *Prosthet Orthot Int* 1994;18:12-17.

27. Thiele B, James U, Stalberg E: Neurophysiological studies on muscle function in the stump of above-knee amputees. *Scand J Rehabil Med* 1973;5: 67-70.

28. James U: Maximal isometric muscle strength in healthy active male unilateral above-knee amputees, with special regard to the hip joint. *Scand J Rehabil Med* 1973;5:55-66.

29. Jaegers SM, Arendzen JH, de Jongh HJ: Changes in hip muscles after above-knee amputation. *Clin Orthop Relat Res* 1995;319:276-284.

30. Jaegers SM, Arendzen JH, de Jongh HJ: An electromyographic study of the hip muscles of transfemoral amputees in walking. *Clin Orthop Relat Res* 1996;328:119-128.

31. Jaegers SM, Arendzen JH, de Jongh HJ: Prosthetic gait of unilateral transfemoral amputees: A kinematic study. *Arch Phys Med Rehabil* 1995; 76:736-743.

32. Pinzur MS, Bowker JH, Smith DG, Gottschalk F: Amputation surgery in peripheral vascular disease. *Instr Course Lect* 1999;48:687-691.

# Malignant Bone Tumors

Kristy Weber, MD
*Timothy A. Damron, MD, FACS
*Frank J. Frassica, MD
Franklin H. Sim, MD

## Abstract

*Malignant bone tumors represent a small percentage of cancers nationwide and also are much less common than malignant soft-tissue tumors. The rarity of the condition makes it imperative that orthopaedic surgeons in nononcologic practices are able to recognize the symptoms that suggest a possible bony malignancy to avoid inappropriate or delayed treatment. The most common primary malignant bone tumors, osteosarcoma and Ewing's sarcoma, occur in childhood. Chondrosarcoma occurs more frequently in older adults. Rare tumors such as chordoma and adamantinoma have anatomic predilections for the sacrum and tibia, respectively. The primary symptom of a patient with a malignant bone tumor is pain, which often occurs at rest or at night. There are also characteristic findings on physical examination such as swelling or decreased joint range of motion. Patients with a likely malignancy require thorough staging to determine the extent of disease and a well-planned biopsy for accurate diagnosis. The biopsy can be an image-guided needle biopsy or an open incisional biopsy. Knowledge of specific tumor characteristics and treatment options for osteosarcoma, Ewing's sarcoma, chondrosarcoma, malignant fibrous histiocytoma, chordoma, and adamantinoma is important. Patients with osteosarcoma and resectable Ewing's sarcoma are treated with chemotherapy followed by surgical resection. Secondary sarcomas can occur in previously benign bone lesions and require aggressive treatment. Specific techniques are available for the resection of malignant bone tumors from the upper extremities, lower extremities, pelvis, and spine. Reconstruction options include the use of allografts, megaprostheses, and vascularized autografts. There has been a trend toward more prosthetic reconstructions because of early complications with allografts. The care of patients with primary malignant bone tumors requires a multidisciplinary approach to treatment. The orthopaedic oncologist is a vital member of a team composed of musculoskeletal radiologists and pathologists, radiation oncologists, medical and pediatric oncologists, and microvascular surgeons.*

**Instr Course Lect 2008;57:673-688.**

*Timothy A. Damron, MD, FACS or the department with which he is affiliated has received research or institutional support from NIH/NCI, Genentech, and Orthovita. Frank J. Frassica, MD is a consultant or employee for SLACK, Inc and Stryker.*

Malignant bone tumors comprise an uncommon and heterogeneous group of cancers. Each year in the United States there are approximately 2,900 new bone sarcomas accounting for less than 1% of new cancer cases.[1] Primary malignant bone tumors may arise within the medullary cavity or on the surface of bones. They are classified along the direction of cell differentiation.[2] Major categories are bone producing, cartilage producing, fibrous, and histiocytic; a few tumors such as Ewing's tumor and adamantinoma have cells of unknown origin. There is also a group of secondary bone sarcomas that occur within irradiated bone or preexisting benign lesions such as Paget's disease, osteochondroma, fibrous dysplasia, or bone infarct.

## General Characteristics
### Grading
Grading of malignant bone tumors is important to guide treatment and predict prognosis. Three grades (low, intermediate, or high) or four grades (well-differentiated, G1; moderately differentiated, G2; poorly differentiated, G3; or undifferentiated, G4) are

most commonly used. Low-grade tumors such as parosteal osteosarcoma, well-differentiated chondrosarcoma, and adamantinoma have a low risk of visceral metastases (< 10%). Intermediate grade tumors such as periosteal osteosarcoma have a risk of metastases of approximately 10% to 25%. High-grade tumors such as osteosarcoma, dedifferentiated chondrosarcoma, or Ewing's tumor have a risk of metastases of 80% to 90%. Adjuvant chemotherapy is used for high-grade malignant tumors when there are effective agents, whereas no adjuvants are used for low-grade tumors.

### Clinical Evaluation

Patients with high-grade malignant bone tumors commonly present with bone pain. At the beginning, pain is often intermittent and progresses to constant pain that is present at rest, at night, and with activity. The pain is often severe enough that it is not responsive to nonsteroidal anti-inflammatory medications or weak narcotics. Physical examination will often reveal a hard, fixed, tender mass. The range of motion of the affected joint is often diminished, and muscle atrophy is a common finding. Fractures occur in 5% to 10% of patients with malignant bone tumors.[3] Patients will often report a history of antecedent pain. These fractures generally occur with minor trauma or with activities of daily living.

### Staging

Staging is an important component in the evaluation of patients with bone malignancies because it enables the clinician to predict prognosis and aids in developing treatment regimens. To determine the stage of a malignant bone tumor, the grade and size of the tumor and whether there are any metastases must be known. Staging studies usually include plain radiographs, MRI of the primary site, technetium bone scan, and CT scan of the chest.

The Enneking system (staging system of the Musculoskeletal Tumor Society) stratifies patients with bone sarcomas into three stages.[4] Stage I is for low-grade lesions, stage II for high-grade lesions, and stage III for patients with metastatic disease. The suffixes A and B are used to denote whether the tumor is contained within the bone or has entered into the soft tissues. The American Joint Committee on Cancer (AJCC) staging system is based on tumor grade, size, and presence or absence of discontinuous tumor or regional/systemic metastases.[5] Low-grade lesions are stage I, high-grade lesions are stage II, a discontinuous tumor (skip metastasis) is stage III, and regional or distant metastases are stage IV. If the tumor is smaller than or equal to 8 cm, the suffix A is used; for tumors larger than 8 cm, the suffix B is used. A patient with regional lymph node metastases has a stage IVA classification, and a patient with distant metastases has a stage IVB classification.

### Biopsy

An appropriately performed biopsy is one of the most important steps in the evaluation and treatment of patients with malignant bone lesions. Mankin and associates[6] have shown that significant complications can occur when the biopsy is not performed correctly. Six major consequences and the incidence of each were identified as follows: major errors in diagnosis, 18%; nonrepresentative tissue, 9%; complications, 17%; altered treatment, 19%; unnecessary amputation, 4%; and adverse outcome, 9%.

Needle and open biopsy are the two major types of biopsy. Needle biopsies have become the dominant method of establishing a diagnosis. Fine-needle aspiration is performed by placing a small needle into the tumor and aspirating cells for analysis. For this technique to be effective, the cytologist must be experienced and have the ability to correlate the cytologic appearance of the cells with the clinical and radiographic findings. Core needle biopsy involves placing a larger bore needle into the tumor and extracting a larger core of tissue. Core needle biopsies must also be read by an experienced surgical pathologist who can correlate the histologic appearance with the clinical and radiographic findings. Open incisional biopsy is a surgical procedure during which the surgeon obtains tissue by incising into the tumor. The incision must be designed to allow excision of the entire biopsy tract at the time of the definitive resection if the tumor is found to be malignant. The incision should be oriented longitudinally and should be as small as possible. In a few anatomic areas a nonlongitudinal incision is used (clavicle, transverse; scapular body, oblique). Soft-tissue flaps are not elevated, and the biopsy is performed directly onto the tumor mass. A frozen section analysis ensures that diagnostic tissue has been obtained. Excisional open biopsy should only be performed when the surgeon is positive that the lesion is benign or when the tumor can be removed with a wide margin if the radiographic appearance supports a malignant diagnosis. Two low-grade malignancies for which an excisional biopsy is sometimes performed include parosteal osteosarcoma and low-grade chondrosarcoma.

## Specific Tumor Types

The four most common bone malignancies are osteosarcoma, Ewing's sarcoma, chondrosarcoma, and malignant fibrous histiocytoma

(MFH). Two other bone sarcomas occur in particular locations—chordoma in the sacrum and adamantinoma in the tibia. Sarcomas also may occur in bone that is abnormal, and these processes are called secondary sarcomas. The most common secondary sarcomas occur in an area of Paget's disease, following irradiation, in a bone infarct, or in a cartilage lesion such as an osteochondroma or enchondroma.

## Osteosarcoma

Osteosarcoma is the most common primary malignant mesenchymal bone tumor.[7] There are two types of intramedullary osteosarcomas: high-grade intramedullary (classic) osteosarcoma and well-differentiated intramedullary osteosarcoma. The three osteosarcomas that occur on the surface of the bone include parosteal osteosarcoma, periosteal osteosarcoma, and high-grade surface osteosarcoma.

High-grade intramedullary osteosarcoma is the most common subtype and is referred to simply as osteosarcoma. Although this high-grade bone tumor most commonly occurs in children and adolescents in the first two decades of life, it also occurs occasionally in older patients. The most common location is around the knee, and patients present with moderate to severe bone pain and a soft-tissue mass. A pathologic fracture occurs in 5% to 10% of patients.[3] Although the radiographic appearance may be variable, the most common findings are a metaphyseal lesion with a combination of bone destruction and bone formation. A mineralized soft-tissue mass is usually present.

Osteosarcoma is treated with preoperative chemotherapy followed by wide surgical resection. Intensive preoperative chemotherapy kills occult micrometastases in the pulmonary system and tumor cells at the primary site. Sterilization of occult pulmonary metastases has markedly improved the survival of patients with osteosarcoma from 20% in historical control subjects to 60% to 70% in patients treated with chemotherapy. The most important prognostic factor is the response to preoperative chemotherapy, which is determined by mapping the resection specimen and determining the percentage of necrosis in the tumor cells. When the tumor cell kill rate exceeds 95%, there is an excellent chance of long-term survival. When the rate of necrosis is less than 90%, the risk of systemic disease is higher. There is also a greater risk of local recurrence when response to preoperative chemotherapy is poor. The presence of metastases, poor response to preoperative chemotherapy, location in the pelvis or spine, and elevated serum alkaline phosphatase or lactate dehydrogenase (controversial) are factors that indicate a poor prognosis in patients with osteosarcoma.

Parosteal osteosarcoma is a low-grade surface osteosarcoma. The most common locations are the metaphysis of the distal femur, the proximal tibia, and the proximal humerus. This lesion is heavily mineralized with a broad attachment to the bone. The treatment of parosteal osteosarcoma is wide surgical resection alone. There is no role for chemotherapy, and the prognosis is excellent. The long-term survival rate with adequate local control is greater than 95%.

Periosteal osteosarcoma is an intermediate-grade sarcoma. In contrast to parosteal osteosarcoma, periosteal osteosarcomas most commonly occur in the diaphysis, and the lesion is not as heavily mineralized as parosteal osteosarcoma. Because the risk of pulmonary me-tastasis is 10% to 15%, patients are generally treated with preoperative chemotherapy and wide resection.

High-grade surface osteosarcomas are rare and treated in the same manner as high-grade intramedullary osteosarcomas. The risk of pulmonary metastases is approximately 50%.

## Ewing's Sarcoma

Ewing's sarcoma or tumor is a high-grade, small cell bone malignancy that also occurs in the first two decades of life.[8] In contrast to osteosarcoma, the tumor does not produce a matrix, and radiographs show lytic bone destruction. Ewing's sarcoma metastasizes early to the pulmonary system and bone. A balanced translocation between chromosome 11 and 22 is present in all patients. Staging studies include a technetium bone scan, a CT of the chest, and a bone marrow biopsy to exclude marrow metastases. Ewing's sarcoma is sensitive to both chemotherapy and external beam irradiation.

Although Ewing's sarcoma was historically treated with external beam irradiation for local control, there has been a shift toward definitive surgical resection. There are no prospective randomized trials comparing wide surgical resection and external beam irradiation as local control modalities. The results of surgical resection are promising in regard to local control and survival. Poor prognostic factors for survival include the presence of pulmonary or bone metastases, poor response to chemotherapy, *p53* mutations, and gene fusion products other than EWS-FLI1.[9]

## Chondrosarcoma

Chondrosarcomas occur predominantly in the medullary cavity.[10] There is a wide spectrum of biologic behavior with approximately two thirds of chondrosarcomas being grade 1 well-differentiated tumors, whereas approximately one third are grade 2 moderately differentiated tumors. Well-differentiated chondrosarcomas seldom metastasize, whereas grade 2 chondrosarcomas spread to the pulmonary system in 20% to 30% of patients. Grade 3 chondrosarcomas rarely occur but have a high risk of pulmonary metastases. Dedifferentiated chondrosarcomas are high-grade malignancies with a substantial risk of pulmonary metastases and a poor prognosis despite chemotherapy. Approximately 10% of chondrosarcomas are dedifferentiated. The histology reveals a bimorphic pattern with a high-grade spindle cell malignancy intimately admixed with a low-grade chondrosarcoma.

Wide surgical resection is the primary modality for the treatment of chondrosarcoma of bone. External beam irradiation is not used, and chemotherapy is not effective. There has been a trend toward intralesional treatment of grade 1 chondrosarcomas in the extremities in instances when no aggressive radiographic features such as frank cortical destruction or a soft-tissue mass are present. Wide resection is necessary for grade 1 chondrosarcomas in the pelvis. Local recurrence of low-grade chondrosarcoma portends a poor prognosis.

### Malignant Fibrous Histiocytoma

MFH is a high-grade malignant bone tumor that primarily occurs in patients older than 40 years of age.[11] This tumor is anaplastic and has been reclassified by the World Health Organization as undifferentiated, high-grade, pleomorphic bone sarcoma. This aggressive neoplasm quickly destroys the cortical bone and extends

into the soft tissues. Plain radiographs show a markedly destructive lytic lesion. Approximately one fourth of MFHs arise in preexisting bone lesions such as Paget's disease, in bone infarcts, and following irradiation. These lesions are treated with wide surgical resection. Most patients are also given adjuvant chemotherapy and are placed on osteosarcoma regimens. Bacci and associates[12] reported a good response rate of only 25% in 65 patients treated with preoperative chemotherapy. Although the response to preoperative chemotherapy was significantly better in patients with osteosarcoma compared with MFH (67% versus 27%), Picci and associates[13] reported similar disease-free survival rates (approximately 65%).

### Adamantinoma

Adamantinoma is a low-grade malignancy that occurs almost exclusively in the diaphysis of the tibia. Patients often have a long history of variable pain and even deformity of the leg. Adamantinoma of bone progresses slowly and is characterized by multiple lucencies with intervening sclerosis. Treatment is wide resection of the bone and intercalary reconstruction. Because this tumor principally involves the diaphysis, the adjacent joints often can be saved. Metastases to the lungs (15%), lymph nodes (7%), and other bones may occur late in the course of the disease.[14] Limb salvage is performed in 90% of patients; however, the risk of local recurrence is almost 20%.

### Chordoma

Chordoma is a rare, low-grade malignancy that arises from notochordal tissue. Because the notochord is a midline structure, chordomas begin centrally and occur primarily in the sacrococcygeal and spheno-occipital

regions. Approximately 10% of chordomas occur in the mobile spine. Sacrococcygeal chordomas grow slowly, and patients often present for treatment with reports of months to years of pelvic pain. As the tumor extends anteriorly, bowel and bladder dysfunction may occur secondary to sacral nerve root compromise. Because this tumor is difficult to detect on plain radiographs, cross-sectional imaging is necessary. Chordomas are treated with wide resection alone. Chemotherapy has no measurable effect, and radiation therapy is reserved for patients with positive margins or unresectable disease. The local failure rate often exceeds 50% at long-term follow-up.[15] Metastases to bone and lungs occur in 5% to 30% of patients in late stages of the disease.

### Secondary Sarcomas

A high-grade sarcoma can develop within a preexisting bone lesion. Examples of common conditions in which a bone sarcoma may develop include Paget's disease, bone infarcts, and following irradiation. Most patients report severe pain for several months' duration. MRI or CT scans are the best modalities to detect the cortical bone destruction present in secondary sarcomas. High-grade osteosarcoma and MFH are the most common histologic diagnoses in patients with secondary osteosarcomas. Patients who can tolerate intensive chemotherapy regimens are treated in the same fashion as those with osteosarcoma. Older patients who have multiple medical comorbidities are treated with wide surgical resection alone.

## Upper Extremity Limb Salvage

Bone sarcomas are less common in the upper extremity than the lower extremity. In the upper extremity, the proximal humerus is the most common site, followed by the scapula.

## Clavicle

No reconstruction is necessary after total resection of the clavicle, and functional outcome is excellent. Most of the literature regarding functional outcome after removal of the clavicle derives from that for thoracic outlet syndrome and vascular access. Reported complications include shoulder drooping, mild weakness, and trapezius dysfunction.

## Scapula

A scapulectomy may be performed as a partial or complete resection, and it may be intra-articular or extra-articular depending on the extent of the tumor. Reconstructive needs differ according to the site of resection. For inferior scapular body resection, the glenohumeral joint is preserved. No bony reconstruction is needed, and appropriate muscle closure should obliterate the dead space. Even when the rotator cuff muscles must be removed, inferior body partial scapulectomy may provide an excellent result if the deltoid is reattached to the remaining scapula and trapezius. For a partial scapulectomy involving glenoid resection, the glenoid can be reconstructed with an osteoarticular allograft or a custom prosthesis, or the humeral head can be left to articulate with the remaining scapular body with or without soft-tissue interposition. Functional outcomes following these rare procedures and their reconstructions are not well documented.

Total scapulectomy patients are commonly left with either a flail shoulder or undergo reconstruction with a scapular prosthesis.[16] In flail shoulder reconstruction, the humeral head is suspended from the clavicle or rib using Dacron (Invista, Wichita, KS) or Mersilene tape (Braun, Tuttligen, Germany) or its equivalent.[17] The purported advantage of a scapular endoprosthesis is the lateralization of the humeral head, which provides a better fulcrum for motion and hence improves function. As long as the proximal humerus is stabilized to another anatomic structure after either a flail or prosthetic reconstruction, the elbow, forearm, wrist, and hand will have near-normal function.[18] In a study by Wittig and associates,[19] the authors reported that the shoulders were consistently stable and that some protraction, retraction, elevation, and abduction of the scapula was restored with use of a constrained scapular prosthesis.

## Proximal Humerus

Proximal humeral resection may be done in an intra-articular or extra-articular fashion with or without maintenance of the deltoid/axillary nerve. This creates four possible types of proximal humeral resection. The best functional outcome is achieved when the deltoid-axillary nerve functional unit is preserved in conjunction with an intra-articular resection. If the deltoid/axillary nerve function is preserved, there is potential for reasonable shoulder function after an extra-articular resection.

When a proximal humeral intra-articular resection is done with preservation of the deltoid/axillary nerve functional unit, options for reconstruction include an osteoarticular allograft (OA), an allograft-prosthetic composite (APC), and a megaprosthesis.

An OA provides the advantage of allowing host rotator cuff repair to tendons remaining on the allograft. Plate fixation is the preferred method of allograft stabilization to host bone. One complication that has discouraged the use of OA in favor of APC has been the occurrence of subchondral collapse a few years after implantation.[20] A potential solution to this complication, which may also decrease the incidence of infection, is the use of an antibiotic cement-loaded allograft.

APC reconstruction offers a solution to allograft fracture complications encountered with OA (Figure 1). Allograft joint collapse is essentially eliminated because of the prosthetic humeral head. Like OA, an APC offers the potential advantage of reattaching the host tendons to the allograft tendons. The allograft is secured with the cemented intramedullary stem of the humeral prosthesis with or without a supplementary plate.

A megaprosthesis also may be used for reconstruction of the proximal humerus. There is less reliable soft-tissue reconstitution into the metallic prosthesis. These prostheses serve as effective spacers, providing a fulcrum for stable function of the distal joints.[18] Malawer and Chou[21] reported the best function (mean, Musculoskeletal Tumor Society score, 26 on a 30-point scale) and lowest complication rate (10% revision, 3 of 29 patients) for proximal humeral megaprosthesis reconstructions compared with all other sites.

Technical considerations when implanting a megaprosthesis include using a 40-mm head size to allow appropriate soft-tissue closure and a minimum 9-mm × 75-mm stem to minimize fatigue failure. The prosthetic head can be suspended by Dacron or Mersilene tape, and an aortic graft sleeve, alloderm, or mesh may be considered for capsular repair to enhance stability. Megaprosthetic

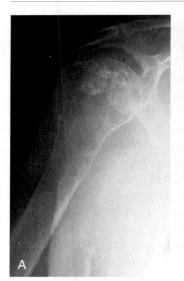 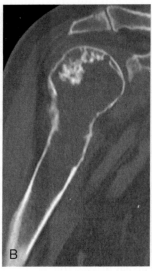 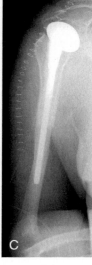

**Figure 1** AP radiograph **(A)** and CT scan **(B)** showing a right proximal humeral grade 2 chondrosarcoma. The segment was resected in an intra-articular fashion with deltoid and axillary nerve preservation and a wide distal margin. An allograft-prosthetic composite reconstruction was chosen, cementing the prosthesis first into the allograft, followed by cementing into the host bone **(C)**.

proximal humeral reconstructions have a low incidence of loosening, but dislocation and instability have been described.[20]

Comparative functional outcomes between the various alternatives have been reported based on clinical outcome and laboratory analysis.[18,20] In a functional laboratory study, OA provided good early strength and range of motion with diminishing function over time if subchondral collapse occurred.[18] In another clinical study originating from the same institution, OA was found to have superior function when compared with early versions of the proximal humeral megaprosthesis when abductor function was preserved.[20]

For those patients in whom the deltoid/axillary nerve unit must be sacrificed, most surgeons limit their alternatives to a suspension procedure, accepting limited shoulder function and focusing on providing a stable shoulder to support distal

function. When an intra-articular resection can be performed, an arthrodesis will potentially provide the patient with the least long-term dysfunction and the strongest extremity.[20] The correct position of abduction is crucial and is described as 20° from neutral, which is achieved by positioning the limb in 50° of abduction relative to the lateral scapular border. However, achieving a successful arthrodesis after proximal humeral resection necessitates using an intercalary allograft, a vascularized fibula, or both. This technically demanding and lengthy procedure has many potential complications, including a high incidence of fracture.[20]

Based on functional laboratory evaluation, it was shown that successful vascularized fibular shoulder arthrodeses, which were generally not done if the rotator cuff and deltoid/axillary nerve could be preserved, resulted in shoulder range of motion that was as good as that

achieved with OA reconstruction, except in rotation. However, shoulder strength after arthrodeses was significantly less than that following OA.[18]

The alternative for patients with no functional deltoid/axillary nerve unit is a functional spacer. A megaprosthesis can be used in this situation, but there are no published functional data to show any advantage over a low-profile suspension device attached to the remaining bone.[18,20] Subluxation may still occur with prosthetic spacers and is generally more prominent when there is no remaining glenoid from which to suspend the prosthesis. In most instances, the subluxation remains asymptomatic apart from the expected poor shoulder function.[20] One additional option is the clavicle pro humero reconstruction in which the medial aspect of the clavicle is released and rotated down to the remaining humerus and affixed there.

When an extra-articular resection is done, most surgeons find there is insufficient bone remaining to articulate either an allograft or prosthesis regardless of the presence of a functional deltoid/axillary nerve. Therefore, the most common alternatives are either arthrodesis or a spacer.

### Humeral Diaphysis

Reconstructive options after resection of the humeral diaphysis include intercalary autogenous bone grafts, allografts, and prostheses. If secure fixation can be achieved, maintenance of normal shoulder and elbow function usually affords the patient an excellent overall functional outcome. Secure fixation for bone grafts requires healing of the graft-host junctions and, for prosthetic spacers, good technique without aseptic loosening.

The most commonly used autogenous graft for this location is the fibula, which may be used in either a nonvascularized or vascularized fashion.[22] Vascularized grafts must generally be 8 cm or longer to preserve the blood supply, but shorter grafts may be harvested in a nonvascularized fashion. Vascularized grafts have the advantage of faster healing times and lower fracture risk than nonvascularized grafts. Dual or "double-barrel" vascularized fibular grafts generally provide adequate stability to allow avoidance of additional fixation. Single fibular grafts, however, may require supplementation with internal fixation.

Intercalary humeral allograft reconstructions require more prolonged healing time than autogenous grafts and should be protected by internal fixation. Plate fixation of humeral allografts should span the entire allograft and should minimize the number of holes in the graft to reduce fracture risk. Allograft contents should be removed to decrease the antigenicity, and consideration should be given to intramedullary antibiotic-loaded cement to minimize the risks of fracture and infection.

A third alternative for humeral shaft reconstruction is a metallic humeral intercalary spacer prosthesis.[23] These spacers are generally reserved for patients with a shortened life expectancy. The intramedullary stems should be cemented. The current lap joint and set screw junction eliminates the need for overdistraction required with earlier models, which had a male-female Morse taper junction.

### Distal Humerus

Reconstructive options for the distal humerus include OA, APC, and dis-

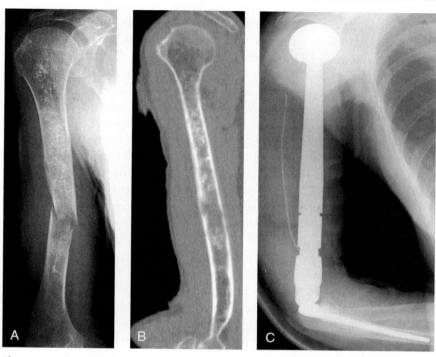

**Figure 2** Radiograph **(A)** of a pathologic fracture of the right humeral diaphysis, which occurred through an extensive grade 1 chondrosarcoma after a preoperative CT scan **(B)** had been performed. **C,** Following total humeral resection, a total humeral endoprosthesis was used for reconstruction along with a synthetic aortic graft sleeve to allow soft-tissue reconstruction and provide stability at the shoulder joint.

tal humeral megaprostheses.[24] However, because there are no important tendinous origins or insertions on the distal humerus, the addition of allograft is generally believed to increase the risk of infection, fracture, and joint mismatch without adding significant function. For this reason, megaprostheses are most often used for this location (Figure 2). Distal humeral modular elbow reconstructions have been reported with complications, including periprosthetic lysis and revision for loosening of the distal humeral components.[24] Total humeral resection requires combining the considerations for both proximal humeral and distal humeral reconstruction. The most commonly used reconstruction in this instance is a total humeral megaprosthesis; approximately 70% of these patients

have been reported to have satisfactory functional outcome.[24]

### Forearm, Wrist, and Hand

Bone sarcomas rarely occur in distal upper extremity locations. After resection of the proximal radius, reconstructive alternatives include a one-bone forearm reconstruction, an autogenous fibular graft, and an allograft. Function after a one-bone forearm reconstruction is excellent because patients usually adapt well to the lack of forearm rotation by positioning their hand in space using the shoulder and elbow. It is the preferred method of reconstruction unless there is enough remaining proximal and distal bone to allow internal fixation of an intercalary bone segment.

Following resection of the distal

radius, articulating wrist reconstructions may be accomplished by use of an osteoarticular allograft or a proximal fibular autograft.[22] The proximal fibula should be harvested with the insertion of the biceps tendon or a portion of the lateral collateral ligament to enhance soft-tissue reconstruction at the wrist joint. Unless the segment of distal radius to be replaced is 8 cm or longer, the fibular graft is implanted in a nonvascularized fashion. Wrist arthrodesis is the other alternative following distal radius resection. Either an intercalary allograft or the proximal fibula may be used in the intervening defect. Proximal ulnar resection usually necessitates a proximal ulnar megaprosthesis with total elbow arthroplasty using a conventional humeral component. For the distal ulna, no reconstruction is needed because it is generally considered an expendable bone.

Bone sarcomas are distinctly rare in the hand. When they occur, wide resection is indicated, and the extent of resection will be dictated by the anatomic location of the tumor. For metacarpal tumors, ray resections are used. Achieving an adequate margin often requires resection of one or both adjacent rays, depending on the extent of soft-tissue extension. Following thumb amputation, function and reconstructive options depend on the level of amputation. For resection at or close to the metacarpophalangeal joint, either distraction-lengthening osteogenesis or microvascular transfers of the great toe or second toe may be used. For phalangeal tumors, the level of amputation is dictated by the tumor location. For distal phalangeal tumors, transmiddle phalangeal amputation is required. For middle or proximal phalangeal tumors, ray resection is recommended.

## Lower Extremity Limb Salvage

Most malignant bone tumors are located in the lower extremities, with the distal femur as the most common site. Because of advances in neoadjuvant chemotherapy and sophisticated biomedical imaging of tumors, it is possible to perform limb-sparing procedures in 90% of patients. It has been shown that overall survival is not compromised in patients who have limb-salvage procedures compared with those who have undergone amputation.[25] Patients treated with successful limb-sparing surgery have improved functional outcomes and a better quality of life; the procedure is also more cost-effective. Other surgical challenges in the treatment of patients with malignant bone tumors include defining an adequate surgical margin and developing biologic and prosthetic reconstructions that match patients' improved life expectancies. The primary methods of reconstruction of a defect following surgical resection of a malignant bone tumor include the use of allografts, autografts, and megaprostheses.

### Allografts

The use of cadaveric allografts was popularized by Mankin and associates[26] in the early years of limb-sparing surgery.[27] The advantages include biologic reconstruction in young patients with the restoration of bone stock in the area where the tumor was resected. Specific options include OAs, APCs, and intercalary allografts.

### Osteoarticular Allograft

The OA was historically most commonly used for reconstruction of the proximal tibia and the distal femur. It was occasionally used to reconstruct the proximal femur; however, the size-matching required for the graft to exactly fit the host acetabulum precluded its use in many patients. The ligaments on the allograft must be meticulously attached to the remaining host ligaments at the hip or knee to ensure joint stability. The host-allograft junction also needs sufficient compression to facilitate healing. The disadvantages of OA reconstruction include the occurrence of graft resorption, subchondral collapse, joint instability with subsequent degenerative changes, and a prolonged healing time. Theoretically, patients receiving chemotherapy have an increased risk of delayed union or nonunion of the allograft-host junction, although this finding remains controversial. Unrelated to the specific joint reconstruction, allografts in general have an increased incidence of fractures (15% to 20%), nonunion (17% to 30%), and infection (8% to 18%).[26] Although some major tumor centers continue to use OA reconstruction for high-grade bone sarcomas, this technique is more commonly used for aggressive benign bone lesions such as giant cell tumor.

### Allograft Prosthetic Composite

An APC allows the advantages of using an allograft without the specific disadvantages related to the joint surface.[28] Compared with a megaprosthesis, the APC's ability to attach the soft tissues of the allograft to those of the host allows improved function. This reconstruction is most commonly used in the proximal tibia and proximal femur, where soft-tissue attachments of the patellar and abductor tendons, respectively, have allowed improved function compared with patients with a megaprosthesis[29] (Figure 3). Postoperatively, braces are usually used to allow tendon healing before starting range-of-motion exercises. There is greater joint stability, especially using constrained-hinged designs about the knee. A long-stemmed prosthesis is placed through the allograft into the distal host bone. Most commonly, the prosthesis is cemented into the allograft and either cemented or press fit into the host bone. Autogenous bone graft or bone graft substitutes can be placed at the allograft-host junction to enhance healing.

### Intercalary Allograft

An intercalary allograft has the distinct advantage of avoiding joint reconstruction. It is used for diaphyseal defects in the femur or tibia. The cartilage deterioration and joint instability complications of the OA are avoided. However, there are two allograft-host junctions and both require meticulous surgical technique to achieve rigid compression and decrease the incidence of nonunion that can occur in up to 30% of patients.[27] Autogenous bone graft can be used at the junctions to enhance healing. Fixation of the allograft can be performed with a plate or intramedullary rod (Figure 4). Newer devices incorporating locking plate technology or compression rod constructs will likely decrease the risk of hardware failure. As previously mentioned, the allograft can be filled with antibiotic-impregnated cement to decrease the incidence of fracture and infection. More recently, surgeons have been making great efforts to preserve the joint surface with transepiphyseal resections, especially in younger patients. This method requires rigid fixation into the subchondral bone. If the growth plate is resected in a very young child, later procedures will be required to equalize leg length. To decrease the incidence of nonunion, some surgeons will sup-

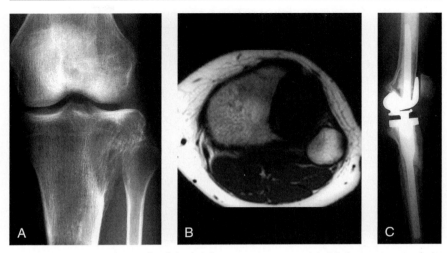

**Figure 3** **A,** AP radiograph of the left knee in a 15-year-old girl shows an osteolytic lesion in the proximal tibia, which was consistent with an MFH after needle biopsy. **B,** An axial MRI further defines the extent of the tumor. **C,** The patient had a wide resection after preoperative chemotherapy and reconstruction using an APC. The patient has full active extension and walks without a limp.

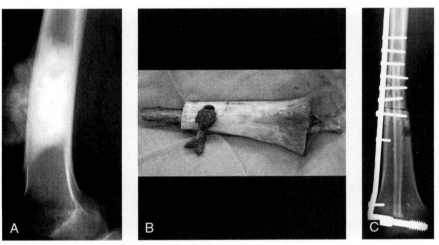

**Figure 4** **A,** Lateral radiograph of the distal femur in an 18-year-old woman shows an osteoblastic lesion consistent with a high-grade osteosarcoma. After preoperative chemotherapy, a joint-sparing resection was performed. **B,** The patient had reconstruction using an intercalary allograft combined with a vascularized fibular graft placed inside the allograft. **C,** The postoperative AP radiograph shows fixation of the allograft using plate fixation.

plement one or both junctions with a vascularized fibular graft. In countries where allografts are not readily available, a cemented metal intercalary spacer similar to that used for diaphyseal humeral reconstruction is used.

### Arthrodesis

Historically, arthrodesis was used more commonly for limb reconstruction after bone tumor resection than it is currently. With the advent of mobile joint arthroplasties, patients often prefer this option that

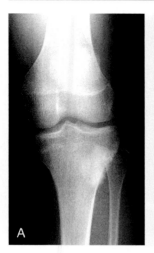
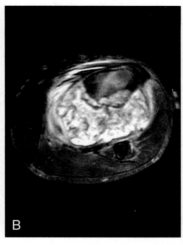
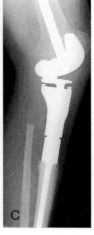

**Figure 5**    **A,** AP radiograph of the knee of a 15-year-old boy shows an osteoblastic lesion consistent with a high-grade osteosarcoma in the proximal tibia. **B,** Axial MRI shows a large soft-tissue mass abutting the fibula. **C,** The patient had a wide resection including the proximal fibula after preoperative chemotherapy and reconstruction with a proximal tibial megaprosthesis with rotating hinge knee replacement.

offers functional knee or hip motion. For arthrodesis about the knee, a slide of the patient's own remaining tibia or femur can be used to fill the defect. More commonly, an intercalary allograft with or without a supplemental vascularized fibular graft is used. With allograft arthrodesis, high complication rates of 20% infection, 25% fracture, and 44% nonunion have been reported. The reconstruction is stabilized with intramedullary or plate fixation. The most common anatomic area where arthrodesis is currently used is the ankle, for patients who have resection of distal tibial malignancies.

### Prosthetic Reconstruction

Advances in the areas of metallurgy, biomaterials, and joint design have made prosthetic reconstruction the mainstay of treatment after periarticular malignant bone tumor resection. The current models are modular so that replacing the exact defect with the correctly sized implant is not difficult. Implants include options for cemented or press-fit stems, porous coating on the surface of the prosthesis at the bone junction, or novel designs that use stable compression to increase osseointegration at the bone-implant interface. The advantages of prosthetic reconstruction in the patient with a tumor include immediate weight bearing (cemented stems); excellent function; increased durability compared with allografts; and few initial complications, which allows resumption of chemotherapy without delay. This quick return to function is especially important for patients with metastasis who have a poorer prognosis. The major disadvantages involve late complications such as loosening. The reconstruction of the patellar tendon or hip abductors directly to the prosthesis is not as solid as tendon-to-tendon fixation; therefore, the patient may have a residual extension lag or limp, respectively. As is the situation with allografts, a major infection involving the prosthesis,

which can occur in up to 13% of patients, can be devastating. Megaprostheses are commonly used for the distal femur, the proximal tibia, and proximal femur and have an overall implant survival rate of 70% to 80% at 10 years[21,30,31] (Figure 5). Outcome studies show implant survival to be highest for proximal femoral replacements and lowest for proximal tibial replacements. A study of 251 patients who had reconstruction with cementless megaprostheses reported a 10-year implant survival of 96% for the proximal femur, 76% for the distal femur, and 85% for the proximal tibia.[32] Megaprostheses are often used to salvage a failed allograft reconstruction with satisfactory results. Revision of distal femoral megaprostheses has similar follow-up failure rates and function as the primary reconstruction.

In the growing child, the challenges of reconstruction are magnified because of the limb-length discrepancies expected after resection of a tumor involving the growth plate. Historically, expandable prostheses allowed equalization of leg lengths and were an alternative to amputation or rotationplasty. However, they required multiple surgeries throughout the growth of the child until skeletal maturity was reached, thereby increasing the risk of infection. Early complications included a high incidence of aseptic failure (from 70% to 100% at 5 years), marked stress shielding, and a high incidence of expansion mechanism failure that made repeat surgeries necessary. Newer designs are available for the hip and knee, allowing cemented or cementless fixation, and involve different types of expansion mechanisms. The recent models involve minimally invasive lengthening that can be done without a major incision. The latest technology allows noninvasive expansion of the prosthesis without anesthesia using electromagnetic induction in both the United States and England.[33] Early results are encouraging and should improve with continued redesign of the implants to minimize failure.

### Vascularized Autografts

The search for better biologic alternatives for limb reconstruction is ongoing. The use of vascularized autografts, primarily the fibula, has a long history of use to stimulate healing of fractures. They are often used for patients with malignant bone tumors to facilitate earlier healing of an allograft or a radiated nonunion site. In young children, vascularized fibular grafts can be used alone as an intercalary segment after tibial or femoral diaphyseal resection. This requires a longer period of protected weight bearing to allow hypertrophy of the vascularized graft. The possibility of vascularized allografts for future use is intriguing but will require more research into safer immunosuppressive agents that could be used in combination with chemotherapeutic agents for appropriate patients.

### Soft-Tissue Advances

After major resection of malignant bone tumors, a large bone and soft-tissue defect remains. Historically, a high incidence of infection associated with allograft or prosthetic reconstruction was caused by compromised blood supply to the surrounding tissues, loss of protective muscle bulk, and low white blood cell counts in patients receiving chemotherapy. The advent of adequate soft-tissue coverage and reconstruction involved the use of local muscle or myocutaneous flaps and free-tissue transfers. This coverage led to a marked decrease in infection rates and is now the standard treatment for patients with large soft-tissue defects. More recently, reinnervated free-muscle transplants can be performed to increase function.[34] A reinnervated latissimus dorsi free flap used to reconstruct loss of the quadriceps muscle allows improvement in active knee extension.

The type of reconstruction used for a particular patient after malignant bone tumor resection depends on many factors, including availability of a particular allograft or prosthesis, the extent of surgery required, the patient's age and expectations, and the surgeon's experience.

## Pelvic and Sacral Limb Salvage

A broad spectrum of tumors involves the pelvis and sacrum, including approximately 25% of chondrosarcomas, 20% of Ewing's sarcomas, and 10% of osteosarcomas.[2] Management of malignant tumors in the pelvis and sacrum remains one of the most difficult challenges in orthopaedic oncology. Diagnosis is often delayed because of the insidious onset of pain, and vague initial symptoms are often attributed to minor trauma, inflammation, or degenerative conditions. The complex regional anatomy and the necessity for wide surgical margins can make surgical treatment demanding.

Historically, most patients with pelvic sarcomas required an external hemipelvectomy, and survival rates were poor. However, in the early 1970s, limb-preserving internal hemipelvectomy was pioneered and has become the standard practice to treat most patients. The development of sophisticated imaging to more clearly delineate the extent of the lesion, effective neoadjuvant chemotherapy, and improved techniques of resection and reconstruction have allowed limb salvage surgery without compromising local control.[35]

### Surgical Considerations

A systematic approach to preoperative evaluation and treatment is essential for patients with pelvic sarcoma. The ability to achieve adequate surgical margins in large lesions that abut adjacent neurovascular and pelvic visceral structures is facilitated by a multidisciplinary team approach.

In planning treatment, the first issue to resolve is whether the lesion can be safely removed using a limb-sparing approach or whether amputation (external hemipelvectomy) is warranted. This decision depends on factors including whether the tumor abuts the critical neurovascular structures and what reconstructive options are available. For surgical planning purposes, special attention must be paid to the relationship of the tumor to the lumbosacral plexus, the femoral neurovascular bundle, and the hip joint. As a general rule, if any two of these three structures can be preserved while safely removing the tumor, a limb-sparing approach is warranted. Otherwise, the functional consequences outweigh the added morbidity of attempts at limb preservation, and amputation should be strongly considered.

### Internal Hemipelvectomy

Internal hemipelvectomy involves removal of a portion of the hemipelvis with preservation of the ipsilateral extremity. Types of resection can be classified based on the area of bone removed, with type I resection involving removal of the iliac wing; type II, removal of the periacetabular region; and type III, resection of the ischiopubic region (Figure 6).

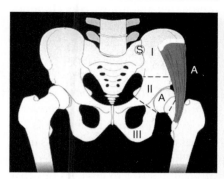

**Figure 6** Schematic diagram illustrating the classification of pelvic tumor location and resection types. Type I involves resection of the iliac wing. Type IS involves removal of the iliac wing along with an adjacent portion of the sacrum. Type IA involves removal of the iliac wing and gluteal musculature. Type II involves resection of the periacetabular region, and type IIA involves resection of the periacetabular region and femoral head (black A). Type III involves resection of the ischiopubic region, and IIIA involves removal of the ischiopubic region with the femoral neurovascular bundle and adjacent muscles. Type IV involves resection of part of the sacrum. (Reproduced with permission from Hugate R Jr, Sim FH: Pelvic reconstruction techniques. *Orthop Clin North Am* 2006;37:85-97.)

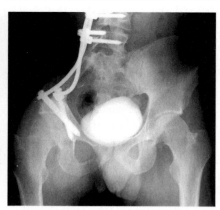

**Figure 7** An example of reconstruction of a defect in the right pelvis after a type I resection using a vascularized fibular autograft supplemented with spinopelvic fixation.

## Pelvic Reconstruction

Pelvic reconstruction following internal hemipelvectomy is indicated when there is loss of pelvic continuity between the acetabulum and sacrum, such that force cannot be transmitted from the lower extremity to the axial skeleton via the pelvis or when the acetabulum is resected (type II). Partial type I resections and complete type III resection typically do not require reconstruction. Adequate reconstruction is the key to a good functional outcome following internal hemipelvectomy. O'Connor and Sim[35] recommended that pelvic reconstruction be individualized and based on the needs of the patient, in-

cluding their age and functional demands as well as the location and extent of the resection.

Complete type I resections are best served by bony reconstruction to reconstitute mechanical continuity of the acetabulum and sacrum.[35] When the distance between the remaining ilium and sacrum is small, a direct appositional iliosacral arthrodesis can be performed. For larger defects, a strut graft must be introduced to span the gap. This may include allograft or autograft fibular struts (Figure 7) or a vascularized iliac wing autograft.

Type II resection involving the acetabulum generally requires reconstruction because of intrinsic loss of mechanical stability, and represents the biggest challenge because of loss of the hip joint. There are a variety of reconstructive options, each with their own advantages and disadvantages. A saddle prosthesis is an expedient procedure to restore function after a long, demanding resection, and patients often can ambulate using a cane (Figure 8, *A*). This reconstruction is

associated with a high incidence of complications, including iliac fracture, dislocation, and infection. Massive pelvic allografts can restore function and maintain limb length (Figure 8, *B*). Early reports showed frequent complications associated with these massive reconstructions, but there has been recent increased interest in acetabular allografts because of improved methods of internal fixation and advances in hip reconstruction.[36]

Custom pelvic prostheses have been popular outside the United States, but there has only been sporadic interest in this country because of the high rate of complications.[37] Iliofemoral arthrodesis is an effective means of reconstruction because it provides durable, stable function; however, it is associated with limb shortening and altered gait (Figure 8, *C*). This procedure is best reserved for young patients with strenuous activity requirements.[35] An iliofemoral pseudarthrosis is less surgically demanding, associated with fewer complications, and often used in older, more sedentary patients (Figure 8, *D*). Fuchs and associates[38] analyzed the functional outcome of 32 patients who had either an iliofemoral arthrodesis or primary pseudarthrosis. Patients with a solid fusion had better function; however, patients with a pseudarthrosis were pleased with their outcome, indicating the importance of individualizing the technique to each patient's situation.

Type III resections generally do not require reconstruction if acetabular stability can be maintained. Although patients have loss of adduction strength, function is usually excellent. Adequate soft-tissue reconstruction, often using a synthetic mesh, will minimize the risk of a perineal hernia.

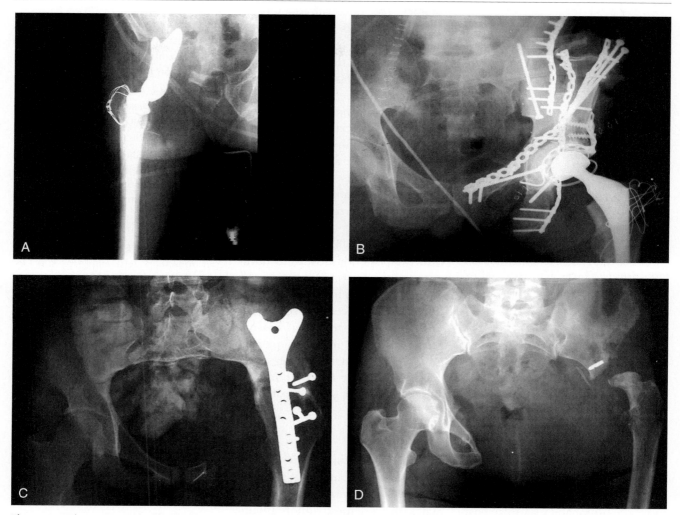

**Figure 8**    There are multiple ways to reconstruct the periacetabular region after a type II pelvic resection, including a saddle prosthesis **(A)**, a massive pelvic allograft with internal fixation **(B)**, iliofemoral arthrodesis **(C)**, and a pseudarthrosis **(D)**.

### Outcome

Significant morbidity and a high incidence of complications are associated with these extensive limb-sparing procedures. In large studies, infection occurred in 23% of patients and local recurrence in 17%.[35] Local recurrence of iliosacral lesions is higher (27%), suggesting the need for more extensive resection for lesions extending along the sacrum and spine. In another study, Fuchs and associates[39] reviewed 18 patients who had an extended iliosacral resection to achieve a clear margin.

An internal hemipelvectomy was achieved in 11 patients, and 13 were surviving at 5-year follow-up with a total of three local recurrences. In most patients with recurrent pelvic chondrosarcoma, more extensive surgery is required. Historically, the outcome of patients with osteosarcoma of the pelvis has been very discouraging, with survival rates reported from 4% to 32%. However, a recent review of 48 pelvic osteosarcomas reported a 5-year survival rate of 48%, with a high rate (31%) of local recurrence.

### Sacrum

With sacral tumors such as chordoma, high local failure rates are reported that influence long-term survival. The reasons for high local recurrence rates include a delay in diagnosis, large tumor volume, and an inaccessible location, which contributes to the difficulty in achieving adequate surgical margins. A recent review of surgical management of 52 patients with sacral chordomas emphasized the need for complete surgical resection.[15] When a wide margin was achieved

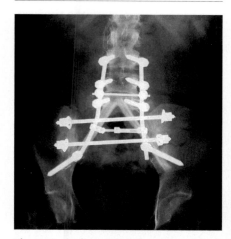

**Figure 9** After a total sacrectomy for a chordoma, a lumboiliac fusion was performed using fibular autografts and extensive spinal fixation.

in 21 patients, there was only 1 recurrence; in 37 patients with less than wide margins, there were 25 recurrences.

### Surgical Considerations

The surgical principles in the treatment of sacral tumors are similar to those of pelvic tumors: safely remove the tumor and maximize postoperative function. The type of sacral resection required to achieve local control varies depending on the location, extent, and type of tumor and can be categorized as either a partial sacrectomy (transverse, sagittal, or combination) or a total sacrectomy. The morbidity associated with sacral resection is related to sacral nerve root sacrifice necessitated by the level of resection. Normal function requires preservation of both S3 nerve roots, whereas there is minimal dysfunction if S3 on one side can be preserved.[40] Hugate and associates[41] recently studied the mechanical effects of partial sacrectomy to determine when reconstruction is necessary. Resections below the S1

foramen had adequate stability to withstand normal static loads. Resection above the S1 foramen significantly decreased the load to failure, and, in this situation, stabilization is recommended.

The surgical approach varies with the location and extent of the tumor. In lesions extending to the S3 segment, a posterior approach is sufficient. For lesions extending above S3, a combined anteroposterior approach is preferred.[15] Before the anterior closure, a vertical rectus abdominis flap is harvested to assist with the posterior closure to minimize wound complications. Although there has been some debate concerning the need for reconstruction following total sacrectomy, recent advances in techniques of lumboiliac fusion have been effective in improving function and the ambulatory status of these patients[42] (Figure 9).

### Summary

Malignant bone tumors are rare and account for less than 1% of new malignancies each year in the United States. Because these tumors are uncommon, it is important that orthopaedic surgeons recognize the clinical presentation of an affected patient. The treatment options vary according to tumor type, but all involve surgical resection and usually require wide margins to achieve local control. Chemotherapy and radiation are used for specific tumor types to prevent systemic metastasis or local recurrence, respectively. There are multiple options for reconstruction of the defect remaining after tumor resection. These include the use of allografts, autografts, or megaprosthetic devices. The most complicated surgical resections and reconstructions involve the pelvis and sacrum.

### References

1. Jemal A, Siegel R, Ward E, et al: Cancer statistics, 2006. *CA Cancer J Clin* 2006;56:106-130.

2. Unni KK: *Dahlin's Bone Tumors: General Aspects and Data on 11,087 Cases*, ed 5. Philadelphia, PA, Lippincott-Raven, 1996.

3. Scully SP, Ghert MA, Zurakowski D, Thompson RC, Gebhardt MC: Pathologic fracture in osteosarcoma: Prognostic importance and treatment implications. *J Bone Joint Surg Am* 2002;84:49-57.

4. Enneking WF: A system of staging musculoskeletal neoplasms. *Clin Orthop Relat Res* 1986;204:9-24.

5. Greene FL, Page DL, Fleming ID, Balch CM, Haller DG, Morrow M: *AJCC Cancer Staging Manual*, ed 6. New York, NY, Springer, 2002, pp 221-228.

6. Mankin HJ, Mankin CJ, Simon MA, et al: The hazards of the biopsy, revisited. *J Bone Joint Surg Am* 1996;78:656-663.

7. Gebhardt MC, Hornicek FJ: Osteosarcoma, in Menendez LR (ed): *Orthopaedic Knowledge Update: Musculoskeletal Tumors*. Rosemont, IL, American Academy of Orthopaedic Surgeons, 2002, pp 175-186.

8. Hornicek FJ: Ewing's sarcoma, in Menendez LR (ed): *Orthopaedic Knowledge Update: Musculoskeletal Tumors*. Rosemont, IL, American Academy of Orthopaedic Surgeons, 2002, pp 195-202.

9. Bacci G, Longhi A, Ferrari S, Mercuri M, Versari M, Bertoni F: Prognostic factors in non-metastatic Ewing's sarcoma tumor of bone: An analysis of 579 patients treated at a single institution with adjuvant or neoadjuvant chemotherapy between 1972 and 1998. *Acta Oncol* 2006;45:469-475.

10. Mankin HJ: Chondrosarcoma of bone, in Menendez LR (ed): *Orthopaedic Knowledge Update: Musculoskeletal Tumors*. Rosemont, IL, American Academy of Orthopaedic Surgeons, 2002, pp 187-194.

11. Quinn RH, Ricci A: Malignant fibrous histiocytoma of bone, in Menendez LR (ed): *Orthopaedic Knowledge Update: Musculoskeletal Tumors.* Rosemont, IL, American Academy of Orthopaedic Surgeons, 2002, pp 203-210.

12. Bacci G, Picci P, Mercuri M, Bertoni F, Ferrari S: Neoadjuvant chemotherapy for high grade malignant fibrous histiocytoma of bone. *Clin Orthop Relat Res* 1998;346:178-179.

13. Picci P, Bacci G, Ferrari S, Mercuri M: Neoadjuvant chemotherapy in malignant fibrous histiocytoma of bone and in osteosarcoma located in the extremities: Analogies and differences between the two tumors. *Ann Oncol* 1997;8:1107-1115.

14. Keeney GL, Unni KK, Beabout JW, Pritchard DJ: Adamantinoma of long bones: A clinicopathologic study of 85 cases. *Cancer* 1989;64:730-737.

15. Fuchs B, Dickey ID, Yaszemki MJ, Inwards CY, Sim FJ: Operative management of sacral chordoma. *J Bone Joint Surg Am* 2005;87:2211-2216.

16. Frassica FJ, Sim FH, Chao EY: Primary malignant bone tumors of the shoulder girdle: Surgical technique of resection and reconstruction. *Am Surg* 1987;53:264-269.

17. Gebhart M, Schlammes H, Colignon A, Lejeune F: Upper extremity function after conservative interscapulothoracic tumor resection. *Eur J Surg Oncol* 1989;15:504-509.

18. Damron TA, Rock MG, O'Connor MI, et al: Functional laboratory assessment after oncologic shoulder joint resections. *Clin Orthop Relat Res* 1998;348:124-134.

19. Wittig JC, Bickels J, Wodajo F, Kellar-Graney KL, Malawer MM: Constrained total scapula reconstruction after resection of a high-grade sarcoma. *Clin Orthop Relat Res* 2002;397:143-155.

20. O'Connor MI, Sim FH, Chao EY: Limb salvage for neoplasms of the shoulder girdle: Intermediate reconstructive and functional results. *J Bone Joint Surg Am* 1996;78:1872-1888.

21. Malawer MM, Chou LB: Prosthetic survival and clinical results with use of large-segment replacements in the treatment of high-grade bone sarcomas. *J Bone Joint Surg Am* 1995;77:1154-1165.

22. Gao YH, Ketch LL, Eladoumikdachi F, Netscher DT: Upper limb salvage with microvascular bone transfer for major long-bone segmental tumor resections. *Ann Plast Surg* 2001;47:240-246.

23. Damron TA, Sim FH, Shives TC, An KN, Rock MG, Pritchard DJ: Intercalary spacers in the treatment of segmentally destructive diaphyseal humeral lesions in disseminated malignancies. *Clin Orthop Relat Res* 1996;324:233-243.

24. Weber KL, Lin PP, Yasko AW: Complex segmental elbow reconstruction after tumor resection. *Clin Orthop Relat Res* 2003;415:31-44.

25. Harris IE, Leff AR, Gitelis S, Simon MA: Function after amputation, arthrodesis, or arthroplasty for tumors about the knee. *J Bone Joint Surg Am* 1990;72:1477-1485.

26. Mankin HJ, Gebhardt MC, Jennings LC, Springfield DS, Tomford WW: Long-term results of allograft replacement in the management of bone tumors. *Clin Orthop Relat Res* 1996;324:86-97.

27. Ortiz-Cruz E, Gebhardt MC, Jennings LC, Springfield DS, Mankin HJ: The results transplantation of intercalary allografts after resection of tumors: A long-term follow-up study. *J Bone Joint Surg Am* 1997;79:97-106.

28. Brien EW, Terek RM, Healey JH, Lane JM: Allograft reconstruction after proximal tibial reconstruction for bone tumors: An analysis of function and outcome comparing allograft prosthetic reconstruction. *Clin Orthop Relat Res* 1994;303:116-127.

29. Zehr RJ, Enneking WF, Scarborough MT: Allograft-prosthesis composite versus megaprosthesis in proximal femoral reconstruction. *Clin Orthop Relat Res* 1996;322:207-223.

30. Eckardt JJ, Eiber FR, Rosen G, et al: Endoprosthetic replacement for stage IIB osteosarcoma. *Clin Orthop Relat Res* 1991;270:202-213.

31. Sharma S, Turcotte RE, Isler MH, Wong C: Cemented rotating hinge endoprosthesis for limb salvage of distal femur tumors. *Clin Orthop Relat Res* 2006;450:28-32.

32. Mittermayer F, Windhager R, Dominkus M, et al: Revision of the Kotz type of tumour endoprosthesis for the lower limb. *J Bone Joint Surg Br* 2002;84:401-406.

33. Neel MD, Wilkins RM, Rao BN, Kelly CM: Early multicenter experience with a noninvasive expandable prosthesis. *Clin Orthop Relat Res* 2003;415:72-81.

34. Doi K, Kuwata N, Kawakami F, Hattori Y, Otsuka K, Ihara K: Limb-sparing surgery with reinnervated free muscle transfer following radical excision of soft tissue sarcoma in the extremity. *Plast Reconstr Surg* 1999;104:1679-1687.

35. O'Connor MI, Sim FH: Salvage of the limb in the treatment of malignant pelvic tumors. *J Bone Joint Surg Am* 1989;71:481-494.

36. Bell RS, Davis AM, Wunder JS, et al: Allograft reconstruction of the acetabulum after resection of stage II-B sarcoma: Intermediate-term results. *J Bone Joint Surg Am* 1997;79:1663-1639.

37. Abudu A, Grimer RJ, Cannon SR, Carter SR, Sneath RS: Reconstruction of the hemipelvis after the excision of malignant tumors: Complications and functional outcome of prostheses. *J Bone Joint Surg Br* 1997;79:773-779.

38. Fuchs B, O'Connor MI, Kaufman KR, et al: Iliofemoral arthrodesis and pseudarthrosis: A long-term functional outcome. *Clin Orthop Relat Res* 2002;397:29-35.

39. Fuchs B, Yaszemski MJ, Sim FH: Combined posterior lumbar spine resection for sarcoma. *Clin Orthop Relat Res* 2002;397:12-18.

40. Todd LT Jr, Yaszemski MJ, Currier BL, Fuchs B, Kim CW, Sim FH: Bowel and bladder function after major sacral resection. *Clin Orthop Relat Res* 2002;397:36-39.

41. Hugate RR Jr, Dickey ID, Phimolsarnti R, Yaszemski MJ, Sim FH: Mechanical effects of partial sacrectomy: When is reconstruction necessary? *Clin Orthop Relat Res* 2006;450:82-88.

42. Dickey ID, Hugate RR Jr, Fuchs B, Yaszemski MJ, Sim FH: Reconstruction after total sacrectomy: Early experience with a new surgical technique. *Clin Orthop Relat Res* 2005;438:42-50.

# Computer-Assisted Surgery: Basic Concepts

*James B. Stiehl, MD
*David A. Heck, MD

## Abstract

*Computer-assisted surgery has been advocated as a significant enabling technology that will enhance the surgical technique of various orthopaedic procedures. The computer becomes a sophisticated measuring tool, determining the three-dimensional spatial orientation of fiducial points, which may be established by a variety of referencing methods. These fiducial points or arrays may define a bone, an instrument, or a prosthesis. Current referencing methods include using segmented computer tomograms; fluoroscopic images; ultrasound images; and imageless, direct anatomic point-picking methods. Tracking technologies use optical cameras and electromagnetic coils. Optical systems have high reliability with errors of less than 0.5 mm. Electromagnetic trackers have a similar capability, but are less reliable because of the distortion of the electromagnetic signal that may result from the complex operating room environment. Accuracy with current CT-referenced systems approximates 1° or 1 mm. Other methods such as fluoroscopy or ultrasound are less precise because of difficulty related to the ability to consistently define a specific anatomic structure. Descriptive measures of outcome include standard deviation and quantification of error. Process capability indices or Six Sigma are suitable methods for comparing outcomes with computer-assisted surgery and can be generalized from various approaches.*

**Instr Course Lect 2008;57:689-697.**

Computer-assisted orthopaedic surgery has recently evolved into an important technical application that offers substantial improvements over conventional, instrumented surgical methods.[1-16] The possibility of using computers in total joint arthroplasty surgery is not a recent discovery. The first successful robotic application for total hip arthroplasty was introduced

by Bargar and Paul in 1987 and was jointly developed with International Business Machines, a company with an extensive research program in applying robotics to medicine.[17] Perhaps the most significant discovery at the time was the capability to refine digital software algorithms to the level of pixel accuracy (20 to 30 $\mu$m). This refinement was required for machining

custom total hip femoral implants, which were being implanted at that time. The next advances occurred in Europe, where computer algorithms were improved to allow intraoperative registration, eliminating the need for preoperative fiducial placement.[18-20] Jaramaz and associates[21] and DiGioia and associates[22] developed the first CT system that could be used to navigate the acetabular component. Actually, this approach was a step backward because the complex robot as introduced by Bargar and Paul was not needed. Imageless total knee applications were an even simpler method because preoperative images were no longer required.[3]

Current computer-assisted orthopaedic surgery systems offer enhanced visualization by displaying a virtual model of the operated anatomy together with relevant information about the position of a surgical instrument or implant. The visual feedback produced on a computer monitor enhances the surgeon's direct visual impression of the surgical field. Important anatomic details, such as femoral neck offset and lower extremity mechanical axis alignment, can be critically measured and the information applied to the surgical technique. The operator's im-

*James B. Stiehl, MD is a consultant or employee for Zimmer. David A. Heck, MD or the department with which he is affiliated has received research or institutional support from Zimmer.*

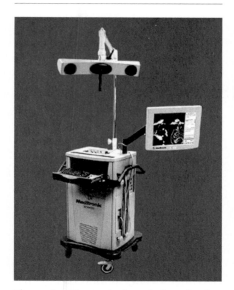

**Figure 1** The typical capital navigation system has a mobile cart containing the computer, monitor, keyboard, and storage space for materials, along with a tower that holds the digital cameras on a boom.

proved visual perception reduces errors that are associated with surgical tasks. Bony procedures such as drilling, reaming, or sawing can be performed more accurately, and implants can be placed with reduced error. These improvements reduce the risks of complications from poorly placed implants or the violation of vital neurovascular structures.

From a purely scientific point of view, the presumed benefits and the proof that these systems increase surgical quality has been straightforward. Studies published to date indicate the potential for improved implant orientation when using computer-assisted techniques compared with conventional mechanical instrumentation.[4-6] These benefits are seen when CT is used to register acetabular component placement and when imageless technologies are used to place femoral and tibial components during total knee arthroplasty.[12,14,23-26] This chapter reviews the basic elements of the technology required for computer-assisted surgery and discusses advantages of certain applications of this technology in joint reconstruction. **(DVD 52.1)**

## Components of a Computer Navigation System

Three elements are required for computer navigation: the computer platform, the tracking system, and the group of dynamic reference bases that constitute the target objects of the navigation procedure. These target objects include the patient's bones, the surgical instruments, and the implants used in the surgical procedure. The surgeon must make important choices regarding each of these components and should have an understanding of standard validation methods. The surgeon should be knowledgeable about possible sources of measurement error in computer navigation systems and should be able to interpret the results of clinical trials that attempt to define performance by measuring the repeatability, reproducibility, and process capability of a given system. Process capability analysis is a particularly valuable framework that has been widely adopted in other industries and is fundamental to quality enhancement.

### The Computer Platform

The most basic component of a computer navigation system is the computer, which coordinates the input data from the surgical field, mathematically interprets the datasets, and displays the resulting information on a monitor. Current systems require hardware capable of robust, real-time calculations, which often result in the pairing of powerful microprocessors and software platforms based on Unix or Linux systems. These base operating systems are considered more responsive and stable for use in mission-critical applications. The measurement system is designed so that the three-dimensional position of objects or targets in the surgical field can be determined with a low rate of error—in a manner similar to that of a global positioning satellite system. Computer platforms may be considered closed or proprietary if the navigation system provides limited support for a specific implant system or surgical technique. An open system that is more general and allows, for example, a software protocol to support the implantation of total knee components from different manufacturers is another option. The advantage of a proprietary system is that more elaborate representations are usually supported, allowing applications such as virtual implant sizing or virtual anatomic reconstruction of the patient's anatomy. These applications may add time and complexity to the surgical procedure and must be balanced against the simplicity of an open system.

A typical capital navigation system includes a rolling cart with computer, keyboard, mouse, liquid crystal display monitor, foot pedal activator, and an optical tracking camera (Figure 1). The optical camera may be placed on a boom or separate tower to allow placement in the appropriate position during the surgical procedure. The optical camera system typically will have two charged-coupled device (CCD) receivers that will pick up laser impulses from an active tracker or a reflected beam from passive balls attached to a passive tracker. Recently, portable systems have been developed with virtually the same hardware and applications as the conven-

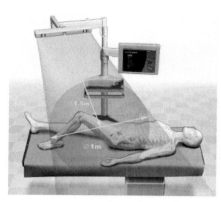

**Figure 2** Illustration showing the typical operating room setup with an optical line of sight system with imaging of the passive dynamic reference bases that are attached to the femur, tibia, and instruments.

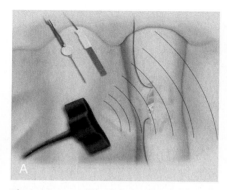
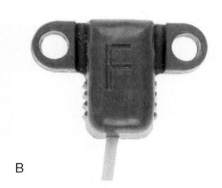

**Figure 3** **A,** Illustration of a typical electromagnetic setup with a coil used for tracking impulses that originate from small trackers placed inside of the knee wound. **B,** Example of a small electromagnetic coil (the size of a dime).

tional systems but with smaller desktop computers, plus cameras and tracking devices that can be quickly assembled from a suitcase. Manufacturers' representatives can bring these portable, full navigation systems to hospitals for limited or one-time use or as a continuing service that may be purchased by the hospital. These systems provide the surgeon with an opportunity to try computer navigation without committing the hospital to an expensive (several hundred thousand dollars) capital system purchase. The portable systems, with technology to perform computer-aided surgery, also are an excellent option for low-volume surgeons and hospitals that may not have resources for the large investment needed for more permanent systems.

### Tracking Technologies

An important element of any computer navigation system is the mechanism or technology chosen to track the target or object. The basic elements are trackers that may be attached to the patient's bones or surgical instruments. These trackers are used in an environment consisting of a camera, an electromagnetic coil, or an ultrasonic probe that will pick up laser or electromagnetic pulses that originate from these trackers. Recently, video monitoring has been added as a real-time tracking option; however, this method has not reached significant clinical application.

Optical tracking systems require two or three CCD cameras to pick up laser impulses from the trackers that are recognized by a minimum of three and possibly four or five active emitters or passive balls (Figure 2). The computer calculates the three-dimensional position of the trackers based on recognizing the spatial footprint of the tracker emitters. The footprint of each tracker is unique and allows differentiation of bones, instruments, and implants. Optical cameras are placed 6 to 8 feet from the object trackers and must have an unobstructed line of sight to the trackers. Operating personnel must be aware of this placement relationship; however, with optimal positioning, the staff can readily adapt to the requirements of the tracking stystem. Clinical validation studies of optical tracking systems have shown high reliability and

accuracy with a typical translational error of 0.25 mm.[27-29] This absolute measurement error increases trigonometrically with increasing distance from the camera position.

Electromagnetic tracking relies on small trackers that create an electromagnetic impulse that is recognized by an electromagnetic coil placed 20 to 30 inches away.[30] These trackers may be placed inside the wound but require small wires that go directly to the computer system for activation (Figure 3). The magnetic coil then measures the interference created by the tracker as it moves in the electromagnetic field. The disadvantage of electromagnetic tracking systems currently in use is distortion of the field created by ferrous metals, which are inherently magnetic; however, any metal (such as brass or copper) and even nonmetals (such as Kevlar) may cause interference. Current computer algorithms have been calibrated to shut down the system if distortion is recognized. However, the electromagnetic approach remains vulnerable to other potential distorting fields found in the typical operating room. Clinical validation studies have identified this problem. Although the electromagnetic system seems to perform with the precision of current

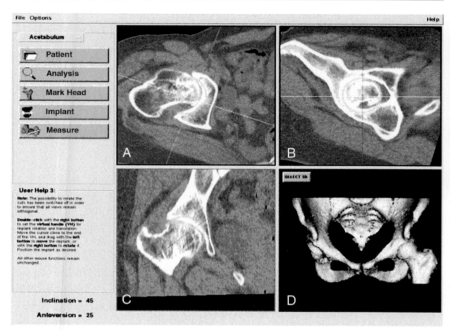

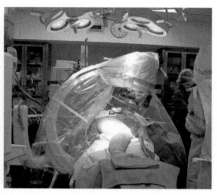

**Figure 5** Operating room setup for video fluoroscopic image-capture during a total hip procedure.

**Figure 4** Segmented CT images showing axial (**A**), sagittal (**B**), and coronal (**C**) slices and the three-dimensional reconstructed CT image (**D**).

optical systems at the 0.5- mm level, occasional outliers may be off by several degrees, making this method less reliable and less process capable.[31-33]

### Referencing Methods

For the surgeon, referencing of the target objects is the most significant challenge and requires a thorough knowledge of both the technology and the desired anatomic points to be matched on the virtual computer model. The process basically involves defining the points in space with a tracker that can be triangulated by the tracking system. For surgical instruments, a referencing tool allows the surgeon to capture the marked instrument such as a pointer probe. The precision of the instrument will be within 250 to 500 $\mu$m of error.[27] The various systems used for computer navigation can be identified by determining the type of referencing used. The earliest system used CT, which required a

series of steps to segment a three-dimensional reconstructed model that could be marked during the surgical procedure (Figure 4). This method has proved to be inherently accurate because bony landmarks are well visualized and can be easily matched by the operator.[14,15,21,22,34,35] A secondary check is possible using the computer algorithm to guarantee that the points can be verified.[34] Studies have shown that a typical CT surgical navigation system for acetabular navigation will have errors of less than 1° or approximately 1 mm.[21,22]

Fluoroscopic referencing uses images captured by a standard surgical fluoroscope, with referencing points chosen directly from the video monitor (Figure 5). To improve precision, a standardization grid is required to account for Earth's magnetic forces. This method allows the use of radiographic images in two planes and can be combined with di-

rect touch point-matching of the anatomic structure. Several authors have shown that this method allows accuracy that approximates that of CT.[36-41] Fluoroscopy is particularly valuable in trauma patients because a virtual live image can be created with the surgeon directing a drill, screw, or intramedullary device into the correct position based on visual cues. Fluoroscopic referencing presents a significant disadvantage for acetabular navigation because the typical field of view is only 9 inches, limiting the ease of capturing an intraoperative pelvic image.

Imageless referencing is possible if the targeted objects are directly visible and is most applicable in total knee arthroplasty. Numerous studies have shown the efficacy of imageless referencing compared with conventional instrumentation for total knee and hip arthroplasty; however, results depend on the surgeon's expertise in choosing the correct reference points.[42-48] Computer algorithms are written with the assumption that the ideal point will be selected. For example, referencing of one universal total knee protocol prescribes that the femoral center is chosen as a point that is under the roof of the intercondylar notch and lies on both the transepicondylar line and the anteroposterior axis of Whiteside. Deviation from this ideal reference point will add error.

Kinematic referencing in total knee arthroplasty has been a novel innovation used to determine the center of the hip and ankle joints, markedly simplifying this procedure.[3] Because the hip joint is not directly visible, a method was needed to accurately reference the hip center. This goal was accomplished by tracking the femur with the optical camera as the femur was rotated in a circular motion. The movement of the tracker described the base of a cone, which when projected to its zenith, closely approximates the center of the hip joint. The computer algorithm calculates either the root mean square error or the standard deviation (SD), which must fall within a limited range for computer acceptance of the hip-center reference point.

A secondary method of referencing is bone morphing, which is a method of selecting hundreds of surface match points by "painting" the bone with the pointer probe.[49,50] This method does not require the segmented three-dimensional model typically used in CT referencing, but uses a virtual model that is then constructed by the computer algorithm. The created virtual image allows enhanced capabilities such as prosthesis sizing, "live" bone resection, and kinematic assessment. However, this additional technology is usually proprietary, adds time and complexity to the surgical procedure, and may limit the surgeon's choice of prosthetic implants.

Ultrasound image capture is a newer method of referencing that is evolving as a potential technique, where multimodal referencing is performed.[51-54] Depending on the frequency and the acoustical properties of the object, point localization is accurate to submillimeter levels with ultrasound, regardless of whether it is two-dimensional, 2.5-dimensional, or three-dimensional in the modality of image capture (on the order of 0.25 to 0.75 mm). Segmentation is possible where this image may be matched with a preoperative CT image or even an intraoperative bone-morphed image. However, clinical applications of ultrasound image capture remain limited for a variety of reasons. Definition of the baseline anatomic points is difficult with ultrasound, which creates an error on the order of 2 to 5 mm; this error level is unacceptable for clinical practice. However, ultrasound is a promising technology because it can be used intraoperatively through the tissues without the need for a skin incision or radiation exposure.

## Validation of Computer Navigation Systems

Because computer navigation is a sophisticated measuring tool, performance assessment is warranted.[55-57] In general terms, the concept of measurement begins with determining the measurable quantity where the value is generally characterized by a unit of measurement. The true value is defined as a given quantity that is obtained from a perfect measurement. True values are considered indeterminant because an infinite number of values are needed to create the true number. Commonly, this problem is solved by creating a "conventional true value," which is considered a better estimate. In some parlance, this could be considered as the baseline, ground truth, or reference value. Measurand is the particular quantity subject to measurement (for example, the inclination of the acetabular component compared with the axial plane of the human body). Influence quantity is the sum of measurements that subtly affect the measurand (in the example, slight variations in assessing the edges of the acetabular component). Accuracy of measurement is the qualitative assessment of the measured value to the true measured value. Accuracy differs from precision, which is defined as the closeness of agreement between independent test results obtained under stipulated conditions that encompass both repeatability and reproducibility. The measure of precision is usually computed as a SD of the test results.

Repeatability is the closeness of measure under the same conditions. Reproducibility is the ability to reproduce the measure when there is a changed condition of measurement, such as using different observers. The error of measurement is the result of the measurement minus the true value of the measurand. Random error is the measurement of a measurand minus the mean after an infinite number of measures. Systematic error is the mean of measurement of the measurand minus the true value of the measurand after an infinite number of measures. Random error is equal to the error minus the systematic error. Systematic error is equal to the error minus the random error. A correction is the value added to the measurement to correct for systematic error. Type A error deals with uncertainties of the statistical measure. Type B error relates to errors other than those determined by statistical measures.

### Descriptive Statistics

The mean, SD (square root of variance), and the experimental SD may be determined for descriptive measures. Equations for descriptive statistics are shown in Figure 6.

Mean:

$$\bar{\chi} = \frac{\chi_1 + \chi_2 + \chi_3 + \ldots + \chi_N}{N} = \frac{1}{N} \sum_{i=1}^{N} \chi_i$$

SD:

$$\sigma = \sqrt{\frac{(\chi_1 - \bar{\chi})^2 + (\chi_2 - \bar{\chi})^2 + \ldots + (\chi_N = \bar{\chi})^2}{N}}$$

$$= \sqrt{\frac{d_1^2 + d_2^2 + \ldots + d_N^2}{N}}$$

$$= \sqrt{\frac{1}{N} \sum_{i=1}^{N} (\chi_i - \bar{\chi})^2} = \sqrt{\frac{1}{N} \sum_{i=1}^{N} d_i^2}$$

Experimental SD:

$$\sigma = \sqrt{\frac{1}{(N-1)} \sum_{i=1}^{N} d_i^2}$$

**Figure 6** Equations for descriptive measures.

## Process Capability Analysis

Process capability analysis is the approach commonly used for process qualification in industrial quality management.[57] In high quality manufacturing, processes are first brought into statistical control. After the process is in control, the process is then characterized mathematically. The process capability index ($C_p$) is mathematically formulated as:

$$C_p = \frac{(USL - LSL)}{6\sigma}$$

In this equation, USL is the upper specification limit, LSL is the lower specification limit, and $\sigma$ is the SD. Commonly, purchasers will require that the supplier be able to produce components with capability indices ($C_p$) of 1.3 or higher. The capability index, however, is limited in its utility because it is an expression of precision that does not address the problem of accuracy. Six Sigma programs, such as that used at Motorola, will frequently require the calculation of the offset capability index or $C_{pk}$. This measure accounts for the random error, where the mean of the measurand differs significantly or is offset from the baseline or "ground truth" mean.

$$C_{pk} = \min\left[ \frac{(USL - \bar{\chi})}{3\sigma}, \frac{(\bar{\chi} - LSL)}{3\sigma} \right]$$

In this equation, USL is the upper specification limit, LSL is the lower specification limit, and $\sigma$ is the SD. Although it is not clear what specific level of quality is appropriate for a specific medical process, very high quality manufacturing is associated with processes that are capable of producing at levels where the $C_{pk}$ exceeds 2.0.

The most important variables in the process capability analysis are the upper and lower control limits, which requires knowledge of the limits or acceptable range of measures that are associated with the outcome(s) of interest. For example, a standard target or "ground truth" could be an accurately measured known quantity, such as the mechanical axis of the lower extremity, which traverses the center of the hip joint, the center of the knee joint, and the center of the ankle joint. A reasonable or acceptable limit of variation must then be determined from this target center beyond which an unacceptable result has occurred. For a total knee replacement, it can be argued that the prosthetic postoperative leg alignment must be placed within 5° of the normal mechanical axis of the leg. If the 5° parameter is exceeded, excessive rates of radiolucencies and joint instability have been identified. For the Six Sigma formulas, the upper and lower specification limits would then be 5°.

Figure 7 shows an example that demonstrates the effect a large or small SD and also the effect of a mean that is offset and does not coincide with the center of the target or desired measurement.

The strength of process capability analysis is the ability to easily compare results from multiple sources or studies with a limited amount of standard data required. The values created using $C_p$ and $C_{pk}$ allow quantitative comparison between techniques or technologies. A basic assumption of process capability analysis is that any isolated value or measurement outside the specified control limits will cause the $C_p$ or $C_{pk}$ to become unacceptable (Table 1). To date, other technology groups have embraced the use of Six Sigma process capability analysis for its

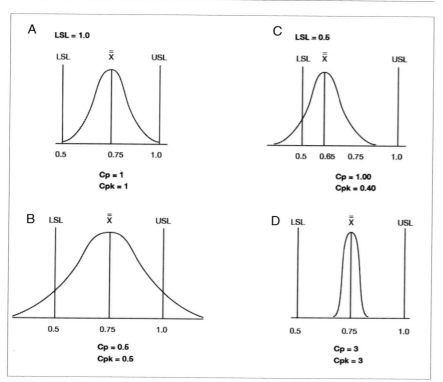

| Table 1 Process Capability Indices: $C_p$ | | |
| --- | --- | --- |
| $C_P$ | % | Parts Per Million (Outliers) |
| 2.00 | 0.02 | 0.002 |
| 1.66 | 0.05 | 0.57 |
| 1.33 | 0.06 | 63 |
| 1.00 | 0.27 | 2,700 |
| 0.66 | 4.55 | 45,500 |
| 0.33 | 31.37 | 317,300 |

Process capability indices that demonstrate the number of outliers with $C_p$ (parts per million). The chance of an outlier above $C_p$ of 1.3 is small.

**Figure 7** Graphs showing the effect of large and small SDs and the effect of a mean that is offset and does not coincide with the center of the target or desired measurement. **A,** Standard bell-shaped curve with normal distribution. **B,** Bell-shaped curve has normal distribution but exceeds specification limits. **C,** Bell-shaped curve is offset as mean does not match true value. **D,** Optimal process capability with mean centered on true value and bell-shaped curve well within specification limits. LSL = lower specification limit, USL = upper specification limit, $C_p$ = process capability index, $C_{pk}$ = offset process capability index.

simplicity and validity in quantifying the capability of a measurement system.

## Summary

For the practicing surgeon, learning about surgical navigation requires interest and time spent to acquire the needed skills for using this technology. This learning experience may require reading available evidence-based medical literature on the subject, practicing referencing in a laboratory setting on cadavers, and visiting a mentor surgeon who has experience with surgical navigation. The belief that computers do not make mistakes is a simplistic analysis of the problem because the human output of this exercise is far more complex than a mere function of the computer. Surgical navigation is a sophisticated tool of measurement that can enhance the quantitative characterization capabilities of the surgical field. The improved information provided by surgical navigation may significantly enhance the surgeon's skills.

## References

1. Langlotz F, Nolte LP: Technical approaches to computer-assisted orthopedic surgery. *Eur J Trauma* 2004;30: 1-11.

2. Nolte LP, Visarius H, Arm E, Langlotz F, Schwarzenbach O, Zamorano L: Computer-aided fixation of spinal implants. *J Image Guid Surg* 1995;1:88-93.

3. Stulberg SD, Picard FD, Saragaglia D: Computer-assisted total knee replacement arthroplasty. *Oper Tech Orthop* 2000;10:25-39.

4. Chauhan SK, Clark GW, Lloyd S, Scott RG, Breidahl W, Sikorski JM: Computer assisted total knee replacement. *J Bone Joint Surg Br* 2004;86: 818-823.

5. Chauhan SK, Scott RG, Breidahl W, Beaver RJ: Computer-assisted knee arthroplasty versus a conventional jig-based technique: A randomised, prospective trial. *J Bone Joint Surg Br* 2004;86:372-377.

6. Decking R, Markmann Y, Fuchs J, Puhl W, Scharf HP: Leg axis after computer-navigated total knee arthroplasty: A prospective randomized trial comparing computer-navigated and manual implantation. *J Arthroplasty* 2005;20:282-288.

7. Stockl B, Nogler M, Rosiek R, Fischer M, Krismer M, Kessler O: Navigation improves accuracy of rotational alignment in total knee arthroplasty. *Clin Orthop Relat Res* 2004;426:180-186.

8. Victor J, Hoste D: Image-based computer-assisted total knee arthroplasty leads to lower variability in coronal alignment. *Clin Orthop Relat Res* 2004;428:131-139.

9. Sparmann M, Wolke B, Czupalla H, Banzer D, Zink A: Positioning of total knee arthroplasty with and without navigation support: A prospective, randomised study. *J Bone Joint Surg Br* 2003;85:830-835.

10. Stulberg SD, Loan P, Sarin V: Computer-assisted navigation in total knee replacement: Results of an initial experience of thirty five patients. *J Bone Joint Surg Am* 2002;84:90-98.

11. Jenny JY, Clemens U, Kohler S, Kiefer H, Konermann W, Miehlke RK: Consistency of implantation of a total knee arthroplasty with a non-image-based navigation system: A case-control study of 235 cases compared with 235 conventionally implanted prostheses. *J Arthroplasty* 2005; 20:832-839.

12. Zheng G, Marx A, Langlotz U, Widmer KH, Buttaro M, Nolte LP: A hybrid CT-free navigation system for total hip arthroplasty. *Comput Aided Surg* 2002;7:129-145.

13. Saragaglia D, Picard F, Chaussard C, et al: Computer-assisted knee arthroplasty: Comparison with a conventional procedure: Results of 50 cases in a prospective, randomized study. *Rev Chir Orthop Reparatrice Appar Mot* 2001;87:18-28.

14. Leenders T, Vandevelde D, Mahieu G, Nuyts R: Reduction in variability of acetabular cup abduction using computer assisted surgery: A prospective and randomized study. *J Comput Aided Surg* 2002;7:99-106.

15. Bernsmann K, Langlotz U, Ansari B, Wiese M: Computer-assisted navigated cup placement of different cup types in hip arthroplasty: A randomised controlled trial. *Z Orthop Ihre Grenzgeb* 2001;139:512-517.

16. Bolognesi M, Hofmann A: Computer navigation versus standard instrumentation for TKA: A single-surgeon experience. *Clin Orthop Relat Res* 2005;440:162-169.

17. Mittelstadt B, Kazanzides P, Zuhars J, et al: The evolution of a surgical robot from prototype t human clinical use, in Taylor RH, Lavallée S, Burdea

GC, Mösges R (eds): *Computer Integrated Surgery*. Cambridge, MA, MIT Press, 1996, pp 397-407.

18. Honl M, Dierk O, Gauck C, et al: Comparison of robotic-assisted and manual implantation of a primary total hip replacement: A prospective study. *J Bone Joint Surg Am* 2003;85: 1470-1478.

19. Jakopec M, Harris SJ, Rodriguez y Baena F, Gomes P, Cobb J, Davies BL: The first clinical application of a "hands-on" robotic knee surgery system. *Comput Aided Surg* 2001;6: 329-339.

20. Paul A: Surgical robot in endoprosthetics: How CASPAR assists on the hip. *MMW Fortschr Med* 1999;141:18.

21. Jaramaz B, DiGioia AM, Blackwell M, Nikou C: Computer assisted measurement of cup placement in total hip replacement. *Clin Orthop Relat Res* 1998;354:70-81.

22. Di Gioia AM, Jamaraz B, Nikou C, LaBarca RS, Moody JE, Colgan S: Surgical navigation for total hip replacement with the use of HipNav. *Oper Tech Orthop* 2000;10:3-8.

23. Anderson KC, Buehler KC, Markel DC: Computer assisted navigation in total knee arthroplasty. *J Arthroplasty* 2005;20:132-138.

24. Bathis H, Perlick L, Tingart M, Luring C, Zurakowski D, Grifka J: Alignment in total knee arthroplasty: A comparison of computer-assisted surgery with the conventional technique. *J Bone Joint Surg Br* 2004;86:682-687.

25. Kim SJ, MacDonald M, Hernandez J, Wixson RL: Computer assisted navigation in total knee arthroplasty: Improved coronal alignment. *J Arthroplasty* 2005;20:123-131.

26. Jolles BM, Genoud P, Hoffmeyer P: Computer-assisted cup placement techniques in total hip replacement improve accuracy of placement. *Clin Orthop Relat Res* 2004;426:174-179.

27. Stiehl JB, Heck DA, Lazzeri M: Accuracy of acetabular component placement with a fluoroscopically referenced CAOS system. *Comput Aided Surg* 2005;10:321-327.

28. Khadem R, Yeh CC, Sadeghi-Tehrani M, et al: Comparative tracking error analysis of five different optical tracking systems. *Comput Aided Surg* 2000; 5:98-107.

29. Wiles AD, Thompson DG, Frantz DD: Accuracy assessment and interpretation for optical tracking systems. *Society of Photo Optical Instrumentation Engineers Proceedings* 2004;5367:1-12.

30. Lionberger R: The attraction of electromagnetic computer-assisted navigation in orthopaedic surgery, in Stiehl JB, Konermann W, Hacker R (eds): *Navigation and MIS in Orthopaedic Surgery*. Heidelberg, Germany, Springer Verlag, 2006, pp 44-53.

31. Frantz DD, Wiles AD, Leis SE, Kirsch SR: Accuracy assessment protocols for electromagnetic tracking systems. *Phys Med Biol* 2003;48:2241-2251.

32. Milne AD, Chess DG, Johnson JA, King GJ: Accuracy of an electromagnetic tracking device: A study of the optimal operating range and metal interference. *J Biomech* 1996;29: 791-793.

33. Glossop N: Accuracy evaluation of the Aurora magnetic tracking system. *Comput Aided Surg* 2001;6:112.

34. Haaker RGA, Tiedgen K, Ottersbach A, Rubenthaler F, Stockheim M, Stiehl JB: Comparison of conventional versus computer-navigated component insertion. *J Arthroplasty* 2007; 22:151-159.

35. Van Hellemondt G, Kleuver M, Kerckhaert A, et al: Computer-assisted pelvic surgery: A in vitro study of two registration protocols. *Clin Orthop Relat Res* 2002;405:287-293.

36. Foley KT, Simon DA, Rampersaud YR: Virtual fluoroscopy: Computer-assisted fluoroscopic navigation. *Spine* 2001;26:347-351.

37. Hinsche AF, Giannoudis PV, Smith RM: Fluoroscopy-based multiplanar image guidance for insertion of sacroiliac screws. *Clin Orthop Relat Res* 2002;395:135-144.

38. Hofstetter R, Slomczykowski M, Sati M, Nolte LP: Fluoroscopy as an im-

aging means for computer assisted surgical navigation. *Comput Aided Surg* 1999;4:65-76.

39. Grutzner PA, Zheng G, Langlotz U, et al: C-arm based navigation in total hip arthroplasty: Background and clinical experience. *Injury* 2004;35 (suppl 1):S-A90-S-A95.

40. Tannast M, Langlotz F, Kubiak-Langer M, Langlotz U, Siebenrock K: Accuracy and potential pitfalls of fluoroscopy-guided acetabular cup placement. *Comput Aided Surg* 2005; 10:329-336.

41. Suhm N: Intraoperative accuracy evaluation of virtual fluoroscopy: A method for application in computer-assisted distal locking. *Comput Aided Surg* 2001;6:221-224.

42. Richolt JA, Effenberg H, Rittmeister ME: How does soft tissue distribution affect anteversion accuracy of the palpation procedure in image-free acetabular cup navigation?: An ultra-sonographic assessment. *Comput Aided Surg* 2005;10:87-92.

43. Yau WP, Leung A, Chiu KY, Tang WM, Ng TP: Intraobserver errors in obtaining visually selected anatomic landmarks during registration process in nonimage-based navigation-assisted total knee arthroplasty: A cadaveric experiment. *J Arthroplasty* 2005;20:591-601.

44. Fuiko R, Kotten B, Zettl R, Ritschl P: The accuracy of palpation from orientation points for the navigated implantation of knee prostheses. *Orthopade* 2004;33:338-343.

45. Siston RA, Patel JJ, Goodman SB, Delp SL, Giori NJ: The variability of femoral rotational alignment in total knee arthroplasty. *J Bone Joint Surg Am* 2005;87:2276-2280.

46. Robinson M, Eckhoff DG, Reinig KD, Bagur MM, Bach JM: Variability of landmark identification in total knee arthroplasty. *Clin Orthop Relat Res* 2006;442:57-62.

47. Pitto RP, Graydon AJ, Bradley L, Malak SF, Walker CG, Anderson IA: Accuracy of computer-assisted navigation system for total knee replacement. *J Bone Joint Surg Am* 2006;88: 601-605.

48. Nogler M, Kessler O, Prassl A, et al: Reduced variability of acetabular cup positioning with use of an imageless navigation system. *Clin Orthop Relat Res* 2004;426:159-163.

49. Stindel E, Briard JL, Merloz P, et al: Bone morphing: 3D morphological data for total knee arthroplasty. *Comput Aided Surg* 2002;7:156-168.

50. Stindel E, Perrin N, Briard JL, Lavallée S, Lefevre C, Troccaz J: Bone morphing: 3D reconstruction without pre- or intra-operative imaging, in Stiehl JB, Konermann W, Hacker R

(eds): *Navigation and MIS in Orthopaedic Surgery*. Heidelberg, Germany, Springer Verlag, 2006, pp 36-43.

51. Huitema RB, Hof AL, Postema K: Ultrasonic motion analysis system—measurement of temporal and spatial gait parameters. *J Biomech* 2002;35: 837-842.

52. Amin DV, Kanade T, DiGioia AM, Jaramaz B: Ultrasound registration of the bone surface for surgical navigation. *Comput Aided Surg* 2003;8:1-16.

53. Chen TK, Abolmaesumi P, Pichora DR, Ellis RE: A system for ultra sound-guided computer-assisted orthopaedic surgery. *Comput Aided Surg* 2005;10:281-292.

54. Kowal J, Amstutz CA, Nolte LP: On B-mode ultrasound-based registration for computer assisted orthopaedic surgery. *Comput Aided Surg* 2001;6:47.

55. ISO: *Guide to the Expression of Uncertainty in Measurement*. Geneva, Switzerland, International Organization for Standardization, 1993.

56. Taylor BN, Kuyatt CE: *Guidelines for Evaluating and Expressing the Uncertainty of NIST Measurement Results: NIST Technical Note 1297*. Gaithersburg, MD, National Institute of Standards and Technology, 1994.

57. Kotz S, Johnson NL: *Process Capability Indices*, New York, NY, Chapman and Hall, 1993.

# Surgical Navigation in Adult Reconstruction Surgery: Techniques and Clinical Experience

Michael A. Rauh, MD
Sandeep Munjal, MD, MCh (Orth)
*Matthew J. Phillips, MD
Kenneth A. Krackow, MD

## Abstract

*A surgeon's first response to the concept of computer-assisted orthopaedic surgery may be a sense of lost autonomy. However, a system need not and should not be designed to this end. Using the computational ability of the computer system to see beyond the human eye to view the knee with full kinematic dimensions, surgeons have recently made progress in the areas of computer-assisted ligament balancing and in using smart tools for minimally invasive surgery.*

*Full comprehension of the use of any navigational system must begin with the understanding that the system can provide feedback that is based on only specifically programmed computer code. In referring to or locating a point or axis, the computer programmer must create an absolutely reliable methodology for determining that point or axis. Expecting the computer to achieve certain functionalities when physicians have no ironclad method to achieve such functionalities exposes the true limitations of any computer-assisted process. Although the computer generates a methodology, the process of computer-assisted surgery requires that the surgeon be constantly vigilant in analyzing the feasibility of these responses. Those instrumental in the development and implementation of computer-assisted surgical techniques must ensure that measurements are valid, precise, and reproducible across subjects and users. Prospective users of computer-assisted techniques must ensure that each of these issues has been addressed before agreeing to use the system in standard practice. Once due consideration has been given to all aspects of use, and the limitations of the system are known, the benefits of computer assistance are easily understood.*

**Instr Course Lect 2008;57:699-706.**

The benefits of computers and similar technologies are evident in society every day. Many people rely heavily on the computational abilities and convenience afforded by standard laptop computers; however, the medical field has been slow to adopt these conveniences. Anesthesiologists use computerized electronics to monitor vital signs, gas concentrations, and heart rhythms, and the nursing staff uses computerized electronics for entering patient information into the hospital database. These sophisticated uses occur at the same time that orthopaedic surgeons routinely use nothing more than rulers, mallets, drills, bovie cords, and oscillating saws as their main surgical tools. Because it is the surgeon's responsibility to accurately plan and execute treatment, some measure of change is needed. The time has come for the orthopaedic surgeon to embrace present-day technology and use its benefits to improve surgical outcomes.

## Computer-Assisted Total Knee Arthroplasty

Successful total knee arthroplasty (TKA) relies heavily on an accurate assessment of alignment from the center of the hip to the center of the knee and through the center of the ankle. Final components must be

*Matthew J. Phillips, MD is a consultant or employee for Stryker.*

implanted correctly in all degrees of freedom because errors at this point are directly related to poor short- and long-term outcomes. For an outcome of functional stability throughout the full range of motion, soft-tissue attachments, capsular structure, and the presence or absence of ligaments need to be accounted for in advance of treatment. Given the capabilities of infrared sensor arrays and the ever-increasing speed and memory capabilities of modern computers, these particular aspects of TKA are perfectly suited for computer assistance.

A review of the literature and the personal experience of orthopaedic surgeons show more than 90% good to excellent clinical results at long-term follow-up for TKAs.[1] Based on this information, many surgeons conclude that mechanical instruments meet current needs. However, errors of component rotation, postoperative instability, and patient dissatisfaction with postoperative range of motion are more common than previously believed. Additionally, many surgeons who perform TKAs indicate that they do not routinely acquire or measure such results as would be provided by postoperative, long-standing, weight-bearing radiographs. In addition, Stulberg and associates[2] showed that long-standing lower extremity films are highly subject to rotational and projectional inaccuracies. Thus, it is impossible to postoperatively determine if axial alignment is as good as it should be.

## Computer Navigation Systems

The term computer-assisted orthopaedic surgery (CAOS) simply infers the assistance of a computer and its computational abilities. Commercial systems also use the term navigation, which infers use of a motion tracking system to guide the performance of a surgical procedure (for example, the placement of hardware, the positioning of screws, and the accuracy of bony cuts). This motion tracking can be provided by an infrared, electromagnetic, or light-emitting tracking device. Computer-assisted navigation includes the important steps of registration, data acquisition, and tracking.[3-9] The initial steps of registration and data acquisition must be performed correctly to obtain high-quality information. When these steps are performed incorrectly, the ability of the computer to accurately track and provide useful information is limited. The computer is only a guide and does not replace the surgeon's ability to use all available information to arrive at informed decisions.

Registration of the distal femoral and proximal tibial anatomy allows the computer, software, and tracking devices to accurately determine the exact tibiofemoral alignment, translation, flexion angles, and rotational alignment of the femur relative to the tibia; all six degrees of freedom can be determined instantly and studied simultaneously. The surgeon can determine axes of flexion-extension movement under varying conditions and plot outlines of clouds of points that allow the surgeon to view surfaces and boundaries on display screens. The computational ability of the system will then analyze motion patterns and provide real-time kinematic feedback to the surgeon.

Surgeons who perform lower extremity reconstructive procedures such as TKAs have traditionally been concerned with optimizing the alignment of the lower extremity and avoiding excessive postoperative varus or valgus deformity. However, as the influence of alignment on survivorship has been delineated, a greater emphasis toward obtaining true neutral alignment and rotational and mediolateral positioning of the components has developed. Experience with navigation systems has already shown an increased ability to position components with the net result of fewer alignment outliers.[2-12] Long-term outcome studies that show true success in computer-assisted TKA are in progress.

## The Stryker Navigation System

The Knee Track Module (Stryker Leibinger, Kalamazoo, MI) was originally developed by the senior author (Kenneth A. Krackow, MD). Although systems developed for clinical use provide assistance in performing TKA, it is incumbent on surgeons to understand the intricacies and limitations of these systems. Navigation systems are tools and devices that can provide a more exact representation of alignment and a better estimation of bony cuts and soft-tissue relationships; these systems are not a substitute for the skill and knowledge of an orthopaedic surgeon.

The Stryker Knee Track Module navigation system uses an infrared sensor array located at the side of the operating room table to localize emitters placed at specific locations on the lower extremity of the patient (Figure 1). In previous versions of this navigation system, it was necessary to place a tracking pin into the ipsilateral iliac crest for the sole purpose of determining the relative femur-to-pelvis motion. This process is no longer necessary because of the development of routines that eliminate this step.

After surgical exposure of the knee, the distal femur and proximal tibial pins, which function as anchors for the infrared tracker-emitters, are placed. A surgeon has the option of using a one-, two-, or three-pin construct for fixation of the tracker devices (Figure 2). With the infrared emitters placed onto the tracking pins, the lower extremity can be manipulated in a circular fashion about the hip. The center of the femoral head is calculated via a mathematical equation, and a subroutine that assumes the head of the femur is spherical. Within a 20-second period, 250 data points are collected as the surgeon moves the lower extremity about the hip joint in a gentle spherical arc. The method of least squares is used to find the best fit sphere given the data points collected.[13] The center estimate is then determined, using an iterative Gauss-Newton algorithm (which runs through 200 iterations to ensure convergence) to solve the true nonlinear system. The center point is then transformed into the femoral reference frame (Figure 3). Using the pointing device, the geometry of the distal femur is digitized[9] (Figure 4). In this process, the surgeon must identify the medial and lateral epicondyles, the center of the knee, the anteroposterior axis of Whiteside, and the condylar surfaces[14] (Figure 5).

The geometry of the proximal tibia is digitized as the surgeon identifies the sulcus between the tibial spines representing the initial center of the proximal tibia, which serves as a vector for neutral anteroposterior tibial rotation, the medial and lateral malleoli, and the center of the ankle; the latter is indicated by direct pointing. The vector of the instrument pointing is projected to the intermalleolar axis because that

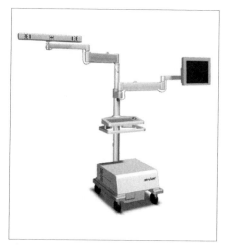

**Figure 1**    The Stryker navigation system.

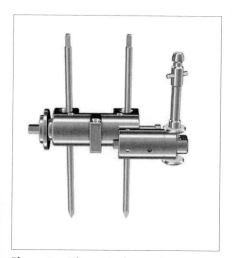

**Figure 2**    The typical two-pin construct for fixation of the tracker device.

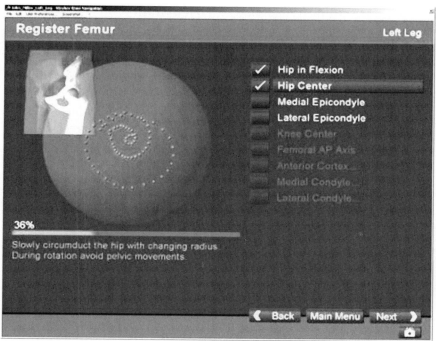

**Figure 3**    Screen-shot of the Knee Track Module of the Stryker navigation system calculating the center of the femoral head.

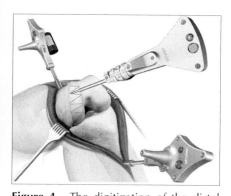

**Figure 4**    The digitization of the distal femoral articular surface with pointing devices.

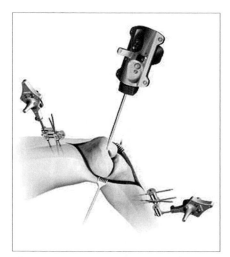

**Figure 5**  An anatomy survey of the distal femur and proximal tibia.

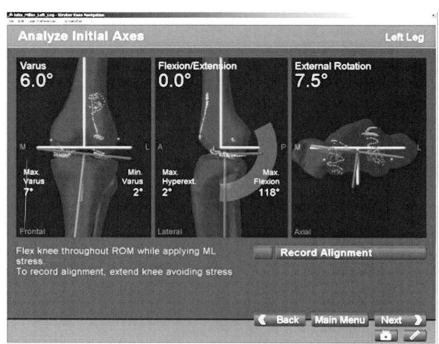

**Figure 6**  Screen-shot. After initial registration, the knee is moved through its maximal ranges of motion to demonstrate alignment deformity and obtain other kinematic data.

axis lies in a plane, including the center point of the proximal tibia together with the points for the two malleoli.

Given all the defined points, the tibiofemoral and mechanical axes can be determined before any bone cuts are made. The navigation system is able to intraoperatively identify the real-time position of the tibia relative to the femur—the surgeon can precisely determine the tibiofemoral angle, the flexion-extension position, and the amount of relative internal or external rotation of the tibia with respect to the femur (Figure 6).

Once the registration process has been performed, the actual positions of the femur and tibia relative to specific total knee components can be determined at any given moment, resulting in greater simplification when assessing the position of a cutting jig, the face of a resulting cut, and the positions of both trial and final components. Because the relative positions of the tibia and the femur are continually determined, the surgeon can follow tibiofemoral gaps throughout the entire flexion-extension cycle. This is helpful to provide information

on gap size and symmetry and allows for more accurate ligament-balancing techniques. All measurements are instantaneous and can be taken without attaching additional mechanical instruments to the bones, which allows the surgeon to obtain a more accurate alignment of the lower extremity than previously obtained.[2,3,7-12,15-18]

The surgeon can use jigs from any specific instrument system to make accurate cuts. The position of the jig is checked, and the position of any resulting cut is also checked (Figure 7). The resting position of the trial and final components can be determined. Routine navigation of the final cementation can verify that the femoral and tibial components are resting at the desired angle and level. Because assessment of the final alignment can be easily determined, this allows for improved outcome analysis (Figure 8).

## Discussion

In the future, the routine use of separately pinning trackers may not be required to obtain alignment data; significant advances are currently being made in this area. A method currently exists in which separate trackers are not required; registration information is acquired from the distal femoral cutting block (Figure 9). However, the limitation of this current iteration is that once the femoral and tibial bony cuts have been made, the surgeon loses the ability to determine alignment and kinematic information. Because this information is necessary throughout the procedure to arrive at an optimal result, separately placed tracker devices are recommended.

Correct placement and alignment of the components and soft-tissue balancing have been cited as the most important aspects of successful

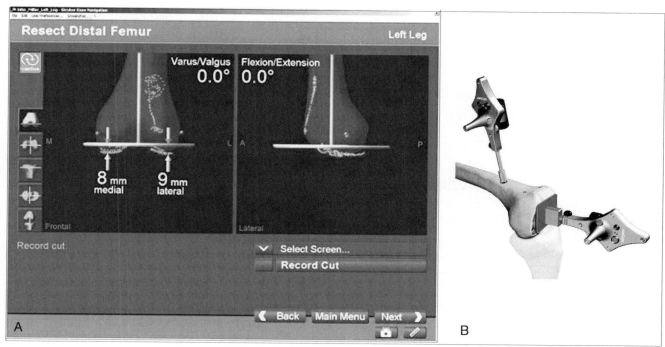

**Figure 7** **A,** Screen-shot showing navigation of bony cuts by jig navigation and reassessment after bony cuts. **B,** The navigated "checking block" to ensure the accuracy of the distal femoral resection.

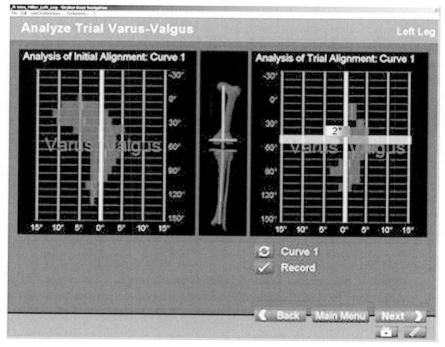

**Figure 8** Screen-shot of the Knee Track Module of the Stryker navigation system demonstrating assessment of final alignment.

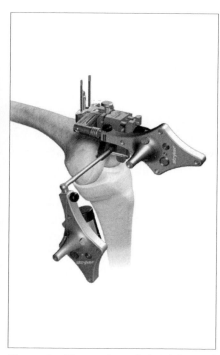

**Figure 9** The navigated distal femoral guide without a separate femoral tracker.

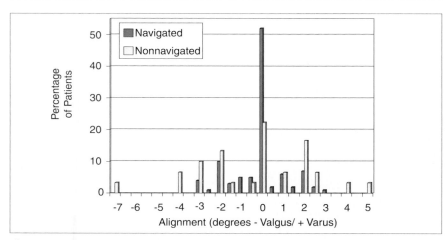

**Figure 10** Postoperative radiographic alignment comparison graph for patients undergoing TKA with and without computer-assisted navigation.

TKA.[19-26] The resulting postoperative alignment depends on many factors, including accurate preoperative planning, accurate assessment of bone morphology, and implantation of the components in an optimal position. Inaccurate alignment, which often leads to abnormal wear, premature mechanical loosening of components, and early failures, can be caused by a variation of any of these factors. Computer navigation of a TKA allows for accurate positioning of jigs, the ability to correctly establish femoral component rotation, instantaneous feedback on overall alignment, and the ability to prevent implantation of malpositioned components. Whereas previously the surgeon relied on knowledge of deformity corrections with various releases, the process now can be monitored with a computer. Exact measurements of flexion extension gaps, varus and valgus deformity, and tibial rotation can be patient specific and can be observed in real time.

Any new surgical technique or protocol needs a period of review. Issues that must be considered in CAOS include the level of risk for infection, bleeding, and postoperative pain, as well as whether the new process adds to or improves on the current methodology. With TKA, improvements in technique or prostheses must also address the issues of proper alignment, durability, accuracy of fit, and surgical reproducibility. In CAOS, achieving improvement in the quality of the surgical procedure is performed through intraoperative feedback to the operating surgeon.

It is critical that the surgeon master the complete description of how a chosen system works (for example, how the system defines bony landmarks and axes). This knowledge will alert the surgeon to potential errors and complications and provides the knowledge to circumvent such problems.

## Outcomes

Although robotic-assisted knee replacement was studied before the 1990s, the first known publication describing the use of an imageless navigation system for TKA was released in 1997.[27,28] A growing number of systems for CAOS from a variety of manufacturers are currently available and are being studied. To date, no long-term studies exist that show that computer assistance in TKA has resulted in an improved implant life span. However, studies have shown that CAOS has resulted in decreased variability and the elimination of outliers[2-7,9,10] (Figure 10). It is believed that as neutral alignment of components is more reliably achieved in TKAs, higher success rates will result, and there will be less need for revision surgery resulting from the adverse effects of malalignment.

Based on the successes of the first studies, potential clinical benefits include faster rehabilitation and improved range of motion.[3] It is anticipated that improvements in computers and the development of procedure-specific software will continue to advance the process of optimizing alignment and will result in improved long-term outcomes.

## Summary

CAOS provides real-time alignment and kinematic data that allow the surgeon to intraoperatively evaluate the accuracy of component implantation and correct errors during surgical treatment that previously may have been imperceptible. It is believed that CAOS will improve the quality of TKA outcomes. Although many surgeons believe that current TKA results are adequate because of improvement in overall alignment, few surgeons routinely obtain and accurately measure those results. Surgeons should look beyond the issue of alignment and recognize the potential for improvements in ligament releasing and in the assessment of ligamentous stability. Placement of the femoral component in the optimum relationship of extension to the functional axis of flexion can be performed to provide maximum range of motion and stability throughout that arc. Navigation equipment also can indicate proper component sizing and placement. Education about and understanding of this new technology will produce better surgeons and provide better outcomes for patients.

## References

1. Saleh KJ, Mulhall KJ, Hofmann AA, Bolognesi MP, Laskin RS: Primary total knee arthroplasty outcomes, in Barrack RL, Booth RE Jr, Lonner JH, McCarthy JC, Mont MA, Rubash HE (eds): *Orthopaedic Knowledge Update: Hip and Knee Reconstruction 3*. Rosemont, IL, American Academy of Orthopaedic Surgeons, 2006, pp 93-110.

2. Stulberg SD, Loan P, Sarin V: Computer-assisted navigation in total knee replacement: Results of an initial experience in thirty-five patients. *J Bone Joint Surg Am* 2002;84-A (suppl 2 ):90-98.

3. Phillips MJ, Mihalko WM, Krackow KA: Computer-assisted total knee replacement: Results of the first 90 cases using the Stryker navigation system, in Bauer A, Miehlke R (eds): *Computer Assisted Orthopaedic Surgery: Proceedings of the 3rd Annual Meeting of CAOS International*. Marbella, Spain, CAOS International, 2003.

4. Rauh MA, Mihalko WM, Krackow KA: Optimizing alignment, in Bellemans J, Ries MD, Victor J (eds): *Total Knee Arthroplasty: A Guide to Get Better Performance*. New York, NY, Springer, 2005, pp 165-169.

5. Rauh MA, Krackow KA: Rationale for computer assisted orthopaedic surgery, in DiGioia AM, Jaramaz B, Picard F, Nolte LP (eds): *Computer and Robotic Assisted Knee and Hip Surgery*. New York, NY, Oxford University Press, 2004, pp 113-126.

6. Munjal S, Krackow KA: Computer assisted total knee replacement, in Scott WN (ed): *Insall and Scott: Surgery of the Knee*. New York, NY, Elsevier, 2005.

7. Krackow KA, Phillips MJ, Bayers-Thering M, Serpe L, Mihalko WM: Computer-assisted total knee arthroplasty: Navigation in TKA. *Orthopedics* 2003;26:1017-1023.

8. Krackow KA: Fine tuning your next total knee: Computer assisted surgery. *Orthopedics* 2003;26:971-972.

9. Krackow KA, Bayers-Thering M, Phillips MJ, Bayers-Thering M, Mihalko WM: A new technique for determining proper mechanical axis alignment during total knee arthroplasty: Progress toward computer-assisted TKA. *Orthopedics* 1999;22: 698-702.

10. Mihalko WM, Krackow KA: Extramedullary, intramedullary and CAS tibial alignments techniques for total knee arthroplasty. *71st Annual Meeting Proceedings*. Rosemont, IL, American Academy of Orthopaedic Surgeons, 2004, p 437.

11. Mihalko WM, Krackow KA, Boyle J, Clark L: Intramedullary and computer navigational femoral alignment in total knee arthroplasty. *71st Annual Meeting Proceedings*. Rosemont, IL, American Academy of Orthopaedic Surgeons, 2004, p 440.

12. Sparmann M, Wolke B, Czupalla H, Banzer D, Zink A: Positioning of total knee arthroplasty with and without navigation support: A prospective, randomised study. *J Bone Joint Surg Br* 2003;85:830-835.

13. Forbes A: Robust circle and sphere fitting by least squares. *National Phys Lab Report* 1989;153:1-22.

14. Whiteside LA, Arima J: The anteroposterior axis for femoral rotational alignment in valgus total knee arthroplasty. *Clin Orthop Relat Res* 1995;321: 168-172.

15. Jenny JY, Boeri C: Computer-assisted implantation of total knee prostheses: A case-control comparative study with classical instrumentation. *Comput Aided Surg* 2001;6:217-220.

16. Jenny JY, Boeri C: Computer-assisted implantation of a total knee arthroplasty: A case-controlled study in comparison with classical instrumen-

tation. *Rev Chir Orthop Reparatrice Appar Mot* 2001;87:645-652.

17. Chauhan SK, Scott RG, Breidahl W, Beaver RJ: Computer-assisted knee arthroplasty versus a conventional jig-based technique: A randomised, prospective trial. *J Bone Joint Surg Br* 2004;86:372-377.

18. Chauhan SK, Schoo RG, Lloyd SJ: A prospective randomized controlled trial of computer assisted versus conventional knee replacement, in Bauer A, Miehlke R (eds): *Computer Assisted Orthopaedic Surgery: Proceedings of the 3rd Annual Meeting of CAOS International*. Marbella, Spain, CAOS International, 2003.

19. Bargren JH, Blaha JD, Freeman MA: Alignment in total knee arthroplasty: Correlated biomechanical and clinical observations. *Clin Orthop Relat Res* 1983;173:178-183.

20. Lotke PA, Ecker ML: Influence of positioning of prosthesis in total knee replacement. *J Bone Joint Surg Am* 1977;59:77-79.

21. Windsor RE, Scuderi GR, Moran MC, Insall JN: Mechanisms of failure of the femoral and tibial components in total knee arthroplasty. *Clin Orthop Relat Res* 1989;248:15-19.

22. Mont MA, Urquhart MA, Hungerford DS, Krackow KA: Intramedullary goniometer can improve alignment in knee arthroplasty surgery. *J Arthroplasty* 1997;12:332-336.

23. Jeffery RS, Morris RW, Denham RA: Coronal alignment after total knee replacement. *J Bone Joint Surg Br* 1991; 73:709-714.

24. Dorr LD, Boiardo RA: Technical considerations in total knee arthroplasty. *Clin Orthop Relat Res* 1986;205: 5-11.

25. Ritter MA, Faris PM, Keating EM, Meding JB: Postoperative alignment of total knee replacement: Its effect on survival. *Clin Orthop Relat Res* 1994;299:153-156.

26. Sharkey PF, Hozack WJ, Rothman RH, Sashtri S, Jacoby SM: Why are total knee arthroplasties failing today? *Clin Orthop Relat Res* 2002;404:7-13.

27. Picard F, Moody JE, DiGioia AM, Jaramaz B, Saragaglia D: History of computer-assisted orthopaedic surgery for hip and knee, in DiGioia AM, Jaramaz B, Picard F, Nolte LP (eds): *Computer and Robotic Assisted Knee and Hip Surgery*. New York, NY, Oxford University Press, 2004, pp 113-126.

28. Delp SL, Stulberg SD, Davies B, Picard F, Leitner F: Computer assisted knee replacement. *Clin Orthop Relat Res* 1998;354:49-56.

# Computer-Assisted Total Hip Navigation

*Richard L. Wixson, MD

## Abstract

*Accurate implant placement in total hip replacement is important in avoiding dislocation, impingement, and edge-loading throughout the patient's postoperative functional range of motion. Current implants and bearing surfaces now provide the potential for prolonged longevity of the reconstruction, which can be compromised by malposition of the components outside of designated "safe zones." Computer-assisted hip navigation offers the potential for more accurate placement of hip components and control of leg length and offset. Systems are now available that allow registration of the bony anatomy based on preoperative CT images, intraoperative fluoroscopic images, or imageless techniques based on palpation of the landmarks. In each of these approaches, cup position has been based on coordinate systems formed by identification of the anterior pelvic frontal plane. All systems have shown improved accuracy of acetabular cup placement compared with conventional manual techniques. Cup anteversion is less accurate than cup abduction with the imageless approach. Measurements made with the use of navigation systems also have shown a large variation in pelvic tilt or pelvic flexion-extension in series of cases, which can affect the appropriate cup position for each patient. The results of computer-assisted navigation in the future may be improved by incorporation of measurements of each patient's pelvic tilt, femoral stem position, and hip kinematics.*

**Instr Course Lect 2008;57:707-720.**

Modern total hip arthroplasty has emerged as one of medicine's most successful operations. Current hip implants and surgical methods routinely result in marked pain relief and restoration of near-normal function in most patients. Compared with earlier generations of total hip replacements, there have been marked improvements in the materials used and the reliability of fixation. Furthermore, total hip replacement is now being performed in younger patients who may aspire to a more active lifestyle and may have significant life expectancy.

In addition to having a stable, well-fixed implant that may have a long period of use, the success of a total hip replacement is also dependent on the surgeon accurately placing the implants in the patient's body. Malposition of an acetabular component may lead to dislocation of the hip or impingement of the neck against the cup or edge of the acetabular liner with premature wear. Restoration of accurate leg length and hip abductor moment arms are important in preventing postoperative limp.

Computer-assisted hip navigation has been introduced as a method to improve the accuracy and reliability of hip implant positioning. The incidence of hip dislocation and neck impingement can be avoided by properly positioning the acetabular cup in a "safe zone." Hip navigation also allows assessment of changes in leg length, offset of the femur from the acetabular cup center, and hip kinematics. Use of hip navigation requires the appropriate equipment and learning new technology. Successful use of hip navigation requires accurate bony registration and incorporation of measures to assess the functional range of motion of the hip.

## Rationale for Hip Navigation

Hip dislocation remains one of the most troubling complications that can occur. Dislocation rates have

*Richard L. Wixson, MD or the department with which he is affiliated has received research or institutional support, miscellaneous nonincome support, commercially-derived honoraria, or other nonresearch-related funding and royalties from Stryker and is a consultant or employee for Stryker.*

varied significantly from 0.5% to 6%.[1-4] Although multifactorial, cup malposition has the largest influence.[5] Lewinnek and associates,[6] using measurements taken from standardized AP radiographs of the pelvis, found that cups positioned outside a "safe" range had a fourfold increase in dislocations. They identified 40° ± 10° of abduction and 15° ± 10° of anteversion as the safe zone. Cups below the 5° of anteversion had posterior dislocations, and cups above 25° of anteversion tended to have anterior dislocations. Similar safe zones have been identified by Barrack[5] as 35° to 55° of abduction and 10° to 30° of anteversion, whereas McCollum and Gray[7] found values of 30° to 50° of abduction and 20° to 40° of anteversion. Nishii and associates,[8] in a CT study of total hip replacements, found that those with dislocation were more frequently positioned with less than 20° of anteversion. In a multivariate analysis of hip dislocations, Jolles and associates[9] found that combined femoral and acetabular anteversion of less than 40° or greater than 60° was associated with a higher incidence of hip dislocations.

In a review of 4,784 hip replacements from their center, Biedermann and associates[10] found a 2.4% incidence of dislocation in primary hips and 4.6% in revisions. For primary hips, those with anterior dislocation had significantly higher amounts of anteversion and abduction than the control group. For those hips with posterior dislocation, there was significantly less anteversion than in the control group. Applying the criteria of Lewinnek and associates,[6] 79% of the control group was within the safe zone, compared with 60% of the dislocation group. By using a safe zone of 45° ± 10° of radiologic abduction

and 15° ± 10° of radiologic anteversion, 93% of the stable group would be included compared with 67% of the dislocation group.

Independent of cup position, the head-neck ratio can affect dislocation rates. The use of larger head sizes, from 22 mm to 32 mm, has not been shown to decrease hip dislocations in a study by Morrey.[11] In the same study, trochanteric migration, reduced offset, and a posterior approach had higher dislocation rates. The increased dislocation rate with posterior approaches has been reduced by surgical repair of the posterior soft tissues,[12] with a meta-analysis by Kwon and associates[13] showing no significant differences in dislocation rates between surgical approaches. Padgett and associates[14] found increased dislocation rates with 22-mm heads compared with 26-mm and 28-mm heads. In a finite element study of a hip dislocation model, Scifert and associates[15] demonstrated the importance of head-neck ratios and component orientation on predisposition to dislocation. Evaluating the effect of larger head sizes in a hip dislocation model, Burroughs and associates[16] found a progressive increase in stability with larger head sizes and changes in acetabular anteversion. Beyond 38-mm diameter, stability was dependent on bone-to-bone contact, not component impingement. Yoshimine[17] described oscillation angles that are specific for each femoral stem and head-neck ratio for specific cups. Only total hip constructs with large oscillation angles avoided impingement with full range of motion in their model.

In addition to dislocation, malposition of the acetabular cup can lead to impingement between the neck of the femoral prosthesis and the edge of the cup. Retrieval analyses have

shown abutment of the neck against the rim of the polyethylene liner with increased damage and wear.[18,19] A cup placed in a more horizontal position (lower abduction) will be prone to impingement with hip flexion. A cup placed with excessive anteversion may undergo impingement with normal activities involving extension and external rotation that occur with toe-off in walking.[19] Crowninshield and associates[20] stressed the importance of proper abduction of cups with large femoral heads to avoid subluxation and increased tensile stress on the polyethylene at the edge of the cup. Kennedy and associates[21] found that cups with increased abduction angles had a higher incidence of wear and foreign-body lytic changes. However, a review by Del Schutte and associates[22] showed no increase in polyethylene wear in a series of cemented cups with increased anteversion.

To achieve the optimal cup position, traditional manual methods of cup placement have emphasized the importance of proper positioning of the cup inside an identified safe zone. Many of the manual techniques for this rely on positioning devices that allow impaction of the cup with alignment guides. Conventionally, these are set so that placement of the guide can be made at a set angle (such as 45° to the table surface) with a guide rod that when placed parallel to the long axis of the body or table edge will place the cup in 20° of anteversion to the body axis.[7,23,24] Ranawat and associates[25] have suggested that a combined anteversion of 25° to 45° of the femur and acetabulum is ideal, with the cup position being guided by the femoral components position. Maruyama and associates[26] found that orienting the cup using a sciatic notch acetabular angle was a reliable guide for cup position. Using preoperative standing lateral radiographs,

McCollum and Gray[7] found that the line from the anterosuperior iliac spine (ASIS) to the sciatic notch identified variation in pelvic tilt between patients and ranged from 0° to 40° to the horizontal. There was a significant change in the patient's pelvic tilt between the standing position and the position of the pelvis on the operating table in the lateral position. By identifying this line intraoperatively on patients in the lateral position, the authors of this study described a method of reproducibly placing the cup in 30° of anteversion (flexion), which they confirmed on postoperative standing lateral radiographs.

Alignment of the cup by manual positioning from the surgeon's estimates of the pelvic and body position can result in variations of the final cup position that may place some hips outside the safe zone. Based on measurements from plain radiographs, Hassan and associates[27] demonstrated that 21 of 50 acetabular cups were outside their target zones for abduction and anteversion. Saxler and associates[28] used CT scans to analyze 105 cups placed with manual methods and found that only 27 cups were inside the safe zone of Lewinnek and associates.[6] They found a mean abduction angle of 46° ± 10° and a mean anteversion angle of 27° ± 15° with large ranges. DiGioia and associates[24] measured the accuracy of a mechanical system with a computer navigation system and found that 54 of 78 cups were outside a desired anteversion range of 20° ± 10°, with significant variation in pelvic tilt.

## Hip Navigation Methods

To improve the accuracy of cup placement, computer-assisted surgical navigation methods have been developed that rely on determina-tion of pelvic bony landmarks to properly orient the cup. These systems rely on a registration process in which the bony landmarks of the pelvis are identified and used to orient the cup. The anterior frontal plane of the pelvis was described by McKibbin[29] as being formed by the most prominent aspects of the right and left ASISs and the right and left pubic tubercles (Figure 1). Lewinnek and associates[6] used this plane to describe in quantitative terms the orientation of the cup in abduction and anteversion.

Once the anterior frontal plane is established, the amount of acetabular cup abduction and anteversion are determined by angles relative to the pelvic plane. Murray[30] described how these angles can vary depending on which coordinate system is used. The angles measured by surgical methods, radiographic measurements, and anatomic measurements vary somewhat because they are based on different planes. Generally, navigation systems use the anatomic definitions of these angles, which are slightly different than the same values chosen at surgery or measured off radiographs. As an example, Lewinnek and associates[6] described their safe zone with a mean of 40° of abduction and 15° of anteversion based on radiographs. Using transformations provided by Murray,[30] these values are 42° of abduction and 23° of anteversion using the anatomic coordinate system with hip navigation.

The use of a preoperative CT scan to identify the pelvic anatomy is commonly referred to as image-based navigation and is based on methods originally developed for intracranial localization. DiGioia and associates[31] and Jaramaz and associates[23] originally described a system in which a preoperative CT

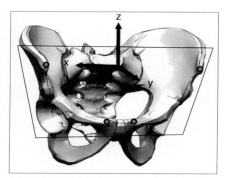

**Figure 1** Anterior frontal plane of the pelvis based on the right and left anterior superior iliac spines and right and left pubic tubercles.

scan was performed on patients before surgery. At surgery, a tracking device was rigidly attached to the pelvis, with other tracking devices attached to the surgical instruments. The movements of markers on the tracking device are followed by a camera system connected to the computer, which identified the position of the tracker in space. Because the tracker was rigidly attached to the pelvis, the position of any point on the pelvis was fixed relative to the tracker. The orientation and position of the pelvis was then determined by a "registration" process, in which various points on the pelvis were marked in a coordinate system defined by the computer. Software in the computer system could then match those points to the saved CT image of the pelvis, resulting in the actual bony pelvis sharing the saved coordinate system with the stored image. From this, the anterior frontal plane of the pelvis could be defined by the known points of the two ASISs and pubic tubercles. With similar trackers attached to the surgical instruments for insertion of the cup, the computer screen displays the cup position with abduction and anteversion

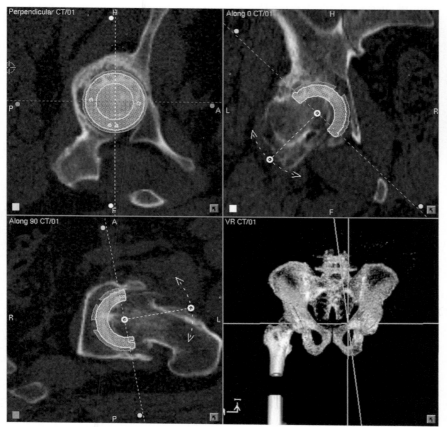

**Figure 2**   Images used to plan cup position for CT-based hip navigation.

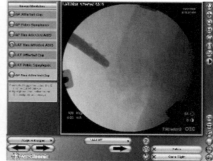

**Figure 3**   Fluoroscopic image identifying the bony landmarks to register the anterior frontal plane of the pelvis. (Courtesy of JB Stiehl, MD)

relative to the frontal plane of the pelvis. In the computer-based navigation approach defined by DiGioia and associates,[24,31] abduction and anteversion were defined relative to the anterior frontal plane using the anatomic coordinate system described by Murray.[30] Other authors have also described systems and results with image-based systems.[28,32-36] Sample preoperative CT images used to plan cup position are shown in Figure 2.

Rather than relying on preoperative CT scans, the pelvic anatomy can also be registered with fluoroscopic methods as another form of image-based registration. Zheng and associates[37] described a system in which a fluoroscopic unit with a reference grid is used to identify the ASISs, pubic tubercles, and femoral anatomy for orienting the hip implants. With tracking devices on the pelvis, femur, and instruments, the cup can be positioned relative to the anterior frontal plane, and the femoral component placed to establish proper leg length and offset. Further descriptions of the use of fluoroscopically based imaging with computer navigation have expanded on this method.[38-41] The positioning of the fluoroscopic unit and navigation system with fluoroscopic images identifies the ASIS in two planes (Figure 3).

Imageless computer-assisted navigation of the hip relies on digitization of the bony landmarks with a pointing device; the position of the device is followed by the camera and computer. As each point is touched by the pointer, a model is developed

of the anatomic relationships for the anterior frontal plane and the native acetabular anatomy. Generally, this is done by placing the pointer on the skin over the bony prominences of the pelvis. Kalteis and associates[42] have described an imageless system with equivalent accuracy to an image-based system, with both navigation systems superior to manual methods.

## Surgical Technique for Imageless Navigation

The author's primary experience has been with imageless navigation, which does not require preoperative or intraoperative imaging. This method can be used with the patient in either a lateral or supine position. The patient is placed in the lateral position with anterior and posterior supports to stabilize the pelvis, chest, and upper body. Following surgical preparation of the skin and draping, percutaneous pins can be placed in the pelvis, usually through the iliac crest. The pins are placed in the thicker area of the ilium at the gluteal tuberosity, approximately 6 to 8 cm posterior to the ASIS. Additional percutaneous pins may be placed in the distal lateral femur for determining leg length, offset, stem

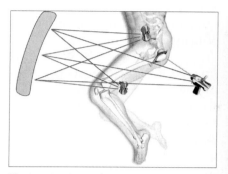

**Figure 4** Imageless navigation in the lateral position, with trackers attached to the femur and pelvis and infrared light-emitting diodes on trackers communicating with the navigation camera.

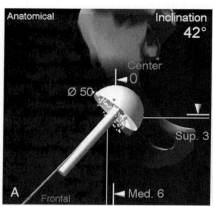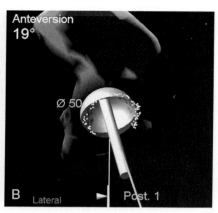

**Figure 5** Computer screen demonstrating the navigated position of the cup for depth of seating and abduction (**A**), and anteversion (**B**).

positioning, and hip kinematics. The trackers are then fixed to the pin attachments so that they face the camera and computer. Depending on the surgical approach, the camera and computer need to be positioned so the trackers are in the camera's field of view. For a lateral position with a posterior approach, the surgeon would be behind the patient, with the camera positioned in front of or above the head of the patient (Figure 4).

Once the pins are solidly fixed to the bone, the registration process begins. In the lateral position, an initial point is picked on the chest in the midaxial line and a second point over the center of the greater trochanter. This creates a line that is roughly parallel to the long axis of the body, which is commonly used in manual alignment methods, and is referred to as the "functional" plane. The pelvic supports are then loosened and the pelvis is allowed to roll back. This facilitates palpation of the lower ASIS. Points are then registered by palpating the two ASISs and the center of the pubic symphysis through the drapes, which creates the coordinate system for the pelvis. Care needs to be taken to push the soft tis-

sue away to get as close to the bone as possible. In the system used by the author, the femur is registered by placing the knee at a 90° angle and recording the center of the Achilles tendon, the medial and lateral epicondyles, and popliteal fossa to establish a knee center. Following surgical exposure, the trochanteric fossa is registered, which creates a femoral axis to the knee and establishes a relationship between the femoral coordinate system and the pelvic coordinate system that was established with determination of the frontal plane. Following removal of the femoral head and neck with exposure of the acetabulum, the anatomy and center of the acetabulum is registered.

An instrument tracker is attached to the handle of the reamer used for preparation of the acetabulum. During the reaming process, the computer monitor displays the depth of reaming and the amount of abduction and anteversion. Following completion of acetabular reaming, the same instrument tracker is attached to the insertion handle for the acetabular cup. As the cup is impacted into place, the depth to full seating (determined by the maximum penetration of the last reamer)

is displayed. The cup is directed to the desired amount of abduction and anteversion as it is impacted to complete seating (Figure 5).

The system can display the abduction and anteversion as measured from the frontal pelvic plane and the functional plane. When the patient has a large amount of pelvic flexion or extension, the functional plane information gives the surgeon an additional guide for judging the appropriate amount of cup anteversion into which to place the cup. Once the cup is impacted into place, its final position is recorded.

Femoral preparation is done in a conventional manner by opening the femoral canal with a series of broaches. Broach handles with attachments for the navigation trackers allow determination of the position of the broach in the femoral canal and the amount of femoral anteversion. The position of the final broach is registered to the femoral coordinate system, and a trial reduction is performed. The navigation system then displays changes in leg length and the amount of femoral offset. A range-of-motion analysis displays the potential range of hip flexion-extension, internal-external

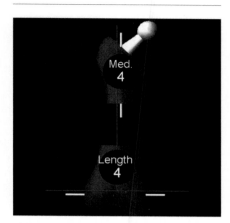

**Figure 6** Computer display showing changes in leg length (+4 mm) and change in offset (medial 4 mm) from the original hip center.

rotation, and abduction-adduction with stability at the extremes of range of motion. A series of trial reductions with different neck and head combinations can be performed until the optimal restoration of leg length, offset, and stability has been achieved (Figure 6).

The femoral stem is then implanted, with or without navigated guidance, until full seating is achieved. In press-fit applications, the fit is determined usually by the bony anatomy and can be recorded by the navigation systems. With cemented stems, the navigation system can be used to accurately position the stem inside the cement. Following stem insertion, a repeat trial reduction is performed, the final head placed, and the ultimate implant position is recorded along with hip kinematics.

## Hip Navigation Results
### Imaged-Based CT
CT-based images for planning and performing navigated total hip replacement were developed and reported by Jaramaz and associates[23] and DiGioia and associates.[24,31] They

were able to develop the hardware and software tools necessary for the surgery as well as the basic principles of applying computer-assisted surgical principles to total hip replacement. In addition to developing the methods used for navigation, they identified limiting issues with variation in pelvic tilt, which affects cup position and limits radiographic analysis. Subsequent comparisons of computer-assisted to manual techniques showed that a significant number of manually positioned hips were outside the desired position, particularly with anteversion.[31] The manual method resulted in 78% of the hips being positioned outside the safe zone defined by Lewinnek and associates.[6] Using their navigation system, with a goal of cup position of 45° abduction and 20° of flexion, they reported acetabular alignment for both groups within 5° of the planned position.[43]

Using navigation systems based on preoperative CT scans, Leenders and associates[34] described a reduction in variability in cup abduction compared to manual methods.

Using an in vitro model with 10 surgeons, Jolles and associates[33] found cup placement with a manual freehand technique to have a mean accuracy of cup anteversion and abduction of 10° and 3.5° (maximum 35°); with a mechanical guide, angles of 8° and 4° (maximum 29.8°); and with computer navigation, angles of 1.5° and 2.5° (maximum 8°). Similar findings were reported by Honl and associates[44] comparing conventional technique to image-based and imageless systems. Other reports on CT-based navigation describe accurate cup placement close to the desired position relative to the frontal pelvic plane in clinical series.[28,38,45] Haaker and associates[32] described improvements in cup alignment with

a preoperative CT-based navigation system in dysplastic hips as well as primary total hip replacement.

### Imaged-Based Fluoroscopy
Although CT-based systems provide accurate registration of the bony landmarks necessary for component positioning, this approach requires the expense and time of preoperative CT, additional time before surgery planning the position of the cup, and increased intraoperative time matching the CT image to the patient's anatomy.[24,37,38] To minimize these issues, fluoroscopic methods to register the bony anatomy have been developed that do not require preoperative imaging or time.

Comparing CT-based and fluoroscopically based cases, Hube and associates[38] described only minimal differences in their accuracy, although both required additional intraoperative time to set up. Stiehl and associates[40] described a fluoroscopic-based, computer-assisted surgery navigation system for hip replacement and documented its accuracy. Tannast and associates[41] also performed a cadaver study and found increased accuracy with a fluoroscopic navigation system compared with manual methods for abduction, but not as improved with anteversion. This finding was attributed to the difficulty of accurately identifying the pubic tubercles in their system, which could introduce error in the determination of cup anteversion. A hybrid method of using fluoroscopy combined with pointer-based percutaneous palpation that avoids the necessity of preoperative CT scans has been described.[37,39] These investigators described reliable cup placement with a maximum error of 5° for inclination (mean 1.5° ± 1.1°) and 6° for anteversion (mean 2.4° ± 1.3°).

## Imageless Navigation

Determination of the anterior frontal plane requires registration of the bony landmarks of the right and left ASIS and right and left pubic tubercles. Because of concerns about the time, cost, and complexity of relying on image-based methods, imageless techniques were developed. These involve the use of a pointing device to identify by percutaneous palpation the underlying bony landmarks. Using a cadaver model, Nogler and associates[46] demonstrated that imageless determination of the anterior frontal plane markedly reduced the variability of cup placement for abduction and anteversion.

Keifer[47] has described an imageless technique using another system. Using this system in a clinical series, Ottersbach and Haaker[48] found that the navigated approach reduced the variation in cup position compared to manual methods. In the navigated group, the standard deviation was 2.8° for abduction and 5.0° for anteversion compared to values of 6.9° and 7.4° for the manual group, respectively. Dorr and associates[49] described an imageless system that also compensates for variation in pelvic tilt, rather than relying solely on the anterior frontal plane. In a randomized, prospective clinical study using imageless navigation, Kalteis and associates[42] compared conventional alignment and image-based and imageless CT navigation. Both navigation techniques were superior to the conventional approach in which only 14 of 30 cups were inside the safe zone defined by Lewinnek and associates.[6] By comparison, 25 of 30 CT-based cups and 28 of 30 imageless cups were inside the safe zone.

The author has used an imageless navigation system in which the bony landmarks of the frontal plane are

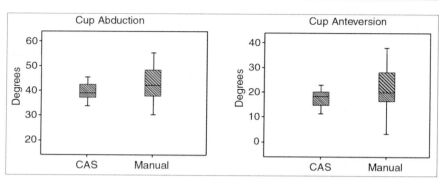

**Figure 7** Box plots comparing imageless computer-assisted (CAS) and manual cases for cup abduction and cup anteversion measured from postoperative CT scans using a radiographic coordinate system. Each box shows the median, quartiles, and extreme values for the two groups.

percutaneously palpated and digitized with a pointing device. A comparison of navigated hips to previously performed total hip replacements done with a conventional technique showed a marked improvement in cup position based on radiographic analysis.[50] A subsequent randomized, prospective clinical study compared conventional (manual) methods with imageless navigation using postoperative CT scans to determine cup position.[51] The surgical procedures were done with the patients in the lateral decubitus position through a posterior approach. The patients were rolled back to allow palpation of the bony landmarks during the registration process. In this study, with 21 navigated cases and 24 manual cases, there was significantly less variation in cup position with navigation than with the manual methods (Figure 7). From an analysis of cup position on the postoperative CT scans, using the radiographic coordinate system for cup abduction, all of the navigated cases were inside the safe zone of 40° ± 10° described by Lewinnek and associates,[6] with 3 of 24 cases in the manual group outside the safe zone ($P = 0.143$). For cup

anteversion, all of the navigated cases were inside the safe zone of 15° ± 10°, compared with only 18 of 24 cases in the manual group ($P = 0.017$). Using the radiographic coordinate system, for abduction, the navigated position at surgery was 40.0° ± 1.6°, the navigated value from the CT scan was 39.9° ± 2.9°, and the manual value for the CT was 43.2° ± 6.2°. For anteversion, the navigated position at surgery was 14.2° ± 1.5°, the navigated value from the CT scan was 17.4° ± 3.4°, and the manual value from the CT scan was 20.0° ± 8.2°.

Although the navigated results were better for anteversion, there was more variability, and there was a mean 3.2° difference between the cup anteversion value recorded at surgery and the results found on the CT scan. In the study, navigation was abandoned during the operation in favor of manual methods when the amount of anteversion appeared inappropriate in three cases. This was believed to be caused by variations in the patients' pelvic tilt (pelvic flexion-extension). Although the amount of pelvic tilt was not measured at surgery, it was found to vary greatly when measured while the patients were supine in the CT scanner postoperatively. Compared with the surface of the CT table, the mean value for pelvic flexion (pubis lower than the two ASISs) was 8.3° ± 8.7° (range, 6° extension to 31° flexion). Thus, while navigation was shown to be more reproducible, the study raised concerns about the accuracy of anteversion of the cup determined by this method and the larger effect of variations in patients' pelvic tilt or pelvic flexion-extension posture.

Several studies have examined the accuracy of imageless techniques. In the analysis of the cup orientation, the cup positions were based on the plane formed by the two ASISs and the pubic tubercles. Abduction is less affected by the accuracy of palpation of the ASIS points in the coronal plane, where the mean distance between the two points is 230 ± 17 mm. Anteversion is affected by changes in the anteroposterior measurement of the pubis in the sagittal plane. With a relatively short distance from the midpoint between the two ASIS points of 91 ± 8 mm, small differences in the palpation of the height of the pubic area can affect the calculated navigated anteversion values.[52] This error is less likely with CT-based imaging systems and more of a problem with fluoroscopic imaging, in which the bony point is selected on the monitor, with imageless systems relying on the surgeon palpating the correct point.

One of the sources of error is the amount of soft tissue that may be on top of the pubis. With palpation, it is necessary to push the soft tissue away to get as close to the bone as possible. Richolt and associates[53,54] investigated the effect of soft tissue in this area. Using ultrasound, they found soft-tissue thickness over the pubis to be 13.6 ± 4.1 mm, which was 5.7 ± 3.4 mm thicker than that over the ASIS, with a range of −2.5 mm to 14.9 mm. This difference would result in a mean underestimation of anteversion of 2.8° ± 1.8°, with a range of −1.2° to 8.0°. Wolf and associates[52] quantified the effect of measurement errors that could be associated with any navigation method, which are much more significant for anteversion.

An issue in the accuracy of imageless navigation is whether the difficulty of accurately finding the bony landmarks is affected by operating in the lateral decubitus position compared with the supine position, where the pelvic points are more accessible. Of 137 operated hips, the pelvic plane was measured in both positions. The mean difference in calculated cup position between the supine and lateral positions for anteversion was 1.2° ± 3.1°, with a range of −3.0° to 10.0°. If an acceptable variation was a range of 8° (−4° to 4°), 25% of the cases were outside this range. By comparison, the calculated cup position difference for abduction between supine and lateral measurements was 0.2° ± 0.9°, with a range of −2.0° to 2.0°. As part of the imageless total hip navigation study conducted by Wixson and associates,[51] CT scans were available in 16 cases in which both measurements were done. There was no significant difference in accuracy of cup anteversion, compared with the CT scan, between digitization in the lateral and supine position. It can be concluded that although imageless navigation is accurate for abduction and better than conventional methods for anteversion, the cup anteversion numbers represent a good approximation rather than an exact value.

The reproducibility of imageless navigation has been studied by Spencer and associates[55] in a cadaver study with eight surgeons. They found significant variation between surgeons, with a standard deviation of 6.3° for abduction and 9.6° for anteversion.

## Pelvic Tilt and Functional Positioning

The basis for much of the work that has been done with hip navigation is the assumption that orienting the cup to the anterior frontal plane will place it in the correct position. Lewinnek and associates' definition of the safe zone (40° ± 10° of abduction and 15° ± 10° of anteversion) was based on this plane.[6] Regardless of whether the navigation is based on images or is imageless, many of the techniques have relied on identifying as accurately as possible the anterior frontal plane for orientation of the acetabular cup. From attempting to interpret radiographs and correlate the navigation values with CT scans, many authors have found that the amount of pelvic tilt or pelvic flexion-extension is a large, unaccounted-for variable with wide variation between patients.[7,24,56-62] Tannast and associates[57] found a range of 27° (−7° to 20°) of pelvic tilt comparing conventional radiographs to measurements from a CT scan.

The variation in pelvic tilt between intraoperative component placement and postoperative evaluation is also dependent on the surgical approach. In the lateral approach, the pelvis can flex forward as the lumbar lordosis straightens out when the patient lies on his or her side. McCollum and Gray[7] found this could range up to 30°. Jaramaz and associates[23] found a range of 0° to 20°.

Measurement of cup position off two-dimensional radiographs, while reasonably accurate for cup abduction, has led to wide variations in the assessment of cup anteversion. Conventionally, abduction is determined by a line drawn across the face of the acetabular cup and its intersection, with a line drawn across the bottom of the ischial tuberosities or the teardrops at the bottom of the acetabulum. Calculations of cup anteversion are generally based on measurements of the size of the ellipse formed by the edges of the cup, with mathematical calculations to convert this to degrees of anteversion.[63,64] These measurements of cup position are better thought of as the amount of abduction and anteversion of the cup relative to the radiographic plate rather than the cup position in the pelvis. Similarly, the assessment of anteversion of acetabular cups on axial CT scans reflects the cup relative to the CT scanner rather than the pelvic anatomy.[59] The appearance on the radiograph is significantly affected by the location of the center of the x-ray beam to the cup and the distance of the x-ray source from the cup and radiographic plate. In their original study, Lewinnek and associates[6] compensated for this; the radiographs were standardized, centered on the pubic symphysis, and a bubble level was used to control pelvic tilt.

Marx and associates[64] reviewed five different methods for calculating the amount of cup anteversion and concluded that all resulted in significant variations from the values found on the CT scan, with the method of Widmer and Grützner[36] being the least inaccurate. Kalteis and associates[65] compared the measurements of cup position measured on plain radiographs using the method of Widmer and Grützner[36] with measurements based on CT scans; they found little difference

with abduction. However, significant differences were found for anteversion, with a mean deviation of 1.8° ± 9.3° and a range of –16.6° to 29.8°. Blendea and associates[58] have described using a CT/radiography matching algorithm to compare different pelvic radiographs and realign them to compensate for the differences in pelvic position and radiographic technique.

Pelvic tilt varies between individuals and changes dynamically between standing, sitting, and supine positions during normal activities of daily living. To assess the effect this may have on proper placement of hip implants, several authors have looked at this variation. Mayr and associates[66] used a digitizer to identify the pelvic frontal plane in 120 volunteers and found a mean inclination of 6.7° in the standing position and 5.6° in the supine position. They concluded that the frontal plane was a valid reference plane for placing the acetabular cup. By contrast, Eddine and associates[56] found significant variation from lying to standing on the basis of lateral pelvic radiographs taken in those positions. They recommended evaluation of the dynamic position of the pelvis in both positions if relying on CT scans for planning of cup position. Pelvic tilt was assessed in 30 normal volunteers by Lembeck and associates[67] using an inclinometer with ultrasound to compensate for soft-tissue thickness. They found pelvic inclination of –4° supine and –8° standing, with a range of –27° to 3°. They concluded that this amount of variation makes navigation systems referring to the pelvic plane inaccurate.

The amount of pelvic tilt has an effect on the anteversion of the cup relative to the anterior pelvic plane compared to the anteversion relative to the long axis of the body, which

can be referred to as the "functional plane." A series of lateral pelvic photographs (Figure 8) show how the apparent forward flexion (anteversion) of the natural acetabulum changes as the pelvis is tilted from an anterior tilt to a posterior tilt. Differences in pelvic tilt between patients are seen with standing lateral radiographs (Figure 9). For patients with increased lumbar lordosis, in which the pelvis tilts anteriorly and the pubis is posterior to the ASIS, the functional position of the cup will be retroverted compared with measurements relative to the frontal plane.

In clinical evaluations, other authors have found similar variations in their patients' pelvic tilt. In analyzing the position of the pelvis on the operating room table before dislocating the hip, DiGioia and associates[24] found that the pelvic plane had a mean difference from the estimated longitudinal axis of the body of 6° of flexion, with a range of –7° to 23°. Nishihara and associates[61] reported on 101 patients with total hip replacements and found a wide range of pelvic flexion-extension that varied between patients for supine, standing, and sitting positions. They found that the preoperative pelvic tilt was maintained at 1 year postoperatively, and the supine and standing positions were relatively equivalent. The mean flexion angle was 5° ± 9°, with a range of –37° to 30°. They concluded that anatomic landmarks may not be appropriate for positioning the acetabular cup, and the functional position of the pelvis, with the patient supine, may be a more reliable guide.

The proper position of the cup is dependent on the motion available and the soft-tissue constraints to create a stable construct and avoid impingement or subluxation with

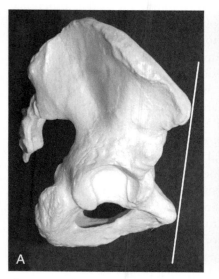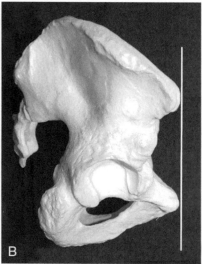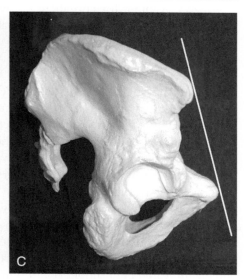

**Figure 8**   Changes in the apparent anteversion or forward flexion of the natural acetabulum with tilting of the pelvis from anterior to posterior. **A,** Anterior tilt effectively causes retroversion of the acetabulum. **B,** Neutral pelvic tilt with normal acetabular anteversion. **C,** Posterior pelvic tilt with increased acetabular anteversion.

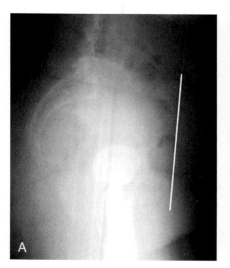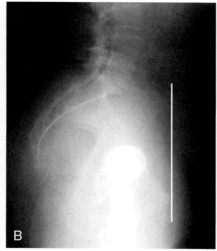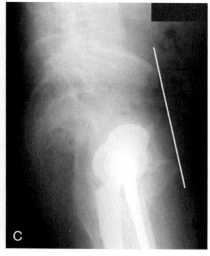

**Figure 9**   Variation in the pelvic tilt of different patients on standing postoperative lateral radiographs. **A,** Anterior pelvic tilt. **B,** Neutral pelvic. **C,** Posterior pelvic tilt.

normal activities. Various recommendations have been made in the past for proper cup position. Charnley[68] recommended 45° of abduction and 0° of anteversion, while Harris[69] advocated 30° of abduction and 20° of anteversion. Lewinnek and associates' study of dislocation patterns resulted in their determination of safe zones.[6]

For each patient's potential hip range of motion, there should be an optimal interplay of cup abduction, cup anteversion, femoral anteversion, femoral stem-neck angle, head diameter, and head-neck ratio.[70] McCollum and Gray[7] advocated adjustment of the amount of anteversion based on preoperative standing lateral radiographs to accommodate variation

of pelvic tilt. With a computer model, D'Lima and associates[71] showed a progressive improvement in potential range of motion without impingement from 35° to 45° to 55° of abduction. They demonstrated that the proper combination of femoral anteversion and acetabular anteversion could produce an optimal range of motion without impingement. Because femoral anteversion is often dictated by femoral bone anatomy, its assessment may provide a valuable guide for acetabular anteversion. Seki and associates[72] described a computer model for acceptable range of motion of the hip without impingement with 30° to 50° of abduction and 10° to 30° of anteversion. They found an inverse relationship between the appropriate cup anteversion and lumbar lordosis and sacral horizontal angle. Widmer and Majewski[70] described how variations in the femoral neck-shaft angle affect the proper cup position to achieve optimal range of motion.

With variation in the ability to accurately locate the anterior pelvic plane and concerns about the validity of the pelvic plane for orienting the acetabular cup, there has been interest in using navigation methods to place the cup on the basis of a functional axis that takes into consideration the individual pelvic tilt of a patient and his or her hip joint kinematics. An imageless hip navigation system has been described by Laffargue and associates[73] in which the principle is to orient the cup in relation to the cone describing the hip joint range of motion, rather than off anatomic bony landmarks. The range of motion and anteversion of the femoral implant was defined and used to orient the cup to allow full motion without impingement or subluxation. Widmer and Zurfluh[45] have outlined an approach of compliant positioning that takes into account cup inclination, cup anteversion, stem anteversion, stem-neck angle, and head-neck ratio where the range of motion of the implant system in any plane is always greater than the available hip range of motion that is controlled by soft tissues and bony constraints. Widmer[74] also has described this approach as a

"stem first" method, in which the cup is positioned after the stem has been placed and the potential hip range of motion determined, so as to avoid impingement or collision between the implants.

## Summary

Although current techniques in total hip replacement using traditional manual instruments have resulted in overall excellent results, there are continuing issues with the accuracy of implant placement and hip dislocation. Computer-assisted hip navigation now provides the tools to measure more accurately the implant's position. By using different types of navigation, both image-based and imageless, hip components can be placed with increased accuracy using the anterior frontal plane of the pelvis as a reference. From this work, a deeper understanding of the variation in pelvic tilt between individual patients has suggested that the ideal cup position may need to vary between patients as well. Future developments with hip navigation will need to continue to improve on the accuracy of the registration of the pelvis and bony landmarks. A more valuable benefit will be the avoidance of abnormal loading, dislocation, or component impingement, with an assessment of the optimum functional positions of the implants to provide full range of motion for each individual patient.

## References

1. Etienne A, Cupic Z, Charnley J: Postoperative dislocation after Charnley low-friction arthroplasty. *Clin Orthop Relat Res* 1978;132:19-23.

2. Ali Khan MA, Brakenbury PH, Reynolds IS: Dislocation following total hip replacement. *J Bone Joint Surg Br* 1981;63:214-218.

3. Woo RY, Morrey BF: Dislocation after total arthroplasty. *J Bone Joint Surg Am* 1982;64:1295-1306.

4. Masonis JL, Bourne RB: Surgical approach, abductor function, and total hip arthroplasty dislocation. *Clin Orthop Relat Res* 2002;405:46-53.

5. Barrack RL: Dislocation after total hip arthroplasty: Implant design and orientation. *J Am Acad Orthop Surg* 2003;11:89-99.

6. Lewinnek GE, Lewis JL, Tarr R, Compere CL, Zimmerman JR: Dislocations after total hip-replacement arthroplasties. *J Bone Joint Surg Am* 1978;60:217-220.

7. McCollum DE, Gray WJ: Dislocations after total hip arthroplasty: Causes and prevention. *Clin Orthop Relat Res* 1990;261:159-170.

8. Nishii T, Sugano N, Miki H, Koyama T, Takao M, Yoshikawa H: Influence of component positions on dislocation: Computed tomographic evaluations in a consecutive series of total hip arthroplasty. *J Arthroplasty* 2004;19:162-166.

9. Jolles BM, Zangger P, Leyvraz PF: Factors predisposing to dislocation after primary total hip arthroplasty: A multivariate analysis. *J Arthroplasty* 2002;17:282-288.

10. Biedermann R, Tonin A, Krismer M, Rachbauer F, Eibl G, Stockl B: Reducing the risk of dislocation after total hip arthroplasty: The effect of orientation of the acetabular component. *J Bone Joint Surg Br* 2005;87:762-769.

11. Morrey BF: Difficult complications after hip joint replacement: Dislocation. *Clin Orthop Relat Res* 1997;344:179-187.

12. Pellicci PM, Bostrom M, Poss R: Posterior approach to total hip replacement using enhanced posterior soft tissue repair. *Clin Orthop Relat Res* 1998;355:224-228.

13. Kwon MS, Kuskowski M, Mulhall KJ, Macaulay W, Brown TE, Saleh KJ: Does surgical approach affect total hip arthroplasty dislocation rates? *Clin Orthop Relat Res* 2006;447:34-38.

14. Padgett DE, Lipman J, Robie B, Nestor BJ: Influence of total hip design on dislocation: A computer model and clinical analysis. *Clin Orthop Relat Res* 2006;447:48-52.

15. Scifert CF, Brown TD, Pedersen DR, Callaghan JJ: A finite element analysis of factors influencing total hip dislocation. *Clin Orthop Relat Res* 1998;355:152-162.

16. Burroughs BR, Hallstrom B, Golladay GJ, Hoeffel D, Harris WH: Range of motion and stability in total hip arthroplasty with 28-, 32-, 38-, and 44-mm femoral head sizes. *J Arthroplasty* 2005;20:11-19.

17. Yoshimine F: The influence of the oscillation angle and the neck anteversion of the prosthesis on the cup safe-zone that fulfills the criteria for range of motion in total hip replacements: The required oscillation angle for an acceptable cup safe-zone. *J Biomech* 2005;38:125-132.

18. Hall RM, Siney P, Unsworth A, et al: Prevalence of impingement in explanted Charnley acetabular components. *J Orthop Sci* 1998;3:204-208.

19. Yamaguchi M, Akisue T, Bauer TW, et al: The spatial location of impingement in total hip arthroplasty. *J Arthroplasty* 2000;15:305-313.

20. Crowninshield RD, Maloney WD, Wentz DH, Humphrey SM, Blanchard CR: Biomechanics of large femoral heads. *Clin Orthop Relat Res* 2004;429:102-107.

21. Kennedy JG, Rogers WB, Soffe KE, Sullivan RJ, Griffen DG, Sheehan LJ: Effect of acetabular component orientation on recurrent, dislocation, pelvic osteolysis, polyethylene wear, and component migration. *J Arthroplasty* 1998;13:530-534.

22. Del Schutte H Jr, Lipman A, Bannar S, Livermore J, Ilstrup D, Morrey B: Effects of acetabular abduction on cup wear rates in total hip arthroplasty. *J Arthroplasty* 1998;13:621-626.

23. Jaramaz B, DiGioia AM III, Blackwell M, Nikou C: Computer assisted measurement of cup placement in total hip replacement. *Clin Orthop Relat Res* 1998;354:70-81.

24. DiGioia AM III, Jaramaz B, Plakseychuk AY, Moody JE Jr, Nikou C, Labarca RS: Comparison of a mechanical acetabular alignment guide with computer placement of the socket. *J Arthroplasty* 2002;17:359-364.

25. Ranawat CS, Maynard MJ, Deshmukh RG: Cemented primary total hip arthroplasty, in Sledge C (ed): *Master Techniques in Orthopaedic Surgery: The Hip*. Philadelphia, PA, Lippincott-Raven, 1998, pp 217-238.

26. Maruyama M, Feinberg JR, Capello WN, D'Antonio JA: Morphologic features of the acetabulum and femur: Anteversion angle and implant positioning. *Clin Orthop Relat Res* 2001;393:52-65.

27. Hassan DM, Johnston GH, Dust WN, Watson G, Dolovich AT: Accuracy of intraoperative assessment of acetabular prosthesis placement. *J Arthroplasty* 1998;13:80-84.

28. Saxler G, Marx A, Vandevelde D, et al: The accuracy of free-hand cup positioning: A CT based measurement of cup placement in 105 total hip arthroplasties. *Int Orthop* 2004;28:198-201.

29. McKibbin B: Anatomical factors in the stability of the hip in the newborn. *J Bone Joint Surg Br* 1970;52:148-159.

30. Murray DW: The definition and measurement of acetabular orientation. *J Bone Joint Surg Br* 1993;75:228-232.

31. DiGioia AM, Jaramaz B, Blackwell M, et al: The Otto Aufranc Award: Image guided navigation system to measure intraoperatively acetabular implant alignment. *Clin Orthop Relat Res* 1998;355:8-22.

32. Haaker R, Tiedjen K, Rubenthaler F, Stockheim M: Computer-assisted navigated cup placement in primary and secondary dysplastic hips. *Z Orthop Ihre Grenzgeb* 2003;141:105-111.

33. Jolles BM, Genoud P, Hoffmeyer P: Computer-assisted cup placement techniques in total hip arthroplasty improve accuracy of placement. *Clin Orthop Relat Res* 2004;426:174-179.

34. Leenders T, Vandevelde D, Mahieu G, Nuyts R: Reduction in variability of acetabular cup abduction using computer assisted surgery: A prospective and randomized study. *Comput Aided Surg* 2002;7:99-106.

35. Sugano N, Sasama T, Sato Y, et al: Accuracy evaluation of surface-based registration methods in a computer navigation system for hip surgery performed through a posterolateral approach. *Comput Aided Surg* 2001;6:195-203.

36. Widmer KH, Grützner PA: Joint replacement-total hip replacement with CT-based navigation. *Injury* 2004;35:S-A84-S-A89.

37. Zheng G, Marx A, Langlotz U, Widmer KH, Buttaro M, Nolte LP: A hybrid CT-free navigation system for total hip arthroplasty. *Comput Aided Surg* 2002;7:129-145.

38. Hube R, Birke A, Hein W, Klima S: CT-based and fluoroscopy-based navigation for cup implantation in total hip arthroplasty (THA). *Surg Technol Int* 2003;11:275-280.

39. Grützner PA, Zheng G, Langlotz U, et al: C-arm based navigation in total hip arthroplasty: Background and clinical experience. *Injury* 2004;35(suppl 1):S-A90-S-A95.

40. Stiehl JB, Heck DA, Lazzeri M: Accuracy of acetabular component positioning with a fluoroscopically referenced CAOS system. *Comput Aided Surg* 2005;10:321-327.

41. Tannast M, Langlotz F, Kubiak-Langer M, Langlotz U, Siebenrock K: Accuracy and potential pitfalls of fluoroscopy-guided acetabular cup placement. *Comput Aided Surg* 2005;10:329-336.

42. Kalteis T, Handel M, Bathis H, Perlick L, Tingart M, Grifka J: Imageless navigation for insertion of the acetabular component in total hip arthroplasty: Is it as accurate as CT-based navigation? *J Bone Joint Surg Br* 2006;88:163-167.

43. DiGioia AM, Plakseychuk AY, Levison TJ, et al: Mini incision technique for total hip arthroplasty with naviga-

tion. *J Arthroplasty* 2003;18:123-128.

44. Honl M, Schwieger K, Salineros M, Jacobs J, Morlock M, Wimmer M: Orientation of the acetabular component: A comparison of five navigation systems with conventional surgical technique. *J Bone Joint Surg Br* 2006; 88:1401-1405.

45. Widmer KH, Zurfluh B: Compliant positioning of total hip components for optimal range of motion. *J Orthop Res* 2004;22:815-821.

46. Nogler M, Kessler O, Prassl A, et al: Reduced variability of acetabular cup positioning with use of an imageless navigation system. *Clin Orthop Relat Res* 2004;426:159-163.

47. Kiefer H: OrthoPilot cup navigation: How to optimise cup positioning? *Int Orthop* 2003;27:S37-S42.

48. Ottersbach A, Haaker R: Optimization of cup positioning in THA: Comparison between conventional mechanical instrumentation and computer-assisted implanted cups by using the ortho pilot navigation system. *Z Orthop Ihre Grenzgeb* 2005; 143:611-615.

49. Dorr LD, Hishiki Y, Wan Z, Newton D, Yun A: Development of imageless computer navigation for acetabular component position in total hip replacement. *Iowa Orthop J* 2005;25:1-9.

50. Wixson RL, MacDonald MA: Total hip arthroplasty through a minimal posterior approach using imageless computer-assisted hip navigation. *J Arthroplasty* 2005;20(7 suppl 3):51-56.

51. Wixson RL, Lim D, Lin F, MacDonald M, Makhsous M: Computer assisted navigation with total hip arthroplasty: A prospective, randomized study. *73rd Annual Meeting Proceedings.* Rosemont, IL, American Academy of Orthopaedic Surgeons, p 482.

52. Wolf A, DiGioia AM III, Mor AB, Jaramaz B: Cup alignment error model for total hip arthroplasty. *Clin Orthop Relat Res* 2005;437:132-137.

53. Richolt JA, Rittmeister ME: Misinterpretation of the anteversion in computer-assisted acetabular cup navigation as a result of a simplified palpation method of the frontal pelvic plane. *Z Orthop Ihre Grenzgeb* 2006; 144:305-310.

54. Richolt JA, Effenberger H, Rittmeister ME: How does soft tissue distribution affect anteversion accuracy of the palpation procedure in image-free acetabular cup navigation? An ultrasonographic assessment. *Comput Aided Surg* 2005;10:87-92.

55. Spencer JMF, Day RE, Sloan KE, Beaver RJ: Computer navigation of the acetabular component: A cadaver reliability study. *J Bone Joint Surg Br* 2006;88:972-975.

56. Eddine TA, Migaud H, Chantelot C, Cotten A, Fontaine C, Duquennoy A: Variations of pelvic anteversion in the lying and standing positions: Analysis of 24 control subjects and implications for CT measurement of position of a prosthetic cup. *Surg Radiol Anat* 2001;23:105-110.

57. Tannast M, Langlotz U, Siebenrock KA, Wiese M, Bernsmann K, Langlotz F: Anatomic referencing of cup orientation in total hip arthroplasty. *Clin Orthop Relat Res* 2005;436: 144-150.

58. Blendea S, Eckman K, Jaramaz B, Levison TJ, Digioia AM III: Measurements of acetabular cup position and pelvic spatial orientation after total hip arthroplasty using computed tomography/radiography matching. *Comput Aided Surg* 2005;10:37-43.

59. Lazennec JY, Charlot N, Gorin M, et al: Hip-spine relationship: A radioanatomical study for optimization in acetabular cup positioning. *Surg Radiol Anat* 2004;26:136-144.

60. Muller O, Lembeck B, Reize P, Wulker N: Quantification and visualization of the influence of pelvic tilt upon measurement of acetabular inclination and anteversion. . *Z Orthop Ihre Grenzgeb* 2005;143:72-78.

61. Nishihara S, Sugano N, Nishii T, Ohzono K, Yoshikawa H: Measurements of pelvic flexion angle using three-dimensional computed tomog-

raphy. *Clin Orthop Relat Res* 2003;411: 140-151.

62. Aubry S, Marinescu A, Forterre O, Runge M, Garbuio P: Definition of a reproducible method for acetabular anteversion measurement at CT. *J Radiol* 2005;86:399-404.

63. Widmer KH: A simplified method to determine acetabular cup anteversion from plain radiographs. *J Arthroplasty* 2004;19:387-390.

64. Marx A, von Knoch M, Pförtner J, Wiese M, Saxler G: Misinterpretation of cup anteversion in total hip arthroplasty using planar radiography. *Arch Orthop Trauma Surg* 2006;126: 487-492.

65. Kalteis T, Handel M, Herold T, Perlick L, Paetzel C, Grifka J: Position of the acetabular cup: Accuracy of radiographic calculation compared to CT-based measurement. *Eur J Radiol* 2006;58:294-300.

66. Mayr E, Kessler O, Prassl A, Rachbauer F, Krismer M, Nogler M: The frontal pelvic plane provides a valid reference system for implantation of the acetabular cup: Spatial orientation of the pelvis in different positions. *Acta Orthop* 2005;76:848-853.

67. Lembeck B, Mueller O, Reize Pand Wuelker N: Pelvic tilt makes acetabular cup navigation inaccurate. *Acta Orthop* 2005;76:517-523.

68. Charnley J: Total hip replacement by low-friction arthroplasty. *Clin Orthop Relat Res* 1970;72:7-21.

69. Harris WH: Advances in surgical technique for total hip replacement: Without and with osteotomy of the greater trochanter. *Clin Orthop Relat Res* 1980;146:188-204.

70. Widmer KH, Majewski M: The impact of the CCD-angle on range of motion and cup positioning in total hip arthroplasty. *Clin Biomech (Bristol, Avon)* 2005;20:723-728.

71. D'Lima DD, Urquhart AG, Buehler KO, Walker RH, Colwell CW: The effect of the orientation of the acetabular and femoral components on the range of motion of the hip at different head-neck ratios. *J Bone Joint*

*Surg Am* 2000;82:315-321.

72. Seki M, Yuasa N, Ohkuni K: Analysis of optimal range of socket orientations in total hip arthroplasty with use of computer-aided design simulation. *J Orthop Res* 1998;16:513-517.

73. Laffargue P, Pinoit Y, Tabutin J, Giraud F, Puget J, Migaud H: Computer-assisted positioning of the acetabular cup for total hip arthroplasty based on joint kinematics without prior imaging: Preliminary results with computed tomographic assessment. *Rev Chir Orthop Reparatrice Appar Mot* 2006;92:316-325.

74. Widmer KH: Stem first: A simplified method for optimized positioning of components in total hip arthroplasty in bioceramics and alternative bearings in joint arthroplasty. *10th Biolox Symposium Proceedings*. Dordrecht, Netherlands, Springer, 2005, pp 137-142.

# 55

# The Current Status of Computer-Assisted High Tibial Osteotomy, Unicompartmental Knee Replacement, and Revision Total Knee Replacement

*Jean-Yves Jenny, MD

## Abstract

*Navigation systems aid in achieving precision and accuracy of surgical steps. Conventional techniques fail to achieve optimal correction in more than 20% of patients undergoing high tibial osteotomy, which is sensitive to the accuracy of limb axis correction. A computer navigation system with dedicated software has been developed to allow the leg axis to be navigated intraoperatively, and the desired correction can be obtained with a corrective device of the appropriate height.*

*Unicompartmental knee replacement also is sensitive to the accuracy of component placement. Standard navigation software has been modified to allow better accuracy when using a minimally invasive surgical approach.*

*Revision total knee replacement is a challenging procedure because most of the standard bony and ligamentous landmarks are lost during the initial implantation. Using the standard navigation technique allows easier restoration of the joint line, adequate limb axis correction, and improved ligamentous stability than can be achieved using a conventional technique. However, standard software does not allow navigation of the stem extensions, which can lead to significant malpositioning of the prosthetic components. Specific software is currently being developed to address this issue.*

**Instr Course Lect 2008;57:721-726.**

The effectiveness of navigation systems for total knee replacement (TKR) has been extensively validated in the literature.[1-4] These techniques can be viewed as a routine method for implanting a total knee prosthesis, even if acceptance of such techniques remains low. It is logical to use computer-assisted navigation in other knee procedures in which the precision and accuracy of surgical steps is relevant, such as high tibial osteotomy (HTO), unicompartmental knee replacement (UKR), and revision TKR.

## High Tibial Osteotomy
### Rationale
HTO is a common procedure for isolated varus gonarthrosis.[5] Short- and long-term results are usually good; however, results are sensitive to the accuracy of limb axis correction.[6] Conventional techniques involve intraoperative control of the limb axis by different methods including fluoroscopic control, alignment jigs, or rods. However, these techniques fail to achieve optimal correction in all patients. It is accepted that approximately 20% of patients will not have an optimal limb axis correction as measured by postoperative radiographs.[7] Navigation systems have proved to be an accurate method for achieving proper lower limb axis correction during TKR. The same algorithms can be used during HTO to achieve optimal correction of the femorotibial angle.

### Surgical Technique
The author uses the OrthoPilot (Aesculap, Tuttlingen, Germany), a non–image-based navigation system. The software for this system is

*Jean-Yves Jenny, MD or the department with which he is affiliated has received royalties from Aesculap and is a consultant or employee for Aesculap.*

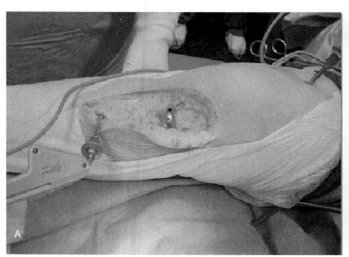
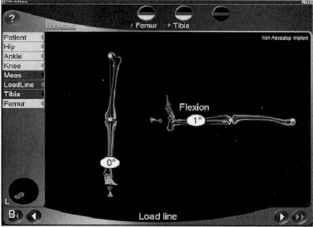

**Figure 1**  **A,** Intraoperative view of a HTO with the corrective device in place. **B,** Intraoperative view of the monitoring screen of the navigation system.

dedicated to the open wedge technique, but another version of the software dedicated to the closing wedge technique is available. Three infrared localizers are implanted on bicortical screws in the distal femur and the proximal tibia and are strapped on the dorsal part of the foot. The relative motion of two adjacent localizers is tracked by an infrared camera (Polaris, Northern Digital, Toronto, Canada). The dedicated software calculates the center of rotation of this movement and thus defines the respective centers of rotation of the hip, knee, and ankle joints. These centers are used to calculate the mechanical axes of the femur and tibia on both coronal and sagittal planes. The coronal mechanical femorotibial angle is measured in full extension, and the amount of knee flexion or extension is measured at full extension.

A medial approach to the proximal tibia is performed, and the level and direction of the osteotomy are defined with the help of an image intensifier. A guidewire is inserted first, and the osteotomy is performed with an oscillating saw, while attempting to preserve the lateral tibia cortex. The osteotomy is opened by hand, and the axis is corrected by placing a metallic corrective device of the appropriate height to obtain the expected correction (Figure 1). The corrected axis is controlled by the navigation system, and the height of the metallic corrective device is changed if necessary. Attention is paid to the maximal extension angle, which should not be changed after insertion of the corrective device to prevent a change in the tibial slope. When the expected correction is achieved, the metallic corrective device is replaced by a trapezoidal-shaped bone substitute of the same height, and the osteotomy is fixed by a plate. At each step, the accuracy of the axial correction can be controlled and adapted if necessary.

### Validation Study
A validation study of this technique was performed by Saragaglia and Roberts.[8] They compared the accuracy of the postoperative axis correction in 28 conventional open wedge HTOs and in 28 procedures using navigated open wedge HTO. The goal of the procedure was to achieve a coronal mechanical femorotibial angle between 2° and 6° of valgus. This goal was achieved in 71% of the conventional HTOs and 96% of the HTOs using navigation ($P <$ 0.0015). This study showed that navigation systems can improve the accuracy of axial correction during HTO, which could improve long-term results and decrease the TKR rate.

## Unicompartmental Knee Replacement
### Rationale
The accuracy of implantation is an established prognostic factor for the long-term survival of UKRs.[9-11] However, most UKR systems offer limited and potentially inaccurate instrumentation that relies substantially on the surgeon's judgment for correct implant positioning. Rates of inaccurate implantations as high as 30% have been reported with conventional, free-hand instrumentation.[12] Intra-

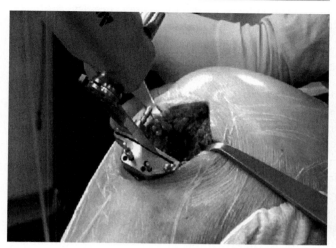

**Figure 2** UKR: tibial resection. The tibial resection guide is screwed onto the proximal tibia under navigation control. The resection is performed with a motorized saw blade.

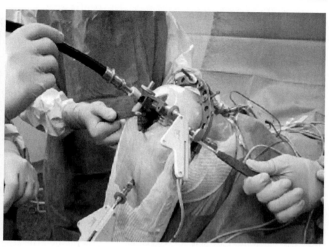

**Figure 3** UKR: femoral resection. The femoral bow is screwed onto the distal femur under navigation control. The femoral reception guide is fixed on the bow and can be moved around the knee flexion axis. Resection is performed with a motorized burr.

medullary femoral-guiding devices can improve these results but do not guarantee reproducible optimal implantation.[13,14] Because computer-assisted systems for TKR have shown higher precision for implant positioning in comparison with conventional instrumentation, it was logical to adapt the TKR technique to UKR.[1-4]

### Surgical Technique

The navigated surgical technique for UKR using the OrthoPilot system was described in the literature in 2003.[15] Since the time of that publication, a navigated, minimally invasive technique has been developed. The navigation system software was modified because the minimally invasive approach does not allow the direct palpation of the lateral femorotibial joint. When using the minimally invasive approach, the positions of the lateral articular points are calculated by the software after radiographic preoperative planning.

The procedure begins with a quadriceps-sparing medial arthrotomy, typically 6 cm in length. Kine-

matic registration is performed in the usual manner. Anatomic registration is limited to the medial femorotibial joint. The tibial resection guide is oriented with a free-hand technique (Figure 2). A navigated bow is fixed by two bicortical screws on the distal femur and oriented along the knee flexion-extension axis. The distal and posterior resection guides are fixed and finely oriented on this bow according to the navigation system but are not fixed directly within the joint (Figure 3).

**Table 1**
**Unicompartmental Knee Replacement: Radiographic Results**

| Criterion | Minimally Invasive Standard Technique | Minimally Invasive Navigated Technique | Significance |
|---|---|---|---|
| Accurate coronal orientation of the femoral component | 93% | 98% | None |
| Accurate sagittal orientation of the femoral component | 49% | 75% | $P < 0.001$ |
| Accurate coronal orientation of the tibial component | 99% | 98% | None |
| Accurate sagittal orientation of the tibial component | 90% | 94% | None |

### Validation Study

Patients who underwent UKR surgery for primary medial osteoarthritis were studied. Using computer-assisted navigation, prostheses were implanted in patients at four different hospitals between October 2005 and April 2006. The control group consisted of patients who underwent conventional implantation of a unicompartmental knee prosthesis in one of the participating hospitals between 1999 and 2005. Forty-eight men and 88 women with a mean age of 65 years (range, 44 to 88 years) were included in the study. All implantations were performed by experienced knee reconstruction surgeons (JY Jenny, MD, unpublished data, 2006).

## Results

The accuracy of implant positioning was determined using standard AP and lateral radiographs. Evaluation was performed according to the manufacturers' specifications. The percentage of implant positions outside the optimal range also was determined.

The accuracy of coronal positioning of the femoral component after minimally invasive navigated implantation was slightly higher than for standard minimally invasive implantation (2% versus 7% outliers). The accuracy of the sagittal positioning of the femoral component after minimally invasive navigated implantation was higher than for the nonnavigated group (25% versus 51% outliers, $P < 0.001$). However, 25% of implants were not in an optimal position. In the first group of patients in the study, preparation of the femoral component was navigated, but the implantation of the femoral component was not navigated. A new instrument was introduced for the last 10 implantations that permitted navigated implantation of the femoral component. With this new device, 9 of 10 femoral components (90%) were in the range of optimal position. For coronal positioning of the tibial component, accuracy was similar in both groups (2% versus 1% outliers). The group treated with navigated implantation had higher accuracy for sagittal positioning of the tibial component than did the nonnavigated group (7% versus 10% outliers). The only significant difference in outcome occurred in the sagittal positioning of the femoral component. Results of this UKR study are summarized in Table 1.

## Conclusion

Minimally invasive, navigated implantation of a UKR using a non–image-based system improved the radiologic accuracy of the implantation without significant inconvenience and with little change in the conventional surgical technique. Outcomes were significantly improved in only one criterion; however, this study involved the learning curve inherent in using a new implant technique in all centers and of the navigation technique in two of the centers. It has been determined that the introduction of a new surgical technique is associated with longer surgical times and poorer accuracy in the first group of patients who undergo surgery with the new technique.[16] Improved results can be expected as surgeons master the techniques of the minimally invasive procedure and the navigation system.

Innovations will probably bring further improvement. Minimally invasive implantation is effective but must be validated in larger studies. Long-term results regarding function and survival time of the prosthesis are needed.

## Revision TKR
### Rationale

The number of revision TKRs has dramatically increased in recent years and may account for 10% of all TKRs.[17] Causes for revision TKR include septic failure, knee instability, and aseptic loosening. Revision TKR is a challenging procedure, mainly because most of the standard bony and ligamentous landmarks are lost during the initial implantation surgery.[18] Restoration of the joint line, adequate limb axis correction, and ligamentous stability are considered critical for the short- and long-term outcomes of revision TKR as they are for primary TKR.

There are no available data about the range of tolerable leg alignments after revision TKR; however, it can be assumed that the range would be the same as for primary TKR ($\pm 3°$ off the neutral alignment). It also can be assumed that the conventional instruments, which rely on visual or anatomic alignments or intramedullary or extramedullary rods, are associated with a significantly higher variation in the leg axis correction. The efficiency of navigation systems for primary TKR makes it logical to adapt this technology for revision TKR.[19]

Perlick and associates[19] hypothesized that significantly better leg alignment and component orientation would be achieved when using a navigation system in comparison with the conventional technique for revision TKR. Two groups of 25 revision TKRs were compared. One group was operated on using a CT-free navigation system and the other with the conventional manual technique. Postoperative leg alignment was measured on long-leg coronal and sagittal radiographs. Significantly better correction of the limb axis was achieved in the navigated group (92%) compared with the conventional group (76%). All navigated femoral components were well aligned in the coronal plane, compared with only 84% in the conventional group ($P < 0.05$). All navigated tibial components were well aligned in the coronal plane, compared with only 94% in the conventional group ($P > 0.05$). The sagittal alignment of both femoral and tibial implants also was improved in the navigation group ($P > 0.05$). The level of the joint line was more accurately restored with help of the navigation system.

### Surgical Technique

The author uses the standard OrthoPilot navigation system for revision TKR, with a few modifications to the standard technique. The reference screws are fixed more proximally on the femur and more distally on the tibia to fit with the expected stem extension. The kinematic and anatomic registration is made in the usual manner, with the index implants in place (placement may be loose). The implants are then removed. Resection of the proximal tibia and the distal femur is controlled with conventional navigated instruments. Navigation of the rotational positioning of the femoral implant is often difficult or impossible because there is no bone remaining on the distal part of the femur to securely fix the appropriate guide. There is no possibility to navigate the stems. The trial implants are placed with the appropriate stem extensions, and restoration of the

limb axis and ligamentous balancing are checked and corrected if necessary. Most knees are perfectly aligned and balanced; however, in some instances there is a significant difference between the expected position of the implant and its actual position, mainly because the direction of the stem extension is not optimal.

### Future Developments

The author's results were basically similar to those of Perlick and associates.[19] Standard navigation software is not perfectly suited for use in revision TKR procedures. Standard software offers no possibility to deal with bone loss, reconstruction of joint-line height, and the direction of the stem extension.[18] Experimental software has been developed specifically for TKR revision surgery. The efficacy of this new software must still be validated in clinical practice (Figures 4 and 5).

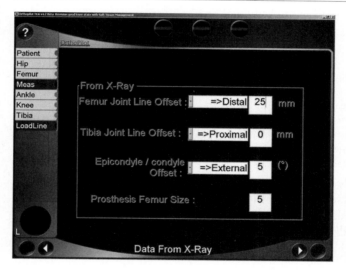

**Figure 4** Experimental OrthoPilot software for restoration of the joint line in TKR revision surgery.

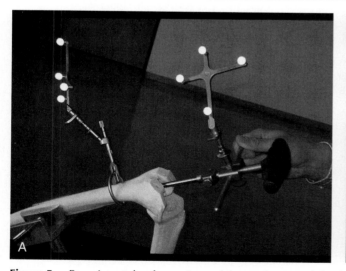

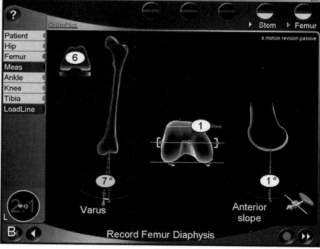

**Figure 5** Experimental software is used for navigation of the femoral stem extension in TKR revision surgery. **A,** The femoral tracker is fixed on the distal femur with a C-clamp with no intramedullary part. **B,** Software is used to navigate the intramedullary rod; its position along the femoral axis simulates the future position of the femoral stem extension.

## Summary

The adaptation of TKR navigation software to HTO and UKR has been successful. The currently available software versions are effective and user-friendly and have improved the accuracy of these procedures. Computer-assisted navigation helps the surgeon perform UKRs with a minimally invasive technique without loss of accuracy. Dedicated navigation software for revision TKR is still being developed but appears to promise better outcomes for patients.

## References

1. Decking R, Markmann Y, Fuchs J, Puhl W, Scharf HP: Leg axis after computer-navigated total knee arthroplasty: A prospective randomized trial comparing computer-navigated and manual implantation. *J Arthroplasty* 2005;20:282-288.

2. Saragaglia D, Picard F, Chaussard C, Montbarbon E, Leitner F, Cinquin P: Computer-assisted knee arthroplasty: Comparison with a conventional procedure: Results of 50 cases in a prospective randomized study. *Rev Chir Orthop Reparatrice Appar Mot* 2001;87: 18-28.

3. Stockl B, Nogler M, Rosiek R, Fischer M, Krismer M, Kessler O: Navigation improves accuracy of rotational alignment in total knee arthroplasty. *Clin Orthop Relat Res* 2004;426:180-186.

4. Victor J, Hoste D: Image-based computer-assisted total knee arthroplasty leads to lower variability in coronal alignment. *Clin Orthop Relat Res* 2004;428:131-139.

5. Flecher X, Parratte S, Aubaniac JM, Argenson JN: A 12-28-year followup study of closing wedge high tibial osteotomy. *Clin Orthop Relat Res* 2006; 452:91-96.

6. Hernigou P, Medevielle D, Debeyre J, Goutallier D: Proximal tibial osteotomy for osteoarthritis with varus deformity: A ten to thirteen-year follow-up study. *J Bone Joint Surg Am* 1987;69:332-354.

7. Jenny JY, Tavan A, Jenny G, Kehr P: Long-term survival rate of tibial osteotomies for valgus gonarthrosis. *Rev Chir Orthop Reparatrice Appar Mot* 1998;84:350-357.

8. Saragaglia D, Roberts J: Navigated osteotomies around the knee in 170 patients with osteoarthritis secondary to genu varum. *Orthopedics* 2005;28 (suppl 10):S1269-S1274.

9. Cartier P, Sanouillier JL, Grelsamer RP: Unicompartmental knee arthroplasty surgery: 10-year minimum follow-up period. *J Arthroplasty* 1996; 11:782-788.

10. Hernigou P, Deschamps G: Unicompartmental knee prosthesis. *Rev Chir Orthop Reparatrice Appar Mot* 1996;82 (suppl 1):23-60.

11. Lootvoet L, Burton P, Himmer O, Piot L, Ghosez JP: A unicompartment knee prosthesis: The effect of the positioning of the tibial plate on the functional results. *Acta Orthop Belg* 1997;63:94-101.

12. Tabor OB Jr, Tabor OB: Unicompartmental arthroplasty: A long-term follow-up study. *J Arthroplasty* 1998; 13:373-379.

13. Argenson JN, Chevrol-Benkeddache Y, Aubaniac JM: Modern unicompartmental knee arthroplasty with cement: A three to ten-year follow-up study. *J Bone Joint Surg Am* 2002;84: 2235-2239.

14. Jenny JY, Boeri C: Accuracy of implantation of a unicompartmental total knee arthroplasty with 2 different instrumentations: A case-controlled comparative study. *J Arthroplasty* 2002;17:1016-1020.

15. Jenny JY, Boeri C: Unicompartmental knee prosthesis implantation with a non-image-based navigation system: Rationale, technique, case-control comparative study with a conventional instrumented implantation. *Knee Surg Sports Traumatol Arthrosc* 2003;11:40-45.

16. King J, Stamper DL, Schaad DC, Leopold SS: Minimally invasive total knee arthroplasty compared with traditional total knee arthroplasty: Assessment of the learning curve and the postoperative recuperative period. *J Bone Joint Surg Am* 2007;89:1497-1503.

17. Knutson K, Lewold S, Robertsson O, Lidgren L: The Swedish knee arthroplasty register: A nation-wide study of 30,003 knees 1976-1992. *Acta Orthop Scand* 1994;65:375-386.

18. Partington PF, Sawhney J, Rorabeck CH, Barrack RL, Moore J: Joint line restoration after revision total knee arthroplasty. *Clin Orthop Relat Res* 1999;367:165-171.

19. Perlick L, Bäthis H, Perlick C, Lüring C, Tingart M, Grifka J: Revision total knee arthroplasty: A comparison of postoperative leg alignment after computer-assisted implantation versus the conventional technique. *Knee Surg Sports Traumatol Arthrosc* 2005;13: 167-173.

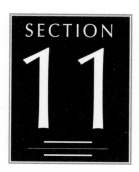

# SECTION 11

# Practice Management

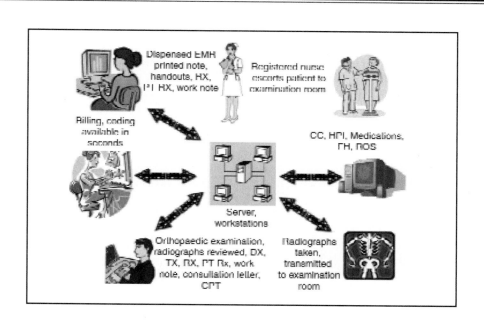

# Selecting and Starting an Orthopaedic Surgery Practice

Allan Mishra, MD
Andrew G. Urquhart, MD
Geoffrey T. Anders, JD, CPA, CHBC

## Abstract

*Every new surgeon is faced with the same question as their residency or fellowship draws to a close: What is next? Few residents or fellows are as well prepared to answer that question as they could be. Most programs do not teach residents how to choose a practice type and location. After formal orthopaedic training, new surgeons must make decisions about their careers that can be nearly as complex and difficult as the decisions they make in the operating room. Career choices have both significant and long-term effects on the physician's financial situation, career satisfaction, and personal life. The physician should be aware of key nonacademic issues that arise when completing a residency program or just beginning the practice of orthopaedic surgery.*

**Instr Course Lect 2008;57:729-736.**

A residency in orthopaedic surgery mandates a specific musculoskeletal curriculum and demands rigorous technical training. There is, however, no requirement to learn the logistic, financial, and legal aspects of the practice of orthopaedic surgery. This lack of exposure to the crucial elements needed for a successful practice can significantly impact the ability of new orthopaedic surgeons to make informed decisions regarding potential career paths.

Few prospective articles are available on how to make employment choices; however, several retrospective survey studies discuss that topic. Graduating surgical residents and fellows are mainly concerned with personal finances, family planning, and the availability of role models.[1] A 2005 study showed that work hours and preferred geographic locations were

predictors of the type of practice selected by ophthalmology residents.[2] Cardiothoracic training programs have recently reported difficulty in achieving suitable job placements for their graduates.[3] The lack of institutional or departmental leadership along with poor financial compensation and limited support for research have been identified as reasons why full-time faculty leave academic practice for private practice. Department leaders who are available and interested in the development of young faculty members are crucial to faculty retention.[4] An extensive literature search revealed no articles that specifically addressed practice selection for orthopaedic surgeons.

This chapter will outline the key nonacademic issues that are vital to graduating orthopaedic residents and surgeons in the first few years of

practice. Practice type and location options will be discussed in the context of call schedules and compensation. The impact of managed care, coding, and contracts on new surgeons will also be summarized. Sources for more detailed information will be provided.

## Selection of Practice Type

Choosing an orthopaedic practice may appear to be a simple choice. However, according to internal informal surveys of instructional course lecturers and other experts at the American Academy of Orthopaedic Surgeons (AAOS), more than one half of new graduates will leave their practice after just a few years, indicating a poor fit with the practice style, the people, or the community. Just as residents have been trained to question patients to obtain a history of illness, there are a set of open-ended questions that can provide perspective on the most suitable practice for an individual physician. Answers to questions of what, where, how, and with whom a physician wants to practice orthopaedics can help in deciding the next step in an orthopaedic surgeon's career.

### What Do You Want to Do?

Many physicians completing a residency program have already made

**Table 1**
**Practice Selection Matrix**

| | Pros | Cons |
|---|---|---|
| Academic practice | Teaching of residents<br>Research potential<br>Coverage of patients by residents<br>Ability to pursue a subspecialty<br>Collaboration with other specialists | Time commitment without reimbursement for teaching<br>Pressure to publish<br>Grant applications<br>Still a need to produce clinically<br>Committee or university responsibilities |
| Private practice Large group (6 to 25+ surgeons) | Better negotiating with managed care insurers<br>More availability for mentor relationships<br>Income may be higher because of ancillary service income<br>Less call coverage but more intense coverage | Too many surgeons may create difficult practice governance<br>May only be able to pursue narrow specialty<br>Internal referrals may be tilted toward older partners |
| Private practice Small group (2 to 5 surgeons) | Right combination of expertise in group may be ideal<br>Easier to make practice decisions<br>Compensation typically better than that of a multispecialty practice<br>Accountability of staff to surgeons | Less negotiating power with managed care insurers<br>Personality conflicts may arise<br>Call coverage more often<br>Internal competition for patients may result |
| Private practice Solo | Ability to make all practice decisions | Need to cover all calls or arrange coverage<br>Difficult contracting for managed care<br>Need to arrange all the business aspects of practice |
| Multispecialty group | Built-in referral base<br>Ability to seek consults from all other medical specialties as needed | Less compensation<br>Likely need to be a general orthopaedist<br>Practice governance usually dominated by primary care physicians |
| Closed HMO | Good starting salaries<br>Busy practice immediately<br>Reasonable call schedules<br>Excellent benefits and pension | Fixed working hours<br>Practiced controlled by HMO<br>No outside patients<br>No equity opportunity<br>Limited ability to benefit from ancillary services |
| Institutional (military/Veterans Administration) | Excellent electronic medical record keeping<br>Serving veterans<br>Immediately busy caseload<br>Potential for travel | Potential for deployment to war zone<br>Lower salaries<br>Highly bureaucratic<br>Very little control over cases or clinics |

HMO = health maintenance organization

the decision to pursue a fellowship. Others are considering a career in an academic practice. However, the decision on practice type and style is not straightforward. Not all academic practices are purely academic. Many have productivity incentives and private practice affiliations. In general, if an orthopaedic surgeon intends to work at an academic practice or wants to serve a larger community, subspecialty training will likely be required. Conversely, if the preference is to serve a rural community in a small group, broad generalist training may be a better fit. AAOS census data indicate there is no major difference in the number of hours spent working in an academic practice compared with a private practice.[5] On average, an orthopaedic practice is a consumptive endeavor, resulting in more than 59 hours per week devoted to the practice. An academic practice may provide the enjoyment of teaching at the expense of accepting a less efficient system, or may provide the joys of academic pursuits and research with the disadvantage of having to allot time for writing grants or working in the laboratory. A general private practice may offer autonomy and independence of governance with the real satisfaction of serving the needs of the patients and community, but may come at the expense of being a jack-of-all-trades and master of none. The fit of a practice is quite personal. Table 1 describes the pros and cons of various types of practices.

### Where Do You Want to Practice?

The location of the practice may be governed by the desired practice style. Working at a major teaching institution or in a major city may necessitate subspecialty training. If the orthopaedic surgeon strongly desires to work in a certain community, choosing a subspecialty that dovetails to the needs of that community may facilitate employment opportunities at that practice location. Where to practice is truly based on individual preference. Fortunately, a large number of resources are available for community comparisons (Table 2). Issues that may play a role in the choice of location include the quality of the schools, lifestyle, nearby recreational facilities/activities, and support available for the physician's spouse, life partner, or family.

An orthopaedic practice is very time consuming. As such, caution should be used in selecting a practice in a less desirable location with the idea that one can travel for recreation. The demands of the practice may limit vacation time. As such, living in an enjoyable community, whether it is close to water, mountains, family, or support structures, is probably more important than the financial aspects of the practice.

## With Whom Do You Want to Practice?

Perhaps most importantly, but equally difficult to judge, is the question of choosing partners. The odds are that an orthopaedic surgeon will spend as much or more time with future business partners as with their own spouse or family. Because an orthopaedic practice is like a marriage, an ill fit between personalities can cause heartache and angst and may eventually result in the breakdown of the practice. It is very important to take time and make many visits to the potential practice to get a real sense of the personalities involved. Time should be spent not only in the office but in the operating room as well. It is wise to visit the hospital personnel, ask many questions, and talk to the referring groups to gain insight into the reputation of the practice and the personalities involved. Be aware that there is a 50% chance of an unsuccessful relationship with partners; therefore, knowledge of the legal aspects and contracting issues involved in a partnership will be valuable in the event of a potential separation.

## Coding and Managed Care

Mastering the complex and constantly changing fields of managed care and medical coding are essential skills for the successful orthopaedic surgeons. These critical subjects, however, are rarely discussed or taught during medical school or res-

**Table 2**
**Websites and References That May Be Helpful in Searching for a Practice**

| Type of Information | Website Address | Description of Information |
|---|---|---|
| Practice | www.aaos.org | Wide variety of information for new surgeons |
| Location/financial | www.bestplaces.net | Discussion of the best locations |
| | www.insurance.com | Average insurance rates |
| | www.census.gov | Median income data |
| | www.uschamber.com | Local business information |
| Housing | www.realtor.com | House-hunting tool |
| | www.realtor.org | Housing statistics and analysis |
| | www.zillow.com | Home value estimator |
| Education | www.greatschools.net | List of award-winning schools |
| | www.census.gov | Includes data such as percentage of students in private schools |
| Quality of life | www.census.gov | Includes health insurance data |
| | www.fbi.gov | Crime statistics |
| Leisure and cultural activities | www.festivals.com | City festivals |
| | www.symphony.org | Orchestras |
| | www.museumlink.com | Museums |
| Outdoor activities | www.trails.com | Hiking trails |
| | www.playgolfamerica.com | Golfing options |
| Zoos, aquariums, gardens | www.aza.org | Listings of zoos, aquariums, and gardens |
| Weather | www.weatherchannel.com | Current weather information |
| Health | www.cdc.gov | Health statistics |
| | www.epa.gov | Air and water quality |
| Legal | www.physiciannews.com/business/405.html | See B. Smith: Claims made versus occurrence malpractice coverage. Physician's News Digest. April, 2005. |
| | www.physiciannews.com/business/303hursh.html | See D. Hursh: Your first employment contract. Physician's News Digest. March, 2003. |
| | www.ama-assn.org/ama/pub/category/print/12716.html | See American Medical Association Office of General Counsel: Restrictive Covenants in Physician Contracts. March 7, 2005. |

idency. It is usually assumed that a new surgeon can easily understand the interface with the health care insurance industry and can appropriately bill for services rendered. That assumption is clearly incorrect.

Billing of almost any office visit or procedure is associated with Current Procedural Terminology (CPT)

codes. These CPT codes must then be correctly paired with an International Classification of Diseases (ICD) number to bill for services. The ninth revision of this classification is commonly known as an ICD-9 code. Books, online references, and handheld devices are available to help surgeons with appropriate coding and billing. The Medicare regulations and managed care contracts associated with the coding process can easily confuse even experts who teach seminars on the subject. Efficient and appropriate coding is a challenge that requires the surgeon's continuing education, and action by a billing office that is willing to challenge payment rejections. Attendance at a coding seminar at least once every 2 years should help surgeons better understand and manage this complex process.

Recognizing the structure of other managed care entities can help surgeons make intelligent financial choices. Some of the most common managed care systems include health maintenance organizations (HMOs), preferred provider organizations (PPOs), independent practice associations (IPAs), physician-hospital organizations (PHOs), and management service organizations (MSOs).[6]

HMOs can be a completely closed system where patients must obtain all of their care within a specified structure (for example, the Kaiser HMO). In this form of managed care, the providers, imaging centers, and hospital choices are highly restricted. PPOs are another pervasive form of managed care. PPOs and some HMOs are networks of hospitals, surgery centers, imaging facilities, and doctors that have been organized by specific insurance companies. Member entities and physicians have agreed to provide services to patients at a discounted rate. Typically, these rates are fixed relative to Medicare reimbursement levels or may be paid at some percentage of billed charges. The compensation paid to surgeons by the insurance companies of HMO and PPO organizations can vary twofold or even threefold.

IPAs are legal structures that allow a group of physicians to collectively negotiate reimbursement rates with HMOs or PPOs. PHOs are collaborations between a group of doctors and a hospital. The group and the hospital then contract together with insurance companies for a comprehensive list of services, including professional fees and facility fees. These contracts are typically negotiated by the hospital and may be tilted in favor of hospital services by discounting the surgeon's professional fees.

Capitation is a less common form of managed care in which an insurance company pays a practice a specified amount of money per patient per year. The practice is then responsible for providing all of the agreed services required by that patient. The practice is given an incentive to control costs because it will keep any money that remains after all necessary services have been provided. Capitation should be avoided by all practices unless the financial structure is clearly in favor of the surgeon, which is rarely the case.

MSOs are companies that provide a specific service to a practice. The most common MSO is a billing company that is responsible for billing and collecting fees for a group of surgeons or an institution. Other MSOs may develop a marketing plan or Website for the practice, which can be quite helpful if expertise is needed in these areas. Recently, companies offering wireless electronic billing or secure electronic mail services have become available but have not yet deeply penetrated the market. Defining the specific financial implications of signing contracts with any of these managed care entities is crucial to the financial success of both private practices and academic institutions. Attempting to stay current on the constantly changing issues associated with managed

care is just one of the many important tasks for new orthopaedic surgeons.

## Compensation and Call

When initially evaluating practice options, residents often focus on compensation and the call schedule. Recruiters typically advertise high initial salaries and tempt new surgeons with seemingly attractive call options. Orthopaedic surgeons rank as the second most sought-after group for these recruiters.[7] However, graduating orthopaedic residents often have little objective information about fair starting salaries or the techniques of negotiating a reasonable call schedule.

The AAOS has collected data on the average salaries of all orthopaedic surgeons but does not have any specific information concerning initial compensation. Surveys of starting wages for orthopaedic surgeons range from $150,000 to more than $300,000, with spine surgeons earning the highest salaries.[8] When selecting a job in a private practice, surgeons may be offered a guaranteed minimum salary with a bonus based on productivity, a straight salary for all services provided, or some percentage of total collections.

In the closed HMO models, a salary based on the number of hours worked is typical. In this practice environment, if the surgeon exceeds the contracted number of hours, compensation will be received in the form of more money or more vacation time. In academic or multispecialty group practices, a formula is often used to calculate compensation. How this formula is devised and executed will significantly impact the net compensation paid. Usually, work is calculated by adding the relative value units in an attempt to measure work across specialties. Most formulas also incorporate research, teaching, and partnership factors. The head of the department or managing partner also may have some discretion regarding final salaries.

Several other potential revenue sources exist for new surgeons and should be part of the initial practice selection discussion. Compensation for "taking call" is increasingly common. The rate varies from a few hundred dollars per night to several thousand dollars. Participation in practice-owned physical therapy, imaging, or surgery centers may be quite lucrative or may represent a poor financial decision. The finances of these ancillary services should be verified with the practice's accountant to confirm income potential. The legality of these auxiliary services varies from state to state and is best evaluated by an attorney.

## Legal Issues

Any employment agreement should be in writing. Important terms should be defined in writing and should not be based on an undocumented verbal agreement; people can be forgetful and may have selective memories, particularly in the event of a dispute. All important terms should be addressed in the final contract because a court will evaluate a dispute based on the terms of the contract. Although the advice of an attorney or consultant is necessary, negotiations should be done directly by the physicians involved. This tactic will enable the physicians to assess their ability to work and deal with each other.[9]

### The Term of Employment

The employment contract should specify a starting date. Term is important as a measuring point for salary, benefit increases, and co-ownership consideration, if applica-

ble. Three types of terms offered in employment agreements are (1) an "at-will" employment term, whereby either party may terminate the employment at any time; (2) a "drop dead" employment term, whereby the employment relationship ends on a specific date (unless a new deal is reached); or (3) an "evergreen" contract, whereby the contract continues for a certain period of time and then automatically renews for successive periods unless either party gives notice to the other party within a set number of days before the end of the employment period.

### Termination

The agreement should state how it can be terminated by each party. The termination provision should explain how the parties may terminate the employment and what type of notice must be given by either party to terminate the agreement.[10] The termination provisions should be mutual; that is, each party's right to terminate the agreement should be the mirror image of the other party's right.[11]

Employment termination "for cause" usually refers to actions that may occur, such as committing a felony, breaching a material part of the contract, or committing any action of similar severity. Ideally, the contract should state that either party may terminate employment immediately only "for cause" (following a provision giving the party the right to cure any alleged breach) or not "for cause" on at least 90 days written notice.[12] This notice provision is important with respect to the bonus provision. The question is whether the employee is entitled to a prorated bonus, and if so, then which date is used for the proration—the date of termination notice or the date of effective termination?[11]

### Compensation

Compensation may consist of salary, bonus, paid business expenses, insurance coverage, paid vacation time, and sick pay. The contract should specify the salary terms for each year in which the physician is a nonowner of the practice. Incremental increases in salary must be spelled out in the contract in specific terms.[13] Bonuses most often are determined by one of three methods: gross production, the net income approach, or full discretionary bonus.[11] Regardless of the method used to determine the bonus, the following issues should be addressed: (1) monthly reports on productivity; (2) how collections will be handled for capitation contracts; and (3) how patients will be allocated. If there is an income threshold for bonus compensation, it is necessary to determine how the amount of the threshold is derived, whether it is achievable, how the practice will help the new physician increase his or her workload, and why the practice is hiring an associate.[11]

### Gross Production

Under the gross production method, the practice pays a bonus based on the cash collections generated by the physician for the practice in excess of a preset amount (required revenues). The gross production method is a good method if income is predictable. However, it may be disadvantageous if there is competition within the practice for patients.

### Net Income Approach

The net income approach states that to the extent the net income (for example, the doctor-owners' salaries, retirement plan contributions, and physician discretionary expenses) in the practice exceeds a percentage of the previous year's net income, the employee is entitled to a share of that excess. This method does not create competition among physicians within the practice. It is important to clarify the expenses that are included in the definition of net income.

### Fully Discretionary Bonus

The fully discretionary bonus method is based on the individual merit of each situation. The contract will offer a salary and a bonus if the board of directors (or managers) deems it appropriate. This method of bonus compensation is increasingly common.

### Business Expenses

Typically, a practice pays all or at least some portion of the general business expenses incurred, including professional liability insurance, society dues, fees for journals and books, staff fees, travel expenses, the cost of continuing medical education, and some costs related to successfully attaining board certification. The practice also pays some or all of noncommuting work-related automobile expenses, the costs of pagers and computers, and for all items necessary for the practice, such as staff, equipment, and the office itself.[10]

### Malpractice Insurance

The two common forms of malpractice insurance are "occurrence" and "claims made." An occurrence policy provides insurance for any actions or omissions as they may occur, regardless of when a claim is brought against the physician. A claims-made policy provides insurance from the day a claim is filed against a physician during the duration of the policy term, as renewed. In some cases, fully matured claims-made policy premiums are only 70% to 80% of the cost of occurrence-based policy premiums.

The cancellation of an occur-rence-type policy incurs no further financial obligation. The cancellation of a claims-made policy requires the physician to purchase additional insurance after the primary coverage ends because the physician is still exposed to the possibility of a future claim. The malpractice insurance company requires the physician to pay a "tail" (a reporting endorsement) to cover claims that may be made after the primary claims-made policy coverage ends.[11]

When negotiating a contract, the physician should attempt to have the employer pay the cost of the tail coverage. If the physician must pay for the tail coverage, it is wise to try to negotiate a provision to pay for tail coverage only in cases in which the physician voluntarily leaves the practice or is terminated for cause. The employer should pay for this coverage if the physician is terminated involuntarily or without cause.[12]

Malpractice insurance is personal to the physician, even though a practice may pay the premiums. Therefore, failure to pay for tail coverage may lead to the loss of the physician's license to practice medicine in the state. Loss of a license in one state may result in a loss in other states. If malpractice insurance is not purchased, it may also lead to having an "unperfected" policy that exposes the physician and practice to personal liability in the event of a lawsuit.[11]

### Employee Fringe Benefits

Fringe benefits may include some combination (or all) of the following benefits: basic and major medical insurance for the physician and physician's family; group term life insurance; payment of disability insurance premiums; coverage under the practice's retirement plan after a waiting period; and relocation expenses. A description for all benefit plans should be obtained, along with information on eligibility.[14] Most of these benefits have tax implications that should be evaluated when comparing contracts from different employers.[11]

### Vacation and Leave of Absence

Generally, new physicians are entitled to 3 to 4 weeks of paid vacation during the first 12 months of employment, and usually at least 1 additional week of absence for continuing medical education, professional society meetings, or to take specialty board examinations.[12] Duration of leave usually increases after the first year of employment. The contract may also address whether unused vacation will be compensated, whether unused vacation may be accrued, and may specify a limitation on the number of days of consecutive absence from the practice.[11]

### Disability and Sick Pay

Typically, physicians receive sick pay for a disability period lasting 15 to 30 days.[11] For longer periods of illness, salary payment will likely stop, but benefits will continue. Pregnancy-related leave is usually treated as a disability under the practice's disability/sick leave policy.[12] Federal laws, such as the Americans with Disabilities Act and the Family Medical Leave Act, may apply if the physician or a family member is sick or disabled.[14]

### Restrictive Covenants

A restrictive covenant is an agreement that a departing employee will not compete with the (former) employer. The covenant offsets the practice's risk in recruiting associates who may leave and take with them practice referral sources, patients, payor contracts, and business contracts. The general law regarding restrictive covenants requires that they be reasonable in duration, scope, and place, and the covenant may not violate the public interest.[15] The following issues should be evaluated: (1) state laws on restrictive covenants; (2) the number of physicians practicing in orthopaedics or any related subspecialty within the restricted area and within a reasonable driving distance; (3) the time period of the restriction; and (4) the applicability of the restriction to working in the emergency department, remaining on the hospital's staff, or maintaining a contractual relationship with third-party payors that the physician joined with the practice.[11]

An attorney or consultant who is familiar with medical practice contracts should review the employment agreement and should explain how the restrictions may be enforced—through an injunction (a court order to stop) or through payment of money (liquidated damages). The attorney should offer negotiation options for the physician.

### Nonsolicitation Agreement

A restriction on soliciting patients, referral sources, or any practice relationship is usually enforceable, even in states where a restrictive covenant may not be enforceable. The purpose of these clauses is to prohibit the employee from soliciting the practice's patients to change to the employee's new practice. The contract should address the following: (1) what information the departing physician can provide to the practice's patients and how this information can be conveyed; (2) what information referral sources and patients will be given when the physician departs; (3) who will care for patients that the departing surgeon was treating; (4) if the physician will

be able to stay on-panel with payors; (5) what remedies are available to the employer if the provision is breached; and (6) who pays the legal expenses in the event of a dispute.

### Senior Doctor's Untimely Death or Disability

The employment contract should address what will happen in the event that a solo physician-owner dies or becomes permanently disabled before the new physician becomes a co-owner of the practice.[11]

### Co-Ownership

The meaning of co-ownership in the practice should be explored and clarified. Usually, co-ownership means gaining some ability to vote on business and practice matters, sharing in financial risks and rewards (including liabilities), and generally enjoying the right to earn what the physician produces (after overhead). The contract should outline the cost and terms for becoming an equal co-owner.

### Discussion

Admittance to a residency program in orthopaedic surgery is difficult to obtain. Completing the residency program and passing the board examinations is even more challenging. Although many resources exist to help medical students select a specialty, there are few resources to help residents and new surgeons deal with what is possibly the most difficult decision of all—selecting and starting an orthopaedic surgery practice.

When selecting a practice, graduating surgeons usually seek counsel from former residents and faculty mentors and consider this advice along with their financial needs and geographic preferences. Physician recruiters often complicate matters by attempting to lure residents with

vague salary and location promises. Residents have difficulty evaluating such enticements and prioritizing their needs. To help residents make informed decisions, orthopaedic residency programs should provide better information and resources that are supported by sound research and statistical analysis.

Patients are constantly studied and evaluated, but no solid data exist on the methods surgeons use to make practice selections. To that end, the authors recommend prospective evaluations of the career decisions made by residents. Specifically, the choices of residents should be tracked with regard to type of practice selected, location, salary, work hours, and specialty. These parameters should then be correlated with short- and long-term career satisfaction outcomes.

### Summary

This chapter has outlined the many disparate practice types that surgeons may choose when completing a residency program. Managed care and coding are important aspects of a practice but are rarely taught in residency programs. Salaries for starting orthopaedic surgeons are highly variable and are based mainly on how difficult it is to fill a position or on the need for an orthopaedic surgeon in a specific geographic region. The legal aspects involved in contracting with a practice are important considerations; it is critical to hire a health care attorney to review an employment contract before committing to a practice.

### References

1. Gabram SG, Hoenig J, Schroeder JV, Mansour A, Gamelli R: What are the primary concerns of recently graduated surgeons and how do they differ

from those of the residency years? *Arch Surg* 2001;136:1109-1114.

2. Gedde SJ, Budenz DL, Haft P, Tielsch JM, Lee Y, Quigley HA: Factors influencing career choices among graduating ophthalmology residents. *Ophthalmology* 2005;112:1247-1254.

3. Salazar JD, Ermis P, Laudito A, Wheatley GH, Paul S, Calhoon J: Cardiothoracic surgery resident education: Update on resident recruitment and job placement. *Ann Thorac Surg* 2006;82:1160-1165.

4. Meals RA: Why orthopaedic surgeons leave full-time academic positions for private practice. *J Bone Joint Surg Am* 2001;83:456-460.

5. Orthopaedic Medical Income in the US 2005-2006. American Academy of Orthopaedic Surgeons Website. Available at: http://www3.aaos.org/research/opus/medinc.cfm. Published 2006. Accessed May 17, 2007.

6. Gottlieb S, Einhorn TA: Beyond HMOs: Understanding the next wave of change in health-care organizations. *J Am Acad Orthop Surg* 1998; 6:75-83.

7. Orthopedic surgeons in demand. *AAOS Bulletin* 2006;54:10. Also available at: American Academy of Orthopaedic Surgeons Website. Available at: http://www2.aaos.org/aaos/archives/bulletin/oct06/fline4.asp. Accessed May 17, 2007.

8. Azevedo D: Your career guide: Surveying the landscape: What they're paying. *Med Econ* 2001;78:29-32.

9. Mangan D: Shape a contract you'll be glad you signed. *Med Econ* 2001;78:79-84.

10. Lee T, Chagala L: *Ten Essential Considerations for Any Employment Agreement.* Corporate Law and Practice Course Handbook Series, New York, NY, Practicing Law Institute, 2004, p 277.

11. *Tools for Practice.* Plymouth Meeting, PA, The Health Care Group, Inc, 1998.

12. Bernick DM: Physician employment contract issues. *Physician's News Digest* Website. Available at: http://www.physiciansnews.com/business/506bernick.html. Accessed September 5, 2006.

13. Darves B: Anatomy of a physician employment contract. *New England Journal of Medicine* Website. NEJM Career Center. September 2002. Available at: http://www.nejmjobs.org/career-resources/physician-job-contract.aspx. Accessed September 5, 2006.

14. American Law Institute: *Restatement of (Second) Contracts.* St. Paul, MN, American Law Institute, 1981.

15. Malsberger BM: *Covenants Not to Compete: A State-by-State Survey,* ed 4. Washington, DC, BNA Books, 2005.

# The Electronic Medical Office: Optimizing Solutions

*Ira H. Kirschenbaum, MD
Jay D. Mabrey, MD
George W. Wood II, MD
A. Herbert Alexander, MD
Charles E. Rhoades, MD
Ian J. Alexander, MD
Gregory J. Golladay, MD
Clifford Wheeless, MD

## Abstract

*Optimizing the care for patients in the orthopaedic clinical setting involves a wide range of issues. Surgical techniques, preoperative and postoperative care, long-term outcomes follow-up, continuing education, and patient communication are a few of the important areas that surgeons deal with on a regular basis. Successful management of this information has an impact on clinical outcomes, direct patient care, financial decisions, and management of the surgeon's time. The development of a comprehensive electronic medical office is a powerful and probably necessary tool to successfully manage such information and achieve the goals of an effective and safe orthopaedic practice.*

**Instr Course Lect 2008;57:737-745.**

There are many choices involved in the development of an electronic-based medical office, and although all of these choices may not apply to each office, there are basic principles and an underlying knowledge base that are helpful in developing a successful information management system. One of the main rationales for changing to electronic medical records (EMRs) and adopting a "paperless" office has much to do with the nature of the current health care delivery system. Patients (especially older patients) often consult with multiple health care providers annually. These providers may order numerous and varied tests, yet it is rare that different offices communicate with each other to exchange information that could prevent a duplication of efforts. Another driving force in the adoption of electronic record keeping is the goal of decreasing medical errors that can occur in a paper environment, especially regarding prescriptions and referrals. In a world where physicians have less time to spend with patients and less revenue to pay for increased staffing, it is becoming more difficult to meet patient needs without the sophistication of electronic tools.[1] The journey to interconnectivity between medical offices and with patients begins with the development of an electronic-based medical office. This chapter details the elements and processes needed for transitioning to an electronic office and also examines the spectrum of work at the national level in the area of health information management.

## The Development of an Electronic Medical Office
### Basic Principles
It is important to determine what type of information will be best

★*Ira H. Kirschenbaum, MD or the department with which he is affiliated has received miscellaneous nonincome support, commercially derived honoraria, or other nonresearch-related funding from ChartLogic, Inc.*

handled electronically by an orthopaedic practice. To make this determination, the type of information that flows into the orthopaedic practice and the method to technically and logistically manage this information should be examined. Key information such as medical records, practice management decisions, and radiographic findings must be communicated and shared between different areas of an office. Key techniques to use information to maximize an individual patient's care must be evaluated. Management of this information may be affected by the clinical setting. In some instances, academic information also must be integrated into the electronic medical office.

## The Nature of Clinical Information

All information that flows into a clinical office can be summarized into four general categories: (1) information generated from the clinical encounter with the patient (for example, EMRs and digital radiographs); (2) information received from outside the office (such as documents and EMRs from another practice or hospital); (3) practice management determinations regarding scheduling and financial information; and (4) electronic information produced by a third party that is involved in the care of the practice's patients or in the management of the practice.

The relationship between medicine and the tools of information management continues to evolve. This relationship includes the consideration of how clinical data are acquired and stored, how data are processed to make a diagnosis, how evidence-based medicine is factored into the therapeutic decision process, and how outcomes are evaluated. Expectations on the acquisition and use of information have been radically changed by the advent of the computer and the wide range of information available on the Internet. Electronic tools make it possible to keep up with this explosion of information by providing an integrated and indexed medical information system.

## Electronic Health Systems: Background

From 1985 to 2002, the number of physicians using practice management systems increased from 10% to almost 95%.[2] Although these systems were fundamentally designed to track patient demographics and insurance and payment information, their real benefit was the electronic printing of patient claims and subsequent electronic transmission of claims to insurers. In 1990, Medicare created new incentives that accelerated the adoption of practice management systems by implementing a policy that reimbursed electronically submitted claims ahead of paper claims.

In the late 1990s, physicians sought better solutions to improve the management of their practices, and the interest in and development of EMRs increased significantly. At the same time, the health care industry began to emphasize medical error reduction and improved clinical documentation, which was highlighted in the first report of the Committee on the Quality of Health Care in America.[3] However, by the end of the decade, a combination of technologic challenges, reimbursement issues, and the difficulty in justifying the capital cost of EMRs kept the number of physician users at only 6% across all practice environments. By 2002, 38% of all university and large medical groups were using EMRs, whereas less than 1% of community-based physicians used EMRs.[1]

It is possible that the industry underestimated the disruption to a medical practice that resulted from the adoption of an EMR system. However, it is likely that physicians will adopt EMRs if such systems are part of an incremental approach toward office automation and can provide improved efficiency and reduced costs with minimal disruption of the existing workflow.

## The Process

Whether a physician is working in a large university setting or a solo practice, there are some unifying features of all electronic medical offices. Real choices need to be made concerning the selection of hardware and software, needed personnel, training, and budgeting. Individual concerns and the goals of associates or interfacing institutions also will play an important role in decision making.

The electronic office functions as more than a medical records repository; it is a complete information management nerve center. Constructing this electronic office must be done in a stepwise fashion. For example, hardware purchases will be followed by software purchase, then training, then reevaluation, and so on. It is a constantly evolving process. As one strives to optimize the electronic office, outmoded software or hardware failures will cause frustration. No single system can support all the physician's needs; therefore, concessions will be necessary.

The development of an electronic medical office demands research by the surgeon and staff. This process should not be delegated to a practice manager nor should the

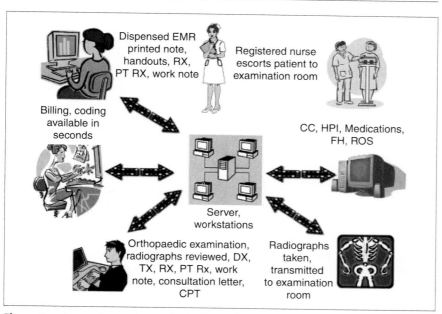

**Figure 1**    In an electronic medical office, all aspects of clinical encounters can be managed electronically. CC = chief complaint, HPI = history of present illness, FH = family history, ROS = review of systems, DX = diagnosis, TX = treatment, RX = medications, PT RX = patient prescription, CPT = current procedural terminology.

**Table 1**
**Features of a Good EMR Program**

Has the ability to import data from any practice management program

Has an intuitive, easy to understand interface

Has multiple templates that are easy to customize; these templates can be transferred within the practice and to other groups

Has multiple options for data entry, such as voice recognition, simultaneous receipt of information from allied staff members, availability to use check box format, ability to use "smarttext" or autotext for data entry

Can import images into the body of the note

Can prioritize information, such as referrals, prescriptions, and other needed actions

Can send and track messages

Allows any member of the office staff to enter International Classification of Disease (ICD) and Current Procedural Terminology (CPT) codes

Allows printing and automatic faxing of prescriptions

Allows design control of the appearance of the note; allows scoring systems to be incorporated into the note; has the ability to fax the note from a computer-based fax server

Allows full reporting functions and data analysis through open architecture programs

Allows completion of any unfinished notes or messages

Allows scanning of documents into the EMR (The office should have an automated multiple document scanner, and each workstation should be equipped with an individual sheet scanner.)

surgeon make decisions without input from key members of the staff; this process should be a group effort. It is advisable to visit several practices that use different programs and methods to learn about the types of systems that are available to address specific issues, such as cost and interconnectivity, and to assess the stability of the program vendor.

## The Electronic Medical Record

The EMR is the backbone of the electronic medical office. Although there are other important components, such as the practice management program, digital radiography, and Internet communications, it is the quality and development of the EMR that will play a central role in the clinical practice of medicine. Features of a good electronic medical records program are summarized in Table 1.

The development of the EMR requires planning regarding the struc-ture of the office work flow, how the actual physical surroundings may need to be modified, the roles of office staff, the development of a working template for clinical notes, and examination of how information is shared within the office. Figure 1 illustrates a general overview of an electronic medical office. All aspects of clinical encounters can be managed electronically. The actual structure of the framework can be managed by as few as two people or by a staff of hundreds—the general principles are the same. The modern electronic office includes various software packages to manage scheduling and billing, develop a clinical note, produce clinical actions from the note, process paper documents sent to the practice, integrate digital radiography into the EMR, communicate with patients, and enable remote access to information.

An example of how this process practically succeeds is detailed by the scenario presented in Table 2. This scenario represents the basic logistics of a simple patient encounter. The endless connections of future messages, prescription renewals, and further office visits all connected together in a web of information can be extrapolated. It is important to note that unlike a paper record, all encounters can be linked to each other, all staff members can view any chart simultaneously, and an accurate chronological record is maintained.

**Table 2**
**Scenario of a Simple Patient Encounter and the Use of an EMR**

| Clinical Event | Use of the EMR |
|---|---|
| The patient registers basic demographics with the front desk. This can be through a paper intake form, a kiosk in the office, or a web-based form that the patient fills out. | Information is keyed into or automatically transferred (web-based) to a practice management software program. This demographic information is then transferred electronically to the EMR/document management program and a digital radiography system. |
| The patient then fills out a comprehensive past medical history form (paper based, kiosk, or web based). | A medical assistant, nurse, or physician's assistant then enters or checks the information and transfers it into the patient's EMR. This is done at any time and on any computer in the office. |
| The patient arrives with important paper-based information from previous medical encounters. | This information is scanned and kept in a document management section of the EMR. |
| The surgeon then interviews and examines the patient (chief symptoms, history of the present illness, and physical examination) and sends the patient to the radiology department. | The surgeon or assistant then enters this information through a variety of means. An effective method is using a combination of voice recognition software and preassembled templates. |
| The patient goes to the radiology department for a digital radiograph. | The demographics of the patient were already transferred to the radiology department so reentry is unnecessary. The digital radiograph is taken and then automatically transferred to a screen in the patient's room or another location for viewing by the surgeon. |
| The surgeon discusses the radiographic finding with the patient and either performs an office treatment (for example, a joint injection), or orders a test (such as a referral for an MRI), or medication (prescription). | The surgeon then notes the treatment or orders the test or medication through the EMR. The treatment is automatically coded in the office. The test request or prescription is printed at the patient exit window and cataloged in the EMR. |
| The patient then exits the practice. | The information on all office treatments (such as radiographs, injection), referrals, and prescriptions has electronically been submitted to the exit staff. They properly counsel the patient and collect all necessary co-pays (for example, for an office visit or radiograph) and discharge the patient. |
| The final note is completed. | The surgeon then enters the impression or other comments (voice recognition or templates). The case is then coded. The information on all past medical history is entered by the assistant at a separate time and location, as well as all treatments entered by staff (injections, radiographs) are brought into the note, completing a comprehensive record. |
| The referring doctor receives a communication. | Once the note is completed and reviewed, the EMR automatically faxes the completed note with a customized cover letter to the referring doctor. This occurs through a computerized fax server. |
| Coding/billing information is transmitted. | The front desk gets an instantaneous superbill for collection. The EMR can then send this information directly to the billing department for review and billing. |
| After the patient leaves, the staff must precertify referrals (such as the MRI). | The staff runs a report on all the patients seen that day, and a printout of all referrals requiring staff intervention is displayed on-screen for the staff to work with. When the precertification number is obtained, it is entered in the EMR chart. |
| The patient calls the next day for the MRI precertification number. | The staff pulls up the record from any screen in the office and gives the patient the number. |
| The patient gets the test, and the MRI facility faxes the report to the office. | This faxed report is scanned into the patient's EMR in the document management section. |
| The patient calls for the MRI result. | A message is left in the patient's EMR that he/she called about MRI results. That message is a permanent part of the EMR, and the surgeon gets the message in his/her message box. |
| The patient discusses the case with the surgeon. | The surgeon, either in the office or remotely from any Internet connection, views the clinical note, the MRI report, or the MRI scan on-screen. The results are discussed with the patient. The discussion particulars are entered on the message and can generate further actions (referrals to specialists, surgical booking, and/or prescriptions) in the EMR. |

Some of the benefits of managing medical information electronically are shown in Table 3. Although the EMR is central to the development of an electronic medical office, two other components also are critical—a practice management program and digital imaging system.

## Practice Management Programs

Practice management programs have been available for many years and are now a commodity, with few differences between various programs. They are used for the simplest functions, such as patient scheduling and billing. Any practice management program should have the ability to share patient demographics with the EMR and digital imaging system used by the practice.

A full-featured practice management program should have the functions outlined in Table 4.

### Digital Imaging Systems

Because radiographs are such an important aspect of orthopaedic surgery, a digital imaging system often serves as the initial entry point to an electronic paperless office. There are many concerns when choosing a digital imaging product, but the most important aspect should be how effectively the digital imaging software integrates into the clinical flow of the practice. For a large multimedical group with staff radiologists, a system that is more appropriate for use by a radiologist than an orthopaedic surgeon may be optimal. To date, the radiologist-based systems are not equipped with all the tools that orthopaedic surgeons generally use.

Digital imaging is performed in one of two ways. Computed radiography uses digital capture cassettes that are read by the computed radiography unit and generally uses the equipment that the practice already has. Each image takes approximately 30 seconds to process. Digital radiography requires the purchase of specialized radiography equipment. This system can capture images immediately, with no processing time. Currently, computed radiography is less expensive than digital radiography. Certain films, such as a scoliosis series, are difficult to obtain with digital radiography and are easier to perform with the more cost-effective computed radiography system.

Digital imaging systems (computed radiography and digital radiography) have many key advantages, such as time savings; the ability to increase the quality of images by changing the contrast and brightness; and increased management options, such as forwarding,

---

**Table 3**
**Advantages of Managing Medical Information Electronically**

Elimination or significant reduction in dictation and transcription (The average annual cost of transcription per provider is about $20,000, and the cost of the time a provider spends dictating charts after hours is priceless.)

Automated evaluation and management coding (For example, clinical data in defined fields can be counted to determine whether requisite bullets for coding at a certain level have been fulfilled or pretemplated.)

Aggregation of clinical data for analysis for research and outcomes purposes

Availability of clinical data to fulfill payer requirements

Availability of information to clinical and business staff

Ability to access the information remotely

---

**Table 4**
**Features of a Good Practice Management Program**

Can store all necessary demographic and insurance data

Has many options for data entry

Has the ability to flag patient charts with information such as copayment requirements, balances owed, and notates patients who are involved in a study

Data can be easily exported to other programs, which eliminates the need to reenter data and allows the selection of different vendors for different services

Permits electronic billing

Permits scheduling for all providers and has the ability to synchronize with a personal scheduler

Has multiple levels of security features

---

e-mailing, and printing of images. Digital imaging systems also allow the use of templating tools such as fracture angulation measurement, Cobb angle and arthroplasty templates; eliminate the need for retakes; eliminate the need for chemicals, labels, storage jackets, and a darkroom; eliminate courier expenses when sending images to other locations; permit compliance with the Health Information Portability and Accountability Act; prevent loss of films; and allow multiple people to view the films simultaneously.

The tools to evaluate a digital radiograph and manage its presentation and flow are facilitated by the system's software. The software programs are all referred to as Picture Archiving and Communications Systems. These systems vary and should be evaluated to determine which system best fits the needs of a particular practice. As previously noted, systems developed for orthopaedic surgeons tend to be more user friendly for the types of applications that are usually performed on a daily basis.

### The Internet

In addition to EMRs, practice management programs, and digital imaging systems, the Internet is also a vital part of an electronic medical office. The Internet can be used for remote access to office and patient information, physician education, patient education by referral to reliable medical Websites, patient education through kiosks within the office, and direct marketing to patients through established Websites accessed by search engines.

### Remote Access

Remote access is one of the most popular features of an electronic medical office. The physician can connect directly to the office from offsite locations and can work as if actually present in the office. This type of system is usually set up by the practice's information technology consultant or can be contracted through a remote access provider. The remote connection should use a virtual private network to allow confidential communications. Another option is the use of a service that permits connection between a specific number of computers within the office. This system is cost effective; however, if many users are allowed to remotely access the system, serious consideration should be given to using a virtual private network.

### Education

The Internet provides a powerful tool for education. Numerous major medical societies and private vendors offer educational material on their Websites. The Internet allows access to current information ranging from prescription data to surgical protocols. Some textbooks are also available on the Internet; in their simplest form, they are the digital re-creations of the printed textbook with some links to related resources. A more ambitious approach is represented by the hypertext Internet textbook, which functions as a search engine for information. This type of book covers a wide range of topics and refers the reader to a vast network of relevant information available for that topic, although the book is generally not edited by any single individual.

Reliable medical Websites also can provide patients with valuable information. Patient education through the physician's own Website can be a powerful tool for communicating with current patients and also prospective patients. The Website can be used to educate patients on diagnoses and treatments. Educational material also can be presented to patients in the waiting room through kiosks established within the office. Having this information on the Internet versus a computer disk allows for easy updating and the ability to present the information at multiple locations.[4,5]

### Marketing

Search engines can direct prospective patients to the physician's Website. This allows the patient to acquire knowledge about the physician and the practice and creates an informed patient. Companies are available that can aid in the development and maintenance of the physician's Website, can provide links to the Website, and can provide keywords that will direct search engines to that site.

### Security

In many ways, electronic information is significantly more secure than paper records. Paper records can be easily stolen, copied, and viewed by others. Paper records can be faxed without a record that the event occurred. A fire or other disaster can destroy paper records that are seldom backed up with duplicate records stored at another location.

Electronic records are easy to back up, the interactions and flow of information can be tracked, and access to the information can be controlled. However, it is important to remember that any health record system is only as secure as the safeguards installed to protect it. A proper security plan is essential to safeguard EMRs (Table 5).

## The National Picture Regarding Health Information Management

The Committee on Quality of Health Care in America issued their second and final report in 2001, which focused on "how the health care delivery system can be designed to innovate and improve care."[3] The committee urged all health care organizations to pursue six major goals: safety, timeliness, effectiveness, efficiency, equity, and patient-centered care (known by the acronym STEEEP). Electronic medical systems are involved in achieving all aspects of these goals. Other national organizations, including the Institute of Medicine (IOM), Health Level Seven, and the Office of the National Coordinator for Health Information Technology, participate in initiatives to improve health by information dissemination and management.

### STEEEP Goals
#### Safety

The concept of safety applies to patients at all times. Based on the definition of the IOM, safety is freedom from accidental injury either through the failure of a planned action to be completed as intended or the use of a wrong plan to achieve an aim.[3] The committee suggested that an automated order entry system (computerized physician order entry or CPOE) could reduce errors in drug prescriptions by contributing to the use of the correct drug and proper dosing regimen.

### Timeliness

Patient care is improved by more timely appointments, and a physician's time is more optimally utilized by an organized surgical schedule. Care is improved when nurses can quickly access test results without contacting the on-call physician. These are just a few of the practical improvements that can be achieved with the use of Internet-based communications and a system that provides immediate access to automated clinical information, diagnostic tests, and treatment results.

### Effectiveness

Effective care is based on the use of systematically acquired evidence to determine whether an intervention or diagnostic test produces better outcomes than alternatives—including the alternative of doing nothing. Automated reminder systems can improve compliance with clinical practice guidelines; some studies suggest that computer-

**Table 5**
**Securing EMRs**

| Feature | Use |
| --- | --- |
| Employee agreement | All employees in your organization, including doctors and partners, should sign an employment agreement that has specific language concerning the protection and use of electronic media and passwords. Specific financial punishment for violation of the agreement should be specified. |
| Lock down computers | The computers of employees should have limited administrator rights. Blocking the downloading or installation of unauthorized programs prevents intrusion from authorized visitors. |
| Encrypted programs | Programs used to store data should have a protected format. It is unwise to develop an EMR using only regular word processing programs and files because these files can be viewed by anyone without password access. |
| Computer monitoring | If the physician owns the office, computer monitoring software can be placed on every computer in the office to monitor and capture e-mail and Websites visited. Screen captures and storage of work performed on each computer also are possible. Employee knowledge that the computers are monitored usually prevents abuse of the system. |
| E-mail protection | Care should be taken when opening attachments from unknown sources, which could contain spy software or viruses. |
| Antispy software | Mini-programs may be installed on your computer when you access certain Websites. Most of these programs attach to the web browser and give feedback to the person whose site you visited about your browsing behavior. Antispy programs are effective in removing most of these threats. |
| Virus protection | No system is complete without a powerful and up-to-date virus protection program. |
| Backup | Having a proper backup protocol is the best protection against tampering and natural disasters. There are many effective protocols in backing up information that include the number of days a week that backup occurs and whether tapes are stored offsite after the system has been backed up. |

assisted diagnosis and management can improve treatment quality.[3]

### Efficiency
The efficiency of providing medical care can be improved by reducing waste and reducing administrative and production costs. The ability to access institutional EMRs can improve efficiency by reducing the number and cost of redundant laboratory tests.

### Equity
Equity in health care depends on universal access to that care. Internet-based health communication can enhance equity by increasing the array of options for physicians to interact among themselves and with their patients.

### Patient-Centered Care
Information technology can contribute to patient-centered care by facilitating access to clinical knowledge through understandable Websites that provide reliable medical information, customized health ed-

ucation, and disease management messages. The Internet can also provide online support groups that bring together patients with a vast range of diseases in widespread geographic locations. Information management may provide a system that can use clinical findings to tailor information according to an individual patient's characteristics, genetic makeup, and specific medical comorbidities.

### IOM: Elimination of Handwritten Clinical Data
The IOM suggested that, "Congress, the executive branch, leaders of health care organizations, public and private purchasers, and health informatics associations and vendors should make a renewed national commitment to building an information infrastructure to support health care delivery, consumer health, quality measurement and improvement, public accountability, clinical and health services research,

and clinical education." It was their recommendation that this commitment would lead to the elimination of most handwritten clinical data by the end of the decade.[3]

The IOM cited three factors that will slow the widespread automation of clinical information. These include the absence of national policies pertaining to privacy, security, and confidentiality; the lack of standards for the coding and exchange of clinical information; and the need for significant financial investment in information technology by large health care organizations. The need to accommodate the hundreds of physicians and thousands of nurses at each major facility, some of whom would be more accepting of change than others, was also noted as another factor that would delay the automation process.

### Health Level Seven
Health Level Seven is an international organization of health care ex-

perts and scientists that works to create standards for the dissemination and management of electronic health care information. The organization takes it name from the highest level (level seven) of the International Organization for Standards communications model for open system interconnection. The seventh level supports such functions as security checks, participant identification, availability checks, exchange mechanism negotiations, and, most importantly, data exchange structuring.[6]

Health Level Seven is one of several American National Standards Institute-accredited organizations that focus on health care concerns. Most of these organizations produce standards for a particular health care domain, such as pharmacy, medical devices, imaging, or insurance transactions. The domain of Health Level Seven is clinical and administrative data and development of interface requirements for the entire health care organization. On an ongoing basis, Health Level Seven develops protocols for its members, such as a widely used standard that enables disparate health care applications to exchange key sets of clinical and administrative data.

### Office of the National Coordinator for Health Information Technology

On April 27, 2004, a presidential executive order established the Office of the National Coordinator for Health Information Technology.[7] The Office focuses on three main missions: (1) to establish a nationwide health information network that allows secure and seamless health information exchange; (2) to develop regional health information organizations by supporting state and other regional projects that help harmonize the privacy and business rules for health information exchange; and (3) to encourage the adoption of EMRs records by reducing the loss and risk physicians face when investing in electronic health record technology. This goal is supported by efforts to ensure that EMR products comply with minimal standards for functionality, security, and interoperability. Multiple contracts have been awarded to multiple vendors to develop the framework of a national health information network. The Office is also charged with helping to provide implementation support to doctors so they can reengineer their business processes using information technology.

## Future Directions: Benefits and Challenges

As has been detailed, establishing an electronic medical office is no small undertaking. Multiple decisions are needed to establish the framework of the system. Once the basic electronic office is operational, there are currently many levels of use for the information, and these uses will continue to expand. In the future, patients will have an online clinical data repository that includes a detailed past medical history and requisite demographic information. This information will reside on commercial, regional health information, organizational, or health system servers. Wherever stored, it will be possible to upload that data to an individual physician's EMR system and then update the server with new information. Patients will routinely enter previsit information via the Internet. Prior to the office visit, the patient will be requested to answer a series of questions with directed single or multiple choice responses regarding their symptoms. Free text fields will allow the unstructured entry of information on the onset of the condition and particulars regarding the progression of symptoms, disease course, treatments, and responses. Electronic data collection will allow a better review of systems; provide pretreatment scoring system data for prospective outcomes studies; and allow the collection of health maintenance, disease, or age-specific information. Point of care mobile computer touch screens will facilitate modification of information on the patient's medical history.

As more health information becomes electronically based, some serious negative concerns will also increase, such as how this information should be managed and archived. Although it is tempting to believe that a single agency will resolve these issues, this is highly improbable because of the many competing interests in medicine (such as physicians, insurance companies, and government agencies) with different priorities. Eventually, market forces will determine standards, which means that dominant and easy-to-use technologies, and those technologies that tie into the revenue stream of medicine are likely to determine the standards.

As more technologies enter the marketplace, the need for standardization grows. Three organizations, the American Health Information Management Association, the Health Information and Management Systems Society, and the National Alliance for Health Information Technology, have joined to develop the Certification Commission for Healthcare Information Technology (CCHIT), which is a voluntary certification process developed for private companies. CCHIT attempts to bring standards to three areas—functionality, interoperability, and security. It is not a true certification agency because it is a voluntary private sector initiative; it makes no evaluations on ease of use, cost, stability, service of the vendor, and other critical issues in choosing an EMR system

The American Society for Testing and Materials International, the Massachusetts Medical Society, the Health Information and Management Systems Society, the American Academy of Family Physicians, and the American Academy of Pediatrics are developing another standard called the Continuity of Care Record.

## Summary

The world of information management is expanding rapidly in medical practices. For the orthopaedic surgeon, the three major areas of practice management, EMRs, and digital imaging are now being augmented by Internet education, direct-to-patient communications, computerized patient education, and remote access to the electronic paperless office. The presence of this increased information also presents the possibility of misuse of such information. Parties can obtain sensitive medical information on large groups of people that will lead to policy changes to protect the public from poorly collected and secured data. Extreme scrutiny of the security standards is needed in all medical practices using electronic information. This responsibility cannot be taken lightly. Although the federal government has laws protecting patients' privacy under the Health Information Portability and Accountability Act, physicians must answer to a higher authority—the relationship between the physician and patient should be justification to protect the privacy and intimacy of all EMRs.

## References

1. Health Care Conference Administrators, LLC Website. Middleton B: AssessingValue/Calculating ROI. HIT Summit Preconference II. Available at: http://www.ehcca.com/presentations/hitsummit1/middleton.ppt. Accessed December 2007.

2. American College of Rheumatology Website: Electronic Medical Records for the Physician's Office. Available at: http://www.rheumatology.org/products/coding/03emr_toc.asp?aud=mem. Accessed December 2007.

3. Committee on Quality Health Care in America: Institute of Medicine: *Crossing the Quality Chasm: A New Health System for the 21st Century.* Washington, DC, National Academy Press, 2001.

4. Biermann JS, Golladay GJ, Clough JF, Schelkun SR, Alexander AH, American Academy of Orthopaedic Surgeons: Orthopaedic information: How to find it fast on the Internet. *J Bone Joint Surg Am* 2006;88:1134-1140.

5. Biermann JS, Golladay GJ, Peters RN: Using the internet to enhance physician-patient communication. *J Am Acad Orthop Surg* 2006;14:136-144.

6. Health Level 7 Website. Available at: www.hl7.org. Accessed December 2007.

7. Health ITW: United States Department of Health and Human Services. Available at: www.hhs.gov/healthit/. Accessed December 2007.

# Index

Page numbers with *f* indicate figures
Page numbers with *t* indicate tables

## M